introduction to
maternal and child health nursing

introduction to maternal and child health nursing

m. christine neff, RN, BSN

Nursing Instructor
Mid-East Vocational School
Zanesville, Ohio

martha spray, RN, BSN, MS

Nursing Instructor
Mid-East Vocational School
Zanesville, Ohio

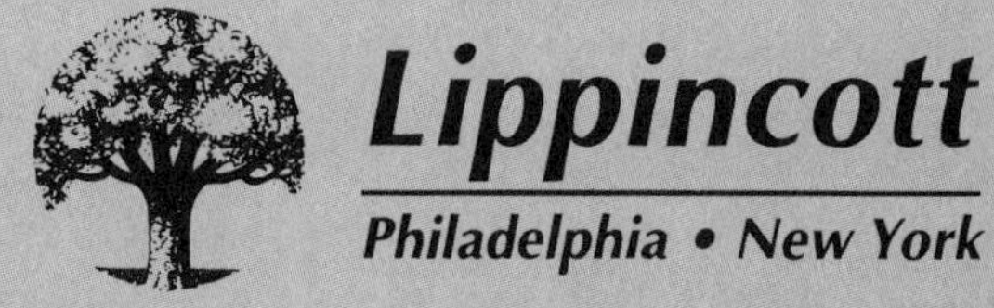

Lippincott
Philadelphia • New York

Acquisitions Editor: Jennifer Brogan
Editorial Assistant: Danielle DiPalma
Project Editor: Barbara Ryalls
Production Manager: Helen Ewan
Production Coordinator: Patricia McCloskey
Design Coordinator: Melissa Olson
Indexer: Katherine Pitcoff

Library of Congress Cataloging-in-Publication Data

Neff, M. Christine.
Introduction to maternal and child health nursing / M. Christine Neff, Martha Spray.
p. cm.
Includes bibliographical references and index.
ISBN 0-397-55025-1
1. Pediatric nursing. 2. Maternity nursing. I. Spray, Martha. II. Title.
[DNLM: 1. Maternal-Child Nursing. WY 157.3 N383i 1996]
RJ245.N44 1996
610.73'62—dc20
DNLM/DLC
for Library of Congress 95-45452
CIP

9 8 7 6 5 4 3 2

To:
my husband, Dave
sons, Augie, Jim, and Chris
daughter-in-law, Sally
grandchildren, David and Tory
and my father, Earl Champagne

—Christine Neff

To:
my husband, Tom
son, Michael
Dr. Jack and Shirley Musick
and their children and grandchildren
and Pete and Jo Ellen Miller
and their children
and my mother, Goldie Benedict

—Martha Spray

contributors

Edna Boyd-Davis, *RN, BSN, MN*
Assistant Professor
School of Nursing and Allied Health
Atlanta, Georgia Unit
Tuskegee University
Atlanta, Georgia

Chapter 27: Nursing Care of the Child and Family During Acute Illness

Linda Calland, *BS, ADN*
Adult PN Instructor
Critical Care Staff Nurse
Good Samaritan Medical
Zanesville, Ohio

Chapter 26: Nursing Administration of Medications and Management of Pain

Glossary

Susan Galea, *RN, MSN, CCRN*
Independent Nurse Consultant
Blue Bell, Pennsylvania
Critical Care Nurse
University of Pennsylvania
Philadelphia, Pennsylvania

Nursing Care Plans

Pat Laing-Arie, *RN*
Instructor, Practical Nursing
Meridian Technology Center
Program of Practical Nursing
Stillwater, Oklahoma

Chapter 16: Nursing Care of the Normal Newborn

Laurie Kaudewitz, *BSN, MSN, RNC*
Assistant Professor of Nursing
East Tennessee State University
Johnson City, Tennessee

Chapter 17: Nursing Care of the Newborn at Risk

Chapter 28: Nursing Care of the Child and Family During Chronic Life-Threatening or Terminal Illness

Chapter 36: The Child with an Alteration in Musculoskeletal Function

Mary Muscari, *PhD, CRNP, CS*
Assistant Professor
University of Scranton
Scranton, Pennsylvania

Chapter 35: The Child with an Alteration in Neurologic or Sensory Function

Tom Spray, *BS, MA*
Guidance Counselor
Zanesville City Schools
Zanesville, Ohio

Chapter 29: Nursing Care of the Child and Family with a Mental Health Problem

reviewers

Diana Bird, RN, BSN
Assistant Professor
Lead Vocational Nursing Instructor
Maric College of Medical Careers
Vista, California

Debbie L. Brown, RN, MSN
LNP Instructor
ACOPNE
Dothan, Alabama

Deborah Cooper Connelly, RNC, MSN, CDE
Chair, Practical Nursing Department
Bishop State Community College, Southwest Campus
Mobile, Alabama

Lynne Hutnik Conrad, RNC, MSN, BSN
Perinatal Clinical Nurse Specialist
Albert Einstein Medical Center
Philadelphia, Pennsylvania

Laurel Danes-Webb, MS, ND, RN
Instructor
Hocking College
Nelsonville, Ohio

Beth Donaher-Wagner, RN, MSN
Women's Center Educator
Lehigh Valley Hospital
Allentown, Pennsylvania

Joyce Harney, RNC, CNA, MSN
Director of Health and Human Services
Ivy Tech State College
Columbus, Indiana

Margrit E. Hayes, BSN, RN
Instructor
Otsego Area School of Practical Nursing
Milford, New York

Margaret Hughes-Towel, RN, BSN
LPN Instructor
Kaw Area Technical School
Topeka, Kansas

Barbara Schoen Johnson, PhD, RN, CS
Assistant Professor
The University of Texas at Arlington
School of Nursing
Arlington, Texas

Mary Meek, RN, MSN
Nursing Faculty
Ivy Tech State College
Indianapolis, Indiana

Kathy S. Newton, RN, MSN
Nursing Faculty
Kellogg Community College
Battle Creek, Michigan

Alice Noquez, RN, BSc
Faculty
Clinical Instructor
Pacific Coast College
Chula Vista, California

Karen A. Paterno, RN, MSN
Associate Professor, Department Chair
Odessa College
Odessa, Texas

Karen Thrasher, BSN
Director of Health
Kentucky Tech, Somerset Campus
Somerset, Kentucky

Bennita Vaughans, BSN, MSN
Nursing Instructor
Trenholm State Technical College
Montgomery, Alabama

Jean E. Wiles
Associate Professor
Riverside Community College–Riverside City Campus
Riverside, California

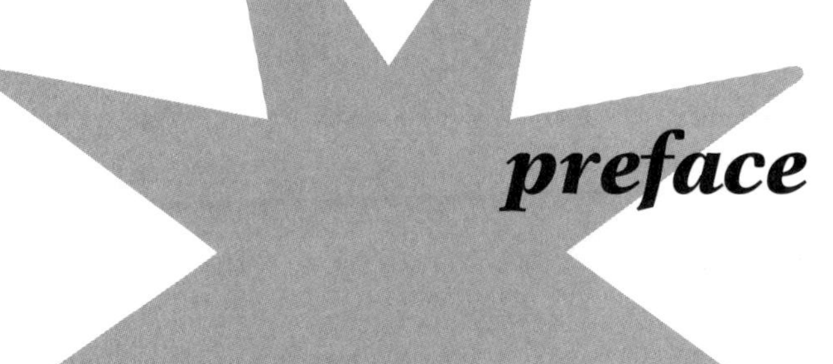

preface

During the years we taught maternity and child health nursing, we witnessed an increase in information at the same time as there was a decrease in classroom time. Contemporary health care concepts, such as family-centered care, home health care, health maintenance, and health promotion were developing. As a result, we adapted our course to reflect these changes. We also empathized with our students, who were concerned about the lack of time they had to read two separate books on maternity and child health. In our search for one book that would combine maternity and child health care in a family-centered approach, we realized the need for a new book that would address current problems and challenges. The book should be not only comprehensive but also concise in its presentation. From this need we developed *Introduction to Maternal and Child Health Nursing.*

Introduction to Maternal and Child Health Nursing is designed to promote student learning in the most efficient way. Maternity and child health nursing combined in one textbook provides a continuum of knowledge and eliminates the redundancy found with two separate texts. For example, care of the neonate is taught in both maternity and child health books. The complete, concise, easy-to-read format of our book helps readers understand a wide range of information and build a solid foundation for quality nursing care. Use of the nursing process increases the student's understanding of nursing assessment, nursing diagnosis, planning and implementation, and evaluation as it applies to the field of maternal-child health care.

organization

Introduction to Maternal and Child Health Nursing follows the family from pregnancy through labor, delivery, and the postpartal period. It then pursues the child and family from care of the neonate, through normal growth and development, and alterations of specific body functions.

The book is organized into eight units:

Unit I: Issues and trends in maternal-child health nursing introduces the student to the profession of contemporary maternal and child health nursing. Chapter 1: Nursing Care of the Family stresses the importance of family on health care. Chapter 2: Issues and Trends in Maternity Care and Chapter 3: Issues and Trends in Child Health Care discuss the sociologic conditions affecting today's families and their health.

Unit II: Reproductive health provides foundational information on reproductive function and women's health. Chapter 5: Family Planning acquaints the student with the latest concepts in contraception and infertility management.

Unit III: The expectant family explores the process of fetal development, through changes during pregnancy and nursing care of the expectant family. After this foundation is established, Chapter 9: Nursing Care During Pregnancy at Risk confronts the issues relevant to high-risk families.

Unit IV: The family during childbirth presents pertinent information on the process of labor and delivery, including special chapters on pain management and nursing care of the family. Chapter 13: Complications and Emergencies During Childbirth concludes the unit with a grounded discussion about care of the high-risk family.

Unit V: The postpartum family addresses the nursing role in caring for the postpartum family and the normal newborn. Chapters on complications and emergencies of the postpartum period and nursing care of the newborn at risk build upon the student's knowledge of normal processes.

Unit VI: Growth and development establishes a framework for child health care. Chapter 18: Theories of Growth and Development offers a complete, concise discussion of theoretical material that serves as a building block. Chapter 19: Health Maintenance and Health Promotion and Chapter 20: Health Protection and Safety examine the impact of growth and development on wellness. Individual chapters detail growth and development from infancy through adolescence. Together these chapters offer a holistic view of growth and development.

Unit VII: The child and family during illness focuses on nuring care of families experiencing acute, long-term, or terminal illnesses. Physical, emotional, and behavioral aspects are described within the chapters. Chapter 29: Nursing Care of the Child and Family with Mental Health Problems is a unique chapter, which adheres to the DSM-IV criteria for child mental health disorders.

Unit VIII: The child with specific alterations in health status uses a systems approach to detail conditions affecting child health. Each chapter reviews pediatric body function and disease pathologies. Furthermore, the chapters discuss specific nursing care for each alteration and considers the family's role in recovery and health maintenance.

The Glossary is a quick reference for the student to clarify terminology used in text. Key terms and additional words are defined in the glossary. Appendices are another handy source to nursing diagnoses, conversion tables, RDAs, excretion of drugs in breast milk, pulse/respiration/blood pressure ranges, growth charts, and teaching considerations.

features

Changes in health care delivery systems demand that nurses understand the value of family dynamics. Families are increasingly responsible for the well-being of the pregnant woman or ill child. The combined approach of this text views the client as both an individual and as part of the family unit. *Family Considerations* and *Nursing Considerations,* located in the beginning of many chapters, highlight information that will help the nurse meet family needs.

Health maintenance and health promotion are concepts in the forefront of health care reform. This wellness approach is reflected in our text so that nurses may guide the family toward healthy living. Two chapters are devoted specifically to this issue.

Nurses and families are required to take on diverse roles because contemporary health care is provided in a variety of settings. Information on home safety, caregiver education, birthing centers, early discharge, home health care, hospice care, and other community-based facilities assist the nurses with understanding their role within the spectrum of continuous care. *Teaching Guidelines,* presented in most chapters, are excellent tools for the nurse who must educate caregivers about their responsibilities in the home.

There are age-specific health concerns relevant across the lifespan. Concerns regarding the pregnant adolescent and the pregnant woman over 35 are presented in the maternity chapters. An understanding of growth and development strengthens the quality of care nurses can offer their young clients. Normal growth and development and age-related factors affecting illness and disease process in children are included in the child health chapters. Additional information incorporated into *Age-Specific Considerations* broaden the nurse's knowledge base.

In a culturally diverse society such as ours, health care workers must be aware of the values, beliefs, and traditions of various cultures. Material integrated throughout the book focuses on an understanding and acceptance of cultural diversity and away from generalizations about specific groups.

A user-friendly design highlights essential information and simplifies reading. Abundant color drawings and numerous photographs allow the student to visualize difficult concepts and procedures. Tables and boxes highlight critical or additional data and provide the student with a ready reference. The reader's retention is improved by the strong chapter pedagogy. Numerous recurring displays enhance theoretical and clinical information.

chapter pedagogy

* ***Chapter outlines*** preview content to be covered and help readers to organize subject matter and to locate topics while reviewing material.
* ***Chapter objectives*** identify the goals of the chapter and allow students to monitor their overall understanding of the chapter.
* ***Key terms*** introduce vocabulary defined within the text. The list of terms help readers verify word comprehension. Each term is italicized the first time it appears in text. These terms are also found in the Glossary.
* NCLEX-style ***Review Questions*** in every chapter help students master course material and prepare for this important test.
* ***Key points,*** placed at the back of each chapter, review major points in the chapter and correspond to chapter objectives.
* An up-to-date ***Bibliography*** at the end of each chapter provides additional resources for the readers to do a more in-depth study of the topics addressed within the chapter.

recurring displays

* ***Family considerations*** introduce concerns of the families and offer practical suggestions. This special heading is found in most nursing care chapters, promoting a thorough understanding of family-centered care.
* ***Nursing considerations*** provide critical information that enriches the nurse's quality of care. The content is discussed in the beginning of many nursing care chapters, emphasizing the importance of efficient, safe, and thoughtful care.
* ***Age-specific considerations*** highlight specific issues nurses should look for in different age groups. This approach focuses on the client as an individual and enhances the nurse's understanding of diverse groups.
* ***Teaching guidelines*** give practical step-by-step information on specific topics. These valuable displays develop the student's ability to educate caregivers.
* ***Nursing alerts,*** strategically placed within a discussion, immediately advise students of urgent information.
* ***Nursing insights,*** also specifically placed, offer helpful hints and observations based on years of experience.
* ***Nursing care plans*** reinforce individualized nursing care. Sample care plans include information and assessment, diagnosis, planning, intervention, and evaluation of the patient or family. Specific situations covered in the care plans address important issues in today's health care system.
* ***What would you do?***, at the end of selected chapters, encourages student interaction and critical thinking through case situations.

instructor's manual/testbank

The Instructor's Manual and Testbank in one convenient text offers helpful teaching strategies, discussion topics, teaching/learning activities, and transparency masters. Each chapter also includes questions and activities for the student to complete. This in-text Study Guide has been printed on perforated pages so it can be copied and distributed to students. The Testbank contains approximately 500 multiple-choice questions to assist in test preparation and measurement of student comprehension.

acknowledgments

We would like to express our sincere appreciation to Nancy Evans, our developmental editor, mentor, and friend and to the staff of Bethesda Hospital in Zanesville, Ohio, including Lea Craig, Librarian, for her help in obtaining research materials, the obstetric and pediatric staff, especially Rhoda King, RN, BSN, and Debra Close, RNC, for their professional consultations. Also to Rambo Memorial Health Center, Southeastern Ohio Otolaryngology Inc., and The Good Samaritan Prenatal Clinic of Zanesville, Ohio, for their assistance in obtaining current information for the care of obstetrical and pediatric clients.

We would like to acknowledge the staff of Lippincott-Raven Publishers who have been especially helpful in the development of this text: Jennifer Brogan, Editor, Danielle DiPalma, Editorial Assistant, Barbara Ryalls, Project Editor, and Sarah Andrus, Developmental Editor. Thanks also to Leo Anton for recognizing our potential as authors.

A special thank-you to Linda Calland, RN, BS, for being a good listener, supporter, and promoter of our work, to Christian Neff for his assistance in obtaining current research data, and finally to Jim Neff for the use of his computer and for sharing his expertise.

contents

introduction to
maternal and child health nursing

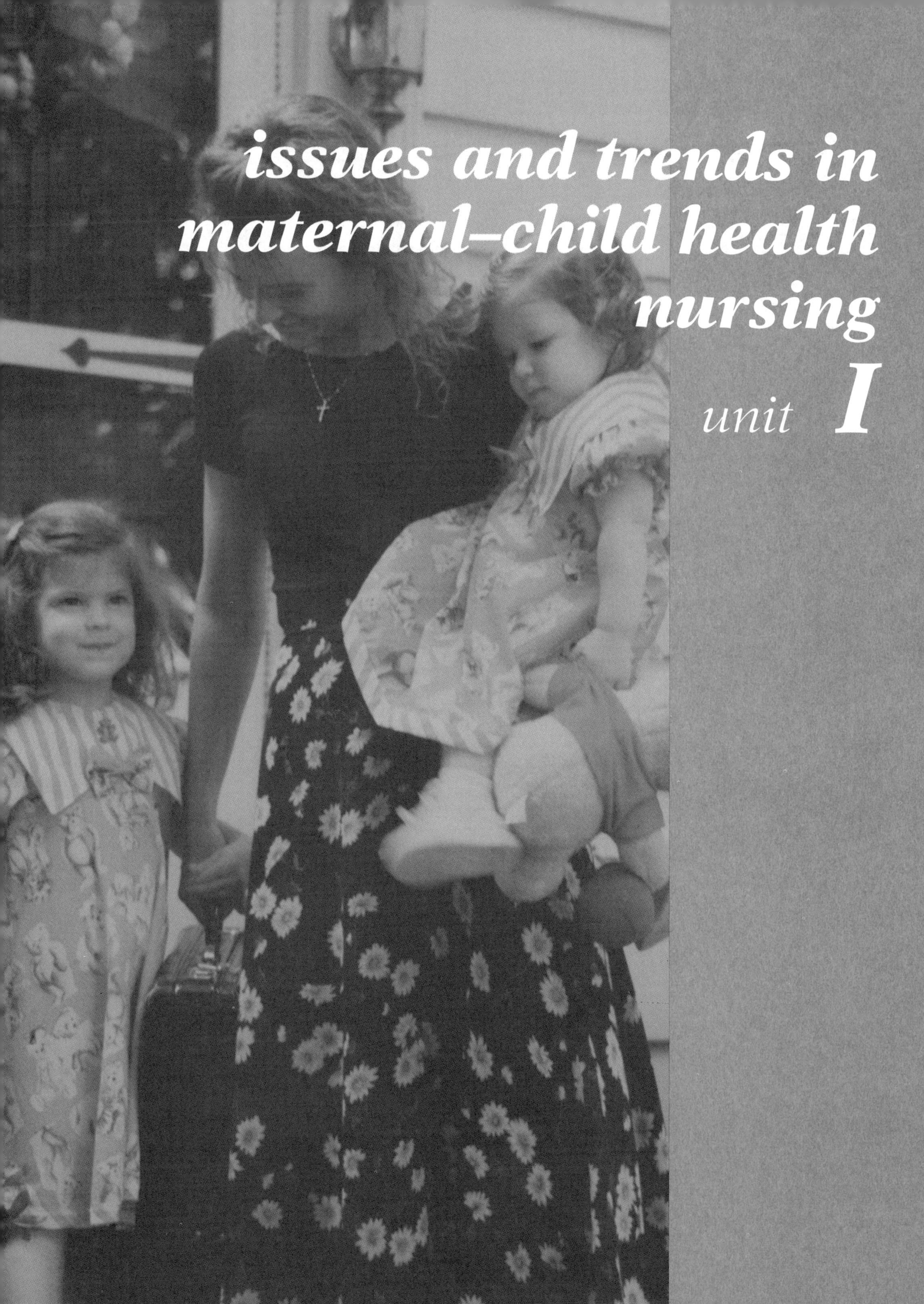

issues and trends in maternal–child health nursing

unit **I**

nursing care of the family

1

outline

objectives

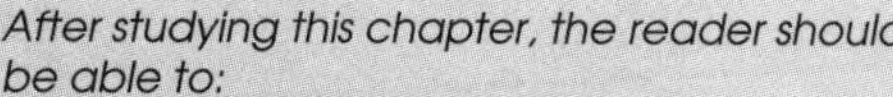

After studying this chapter, the reader should be able to:

- ✳ Discuss the role of a family.
- ✳ Describe how parenting is learned.
- ✳ Describe the difference between functional and dysfunctional families.
- ✳ List at least three different types of families.
- ✳ Discuss the sociocultural considerations in family health care.
- ✳ Describe the steps of the nursing process.
- ✳ Describe the application of the nursing process in family-centered care.

key terms

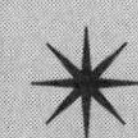

acculturation
adoptive family
assessment
blended family
cohabitation family
communal family
culture
ethnic group
evaluation
extended family
family
implementation
nuclear family
nursing diagnosis
nursing process
objective data
parent
planning
race
single-parent family
subjective data

The family is society's oldest, most basic unit; it is there that people learn what it means to be human, to be male or female, and to be part of a culture. Although family structure varies among different cultures, family functions related to children are similar: to provide physical care, education and training, and protection for children's psychological and emotional health. Every child born into a family influences and is influenced by other family members. In addition, family members are individually and collectively affected by the larger community around them. The health and well-being of families directly affect the health of a society.

the family approach to health care

A family approach to health care begins with care of the pregnant woman, her partner, and other family members during the months before birth. With time, as family members age, the health needs of each member also change. As children engage in school and other activities outside the family, these activities also influence the health of the family. Thus, a family approach to health care considers each individual as part of the family and of the larger community. It means understanding the normal patterns of physical, psychological, social, intellectual, and spiritual growth and development and the cultural customs, beliefs, and values of the family and community. A family approach to health care also means appreciating the uniqueness of each child and family.

table 1-1 stages of family development

Stage	*Health Concerns*
Beginning family	Marital and sexual adjustment Developing communication patterns Adjusting to new roles Family planning
Early childbearing family	Prenatal care Infant care Child development Safety
Family with preschool children	Growth and development Accidents Communicable diseases
Family with school-age children	Behavioral problems Physical or emotional disabilities Communicable diseases
Family with teenagers	Struggle for independence Biologic and emotional changes of puberty Peer pressure Sexually transmitted diseases Substance abuse

Duvall, E. (1977). *Marriage and family development* (5th ed.). Philadelphia: J. B. Lippincott and Aldous, J. (1975). *The developmental approach to family analyses*. Minneapolis: University of Minnesota Press.

the family and parenting

A family can be defined as two or more people living in the same household; sharing common emotional bonds; having a caring, long-term commitment; providing for individual growth of each family member; and interacting in social activities. The family is the primary nurturing and socializing influence for children. Children often mimic the attitudes, values, communication styles, and reaction patterns of their parents. The bond between parents and children develops a relationship of mutual giving and receiving. This relationship strengthens the concept of the family as a system in which each member affects the others.

developmental stages of the family

Caring for the health of children and families requires understanding the various stages of family development. Duvall in her classic work, *Marriage and Family Development* (1977), described the development of families in eight stages (Table 1-1). This book considers the first five stages: beginning family, early childbearing family, the family with preschool children, the family with school-age children, and the family with teenagers. In each stage of development, families may confront change, stress, and crises that can affect the health of one or more family members.

parenting

Parenting is not intuitive; we learn how to parent, first from our own parents, then from observing parenting skills in others, and finally from reading and listening to others (Fig. 1-1). *Parent* is defined as the person(s) who establishes a parent–child relationship by caring for a child and providing the physical, social, spiritual, and emotional support necessary for normal growth and development. The health of the family is partially reflected in parents' attitudes toward their expected roles and responsibilities.

functional and dysfunctional families

As stated previously, the functions of a family in relation to children are to provide physical care of children, education and training, and protection for children's physical, psychological, and emotional health. The family who effectively performs these functions is said to be functional. Unfortunately, for a variety of reasons, some families fail to perform one or more of these functions and thus are described as dysfunctional.

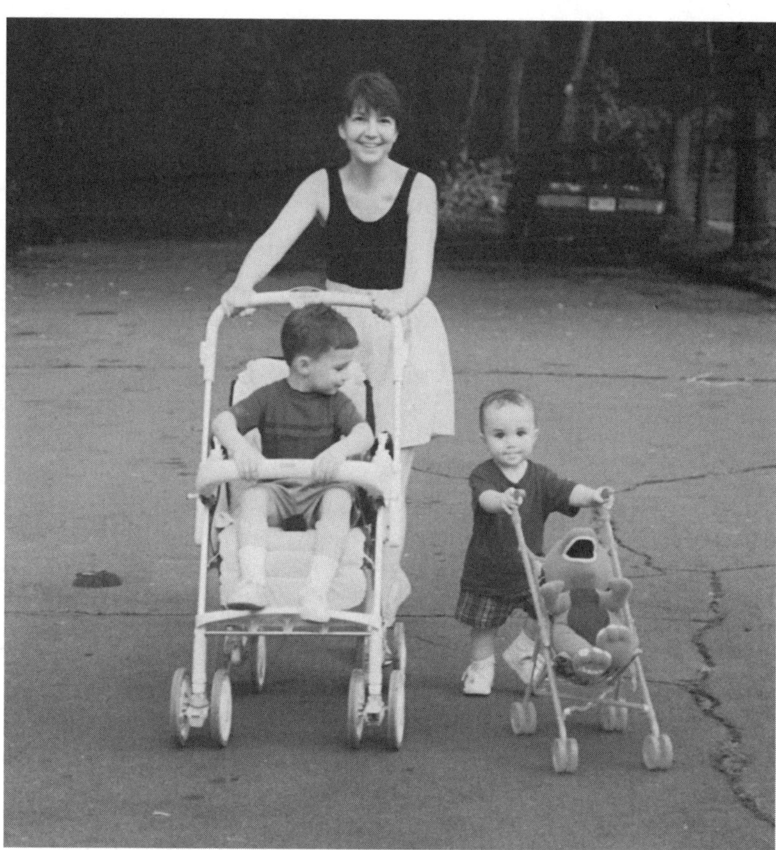

figure 1-1 *Children learn at a very young age to parent by mimicking their own parents. (Photo by Elise Dinerman.)*

functional families

In the healthy functioning family, no single participant dominates another. There is consideration for each family member. Parents share control (or in the case of a single parent, take control) to establish a sense of order rather than a sense of power. Children are permitted to voice opinions, and constructive communication methods are dominant in working out differences of opinion.

Positive family interactions enable family members to develop a sense of self-worth and positive self-esteem. Positive self-esteem increases an individual's productivity in society. The functional family recognizes the need of each child to progress through stages of development, just as the family needs to progress through stages of development. These stages include bonding or attachment, independence, separation, and individualization. Although personal independence is a positive attribute, it need not occur at the expense of the family as a unit.

dysfunctional families

Families can be *dysfunctional* in different ways. For example, well-meaning, loving parents may fail to teach their children habits that contribute to a healthy lifestyle (eg, regular meals, breakfast every day, exercise, regular bedtime) because they lack that knowledge themselves. Parents who are loving but overprotective may fail to teach their children to live in society. Family dysfunction may be related to issues of power and power struggles. This could mean that the family has no clearly identified leader or parent taking control or establishing a sense of order. On the other hand, it could mean that one parent controls all the power and makes all decisions without consulting other family members. If communication is not open or honest, family members may give and receive mixed messages. Dysfunctional families may have a limited or distorted understanding of normal childhood growth and development. This lack of understanding can create unreasonable expectations and responsibilities for children within the family unit. Family function can improve when members show genuine concern and respect for feelings and needs of each other.

Parents in a dysfunctional family often lack effective parenting skills, perhaps because their own parents were poor role models. Without these skills, parents become overwhelmed with the task of parenting. They are at high risk for becoming abusive or neglectful parents if appropriate interventions are not made.

types of family structure

The word "family" can describe many different types of family structure. This chapter discusses the following family types: nuclear, extended, single-parent, blended, communal, cohabitation, adoptive, homosexual, foster, and homeless. Family structure changes with time as it is modified by birth, death, work, divorce, and the growth and development of each family member. The nurse needs to be aware of the differences in family types to assess family function.

nuclear family

A *nuclear family* consists of a husband, wife, and one or more children. The nuclear family provides strong support to its members and promotes the family's value system within each family member. Any crisis affecting one family member also can have a serious impact on all others in the family.

extended family (multigenerational)

An *extended family* includes the nuclear family and other family members, such as grandmothers, grandfathers, aunts, uncles, cousins, and grandchildren. The relatives who surround the nuclear family can be resources during crisis. They also provide additional role models for behavior and learning values. On the other hand, additional people can be a financial burden.

Extended families are common to several ethnic groups. Although there is wide variation among Asian American cultural groups, many Asian Americans live in extended families, particularly first-generation immigrants. These families reflect a deep sense of obligation toward parents and elders. African Americans, the largest minority group in the United States, also may live in multigenerational families, often headed by women; grandmothers may take responsibility for child care. Extended families are common among some Latino American cultural groups, such as Mexican Americans.

single-parent family

The *single-parent family* is becoming increasingly common. This trend results from a variety of factors, including a high divorce rate, an increasing number of teenage mothers who choose to become single mothers, and a growing number of women choosing to raise children outside of marriage. Growing up in a single-parent family can help a child to become independent and self-reliant. On the other hand, because most single-parent families are headed by women, it often means a lower standard of living because women's incomes are generally lower than men's. The person heading a single-parent family bears all the responsibilities usually shared by two people and lacks physical and emotional support when children are ill. Whether male or female, the single parent must learn and perform the tasks of both mother and father, a challenging job (Fig. 1-2).

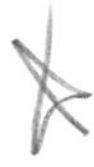

blended family

The *blended family* consists of divorced or widowed people, each of whom may have children from a previous marriage, plus children from the current marriage. An ad-

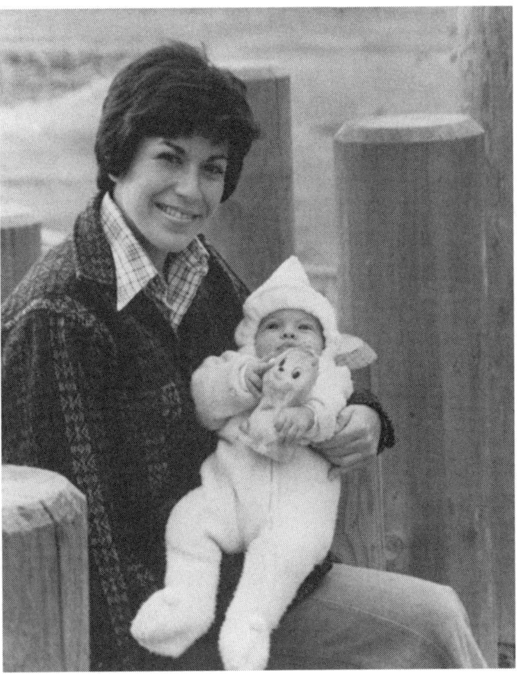

figure 1-2 *It is important for single parents to take time to relax with their children.*

vantage to this type of family is the exposure to other siblings; however, there may be difficulties concerning childrearing and discipline issues. Rivalry can be common as children compete for attention. Financial problems can occur if one of the parents has to pay child support for offspring of a previous marriage.

communal family

The *communal family* is made up of people who have chosen to live together because of common social values or interests or by economic necessity. This type of family may be unrelated by kinship. A communal family approach is found in some of the 200 Native American tribes. In the Cherokee nation, for example, the children of the tribe belong to all members of the community. Depending on their cultural make-up, the communal family may differ from mainstream society in their views on health care.

cohabitation family

Families in *cohabitation* consist of couples who live together with their children but remain unmarried. The cohabitation family may be temporary or long-lasting. Family stability is enhanced when the relationships are long lasting.

adoptive family

The *adoptive family* consists of one or both parents with no biologic claim to their child or children. Children may be adopted at any age from birth to the teenage years, from private, church-affiliated, or state agencies after the biologic parent(s) have legally given up all claims. Adopted children are entitled to know they are adopted. Parents have an obligation to introduce and discuss the topic on a regular basis as the child matures.

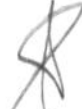

homosexual family

The homosexual family consists of individuals of the same sex living together as married partners. Some homosexual families include children from a previous marriage. Some lesbian couples have chosen to bear children by artificial insemination. In many ways, the homosexual family can function much like the nuclear family.

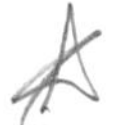

foster family

The foster family includes children whose parents are unable to care for them and foster parents who may or may not have children of their own. Placement of children in a foster family is often temporary and under the supervision of the state. It is important to assess who has legal responsibility for the child when providing health care services.

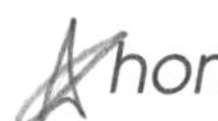

homeless family

Homeless families are those without any form of housing or the resources to pay for housing. They may be mobile, such as migrant families, or less mobile, such as urban and rural poor families. Poverty and unemployment create health problems, such as malnutrition, diabetes, tuberculosis, depression, suicide, homicide, and lack of health maintenance. Homeless families are often unfamiliar with health resources available in a community. Young children in these families may not have access to immunizations or regular physical and dental examinations (Fig. 1-3).

sociocultural considerations in family health care

Almost every family is part of a larger social network: the neighborhood, town, city, or rural community; state or province; and country. Effective care of children and families must take into account how the larger social network affects and is affected by the health of clients.

racial, ethnic, and cultural factors

Caring for children and families includes understanding of and sensitivity to different *racial, ethnic,* and *cultural* differences. *Race* is a system of classifying people into groups according to physical features, such as skin color, facial features, and texture of body hair. *Culture* is an individual's way of looking at life. It encompasses the person's feelings, beliefs and attitudes, and practices in dealing with family, community, and social practices. Culture affects how the individual views health, nutrition, and health practices. An *ethnic* group is a collection of people who share the same cultural and social beliefs that have been passed from one generation to another. An individual's cultural patterns can be altered by the society in which he or she lives, a process called *acculturation.*

The United States and Canada have a rich diversity of racial, ethnic, and cultural traditions. The earliest settlers in North America were white Anglo-Saxon Christians. During the 1700s, however, the slave trade brought large

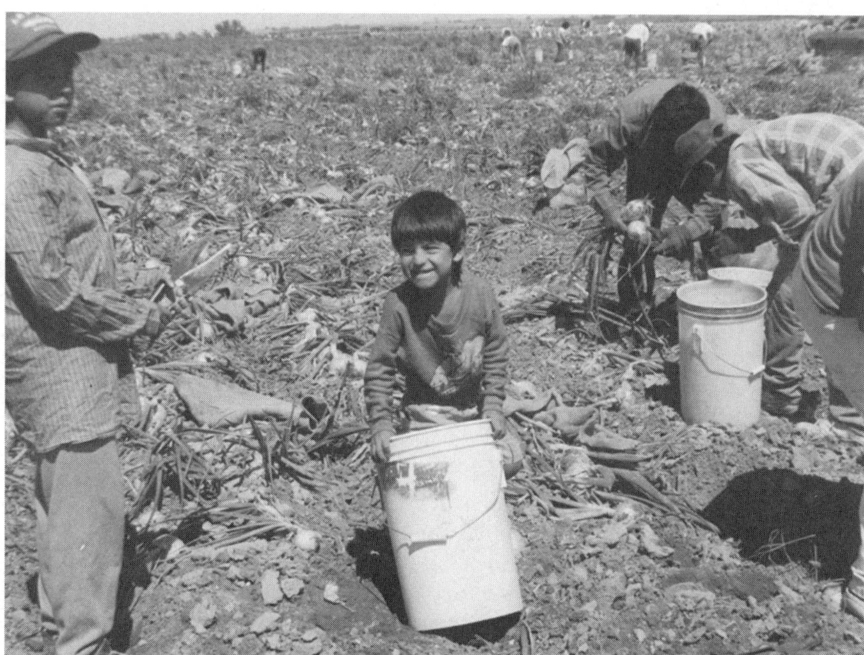

figure 1-3 *Young children in migrant families are at a heightened risk for poor health.*

numbers of Africans into the United States, and African Americans remain the largest minority group in this country. Though the U.S. population is 80% white, racial, ethnic, and cultural diversity is increasing. Latino Americans are the second largest minority group in the United States and are predicted to be the largest by the year 2000. Asian American and Arab American populations also are increasing. To be effective caregivers, nurses need to become familiar with the various health practices, dietary patterns, and basic beliefs of the families in their care. For example, families in some cultural groups may request the presence of the entire family during hospitalization of one member.

the health care culture

Each nurse has his or her own cultural beliefs, attitudes, and practices just as does each client. Some of the nurse's cultural patterns come from the health care culture itself. The health care professions have their own cultural patterns with their own language. One example is the "formula" infants may be fed. The word formula denotes some mysterious concoction, when it is only a preparation of milk with added vitamins and other nutrients. The client may not understand the language of health care and thus needs instructions and explanations in understandable terms.

The nurse must show respect and a nonjudgmental attitude when dealing with cultural beliefs different from his or her own. Each client is an individual who has his or her own set of beliefs. Once a nurse has developed rapport with the client, specific questions may be asked of the client to understand better the needs to be met. The following types of questions may be appropriate:

- "Do you avoid particular kinds of food?"
- "When there is a hospitalization for illness in your family, do you prefer to have someone of your faith contacted?"
- "Who makes decisions in your family?"
- "Do you obtain immunizations for your family?"
- "How may I help you in meeting your needs?"

Regardless of the cultural background of the client, he or she must deal with today's Western health care system. The nurse can help the client successfully bridge the cultural gap.

spiritual factors

The spiritual aspect of maternal and child health nursing must not be overlooked. The family in crisis may depend heavily on their spirituality as a coping mechanism. The client's ethnic background, culture, and spiritual beliefs may intertwine. Beliefs about life, death, childrearing, and crisis management are based on their own experience as part of the family unit. To be effective, the nurse respects the client's beliefs, remains nonjudgmental, and encourages clients to express their desire for visits from their minister, rabbi, priest, or church members.

economic and environmental factors

Many changes have occurred in North American society since 1960 that affect family health care. Many young adults continue to live with their parents for longer periods. People are delaying marriage, sometimes choosing to live as a couple without marriage. Many women delay childbearing to establish a career. Nearly 60% of all women work outside the home; most of them are married (Killien, 1993). The percentage of families with three or more children has dropped by 50% since 1970 (Holland & Peterson, 1993).

Due to economic demands, a large number of mothers with preschool children are in the workforce. These women are juggling many roles: parent, wife, homemaker, and career woman. Support from the extended family may be weak because of the distance separating some families. Child care options may be limited and expensive.

For the first time in United States history, 37 million people are without health care insurance (Holland & Peterson, 1993). Lack of financial resources increases the chance of illness. Because preventive care usually is not part of the family budget, medical care may be delayed until illness is life-threatening. Clients living in rural areas may not have access to medical facilities. In addition, lack of proper sanitation facilities may contribute to development of infectious diseases.

Poverty, drug addiction, alcoholism, and homelessness are problems in many places. For example, approximately 20% of American children live in poverty. Among African Americans, nearly half (44%) of all children live in poverty (Holland & Peterson, 1993). African American infants are more than twice as likely as white infants to die in their first year of life (Centers for Disease Control, 1993).

Nurses have a responsibility to be patient care advocates, to participate in cost-containment programs, and to advocate health promotion and illness prevention programs, such as well-baby clinics, immunizations, and screening (Table 1-2). Teaching the family about the importance of health maintenance may decrease health care costs in the long run.

dietary factors

Dietary practices are closely linked with family beliefs and cultural patterns. The nurse needs to be familiar with clients' food patterns to determine if their nutritional needs are being met. For example, rice is the staple of some Asian American diets. Mexican Americans may have a limited intake of protein and rely heavily on the use of corn, beans, rice, and hot spicy foods. African American diets may include much protein, such as pork, chicken, and fish, but include a limited intake of dairy products. Working closely with the dietitian, the nurse assists the family in meeting nutritional needs while staying within the cultural and financial bounds of the family. Also, not all members of a cultural group follow the typical dietary practices.

table 1-2 nursing interventions to promote family health and wellness

Family Developmental Level	*Nursing Interventions*
Beginning family	Family planning clinics
Early childbearing family	Prenatal classes Infant care classes Immunization information Poison prevention and other safety information
Family with preschool and school-age children	Vision and hearing screenings Dental health information Parent support groups Communicable disease control
Family with teenagers	Substance abuse information Accident prevention programs Sex education Mental health programs

overview of the nursing process

The nursing process is a scientific, systematic, problem-solving approach to safe, consistent nursing care. It may be used in the care of individuals, families, or whole communities. It consists of five steps: assessment, nursing diagnosis, planning, implementation, and evaluation.

Although the nursing process is presented as five distinct steps, it also is a dynamic, ongoing, overlapping process. Each step may occur independently or simultaneously with the other steps. In complex family situations, such as child abuse, drug abuse, or alcoholism, the nurse may work slowly and tediously through each step of the process in helping the family to resolve their problems. In an emergency situation, for example, a patient bleeding from an incision site, the nurse identifies the problem, takes rapid steps to slow or stop the bleeding, and evaluates whether the interventions have been successful. In both situations, the nurse uses the nursing process to arrive at safe, consistent nursing care.

assessment

Assessment is the first step of the nursing process. It involves the collection of information (*data*) and interpretation (*analysis*) of the information obtained. Two types of data, subjective and objective, are collected.

Subjective data include information obtained by interviewing the client and family. It includes what the patient tells you, such as reports of pain, illness, and feelings.

Objective data are obtained by physical inspection and examination of the patient. Laboratory tests, x-rays, and diagnostic reports also are reviewed (Fig. 1-4). It includes observable and measurable information, or what the nurse sees.

Once the nurse has gathered and examined the available data, he or she prepares a problem list. This information is shared with the patient to confirm or deny the problems or potential problems that may exist. At this point, the nurse can formulate the nursing diagnosis.

nursing diagnosis

"Nursing diagnosis is a clinical judgment about individual, family, or community responses to actual or potential health problems/life processes. Nursing diagnosis provides the basis for selection of nursing intervention to achieve outcome for which the nurse is accountable" (NANDA, Editorial, 1990). The North American Nursing Diagnosis Association (NANDA), the national group responsible for formulating nursing diagnoses, has prepared and approved a list of acceptable nursing diagnoses for use by the maternal–child nurse (see Appendix).

Selection of the appropriate nursing diagnoses is vital to the planning stage of care for the client. It identifies spe-

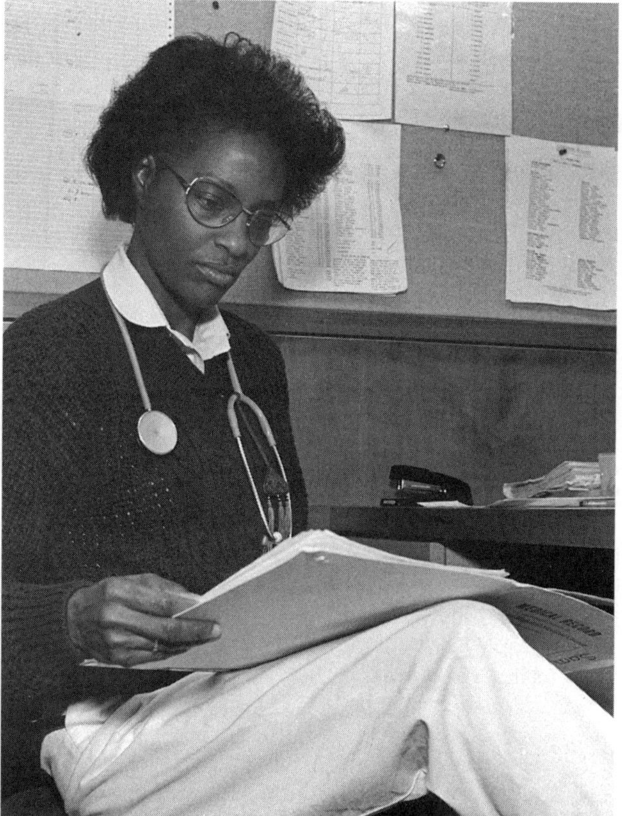

figure 1-4 *The nurse reviews records, notes, physician's orders, and other documentation before interviewing or performing a physical examination on the child. (Photo by Kathy Sloane.)*

cific problems or potential problems the client may have and thus helps the nurse individualize the care for each patient.

planning

Once the nursing diagnoses have been identified, the nurse then prepares a plan to meet the needs that have been identified by the nurse and the client. These plans include setting priorities, establishing goals, and selecting the appropriate nursing interventions.

During the planning phase, the nurse describes desired outcomes or patient goals. These are descriptions of mutually desired behaviors that are expected following the nursing interventions. For example, "After viewing the baby bath video, the mother will successfully demonstrate bathing her own infant." This statement reflects the client's behavior, not the nurse's behavior.

implementation

Implementation, the fourth phase of the nursing process, is the action or doing phase of the process. During this phase, the nurse carries out the selected plans for patient care. While implementing the plans, the nurse continually assesses and evaluates the patient's responses to the actions. This phase requires accurate charting and documentation of the interventions performed, the patient's responses to the interventions, and any progress toward the ultimate goals.

evaluation

Evaluation, the final phase, determines the effectiveness of the plans and interventions used to meet the goals. During the evaluation process, the nurse may discover that some goals were met or partially met. During this time, new problems may be identified, which will lead to new goal setting, planning, and implementation. Thus, the nursing process continues until the patient reaches the optimum level of wellness.

✳ nursing process in family-centered care

Caring for children and families begins with understanding the family, its overall strengths and weaknesses, and how those strengths and weaknesses affect the individual and collective health of the family. The nursing process offers a useful framework for this evaluation.

assessment

Nurses assess family relationships and interactions to evaluate how they will affect and be affected by pregnancy, childbirth, or the illness of a child. Assessment begins with collection of subjective and objective data. This involves interviews, questionnaires, and careful nursing observation of family interactions.

Many family assessments are made when the family is in crisis. The crisis may be related to the birth of a child, a sick child, impending surgery, emergency care, or terminal illness. Crisis interactions can differ from everyday interactions and thus fail to reflect the typical interaction patterns of the family unit. During times of crisis, the nurse may need to use "gut" (intuitive) feelings concerning the effectiveness of family interactions until more typical communication patterns can be observed. The assessment factors listed in Display 1-1 will yield subjective and objective data.

nursing diagnoses

The nursing diagnoses used in association with family concerns direct attention to how the family handles stress. The following nursing diagnoses address maternity and child care concerns.

The nurse working with the family of a high-risk newborn may need to address the following nursing diagnoses:

- Anticipatory Grieving, related to possible future death of the infant
- Altered Family Processes, related to the infant's extended hospitalization and its emotional and financial impact
- Anxiety, related to unpredictable prognosis
- Altered Parenting, related to inadequate attachment secondary to parent–child separation or failure to accept impaired child
- Parental Role Conflict, related to feelings of inability to provide for infant's physical and emotional needs
- Impaired Social Interaction, related to demands of caring for infant's needs.

A family who demonstrates dysfunctional behavior patterns in response to managing stressors can neglect the care of a child. The decisions or actions made are often destructive to economic and social well-being. One nursing diagnosis appropriate for this type of family is Ineffective Family Coping, related to single or adolescent parent(s), abuse of alcohol or other drugs, mental illness, dysfunctional relationship with own parent, unrealistic expectations of child by parent, or unmet psychosocial needs of child or parent.

display 1-1
factors in family assessment

Family structure
Health status of family members
Communication patterns
Parents' understanding of growth and development
Spiritual beliefs
Cultural values and beliefs related to child care
Socioeconomic status

Even though families are functional and healthy, a crisis can threaten the equilibrium of the family. The following nursing diagnoses may be appropriate to use in such cases.

* Altered Family Processes, related to illness of family member; discomforts related to the symptoms of the illness; change in the family member's ability to function; time-consuming, expensive treatments; loss of body part or function, and surgery
* Family Coping: Potential for Growth, related to family members' attempting to describe the growth impact of a crisis on their own values, priorities, goals, or relationships
* Ineffective Family Coping: Compromised, related to concern about significant other's response to health problems, anticipatory grief, guilt, anxiety about child's illness or disability, inadequate knowledge to provide supportive behaviors

planning

Family-centered care requires an individualized plan based on needs that have been prioritized by the family and nurse and on the family's strengths and weaknesses. The most effective nursing care plans enable family members to gain independence and control over their situation. The nurse does not try to take over the family's problem(s) but helps them learn problem-solving skills they can use. Economic, environmental, and safety factors should be considered in the plan. The following factors need to be considered when planning with families:

* How safe are the neighborhood playgrounds or park for playing and walking?
* How close is the nearest prenatal clinic?
* Does the pregnant woman have suitable clothing to wear to a clinic or doctor's office?
* What is the main source of transportation for the family?
* What is the cost of public transportation in the community (eg, fares for subway, bus, taxi)?
* What is the cost of babysitting services in the community?
* Does the school have a program whereby children can stay after school until their parents arrive?
* Who could be used as a back-up babysitter if the primary sitter is ill or unavailable?

implementation

A major goal when working with families is to promote positive changes in the family by focusing on family strengths. Any change, positive or negative, creates a degree of stress. Change and stress often begin when a couple realizes the woman is pregnant and continue throughout the life cycle of the child. The needs of each developmental phase must be considered in the life cycle because they differ from infancy to adolescence, as does the degree of stress brought about by the changes. Family developmental levels and interventions for health promotion are included in Table 1-2.

evaluation

The evaluation phase of the nursing process is to measure the outcome of nursing interventions. When applying this phase to family interactions, the following must be considered:

* The family identifies responses that are neglectful or harmful.
* The family members verbalize the need for assistance with a stated problem.
* The family uses available community resources.

key points ✳

* A family is defined as two or more people living in the same household, sharing common emotional bonds, and providing for the basic needs of life.
* A parent is defined as the person(s) establishing a parent–child relationship by caring for the child and providing the physical, social, and emotional requirements necessary for normal growth and development.
* Parenting is not intuitive but learned from family interactions.
* Dysfunctional family relationships can result from a limited or distorted understanding of normal growth and development in children and foster child abuse or neglect.
* The nuclear family, consisting of husband, wife, and children, is no longer the typical family type as the number of single-parent families continues to increase.
* Culture includes feelings, beliefs, attitudes, and practices passed down from generation to generation.
* Nurses need to be familiar with and sensitive to the spiritual and cultural practices of clients.
* Nurses must be client advocates to ensure meeting health care needs.
* The most effective nursing care plans enable family members to gain independence and control over their situation by providing them with problem-solving skills.

review questions ✳

1. The Rolland family consists of a husband, wife, and two children. The nurse understands this family type to be
   a. nuclear.
   b. extended.
   c. multigenerational.
   d. single family.
2. Select the most appropriate response to concerns about parenting skills.

   a. Parenting is a natural instinct based on human needs.
   b. Parenting skills are learned from observing parents and others, reading, and listening to other parents.
   c. Parenting skills are less effective when shared with another family member.
   d. Parenting is a personal issue involving mostly physical care, such as bathing, feeding, and clothing, throughout childhood.
3. Select the most appropriate statement concerning interacting with families having different cultural customs.
   a. Culture is not an important issue when caring for clients.
   b. Basically, all families have the same needs.
   c. The nurse can help families deal with today's Western health care system by bridging cultural gaps.
   d. A family's set of beliefs is significant if they conflict with the value system of the nurse.
4. Select the most appropriate statement concerning the nursing process.
   a. It is a scientific, systematic, problem-solving approach to safe, consistent nursing care.
   b. It is most effective for the client experiencing an acute crisis or emergency situation, such as potential loss of a baby.
   c. The nursing process consists of assessment, planning, and evaluation.
   d. The nursing process is based on the medical or surgical diagnosis and relates to the physician's orders.
5. Jenna is 6 months pregnant and is being seen in the clinic for a routine check-up. Nursing tasks include checking the vital signs, weight, and presence of edema. These tasks represent which step of the nursing process?
   a. Planning
   b. Implementation
   c. Evaluation
   d. Assessment

references

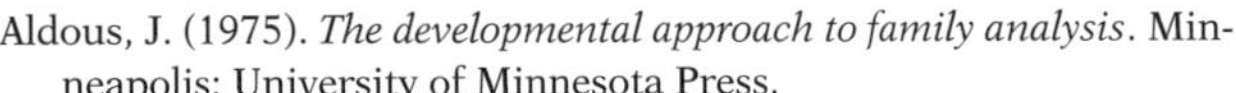

Aldous, J. (1975). *The developmental approach to family analysis*. Minneapolis: University of Minnesota Press.

Centers for Disease Control (1993). Infant mortality—U.S., 1991. *Morbidity and Mortality Weekly Report, 42*, 926–930.

Duvall, E. *Marriage and family development* (5th ed.). Philadelphia: J. B. Lippincott. (1977).

Holland, S., & Peterson, K. (1993). The health care titanic: Women and children first? *Second opinion, 1*, 11–27.

Killien, M. G. (1993). Returning to work after childbirth: Considerations for health policy. *Nursing outlook, 41*(2), 74–78.

bibliography

Campbell, T., Doherty, W., & Mooney, A. (1992). Reaching out to the family in crisis. *Patient Care, 4*, 125–136.

Castiglia, P., & Harbin, R. (1992). *Child health care: Process and practice*. Philadelphia: J.B. Lippincott.

Corrine, F., Bailey, V., Valentin, M., Morantus, E., & Lillian S. (1992). Spiritual interventions in maternal-child health. *MCN, 17*, 141–145.

Craft, M., & Willadsen, J. (1992). Interventions related to family. *Nursing Clinics of North America, 2*, 517–527.

Editorial (1990). NANDA definition. *Nursing Diagnosis, 1*(2), 50.

Ellis, J., & Nowlis, E. (1995). *Nursing: A human needs approach* (5th ed.). Boston: Houghton Mifflin.

Eschleman, M. M. (1996). *Introductory nutrition and diet therapy* (3rd ed.). Philadelphia: Lippincott-Raven.

Magnet, M. (1992). The American family. *Fortune, 10*, 42–48.

McCool, W., Tuttle, J., & Crowley, A. (1992). Overview of contemporary families. *Critical Care Nursing Clinics of North America, 4*, 549–557.

McCormick, J., & Wingert, P. (1991). Whose child am I anyway? *Newsweek, Summer*, 58–60.

Oermann, M. H. (1991). *Professional nursing practice—A conceptual approach*. Philadelphia: J.B. Lippincott.

Pillitteri, A. (1995). *Maternal and child health* (2nd ed.). Philadelphia: J.B. Lippincott.

Reeder, S. J., Martin, L. L., & Koniak, D. (1992). *Maternity nursing: Family, newborn, and women's health care* (17th ed.). Philadelphia: J.B. Lippincott.

Shives, L. (1994). *Basic concepts of psychiatric-mental health nursing* (3rd ed.). Philadelphia: J.B. Lippincott.

Stanhope, M., & Lancaster, J. (1992). *Community health nursing* (3rd ed.). St. Louis: C.V. Mosby.

Taylor, C., Lillis, C., & LeMone, P. (1993). *Fundamentals of nursing* (2nd ed.). Philadelphia: J.B. Lippincott.

issues and trends in maternity care

2

outline ✳

objectives ✳

After studying this chapter, the reader should be able to:

- ✳ Discuss the evolution of maternal–newborn nursing.
- ✳ Discuss the factors that brought about family-centered maternity nursing.
- ✳ Define statistical terms used in family health care.
- ✳ Discuss the importance of adequate prenatal care.
- ✳ Discuss the factors that the U.S. Public Health Service recommends for adequate prenatal care programs.
- ✳ Describe the cost factors that are considered in the delivery of maternal–newborn health care.
- ✳ Discuss the issues of drug and alcohol abuse, domestic violence, single parents, maternal age, and infertility.
- ✳ Explain the impact of legal issues in maternal–newborn nursing.

key terms 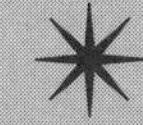

birthing rooms
birth rate
case management
childhood mortality
family-centered maternity care
fertility rate
fetal mortality rate
infant mortality rate
LDRP
maternal mortality rate
midwifery
neonatal mortality rate
perinatal mortality rate

Care of the childbearing family has undergone major changes during the last 25 years. Many pregnant women have a choice of how and where to give birth—in a hospital with single-room maternity care or birthing rooms, a free-standing birthing center, or at home. They may be attended by a nurse-midwife or an obstetrician. Depending on the location, their partner, other support person, and even friends or older children may be present. Women with health insurance have access to prenatal care and postpartum care for themselves and their infants. However, a growing number of American women have limited access to prenatal care and few choices about where and how their children are born. This lack of access to adequate care jeopardizes their own well-being and the life and health of their newborns.

Nurses have a key role in caring for the childbearing family, from the first prenatal visit through the birth and postpartum period. They are educators, caregivers, and comforters to women and their families. Many nurses today function in expanded roles, such as certified nurse-midwives (CNMs) and family nurse practitioners. To be effective in their various roles, nurses need an understanding of the current issues and trends in maternal–newborn nursing.

the evolution of maternal–newborn nursing

From the 1700s to the 1900s, pregnant women received no prenatal care, and birth occurred in the home, usually attended by a midwife. These midwives were not formally trained but learned by attending and assisting births with other women who had more experience with the birthing process. Physicians were only in attendance if the health of the mother seemed to be in jeopardy. Despite these practices, however, maternal mortality was relatively low because women received plenty of fresh air, fresh foods, and exercise. Childhood mortality was high, however. Only 15% to 25% of children born in the American colonies survived to their 21st birthday, probably because of lack of immunizations against life-threatening childhood diseases, antibiotics, and surgical and medical interventions.

With the arrival of the 20th century and the industrial revolution, many rural families flocked to the cities seeking factory work. As this trend continued, women began to be hospitalized for birth, which was attended by physicians. The use of anesthetics was widespread. The woman was "asleep" during much of labor and delivery. Newborn and mother were groggy in the immediate postdelivery phase, making early maternal–newborn attachment difficult. As physicians took control of the birth process, midwifery was outlawed in several states.

Once childbirth moved into the hospital, the experience was barraged by rules and restrictions. The woman was isolated from her family for labor and delivery. She was transported to a delivery room that resembled an operating room. When the newborn was delivered, he or she was shown briefly to the mother and then taken to the communal nursery, with only limited, scheduled visits with the new mother. All family members, including siblings and grandparents, were denied visitation. The father, after scrubbing, masking, and gowning, was permitted a brief visit if it did not interfere with hospital routine. All family contact with the newborn was limited to a scheduled viewing through the window of the newborn nursery. The new mother and infant were hospitalized for 1 week or more. The labor, delivery, and postrecovery were managed according to a medical regimen as though the mother and newborn were sick patients rather than participants in a normal physiologic life event.

contemporary maternal–newborn nursing

In the 1940s, a group of families, health care providers, and other concerned citizens recognized that birthing policies and practices failed to meet the needs of the family. Pregnancy began to be viewed not as an illness but as

display 2-1
summary of influence of governmental programs

Year	*Program*
1935	Title V of the Social Security Act was amended to provide funding for maternal–child health programs.
1962	The National Institute of Child Health and Human Development was instituted to support research and training in special needs of mothers and children, including prenatal care.
1964	The title V amendment to the Public Health Service Act established the Maternal and Infant Care projects to provide comprehensive prenatal and infant care in public centers.
1969	The National Center for Family Planning was established to serve as a clearing house for contraceptive information.
1975	The Women, Infants, and Children program was established to provide supplemental food and nutrition education for low-income families.
1987	The National Commission to Prevent Infant Mortality was established to work with Congress on legislation to improve the national infant mortality rate and to build a national infrastructure to coordinate and integrate services to pregnant women.

a normal physiologic process. The practices and beliefs of Fernand Lamaze, Grantley Dick-Read, and Robert Bradley encouraged the participation of awake, alert mothers and partners for the birth process. These were the first rumblings of the need and desire for family-centered maternity care. Display 2-1 summarizes Federal government programs that affect maternal–child care.

changes in hospital childbirth practices

In 1950, the first family-centered maternity care program was established in Evansville, Indiana. By the 1970s, prepared childbirth with husband or partner participation was widely accepted. Today, family-centered maternity care is well established throughout the United States. Most hospitals allow partner participation in the birthing process and unlimited family visitation with mother and newborn. The newborn generally stays with the mother, and the nurse performs daily care for the newborn at the bedside, providing an excellent opportunity for parent teaching. This relaxed atmosphere encourages the mother to ask questions and receive information in a nonthreatening environment (Fig. 2-1).

Family-centered care encourages attendance at prenatal classes and family participation in the birthing experience from admission to discharge; it provides a homelike, relaxed environment. The family is viewed as active, prepared participants who have a role in decision-making about the birthing event.

In many of today's hospitals, the traditional delivery suite has been replaced by birthing rooms or labor, delivery, recovery, postpartum rooms (LDRPs or multipurpose rooms). The birthing room concept allows the woman to

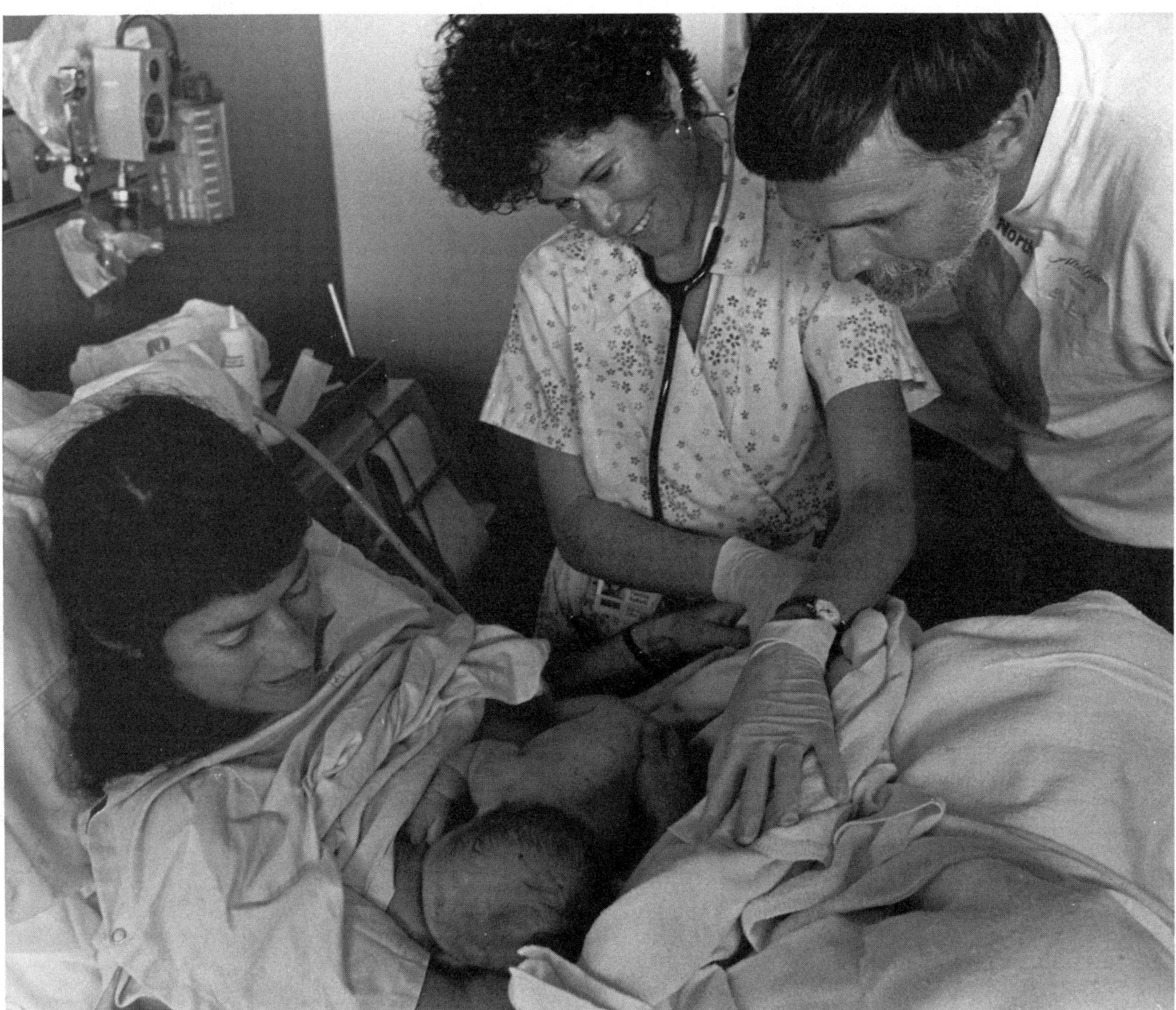

figure 2-1 *Contemporary family-centered maternity nursing encourages immediate care and education of the family together in the hospital room. (Photo © Kathy Sloane.)*

labor and deliver in a homelike setting and then transfer to a postpartum room for the remainder of her stay. The LDRP concept is based on single-room maternity care, in which the woman remains in a homelike setting for the entire process. This practice benefits the family and the hospital because it avoids multiple transfer from labor to delivery to postpartum and recovery areas, reduces the risk of infection, and provides a more relaxed atmosphere for the woman and family. The newborn stays with the mother and other family members. Visiting hours are not restricted, and other than good handwashing, no special ritual is maintained.

Midwives have again become part of the birth process, evolving from the local volunteer to registered nurses who have acquired additional specialized education to become certified nurse midwives (CNMs). There are 4,500 CNMs practicing in the United States (Lucas, 1993). Some have private practices; others are employed by hospitals or birthing centers or participate and direct home deliveries. According to the nurse practice acts, CNMs function under the direction of a physician but have a great deal of freedom to care for the woman during her pregnancy and delivery.

home birth

When consumers began to challenge the technical atmosphere of hospital birth, home birth gained popularity. Some couples decided to experience the birth process in their own home, feeling that birth at home meant more personal comfort and convenience. Home birth gives couples more control over the decision-making process, such as who can attend the birth, positions for labor and delivery, and the presence or absence of older siblings. These couples express a strong desire to experience the event in familiar surroundings.

Most home births are attended by CNMs; physicians rarely are present. In some areas of the United States, home births can be medically supervised and assisted in a mobile van that is fully equipped with the latest technology. The woman calls when labor starts and the fully staffed van pulls up outside the home for convenience (Hyde-Robertson, 1992). Couples planning a home birth need to check the credentials of the CNM and make plans for transportation to the hospital if an emergency occurs. Attending prenatal classes is recommended.

birthing centers

Another popular alternative to hospital childbirth is a birthing center. Up to 4% of all births take place in one of the 135 birthing centers located in the United States (Lucas, 1993). The woman is attended by registered nurses and CNMs and receives prenatal care and instructions at the center. The woman and her family are encouraged to be active planners and participants in the birthing process (Fig. 2-2). Many birthing centers are part of the local hospital complex or are located within 30 minutes of the hospital for ease of transfer in case the woman experiences an emergency requiring medical or surgical intervention.

> ✳ **nursing insight**
> *Women who have high-risk pregnancies (at high risk for severe life-threatening maternal or fetal emergencies) have limited birthing options. They need early prenatal care and should plan to deliver in the hospital where emergency equipment and personnel are readily available.*

statistics used in family health care

The numeric collection of data used to describe or analyze a given population is called *statistics*. Worldwide statistics concerning maternal and child health are collected to help identify health needs and population trends as a basis for health management decisions. These statistics have become standardized so that they can be used for international comparisons. Table 2-1 summarizes definitions of these terms.

The populations of the United States and Canada have increased dramatically since 1940. The population in the United States has reached approximately 260 million and Canada has more than 26 million people. The world population now totals more than 5 billion.

birth rate

The *birth rate* is affected by several factors, including the number of women of childbearing age, social attitudes toward childbearing, legalized abortion, religious beliefs, and availability of family planning methods. The current birth rate is approximately 16 to 17 live births per 1,000 population. Slightly more boys are born than girls (1,053 boys to 1,000 girls).

fertility rate

The *fertility rate* reflects the number of women of childbearing age who are actually giving birth. Childbearing age is generally said to be between 14 and 44 years; however, there are always exceptions. The current fertility rate is 71 live births per 1,000 women of childbearing age.

fetal mortality rate

Fetal mortality rate refers to the number of fetuses that die in utero after 20 or more weeks' gestation; these fetuses also are called *stillborn*. After 20 weeks, the fetus is capable of living outside the uterus; this point in development is also called the age of *viability*. The fetal mortality rate indirectly provides information about the quality and availability of prenatal care for the pregnant woman. Fetal death occurs for a variety of reasons, including poor prenatal care, maternal complications or illnesses, and other unknown causes. The fetal mortality rate in 1994 for the United States was 7.5 per 1,000 live births, down from 14.2 in 1970 (U.S. Bureau of Vital Statistics, 1994).

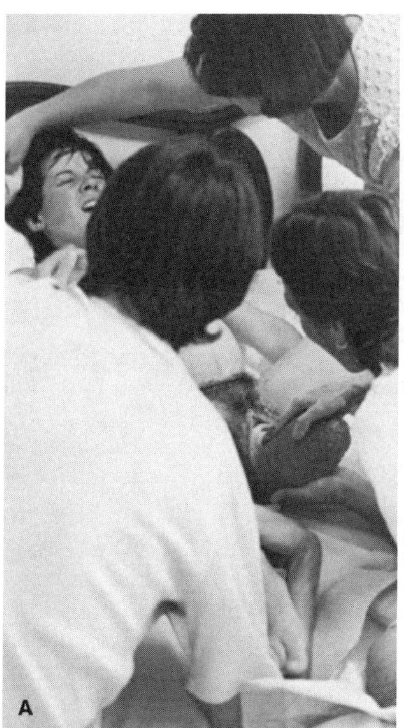

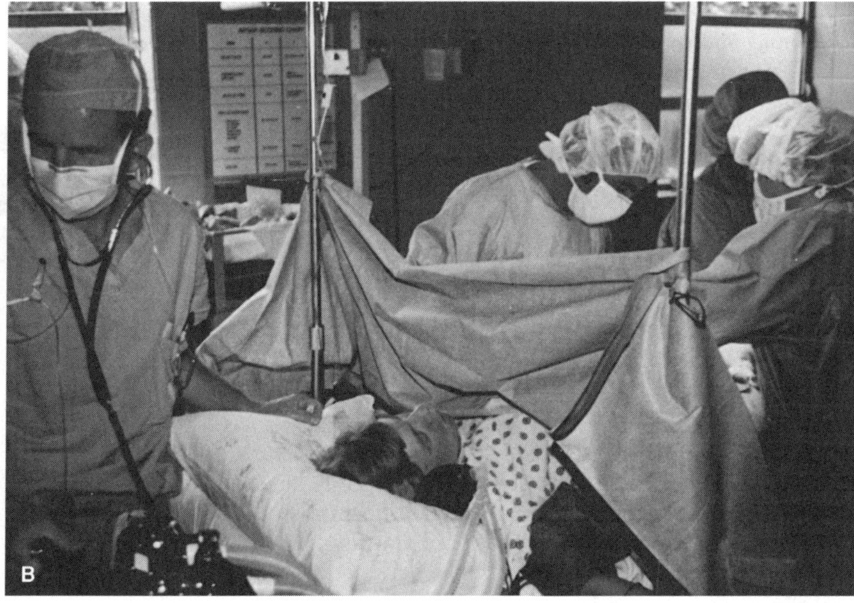

figure 2-2 ***(A)*** *Today the trend is toward a homelike birthing unit where the woman and family members take an active part in the birth. (Photo by Lyn Jones.)* ***(B)*** *Traditional hospital operating rooms, located near the birthing unit, are reserved for emergencies.*

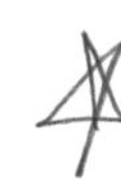

table 2-1 *summary of statistical terms for population studies*

Term	*Definition*
Birth rate	The number of births per 1,000 population
Fertility rate	The number of births per 1,000 women 15 through 44 years
Fetal mortality rate	The number of fetuses that die in utero after 20 weeks
Neonatal mortality rate	The number of neonatal deaths per 1,000 live births
Perinatal mortality rate	All stillborn infants whose gestational age is 28 weeks or more, plus all neonatal deaths less than 7 days per 1,000 births
Maternal mortality rate	The number of maternal deaths per 100,00
Infant mortality rate	The number of deaths occurring before the first birthday per 1,000 births
Childhood mortality rate	The number of deaths from birth until puberty

neonatal mortality rate

For the first 28 days after birth, the infant is called a *neonate*. The number of deaths per 1,000 live births during this period is the *neonatal mortality rate.* Premature birth and resulting low birth weight are the leading causes of neonatal mortality. The neonatal mortality rate for 1991 was 5.6 per 1,000 live births, down from 15.1 in 1970 (U.S. Bureau of Vital Statistics, 1994). This improvement is largely due to technology that has made it possible to save the lives of low–birth-weight newborns who would otherwise have died.

perinatal mortality rate

The *perinatal mortality rate* combines the fetal and neonatal mortality figures, that is, the number of deaths of fetuses weighing more than 500 g and the number of neonates who die within 28 days after birth.

maternal mortality rate

Maternal mortality is the number of maternal deaths directly related to the process of reproduction per 100,000 live births. This rate has decreased from 600 deaths per 100,000 live births in the early 1900s to the current rate of 7.9 deaths per 100,000 live births. This drop in maternal mortality can be attributed to a better understanding of bacteriology and infection control, improvement in health technology, and better prenatal care. The three major causes of maternal mortality are hemorrhage, infection, and pregnancy-induced hypertension.

infant mortality rate

Infant mortality refers to the number of deaths occurring before the first birthday of the infant. Two thirds of infant deaths are the result of low birth weight. The United States ranks 24th in infant mortality among other developed countries of the world, despite advanced technology and state-of-the-art health care systems. Some of the reasons for this high rate are limited access to prenatal care for women without insurance, the high number of adolescent mothers (twice that of France, Germany, and the United Kingdom), and the high percentage of cesarean births in this country compared with other countries.

childhood mortality

Childhood mortality is a broad term that includes the number of deaths that occur from birth until puberty. The death rate is higher in the first year of life than any other period until after age 55. Adolescents have the next highest incidence of death, attributed largely to motor vehicle accidents and suicides.

issues and concerns of maternal–newborn nursing

Many complex issues confront today's maternity nurse, including lack of prenatal care, cost factors, maternal substance abuse, maternal age, single-parent families, domestic violence, infertility, and assisted reproductive technologies. These issues are related to larger problems of society and have long-term implications for the future of nursing and the nation.

delivery of prenatal care

Adequate prenatal care to decrease the infant mortality rate and increase the number of healthy term infants remains one of the most important issues in maternity nursing. Studies have shown that prenatal care improves birth weight and lowers the risk of preterm delivery. Prenatal care is the most important step in providing adequate maternal–infant care. Early prenatal care decreases the infant mortality rate by providing assistance and interventions that deal with medical care and with the social, economic, and environmental needs of the pregnant woman.

Most industrialized countries have national health care systems, making prenatal care free and readily available. Sweden awards a monetary bonus to its mothers for early participation in prenatal care. However, only 75% of pregnant women in the United States begin prenatal care in the first trimester. The greatest barriers to prenatal care follow:

1. Lack of access to care in rural districts and inner-city areas due to finances and transportation costs
2. Inadequate maternal understanding of the importance of prenatal care due to lack of education
3. Shortage of health care providers in financially deprived areas probably due to low wages, poorly equipped facilities, and lack of educational and social opportunities for themselves and their family members

The U.S. Public Health Service recommends that prenatal care become more accessible and include the following:

* Support of preconception care
* Evaluation of the woman during the first trimester to determine frequency and type of visits needed
* Appropriate psychosocial assessment to evaluate for intervention
* Individualized care during prenatal visits, including nutritional, physical, and psychosocial interventions
* Evaluation of suitability of personalized home visits, follow-up telephone contacts, and provision of care availability in locations of easy access (eg, shopping malls; Stevens & O'Connell, 1994)

cost factors

The cost of maternity care has increased dramatically; from 1986 to 1989 it increased by 25% (Stevens, 1992). More than 50 million women of childbearing age have inadequate insurance to meet their needs, while another 25% of the female population is without any insurance coverage, public or private. Those on public assistance have difficulty finding a care provider. Many physicians will take a limited number of Medicaid clients, while others refuse to take any.

Many obstetricians are leaving their practices due to the high cost of malpractice insurance and the high rate of litigation. This has resulted in a shortage of care providers and an increase in costs.

Transportation to available care also is a concern. Many living in rural areas must travel long distances to reach appropriate facilities. Others may be within traveling distance but lack personal transportation or funds for public transportation.

In an effort to restrain the escalating cost of health care delivery, several plans or systems have been developed. Health maintenance organizations (HMOs) are prepaid health insurance plans that provide comprehensive health care for an annual fixed fee. Nurses and CNMs are readily employed by HMOs because they provide competent care while keeping the costs down. Because the focus of most HMOs is preventive care, prenatal and maternity care are emphasized to keep the cost of complications to a minimum.

Prospective payment programs have been developed and refined through the use of diagnosed-related groups (DRGs). Prospective payment means the institution has agreed to pay a fee for a type of care based on the DRG, regardless of the actual cost. This plan was first introduced by Medicare in 1987. Today, it is universal and used by all insurance companies. The DRG determines a length of stay for a particular diagnosis, for example, vaginal delivery without complications (24 hours postdelivery). The DRG is assigned a code number that is used for billing purposes (Display 2-2). The hospital is reimbursed for the length of stay that is expected. If the client stays longer, the hospital assumes the cost. If the client is discharged earlier, the hospital still receives the same payment. This makes it advantageous to the hospital to provide excellent care and to minimize complications that could result in a longer stay. Reduced lengths of stay result in greater profit for the institution.

Many hospitals have begun to use case management to deliver more organized care and to reduce length of stay. This system of care provides a patient care advocate who assists the patient in obtaining satisfactory care. The client has a team of health providers with a registered nurse coordinating and planning the care. This includes actual care, teaching, and referrals to other members of the health care team; this is an attempt to decrease the fragmentation of health care (Fig. 2-3).

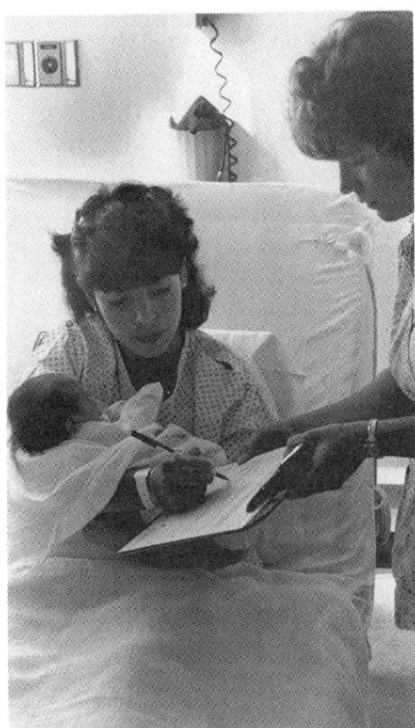

figure 2-3 *Among many other duties, nurse case managers assist the client with confusing and detailed health insurance forms. (Photo by Lyn Jones.)*

drug and alcohol abuse

It is estimated that approximately 11% or 375,000 infants born in the United States each year are victims of drug abuse, with cocaine being the drug of choice for many drug-dependent women (Kelly, Walsh, & Thompson, 1991). According to the U.S. Department of Health, the number of American-born "crack babies" will exceed 1 million by the year 2000.

Maternal cocaine use results in spontaneous abortion, premature separation of the placenta, premature labor and delivery, low birth weights, and small-for-gestational-age newborns. If the mother used cocaine during the first trimester, especially when the fetal brain is forming, the nervous system message pathways may be damaged. Research indicates that the pleasure-reward pathway is particularly vulnerable and explains why these newborns exhibit a general lack of emotion.

It is estimated that more than half the women in America consume some form of alcohol during the first trimester of pregnancy, with at least 10% continuing to drink throughout their pregnancy. Alcohol contains many chemicals that are toxic to the fetus and result in fetal anomalies and growth retardation. Alcoholism can result in fetal death.

The most serious alcohol-related fetal complication is called *fetal alcohol syndrome* (FAS), which results in physical, developmental, and intellectual abnormalities. FAS is produced by continual maternal ingestion of five or more drinks per day. Because the effects on the fetus of low levels of maternal alcohol ingestion have not been determined, the pregnant woman is advised to abstain from the use of alcohol during pregnancy. Women who have been identified as alcoholics need nonjudgmental support and intervention during their pregnancy.

display 2-2
examples of maternity-related diagnosis-related groups with code number

370 Cesarean section with complications
371 Cesarean section without complications
372 Vaginal delivery with complications
373 Vaginal delivery without complications
374 Vaginal delivery with sterilization or dilatation and curettage
375 Vaginal delivery with operative procedures
376 Postpartum diagnosis without operative procedure
377 Postpartum diagnosis with operative procedure
378 Ectopic pregnancy
379 Therapeutic abortion
380 Abortion without dilation and curettage
381 Abortion with dilation and curettage
382 False labor
383 Other antepartum diagnosis with medical complications
384 Other antepartum diagnosis without medical com-plication
385 Neonatal death or transfer

> **✳ nursing insight**
> *Educational materials for patient teaching may be obtained from National Clearinghouse for Alcohol and Drug Information Services, P.O. Box 2345, Rockville, MD 20852.*

domestic violence

Domestic violence is an area of increasing concern in America. Recent studies have shown that 11% to 23% of women of childbearing age have been physically abused. This violent behavior may continue or even increase during pregnancy. More than 25% of battered women have reported being hit in the abdomen during their pregnancy (Bersenson, Wiemann, Wilkinson, Jones, & Anderson, 1994). This may result in injury to the woman and to the unborn child. Preliminary reports indicate these women are twice as likely to experience preterm labor resulting in premature birth.

single-parent families

The number of "traditional" families is slowly decreasing, while the number of single-parent families is increasing. The single-parent family results from divorce, abandonment, death of a spouse, or the choice of remaining single while parenting a child.

Many single-female parents have limited support systems and live at or below the poverty level. Nearly 80% of the poor in the United States are women and their children. The fastest growing group of homeless are single mothers and their children.

For a variety of reasons, single pregnant women often seek prenatal care late in their pregnancy. The reasons may include denial of the pregnancy, lack of transportation, lack of support, or indecision about whether to continue or terminate the pregnancy. A supportive and nonjudgmental attitude must be maintained when caring for the single parent. Information about obtaining public assistance through various programs, such as Women, Infants, and Children and Aid to Dependent Children may alleviate some of the financial burden of these clients. Parenting programs, prenatal care classes, and future birth control planning also may assist the single parent.

maternal age

Pregnancy at either end of the age continuum presents its own joys and trials. More teens and women older than 35 are becoming pregnant, giving birth, and raising their newborns.

Adolescent pregnancy is more prevalent in the United States than most industrialized countries. Approximately 1,000,000 teenagers become pregnant each year in the United States, resulting in more than 500,000 live births (Quimby, 1994). Ninety-five percent of these teens become single parents and raise their newborns. Some have two or more infants during their teenage years.

Teenage pregnancy puts the adolescent at risk for decreased weight gain, urinary tract infections, sexually transmitted diseases, iron deficiency anemia, and prolonged labor. Teen pregnancy results in twice the likelihood of delivering a low–birth-weight infant (see Chap. 9).

Delaying pregnancy until 35 or beyond is becoming more frequent in this country. Approximately 61,000 American women 35 or older gave birth to their first child in 1988, and the trend is increasing (Aldous & Edmonson, 1993). Most of these women are white, married, middle class, college educated, and in good to excellent physical health.

The threat of the "biological clock" ticking is no longer as serious as before due to the advance of reproductive technologies. Thus, women feel more comfortable delaying childbirth while they pursue education, careers, and other interests. Many delay pregnancy while they decide if they really want to parent and if they want the added responsibility of a child. Others delay pregnancy due to divorce, remarriage, or concern about the stability of their marriage. Finally, others have infertility problems that may not have been diagnosed until later in life (see Chap. 9).

infertility and assisted reproductive technologies

Infertility may be defined as the inability to conceive after 1 year of unprotected sexual intercourse. The diagnosis and crude attempts at the cure of infertility were discussed as early as 2000 BC in the Kahoun Papyrus. The United States reports approximately 2.4 million married couples experience infertility (Awadalla & Drake, 1993).

The three most common causes of infertility are abnormalities in sperm production, scarring of the fallopian tubes, and problems with ovulation. Approximately 60% to 70% of couples seeking assistance in conceiving a child will have a successful outcome. This may be through routine treatment, such as surgical intervention or medication, or through the use of assisted reproductive technologies.

Assisted reproductive technology is costly, and many insurance companies do not cover the cost of treatment. The couple may face other concerns, including questions of paternity if donor sperm is used, the possibility of multiple pregnancy, and what happens to any embryos not implanted. (See Chap. 5 for further discussion of infertility, treatment, and interventions.)

legal issues in maternal–newborn nursing

Maternal–newborn nursing care requires comprehensive assessment and appropriate nursing interventions to ensure the safety of the mother and the fetus and newborn. Seventy-five percent of all obstetricians/gynecologists in the United States have been sued, and joint actions

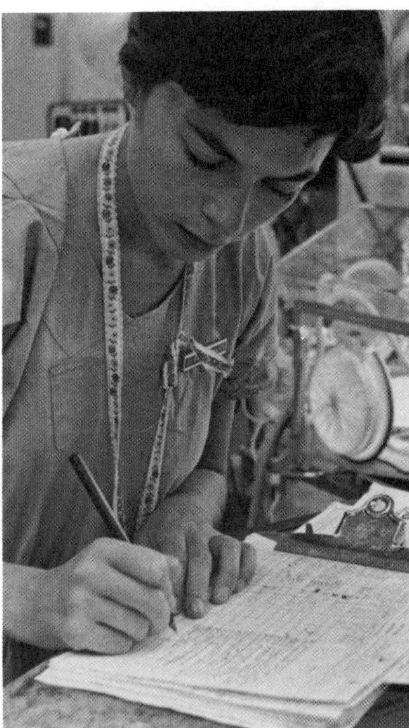

figure 2-4 *Taking time from a hectic schedule to make clear, accurate, and descriptive documentation helps protect the nurse during a later lawsuit.*

against the physician and the nurse are common. The majority of lawsuits claim substandard care resulting in injury; unavailability of the physician, particularly in an emergency; or severe birth injury that will require lifelong care. This has resulted in increased premiums for liability insurance for physicians and nurses caring for the childbearing family.

Nurses may best safeguard themselves by ensuring that they have a sound knowledge base, documenting nursing care completely, and keeping current on nursing care, trends, and issues in maternal–newborn nursing (Fig. 2-4).

key points ✳

- **Before the 20th century, women delivered their babies at home with a midwife who received "on the job training." Childbirth was viewed as a normal physiologic event.**
- **With the arrival of the 20th century and the industrial revolution, women were hospitalized for childbirth, anesthetics were used, and a physician was always in attendance.**
- **In 1950, the first family-centered maternity care program was established in response to families' and health care providers' concerns. Family-centered care encourages attendance at prenatal classes, family participation in the birthing experience from admission to discharge, and the use of a relaxed, homelike atmosphere.**
- **Midwifery has evolved from a home-trained individual to a registered nurse with specialized training.**
- **Births today take place in a variety of settings in the hospital, birthing centers, and at home. Women are demanding the right to have control over their labor and delivery.**
- **Worldwide statistics concerning maternal and child health are collected to help identify health needs and population trends as a basis for health management decisions.**
- **Statistics collected for maternal and child health include birth rate, fertility rate, fetal mortality rate, neonatal mortality rate, perinatal mortality rate, maternal mortality rate, infant mortality rate, and childhood mortality.**
- **Prenatal care is the most important factor identified to decrease infant mortality rate and to increase the number of healthy term infants.**
- **Major issues and concern of maternal–newborn nursing include prenatal care delivery, cost factors, drug and alcohol abuse, domestic violence, the rise in single-parent families, maternal age, infertility, and assisted reproductive technologies.**
- **The majority of lawsuits in maternal–newborn nursing claim substandard care resulting in injury, unavailability of the physician, or severe birth injury that will require lifelong care.**

review questions 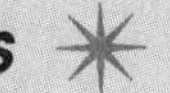

1. Mona El Safy tells her friend that she plans to have a home birth with a midwife in attendance. The nurse knows that
   a. midwives are no longer used.
   b. a physician must be in attendance.
   c. midwives are registered nurses with specialized training.
   d. home births are no longer permitted.
2. The nurse realizes that the most important change in the last century that has improved the maternal and neonatal birth rate is
   a. good nutrition.
   b. prenatal care.
   c. plenty of rest.
   d. birthing in a hospital setting.
3. The rate that refers to the number of women of childbearing age who are actually giving birth is
   a. fertility rate.
   b. maternal mortality rate.
   c. childhood mortality.
   d. neonatal mortality rate.
4. Prepaid health insurance plans that provide comprehensive health care for an annual fixed fee are called
   a. DRGs.
   b. managed care.
   c. HMOs.
   d. general health insurance plans.

5. Domestic violence during pregnancy is on the increase. Women who have received a blow to the abdomen are twice as likely to experience
   a. infertility.
   b. preterm labor.
   c. death of the fetus.
   d. low–birth-weight infants.

references 

Aldous, M. B., & Edmonson, M. B. (1993). Maternal age at first childbirth and risk of low birth weight and preterm delivery in washington state. *JAMA, 270*(21), 2574–2577.

Awadalla, S. G. & Drake, L. (1993). *Infertility update.*

Bersenson, A. B., Wiemann, C. M., Wilkinson, G. S., Jones, W. A., & Anderson, G. D., (1994). Perinatal morbidity associated with violence experienced by pregnant women. *American Journal of Obstetrics Gynecology, 170*(6), 1760–1765.

Hyde-Robertson, B. L. (1992). The necessity for maternal-infant perinatal home care. *Caring magazine*, 26–29.

Kelly, S. J., Walsh, J. H., & Thompson, K. (1991). Birth outcomes, health problems, and neglect with prenatal exposure to cocaine. *Pediatric Nursing, 17*(2), 130–135.

Lucas, V. A. (1993). Birth: Nursing's role in today's choices. *RN, 56*(6), 38–44.

Quimby, C. H. (1994). Women and the family of the future. *Journal of Obstetric, Gynecologic, and Neonatal Nursing, 23*(2), 113–122.

Stevens, K. A., & O'Connell, M. L. (1992). The problem of access: Meeting needs of pregnant women. *The Journal of Perinatal Education, 1*(2), 1–11.

U.S. Bureau of the Census (1994). *Statistical abstract of the United States: 1994* (114th ed.). Washington, D.C.: U.S. Bureau of Statistics.

bibliography

Burnhill, S. M. (1994). Adolescent pregnancy rates in the US. *Contemporary OB/GYN, 39*(2), 26–30.

Cardale, P. (1994). Changing role for midwives. *Nursing Times, 90*(28), 60–62.

Casey Foundation (1995). Trend toward fatherless households goes unchecked. *Ohio Schools, 73*(6), 18–19.

Department of Health and Human Services (DHHS). (1990). *Healthy people 2000: National health promotion and disease prevention objectives.* Washington, D.C.: Public Health Service.

Elmer-Dewitt, P. (1991). Making babies. *Time*, 56–63.

Forsman, I. (1994). Evolution of the nursing role in genetics. *Journal of Obstetric, Gynecologic, and Neonatal Nursing*, 481–485.

Jones, H. W., & Toner, J. P. (1993). The infertile couple. *New England Journal of Medicine, 329*(23), 1710–1714.

Klerman, L. V. (1994). Perinatal health care policy: How it will affect the family in the 21st century. *Journal of Obstetric, Gynecologic, and Neonatal Nursing, 23*(2), 124–128.

(1996). *Lippincott's review series: Maternal-newborn nursing.* (2nd ed.). Philadelphia: Lippincott-Raven.

Liu, D. T., Jevons, B., & Thwaites, P. (1992). Antenatal care towards the year 2000. *Midwives chronicle*, 388–390.

Malloy, C. (1992). Children and poverty:america's future at risk. *Pediatric Nursing, 18*(6), 553–557.

May, K. A., & Mahlmeister, L. R. (1994). *Maternal and neonatal nursing* (3rd ed.). Philadelphia: J.B. Lippincott.

Norwood, S. (1994). First steps: Participants and outcomes of a maternity support services program. *Journal of Obstetric, Gynecologic, and Neonatal Nursing, 23*(6), 467–473.

Old, S. B., London, M. L., & Ladewig, P. W. (1992). *Maternal-newborn nursing: A family-centered approach* (4th ed.). Redwood City, CA: Addison-Wesley Nursing.

Sharp, N. (1993). Mothers, infants, and children: What's happening now? *Nursing Management, 24*(2), 17–20.

Stolte, K., Myers, S. T., & Owen, W. L. (1994). Changes in maternity care and the impact on nurses and nursing practice. *Journal of Obstetric, Gynecologic, and Neonatal Nursing, 23*(7), 603–608.

Taffel, S. M., Placek, P. J., & Kosary, C. L. (1992). U.S. cesarean section rates 1990: An update. *Birth, 19*(1), 21–22.

Winston, R. M., & Handyside, A. H. (1993). New challenges in human in vitro fertilization. *Science, 260*, 932–936.

issues and trends in child health care

3

outline

objectives 

After studying this chapter, the reader should be able to:

- Define the terms pediatrics and pediatrician.
- Discuss the concept of family-centered child care.
- List at least two factors impacting the future of children.
- Discuss how a lack of health insurance affects child health care.
- State the largest public source of health care financing for pregnant women and children.
- Discuss how health risks for children increase when mothers work outside the home.
- Describe at least five health risks involving homeless children.
- Discuss the impact of medical technology on child care.
- List at least five health care goals for the year 2000.

key terms 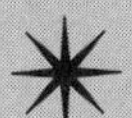

acupuncture
alternative therapy
family-centered care
mainstreaming
meditation
pediatrician
pediatrics
pedophiles
technology

Child health nursing involves health promotion, health maintenance, health restoration, and health rehabilitation based on a family-centered approach. Family-centered child health nursing recognizes the child as an integral part of the family and acknowledges racial, ethnic, cultural, and socioeconomic diversity. Health teaching is a major component of child health nursing based on understanding child development as a process of individual and family growth.

Pediatrics is the medical science relating to the care of children and treatment of their diseases. A *pediatrician* is a physician who specializes in the medical treatment of children. Accessibility and availability of health care play a major role in the growth and development of children and in the health of society in the future. Programs seeking to promote healthy development of children by strengthening families are gaining momentum. Family-centered care programs are reshaping traditional approaches to families and children, and are becoming important incentives for change in health care delivery.

evolution of child health nursing

Throughout history, major health problems for children have resulted from poverty. Overcrowded, unsanitary, and substandard living arrangements existed in the early 1900s and continue to be a critical factor in child health as 2000 approaches.

Before pasteurization, contaminated milk led to serious intestinal disorders among infants and children. Today, however, milk and other foods are contaminated with hormones injected into animals and into milk, agricultural pesticides, acid rain, and waste products of technology.

government programs affecting child health

Concern about child health and welfare led to two important historic events that have affected the health of children over several decades: the 1909 White House Conference on Dependent Children and establishment of the Children's Bureau in 1912. Child health continues to be advanced by both organizations. National efforts to improve child health are summarized in Table 3-1.

white house conferences

The White House Conference on Children originated in 1909 to advance and safeguard the well-being of children. The White House Conference on Children and Youth was convened every 10 years until 1970, keeping channels of communication open among the specialists, practitioners, and research workers in children's services and parents, citizens, and youth.

children's bureau

The Children's Bureau was established in 1912 by Lillian Wald, founder of the Henry Street Settlement in New York City, and Mrs. Florence Kelley of the National Consumers' League to improve general care of children. The Bureau continued its work until 1969 when the work was reassigned to other agencies of the federal government.

world health organization

The World Health Organization (WHO) was established as a specialized agency of the United Nations in 1948 and is located in Geneva, Switzerland. The organization acts as a director and authoritative coordinator of international health work, establishing and maintaining effective collaboration with governments and other interested groups (Display 3-1).

united nations international children's emergency fund

United Nations International Children's Emergency Fund (UNICEF) was created by the United Nations in 1946 to meet the emergency needs of children throughout the world in times of war or other disasters. Voluntary contributions from governments, groups, and individuals provide the financing for UNICEF.

national association of pediatric nurses associates and practitioners

The National Association of Pediatric Nurse Associates and Practitioners was founded to enhance the quality of health care for infants, children, and adolescents. This organization believes that health care systems must incorporate changes that focus on the promotion of health and prevention of disease. Preventive health care includes activities that promote responsible behavior and adoption of healthy lifestyles.

Primary care includes the child or family's first contact with a health care agency, pediatrician, pediatric nurse practitioner, or pediatric nurse. Nurse practitioners are primary health care providers involved in the maintenance of health, treatment of minor illness, and management of chronic illness conditions.

display 3-1
world health organization responsibilities

World Health Organization furnishes assistance to countries by providing the following:

- **Health information, including technical, educational, and other health-related services.**
- **Evaluation of a country's health problems when requested**
- **Encouragement and promotion of work to eradicate diseases and prevent injuries**
- **Pertinent information about nutrition, housing, sanitation, and environmental hygiene pertinent to a country's resources**
- **Aid in control of communicable diseases**

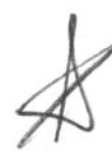

table 3-1 government assistance programs for children

Assistance Program	*Age Group*	*Health Care Benefits*
Medicaid	Any age	Health care paid by state to health care provider
Early and periodic screening diagnosis and treatment	Children on Medicaid; birth to 21 y	Early detection and treatment of health problems through regular medical, dental, vision, and hearing examinations
Aid to Families with Dependent Children	Children living in poverty	Cash vouchers given to a parent of a child who qualifies to spend on clothes and shelter
Children with Special Health Care Needs; Title V	Birth to 21 y with special health needs	Helps pay child's medical bills
Head Start	3–5 y	Addresses health and educational needs of the economically disadvantaged
Special Supplemental Food Program for Women, Infants, and Children (WIC)	Pregnant, breast-feeding women, infants, children younger than 5 y with special nutritional needs	Provides nutritious food to people at risk based on medical assessment
Food Stamps, Commodity Supplemental Food Program (CSFP)	Families living in poverty	Provides vouchers to buy food; CSFP provides nutritionally prescribed package for infants and children
Education of All Handicapped Children Act of 1975	5–21 y	Mainstream children with disabilities
The Education of The Handicapped Amendments of 1986	0–5 y	Early intervention to reinforce development
The Individual with Disabilities Education Act (IDEA)	0–21 y	Specifically addresses transition issues of children with disabilities
Child Identification Process	0–21 y with developmental delays	Aids in finding children eligible to receive services
Individualized Education Plan (IEP)	5–21 y	Sets educational goals
Individualized Family Service/Support Plan (IFSP)	0–5 y	Authorizes families to participate in planning child's health care needs

Adapted from Burns, M. (1993) Broadening the scope of nursing practice: Federal programs for children. *Pediatric Nursing, 19*(6), 549.

health care trends

Health care trends are influenced by many social forces, including economics, politics, science, culture, and population demographics. These social forces are complex and rapidly changing. Among the social forces shaping the health of children in the United States are continued advancement of health-related technology, increased accessibility to information through state-of-the-art computer systems, a widening gap between rich and poor, and the rising cost of health care. Trends are summarized in Display 3-2.

health promotion and disease prevention

The focus of child health nursing has shifted from treatment of illness to promotion of health and prevention of disease. The pediatric nurse needs to be prepared to care for the healthy child and the child with short-term acute illness or chronic illness. Nursing care based on family-centered goals includes assisting children, parents, siblings, and other care providers to develop and function at their optimal level of ability.

goals for the year 2000

Improving access to health care for children from birth through 17 years is identified as a major goal of *Healthy People 2000* (Department of Health and Human Services, 1990). Health care goals for the year 2000 include the following:

* Administration of the basic immunization series to at least 90% of children younger than 2 years
* Elimination of measles and rubella; decrease in incidence of mumps to less than 500 cases per year and of pertussis to less than 1,000 cases per year
* Promotion of physical fitness and good nutritional sta-

display 3-2
acronym summarizing trends in child care

Relationships with family
Economy, exercise, ethics, educational mainstreaming
Alternative health care, ambulatory services
Control of infectious diseases, obesity in teens, drug abuse, violence; children with disabilities, children living in poverty, culture, community
Home health, health promotion

tus; reduction in the incidence of overweight adolescents; management of weight in at least 50% of children 12 years or older through sound dietary practices; promotion of regular physical activity to attain an appropriate body weight; and reduction of unhealthy weight loss behaviors, such as fasting diets, skipping meals, taking diet pills, vomiting, and taking laxatives

* Individualization of care according to sociocultural uniqueness
* Awareness of health care costs
* Emphasis on preventive care (especially accident prevention)
* Promotion of family-centered care
* Empowerment of health care consumers
* Reduction in incidence of sexually transmitted diseases (STDs)
* Reduction in violence, drug abuse, and drug addiction

immunization

Immunization decreases the child's risk of contracting communicable childhood diseases. Although immunization is available for most of the common communicable diseases of childhood, some children do not receive these immunizations as recommended. Since 1990, for example, measles outbreaks have been reported in 25 states. Many school districts now require a measles, mumps, and rubella booster for children entering kindergarten. The Centers for Disease Control and Prevention (CDC) suggest that health care workers without a clear history of natural immunity to rubella need a rubella booster unless they have already had one or know they have a positive rubella blood titer. The nurse needs to teach caregivers about the importance of immunization in preventing serious and even life-threatening illness. (For more information on childhood immunization, see Chapter 20.)

The benefits of childhood immunization greatly outweigh the risk of serious side effects. Nonetheless, the Vaccine Injury Compensation Act of 1988 requires a record of the manufacturer, expiration date, and lot number of every vaccine; the signature and title of the person administering the vaccine; and the date of administration. This federal law recognizes warranted malpractice claims and provisions for monetary compensation of the small percentage of children who suffer from serious adverse reactions. The law orders agencies to report severe vaccine-induced reactions to the Food and Drug Administration on forms available through state health departments (Jurgrau, 1990).

Preventable infectious diseases cause 6 to 8 million childhood deaths each year. Researchers are working on a single-dose vaccine that could change vaccine administration. The vaccine, projected to be available within 5 years, would protect infants against all major childhood diseases. A booster could be added to protect against regional scourges, such as malaria. Scientists expect the vaccine to provide lifetime immunity with a single dose; to be easy to administer, store, and transport; and to be effective at any time after birth.

physical fitness and nutritional status

Television, fast food, and labor-saving devices have contributed to an inactive lifestyle for many Americans, making obesity a national problem. Obesity often begins in childhood, when lifetime eating habits are formed. Unless children learn the value of good nutrition and regular exercise, they are likely to experience serious health problems throughout life. A recent survey (Wynder, 1994) suggests that schoolchildren need better education about healthy ways of living (Display 3-3). Nurses can help teach families the importance of adopting healthy behaviors, such as eating a diet high in fiber and low in fat, getting regular exercise, and avoiding alcohol and tobacco products.

Nutrition programs available to all children based on the family's financial eligibility or the child's nutritional

display 3-3
why children need better health education

A 1994 survey of American children, grades 2 through 6 revealed the following:

* 50% thought apple juice had more fat than whole milk
* 24% had eaten no fruit and 25% had eaten no vegetables the previous day
* 24% did not brush their teeth the night before
* 36% said watermelon has more fat than American cheese
* 59% did not wear a helmet the last time they rode a bicycle
* 12% did not believe acquired immunodeficiency syndrome could be passed from person to person
* 7% planned to smoke cigarettes; 15% were not sure; 11% of 6th graders had already smoked; 34% had tried alcohol.

The study was conducted by American Health Foundation, a private New York research organization, and Scholastic Inc, a publisher, and presented at a conference sponsored by the American Cancer Society in New Orleans, March 28, 1995.

risk are food stamps; Special Supplemental Food Program for Women, Infants, and Children (WIC) and Commodity Supplemental Food Program (CSFP). All three programs originate in the Department of Agriculture and are state-administered programs. Food stamps are allotted monthly according to financial need; CSFP and WIC programs focus on improving basic nutrition through counseling.

The President's Challenge Physical Fitness Program (1994) was established to motivate school-age children to achieve a basic but challenging level of fitness through program participation. Students who participate must score at or above the 50th percentile on all five items outlined in the program. Students completing the President's Challenge are eligible to receive the National Physical Fitness Award. A special program is provided for physically handicapped students. Information about the program can be obtained by writing to President's Challenge, Poplars Research Center, 400 East 7th Street, Bloomington, IN, 61704 or calling 1-800-258-8146.

diversity and cultural uniqueness

The population of the United States is becoming increasingly diverse. In 1986, immigration in the United States reached the highest point in more than 50 years. A 1990 Census Bureau report showed that 14% of U.S. residents spoke a language other than English at home. Each racial, ethnic, and cultural group has its own set of values that influences health practices and compliance.

Individuals learn ways to relate to the world through their culture, and this includes the world of health care. Culture plays a major role in family-centered child care. The nurse's understanding of cultural values promotes acceptance of cultural differences seen in others and aids in the individualization of nursing care according to sociocultural uniqueness. Nursing care that is sensitive to cultural factors promotes health care compliance. Cultural beliefs can be incorporated into nursing practice by listening, exploring cultural differences, and learning more about different cultures:

* In Hawaiian culture, life centers around the family or "ohna," with a high rate of children adopted interfamily, promoting a belief that all children are wanted and loved.
* Communication styles, such as saying "Oh, my God" when surprised or excited, may be offensive to cultures who see that expression as taking the Lord's name in vain.
* Japanese divide the world into two spheres, a public world and a private world, using a different communication pattern for each. Thoughts and feelings concerning the private self are shared with a select few. In contrast, Americans tend to expose their private selves more often and to people who are not necessarily intimate.
* Some cultures view deadlines or appointment times as inflexible and serious, while clocks or the concept of time constraints are nonexistent in other cultures.
* Some Hispanic girls learn that showering or bathing while they are menstruating can cause *pasmo* (pain). For the same reason, women who have given birth may not shower for 7 to 10 days.
* Trusted home remedies are often based on ancient traditions or folklore. For example, a Hispanic mother may rub *alcoholado* (a mixture of rubbing alcohol, eucalyptol, and eucalyptus leaves) on her feverish child's body or feet to keep the fever from increasing (Gilbert-Diaz, 1993).
* Stress-related issues in groups such as Native Americans, African Americans, Hispanics, and white Americans living in Appalachia and other parts of the United States are often related to poverty and involve hypertension, alcoholism, and family violence.

promotion of family-centered care

Programs based on self-help and child and parent education increase families' ability to overcome discrimination and other social ills. Family Resource Coalition has grown rapidly as a leadership organization and national clearinghouse for family support programs since 1981. Recently it was funded by the United States Department of Health and Human Services to establish a National Resource Center for Family Support Programs (Thomas, 1994). The resource center's aim is to build support and resources within communities to strengthen and empower families, enhance the capacities of parents, and foster optimal development of children and youth. (see Display 3–4.)

A strong characteristic of family support programs is their ability to deal with a wide variety of family needs. Typical program activities include education about par-

display 3-4
family support group organizations

* **Family Resource Coalition, 200 South Michigan Ave., Suite 1520, Chicago, IL 60604. Offers consultation, technical assistance, training, conferences, publications. Membership fee required.**
* **Parent Action, 2 N. Charles St., Suite 960, Baltimore, MD 21201. Nonprofit organization representing the nation's special interests of parents. Involved with policy and workplace initiatives, public education, community outreach, media projects, newsletter. Membership fee required.**
* **Children's Defense Fund, 25 E. Street N.W., Washington, DC 20001. Private, nonprofit research organization that monitors state and federal policy, gathers and disseminates data, offers extensive publications.**

Adapted from Thomas, H. (1994). Conceptual underpinnings of the family support movement, *Journal of Pediatric Health Care, 8*(2), 57–62.

enting and other life skills, parent support and self-help groups, joint parent and child activities, health and developmental screenings, child care to allow involvement in program activities, and information about referral to other services in the community.

Family support programs are oriented toward primary and secondary prevention rather than treatment or remediation. Services are oriented to the child, family, and community rather than solely to individual children.

lack of access to health care

The United States spends more on health care than any industrialized country in the world, nearly $800 billion annually. However, as many as 30 million Americans (15% of the population) have limited or no access to health care because they have no health insurance. Unlike other industrialized countries, the United States has no national health insurance program. Thus, economics is the most significant influence on child health care in the 1990s.

Families without health insurance often delay care until problems become serious. Conditions that could be effectively and economically treated on an outpatient basis remain untreated until hospitalization is required. Families of children with special needs often require help to access community health care. Nurses can provide the crucial link between families in need and the community resources available.

Federal programs for children do not ensure a child's access to health, education, and related services. Early identification of a child with special needs is especially critical when a family lacks financial resources; otherwise, care may be delayed unnecessarily.

medicaid

Medicaid is the largest single public source of health care financing for pregnant women and children. Early Periodic Screening Diagnosis and Treatment, legislated in 1967, is a special health care program within Medicaid for people from birth to 21 years, providing early detection and treatment of health problems through regular medical, dental, vision, and hearing check-ups. States are required to provide all medically necessary treatments identified in this process.

aid to families with dependent children

Aid to Families With Dependent Children recognizes special financial needs of families headed by single parents. Programs for children with special health care needs vary from state to state, but generally programs pay expenses not covered by private health insurance carriers or Medicaid. Enrollment of children from birth to 21 years is based on medical and financial income criteria outlined by each state.

cost containment

Hospitals and other health care agencies have made many changes to help control the escalating costs of health care. Some of these changes, such as health maintenance organizations and prospective payment using diagnosis-related groups, are discussed in Chapter 2. Regionalization of health care is another trend based on cost containment and community demand for quality health care. Costly physical facilities and medical and nursing personnel can no longer be duplicated in agencies that are in close proximity to each other. Small pediatric units in general hospitals are closing because a surplus of pediatric beds has made some departments uneconomical.

ambulatory care

More children who might have been admitted to a hospital are now receiving care in ambulatory clinics or at home. Many hospitals perform children's surgery, such as tonsillectomy or hernia repair, without requiring an overnight stay. The child arrives at the hospital, receives preoperative care, is sent to surgery, is observed in the recovery room, and if no complications arise, is dismissed.

Short-term hospitalization requires intensive health teaching by the nursing staff to ensure that family members are competent in performing special treatments or administering medications.

home health care

Home health care is one of the fastest growing components of health care spending, especially pediatrics. Home health care nursing requires an understanding and use of community resources (Fig. 3-1).

Families of infants and children with chronic conditions dependent on medical technology have found care at home possible because of advances in technical equipment designed or adapted for home use, such as home oxygen use. Children who are ventilator dependent or require prolonged nutritional support are receiving care and being monitored by parents, caregivers, visiting nurse associations, private-duty service agencies, and hospital-based home care organizations. A spectrum of services has been designed to target specific needs of the child, including intravenous medications, parenteral nutrition, nasogastric or enterostomy feedings, peritoneal dialysis, oxygen administration, ventilator support, and physical, occupational, and speech therapies.

school-based health centers

School-based health centers can help low-income young people gain access to clinical care. These health centers play a key role in supporting health-promoting behaviors among students, providing early intervention, interacting with the curriculum, and creating healthier student environments. Many high schools provide child care while single parents attend classes, helping them to stay in school instead of dropping out.

health care technology

Modern technology offers many lifesaving benefits to children and adults. Technology has made possible the identification of genes responsible for many inherited diseases. This provides the opportunity for early intervention and reduction of serious complications. For example, isolation

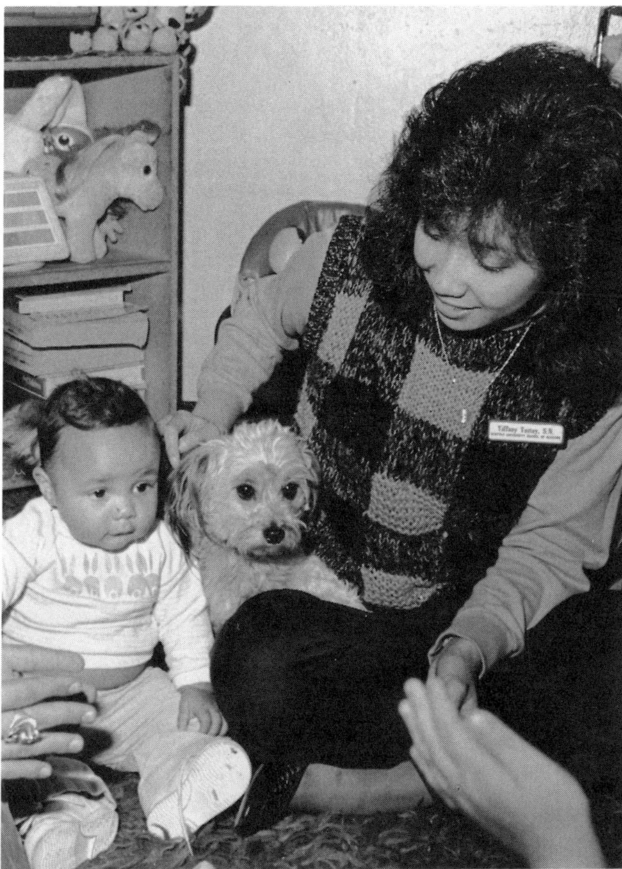

figure 3-1 *The nursing student learns about the individual, family, and community during a family home health care visit. (Courtesy of Seattle University.)*

of the gene responsible for cystic fibrosis provides a way to treat the disease, reduces costly interventions, and decreases life-threatening complications (see Chap. 30).

The long-term effects of technical interventions are not fully understood. However, the technology that makes possible the survival of tiny premature babies has led to a generation of disabled children who are often retarded, severely nearsighted, unable to walk, and inattentive to learning. These children are at increased risk of developing heart disease, hypertension, and diabetes during adult life (Barker, 1994). Many of these children have complex chronic conditions requiring continuing care. For example, ventilator care may be necessary for children with bronchopulmonary dysplasia, a chronic complication of very low birth weight and prematurity.

alternative health care

Use of alternative or complementary forms of therapy is increasing in pediatric nursing, resulting in part from cultural practices. For example, acupuncture, meditation, and therapeutic touch are common in many Asian cultures. Nurses have an increasing obligation to be aware of alternative therapies and health care agency policies regarding specific therapies. When an alternative form of care can be incorporated in the nursing plan, child and family compliance with the care plan is enhanced. For example, meditation or visualization can be used to decrease a child's discomfort before a painful or frightening procedure, empowering the child to maintain self-control.

Attempts to help children cope with the distress and anxiety associated with their hospitalization have involved the use of a combination of relaxation, distraction (visual imagery), and comforting self-talk beginning as young as 2 years. Nurses can teach positive self-talk skills useful during procedures. Coping interventions that bolster a child's feelings of personal control help build self-confidence needed during a hospital experience.

working families and child care

During the last 30 years, the number of mothers employed outside the home has risen rapidly and steadily. The U.S. Bureau of Census in 1990 reported that 60% of working mothers had children younger than 5 years, and 70% of working mothers had school-age children, which increases the need for child care outside of the home (Fig. 3-2). Care for school-age children can involve self-care before and after school, increasing the child's responsibilities for self and siblings.

The cost of child care is a burden to many working families, especially those headed by single mothers. Although some programs of subsidized child care exist for the poorest families, many middle-class families cannot afford quality child care.

Child care outside the home is not without risks, including exposure to infectious diseases from other children and child care workers and increased danger of physical and sexual abuse. In 1993, the Ohio Senate passed Senate Bill 38 (Ohio Revised Code, 1993) making it mandatory for people working with children to undergo a criminal background check including fingerprinting in an attempt to reduce the risk of exposing children to known *pedophiles* (people with an unnatural desire for sexual relations with children) or people convicted of child abuse.

challenging issues in child health

The value of children to society exists in their potential worth as adults, parents, citizens, contributors to the national economy, and promoters of the arts and sciences. Therefore, healthy children are a priceless asset to their community and their nation. Many indicators suggest that the United States is neglecting this priceless asset, allowing the general health of its youngest citizens to decline.

The Fordham University Institute for Innovation in Social Policy monitors the social health of children, using statistics from six problem areas: child abuse, children living in poverty, teenage suicide, teenage drug abuse, high school dropouts, and infant mortality. As Figure 3-3

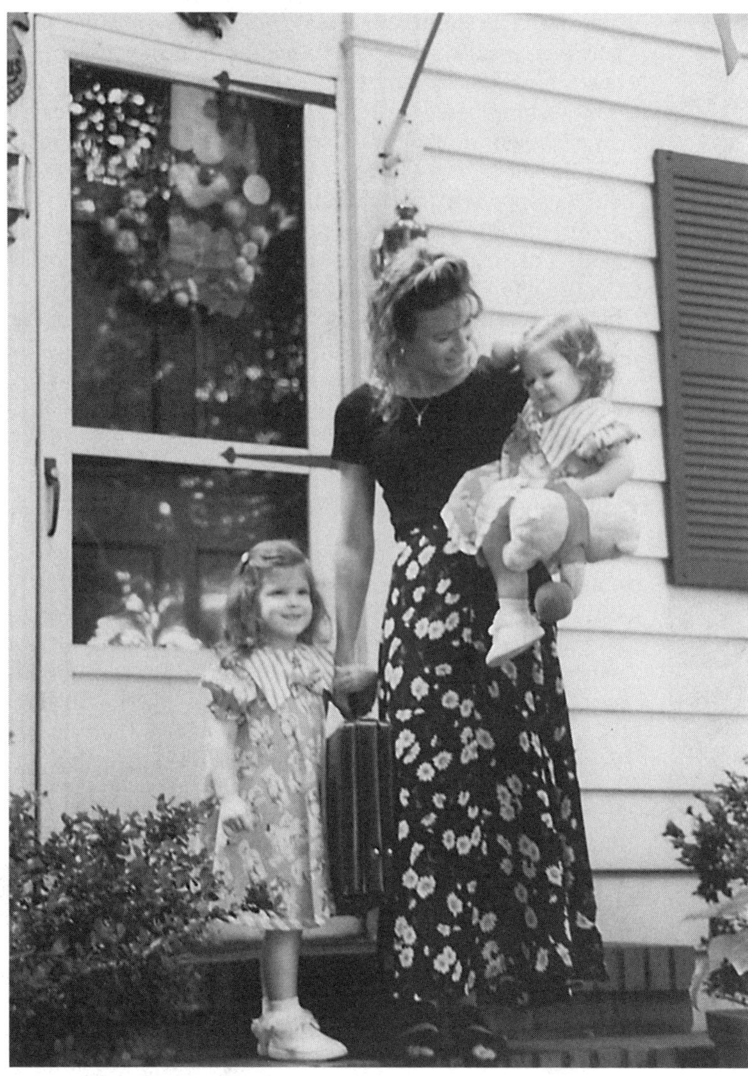

figure 3-2 *Today it is often necessary to juggle work and parenthood.*

shows, the social health index of children in the United States has declined substantially since 1970.

poverty and homelessness

Although America's health care costs exceed 11% of our gross national product, the health status of American children is declining. The Census Bureau listed 44.8 million, or 18% of the population, as being poor in 1990 (U.S. Bureau of Census, 1992). Although children make up only 27% of the nation's population, they make up 40% of the people living in poverty. During the last 20 years, the poverty growth rate for children younger than 6 years has been several percentage points higher than that of any other age group (Perry & Perry, 1994).

Poverty occurs more frequently among people of color. For example, more African Americans and Hispanics live in poverty than white Americans (Fig. 3-4).

In households with children headed by a caregiver younger than 30 years, 40% of the children live in poverty (Children's Defense Fund, 1992). Economic dilemmas can overwhelm young families.

Children living in poverty are often deprived of their most basic needs for safety, food, stability, support, and a healthy future (Display 3-5). Poor children often have difficulty developing a sense of trust, especially when their environment lacks basic nurturing. A 1995 study by the CDC reports that children born to poor, uneducated mothers are more likely than others to be mildly retarded (intelligence scores between 50 and 70; Satcher, 1995). As a result of this study, special pilot programs in child development have been started to determine whether early intervention can help improve the skills of these children before they reach school age.

homeless children

Children now constitute the largest segment of the population of homeless people. Their health problems are similar but more severe than those of other children living in

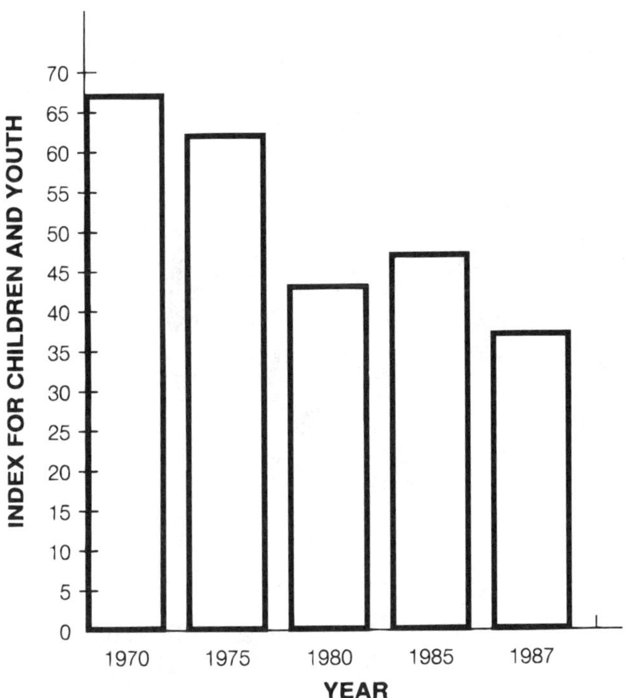

figure 3-3 *Index for social health for children and youth, 1970 to 1987. This is a composite measure based on figures from six problem areas (child abuse, children living in poverty, teenage suicide, teenage drug abuse, high school drop-outs, and infant mortality). (Data from Fordham Institute for Innovation in Social Policy, The Index of Social Health: 1989.)*

display 3-5
profile of american children living in poverty

CAUSES

* Inadequate financial resources in parent or caregiver earnings related to unemployment, low wages, trend toward part-time employment, and lack of training
* Family breakdown related to increases in teenage pregnancies, family dissolution, and child abandonment by fathers and mothers
* Inadequate governmental child support policies

BARRIERS TO HEALTH

* Lack of adequate health insurance coverage
* Critical shortage of health care providers and services (80% of pediatricians treat children covered by Medicaid, but more than half limit the number of cases accepted)
* Overloaded public health system
* Unavailable health care education

Adapted from Malloy, C. (1992). Children and poverty: America's future at risk. *Pediatric Nursing,* 18(6), 553–557.

poverty. For example, reports indicate that homeless children have three or more times the number of developmental delays than other poor children. Homeless families live in a chaotic and inconsistent environment with little or no financial resources. Temporary living conditions often require shared cooking and bathroom space, increasing the risk of contracting diseases and infections. Family problems, physical abuse, and lack of financial resources are among the leading causes of homelessness identified by shelter directors (Barge & Norr, 1991).

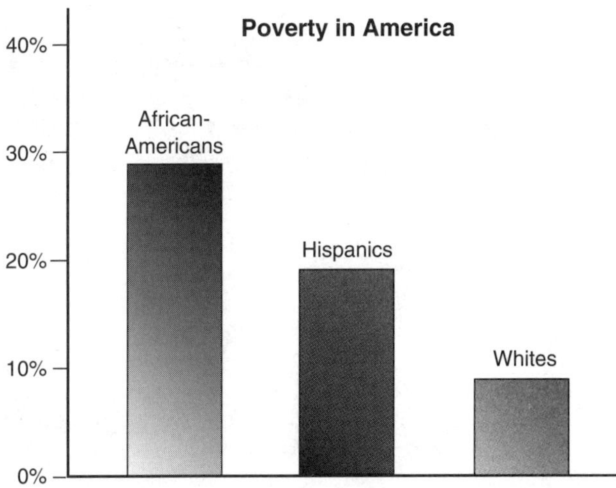

figure 3-4 *Poverty in America. Percentage of specific groups living below the poverty level.*

tuberculosis

Long regarded as a disease of poverty, tuberculosis among childbearing families has risen to epidemic proportions, bringing new challenges to pediatric nurses. The return of tuberculosis in the United States has been attributed to migration of families into the United States from high-prevalence areas in Asia, Africa, and Latin America; increased numbers of families living in poverty and crowded conditions with limited access to health care; and increased incidence of acquired immunodeficiency syndrome (AIDS). (For more information on tuberculosis, see Chapter 30.)

human immunodeficiency virus and acquired immunodeficiency syndrome

The latest figures from the WHO suggest that there are about 500,000 children with AIDS worldwide. Children make up about 1 million of the estimated 13 million people infected with human immunodeficiency virus (HIV). Based on these figures, experts speculate by 2000, 10 million infants and children will be infected with HIV, and most will die before their fifth birthday (WHO, 1993). Children infected with HIV experience recurrent illness, disrupting family life and ultimately leading to death and grief.

Most cases of HIV and AIDS in children younger than 13 years are the result of transmission of the virus during childbirth (from an infected mother) or during blood transfusions. About 25% of HIV- or AIDS-infected women are between 20 and 29 years old, suggesting that the infection was transmitted during adolescence. As adolescents become sexually active at earlier ages, education aimed at preventing AIDS and other STDs is essential to avoid tragic, needless loss of life.

drug addicted and HIV-positive newborns

Infants born to mothers with substance abuse problems (especially crack cocaine) or AIDS may spend extended time in hospitals because no one is available to care for them. Most of these babies could receive home care, but fear, prejudice, and increased demands relative to the child's problem make finding foster homes difficult. Crack-addicted babies have health problems beyond the newborn period, including small stature and *hypertonia* (abnormal tension of arteries and muscles), neurobehavioral abnormalities that put the child at risk for developmental problems because of easy overstimulation, difficult and unfulfilling interactions, and sleep disturbances (Kelly, Walsh, & Thompson, 1991).

Drug-addicted and HIV-positive babies have already affected hospitals in cities with large populations of drug addicts, such as Newark, New Jersey; New York City; and Miami Beach, Florida. The problem is spreading to other cities, such as Boston and Washington, D.C., and is projected to affect smaller communities unless substance abuse decreases.

cancer

Cancer is the leading cause of death by disease in children between 1 and 14 years. Although the incidence of childhood cancers increased 1.3% between 1950 and 1990, mortality decreased nearly 60% in the same period due to more effective treatments. New cases of childhood cancer in 1994 were estimated at 8,200; deaths from childhood cancer totaled 1,600, about one third of them from leukemia. Common sites of childhood cancer include the blood and bone marrow, bone, lymph nodes, brain, nervous system, kidneys, and soft tissues. Acute lymphocytic leukemia accounts for approximately 2,000 cases of leukemia among children (see Chap. 32). Although cancer mortality is higher among African American children, it is believed to be due to lack of access to quality health care rather than to racial differences. With equal access to state-of-the-art treatment in a pediatric oncology center, African American children fare as well as white children (Pui, 1995).

display 3-6
data on children with disabilities

The number of children with specific disabilities in the United States includes the following:

- **2.5 million developmental or growth delays (temporary or long-standing)**
- **3.4 million learning disabilities**
- **6.6 million behavioral and emotional problems, including attention deficiency disorder, phobias, anxiety disorders, and childhood depression**

Adapted from Feeney, D. & Kaufman, J. (1994). Caring for children with special health needs. *Caring Magazine, XIII*(12), 12–16.

chronic illness and disabilities

Children with chronic illness or disability constitute almost one fourth of the total population of American children (Display 3-6). From 6% to 12% of all American children from birth to 21 years have some form of disability. Of the 20 to 35 million children in the United States with chronic health conditions, 10% to 15% have problems severe enough to interfere with everyday activities requiring daily assistance (Ekvall, 1993). Children with disabling conditions can attend school regularly but typically do not participate in sports or other physically demanding activities. Chronic disabling conditions are most common among poor adolescent boys. These children are at particular risk for abuse by parents or other caregivers.

Many disabilities are the result of birth defects or lack of prenatal care. Birth defects continue to increase. A 1990 report from the CDC indicates that 29 out of 38 types of birth defects are increasing (Edmonds, et al., 1990). Some authorities believe that this increase is due to toxic chemicals in the air, food, and water.

mainstreaming

The U.S. Justice system has successfully applied the premise that "separate is not equal," favoring the integration of students with disabilities into regular public schools, referred to as *mainstreaming* (Fig. 3-5). In 1990, the Supreme Court ruled that a separate set of standards had to be developed for children with disabilities, based on an evaluation of the child's level of function and ability to walk, eat, dress, and perform other normal daily activities compared with those of a child of the same age.

The Education for All Handicapped Children Act (EHCA) of 1975, amended in 1986, deals with mainstreaming previously institutionalized children into public education settings. Schools are directed to write an Individualized Educational Program (IEP) for each student with special needs, respecting the child as part of a larger family unit. School nurses need to be part of the IEP process, contributing their findings and recommendations from a health assessment perspective.

The EHCA law establishes interagency and interdisciplinary collaboration, a child identification system, a family-designated case manager, and a definition of specific developmental delays. Children with delays in physical, cognitive, language and speech, psychosocial, or self-help skills are eligible for early intervention services. Conditions known to put the child at risk for developmental delays are often enough to make the child eligible for intervention. Health care providers, educators, and parents can refer children for screening, evaluation, and service recommendations.

Although parents often recognize a potential problem in a child, they sometimes wait for physicians, nurses, or social workers to confirm their fears and make the diagnosis "official." Eligible children receive services that contribute to educational and developmental success of the child, such as occupational therapy, speech therapy, physical therapy, and infant stimulation programs. Head Start is an example of an early intervention program geared to help at-risk preschool children.

asthma and other respiratory diseases

The incidence and mortality rates of asthma and other respiratory diseases have increased dramatically during the last 2 decades in the United States and all industrialized countries (Rachelefsky, 1995). Respiratory diseases are a major cause of hospitalization for children ages 1 to 9 years. Deaths from asthma increased 31% between 1980 and 1987. A chronic disease with acute episodes, asthma is a disorder that children and caregivers can learn to manage; however, children without adequate health care and family support have a poor prognosis.

educational inequity

Research consistently shows that well-educated people enjoy better health throughout life than those who lack education. This direct relationship between education and health is important to every child. The quality of educational opportunity available to the children in America's public schools varies from excellent to poor, depending on the human and financial resources invested. For example, schools in Great Neck, New York, an affluent Long Island suburb, invested $15,594 per pupil in the 1989 to 1990 school year. In contrast, New York City schools invested only $7,299 per pupil in the same year (New York State Board of Education, 1989). Greater financial investment in education usually means better teachers, better educational materials, and an environment more conducive to learning; it also reflects greater parental and community support of education, an essential element in educational success.

Staying in school serves many functions, including general education, vocational and life skills, and socialization. The consequences of dropping out of school can be severe. Youth who do not complete high school are far more susceptible to health, economic, and social problems (Lewit, 1992).

violence and child abuse

American society is becoming increasingly violent. Research studies published during 1994 indicate that one in four children ages 10 to 16 years reported being assaulted or abused within the previous year and 1 in 10 reported being sexually abused or assaulted. Among teenagers in suburban Colorado and Ohio, 14% of girls and 44% of boys reported being hit or punched at school, indicating that violence is not just an inner-city problem (Wilson & Joffe, 1995).

One of the most shocking public health problems in the country is the increase in gun violence among children. Every day in America, 14 children 19 years and younger are killed in gun-related accidents, suicides, and homicides. Many more are wounded. One in five Americans

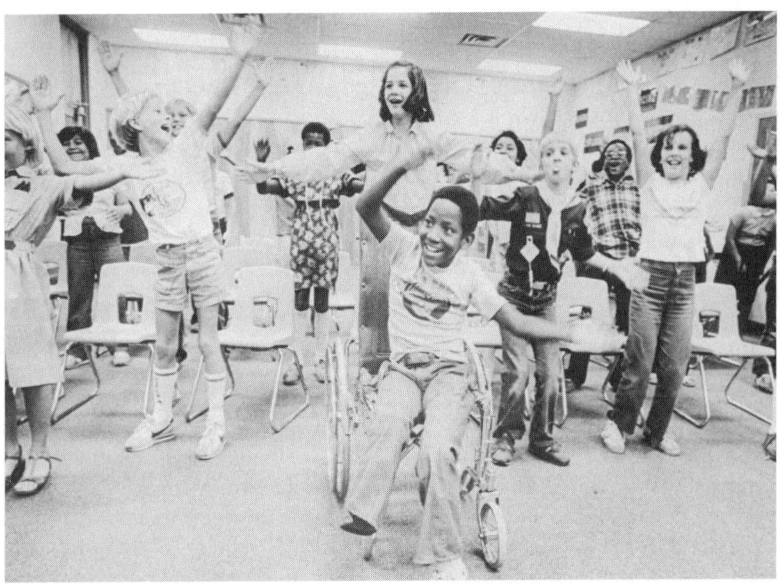

figure 3-5 *Mainstreamed children enjoy the education, facilities, and activities of public schools. (© Bob Deammrich/Stock Boston.)*

knows a child who has been shot by another child (Kohl, 1993).

The Youth Handgun Safety Act of 1993 makes it a federal crime to sell or transfer a handgun to a person younger than 18 years or for the minor to possess the gun. Firearm education must be included as a routine part of anticipatory guidance for all children and their parents. Youth violence and firearm injury are two tragedies that are linked and preventable.

Reports of suspected physical and sexual child abuse and neglect rose to 2.9 million in 1992. More than 1,000 children a year die as a result of abuse or neglect. Nationally, 1,383 children were officially registered as fatal victims of maltreatment in 1991. This figure represents a 10% increase over 1990. More than 75% of the victims were younger than 5 years; more than half were 1 year or younger (Ohio State Medical Association, 1992).

All 50 states have laws that mandate reporting suspected child abuse. These laws protect health care professionals from any liability that might result from reporting suspected abuse in good faith. If the nurse suspects a child has been physically abused, it is a legal and professional obligation to report the suspicions to local protection agencies and file a Suspected Child Abuse or Neglect form, following health care agency policies. By correctly identifying and reporting child abuse, the nurse is taking the first step in getting help for a dysfunctional family (Devlin & Reynolds, 1994).

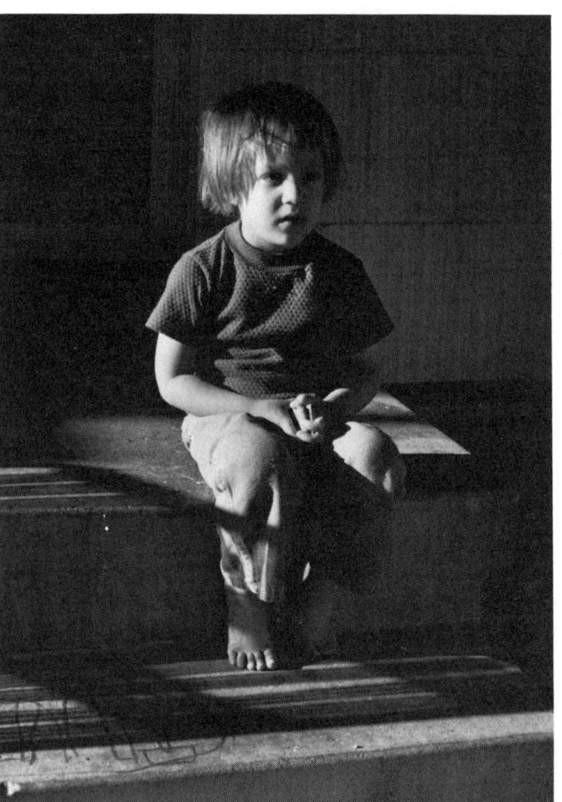

figure 3-6 *The fear, vulnerability, and isolation an abuse victim knows as a child may haunt her well into adulthood.*

✳ nursing insight

A national child abuse hotline can be reached by calling 1-800-4-A-CHILD (1-800-422-4453), providing 24-hour-a-day service.

Studies show that childhood abuse may have far-reaching consequences for women's mental health. Violent sexual abuse often has the strongest long-term consequences. Severe physical abuse in childhood is associated with higher depressive symptoms in adulthood (Fig. 3-6). Combined with risk factors of low income, gender, single-parent status, and presence of young children, the additional risk factor of childhood abuse may have a major effect on a woman's mental health. Early identification and preventive intervention with mothers at high risk are critical for improving their mental health and reducing the potential of adverse outcomes for their children (Hall, Sachs, Rayens, & Lutenbacher, 1993).

health issues affecting adolescents

Many major health care issues converge during adolescence, making this period one of the most difficult challenges for the client, caregivers, and nurses. The health of adolescents in the United States has been declining for several decades and is expected to continue to decline (Wilson & Joffe, 1995).

The health and well-being of adolescents are closely related to their physical and psychosocial development, which are jeopardized by sexual and reproductive health hazards increasing throughout the world. Earlier sexual maturity, later marriage, decreasing influence of the family, and continued exposure to sexual stimuli through mass media have resulted in risky sexual behavior, early pregnancy, and an epidemic of STDs (Friedman, 1992; WHO, 1994).

At least 50% of American youth are at risk for drug abuse, STDs, teenage pregnancy, and injury or death from interpersonal violence and accidents. Health promotion programs concentrate on participants' gaining knowledge, changing attitudes, and practicing healthy behaviors (Giordano & Igoe, 1991).

sexually transmitted diseases

Nearly 13 million Americans are infected each year with STDs; the majority of these are 24 years old or younger. The incidence of *Chlamydia*, gonorrhea, and pelvic inflammatory disease is highest among adolescents.

The hazards of unprotected sexual intercourse are no longer limited to unplanned pregnancy but include HIV, AIDS, and other STDs. Thus, adolescents engaging in high-risk sexual behaviors may face long-term and even fatal consequences. Adolescent girls are at particular risk because they are more easily infected than boys, STDs tend to be asymptomatic in girls, and they have the potential to infect their offspring. Many STDs can result in pelvic inflammatory disease, ectopic pregnancy, infertility, chronic pelvic pain, and cervical cancer (Hatcher, 1994).

substance abuse

Use of alcohol and other drugs is increasing among American adolescents, according to 1994 government statistics. For example, marijuana use among eighth graders has more than doubled since 1991 (Johnston, et al., 1994). Substance abuse among homeless adolescents and other low socioeconomic groups is more prevalent than in the general population (Kipke, et al., 1993).

tobacco

Beginning in 1967, tobacco advertising targeted young women, resulting in an increase in smoking among adolescent women. Since 1980, however, smoking among adolescents has declined, particularly among African Americans; however, the rate of decline has slowed since 1985. This reflects the effect of tobacco company advertisements and promotions directed at young people and the need for more effective antitobacco education.

suicide

Suicide is the second leading cause of death among teenagers 15 to 19 years old; the incidence of teenage suicide has tripled in the last 30 years. Undiagnosed major depression (unipolar disorder) contributes to many of these deaths (Jaffe, 1991). Sexual abuse or assault also is linked to an increased incidence of suicide.

legal issues

Malpractice lawsuits concerning child care can be filed by children or families up to and including the age of 21 years. Nurses need to be conscientious about obtaining informed consent from the child's legal guardian for all invasive procedures. Legal guardianship in divorced or blended families is established by identifying who has the legal right to give consent for health care.

Additional health care concerns include resuscitation questions, such as how much and how long. The nurse and parents should determine how many procedures and how much pain a child can be asked to endure, and a reasonable balance between modern technology and quality of life. Guidelines for responsible child care are included in the United Nations Declaration of Rights of the Child (see Appendix).

The increase of physically handicapped children mainstreamed into public school systems has created concerns for nurses and teachers about issues involving cardiopulmonary resuscitation. A new National Education Association policy on do not resuscitate (DNR) orders adopted the following guidelines, stating school districts should not grant a DNR request unless the following minimum conditions have been met:

- Parent's request and pediatrician's orders are in writing.
- School district has established a team whose members include the student's parent(s), doctor, teachers, appropriate support staff, superintendent, and school nurse to seek alternatives to a DNR; if they fail to obtain the parent's agreement, the team will specify what actions school staff should take if a life-threatening emergency occurs.
- School staff members are given necessary training, and counseling is provided for staff and students in the event of the death of a student (NEA Debate, 1994).

ethical issues

The growing ability of scientists to identify disease-causing genes before the disease develops has generated a variety of ethical issues. For example, the ethical issue of who has ownership of genetic-related information and to what extent the information can be used has not yet been clarified in any legislation.

The United Nations Educational, Scientific, and Cultural Organization has mandated a committee of experts to explore bioethical principles for medical research internationally. The recent progress in genetic research has prompted concern about possible abuse by unethical scientist seeking to "improve" the human race by gene manipulation.

organ donation

Because many healthy children die from injury accidents, their organs are priceless gifts that can enable another person's life to continue. Donation and transplantation of vital organs, such as the heart, lungs, liver, kidneys, and pancreas, are increasingly common.

Organs can be donated when a child has been declared brain dead and is maintained by life-support systems promoting circulation to body organs. Laws concerning organ donation specify the priority order for consulting next of kin and include either parent, guardian at the time of death, and any other person authorized or under obligation to dispose of the body.

key points ✳

- Pediatrics is the medical science relating to the care of children and treatment of their diseases; a pediatrician is a physician who specializes in the treatment of children. Family-centered child health care considers the child an integral part of the family.
- Family-centered maternal and child health recognizes racial, ethnic, cultural, and socioeconomic diversity, promoting programs that encourage healthy develop-

ment of children by strengthening families and reshaping traditional approaches to health promotion, health maintenance, health restoration, and health rehabilitation.

- ✳ The future of our children depends greatly on health care accessibility and availability of resources with a growing trend toward regionalization of health care, ambulatory care systems, and home health services.
- ✳ Pediatric health care in the 1990s is influenced by a lack of health insurance benefits, making health care costs a major factor in seeking preventive and restorative child care.
- ✳ Medicaid is the largest single public source of health care financing for pregnant women and children (from birth to 21 years); Aid to Families with Dependent Children recognizes special financial needs of families headed by single parents. Both programs vary from state to state.
- ✳ The increase of working mothers with children expands the need for child care outside the home, creating risks that include exposure of children to infectious diseases from other children and workers and increased danger of physical and sexual abuse.
- ✳ Children now constitute the largest segment of the population of homeless people, resulting in multiple health risks. These risks include increased number of developmental delays compared with other poor children, living in chaotic and inconsistent environments with parents or caregivers who often suffer from chronic mental illness, acute alcoholism, social isolation, and diseases contracted from sharing cooking and bathroom space.
- ✳ A new population of children has emerged as a result of medical technology; these children have complex chronic conditions.
- ✳ Health care goals for the year 2000 include immunization administration; promotion of physical fitness and good nutritional status; safe weight reduction in overweight adolescents through dietary practices and regular physical activity, reduction of unhealthy behaviors to manage weight, such as fasting diets, skipping meals, taking diet pills, vomiting, and taking laxatives; individualization of care according to sociocultural uniqueness; awareness of health care costs with an emphasis on preventive care (especially accident prevention); promotion of family-centered care; empowerment of health care consumers; reduction of violence and drug abuse; and reduction of STDs.

review questions ✳

1. Select the most accurate response for describing family-centered child care.
   a. Nursing care involving the health promotion of children
   b. The medical science relating to the care of children
   c. Advances in medical technology enabling children with serious disabilities to have expanded lifestyles through home health
   d. Nursing care involving culture, health promotion, health maintenance, health restoration, and rehabilitation of the child and family
2. The social and economic impact on children in the 1990s has created
   a. improved accessibility to health care.
   b. increased numbers of poor and homeless children.
   c. a decrease in health problems associated with infections.
   d. a decline in physical disabilities.
3. Nursing care appropriate for Healthy People 2000 includes
   a. discussing the importance of eating a balanced diet and increasing exercise as a weight control measure.
   b. describing pedophiles.
   c. stating legal protocol concerning "do not resuscitate orders."
   d. increasing guidelines set up by the White House Conference for Children.
4. Select the most appropriate legal concern for pediatric nurses.
   a. Genetic information restricting a family's insurance coverage
   b. Failure to get authorized consent for treatment from the parent providing emotional support to the child
   c. Failure to collect data for a genogram
   d. Failure to report known physical or sexual child abuse
5. Select the most accurate statement about HIV-positive children.
   a. Increased knowledge of HIV/AIDS has opened the doors of many foster parents to HIV-positive infants.
   b. There are one million children with AIDS worldwide.
   c. Transmission of the HIV virus during childbirth is one of the most common causes of HIV/AIDS in children under 13.
   d. HIV-positive newborns present with tuberculosis or diabetes.

references ✳

Barker, D. J. (1994). Outcome of low birthweight. *Hormone Research, 42*(4–5), 223–230.

Barge, F., & Norr, K. (1991). Homeless shelter policies for women in an urban environment. *IMAGE, Journal of Nursing Scholarship, 23*(3), 145–149.

Children's Defense Fund (1992). Economic plight crushes young families. *Children's Defense Fund Reports, 13*(6), 1–3.

Department of Health and Human Services (1990). *Healthy people 2000: National health promotion and disease prevention objectives.* Washington, DC: Public Health Service.

Devlin, K., & Reynolds, E. (1994). Child abuse how to recognize it, how to intervene. *American Journal of Nursing, March*, 26–31.

Ekvall, S. (1993). *Pediatric nutrition in chronic diseases and developmental disorders.* New York: Oxford University Press.

Friedman, H. L. (1992). Changing patterns of adolescent sexual behavior: Consequences for health and development. *Journal of Adolescent Health, 13*(5), 345–350.

Gilbert-Diaz, M. (1993). Caring for culturally diverse patients. *Nursing 93, October,* 44–45.

Giordano, B., & Igoe, J. (1991). Health promotion: The new frontier. *Pediatric Nursing, 17*(5), 490–491.

Hall, L., Sachs, B., Rayens, M., & Lutenbacher, M. (1993). Childhood physical and sexual abuse: Their relationship with depressive symptoms in adulthood. *IMAGE, Journal of Nursing Scholarship, 25*(4), 317–323.

Jaffe, E. (1991). Working with troubled teens. *RN, February,* 58–62.

Johnston, L. D., et al. (1994). *National survey results on drug use from the monitoring the future study, 1975–1993.* Rockville MD: National Institute on Drug Abuse. Publication 94-3809.

Jurgrau, A. (1990). Why aren't we protecting our children? *RN, November,* 30–34.

Kelly, S., Walsh, J., & Thompson, K. (1991). Birth outcomes, health problems, and neglect with prenatal exposure to cocaine. *Pediatric Nursing, 17*(2), 130–135.

Kipke, M. D., et al. (1993). Substance use among youth seen at a community-based health clinic. *Journal of Adolescent Health, 14*(4), 289–294.

Kohl, H. (1993). Opening statement before U.S. Senate committee on the Judiciary, Subcommittee on Juvenile Justice.

Lewit, E. (1992). Dropout rates for high school students. *The Future of Children, 2*(1), 127–130.

NEA Debate (1994). Should schools honor do-not-resuscitate orders? *NEA Today, October.*

New York State Department of Education (1989). *Statistical profiles of school districts.* Albany, NY: National Education Association.

Ohio State Medical Association (1992). *Ohio physicians' child abuse prevention project: Trust talk.* Columbus, OH: Author.

Perry, J., & Perry, E. (1994). *Contemporary society, an introduction to social science* (7th ed.). New York: Harper Collins.

Pui, C. H. (1995). Race no factor in cancer. *Journal of the American Medical Association, 273*(8), 633–637.

Rachelefsky, G. S. (1995). Asthma update: New approaches and partnerships. *Journal of pediatric health care, 9*(1), 12–21.

Satcher, D. (1995). The sociodemographic correlates of Mental Retardation. *American Journal of Public Health, 85*(3), 304–306.

Thomas, H. (1994). Conceptual underpinnings of the family support movement. *Journal of Pediatric Health Care, 8*(2), 57–62.

U.S. Bureau of Census (1990). *Statistical abstracts of the United States: 1990* (110th ed.). Washington, D.C.: U.S. Government Printing Office.

Wilson, M., & Joffe, A. (1995). Adolescent medicine. *Journal of the American Medical Association, 273*(21), 1657–1659.

World Health Organization (1993). *Thirteen million HIV-positive women by 2000.* Geneva: Author.

World Health Organization (1994). *World health statistics quarterly, 47*(1), 31–35.

Wynder, E. L. (1995). A survey of nutrition and health education: Grades 2–6. Presented at American Cancer Society conference, March 28, 1995, New Orleans.

bibliography ✳

American Thoracic Society (1992). Control of tuberculosis in the United States. *American Review of Respiratory Disease, 146*(6), 1623–1633.

Burns, M., & Thornam, C. (1993). Broadening the scope of nursing practice: Federal programs for children. *Pediatric Nursing, 19*(6), 546–552.

American Cancer Society (1994). *Cancer facts and figures.* Atlanta, GA: Author.

Centers for Disease Control (1992). Body-weight perceptions and selected weight-management goals and practices of high school students—United States, 1990. *Morbidity and Mortality Weekly Report, 40,* 741, 747–750.

Feeney, D., & Kaufman, J. (1994). Caring for children with special health care needs. *Caring Magazine, XIII*(12), 12–16.

Goldberg, A., Gardner, G., & Gibson, L. (1993). Home care: The next frontier of pediatric practice. *Journal of Pediatrics, 125*(5), 686–690.

Igoe, J., & Giordano, B. (1992). Health promotion and disease prevention: Secrets of success. *Pediatric Nursing, 18*(1), 61–62.

Kellerman, A., et al. (1993). Gun ownership as a risk factor for homicide in the home. *New England Journal of Medicine, 329,* 1084–1091.

Keltner, B. (1992). Family influences on child health status. *Pediatric Nursing, 18*(2), 128–131.

Lear, J. (1993). Building a health/education partnership: The role of school-based health centers. *Pediatric Nursing, 18*(2), 172–173.

Malloy, C. (1992). Children and poverty: America's Future at Risk. *Pediatric Nursing, 18*(6). 553–557.

Nugent, K., Hughes, R., Ball, B., & Davis, K. (1992). A practice model for a parent support group. *Pediatric Nursing, 18*(1), 11–16.

Pittman, K. (1992). Awakening child consumerism in health care. *Pediatric Nursing, 18*(2), 132–136.

Portelance, D. (1994). Pediatric update. *Nursing 94, August,* 45–47.

(1994). Policy and position statement. *Journal of Pediatric Health Care, 7*(5), 242–244.

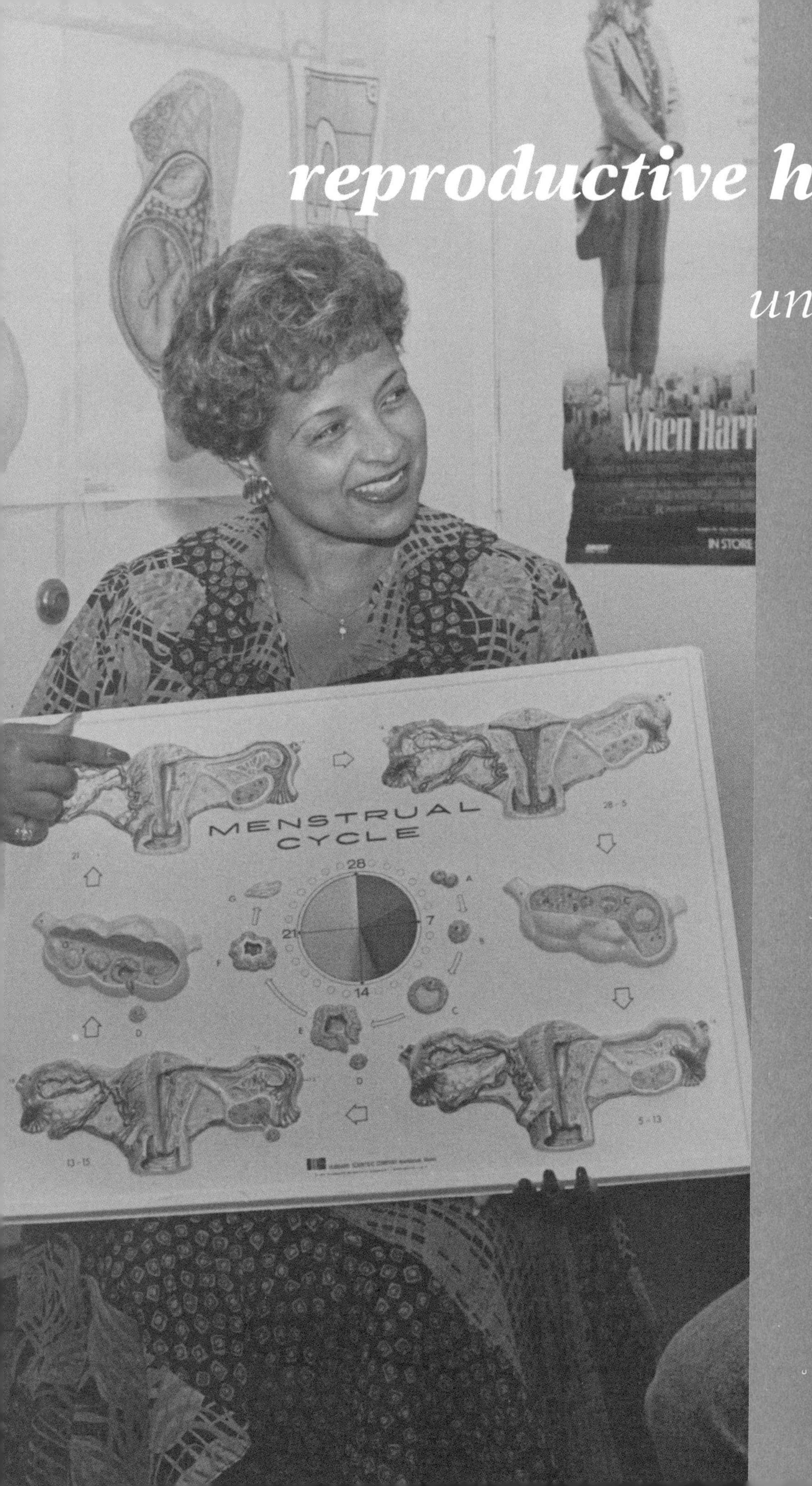

reproductive health

unit II

reproductive function and sexuality

4

outline

objectives

After studying this chapter, the reader should be able to:

- Identify the structures and functions of the female reproductive system.
- Discuss the structure and function of the female breast.
- Discuss the various hormones and their functions in the menstrual cycle.
- Differentiate menarche and menopause.
- Identify the structures and functions of the male reproductive system.
- Describe the process of semen production.
- Discuss human sexuality and its role in human development.

key terms

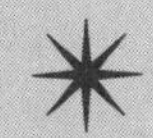

coitus
copulation
estrogen
false pelvis
gamete
menarche
menopause
menstrual cycle
ovum
progesterone
puberty
seminal fluid
sexual response cycle
sperm
testosterone
true pelvis

Neff C & Spray M. *Introduction to Maternal and Child Health Nursing*,

Human reproduction normally begins with sexual intercourse between a male and a female. After 9 months of pregnancy, the process ends when the baby is born. This process is universal and yet unique to each couple and each child.

To care for the childbearing family effectively, the nurse needs to understand human reproduction: conception, pregnancy, labor, birth, and human sexuality. This chapter reviews the anatomy and physiology of the male and female reproductive systems and the basics of male and female sexuality. This information will help prepare the nurse to explain and discuss reproduction and sexuality with the woman and her family. By answering questions and giving accurate information to the client, the nurse dispels myths and misinformation that can cause undue stress and anxiety.

The male and female reproductive systems vary in structure and function, yet they are basically similar in many ways. Both systems develop from similar structures during the first 8 weeks after conception. The primary function of both systems is to produce sex cells, called *gametes*, and to transport those cells to a place where they can unite and form the beginning of a new human.

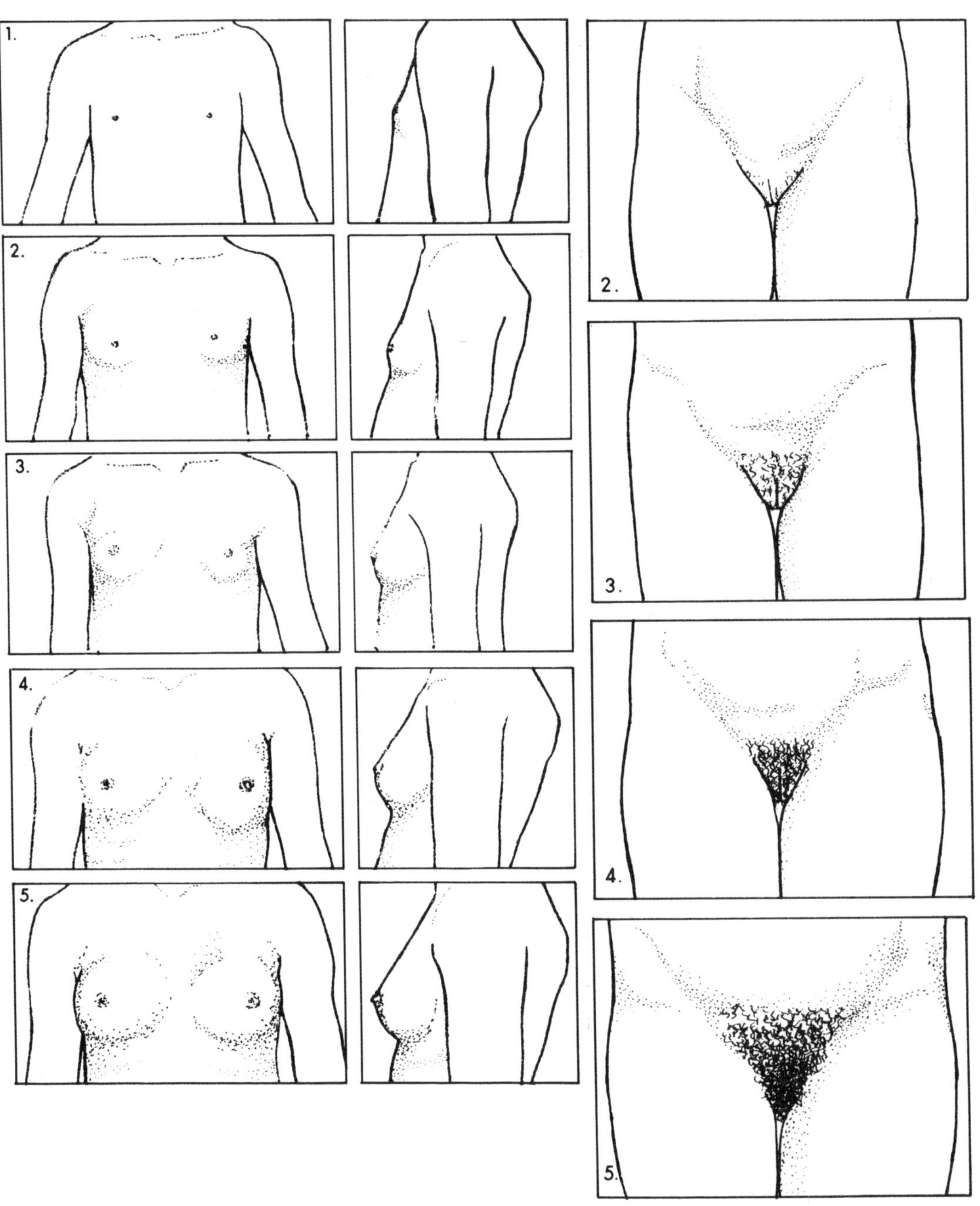

figure 4-1 *(A) Development of the breasts and pubic hair during adolescence.* ***(continued)***

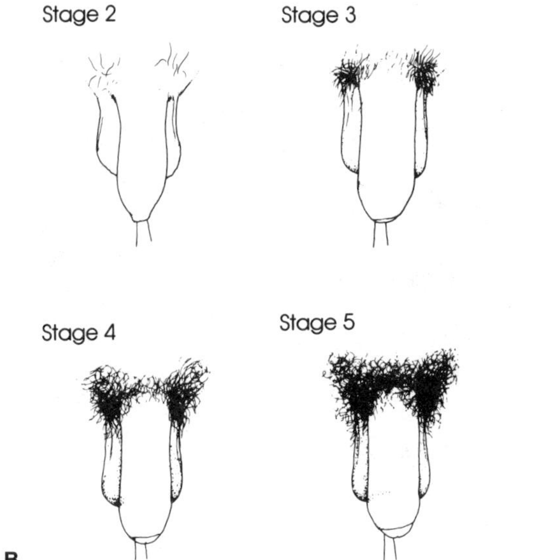

figure 4-1 ***(continued)*** *(B) Development of the penis, scrotum, testes, and pubic hair during adolescence.*

puberty

Puberty is the stage of the life cycle when boys and girls reach sexual maturity and become capable of reproduction. At puberty, boys and girls experience a growth spurt. A girl's breasts begin to develop, and hair starts to appear in the pubic and underarm areas. A boy's penis, testes, and scrotum enlarge, and pubic hair appears, followed by facial and underarm hair. Muscle strength and coordination develop rapidly. The male voice becomes deeper. Girls reach puberty at an earlier age than boys; however, the timing of puberty varies with each individual (Fig. 4-1).

female reproductive system

Like the male reproductive system, the female reproductive system includes internal, external, and accessory structures (Display 4-1). Because the developing child grows within the female body, it is important to understand the bony structure of the female pelvis and the action of female hormones on conception, pregnancy, labor, and birth.

external structures

The external structures of the female reproductive system include the *mons pubis, labia majora, labia minora, clitoris, vestibule, hymen*, and *perineum* and are collectively called the vulva (Fig. 4-2).

mons pubis

The *mons pubis* is a fatty pad that covers the anterior portion of the pubic bone joint. It is covered with coarse, curly hair and protects the pubic joint from trauma or injury.

labia majora

The *labia majora* are two longitudinal folds of skin that lie posterior to the mons pubis. They extend posteriorly to the anterior portion of the perineum (the area between the *labia minora* and the opening to the rectum). They are composed of adipose tissue, covered on the the outer edges with pubic hair, and lined with moist mucous membrane. The main function of the labia majora is to protect the underlying structures, including the *pudendal arteries*, which form an extensive blood supply. This highly vascular tissue may be bruised during childbirth.

labia minora

The *labia minora* lie directly under the labia majora and are composed of erectile connective tissue, blood vessels, and muscle tissue. Situated within the labia minora are sebaceous glands that lubricate and protect the area. They extend posteriorly and join with the labia majora to form the *fourchette*, a ridge of tissue that is sometimes cut to enlarge the opening during childbirth.

clitoris

The *clitoris* is situated between the anterior folds of the labia minora, partially covered by a thin fold of tissue called the *prepuce*. Like the male penis, the clitoris is composed of erectile tissue and is the area of sexual pleasure in the female.

vestibule

The *vestibule* is a flattened oblong space between the labia minora that contains the opening to the vagina (*introitus*)

display 4-1
summary of female reproductive system

EXTERNAL STRUCTURES

* Mons pubis
* Labia majora
* Labia minora
* Clitoris
* Vestibule
* Hymen
* Perineum

INTERNAL STRUCTURES

* Ovaries
* Fallopian tubes
* Uterus
* Uterine ligaments
* Vagina

ACCESSORY STRUCTURES

* Bartholin's glands
* Skene's glands
* Mammary glands

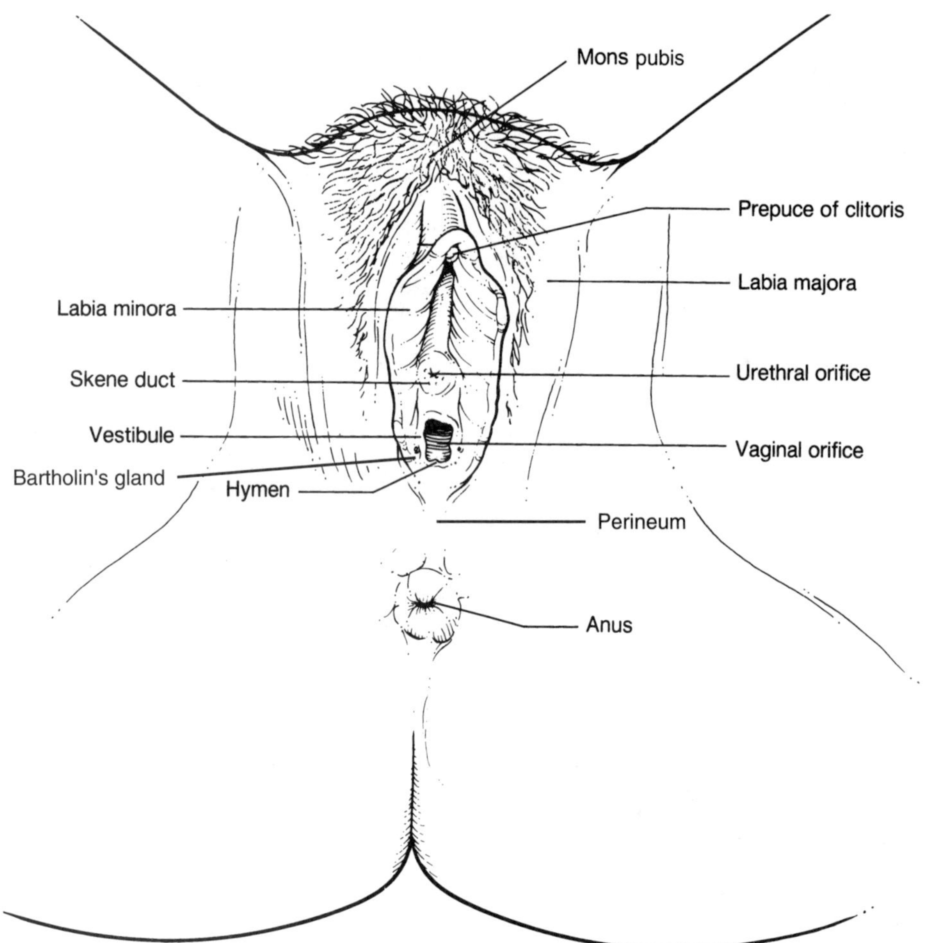

figure 4-2 *External structures of the female reproductive system.*

and the *urinary meatus*. In childhood, the vaginal opening may be covered by a thin elastic mucous membrane, the *hymen*. The hymen may be torn by strenuous physical exercise, the use of tampons, masturbation, or other sexual activity.

perineum

The *perineum* is a fibromuscular tissue extending from the fourchette of the vulva to the anus. The perineum stretches during childbirth to allow birth of the infant. Sometimes, however, this area may tear or may be surgically cut (*episiotomy*) during childbirth.

internal structures

The internal structures of the female reproductive system are the vagina, uterus, fallopian tubes, and ovaries (Fig. 4-3).

vagina

The *vagina* is a muscular canal leading from the outside of the body to the *uterus* (womb). It is approximately 10 cm (5 in) long and lined with mucous membrane. The vagina is the soft portion of the birth canal, the passage for menstrual flow, and a receptacle for the penis during sexual intercourse. The walls of the vagina are moist and contain folds (*rugae*) of muscle tissue that permit stretching during childbirth.

uterus

The *uterus* is a hollow, pear-shaped muscular organ that contains the fetus during pregnancy. It lies low in the pelvis, behind the bladder, in front of the rectum, and above the vagina. In the nonpregnant woman, the uterus measures about 7.5 cm (3 in) long, 5 cm (2 in) wide, and 2.5 cm (1 in) in diameter. During pregnancy, the uterus expands greatly to 30 cm (12 in) long. The uterus is composed of three sections:

- The lower portion, or neck, called the *cervix*, which protrudes down into the upper part of the vagina
- The central portion called the body or *corpus*
- The upper dome-shaped portion, called the *fundus*, which is located between the insertion of the *fallopian tubes*

The upper opening of the cervix, the *internal os*, leads into the uterine cavity. The lower opening, the *external os*, leads into the vagina.

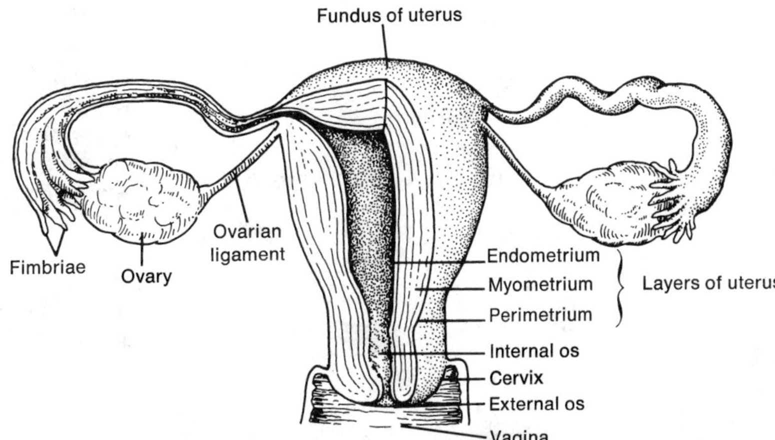

figure 4-3 *Internal structures of the female reproductive system*

The uterine corpus is composed of three layers of tissue:

* The *perimetrium*, the thin outer layer, consists of *peritoneum*, the same serous membrane that lines the entire pelvic and abdominal cavity.
* The *myometrium*, the middle layer of uterine tissue, is actually a three-layer network of involuntary smooth muscle fibers (Fig. 4-4*A*). The muscles in the outer layer are principally in the fundus area and run from top to bottom. The middle layer of fibers is arranged in an interlacing figure eight pattern around the major blood vessels, helping to prevent hemorrhage by contracting after delivery. The innermost layer contains circular muscle fibers that form sphincters at the insertion site of the fallopian tubes and at the internal os. The sphincter at the internal os helps prevent expulsion of the fetus during pregnancy but stretches during labor as the cervix dilates. The sphincter at the fallopian tube openings prevents menstrual discharge from flowing back into the fallopian tubes. This thick muscular network makes the uterus very strong; it contracts forcefully during labor to expel the fetus and reduces the risk of hemorrhage by contracting after delivery (see Fig. 4-4*B*).
* The *endometrium*, the inner layer or lining of the uterus, is composed of mucous membrane that thickens and becomes more vascular each month in preparation for pregnancy. If pregnancy does not occur, the excess thickness is sloughed off as "menstrual flow."

uterine ligaments

The uterus is supported on either side by ligaments and by the muscles of the pelvic floor. The supporting ligaments include the broad ligaments, the round ligaments, and the uterosacral ligaments.

ovaries

The *ovaries* are two grayish white, almond-shaped glands approximately 2.5 cm (1 in) wide and 2 to 5 cm (1–2 in) long. They are located in the upper portion of the pelvic cavity close to either side of the uterus (see Fig. 4-3).

The ovaries are composed of three layers of tissue, each with a distinct function:

* Outer layer (*epithelium*), which protects the contents of the ovary
* Middle layer (*cortex*), which contains *ova* (female sex cells or gametes)

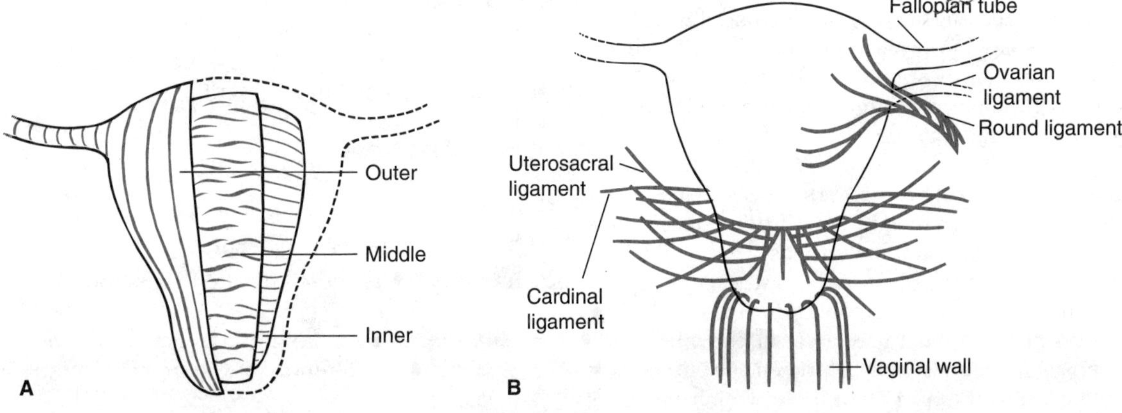

figure 4-4 *Uterine muscle layers. **(A)** Muscle fiber placement. **(B)** Interlacing of uterine muscle layers.*

* Inner layer (*medulla*), which contains nerves and blood vessels

The function of the ovaries corresponds to that of their male counterpart, the testes. They are responsible for the monthly maturation and release of an ovum and the development and release of the female hormones, *estrogen* and *progesterone*.

Unlike the testes, which produce sperm throughout a male's life cycle, the ovaries contain all of a female's egg cells (*follicles*) at birth. The ovaries normally contain several hundred thousand follicles; no more are produced during a woman's lifetime.

fallopian tubes

The *fallopian tubes* are slender muscular tubes that extend outward from the upper portion of the uterine corpus. They are approximately 10 cm (4 in) long and flared at the distal end into hairy (*ciliated*) finger-like projections called *fimbriae*; see Fig. 4-3. When the ovum is released from the ovary, the wavy motions of the cilia and fimbriae sweep the recently released ovum into the fallopian tube, where fertilization may occur.

accessory structures

bartholin's glands

The *Bartholin glands* (greater vestibular glands) are located at either side of the vagina. Their ducts open near the distal portion of the vagina and lubricate the vulva during sexual intercourse.

skene's glands

The *Skene glands* (paraurethral glands) are tiny mucus-secreting glands located at either side of the urinary meatus. Their main function is to keep the vestibule lubricated during sexual intercourse.

breasts

Breast tissue is present in men and women. However, only the female breast is capable of producing milk to nourish the newborn and infant.

The *breasts* (mammary glands) are located bilaterally between the second and sixth ribs on the anterior surface of the chest wall and slightly extend bilaterally into the underarm (axillary) region. The breasts consist of glandular and adipose tissue, supported by suspensory ligaments. The breast is abundantly supplied with nerves and blood vessels and in the lateral portion near the axilla, also is supplied with lymphatic tissue.

Development of the breast occurs during puberty and is stimulated by estrogen. The size of the breast depends on the amount of adipose tissue present; thus, breast size has no bearing on a woman's ability to breast-feed.

Smooth skin covers most of the breast, except for the circular pigmented area (*areola*) containing the nipple. The areola is covered with small raised areas (*Montgomery's tubercles*), sebaceous glands that help keep the nipple soft and supple during nursing. The nipple, which becomes erect with stimulation, enables the infant to suckle.

Internally, each breast contains 15 to 20 lobes, each consisting of several lobules. These lobules contain the *alveoli*. The alveoli contain the milk-secreting cells, the *acini*, and connect to the ducts that open onto the surface of the nipple. When the milk is produced, it is secreted into the lobules and stored in an enlarged portion of the lobule (*ampulla*) just behind to the nipple (Fig. 4-5).

female bony pelvis

The female *bony pelvis* supports and protects the pelvic organs and forms the fixed, rigid portion of the birth canal. The bony pelvis consists of four bones that form a bowl-like structure: the two hip bones (*innominate bones*) located on either side, and the *sacrum* and *coccyx*, located at the back. The pelvic bowl is lined with fibrous cartilage and held together by ligaments. The four bones of the pelvis are joined at the *symphysis pubis* (pubic bone) and the *sacroiliac* and *sacrococcygeal joints* (Fig. 4-6).

The hip bones consist of three sections (see Fig. 4-6):

* The *ilium*, the superior and posterior portion of the pelvis
* The *ischium*, the posterior portion (The *ischial spines*, located near the junction of the ischium and the ilium, are important landmarks used to determine the descent of the fetus through the birth canal during labor; this is the shortest diameter of the bony pelvis.)
* The *pubis*, the anterior portion of the pelvis

These three sections become fused by adulthood.

The pelvis contains four joints: two sacroiliac joints, the symphysis pubis joint, and the sacrococcygeal joint. These joints become increasingly mobile during pregnancy as the fibrocartilage lining the joints and ligaments softens to allow for delivery of the fetus. These structural changes can cause discomfort in the mother's back and legs.

true pelvis and false pelvis

The pelvis is further divided into the *true pelvis* and the *false pelvis* (Fig. 4-7). The *false pelvis* is formed by the upper portions of the ilium. It supports the growing fetus and during labor, guides the fetus into the true pelvis. The *true pelvis* is the inferior portion of the pelvis. The linea terminalis separates the false and true pelves. The fetus must pass through the *pelvic inlet* (superior portion), the *pelvic cavity* (midportion), and the *pelvic outlet* (inferior portion). The importance of these parts and their measurement are discussed in Chapter 9.

types of pelves

The shape and size of the pelvis is unique in every woman; however, four general types of pelvis have been identified (Fig. 4-8):

* *Gynecoid*, the most common type and best suited to childbearing
* *Anthropoid*, more common in nonwhite women
* *Android*, less common and more problematic in childbearing
* *Platypelloid*, least common

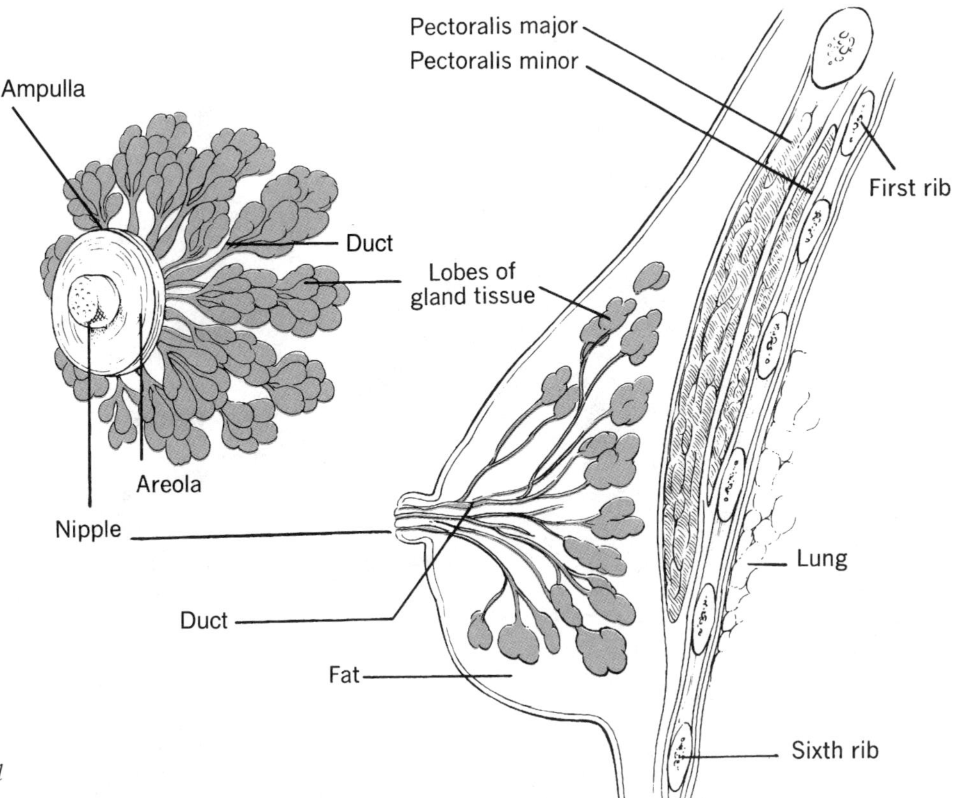

figure 4-5 *Glandular tissue and ducts of the breast.*

The type of pelvis affects all dimensions of the birth canal and the degree of difficulty that can be expected during labor and delivery.

hormonal regulation of female reproductive function

Female reproductive function is regulated by the secretion of hormones, primarily by the pituitary gland and the ovaries. At puberty, the hypothalamus senses the readiness of the female body to begin menstruation. The hypothalamus sends a signal to the pituitary gland to begin the cycle of menstruation and ovulation.

The *pituitary gland* releases two hormones that affect the menstrual cycle: *follicle-stimulating hormone (FSH)* and *luteinizing hormone (LH)*. The ovaries, in turn, release *estrogen* and *progesterone*. The interplay of these hormones regulates menstruation, ovulation, and fertility.

menstruation

Menstruation is a cycle of regular uterine bleeding that begins with puberty and ends with menopause (Table 4-1). It occurs each month except during pregnancy. The *menstrual cycle* is initiated in response to the interactions between the reproductive and endocrine systems. It is interrupted by pregnancy and can be disrupted by other factors, such as illness, stress, or excessive weight loss.

menarche

The first cycle (*menarche*) normally occurs between the ages of 9 and 16 years, with 12 to 13 years of age the most common time. Menarche signals the final stages of puberty and maturity of the reproductive organs. Many factors affect menarche, including heredity, environment, nutritional status, and race.

ovulation

After puberty, about 20 of the several hundred thousand egg cells (*follicles*) begin to ripen each month, but usually only one matures sufficiently to break through the wall of the ovary. Once the follicle has reached the surface of the ovary, it ruptures, releasing the egg near the fallopian tube. This process is called *ovulation*.

Ovulation occurs approximately 14 days before the beginning of a woman's menstrual period. Ovulation occurs monthly, except during pregnancy, from menarche until menopause, or approximately between the ages of 14 and 55.

At ovulation, the fimbriae sweep the egg into the tube, where it may be fertilized by a sperm and move on to implant in the uterus. If fertilization does not occur within 24 hours after release of the egg from the ovary, the egg will no longer be viable, and conception cannot take place. The excess endometrium is shed through the vagina as menstrual flow.

The average menstrual cycle is every 28 days, but ranges of 25 to 40 days are not uncommon. The cycle can

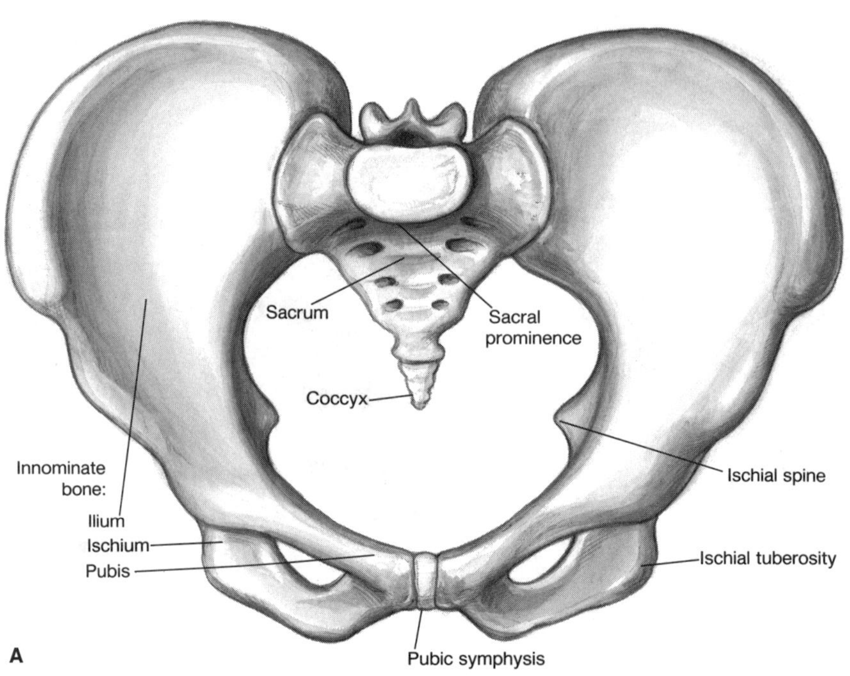

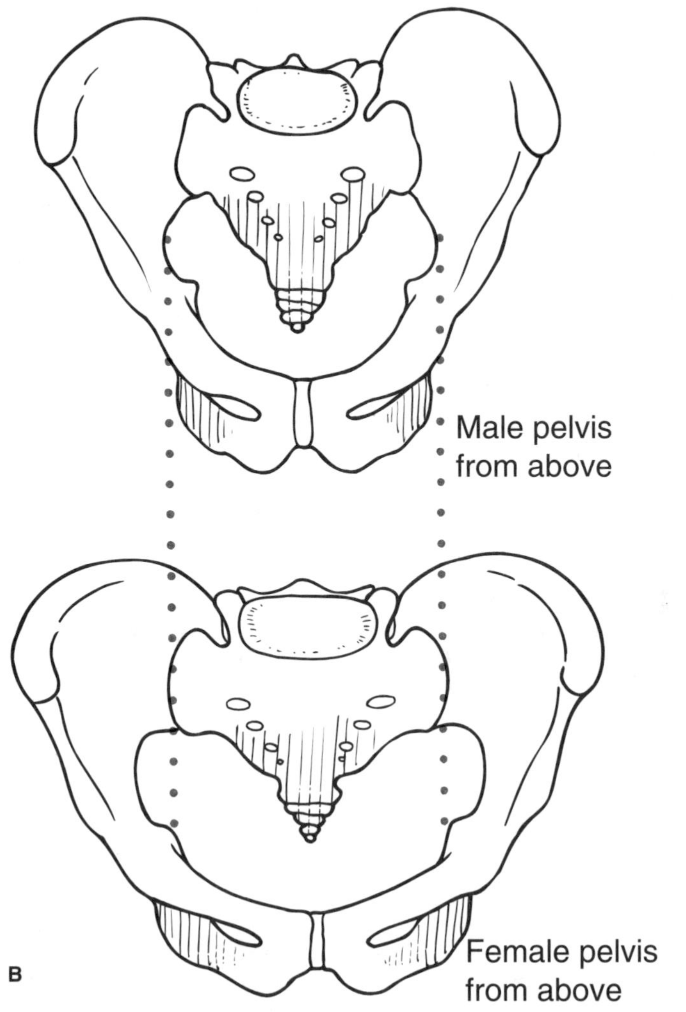

figure 4-6 *(**A**) Anterior of the pelvis, showing major bones and joints. (**B**) Pelvic girdle showing male pelvis and female pelvis.*

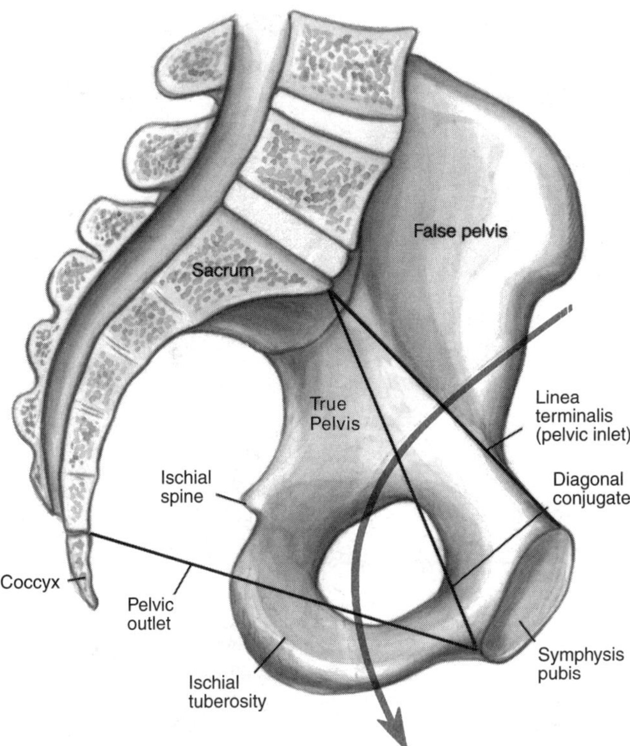

figure 4-7 *True and false pelvis. Portion above linea terminalis is false pelvis. Portion below is true pelvis. Arrow shows "stovepipe" curve that the fetus must follow to deliver.*

be viewed in three phases: *menstrual, proliferative,* and *secretory* (Fig. 4-9).

menstrual phase

The *menstrual phase* consists of days 1 through 5 of the cycle when estrogen and progesterone are at low levels. During this time, the menstrual flow (*menses*) has been initiated. Usually, 25 to 150 mL (1–5 oz) of dark red bloody discharge is secreted from the vagina. This discharge consists of endometrial cells sloughed (shed) from the uterine lining (endometrium), mucus, and blood. Normal menstrual flow has a musty, not foul, odor.

The menstrual phase is the culmination of a series of month-long preparations but is discussed first because it is an outward, measurable sign. It enables the nurse to follow the menstrual history of the client.

proliferative phase

Immediately following the sloughing of the endometrium, the pituitary gland releases FSH, which stimulates the ovary to prepare and mature an ovum in a saclike structure, the *graafian follicle*. The graafian follicle then releases estrogen, which prepares the endometrium for possible implantation of an embryo. Under the influence of estrogen, the endometrium becomes thicker and more vascular to meet the nutritional needs of the embryo.

The proliferative and secretory phases are divided by a special event called *ovulation*, described previously. Ovulation occurs 14 days before the onset of the next menses. The graafian follicle, approximately 0.5 in in diameter, can been seen on the surface of the ovary.

A surge of LH from the pituitary gland causes the graafian follicle to rupture and release its mature ovum. The motion of the fimbriae sweeps the ovum into the fallopian tube.

secretory phase

The secretory phase begins with the formation of a yellow scarred area (*corpus luteum*) where the graafian follicle has ruptured. The corpus luteum secretes estrogen and progesterone to maintain the vascular lining of the uterus until the placenta can form. If fertilization does not occur, the corpus luteum survives only 8 days and then disintegrates. This causes the levels of estrogen and progesterone to fall, resulting in menstruation.

menstrual problems

Between menarche and menopause, women may experience menstrual cycle problems. Painful menstruation (*dysmenorrhea*) may have no known cause or may be the result of a medical problem, such as displacement or tilting of the uterus or narrowing of the cervical canal. Absence of menstrual flow (*amenorrhea*) or infrequent menses (*oligomenorrhea*) may be the result of hormonal imbalance. Excessive menstrual flow (*menorrhagia*) may be caused endocrine imbalance, stress, tumors, polyps, or decreased coagulation time. Breakthrough bleeding or bleeding at various times during the cycle (*metrorrhagia*) may be caused by hormonal imbalances, structural abnormalities, tumors, or infections.

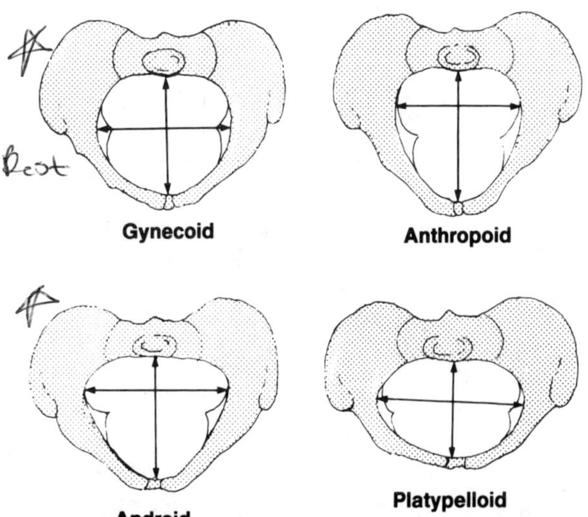

figure 4-8 *Pelvic types: **(A)** Anthropoid. **(B)** Gynecoid. **(C)** Android. **(D)** Platypelloid (flat).*

table 4-1 summary of normal menstruation

Characteristics	Description	Range
Menarche	First menstrual cycle; signals reproductive organs are mature	9–16 y average—12 y
Length of cycle	Period of time from beginning to end of the cycle	25–35 d average—28 d
Duration of menses (flow)	Number of days the uterus sheds its endometrial lining	1–9 d average—3–5 d
Amount of menstrual flow	Should be dark red, without clots, and have a musty odor	25–150 mL Saturation of pad in less than 1 h considered excessive
Menopause	Cessation of the menses with a decrease in ovarian activity	45–55 y average—50 y

✶ nursing considerations

The nurse discusses the client's attitude toward menstruation to assess her level of understanding and any misconceptions. The adolescent may feel embarrassment, shame, or low self-esteem. The nurse can educate and promote a positive self-image by emphasizing that menstruation is a normal physiologic response to maturation.

The nurse offers suggestions to control menstrual discomfort as needed. Measures that may be helpful include use of a heating pad to the lower abdomen (which increases the blood flow and decreases any muscle spasms), use of over-the-counter analgesics (ibuprofen products are particularly helpful), and the importance of exercise three times per week for 30 minutes (to build abdominal muscle tone).

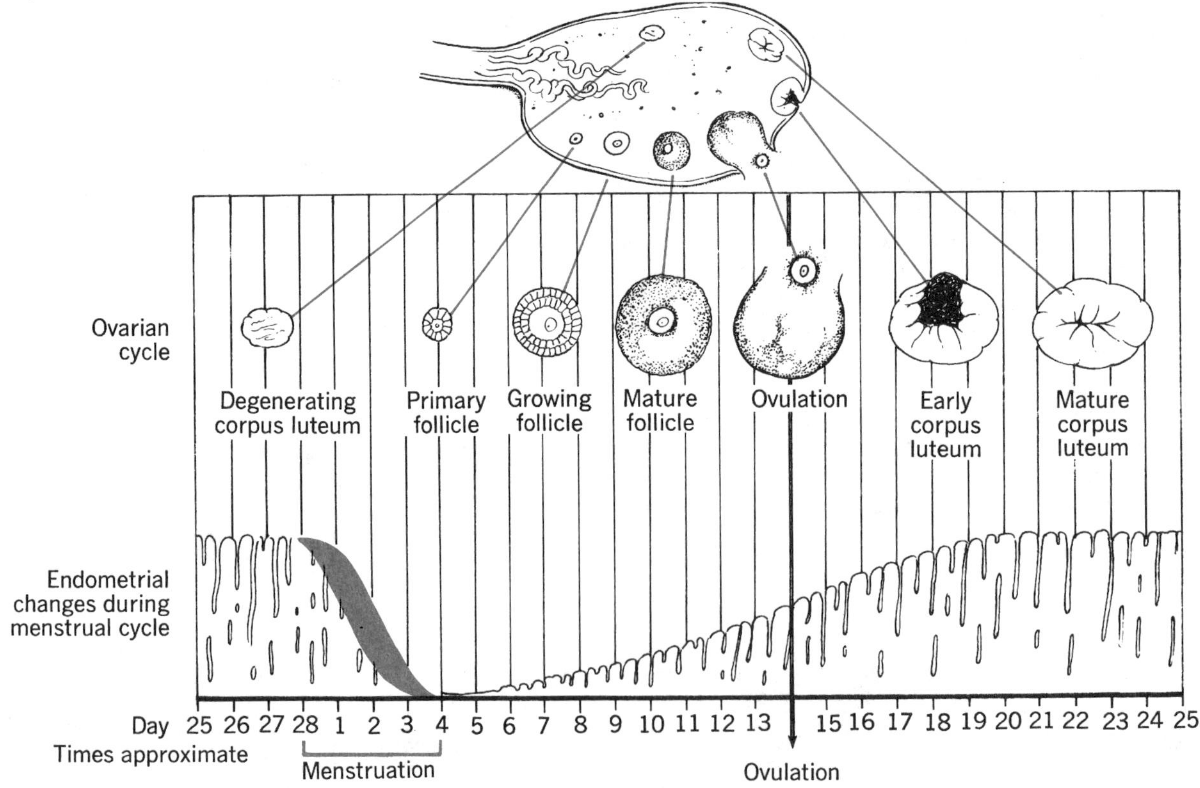

figure 4-9 *Schematic representation of one ovarian cycle and the corresponding changes in thickness of the endometrium. It is thickest just before menstruation begins and thinnest just as menstruation ends.*

The nurse also assesses the nutritional status of the client. Adequate nutrition, including iron, is important due to the loss of 0.5 to 1.0 mg of iron per day during menses.

menopause

Menopause is the cessation of menses and reproductive capability in the older adult woman, usually occurring at around age 50. Many physiologic and psychological changes occur during this time. Menopause is discussed briefly here because it is the culmination of the reproductive cycle of the woman.

Menopause occurs because ovarian activity slows, and the amount of circulating estrogen decreases dramatically. The term *climacteric* characterizes all of the signs and symptoms, both physical and psychological, that occur during this time.

Physical changes during menopause include atrophy (shrinking) of the vagina and vulva, causing the client to experience vaginal burning or itching (*pruritus*). She also may experience "night sweats," sleep disturbances, "hot flashes," and occasional chills. Heart palpitations, dizzy spells, and joint pain also are common symptoms in menopause.

Psychological changes during menopause include mood swings, depression, anxiety, and possible loss of self-esteem. The ability to deal with these changes varies from woman to woman and is based on many factors, including self-concept, cultural beliefs, and support systems.

The nurse can offer accurate information, understanding, support, and empathy.

Decrease in estrogen can increase susceptibility to coronary heart disease and osteoporosis in some women. The physician may recommend estrogen replacement therapy (ERT); however, women need to know the possible side effects of ERT, including increased risk of breast cancer. A diet rich in calcium or calcium supplements also may help prevent osteoporosis.

male reproductive system

The male reproductive system consists of several structures that can be grouped according to their anatomic position. They are external, internal, and accessory structures (Display 4-2). Figure 4-10 illustrates male reproductive anatomy.

external structures

The *penis* and *scrotum* are located between the thighs and are attached to the abdominal wall (see Fig. 4-10).

penis

The penis is an elongated structure (*shaft*) with a sensitive dome-shaped end (*glans*). It is covered by a retractable layer of skin (*prepuce* or *foreskin*), which may be trimmed off by circumcision. Until recently circumcision was a conventional practice for religous or social custom or to prevent tightening of the skin over the glans (*phimosis*).

The penis contains three spongy, cylindric columns of erectile tissue that become engorged with blood during sexual stimulation. An *erection* results, which enables the man to insert the penis into the woman's vagina.

The man's urethra passes through the penis, forming a passageway for urine and seminal fluid (*semen*), which is the fluid containing *sperm*, the male sex cells.

scrotum

The *scrotum* is the sac containing the *testes* (testicles; Fig. 4-11). It consists of two layers, an outer wrinkled layer of skin and an inner layer of muscle tissue. The layer of muscle tissue can contract and pull the testicles close to the body to provide warmth, or it can relax and allow the testicles to descend to allow for cooling. This mechanism provides a constant temperature of approximately 3°F lower than normal body temperature. This lower temperature is necessary for the production of normal healthy sperm (*spermatogenesis*).

internal structures

The internal structures of the male reproductive system include the testes, epididymis, vas deferens, ejaculatory duct, and urethra. All are involved in the production or transport of sperm (Fig. 4-12); the urethra also is a passageway for urine.

testes (testicles)

The *testes* are oval, egg-shaped glandular organs, each weighing 10 to 15 g. Each testis is divided into 250 to 400 partitions or *lobules*. Each lobule contains two important anatomic structures:

* The *seminiferous tubules*, where sperm are produced
* The *cells of Leydig*, which secrete male hormones (*androgens*)

display 4-2
summary of male reproductive system

EXTERNAL STRUCTURES

* **Penis**
* **Scrotum**

INTERNAL STRUCTURES

* **Testes**
* **Epididymis**
* **Vas deferens**
* **Ejaculatory ducts**
* **Urethra**

ACCESSORY STRUCTURES

* **Seminal vesicles**
* **Prostate gland**
* **Bulbourethral glands**

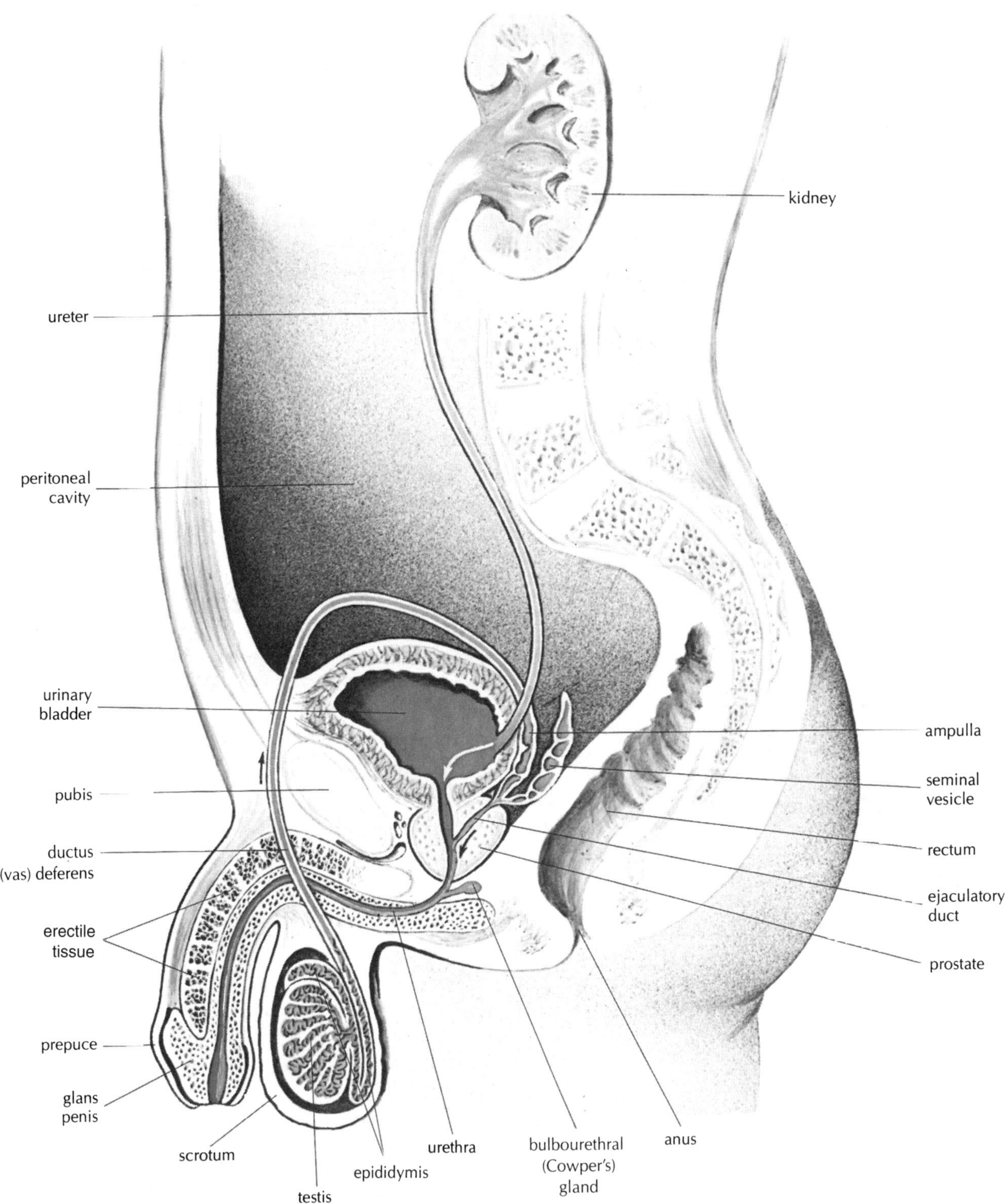

figure 4-10 *Internal and external structures of the male reproductive system.*

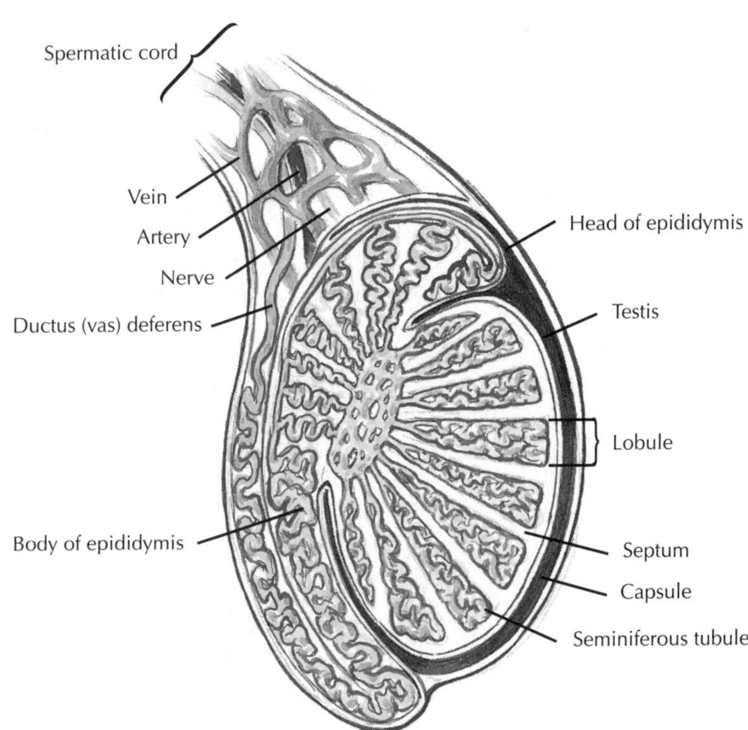

figure 4-11 *Scrotum.*

The principal male hormone is *testosterone*, essential to the formation of sperm and the development of male *secondary sex characteristics* (pubic and facial hair, deep voice, and a more muscular body).

epididymis

The *epididymis* is a thin, coiled tube approximately 6 m (20 ft) in length located on each testis, connecting the testes to the *vas deferens* (see Fig. 4-10). Sperm are stored in the epididymis for 2 to 3 weeks, where they mature and develop *motility*, the ability to move through fluid.

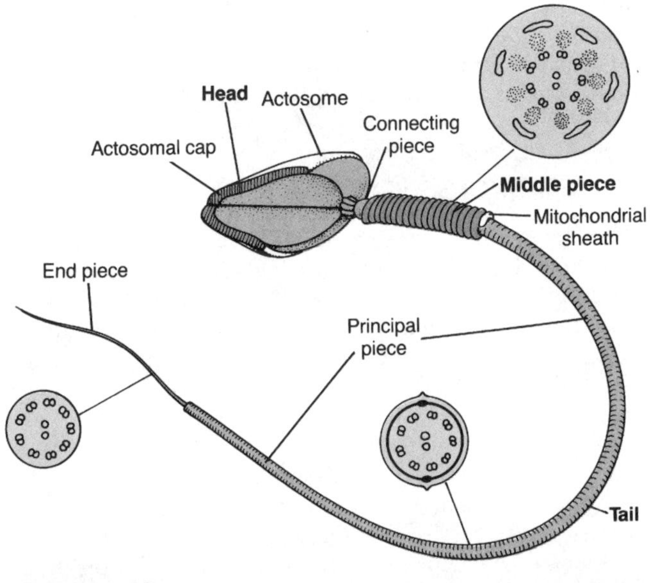

vas deferens

The *vas deferens* is a straight duct approximately 45 cm (18 in) long that connects to the epididymis, extends through the inguinal canal in the abdominal wall, and curves behind the urinary bladder (see Fig. 4-10). The vas deferens is surrounded by arteries and veins and is protected by fibromuscular tissue.

ejaculatory duct

The vas deferens joins with the seminal vesicle (a gland) to form the *ejaculatory duct*, a tube approximately 2.5 cm long (1 in). Semen is released through the *ejaculatory duct*, passing through the *prostate gland*, the *urethra*, and out the end of the penis.

urethra

The male *urethra* is a tube approximately 20 cm (8 in) long, lined with mucous membrane, leading from the urinary bladder through the prostate to the urinary meatus at the tip of the glans penis. Both semen and urine exit the penis through the urethra.

accessory structures

seminal vesicles

The *seminal vesicles* are two muscular saclike glands approximately 7.5 cm (3 in) long. They are located above the base of the prostate gland between the urinary bladder and the rectum. Connected to the ejaculatory duct, the seminal vesicles secrete a thick, yellow, alkaline fluid con-

figure 4-12 *Schematic representation of a mature spermatozoon.*

taining fructose and protein. This fluid makes up more than half the volume of semen and energizes and greatly increases the motility of sperm.

prostate gland

The *prostate gland* is a walnut-sized gland approximately 5 cm (2 in) in diameter. Enclosed in a fibrous capsule, the prostate surrounds the male urethra much like a doughnut. During ejaculation, the prostate releases an alkaline fluid into the urethra. This fluid helps neutralize acidic fluid in the male urethra and the female vagina.

bulbourethral glands (cowper's glands)

The *bulbourethral (Cowper's) glands* are two pea-sized glands located just below the prostate gland. They secrete a clear, thick alkaline mucus into the male urethra that helps neutralize acidity and lubricates the tip of the penis.

sperm production and ejaculation

Sperm (*spermatozoa*) are the male gametes; they are microscopic, and each is made up of a head and a tail (see Fig. 4-12). The head of the sperm contains the nucleus, in which the *chromosomes* (genetic material) are located. The head of the sperm is covered by a caplike structure called the *acrosome*. The acrosome contains two enzymes that help the sperm break through the covering of the *ovum* (female sex cell or egg) so that fertilization can occur.

The tail (*flagellum*) of the sperm is necessary for motility. Its back-and-forth sweeping motion maneuvers the sperm through the vagina and into the fallopian tube to fertilize the female ovum.

Sperm production begins at puberty in the boy and continues throughout the man's lifespan. A man produces approximately 30 million new sperm each day. The average ejaculation of 5 mL of seminal fluid contains 200 million spermatozoa.

nursing alert

The man should avoid tight clothing, such as briefs, and hot baths to prevent damage or death to the sperm, due to increased temperature.

The journey of the sperm begins in the seminiferous tubules within the testes where sperm are produced. They then travel to the epididymis, where they remain for 2 to 3 weeks until they mature. During sexual stimulation, sperm move into the ejaculatory duct, through the prostate, and into the urethra. Along the way, they mix with secretions of the seminal vesicles, prostate, and bulbourethral glands, forming *seminal fluid*, which is ejaculated through the tip of the penis. Because of sperm's motility, ejaculation in or near the vagina may result in fertilization of the ovum, the beginning of pregnancy.

sexuality

All humans are sexual beings. An individual's *sexuality* includes many components, among which are biologic gender, sexual identity, physical characteristics, attitudes, emotions, behaviors, and cultural beliefs. Roles in society are based on one's interpretation of that sexuality.

Biologic gender is the anatomic determination of physical traits, the outward manifestation of being male or female. This determination is based on the combination of chromosomes at conception. The male sex chromosome combination is XY and the female sex chromosome combination is XX.

Sexual identity, also called *gender identity*, describes the person's inner feelings or beliefs about being male or female. This may differ from the biologic gender or anatomic characteristics; however, it is not clear whether there are biologic influences on sexual identity. Sexual identity is established early in life, usually between ages 3 and 4 years and determines what sex role, masculine or feminine, one assumes in society. It is influenced by interactions with family and peers and by cultural customs, the media, and society. Sexual identity affects sexual behavior, including one's preference in a sexual partner (*sexual orientation*) and practices chosen to provide sexual pleasure.

sexual orientation

An individual's *sexual orientation* refers to that person's preference in a sexual partner. If the person prefers a partner of the opposite sex, the sexual orientation is said to be *heterosexual*. If a partner of the same sex is preferred, the sexual orientation is termed *homosexual*. When someone enjoys sexual activities with partners of either sex, the orientation is called *bisexual*.

Sexual orientation is a major influence in each individual's life. Sometimes the client's sexual orientation may differ from that of the nurse; for example, a pregnant client may be in a lesbian relationship. The nurse must remain nonjudgmental when approaching all clients and their families, acknowledging their uniqueness and valuing their humanity.

sexual expression

The expression of one's sexuality as sexual pleasure may be achieved in a variety of ways, including intercourse between a male and female (*coitus, copulation*), masturbation (manual stimulation of the genitals, alone or with a partner), oral-genital intercourse (stimulation of the genitals with the mouth), fantasy (movies, books, daydreaming), or other activities. Any of these sexual activities may result in an *orgasm*, intense sexual pleasure that releases muscle tension and vasocongestion.

Although sexual expression is a personal and private matter, it also carries a potential health risk. Nurses need to educate all clients about the importance of protection against sexually transmitted diseases (STDs), such as the human immunodeficiency virus (HIV). These infectious diseases can be spread by oral-genital, vaginal, or anal intercourse or other sexual activities involving an exchange of body fluids.

sexual response cycle

The body's response to sexual stimulation follows a similar pattern or cycle in both sexes, called the *sexual response cycle*. The cycle is divided into four phases: 1) *excitement*, 2) *plateau*, 3) *orgasm*, and 4) *resolution*.

excitement

The *excitement* phase is initiated by erotic suggestions, thoughts, feelings, or sights. During this time, the arteries dilate and the veins constrict, resulting in congestion of erectile tissue and rising muscle tension in the genital region. The vital signs (blood pressure, pulse, and respirations) increase in both sexes.

In the male, the penis becomes erect, the scrotum enlarges, and the testes contract close to the abdominal wall. Drops of seminal fluid may been seen on the urinary meatus.

In the female, the clitoris becomes erect, the vagina widens approximately 1 cm, and vaginal secretions increase. The labia majora and minora swell, the cervix slightly dilates, and the nipples of the breast become erect.

plateau

The *plateau* phase usually results from penal thrusts within the vagina. It is the period immediately preceding orgasm.

In the man, the testes remain close to the body and enlarge; the urethra becomes distended with semen. The heart rate may be as high as 175 beats/min and the respirations 40 per minute.

In the woman, the clitoris remains erect but is covered by surrounding tissue (prepuce), the distal one third of the vagina becomes swollen, forming an orgasmic platform. The uterus retracts and pulls the cervix forward, providing more space in the vaginal area and a more favorable environment for conception to occur.

orgasm

Orgasm is the release of sexual tension, an individual experience described in many different ways. Both sexes describe orgasm as a very pleasurable experience that involves the whole body, not just the pelvic area.

In the man, the penis contracts, releasing the seminal fluid in three or more spurts. This sudden release of semen is caused by involuntary muscle contractions.

In the woman, the pelvic region, particularly the clitoris and vagina, experience rhythmic involuntary muscle contractions.

resolution

The *resolution* phase is a resting phase in which the male and female reproductive organs return to pre-excitement state.

The penis becomes flaccid, and the congestion dissipates. During this time, it is not possible for the male to experience another erection.

Unlike the man, the woman is capable of multiple repeated orgasms without the interruption of a resolution phase. When she does enter the resolution phase, the reproductive organs return to their prearousal state.

pregnancy and sexuality

The individual's attitudes and beliefs about sexuality develop gradually throughout childhood, adolescence, and into adulthood. During pregnancy, the woman's sexuality may be influenced by the many physical and emotional changes that occur. Miscommunication between the partners may lead to stress on the relationship. Myths and misconceptions are not uncommon. Sex education is important to prevent guilt, myths, shame, and fear about the couple's sexual practices. The maternity nurse has a responsibility to promote positive sexual health. He or she may prepare the couple by giving accurate information and promoting an open atmosphere that makes the couple feel comfortable to discuss their concerns.

key points ✳

- **The female reproductive system consists of external structures (mons pubis, labia majora, labia minora, clitoris, vestibule, hymen, and perineum), internal structures (ovaries, fallopian tubes, uterus, uterine ligaments, and vagina), and accessory structures (Bartholin's glands, Skene's glands, and mammary glands).**
- **The vagina is the soft portion of the birth canal, a passageway for menstrual flow, and a receptacle for the penis during sexual intercourse.**
- **Estrogen is the female hormone responsible for the increased vascularity of the uterine lining and for the female secondary sex characteristics.**
- **The size of the breast is determined by the amount of adipose tissue and therefore has no bearing on the woman's ability to breast-feed.**
- **The true pelvis is the rigid part of the birth canal and must be large enough to allow safe passage of the fetus during labor and birth.**
- **Menarche marks the beginning of menstruation and reproductive capability; menopause signals the end of menstruation and reproduction.**
- **The menstrual cycle is divided into three phases: menstrual, proliferative, and secretory.**
- **The male reproductive system consists of external structures (penis and scrotum), internal structures (testes, epididymis, vas deferens, ejaculatory ducts, and urethra), and accessory structures (seminal vesicles, prostate gland, and bulbourethral gland).**
- **The penis is the male organ used in sexual intercourse (copulation, coitus).**
- **Testosterone is the male hormone responsible for the formation of sperm and the secondary sex characteristics.**
- **Sexuality includes many components, including biologic gender, sexual identity, physical characteristics, attitudes, behaviors, and cultural beliefs.**

review questions

1. What is the name of the hormone responsible for the production of sperm and the development of secondary sex characteristics in the male?
   a. Progesterone
   b. Prolactin
   c. Testosterone
   d. Estrogen
2. What structure is responsible for the release of the hormones estrogen and progesterone following ovulation?
   a. Hymen
   b. Fourchette
   c. Mons pubis
   d. Corpus luteum
3. Juanita Morez, age 18, tells you the physician has done a physical examination and told her that the hymen is not in place. She does not understand this because she has never been sexually active. Your best response would be,
   a. "Ask your doctor to explain this."
   b. "The hymen may be torn by physical activity, such as horseback riding and track and field athletics, or by using tampons."
   c. "Discuss this with your mother."
   d. "Not all girls are born with the hymen in place."
4. Janelle Brown, age 50, tells you she has been experiencing "hot flashes" and mood swings. She is concerned that she is mentally unstable. Your best response would be,
   a. "You are ok."
   b. "You may be experiencing menopausal symptoms; perhaps a visit with your physician might be helpful."
   c. "Many women your age experience this; it will go away—just ignore it."
   d. "Perhaps you need to see a psychiatrist."
5. Biologic gender refers to
   a. sexual preference.
   b. feelings or emotions one experiences.
   c. anatomic structure of the reproductive system.
   d. cultural beliefs of a society of men or women

bibliography

Bullock, B. L. (1996). *Pathophysiology* (4th ed.). Philadelphia: Lippincott–Raven.

Cumming, D. C., Cumming, C.E., & Kiernan, D.K. (1991). Menstrual mythology and sources of information about menstruation. *American Journal of Obstetrics and Gynecology*, 164, 472.

Kenner, C. A., & Mac Laren, A. (1993). *Essentials of maternal and neonatal nursing.* Springhouse: Springhouse Corporation.

Masters, W. H., & Johnson, V. E. (1966). *Human sexual response.* Boston: Little, Brown.

Pillitteri, A. (1995). *Maternal and child health nursing* (2nd ed.). Philadelphia: J.B. Lippincott.

Reeder, S. J., Martin, L. L., & Koniak, D. (1992). *Maternity nursing: Family, newborn, and women's health care* (17th ed.). Philadelphia: J.B. Lippincott.

Spence, A. P., & Mason, E. B. (1992). *Human anatomy and physiology* (4th ed.). St. Paul: West Publishing.

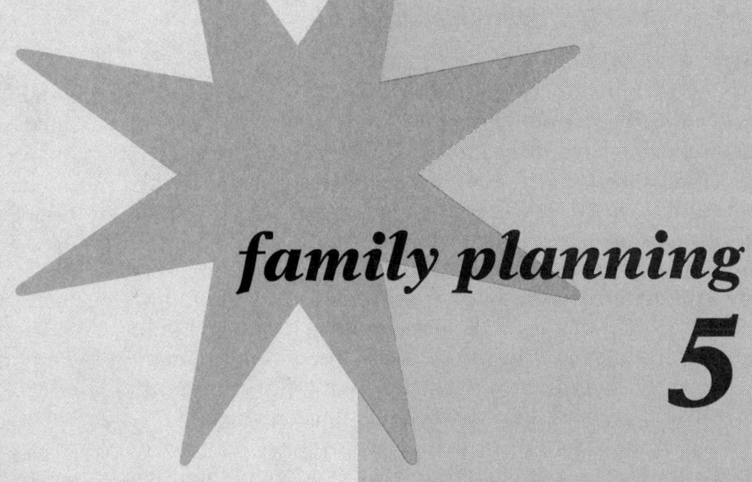

family planning 5

outline

objectives 

After studying this chapter, the reader should be able to:

* List the hormonal, chemical, and mechanical methods of birth control.
* Instruct the client in the use of available birth control methods.
* Assist the client in making reasonable, informed choices of birth control methods.
* Discuss some of the common reproductive myths.
* Define the various methods of elective abortion.
* Explain the three most common causes of male infertility.
* Explain the three most common causes of female infertility.
* Discuss some of the common myths of infertility.
* Describe the difference between open and closed adoption.
* Discuss the nursing goals used in genetic counseling.

key terms 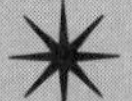

anovulation
chemical barrier method
closed adoption
contraception
elective abortion
endometriosis
genetic counseling
hormonal method
impotence
infertility
mechanical barrier method
natural family planning
open adoption
tubal ligation
vasectomy

Couples have many options from which to choose for planning the size of their family. Many *contraceptive* (birth control) methods make it possible to delay childbearing or to limit or space the number of children in the family. Abortion may be the choice when pregnancy is not desirable. At some point, a couple may choose sterilization to terminate further fertility.

Although many couples use contraceptives to plan the number and spacing of their children, an increasing number of couples are having difficulty becoming pregnant. More than 1 million couples (one out of every six) in the United States seek infertility treatment each year.

Adoption also may be considered by some couples, either because they are unable to have children of their own or because they want to give a child the advantages of a stable family environment.

✳ family considerations

To make successful choices in planning their family, a couple needs to consider the following concerns:

- Compatibility of each other's cultural background and values
- Compatibility of each other's religious beliefs
- Desirability of having children, how many, and within what time span
- Frequency of sexual contact versus the cost of the birth control
- Acceptability of the birth control or fertility awareness method to both partners
- Physical health of the partners

contraceptive (birth control) methods

To simplify the study of contraceptive (birth control) methods, they can be categorized as hormonal, mechanical barrier, chemical barrier, and natural family planning methods.

hormonal methods

Hormonal methods of contraception include birth control pills, "morning after" pills, medroxyprogesterone acetate (Depo-Provera), and Norplant. These medications contain hormones that prevent ovulation or prevent implantation of a fertilized ovum. Although these drugs can prevent pregnancy, they offer *no* protection against sexually transmitted diseases (STDs), such as acquired immunodeficiency syndrome (AIDS), chlamydia, and gonorrhea.

oral contraceptives

Oral contraceptives were introduced in the early 1960s and have become one of the most popular forms of birth control in the United States. Today, more that 10 million American women use "the pill" (Fig. 5-1*A*).

There are two broad categories of oral contraceptives: the combination pill and the "mini-pill." The most commonly used is the combination pill, which contains the hormones estrogen and progesterone. Estrogen prevents the production of the pituitary hormones follicle-stimulating hormone and luteinizing hormone, which halts ovulation. Progesterone prevents the build-up of the uterine lining, decreases sperm motility, and thickens cervical mucus, making it difficult for the sperm to travel through the female reproductive tract.

The first combination pills, released in the early 1960s, contained high doses of estrogen, which led to serious side effects in some women. With time, the manufacturers have decreased the amount of estrogen in the combination pill, reducing the severity of side effects yet still effectively preventing pregnancy. Since the 1980s, three types of combination pills have been available (Display 5-1):

- **Monophasic**—releasing a constant amount of the hormones throughout the cycle
- **Biphasic**—releasing a constant amount of estrogen and an increasing amount of progesterone
- **Triphasic**—releasing three different dosages of estrogen and progesterone at different parts of the cycle

These newer combinations allow the physician to tailor the prescription to each woman to prevent side effects, such as breakthrough bleeding (bleeding during the cycle), fluid retention, and headaches.

The second broad category is the "mini pill," first made available in the early 1970s; it is composed of the single hormone progesterone. These pills are reserved for women who are unable to tolerate estrogen and who have a strong desire to use this form of contraception. Problems encountered with the "mini pill" include breakthrough bleeding and absence of menses (amenorrhea).

The pill is dispensed in packages of 21 or 28 pills and range in cost from $5 to $20 a month. (Agencies such as Planned Parenthood will make the pills available without charge for women who cannot afford to pay.) The difference in the number of pills is merely one of convenience. The 28-day pack contains seven "empty" pills (placebos). This packaging allows the woman to maintain the routine of taking one pill a day and not skip a dose. If she chooses the 21-day pack, she takes one pill a day for 21 days, then waits 7 days before starting the next pack. With either method, the menstrual period usually starts within a day or two after 21 pills have been taken. (See Teaching Guidelines: safe and effective use of oral contraceptives)

depo-provera®

Late in 1992, the FDA approved a contraceptive injection called Depo-Provera. A synthetic progesterone, Depo-Provera has been used for 30 years in approximately 90 other countries, with many of the women using it for 10 years. During the first year of use, the woman may notice changes in her menstrual period, including breakthrough bleeding, an increase or decrease in the menstrual flow, or absence of menses. Once the woman ceases the use of Depo-Provera, normal menstrual periods return within 3 to 10 months, and within 15 months, conception can usually occur without difficulty.

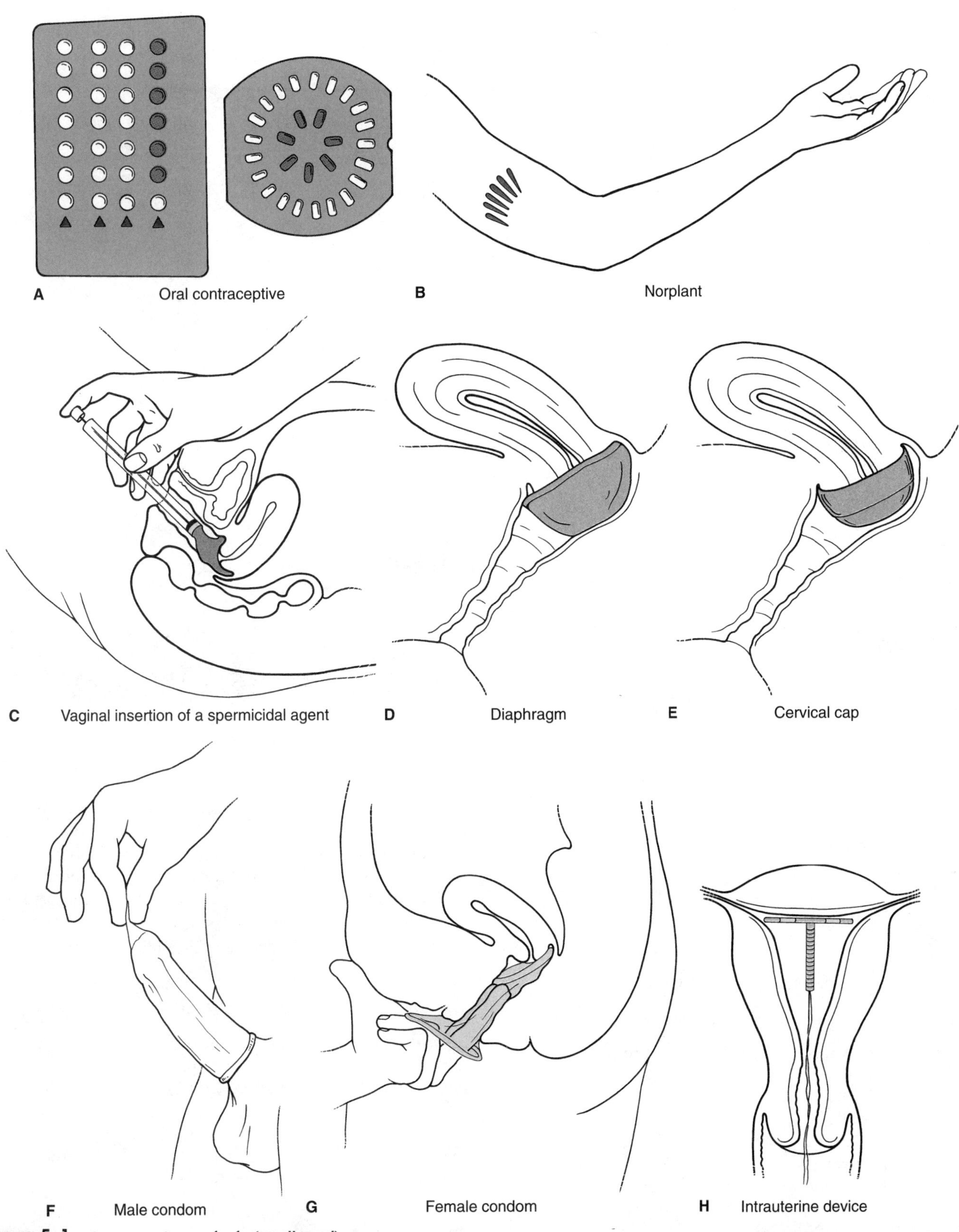

figure 5-1 *Contraceptive methods* ***(continued)***

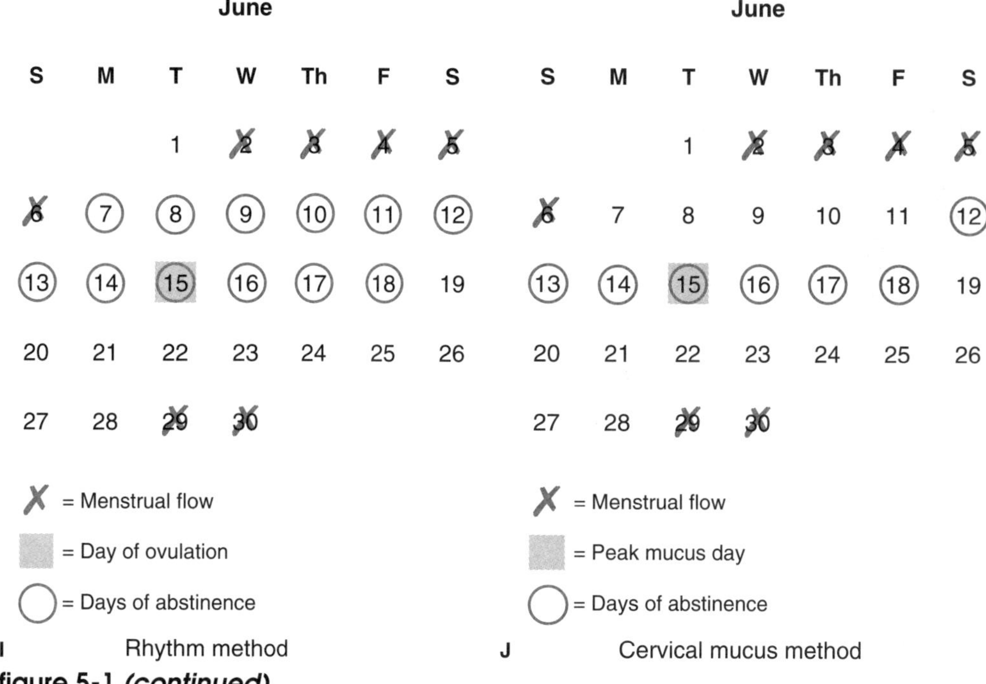

figure 5-1 ***(continued)***

Depo-Provera is injected intramuscularly (in the arm or buttock) once every 3 months, preventing ovulation and the normal menstrual cycle changes that occur in the uterus. It is rated as 99.7% effective, similar to the effective rate of oral contraceptives but without the necessity of taking a daily pill.

Once the woman has made the decision to use Depo-Provera, she is given an injection within 5 days after the beginning of her menses. If she has recently given birth and is not breast-feeding, she may have the injection during the first 5 days after the birth. If she is breast-feeding, however, she must wait 6 weeks before receiving the first injection. (See Teaching Guidelines: safe and effective use of Depo-Provera®)

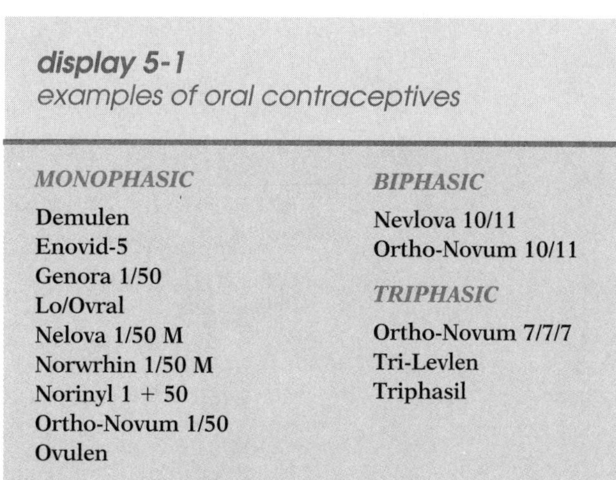

display 5-1
examples of oral contraceptives

MONOPHASIC	BIPHASIC
Demulen	Nevlova 10/11
Enovid-5	Ortho-Novum 10/11
Genora 1/50	**TRIPHASIC**
Lo/Ovral	Ortho-Novum 7/7/7
Nelova 1/50 M	Tri-Levlen
Norwrhin 1/50 M	Triphasil
Norinyl 1 + 50	
Ortho-Novum 1/50	
Ovulen	

norplant

The Norplant system was introduced in the United States in 1991. It consists of six tiny silastic capsule-like membranes that deliver a constant low dose of progesterone over 5 years. The physician inserts the tiny capsules in the inner aspect of the upper arm in a fanlike configuration (see Fig. 5-1*B*). The procedure takes approximately 10 minutes and generally requires only a local anesthetic. Once inserted, they are usually not visible but can be palpated with the fingers. The cost is about $350 for the kit, plus physician fees for insertion and removal.

Norplant is a viable alternative to oral contraceptives for teenagers and women older than 35 years who prefer not to use estrogen-containing contraception. The capsules are inserted during the first 7 days of the menstrual cycle, immediately following an elective or spontaneous abortion, or 6 weeks after delivery. (See Teaching Guidelines: safe and effective use of the Norplant)

chemical barrier methods

Chemical barrier methods of contraception include products that are inserted into the vagina before sexual contact to kill the sperm (spermicidal) and neutralize the vaginal secretions, preventing the sperm from traveling to the fallopian tubes. Included in this group are the spermicides: aerosol foams, creams, jellies, tablets, and suppositories.

spermicides

Spermicidal agents are readily available without a prescription (see Fig. 5-1*C*). The nurse must instruct the client

teaching guidelines
safe and effective use of oral contraceptives

- If the client misses a dose, she should take it as soon as she remembers. If more than one dose has been missed, an alternate form of contraception should be used for the remainder of the 28-day period.
- Breakthrough bleeding may occur with some antibiotics, such as tetracycline, ampicillin, penicillin V, and antihistamines.
- The pill should be discontinued 4 top 8 weeks before any planned surgery to decrease the risks of blood clots.
- The pill should be discontinued 3 to 4 months before a planned pregnancy to allow the hormone levels to return to normal.

ADVANTAGES

- 98% to 100% effective if taken appropriately
- No precautions needed previous to sexual contact
- No precautions needed previous to sexual contact
- Decrease in the risk of cancer of the female reproductive system (eg, endomedtrium, ovaries)
- Decrease or elimination of premenstrual tension

SIDE EFFECTS

- Irregular bleeding patterns (breakthrough bleeding)
- Headaches—possible migraine
- Weight gain or loss
- Breast tenderness
- Slight increase in risk of breast cancer
- Depression
- Decreased sex drive (libido)
- Increased incidence of vaginal yeast infections
- Hypertension

CONTRAINDICATIONS

- Bleeding and clotting disorders
- Thrombophlebitis
- Cerebrovascular accident
- Heart disease
- Impaired liver function
- Pregnancy
- Smoking
- Cancer of the reproductive system
- Diabetes

to read the package carefully to make sure she has a spermicidal agent and not a feminine hygiene product.

Spermicidal creams and jellies are used in conjunction with another method, such as the cervical cap or diaphragm. The foam products may be used alone but have a higher effectiveness rate if used with a condom. The effectiveness rate is 85% to 98% and depends largely on the compliance of the couple. Although spermicides offer some protection against the human immunodeficiency virus and other STDs, the best protection against these diseases is a condom. (See the Teaching Guideline: safe and effective use of spermicide)

teaching guidelines
safe and effective use of Depo-Provera®

- Report any signs of injection site infection, including redness, tenderness, and pain.
- Report any serious side effects, such as chest pain (possible pulmonary emboli), heavy vaginal bleeding (possible hemorrhage), and severe pain or swelling in the calf of the leg (possible blood clot).

ADVANTAGES

- 99.7% effective
- Does not contain estrogen; therefore, has less side effects
- No daily pills or special preparations for sexual contact
- No increased risk of cancer of the reproductive organs

SIDE EFFECTS

- Decrease in the amount of stored minerals in the bones, which could lead to fractures
- Amenorrhea
- Weight gain
- Headaches
- Abdominal cramps
- Depression
- Fatigue
- Decreased libido
- Edema

CONTRAINDICATIONS

- Pregnancy
- Cancer of the reproductive organs
- History of cardiovascular disease
- Liver disease
- Diabetes

teaching guidelines
safe and effective use of the Norplant

* Breakthrough bleeding and irregular menses are not uncommon during the first year. (Clients should understand this because it is one of the most common reasons for early requests for removal.)
* Signs and symptoms of infection should be reported to the physician. (One of the side effects is insertion site infection.)
* Reasons for early removal include severe headaches, visual disturbances, hypertension, onset of liver disease, pregnancy, or the development of infection at the insertion site.

ADVANTAGES

* 99.8% effective rate
* May be used for teens and woman older than 35 years
* No daily pills to remember or special preparations prior to sexual contact

SIDE EFFECTS

* Breakthrough bleeding
* Amenorrhea
* Acne
* Weight gain or loss
* Water retention
* Hypertension
* Injection site infection

CONTRAINDICATIONS

* Thrombophlebitis
* Abnormal uterine bleeding
* Pregnancy
* Liver disease
* Breast cancer

mechanical barrier methods

Mechanical barrier methods of contraception prevent contact of the penis with the cervix, blocking the sperm from entering the uterus. These methods include the diaphragm, the cervical cap, and the condom. Only the condom offers protection against STDs.

diaphragm

The diaphragm is a flexible rubber dome-shaped device with a spring rim that fits over the cervix (see Fig. 5-1*D*). Its effectiveness ranges from 82% to 98%, and prices start at $50. The physician must measure the cervix to ensure a proper fit. Once the proper size has been selected, the client must be instructed in the correct procedure for use. It may be helpful to let the client practice insertion and verbalize understanding of the method. Noncompliance seems to be one of the major reasons for a higher pregnancy rate with the diaphragm; either the woman does not use it properly or fails to use it at all. The Teaching Guidelines display explains the proper use of the diaphragm.

cervical cap

The cervical cap is similar to the diaphragm except it is held in place by a natural suction because it is smaller and fits more snugly over the cervix (see Fig. 5-1*E*). Its effectiveness ranges from 82% to 93%; the cap is slightly more expensive than the diaphragm. The Teaching Guidelines display offers instructions for use of the cervical cap.

male condom

The male condom is one of the oldest methods of contraception, dating back to the 16th century. Originally condoms were designed to prevent the spread of STDs but were promptly recognized for their ability to prevent pregnancy. Condoms are made of latex, collagenous material,

teaching guidelines
safe and effecitve use of spermicide

* Spermicidal agents must be inserted before each sexual contact. This may be done up to 1 hour before contact.
* For insertion of the spermicide, the woman should be in a recumbent position, and the spermicide should be placed high in the vagina, near the cervix.
* The male partner may insert the spermicide as part of the preliminary touching.
* Containers of foam should be shaken well before filling the applicator.
* Wait at least 8 hours after intercourse before douching.

ADVANTAGES

* May be purchased over-the-counter
* No hormonal side effects

SIDE EFFECTS

* May be messy to use
* Local skin irritation may be a problem—may try another brand
* May interfere with spontaneity

CONTRAINDICATIONS

* None

teaching guidelines
safe and effective use of the diaphragm

* Before insertion, 1 teaspoon of spermicidal jelly or cream must be placed inside and along the rim of the diaphragm.
* The position of the diaphragm must be checked with the fingers to make sure it is totally covering the cervix.
* If inserted more than 2 hours before sexual intercourse, an additional dose of spermicidal jelly or cream must be inserted into the vagina with an applicator.
* The diaphragm must be left in place for 6 to 8 hours following sexual intercourse.
* With a gain or loss of 10 lb, birth of a child, or pelvic surgery, the diaphragm should be refitted and possibly replaced to ensure proper fit and effectiveness.

ADVANTAGES

* 82% to 100% effective
* No hormonal side effects
* Ideal for individual who has infrequent sexual contact

SIDE EFFECTS

* Cramping
* Vaginal ulceration
* Allergies to rubber or spermicidal agent

CONTRAINDICATIONS

* History of toxic shock syndrome
* Recurrent urinary tract infections
* Uterine prolapse
* Cystocele
* Rectocele

or sheep's intestines. Those made of latex are the most effective for preventing pregnancy and STDs.

The condom is slipped over the erect penis, leaving a small space at the tip to act as a reservoir for the ejaculated semen (see Fig. 5-1*F*). Condoms are relatively inexpensive (1–2 dollars apiece) with an 85% to 95% effectiveness rate. This rate can be increased to 100% if the woman uses a spermicidal agent. Some guidelines for safe and effective use of the condom are provided in the Teaching Guidelines display.

nursing alert

The condom must have adequate space at the tip of the penis to allow for collection of the ejaculate. If the condom fits too tightly, the ejaculate may be pushed along the sides of the condom and escape into the vagina during sexual intercourse.

female condom

A company called Reality is marketing a female condom made of polyurethane (see Fig. 5-1*G*). It is a loose-fitting sheath with a flexible ring on either end. The inner ring near the closed end of the condom is used to anchor it internally near the cervix. For insertion, the inner ring is squeezed and placed into the vagina, much the same as a diaphragm would be inserted. The outer ring and approximately 1 in of the sheath remain outside the vagina, near the labia. It may be inserted up to 8 hours before sexual contact.

Following intercourse, the woman should twist the outer rim to close the sheath and then remove it from the vagina. This twisting of the outer rim seals the semen inside the sheath to prevent spillage into the vagina. With correct and consistent use, the female condom is 94% effective. The Teaching Guidelines display provides educational information regarding the female condom.

teaching guidelines

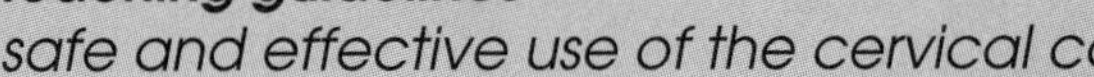

safe and effective use of the cervical cap

The instructions are similar to those for the diaphragm with the following exceptions:

* The cap must be filled one-third full of spermicidal jelly or cream, making sure that none is on the rim.
* The cap must be left in place for 6 hours but no more than 48 hours.
* No extra spermicidal jelly or cream needs to be added for repeated sexual contact during the time the cap is left in place.

ADVANTAGES

* No hormonal side effects
* May be left in longer than the diaphragm and no repeated applications of spermicidal jelly needed

SIDE EFFECTS

* Increased risk of cervicitis
* May cause toxic shock syndrome
* Slight chance of vaginal lacerations
* May cause strong odor if left in place more than 1 day

CONTRAINDICATIONS

* History of toxic shock syndrome
* Acute cervicitis
* Abnormal Pap smears

teaching guidelines
safe and effective use of the male condom

* Care should be exercised when removing the penis from the vagina to prevent tearing or slipping of the condom, which would permit semen to come in contact with the vagina.
* Condoms are meant for a single act of intercourse and should not be reused.
* If a vaginal lubricant is needed, it should be water soluble, such as KY jelly. Petroleum jelly dissolves the latex.
* Heat can destroy condoms, so they should be stored in a cool, dry place, never in the glove compartment of the car or in a wallet.

ADVANTAGES	*SIDE EFFECTS*	*CONTRAINDICATIONS*
* No health risks from hormones * Protects from sexually transmitted diseases	* Occasional allergies to rubber or latex * May break during use * May decrease sexual sensation for the male	* None

intrauterine device

The intrauterine device (IUD) is a small T-shaped plastic device (coated with barium for visibility on x-ray) that is inserted into the uterus to prevent pregnancy (see Fig. 5-1*H*). Only two types of IUD are available in the United States: 1) Progestasert T and 2) the ParaGard. Many other types introduced in the 1960s were removed from the market because of legal issues regarding their safety.

The Progestasert T releases a continuous low dose of progesterone over 1 year; at the end of that time, it must be replaced to be effective. The progesterone stops the buildup of the endometrium and prevents the fertilized egg from embedding (implanting) in the uterine lining. This may result in a higher incidence of ectopic pregnancy.

The ParaGard is coated with copper wire, which acts as a spermicidal agent. Yearly vaginal examinations and Pap smears are required. The device is effective for 4 years and must be replaced after 4 years if continued contraception is desired.

The IUD is placed in the uterus in a collapsed position using an insertion device that resembles a long hollow straw. When the insertion device is removed, the IUD stretches out to its T-shape position. The IUD is inserted during the first 7 days of the menstrual cycle while the cervix is slightly dilated; thus, insertion causes less discomfort. Once the IUD is in place, a small string hangs down into the vagina.

If pregnancy should occur while an IUD is in place, the physician probably will attempt to remove the device. Removal carries a 25% risk of spontaneous abortion; leaving the device in place, however, doubles the risk to 50% and carries a high risk of uterine infection. The advantages, side effects, and contraindications of the IUD are described in the Teaching Guidelines display.

natural family planning methods

Many couples choose *natural family planning* methods, either because of religious beliefs or personal preference. These methods rely on the couple's ability to abstain from sexual contact on the fertile days of the menstrual cycle; these methods include the rhythm (calendar) method, the

teaching guidelines
safe and effective use of the female condom

* Like the male condom, the female condom is intended for one-time use.
* Condoms are the most effective method (other than abstinence) of preventing transmission of human immunodeficiency virus, cytomegalovirus, hepatitis B virus, and other sexually transmitted diseases.

ADVANTAGES	*SIDE EFFECTS*	*CONTRAINDICATIONS*
* The woman controls its use * Because of the condom's loose fit, the penis may penetrate the vagina before complete erection * Less chance of tearing than the male condom because it is much stronger * Does not require immediate removal of the penis following orgasm like the male condom	* None	* None

teaching guidelines
safe and effective use of the intrauterine device

- Check for placement of the IUD by feeling the string.
- Wait at least 3 months after removal of the IUD to allow the uterine environment to return to normal before attempting to conceive.

ADVANTAGES

- Once inserted, no other preparation for sexual contact is needed

SIDE EFFECTS

- Slight pain during insertion
- Backache
- Vaginal bleeding
- Perforation of the uterus
- Risk of infertility

CONTRAINDICATIONS

- Nulliparas (no previous pregnancy
- Uterine abnormalities
- History of heavy vaginal bleeding
- Anemia

basal body temperature (BBT) method, and the cervical mucus (Billing's or ovulation) method. Also included in this group is an ancient, unreliable, but "better than nothing" method, *coitus interruptus*. Except for coitus interruptus, these methods also are called *fertility awareness methods* and may be used in infertility treatment to encourage conception rather than to prevent it. Even when these methods are effective in preventing pregnancy, they offer *no* protection against STDs.

rhythm (calendar) method

The least reliable method of family planning, the rhythm method, requires the woman to record the pattern of 6 to 8 menstrual cycles, calculate her fertile days, and avoid intercourse on those days. She should subtract the number 18 from her shortest cycle (this gives her the first fertile day) and subtract the number 11 from her longest cycle (this gives her the last fertile day). Refer to Chapter 4 for a discussion of ovulation. For example, if her cycles ranged from 28 to 32 days, her fertile days would be days 10 through 21. For this method to be effective, she would avoid sexual contact on days 10 through 21 during all of her cycles (see Fig. 5-1*I*).

basal body temperature method

This method requires the woman to take her temperature every morning before arising and record the pattern for at least 6 months to identify the pattern. The BBT is the temperature of a normal healthy body that is awake but inactive. She must use a basal body thermometer that measures body temperature in one-tenth increments rather than the standard thermometer that measures in two-tenths increments. The woman's body temperature will drop slightly (0.2°F) immediately preceding ovulation and rise abruptly (0.4°–0.8°F) 24 to 72 hours after ovulation. Sexual contact should be avoided from the first day of her menses to the third day of temperature elevation.

Although more effective than the rhythm method, the BBT method is still highly unreliable, even for women with regular menstrual cycles. Such factors as a cold or other infection, fever, stress, or fatigue can cause changes in body temperature that are unrelated to ovulation.

The BBT method may be further refined by using the symptothermal method, which watches for signs of ovulation in addition to the temperature changes. These signs include the following:

- Pelvic bloating or fullness
- Increased libido (sex drive)
- Midcycle spotting
- Lower quadrant pain experienced from the rupture of the ovarian follicle (mittelschmerz)

cervical mucus method (billing's or ovulation method)

This method requires the woman to examine her cervical mucus for changes that occur in response to ovulation (see Fig. 5-1*J*). Normally, cervical mucus is yellow-white, sticky, and thick. Just before ovulation, mucus secretion increases, and when ovulation begins, the mucus becomes clear, thin, and very elastic, resembling raw egg white. This elasticity (called spinnbarkeit) may be checked by stretching it between the thumb and index finger (Fig. 5-2). The mucus will stretch from 2 to 5 in. This stretchability of the vaginal mucus helps the sperm swim up into the fallopian tubes, a journey of only a few seconds under ideal conditions. Guidelines for the cervical mucus method are highlighted in the Teaching Guidelines display.

coitus interruptus

Coitus interruptus is a form of unprotected sexual intercourse that requires the man to remove the penis from the vagina just before ejaculation. It is an unreliable method for two reasons: It requires a great deal of self-control during the height of passion. The man's pre-ejaculatory secretions contain thousands of sperm capable of fertilization.

Few Americans, probably less than 2%, use this method, but it is used widely throughout developing countries. It has a less than 75% effectiveness rate, but it requires no special preparation or cost.

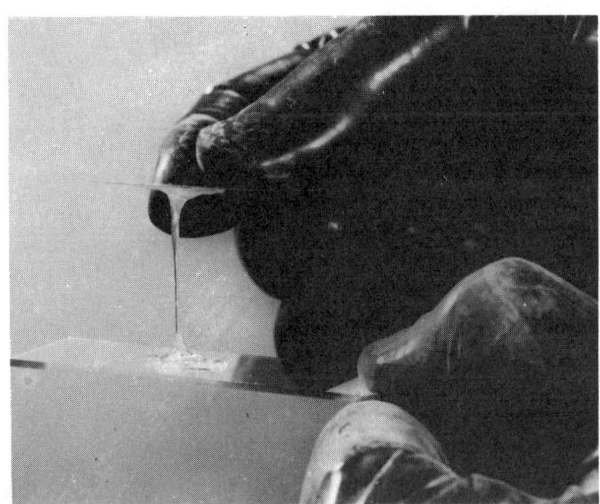

figure 5-2 *Spinnbarkeit (elasticity).*

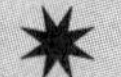 **nursing insight**

Natural family planning methods require considerable time, effort, and commitment from both partners for the chosen method to be successful.

elective abortion

Elective abortion is the intentional interruption or termination of pregnancy. In 1973, the United States Supreme Court (Roe v. Wade) legalized elective abortion. Individual states were charged with formulating policies, such as the need for permission from the husband or from the parent of a minor, during what term of the pregnancy the abortion may be performed, what type of health care facility may be used, and any special circumstances that limit or permit abortion. For example, some states require preabortion counseling about the growth and development of the embryo, followed by a specified waiting period.

In 1976, the United States Congress passed the Hyde Amendment that prohibits the use of federal funds for abortions except in extenuating circumstances in which the continuation of the pregnancy is life-threatening to the mother or is the result of incest or rape. Some states also have policies regarding the use of state funds for abortions.

Elective abortion is an emotionally charged issue and has polarized the country into two large factions. The "pro-life" group believes that abortion should not be legal because the embryo or fetus is a human being and has a right to life. The "pro-choice" group believes that the woman has the right to control her own body and bodily functions. Nurses have a moral, ethical, and legal responsibility to remain nonjudgmental and supportive of their clients and to provide factual information. If the nurse has a problem dealing with clients seeking abortion information, it is best to seek another colleague to assist the client. If this is not possible, the nurse needs to reconsider his or her position with the institution and seek employment elsewhere, because clients' welfare and right to make their own decisions must come first.

dilatation and curettage

This procedure may be done during the first 12 weeks of pregnancy. The cervix is dilated with surgical instruments, and then a sharp curette is used to scrape the endometrium and remove the products of conception. A small compressed piece of sterile seaweed (*Laminaria*) may be inserted into the cervix to assist with dilation. The *Laminaria* expands slowly (up to 6 hours), making cervical dilatation less painful and preventing cervical laceration. A general or local anesthetic may be used during the procedure, and the woman can expect mild bleeding and abdominal cramping during the first 24 hours following the procedure.

teaching guidelines ✷

safe and effective use of the cervical mucus method

* Natural family planning methods may be altered by illness, stress, fatigue, or infection.
* Care must be taken to ensure that the cervical mucus being examined is not mixed with spermicides, lubricants, semen, or other products that could alter evaluation.
* Sexual contact should be avoided when the cervical mucus begins to change until 3 days past ovulation.

ADVANTAGES	*SIDE EFFECTS*	*CONTRAINDICATIONS*
✷ Accepted by religious groups ✷ Requires little or no supplies and therefore is inexpensive ✷ Encourages both partners to be active participants in the family planning regimen	✷ Cycle is affected by infections, stress, and environmental changes	✷ None

vacuum extraction

This procedure may be performed during the first 12 weeks of pregnancy. After the cervix is dilated slightly using *Laminaria*, a special suction catheter is passed into the uterus, and the products of conception are slowly removed (aspirated). This procedure appears to be less traumatic to the cervix and uterus than dilatation and curettage. The woman will still receive a general or local anesthetic and experience mild bleeding and abdominal cramping.

prostaglandins

Prostaglandins are fatty acids originally discovered in semen. Used to induce abortion primarily during the 12th to 16th week of pregnancy, a prostaglandin may be administered as a vaginal suppository or intramuscularly, intravenously, or transabdominally into the amniotic sac. It causes the uterus to contract and the cervix to dilate, resulting in evacuation of the uterine contents within a few hours. The woman may suffer side effects, such as mild nausea, vomiting, and diarrhea. The nurse monitors the woman for complaints of labor pain and administers pain medication as needed. Emotional support is vital during and after the procedure.

nursing alert

Oral administration of prostaglandin is prohibited due to severe side effects, such as nausea, vomiting, diarrhea, chills, and fever.

hypertonic saline abortion (amnioinfusion)

When the pregnancy has progressed to between 12 and 20 weeks, a hypertonic saline abortion may be performed. A needle is passed through the abdominal wall into the amniotic sac and a few milliliters of amniotic fluid are withdrawn. Using the same needle, a 200-mL infusion of 20% hypertonic saline is instilled slowly, and within a few hours, uterine contractions begin. Fetal death in utero usually occurs almost immediately after instillation of the saline. The mother may need pain medication for the labor contractions and considerable emotional support from the nurse during this time. In some areas, hyperosmotic urea (30%–40%) in 5% dextrose solution is used instead of saline because of the potential for complications from the high concentrations of saline. A slow IV drip of oxytocin is used with the urea to enhance the uterine contractions.

hysterotomy (mini-cesarean)

A hysterotomy is performed either through an abdominal incision similar to a cesarean delivery or through the vagina. It is reserved for late second-trimester or early third-trimester abortions when other methods are contraindicated and requires preoperative and postoperative care along with general or spinal anesthesia. Delivery of a fully formed fetus who may still be alive means that the woman will need special emotional support, pain medication, and routine postoperative care.

mifepristone (ru-486)

Though widely accepted in Europe, mifepristone (RU-486), the world-renowned French "abortion pill" was banned in the United States until 1993 because of political pressure from anti-choice groups. In April of that year, an agreement was signed by the U.S. Population Council and the manufacturer, Roussel Uclaf, to allow clinical trials of RU-486 in the United States. Oregon and New Hampshire were the first states to volunteer as test sites. At least 2000 American women will have access to the pill during the clinical trials. Approval of RU-486 for general use could come by 1996 or 1997.

Ru-486 is a progesterone-blocking agent that prevents the embryo from implanting in the uterine lining. It must be taken during the first 7 weeks of pregnancy and is followed by a dose of misoprostol (Cytotec) 2 days later. Cytotec has properties similar to prostaglandin, and it causes uterine contractions and dilation of the cervix, resulting in expulsion of the embryo. RU-486 is reported to be 97% effective.

In 1991 in France, a woman who was a heavy smoker attempted to abort her 13th pregnancy and died of a heart attack. Following this incident, RU-486 was contraindicated in certain groups, including heavy smokers, women older than 35 years, and those who are at high risk for complications.

RU-486 also has shown promise in the therapy of diseases unrelated to pregnancy. These include endometriosis, fibroid tumors, premenstrual syndrome, breast cancer, and adrenal cancer.

sterilization

Sterilization is a permanent form of contraception that ends the reproductive capabilities of the individual. This method is usually chosen when a woman or couple decides they do not want any additional children or wishes to remain childless. When counseling the client and family on methods of sterilization, the teaching guidelines in the accompanying display are useful.

female sterilization

There are several techniques and approaches to female sterilization (*tubal ligation*). Regardless of the procedure performed (severing, plugging, ligating, banding, or cauterizing), the pathway through the fallopian tubes is interrupted, preventing the sperm from reaching the egg.

A *laparoscopy*, frequently called "Band-aid surgery," requires 1 or 2 small incisions in the abdominal wall. The abdomen is filled with carbon dioxide to move the intestines to one side and aid visualization of the fallopian

teaching guidelines
preparing the client and family for sterilization

- All reversible types of family planning measures should be reviewed to make sure the individual is comfortable with his or her decision for permament sterilization
- A thorough explanation of the sterilization procedure and answers to all the questions the client may ask are necessary.
- A surgical consent form must be signed prior to surgery.
- The individual to be sterilized has the legal right to make the decision; it is not necessary to obtain partner or spousal consent. If federal funds are used to pay for the procedure, the client must be 21 years old, mentally competent, and must wait 30 days after signing a consent form before the procedure can be performed.
- Reversal may be attempted, but it is costly, requres additional surgery, and may not be successful.

tubes. The laparoscope is passed into the abdomen and the tubes severed. The procedure is usually performed under a regional or local anesthetic on an outpatient basis. Recovery from this minor procedure usually takes only a couple of days.

An *abdominal laparotomy* requires a small abdominal incision near the suprapubic region. The tubes are identified and severed. A general anesthetic is administered, and the woman is kept in the hospital overnight for observation. Recovery time ranges from 1 to 3 weeks. This procedure may be performed anytime, including 1 to 3 days postpartum. A vaginal approach also may be used to prevent any abdominal scarring, but this has a higher incidence of infection and is rarely used.

Complications that may be seen following a tubal ligation include wound infection, hemorrhage, bowel or bladder perforation, and possible anesthetic reactions, such as nausea and vomiting. The woman who has a laparoscopic tubal ligation also may have abdominal cramping due to the inflation of the abdomen with carbon dioxide; this usually subsides within 24 hours (Fig. 5-3a).

male sterilization

Male sterilization is performed by *vasectomy*, a minor procedure in which the vas deferens is severed to prevent sperm from entering the seminal fluid. Sperm are still produced, but they die and are absorbed into the body. This procedure does not affect testosterone levels and therefore does not alter secondary sexual characteristics or the ability to have an erection or to urinate. Vasectomy is often done as an outpatient procedure or in the physician's office. The man is given a local anesthetic, and two small incisions are made (1.5–3 cm in length) over the vas deferens. The vas deferens are exposed and severed, cauterized, or banded. The skin is then closed with absorbable suture material (see Fig. 5-3b). The procedure usually takes 15 minutes or less. The client is advised to wear a scrotal support and to apply ice packs to the affected area, especially for the first 24 to 48 hours. He should be instructed to use an alternate method of contraception until he has two to three semen samples that are negative for viable sperm.

Complications that may been seen following a vasectomy include edema of the scrotum, pain, and localized infection.

infertility

Infertility may be defined as the absence of conception after 1 year of unprotected sexual intercourse (the time span is shortened to 6 months for older couples). The percentage of couples seeking infertility treatment has tripled in the last 25 years. Today, as many as one in six couples may seek infertility intervention.

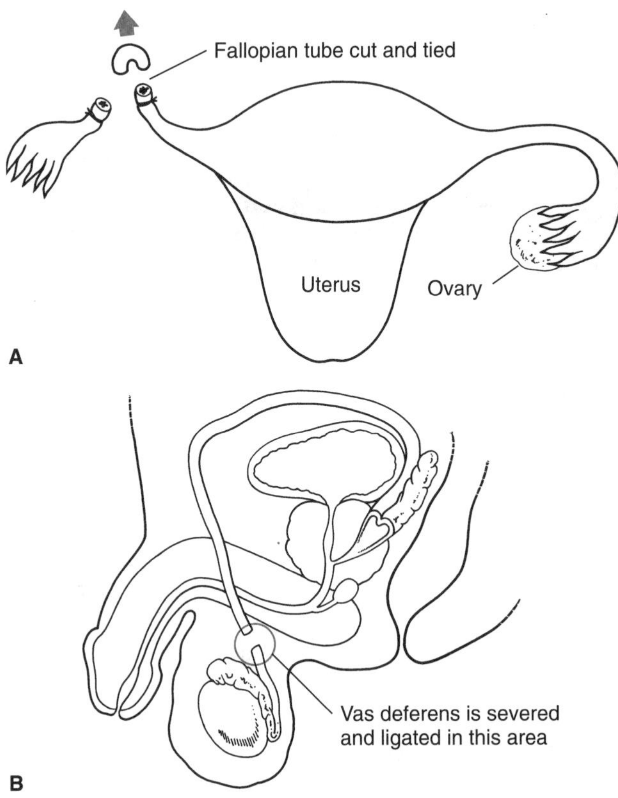

figure 5-3 *(**A**) Female tubal ligation. (**B**) Male vasectomy.*

The infertility rates according to sex are 30% male problems, 40% to 50% female problems, and 20% to 30% a combination of problems from a specific couple (for example, low sperm count and "hostile" cervical mucus).

Four main factors are believed responsible for the rise in infertility:

1. The incidence of STDs has increased, which causes blocking and scarring of the reproductive tracts of both sexes.
2. Childbearing is increasingly delayed until the woman is in her 30s or 40s, when fertility may be as low as 25% of original capability.
3. Malformation of the reproductive tract in thousands of women and men of childbearing age, the result of their mother's ingestion of diethystilbestrol (DES). From 1941 to 1971, DES was used to prevent miscarriage (spontaneous abortion). It was found to cause vaginal cancer in daughters of women taking it and reproductive tract abnormalities in offspring of both sexes.
4. Sperm count in men in the United States and 20 other countries has dropped an average of 50% since 1938, perhaps due to exposure to estrogen-like chemicals (such as pesticides) in their mothers' blood and milk.

Determining the causes of infertility begins with interviewing the couple and obtaining a complete health history (see Display 5-9 later in this chapter). Careful attention is paid to the basic functioning of the reproductive tract (Displays 5-2 and 5-3). When conducting the interview, many of the questions and discussions can be embarrassing for the nurse and the couple. The nurse must be comfortable with his or her own sexuality before assisting a couple to deal with their discomfort during the interview process.

male infertility

Four types of male infertility have been identified: 1) low sperm count and poor-quality sperm; 2) infections and scarring of the reproductive tract; 3) inability to deposit the sperm in the vagina; and 4) impotence.

Following the physical examination, the man will have a laboratory sperm count performed. A normal sperm count contains 20 to 250 million/mL of live sperm; 50% of these should have normal shape and motility.

display 5-2
female reproductive function necessary for conception

1. **The vaginal mucus must be receptive to sperm.**
2. **The fallopian tubes must be patent (open).**
3. **The ovaries must be capable of releasing a healthy ovum.**
4. **The uterine lining must be capable of supporting the implantation, growth, and development of the embryo.**

display 5-3
male reproductive function necessary for conception

1. **The duct system must be patent.**
2. **The testes must produce an adequate number of normal sperm.**
3. **The accessory glands must produce adequate seminal fluid.**
4. **The man must be able to deposit the sperm into the vagina.**

If the sperm count or quality is poor, the client is counseled to avoid any sources of excess heat (saunas, hot tubs, working in extremely hot environment), to avoid the use of alcohol or drugs, and to eat a nutritionally adequate diet. These measures usually promote the production of normal sperm within 3 months of compliance. If the count is low due to a medical condition, for example, an undescended testicle, there is no known intervention.

Infections usually respond to antibiotic therapy, but scarring or blockage requires surgical intervention. Twisted or swollen veins in the scrotum (*varicocele*) or excess fluid in the scrotum (*hydrocele*) are the two most common conditions related to male infertility that can be surgically corrected.

The inability to deposit the sperm high enough in the vagina to reach the cervix may result from a congenital defect. The most common defects are the positioning of the meatus under the penis (*hypospadias*) or on top of the penis (*epispadias*). These conditions may be corrected by surgery. Morbid obesity can occasionally prevent the male from inserting the penis into the vagina; weight loss could resolve this problem.

A man is *impotent* if he is unable to sustain an erection for sexual intercourse. If the problem is psychological, counseling may achieve positive results. Other causes and treatments include the following:

1. Hormonal imbalance, corrected by hormonal supplementation
2. Impairment of blood supply to the penis (from diabetic changes or pelvic surgery), corrected by vascular surgery or the surgical insertion of a penile implant
3. Medications (high blood pressure medications, tranquilizers, or barbiturates), corrected by changing the dosage or substituting another medication

female infertility

Three types of female infertility have been identified: 1) ovulation disorders, 2) tubal blockage, and 3) uterine disorders.

Failure to ovulate (*anovulation*) is the most common cause of female infertility. For regular monthly ovulation to occur, the hormones must be in perfect balance (see

Chap. 4 for review of the menstrual cycle). Other conditions that may prevent ovulation are ovarian cysts or tumors, poor physical and nutritional status, and repeated exposure to radioactive materials. Medications may be administered to correct the hormonal balance. Clomiphene citrate (Clomid) and human menopausal gonadotropin (Pergonal) are two drugs commonly used to induce ovulation. These drugs can cause multiple ovulation, which may result in multiple births.

Infection is the primary cause of tubal blockage. The most common causes are chlamydia, syphilis, and gonorrhea. These bacteria cause tissue damage and scarring that prevent the fertilized ovum from traveling to the uterus. Scarred tubes may be treated with microsurgery. The physician can remove the scar tissue or remove the scarred portion of the tube and reconnect the remaining portion to the uterus, permitting safe passage of the ovum.

Two major uterine problems causing infertility are *endometriosis* and *hostile cervical mucus.* Endometriosis occurs when endometrial tissue (the tissue lining the uterus) is transplanted outside the uterine cavity. During the normal menstrual cycle, the endometrial lining of the uterus thickens, then sloughs off and bleeds. Any endometrial tissue outside the uterus responds the same way but without a natural outlet (see Fig. 5-4 for common sites of endometriosis). This causes pain and formation of scar tissue. To treat the condition, the physician may order oral contraceptives or danazol (Danocrine) to atrophy the external endometrial tissue and laparoscopic surgery to cauterize the affected areas and restore fertility.

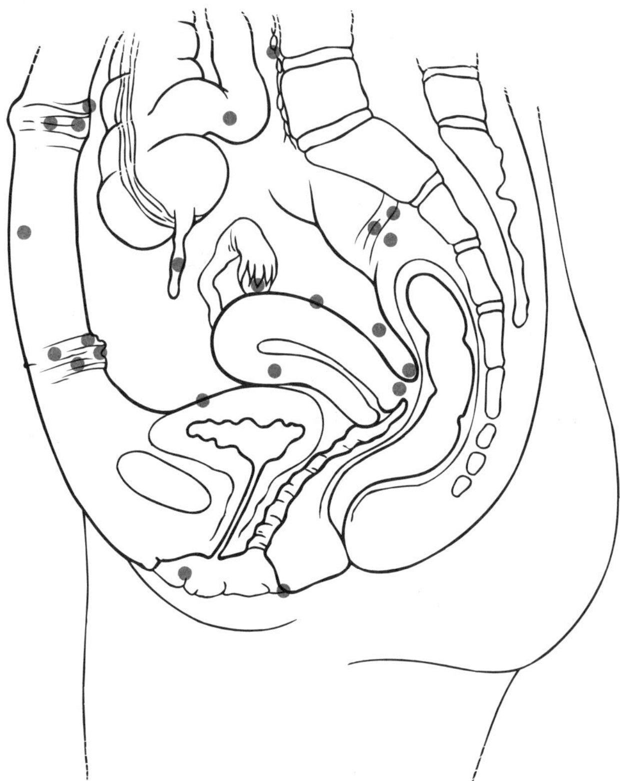

figure 5-4 *Common sites of endometriosis.*

display 5-4
assisted reproductive technologies (ART) for infertile couples

IN VITRO FERTILIZATION-EMBRYO TRANSFER (IVF-ET)

Step 1: A ripe ovum is obtained from the female, and semen is obtained from the male.

Step 2: They are placed in a special medium, which allows fertilization to take place in the laboratory.

Step 3: A catheter is inserted into the uterine cavity, and the embryos are transferred there.

GAMETE INTRAFALLOPIAN TRANSFER (GIFT)

In this procedure, fertilization takes place in the woman's body. The ovum is obtained, and a semen sample is obtained. The ovum and sperm are loaded into a catheter and placed in the woman's fallopian tube with the use of a laparoscope.

ZYGOTE INTRAFALLOPIAN TRANSFER

This procedure combines IVF and GIFT techniques to transplant the fertilized ovum into the fallopian tube.

For the cervical mucus to be receptive to sperm, it must become thin and stretchy (spinnbarkeit) during ovulation. Cervical infections and decreased estrogen can prevent this from happening, a condition called *hostile cervical mucus.* If the mucus remains thick, the sperm cannot travel through it to reach the fallopian tube for contact with the ovum. The physician may order antibiotics to clear the infection and estrogen supplements to improve the quality of the cervical mucus, usually increasing fertility.

Infertility treatments are very costly, both emotionally and financially; each attempt may cost more than $10,000. Each unsuccessful attempt takes a heavy emotional toll on the couple. However, new procedures have given hope to couples who in the past might have had to remain childless (Display 5-4) (Figure 5-5). The nurse can be the mainstay throughout all the medical and laboratory testing, charts and records, histories and physical examinations. The nurse's role as teacher, listener, counselor, and advocate cannot be overemphasized. A great deal of compassion and understanding is required for these clients.

genetic counseling

Genetic counseling provides a family with information about diseases and disorders that may be inherited by transmission of either a dominant or recessive trait. (See Chap. 6 for a review of genetic inheritance.) The genetic counseling team may include medical specialists, counselors, social workers, and specially prepared nurses. The team offers the family testing, education about specific disorders, and psychological support as needed. Strict confi-

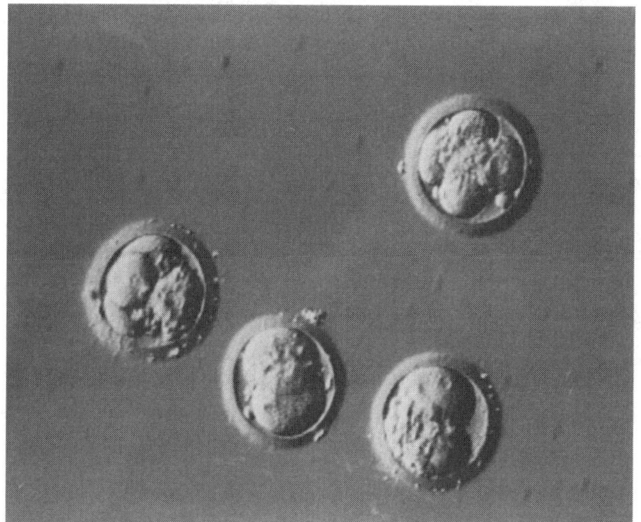

figure 5-5 *Fertilized eggs awaiting transfer to the mother.*

display 5-6
nursing goals of genetic counseling

1. Ensure confidentiality; develop therapeutic relationship.
2. Describe and discuss the purpose of genetic counseling.
3. Describe factors that put the fetus at risk (family history, exposure to drugs and alcohol).
4. Explain all diagnostic procedures and their cost.
5. Provide emotional support for the family at risk.
6. Assist families to list all possible courses of action (termination of pregnancy, care and treatment of a child with a genetic disorder).
7. Provide a nonjudgmental atmosphere that allows family to problem solve.

dentiality must be maintained to protect the family's privacy.

The goals of genetic counseling are to diagnose genetic conditions, determine the probability of a genetic condition through investigation of the family history and laboratory tests, and offer counseling and support to families affected by genetic conditions. (See Display 5-5 for a list of disorders currently detectable.) Examples of clients who seek genetic counseling include those with the following:

* Family history of genetic diseases or disorders
* Family history of birth defects
* Family history of infertility
* Clients older than 35 years who are pregnant or planning a pregnancy
* Clients with history of spontaneous abortions or stillbirths

A nurse may be the family's first contact when seeking information. This may occur in the hospital following a birth or miscarriage, in a physician's office following a visit for care of a genetic disease, or in a school following a nurse's screening exam.

display 5-5
disorders currently detectable through genetic testing

Thalassemia
Muscular dystrophy
Cystic fibrosis
Hemophilia
Huntington chorea
Neurofibromatosis
Phenylketonuria
Polycystic kidney disease
Retinoblastoma
Sickle-cell anemia

Once the diagnosis has been made, families with genetic disorders may experience a variety of emotions, such as anger, denial, and extreme grief. The nurse may need to use all his or her skills to assist the family with coping. (See Display 5-6 for goals of the nurse in genetic counseling.)

adoption

Adoption is a way for some couples to parent a child. The road to adoption can be long and frustrating, but it offers a way to enjoy the real satisfaction of parenthood. Frustrations encountered by the adoptive parents include questions about their personal lives, home visits by the social worker to assess the home environment and their suitability as parents, the waiting period, and the cost. A couple wanting to adopt an infant may encounter a waiting period of 1 to 5 years and costs as high as $15,000.

Couples seeking to adopt a sibling group or an older child may have a much shorter waiting period. Adoptions of children from foreign countries also are possible but require special legal intervention, which may add to the cost. Sometimes single people may adopt a child if they meet the criteria of the adoption agency.

The goal of a successful adoption is to provide a safe and loving environment for the child. The process begins with a personal interview and a client profile by the adoption agency or the representative of the biologic mother. If the father of the child has been named, his permission for adoption must be secured.

In an open adoption, the prospective parents may sometimes attend the labor and delivery of the newborn and within hours may be caring for their child. In a closed adoption, the adoptive couple may receive the child within 1 to 2 days of the birth. If all parties, including the child,

display 5-7
common reproductive myths

* Lack of female orgasm prevents pregnancy.
* Having intercourse close to menses prevents pregnancy.
* Standing while having intercourse prevents pregnancy.
* Douching after intercourse prevents pregnancy.
* It is impossible to get pregnant while breastfeeding.
* Voiding after intercourse prevents pregnancy.
* Plastic wrap may be substituted for a condom.
* Having sexual intercourse in bathwater prevents pregnancy.
* Sterilization makes a person overweight.
* Sterilization destroys sex drive.

are satisfied, the adoption may be finalized within 6 months.

✳ nursing considerations

The nurse has a responsibility to be knowledgeable about available family planning methods and their effectiveness, cost, and proper use. The client's choices may change during the childbearing years, and the nurse should be prepared to offer alternatives and new information as the need arises.

Prevention of STDs such as AIDS also may be a concern, and the nurse should be prepared to discuss the potential of the various birth control methods to prevent disease transmission. Again, the nurse needs to be ready to give current, correct information to dispel any myths or misinformation. (See Display 5-7 for list of common reproductive myths.)

When elective abortion is a possible choice, the nurse can be instrumental in counseling and educating the family to assist them in making an informed, comfortable decision. The client seeking information about an abortion may be overwhelmed, and the nurse can be most helpful by lending an empathetic ear.

If the client chooses sterilization, the nurse must be prepared to discuss the procedure, preoperative and postoperative care, and discharge instructions for self-care at home. The nurse should emphasize the fact that the procedure renders the individual permanently sterile (even though there has been some success with surgical reversal of sterilization). Finally, the nurse should make certain that a surgical consent form has been signed prior to the procedure.

The family dealing with the issue of infertility requires support, compassion, empathy, and accurate information on which to base their decisions. The nurse can provide all this and can dispel common misinformation. (See Display 5-8 for list of common infertility myths.) The couple dealing with infertility commonly feels helpless in their efforts to have a child of their own. Many times they are overwhelmed with scheduled intercourse, charts, options, and procedures. The nurse can be a valuable advocate, someone with whom they can share their fears and concerns and openly discuss their options.

If the family has chosen adoption, the nurse can help them find the appropriate agencies to assist in pursuing their goal. If the family chooses an *open adoption*, the biologic mother works with a physician and an attorney to select the adoptive families. If the family chooses a *closed adoption*, they work through a church or government-operated adoption agency, and there is no contact with the

display 5-8
common infertility myths

1. If a couple adopts a child, pregnancy will follow.
2. Infertility is usually the fault of the female.
3. Infertility is psychological, not physical.
4. Infertility is incurable.

display 5-9
health history

VITAL STATISTICS

* Age
* Sex
* Weight
* Height

MEDICAL HISTORY

* Family history of cardiac disease, respiratory disease, diabetes, epilepsy, cancer, or other serious disease
* Personal history of cardiac disease, respiratory disease, diabetes, epilepsy, cancer, or other serious disease
* Any history of sexually transmitted disease
* Name of any medications currently taking
* Any history of genetic disorders
* Exposure to teratogens at work
* Any injuries to reproductive organs
* Any history of drug, tobacco, or alcohol use

OBSTETRIC HISTORY

* Age menses started
* Last menstrual period
* Any difficulties with menstrual periods (eg, irregularity, heavy flow, clotting, severe abdominal cramping)
* Any previous pregnancies

biologic mother. Once a closed adoption process is complete, all records are sealed to prevent tracing the biologic parents.

Regardless of which family planning method the family chooses, the nurse needs to understand the issues to be discussed. He or she must strive to develop rapport with the woman and her partner, especially because of the natural embarrassment that may occur with such sensitive personal topics. The nurse must obtain a complete health history, which will provide information to formulate the care and instructions. (See Display 5-9 for a sample health history.) Finally, the nurse must ensure the client that confidentiality will be maintained throughout the process.

key points

- **The family planning methods a woman or couple choose may change throughout the life span, depending on individual needs and circumstances, cultural background, values, and religious beliefs.**
- **Sterilization is a permanent form of birth control that ends the reproductive capabilities of the individual. There has been limited success with reversal procedures, but this is costly, and there are no guarantees.**
- **The U.S. Supreme Court legalized abortion in 1973 in the Roe v. Wade case; however, individual states can legislate waiting periods, requirements for parental or spousal permission, and other regulations.**
- **The French "abortion pill," RU-486 is in clinical trials in the United States.**
- **Four possible factors have contributed to the rise in infertility: 1) a rise in STDs; 2) a delay of childbearing until later in life; 3) the use of DES from 1941 to 1971, which caused malformations of the reproductive tract in today's childbearing generation; and 4) drop in male sperm count since 1938, possibly related to exposure to estrogen-like chemicals in maternal blood or breast milk.**
- **Female infertility is caused by anovulation, tubal blockage, or uterine problems.**
- **Male infertility is caused by low sperm count or poor quality sperm, infections and scarring of the reproductive tract, inability to deposit the sperm in the vagina, or impotence.**
- **The nurse is often the first person to have contact with the family needing genetic counseling. He or she can be instrumental in assisting the family to cope with the diagnosis.**
- **Adoption is an alternative for some couples to parent a child. An adoption may be closed, with sealed records, or open, with the biologic and adoptive parents participating in the birth process.**
- **The nurse should understand the types of birth control available and their effectiveness and proper use to educate his or her clients.**

review questions 

1. Mrs. Sanchez, age 31, has five children ranging in age from 3 to 15 years. She is requesting information about a permanent form of birth control. She tells the nurse she cannot stay in the hospital and wants to know if there is an outpatient procedure. About what procedure would the nurse tell her as a possible option?
   a. Hysterectomy
   b. Vasectomy
   c. GIFT procedure
   d. Laparoscopic tubal ligation
2. Mrs. Sanchez furthers explains that she is divorced but planning to remarry in a few months and may want to reverse the procedure to have a child with her new husband. The nurse would tell her that
   a. that sounds like a wonderful idea.
   b. she should consider sterilization as a permanent method and may want to choose another birth control method until she is certain she does not want any more children.
   c. she should consider adoption because she is already 31 and wants to be sterilized.
   d. she already has a nice family and really should consider the financial burden of having additional children.
3. Tina Brown is currently breast-feeding her 3-month-old infant. She tells the nurse her mother said as long as she breast-feeds, she can't get pregnant. The nurse's best response would be,
   a. "Women cannot conceive while they are breast-feeding."
   b. "Women ovulate while breast-feeding but are infertile."
   c. "Breast-feeding does not prevent pregnancy, but it sometimes delays ovulation."
   d. "Ask your physician."
4. Elaine Levy is 7 weeks pregnant and has decided to have an abortion. She asks the nurse what type of procedure she may expect. The nurse would respond:
   a. A vacuum aspiration
   b. A hysterectomy
   c. RU-486
   d. A saline abortion
5. Mr. and Mrs. Moore have decided to adopt a child and have asked the nurse what they should do first. She would reply:
   a. "Let me make an appointment for you with financial counseling services."
   b. "Let me make an appointment for you with children's services to explore your options."
   c. "Let me make an appointment for you with your physician to explore your options."
   d. "Let me make an appointment with a genetic counseling service to explore your options."

bibliography ✳

Asch, R. H., & Marrs, R. P. (1992). *ART-assisted reproductive technologies*. Norwell, MA: Serono Laboratories.

Bartholet, E. (1993). *Family bonds—adoption and the politics of parenting*. New York: Houghton Mifflin.

Brill, M. T., & Amon, E. (1991). *Infertility and you*. Chicago: Budlong Press.

Cunningham, F. G., McDonald, P. C., Leveno, K.J., Gant, N.F., & Gilstrap, L.C. (1993). *Williams obstetrics* (19th ed.). Norwalk, CT: Appleton & Lange.

Elmer-Dewitt, P. (1991). Making babies. *Time*, 56–63.

Kenner, C. A., & MacLaren, A. (1993). *Essentials of maternal and neonatal nursing*. Springhouse, PA: Springhouse.

King, J. (1992). Helping patients choose an appropriate method of birth control. *The American Journal of Maternal Child Nursing, 17*, 91–95.

Pernoll, M. L. (1991). *Current obstetric and gynecologic diagnosis and treatment* (7th ed.). Norwalk, CT: Appleton & Lange.

Smolowe, J. (1993). New, improved and ready for battle. *Time*, 48–51.

Upjohn (1992). *Depo-Provera, contraceptive injection.*

Williams, J. K. (1993). New genetic discoveries increase counseling opportunities. *The American Journal of Maternal Child Nursing, 18*, 218–222.

Weiss, B. D., Brassford, T., & Davis, T. (1991). The cervical cap. *American Family Practice*, *43*(2), 517–523.

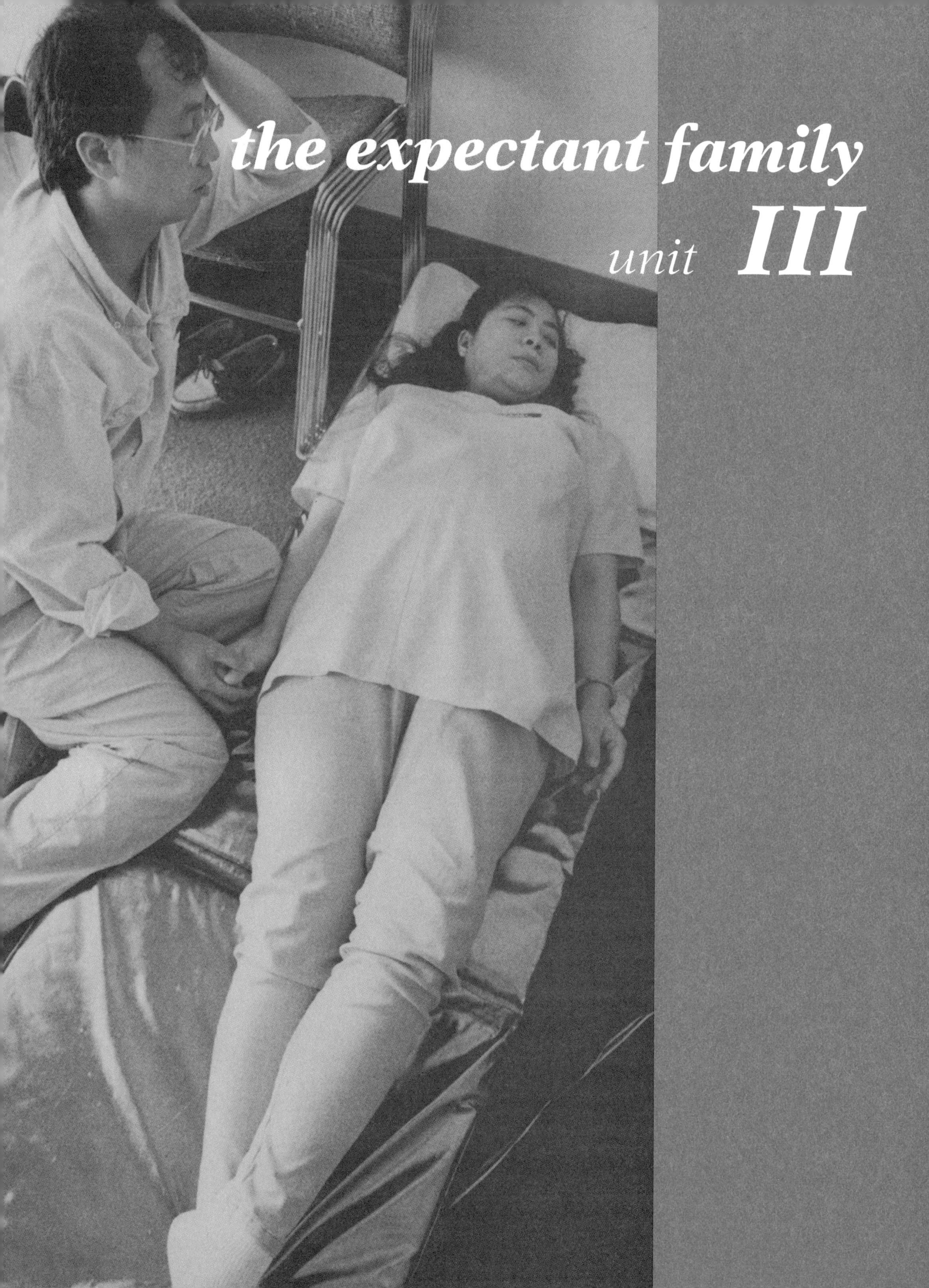

the expectant family

unit III

embryology and fetal development

6

outline

objectives

After studying this chapter, the reader should be able to:

* Discuss how physical characteristics are inherited.
* Describe the events that occur during fertilization and implantation.
* List the supportive structures necessary for growth of the embryo and fetus.
* List the placental hormones and their functions.
* Discuss normal fetal growth and development.
* Discuss fetal circulation and how it differs from adult circulation.
* Discuss the diagnostic tests used in fetal assessment.

key terms

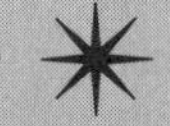

amniocentesis
amnion
autosome
chorion
chorionic villi
chromosome
decidua
ductus arteriosus
ductus venosus
ectoderm
endoderm
fertilization
foramen ovale
gene
human chorionic gonadotropin
implantation
karyotype
mesoderm
multifactorial inheritance
teratogen
Wharton's jelly
zygote

Neff C & Spray M. *Introduction to Maternal and Child Health Nursing,*

The process of human reproduction begins with the fertilization of a mature ovum by a mature sperm. Fertilization also is called *conception.* The new cell formed from this union is called a *zygote,* and approximately 9 months later, this single cell has grown and developed into a newborn.

The union of ovum and sperm creates a blueprint of inherited characteristics from the mother and the father. Through the ages, people have observed that children resemble their parents. Thanks to the work of a 19th century Austrian monk, Gregor Mendel, we now understand why this happens. Mendel studied garden peas and their ability to pass certain traits from one generation to another; this formed the basis for modern *genetics*, the study of heredity. This field of study continues to advance our understanding of inherited diseases.

cells, chromosomes, and genes

There are two types of cells within the human body: *somatic cells* (body cells) and *sex cells* (also called *germ cells* or *gametes*). Within the nucleus of each cell, deoxyribonucleic acid (DNA) forms rodlike structures called *chromosomes*, which are responsible for the transmission of genetic information, instructions contained in the *genes*. The gene is the unit of hereditary information. Thousands of *genes* are arranged in a specific order along the sides of the chromosomes and are responsible for the biologic and behavioral characteristics (traits) of the individual.

Each body cell contains 46 chromosomes, arranged in 23 pairs. The first 22 pairs are called *autosomes* and transmit characteristics that are not sex linked. The remaining pair are the *sex chromosomes*, which are designated as X and Y chromosomes. The female has two X chromosomes, and the male has one X and one Y chromosome.

For life to continue, the somatic cells and the sex cells must divide. Each of the two types of cell divides through a different process. The somatic cell continually divides and reproduces itself to allow for growth and development of the individual, a process called *mitosis*. During mitosis, each somatic cell produces two daughter cells with identical characteristics of the original cell.

The sex cells must go through a special process to reduce their chromosome number so that the fertilized egg (*zygote*) can receive one half of its chromosomes from each parent. This division process is called *meiosis*. Meiosis is part of a larger process called *gametogenesis*, the process in which gametes (sex cells) are produced. In the female, this process is called *oogenesis* and occurs in the *graafian follicle* of the ovary. Gametogenesis in the male is called *spermatogenesis* and occurs in the seminiferous tubules of the testes.

Following meiosis, the ovum (XX) can offer only an X chromosome for fertilization. The sperm can offer either an X or a Y chromosome (Fig. 6-1); thus, the male chromosome determines the sex of the baby. The Y chromosome is slightly smaller than the X chromosome and is responsible for sex determination but contains very few other traits. The X chromosome is responsible for female characteristics in addition to several other inherited traits, such as traits for color blindness, certain blood disorders, metabolic disorders, and some forms of male baldness.

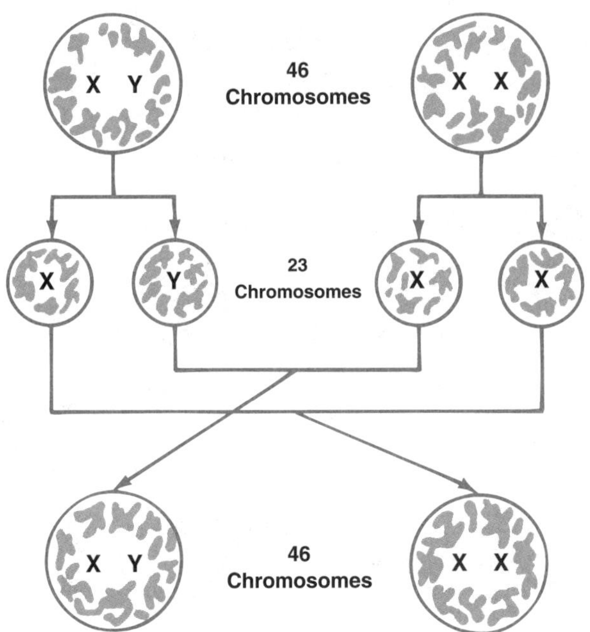

figure 6-1 *If an X chromosome from a male unites with an X chromosome from a female, the child is female; if a Y chromosome from a male unites with an X chromosome from a female, the child is male.*

dominant and recessive genes

When fertilization occurs, the inherited chromosomes from each parent line up, and the corresponding genes are matched together. The zygote then receives its genetic blueprint for life. Genes may be *dominant* or *recessive*, which accounts for the wide variations of skin, eye, and hair color and other inherited physical characteristics evident in families. A *dominant* gene will exert its message for characteristics, regardless of its matching counterpart. The zygote needs to receive the dominant gene from only one parent for a particular characteristic to appear. A *recessive* gene will not exert its message for characteristics unless its matching counterpart also is recessive. The zygote can be a *carrier* for a recessive gene if it has received both a dominant and recessive gene. The dominant gene will be expressed and the recessive gene passed on to future generations, even though it does not express itself during the current generation.

Many human characteristics, including most genetic diseases, are determined by a single pair of genes. Other physical traits, such as body structure, height, weight, and life span, are a result of two or more pairs of genes working together and of environmental influences. This is called *multifactorial inheritance*. Multifactorial inheritance explains the wide variations of individuals within a population.

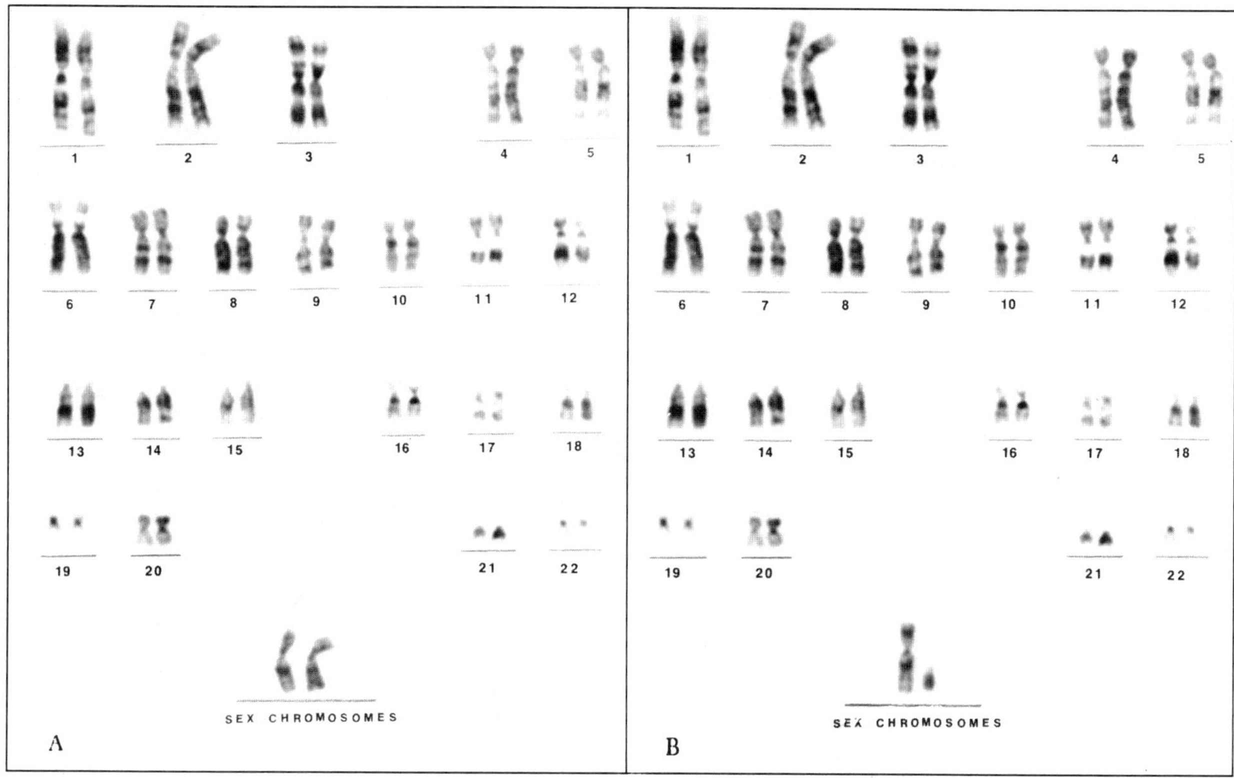

figure 6-2 *Karyotypes—photomicrographs of human chromosomes.* ***(A)*** *Normal female karyotype.* ***(B)*** *Normal male karyotype.*

karyotypes

A picture of the chromosome pattern of an individual is called a *karyotype* and may be prepared by obtaining cells from blood or mucous membranes. These cells are stained, specially prepared, and placed under a microscope where the cell nucleus is photographed. The chromosomes are then arranged in pairs according to their size and structure, creating a karyotype (Fig. 6-2). This procedure can be used to detect abnormalities in the number or structure of chromosomes.

nursing alert

Be prepared to offer emotional support to parents who receive a report showing chromosomal abnormalities, either in themselves or in their offspring. This information can be devastating.

fertilization

After ovulation has occurred, the finger-like projections (*fimbriae*) of the fallopian tube sweep the egg into the outer third of the tube, where fertilization normally takes place. Mature sperm that have entered the uterine cavity swim to this area and attempt to fertilize the ovum. If the attempt is not successful within 24 to 48 hours, the ovum dies. The mature sperm live 48 to 72 hours.

It takes thousands of the sperm to break through the outer layer of the ovum, but once accomplished, only one sperm enters. A physiologic barrier prevents the remaining sperm from entering the egg.

stages of growth and development

Three major stages of development occur after conception: *pre-embryonic, embryonic,* and *fetal.* The developmental process is vulnerable to internal and external influences throughout pregnancy, but it is most vulnerable in the earliest stages before a woman realizes that she is pregnant. Thus, it is important for women who are trying to become pregnant to avoid any substances, such as alcohol or other drugs, that might jeopardize the developmental process.

pre-embryonic (germinal or zygotic) stage

The first 2 weeks following conception are a period of rapid growth and change. This period is called the *pre-embryonic, germinal,* or *zygotic* stage. Immediately after fertilization, the nuclei of the sperm and ovum unite to form a zygote with a full complement of 46 chromosomes, 23 from the sperm and 23 from the egg. At this time, the sex of the zygote is determined, depending on whether the male contributed an X or a Y chromosome. Cell division (*mitosis*) begins and forms a mulberry-like structure called a *morula*. Although the number of cells increases, the size of the structure remains the same.

During the next 4 days, the morula continues its journey down the fallopian tube. Fluid develops in the center of the structure and pushes the cells toward the outer walls. The cells then develop into two specialized layers. The outermost layer is called the feeding layer (*trophoblast*) and is responsible for nourishing the inner layer (*blastocyst*) from which the embryo and an embryonic membrane (*amnion*) will develop. Eventually, the trophoblast also develops an embryonic membrane called the *chorion* (Fig. 6-3).

implantation

For the next 3 days, the morula floats in a nutrient-rich fluid in the uterus while preparing for attachment. During this time, the trophoblast begins to secrete an enzyme that will help the blastocyst embed in the uterine lining, a process called *implantation*. The total time from conception to implantation is about 7 days. Because ovulation occurs on the 14th day of a typical 28-day menstrual cycle and an additional 7 days have lapsed, it is now about the 21st day of the cycle, and the uterine lining (*endometrium*) is very thick and vascular.

The blastocyst burrows into the rich, vascular endometrium until it is completely covered and implants or attaches itself, usually in the upper posterior portion of the uterus. Once implantation has taken place, the endometrium is called the *decidua*. After implantation, the decidua continues to thicken under the implanted blastocyst, and the trophoblast develops finger-like projections called *chorionic villi*. The chorionic villi, which contain the blood of the developing zygote, admit oxygen and nutrition from the mother's blood vessel walls through the processes of osmosis and diffusion (Fig. 6-4).

embryonic stage

Weeks 3 through 8 encompass the *embryonic stage*, the period when the cells of the embryo continue to multiply and begin to differentiate to form the various body tissues and organs (Table 6-1). During this time the external features of the embryo also begin to develop. This is a critical time when drugs, viral or bacterial infections, and other outside influences can cause congenital abnormalities in the developing embryo. These harmful influences are called *teratogens*. By the end of the embryonic stage, circulation is established, and the embryo has begun to take on human appearance with the formation of arms, legs, and a disproportionately large head.

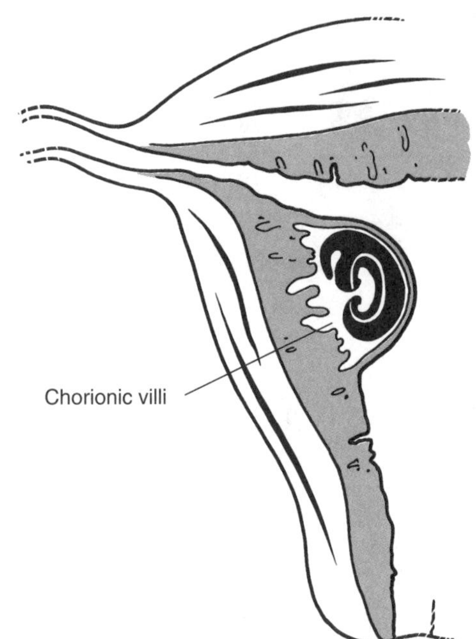

figure 6-4 *The decidua: chorionic villi reach out to the endometrium for oxygen and nutrients*

germ layers

As the embryo is forming, the cells develop into three specialized layers (*germ layers*) that will eventually form all the major fetal organs. These germ layers are called the *endoderm* (inner layer), *mesoderm* (middle layer), and *ectoderm* (outer layer). It is helpful to understand what systems and structures arise from each germ layer, especially if congenital defects are present at birth. Generally, there is more than one defect, and they usually come from the same germ layer. For example, it is common for a newborn with a heart defect also to have kidney problems because both of these organs arise from the mesoderm. Table 6-2 lists germ layers and the body systems that arise from each.

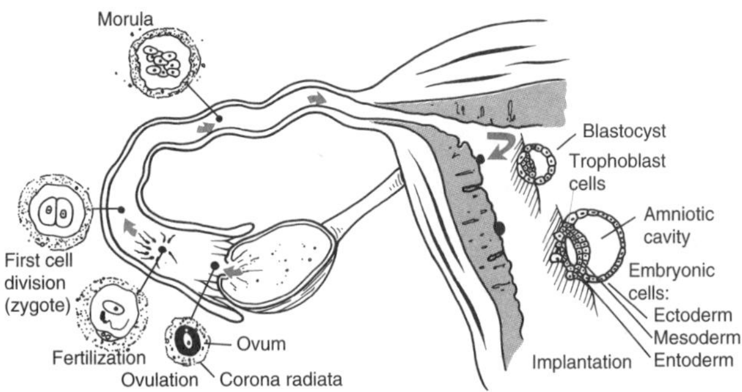

figure 6-3 *Ovulation, fertilization, and implantation.*

> **nursing alert**
>
> *Reinforce the importance of abstaining from the use of tobacco, alcohol and other drugs, and other known teratogens during pregnancy, particularly in this critical phase of development.*

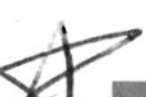

table 6-1 fetal growth calendar

Age	*Growth*	*Length/Weight*	*Picture*
4 weeks	✶ Trophoblast imbeds. ✶ Chorionic villi form. ✶ Buds of arms and legs form. ✶ Eyes, ears, and nose begin to form. ✶ Central nervous system, genitourinary system, bones, lungs begin to form.	Length: 0.75 cm or ⅓ in Weight: negligible	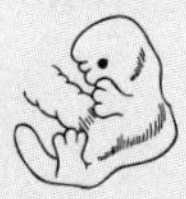
8 weeks	✶ Fetus is bent with large head. ✶ Septum and valves of heart have formed.. ✶ Extremities have developed. ✶ Sex differentiation begins but is unable to be determined with naked eye.	Length: 2.54 cm or 1 in Weight: 4 g or 1/30 oz	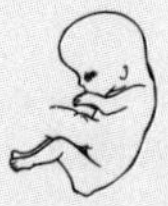
12 weeks	✶ Finger and toes are formed. ✶ Nail beds begin to form. ✶ Placenta is totally formed and fully functioning. ✶ Tooth buds are present. ✶ Sex of fetus is apparent with naked eye. ✶ Heart beat is audible with electronic Doppler.	Length: 9 cm or 3½ in Weight: 28 g or 1 oz	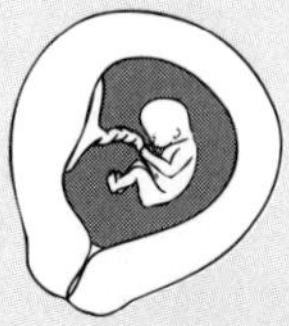
16 weeks	✶ Palate and nasal septum close. ✶ Heartbeat may be heard with stethoscope. ✶ Swallows amniotic fluid and excretes urine. ✶ Lanugo (downy soft hair) forms over body.	Length: 17 cm or 6½ in Weight: 55 to 120 g or 4 oz	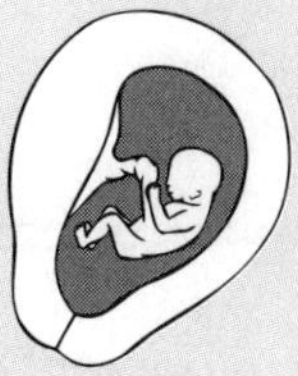
20 weeks	✶ Movement of fetus can be felt by mother (quickening). ✶ Considered the age of viability because some infants have survived at this age.	Length: 25 cm or 10 in Weight: 220 to 280 g or 8 to 10 oz	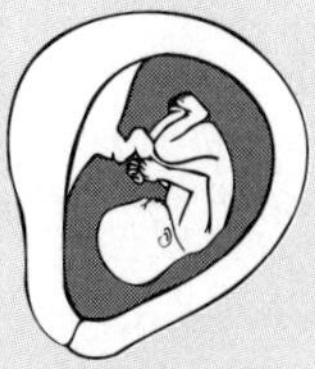
24 weeks	✶ Cheesy substance (vernix caseosa) protects the skin. ✶ Eyebrows and eye lashes are formed. ✶ Eyes can open and pupils able to react to light.	Length: 36 cm or 14 in Weight: 680 g or 1½ lb	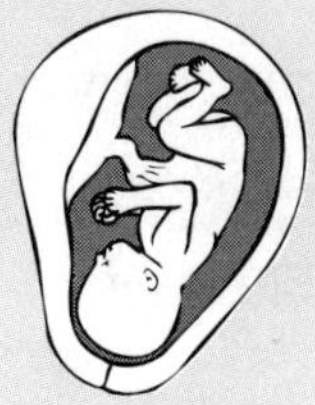
28 weeks	✶ Air sacs (alveoli) in lungs begin to mature. ✶ Skin is wrinkled. ✶ Subcutaneous fat begins to form.	Length: 38 cm or 15 in Weight: 1100 to 1200 g or 2½ lb	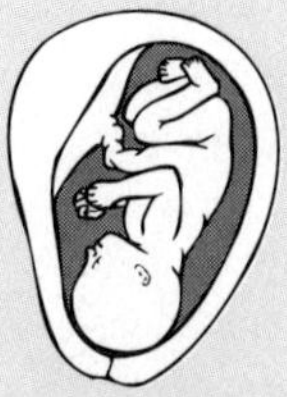

(continued)

table 6-1 fetal growth calendar (continued)

Age	Growth	Length/Weight	Picture
32 weeks	✳ Fingerprints begin to form. ✳ Areola of breast visible but flat. ✳ Skin is pink. ✳ Fetal movement is vigorous.	Length: 43 cm or 17 in Weight: 1700 g or 3½ to 4 lb	
36 weeks	✳ Lanugo is disappearing. ✳ Breast tissue further develops. ✳ Body begins to look plump and rounded.	Length: 49 cm or 19 in Weight: 2240 to 2270 g or 5 to 6 lb	
40 weeks	✳ Infant is full-term. ✳ Skin is smooth; lanugo is gone from face and extremities. ✳ Eye color established (blue-slate gray). ✳ Head is erect. ✳ Fingernails are fully formed and extend to ends of fingers.	Length: 50 cm or 20 in Weight: 3100 to 3360 g or 7 to 7½ lb	

development of supportive structures

During the growth and development of the embryo, certain structures also develop to support and maintain the new life throughout the pregnancy. These structures are the *embryonic or fetal membranes* (*amnion* and *chorion*), the *placenta*, and the *umbilical cord*.

embryonic or fetal membranes (amnion and chorion) A sac made up of two membranes, the *amnion* and the *chorion*, forms to protect and support the embryo. The *amnion* is the innermost membrane and contains amniotic fluid and the growing embryo. Eventually it also will contain fetal urine, sebaceous material, epithelial cells, and fetal hair. Amniotic fluid is a clear fluid that is approximately 98% water. Amniotic fluid has five major functions:

1. It prevents the amnion from adhering to the developing embryo or fetus.
2. It permits free movement of the embryo or fetus within the amniotic sac.
3. It aids in maintaining a constant normal body temperature for the embryo or fetus.
4. It helps protect the embryo or fetus from external injury.
5. It provides nourishment; a mature fetus may drink 6 to 7 oz of the fluid daily.

At term, the amniotic sac contains 500 to 1000 mL of amniotic fluid and is sometimes called the "bag of waters." If the amniotic fluid is significantly less than 500 mL, it is called *oligohydramnios*. If it is significantly increased (more than 2,000 mL at term), it is called *hydramnios* or *polyhydramnios*. Both of these conditions are associated with fetal abnormalities, such as *spina bifida* (open spine) or *anencephaly* (without a brain). The amniotic fluid may

table 6-2 germ layers

Mesoderm	Endoderm	Ectoderm
Connective tissue Bones Muscles Kidneys and ureters Reproductive system Heart Circulatory system	Bladder and urethra Lining of respiratory tract Liver and pancreas	Nervous system Skin Eyes Ears Hair follicles Nasal cavity Mammary glands

be aspirated (*amniocentesis*) and analyzed to provide the physician with important diagnostic information.

The outermost membrane of the bag of waters is the *chorion,* a thick layer with finger-like projections, *chorionic villi*, that extend outward. These villi embed in the decidua and will eventually develop into the *placenta*. Following the third month of pregnancy, as growth and development continue, the amnion and chorion are so close together they appear fused.

placenta The *placenta* is a temporary structure that functions as an organ and an endocrine gland. As an organ, the placenta is responsible for metabolism and transfer of nutrients and wastes between the woman and embryo or fetus. As an endocrine gland, the placenta secretes the various hormones of pregnancy. The placenta is shared by the embryo or fetus and the woman and is fully functional by the 12th week of pregnancy.

As the chorionic villi grow into the decidua, embryonic or fetal blood vessels grow into each villus. Maternal blood flows into the spaces between villi (*intervillous spaces*), allowing for diffusion of oxygen and nutrition to the fetus and return of fetal waste products by diffusion to the maternal circulation (Fig. 6-5). The maternal and fetal blood do not mix except when a chorionic villus ruptures and permits leakage of fetal red blood cells into the woman's circulation.

During pregnancy, the ovaries become relatively inactive, and the placenta functions as an endocrine gland, secreting hormones essential to maintain pregnancy. The hormones of pregnancy include estrogen; progesterone; human chorionic gonadotropin (HCG); human placental lactogen (HPL), also called human chorionic somatomammotropin; and relaxin. The functions of each of these hormones are summarized in Table 6-3.

At term, the placenta is oval, about 6 to 8 in in diameter and about 1 in thick, weighing about one sixth as much as the fetus. The maternal side of the placenta is covered with rough, bumpy structures called *cotyledons*. The fetal side is shiny and smooth, covered by the amnion and the chorion,

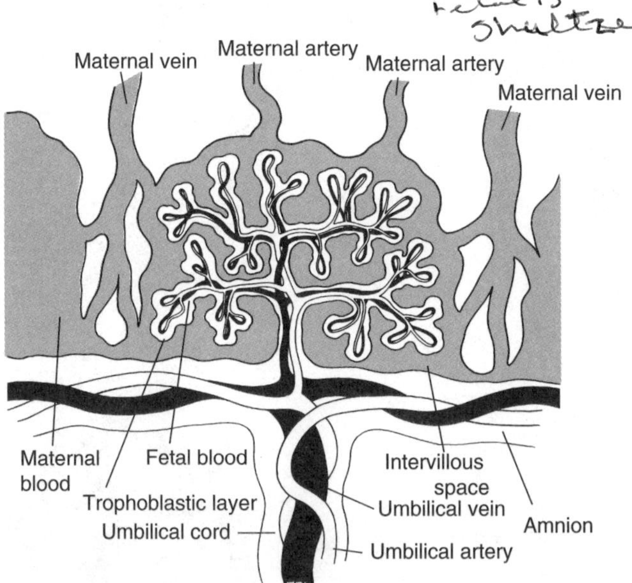

figure 6-5 *Placental circulation.*

with the umbilical cord extending from the center of the placenta to the fetus.

umbilical cord The lifeline between the placenta and the fetus is the *umbilical cord*. It contains three vessels: one large vein that brings oxygenated blood and nutrients to the fetus and two arteries that return nonoxygenated blood, carbon dioxide, and other fetal waste products to the placenta.

The three vessels within the umbilical cord are surrounded by a gelatinous material called *Wharton's jelly*. This substance protects the vessels and prevents them from kinking, twisting, or collapsing. At birth, the umbilical cord is approximately 18 to 20 in long (Fig. 6-6).

fetal stage

Weeks 9 through 40 comprise the *fetal stage,* the final stage of intrauterine growth and development; this is a time of growth and refinement of existing structures and organs. The fetus begins to take on the characteristics of an infant, and increases in weight and length until it reaches full term (see Table 6-1). Until this time, the woman may not be consciously aware of the pregnancy, but during this period of growth, her abdomen will steadily increase in size. Between 18 and 20 weeks' gestation, the first fetal movements may be felt (*quickening*). At about 20 weeks, she can hear the fetal heartbeat through a stethoscope.

fetal circulation

Fetal circulation (circulation in utero) differs from infant or adult circulation (extrauterine circulation) because the fetus depends on the placenta to meet its oxygen needs while it is still forming its organs, such as the liver and lungs (Fig. 6-7). Oxygenated blood flows from the placenta to the fetus through the large vein of the umbilical cord. It flows into the *inferior vena cava* through a small vessel called the *ductus venosus*. A small amount of blood is routed to the growing liver to meet its needs. (This constant small supply of fresh blood from the umbilical cord straight to the liver is thought to be the reason the newborn has such a large liver in proportion to its body size.)

The blood continues to travel up the inferior vena cava and empties into the right atrium of the heart. It then passes to the left atrium through a small opening in the septum called the *foramen ovale*, almost completely bypassing the nonfunctioning lungs.

The blood then travels to the left ventricle, where it is pumped into the aorta, circulates to the upper extremities, and returns to the right atrium. Next it flows to the right ventricle and into the pulmonary arteries. A small amount travels to the growing lungs. Because the lungs are not functioning, most of the blood is shunted from the pulmonary arteries through a small vessel, the *ductus arteriosus*, into the aorta. The blood then returns through the two umbilical arteries to the placenta where it will be resupplied with oxygen.

The special structures involved in fetal circulation are summarized in Table 6-4.

conversion of fetal circulation to infant circulation

At birth, the change from intrauterine life to atmospheric pressure causes to the lungs to inflate. Once the umbilical

table 6-3 *hormonal influences during pregnancy*

Hormone	Influence
Estrogen	Promotes growth and enlargement of the uterus
	Promotes vascularity of the mother's body, particularly in the reproductive organs
	Promotes development of the ducts and nipples of the breast
	Stimulates melanin production, causing pigmentation changes in the pregnant woman
	Contributes to formation of stretch marks (striae gravidarum)
	Thought to be responsible for mood swings and changes in libido
	Promotes retention of sodium and water
Progesterone	Promotes development of the decidua
	Prevents premature labor by decreasing contractility of the uterus
	Promotes fat storage to prevent starvation of the woman and the fetus (7½ lb or more)
	Causes a decrease in gastric motility, which may cause consti-pation and hemorrhoids
	Causes decrease in bladder and ureter tone, increasing the changes for urinary tract during pregnancy
Human chorionic gonadotropin	Stimulates the corpus luteum to release estrogen and progesterone until the placenta is fully func-tional
	Helps prevent the woman's body from rejecting the newly forming placenta
	Stimulates the male fetus to release testosterone from the testes, aiding in intrauterine development of the male reproductive tract
	Offers a presumptive sign of pregnancy when present in the urine; basis for pregnancy tests
Human placental lactogen	Stimulates changes in the mother's metabolism that make more protein, glucose, and minerals available for the fetus
	Contributes to breast enlargement
Relaxin	Promotes relaxation of the sacroiliac, sacroccygeal, and pubic joints
	Helps prevent premature labor contractions
	Promotes softening of the cervix

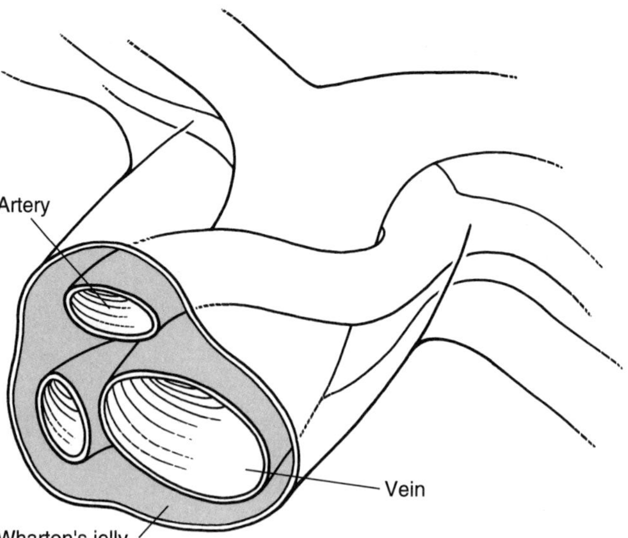

figure 6-6 *Cross-section of umbilical cord containing one large vein and two smaller arteries. The vessels are surrounded by Wharton's jelly.*

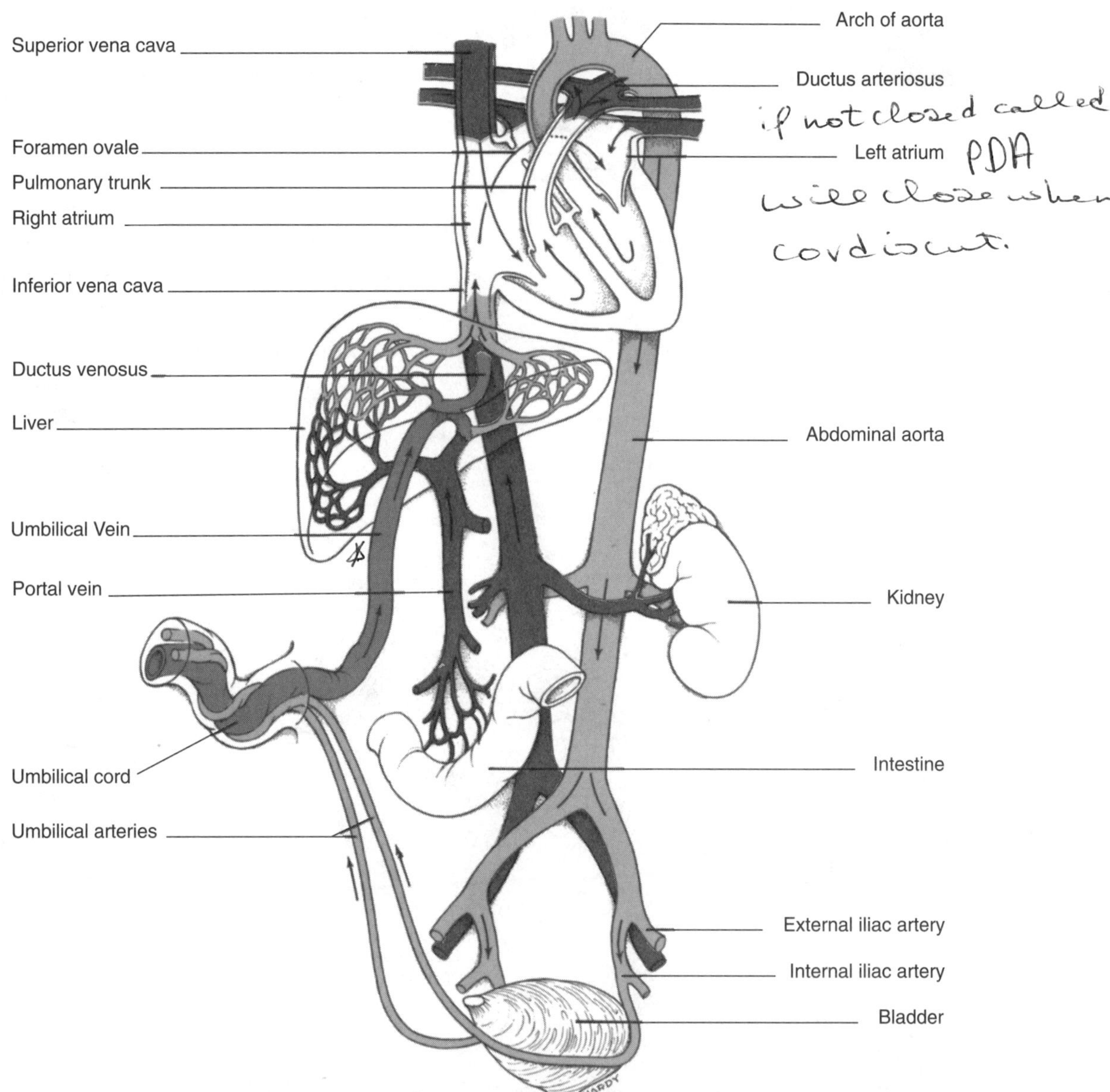

figure 6-7 *Fetal circulation.*

cord is clamped and cut, the umbilical arteries begin to atrophy, and the umbilical vein eventually becomes a fibrous support ligament of the liver. Normally, the foramen ovale, ductus arteriosus, and ductus venosus close, atrophy, and become fibrous ligaments.

multiple pregnancy

Multiple pregnancy, the conception of twins, triplets, quadruplets, and so forth, results from one of two different processes that occurs at fertilization. Twins may result from the sudden complete division of the fertilized egg, resulting in two separate embryos (*monozygotic twins*) or the fertilization of two separate eggs with two separate sperm (*dizygotic twins*; Fig. 6-8).

The incidence of twins is greater in nonwhite people than in white people. The use of fertility drugs also increases the incidence of twins or other multiple pregnancy.

monozygotic twins

Monozygotic twins share the same placenta and chorion but have two separate amnions and umbilical cords. They share an identical genetic make-up and are always the same sex; thus, they are called *identical twins*. Conception of monozygotic twins seems to be a random event unrelated to hereditary factors.

dizygotic twins

Dizygotic twins are two separate individuals with differing genetic make-up, two siblings that share the same birth

table 6-4 specialized structures of fetal circulation

Structure	*Function*
Umbilical vein	Brings oxygenated blood from the placenta to the fetus
Umbilical arteries	Brings deoxygenated blood from the fetus to the placenta
Ductus venosus	Bypasses the liver
Foramen ovale	Shunts blood from the right atrium to the left atrium
Ductus arteriosus	Bypasses the lungs

date. They have two placentas, two chorions, two amnions, and two umbilical cords. They may be the same sex or different sexes and are called *fraternal twins*. Conception of dizygotic twins may be related to a hereditary factor; however, the incidence also increases with the number of pregnancies (*parity*) and the woman's age.

✳ family considerations

dealing with multiple pregnancy

Once the diagnosis of multiple pregnancy has been made, the family faces many issues:

✳ The idea that they may be bringing home more than one infant

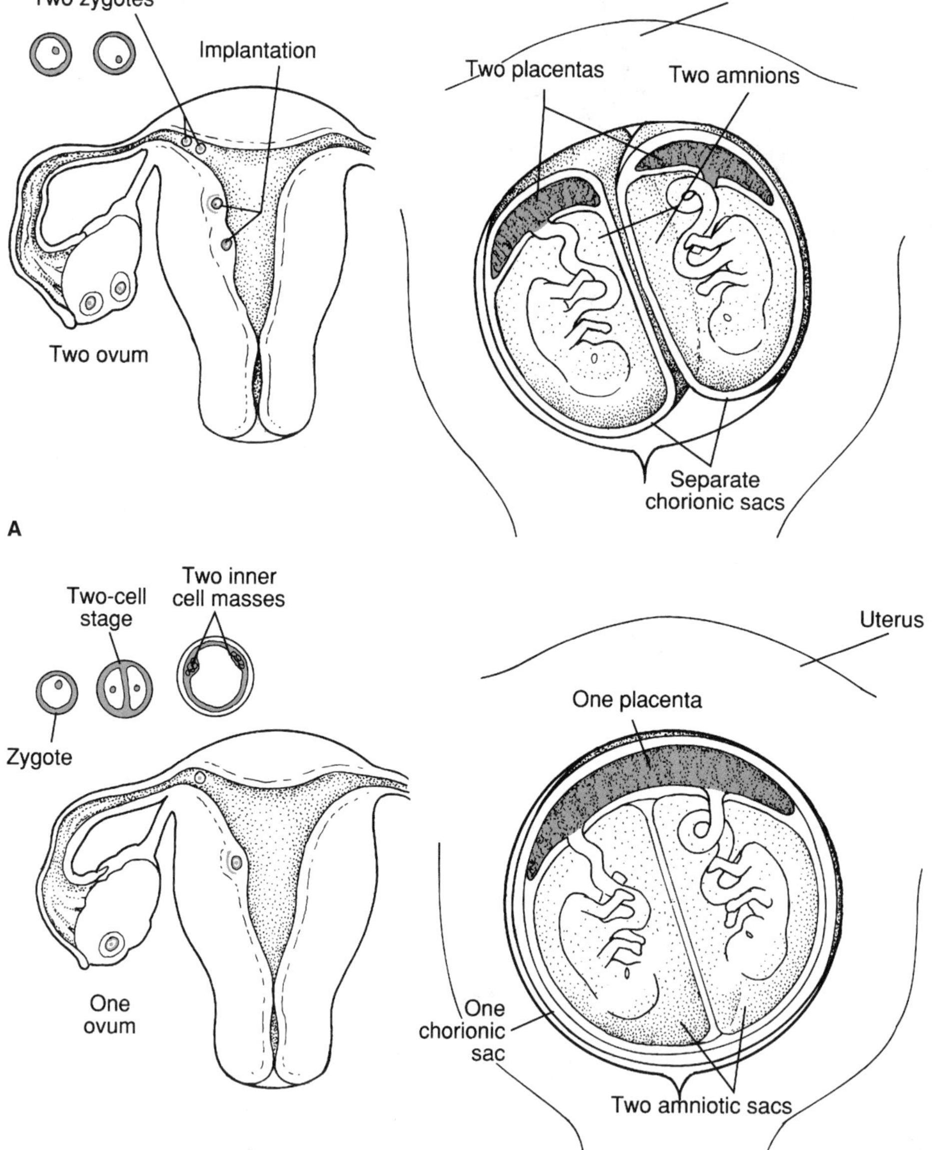

figure 6-8 *Twin pregnancy: **(A)** Fraternal (dizygotic) twins. **(B)** Identical (monozygotic) twins.*

- The necessity for close monitoring by the physician during the pregnancy: frequent visits, the possibility of extra diagnostic testing (eg, repeated ultrasound examinations, amniocentesis)
- Determining whether enough space is available in the home environment for these new family members.
- Determining whether income will be sufficient, and if the woman works outside the home, whether she can continue
- The impact on other children

Parents will need to call on all their coping mechanisms to deal with these concerns. Other family members and friends may lend support in helping the family cope.

assessment of fetal growth and development

Prenatal care includes a variety of assessments and tests used to monitor the growth and development of the fetus and the health of the woman. The pregnant woman is seen frequently throughout the pregnancy, and her weight gain, the growth of her uterus, fetal growth and activity, and the fetal heart rate are monitored. In approximately 20% of all pregnancies, further assessment studies are needed, including electronic fetal monitoring (EFM). Tests that include EFM are discussed in Chapter 7. The nurse has an important teaching role in preparing a woman for prenatal tests (see Teaching Guidelines: The Client Undergoing Prenatal Diagnostic Tests).

teaching guidelines
the client undergoing prenatal diagnostic tests

Teaching is aimed at reducing pain and anxiety through proper preparation of the woman. This may be accomplished by the following:

- Explaining the procedure, step by step, in easy to understand terminology
- Having the client verbalize her understanding to avoid misinformation
- Allowing time for questions and answers in a nonstressful environment
- Using pictures and diagrams to assist the woman in her understanding of the procedure
- Assisting the woman into a comfortable supine position in preparation for the testing
- Holding the woman's hand or touching her shoulder during the procedure to provide comfort

fetal heart rate

As early as 10 to 12 weeks' gestation the fetal heart rate may be heard in the suprapubic region of the abdomen using an electronic Doppler. The normal fetal heart rate (FHR) ranges from 120 to 160 beats/min. The FHR may be heard with a obstetric stethoscope (fetoscope) after 20 weeks' gestation.

When assessing FHR, it is important to distinguish it from the woman's heart rate. A simple way to differentiate is to check the woman's radial pulse while listening to the FHR. Occasionally, the nurse may hear the blood rushing through the large vessels of the uterus. This is called *uterine souffle* and again may be distinguished from the FHR by palpating the radial pulse of the woman. The uterine souffle and the radial pulse are the same.

If FHR cannot be heard, it may be due to the following reasons:

- Environmental noise or defective fetoscope or Doppler
- Earlier gestational age than calculated
- Maternal obesity
- Hydramnios
- Fetal death

fundal height (mcdonald's technique)

Once the woman has reached her 20th week of pregnancy, it is possible to estimate the length of the fetus by measuring the height of the uterine fundus using McDonald's technique. The woman is instructed to empty her bladder and lie in a supine position. A flexible tape measure (paper or plastic) is used to measure in centimeters the distance from the upper edge of the symphysis pubis to the top of the uterine fundus. This measurement should correspond to the number of weeks of the pregnancy; for example, at 22 weeks, the measurement should be about 22 cm. A difference of plus or minus 1 to 2 cm may be due to the height or body build of the woman. A difference of 3 cm or greater is cause for further investigation. Greater-than-normal fundal height may be related to multiple gestation, an excess of amniotic fluid (polyhydramnios), or an abnormally large fetus. Some causes of less-than-normal fundal height may be growth retardation of the fetus, congenital abnormalities, an abnormal position of the developing fetus, or an abnormally small amount of amniotic fluid (oligohydramnios).

fetal movement (quickening)

The first movements of the fetus felt by the woman are called *quickening*. She may describe these movements as a soft fluttery sensation. These movements are usually felt between 18 and 20 weeks' gestation but may be felt as early as 16 weeks' gestation by the woman who has had previous pregnancies. Quickening is exciting for family members because it is the first time the fetus may be seen as an independent being within the woman's womb.

ultrasonography

Ultrasonography is a technology that uses sound waves to provide an image, called a *sonogram*, of the fetus, uterus, and placenta. Ultrasound examination provides a moving image that assists the physician in the diagnosis of pregnancy and the health and well-being of the growing fetus. As the scanner moves over the woman's abdomen, the parents can see their infant in motion. They may be able to see the head, extremities, general body position, and sometimes the sex of the fetus (Fig. 6-9). The parents are always asked if they want to know the sex of the infant or would rather wait for the birth.

To prepare for an ultrasound test, it may be necessary for the woman to have a full bladder. As the bladder fills, it pushes the uterus up and out of the pelvis and offers better visualization of the uterine contents. The woman is instructed to drink a quart (1 L) of water 1 to 2 hours before the procedure.

During the procedure, the woman is placed on her back, and a transducer gel is spread on the abdomen. The gel reduces friction as the transducer (a hand-held device that transmits the sound waves) is moved over the abdomen. If the transcervical approach is used, the woman is positioned the same, but the transducer is introduced into the vagina. Either method produces the same information. This procedure may be performed periodically throughout pregnancy for the following reasons:

* Assessment of gestational age
* Evaluation of vaginal bleeding
* Evaluation of congenital anomalies
* Assessment of placental location
* Diagnosis of multiple gestation
* Estimation of fetal size
* Determination of fetal position
* Preparation for other diagnostic tests

amniocentesis

Amniocentesis is the withdrawal and analysis of fluid from the amniotic sac. The fluid is withdrawn through the abdominal wall of the woman. *Amniocentesis* may be performed in a hospital or in the physician's office any time after the amnion has produced sufficient fluid, usually after 14 weeks. The amniotic fluid is analyzed for chromosomal pattern and a variety of other tests, depending on the risk factors involved.

The woman is placed in a supine position, and ultrasound is used to locate the fetus and the placenta to avoid puncturing these areas. A large needle is then inserted through the abdominal and uterine walls, and a sample of amniotic fluid is aspirated. Following the procedure, the woman is instructed to notify the physician if she has abdominal cramping, fever, chills, vaginal bleeding, or leaking of amniotic fluid.

chorionic villus sampling

Chorionic villus sampling (CVS) is a procedure involving removal of a small amount of chorionic villi cells for assessment and diagnosis. It is used to detect such genetic defects as Down syndrome, Tay-Sachs disease, or sickle cell anemia. This test may be performed as early as 9 weeks' gestation in the physician's office or in the hospital. Using ultrasound to locate the placenta and chorionic villi, the physician removes the cells either by inserting a small tube through the vagina into the uterus and applying gentle suction or by inserting a needle through the abdominal wall into the uterus and aspirating the cells (Fig. 6-10). Following the procedure, the woman is instructed to notify the physician if she has any abdominal cramping,

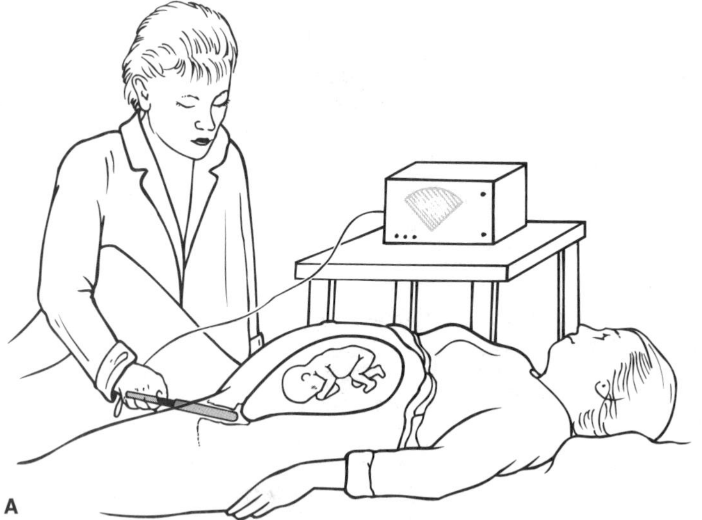

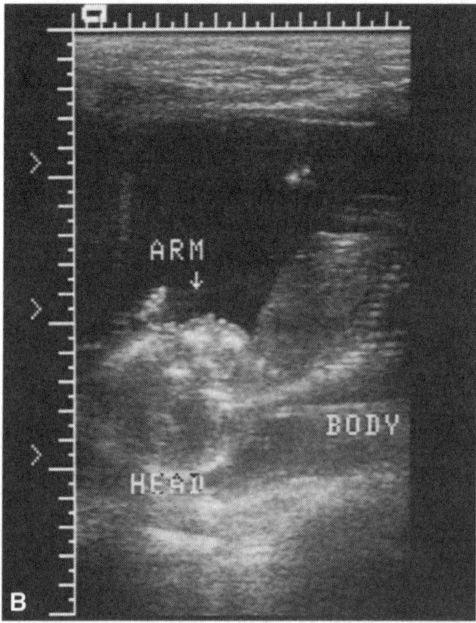

figure 6-9 *(A) Transvaginal ultrasound. (B) Ultrasound image taken at 20 weeks' gestation.*

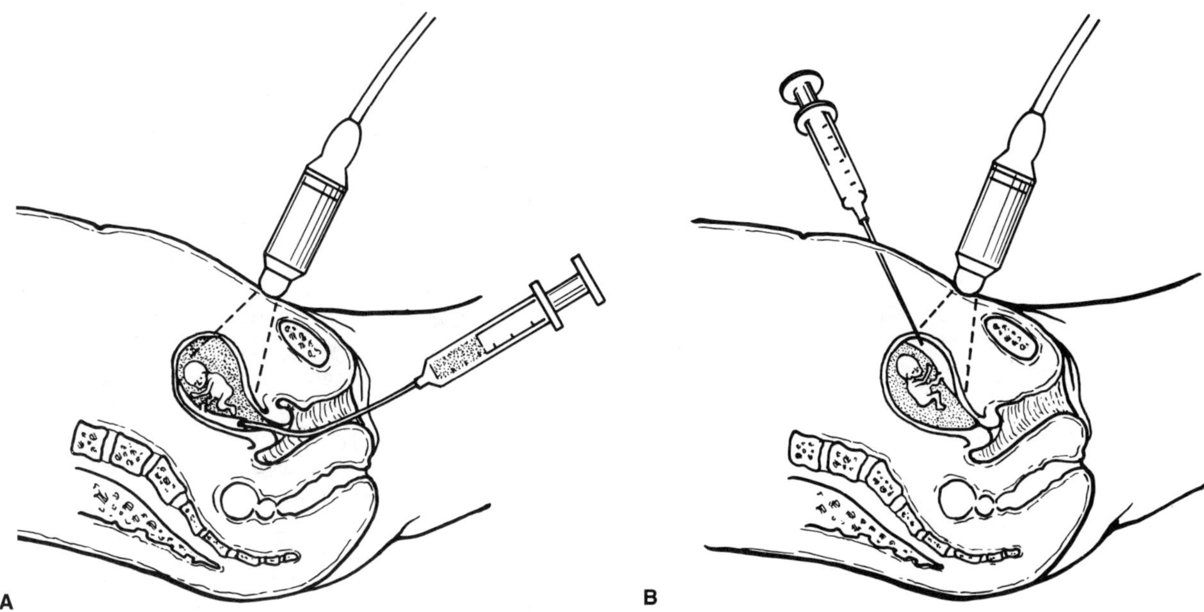

figure 6-10 *(**A**) Transvaginal chorionic villus sampling. (**B**) Transabdominal chorionic villus sampling.*

vaginal bleeding, fever, chills, or leaking of amniotic fluid (see Fig. 6-8).

The major advantage of CVS is that it can be performed 6 to 9 weeks earlier than amniocentesis; if serious genetic defects are present, the woman has an opportunity to decide earlier about possible termination of the pregnancy. A recent study indicates that CVS increases by six times an infant's chances of missing fingers or toes. CVS also carries a slightly higher risk of spontaneous abortion than amniocentesis.

✳ nursing considerations

The nurse dealing with expectant parents needs to be attuned to their desire to learn about their developing child. Every attempt should be made to answer their questions and provide them with the knowledge needed to guide them through a safe pregnancy. Charts and diagrams may be helpful when explaining the growth and development of the fetus.

The nurse needs to emphasize the importance of a balanced diet, adequate physical exercise, plenty of rest, and avoidance of tobacco, alcohol, and any drugs not prescribed by the physician managing the pregnancy.

Clients needing special diagnostic tests, such as amniocentesis, may be fearful. Often they will feel more comfortable with the nurse and will share information and concerns that they may not share with the physician. The nurse needs to be available for clients and offer complete instructions and explanations.

When preparing the client for these tests the nurse needs to do the following:

* Be sure the consent form has been signed.
* Position the woman appropriately, making her as comfortable as possible; usually she will be in the supine position.
* Obtain vital signs and fetal heart rate before and after the test is performed.
* Have the woman empty her bladder prior to the test (except for amniocentesis, for which a full bladder may be required).

key points ✳

* **The sex of an embryo is determined by the male, based on whether he contributes an X or a Y chromosome.**
* **Intrauterine growth and development may be divided into three stages: pre-embryonic, embryonic, and fetal.**
* **All organs of the fetus are derived from three embryonic germ layers: endoderm, mesoderm, and ectoderm.**
* **The supporting structures responsible for maintaining the pregnancy are the amnion, chorion, placenta, and the umbilical cord.**
* **The specialized structures necessary for fetal circulation are the umbilical vein, the two umbilical arteries, the ductus venosus, formen ovale, and ductus arteriosus. At birth, the infant converts to adult circulation, and the structures no longer function.**
* **During pregnancy, the placenta functions as an endocrine gland and secretes the hormones estrogen, progesterone, relaxin, HCG, and HPL.**

* **Growth, development, and health status of the fetus are monitored throughout pregnancy using such assessments as fetal heart rate, fundal height, fetal movement, ultrasonography, chorionic villus sampling, and amniocentesis.**
* **Twins may be monozygotic, arising from the same ovum and sperm, or dizygotic, arising from two separate sperm and ova.**

review questions

1. Louisa Gonzales has three boys and is now 3 months pregnant. She wants to know what she can do to ensure that this pregnancy results in the delivery of a girl. The nurse should respond,
   a. "Eat plenty of protein during your pregnancy to increase the chances of a girl."
   b. "The sex of the child is determined at conception."
   c. "Ask you doctor for this advice."
   d. "We will know the sex of the child in 4 more months."
2. Anita Jenkins is 6 weeks pregnant and is concerned because she has not felt the baby move yet. The nurse should respond,
   a. "You should discuss this with your doctor.
   b. "Don't worry; it wil move when it's ready.
   c. "You probably will not feel your baby move until the 18th to 20th week."
   d. "Your baby must be much larger to move."
3. Sandra Raivitch has come to the clinic for her 5-month check-up. She is crying and upset and tells the nurse that her neighbor said that babies have a hole in their heart during the length of the pregnancy. The nurse's best response would be,
   a. "Yes this is true because the fetal circulation is not the same as the adult circulation, but the opening closes at birth when the baby's circulation changes to adult circulation."
   b. "This is not true, and you shouldn't listen to neighborhood gossip—it only upsets you."
   c. "You may want to discuss this with your doctor; I'm sure she will be able to answer your questions."
   d. "Yes this is true; your baby doesn't use his heart during pregnancy."
4. Rochelle Myers must have an ultrasound, and she is concerned that she will not be able to drink all the water that is needed to prepare for the test. The nurse's best response would be,
   a. "It is not necessary for you to drink any water if you choose not to; just let the doctor know your choice."
   b. "You do not have to drink it all at once; sipping it over a short period of time may be easier, and you do not have to drink it until shortly before the test."
   c. "This test is very costly, and you must prepare for it properly or you are wasting your time."
   d. "It is not necessary to drink water for an ultrasound; that is a requirement for an amniocentesis."
5. Jane Dorsey is to be positioned for an ultrasound. The nurse would place her
   a. in dorsal recumbent.
   b. in dorsal lithotomy.
   c. supine.
   d. prone.

bibliography

Bullock, B. L. (1996). *Pathophysiology* (4th ed.). Philadelphia: Lippincott–Raven.

Gebauer, C. L., & Lowe, N. K. (1993). The biophysical profile: antepartal assessment of fetal well-being. *Journal of Obstetric, Gynecologic, and Neonatal Nursing, 22*(2) 115–123.

Gregor, C. L., & Paine, L. L. (1992). Antepartum fetal assessment techniques: An update for today's perinatal nurse. *Journal of Perinatal Neonatal Nursing*, 1–13.

Kenner, C. A., & Mac Laren, A. (1993). *Essentials of maternal and neonatal nursing.* Springhouse: Springhouse Corporation.

May, K. A., & Mahlmeister, L. R. (1994). *Maternal and neonatal nursing* (3rd ed.). Philadelphia: J.B. Lippincott.

Olds, S. B., London, M. L., & Ladewig, P. W. (1992). *Maternal newborn nursing* (4th ed.). Redwood City: Addison-Wesley Nursing.

Pillitteri, A. (1995). *Maternal and child health nursing* (2nd ed.). Philadelphia: J.B. Lippincott.

Reeder, S. J. et al. (1992). *Maternity Nursing* (17th ed.). Philadelphia: J.B. Lippincott.

Sloan, E. (1993). *Biology of Women* (3rd ed.). New York: Delmar.

outline

physiologic and psychosocial changes during pregnancy

7

objectives

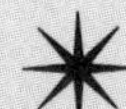

After studying this chapter, the reader should be able to:

- ✳ *Define the medical terminology used to describe pregnancy.*
- ✳ *Calculate the due date of pregnancies using Nägele's rule.*
- ✳ *Discuss the presumptive, probable, and positive signs of pregnancy.*
- ✳ *Discuss the changes that occur in the body systems during pregnancy.*
- ✳ *Identify the developmental tasks of pregnancy.*

key terms

Braxton Hicks contractions
Chadwick's sign
chloasma
couvade
funic souffle
Goodell's sign
gravida
Hegar's sign
linea nigra
Nägele's rule
oxytocin
para
prolactin
quickening
relaxin
striae gravidarum
TPAL
uterine souffle

Neff C & Spray M. *Introduction to Maternal and Child Health Nursing,*

The nurse and the family must recognize that pregnancy is a normal physiologic process, not an illness. The woman's body is designed for pregnancy and childbirth. She can expect to experience physical and psychological changes during pregnancy. This chapter discusses those changes and how they affect the woman and her family.

description of pregnancy

The average length of pregnancy is 280 days, approximately 9 calendar months, or 40 weeks. The pregnancy also may be divided into 10 *lunar* months (a lunar month is 28 days; 28 × 10 = 280). Pregnancy is considered as three trimesters of three calendar months each.

Not all pregnancies last exactly 280 days. If the fetus is expelled before the age of viability (20 weeks), it cannot survive; this is called a *spontaneous abortion*. If the fetus is born after 20 weeks but prior to the completion of the 37th week, the fetus is called a *premature infant*. One born after 42 weeks' gestation is called a *postmature infant*.

terminology

To understand the language used in the care of the pregnant woman the nurse must understand some common obstetric terms:

- Antepartum: the period of pregnancy up to delivery
- Estimated date of delivery (EDD): the calendar date that estimates 280 days of pregnancy; also may be called estimated date of confinement (EDC)
- Gestation: the length of time between conception and birth
- Gravida: suffix (ending) meaning pregnant or the number of pregnancies the woman had
- Multigravida: pregnant woman with history of previous pregnancies
- Multipara: a woman who has delivered a fetus previously (the fetus may have been alive or dead at birth)
- Nulligravida: a woman who has never experienced pregnancy
- Nägele's rule: a guide used to determine the EDD. Add 7 days to the first day of the last menstrual period, and count back 3 months.
- Para: a woman who has delivered a viable infant; term may be used with a number to denote the number of viable births
- Primigravida: a woman pregnant for the first time
- Primipara: a woman in labor for the first time or who has just given birth for the first time
- TPAL: an abbreviation sometimes used when taking an obstetric history:
    - T: number of term pregnancies
    - P: number of premature infants delivered
    - A: number of abortions, miscarriages
    - L: number of living children

The term *gravida* refers to the number of times a woman has been pregnant (including this pregnancy); the term *para* is used to denote the number of births that occurred after the age of viability.

For example, Mrs. Grable has three children, delivered at term. She had one miscarriage at 6 weeks. She is now pregnant for the fifth time. She is gravida V, para III.

Using this method, it is necessary to make extra notations to refer to interruption of pregnancy before the age of viability was reached. The pregnancy is listed as gravida, but the nurse has no way of knowing what happened with that pregnancy without additional written information. Multiple births present another problem with this system. The pregnancy is listed as gravida I, but depending on the institutional policy, the para may be listed as I (for one birth) or II or III if there were twins or triplets.

A newer obstetric notation has been developed for classifying obstetric history. It is more inclusive, just as easy to use, and eliminates the need for extra written information. This system is abbreviated TPAL. The *T* denotes the number of pregnancies; *P*, the number of preterm infants (those born before 37 weeks' gestation); *A*, the number of spontaneous or induced abortions; and *L*, the number of living children. Using this system, the example of Mrs. Grable would be listed as T-III, P-O, A-I, L-III.

To determine the due date, using the first day of the last menstrual period, the nurse adds 7 days and counts back 3 months (Nägele's rule). For example, Mrs. Grable's last menstrual cycle began on February first.

Step one: add 7 days (1 + 7 = 8).
Step two: Count back 3 months (to November).
Step three: This child is due on November 8.

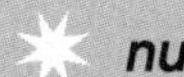

nursing alert

Gravida and para always refer to the number of pregnancies or births, not the number of fetuses.

signs of pregnancy

The signs of pregnancy are a group of symptoms and observations made by the woman and the physician or nurse that lead to the positive diagnosis of pregnancy. These signs and symptoms are grouped in three major categories (Table 7-1): *presumptive signs* (early but unreliable; generally subjective), *probable signs* (stronger indicators but still not reliable; generally objective), and *positive signs* (definite).

presumptive signs

The *presumptive signs* of pregnancy occur early but may be caused by other medical conditions. They are subjective, that is, perceived by the woman. They include amenorrhea, nausea and vomiting, urinary frequency, breast changes, fatigue, and quickening (fetal movement).

amenorrhea

Amenorrhea (absence of menses) is usually the first indication of possible pregnancy. This results from the rising

table 7-1 signs of pregnancy

PRESUMPTIVE SIGNS (SUBJECTIVE; EARLY BUT UNRELIABLE)
Amenorrhea
Nausea and vomiting
Urinary frequency
Fatigue
Quickening
PROBABLE SIGNS (OBJECTIVE BUT NOT CONCLUSIVE)
Hegar's sign
Goodell's sign
Chadwick's sign
Abdominal enlargement
Braxton Hicks contractions
Ballottement
Fetal outline
Pregnancy tests
Skin pigmentation changes
POSITIVE SIGNS (DIAGNOSTIC; 100% ACCURATE)
Fetal heart beat
Movement of fetus felt by examiner
Ultrasound
X-ray

levels of *human chorionic gonadotropin* (HCG), a hormone secreted on the surface of the embryonic placental membrane.

Many other factors can cause amenorrhea. The woman may have stopped ovulating, may be nursing an infant, or may be going through menopause. Other causes may include stress, excessive weight loss or vigorous exercise, malnutrition, or certain medications, for example, the phenothiazines (Thorazine, Compazine)

nausea and vomiting

Nausea and vomiting (called "morning sickness," even though it may occur throughout the day or night) may begin about the fourth week of pregnancy and continue throughout the first trimester. Morning sickness is caused by rising levels of HCG and estrogen, slowed gastrointestinal function, and occasionally, emotional stress.

Nausea and vomiting may be related to many other factors, such as gastric disorders; influenza; food poisoning; allergies; or some systemic infections. In addition, stress or eating disorders, such as *anorexia nervosa*, can lead to nausea and vomiting.

urinary frequency

Urinary frequency occurs during the first and third trimesters. In the first trimester, the uterus begins to enlarge while low in the pelvic cavity, putting pressure on the bladder. This causes the woman to feel the need to urinate frequently. As the uterus rises during the second trimester, urinary frequency subsides. By the third trimester, the enlarged uterus again presses on the urinary bladder, and urinary frequency returns.

Many other medical conditions can cause urinary frequency, such as urinary tract infection, a pelvic tumor, or renal disease. Again, stress may be a factor.

breast changes

During the first trimester, the breasts begin to enlarge and may feel tender. The woman also may experience a feeling of fullness and tingling in the breast tissue. The nipples enlarge and elongate and may feel tender. The areola widens, and the veins beneath the skin of the breast become more visible. These changes are caused by hormonal influences that help prepare the ducts, nipples, and glandular tissue for breast-feeding.

Other medical conditions that may cause similar changes in the breast include premenstrual syndrome (PMS), pituitary tumors, breast tumors or cysts, and infection. Some drugs, particularly certain tranquilizers (Thorazine and Trilafon), also may cause breast tenderness.

fatigue

A frequent symptom experienced in early pregnancy is *fatigue*. The woman may report that she wants to sleep all the time and has no energy. Getting through the normal day may be a struggle. The exact cause of the fatigue is unknown, but it may be the hormonal changes occurring in the body, particularly the levels of progesterone.

Fatigue can result from many conditions other than pregnancy. Any chronic illness may cause fatigue. In addition, chronic fatigue syndrome or anemia should be considered.

quickening

The first "fluttering" fetal movements felt by the mother are called *quickening*. This occurs sometime between the 16th and 20th week of pregnancy. Medical conditions that may cause similar symptoms are excessive flatus or increased peristalsis.

probable signs

Probable signs of pregnancy are objective signs that can be observed by the examining care provider. Probable signs suggest more strongly that the woman is pregnant but are not conclusive. The probable signs of pregnancy include Hegar's sign, Goodell's sign, Chadwick's sign, abdominal enlargement, Braxton Hicks contractions, ballottement, palpable fetal outline, positive pregnancy tests, and skin pigmentation changes.

hegar's sign

Hegar's sign is the softening of the lower uterine segment that can be felt during a vaginal examination. This sign usually occurs by the sixth to the eighth week of pregnancy and is caused by increased blood flow to the reproductive organs. Hegar's sign is only a probable sign because some women may have very weak or soft uterine walls even when not pregnant.

goodell's sign

Goodell's sign is the softening of the cervix, which is normally very firm. This may be felt by the examining clinician as early as 6 to 8 weeks' gestation and results from increased blood flow to the reproductive organs. Because oral contraceptives also may cause this phenomenon, Goodell's sign is only a probable sign of pregnancy.

chadwick's sign

As early as 6 to 8 weeks' gestation, the mucous membranes of the cervix, vagina, and vulva become bluish; this phenomenon is called *Chadwick's sign*. Increased vascularization (development of additional blood vessels) of the reproductive organs causes the blood to show through the thin mucous membrane. Chadwick's sign is probable because some nonpregnant women have pelvic congestion or increased blood flow to the area.

abdominal enlargement

During pregnancy, as the contents of the uterus enlarge, so does the abdomen. By the end of the third month, the uterus has reached the height of the symphysis pubis; by the end of the fifth month, it is at the level of the umbilicus. Many other factors may cause abdominal enlargement, such as tumors, obesity, or fluid retention; thus, this is only a probable sign of pregnancy.

braxton hicks contractions

Braxton Hicks contractions are irregular, usually painless contractions of the uterus that occur sporadically throughout pregnancy. These contractions stimulate blood flow through the placenta and enable the uterus to maintain muscle tone and accommodate the enlarging fetus. Most of the time the woman is unaware of these contractions, but in the later stages of pregnancy, they may become stronger, causing the woman to mistake them for labor contractions (false labor).

ballottement

During the fourth or fifth month when the fetus is small in relation to the volume of amniotic fluid, a gentle push or tap of the uterus will cause the fetus to float away and then rebound, touching the clinician's hand (Fig. 7-1). Other medical conditions that may create this sensation are excessive fluid accumulation in the abdomen (ascites) or uterine tumors.

palpable fetal outline

Around the sixth month of pregnancy, the examiner may be able to palpate the legs, arms, head, and trunk of the fetus. As the pregnancy continues, the outline becomes even easier to detect. Although this seems fairly sound evidence of pregnancy, in rare cases, a tumor can resemble the shape of a fetus.

positive pregnancy tests

Pregnancy tests work by detecting the presence of HCG in maternal serum or urine. HCG is a hormone secreted early in pregnancy by the chorionic villi of the placenta. Using immunologic methods, such as *radioimmunoassay*, these tests can detect pregnancy as early as 8 to 10 days following conception.

To obtain the most accurate results when testing urine, the woman should use the first voided specimen in the morning because it contains the highest concentration of HCG. Using proper technique can give accurate results up to 97% of the time. Pregnancy tests may be inaccurate for a variety of reasons, including failure to follow instructions, presence of certain medications (phenothiazines, such as Thorazine, Trilafon, and Phenergan), or improper handling of the urine specimen (it should be refrigerated if

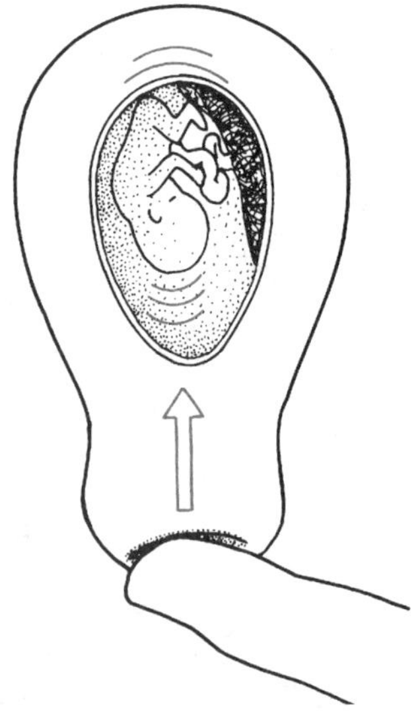

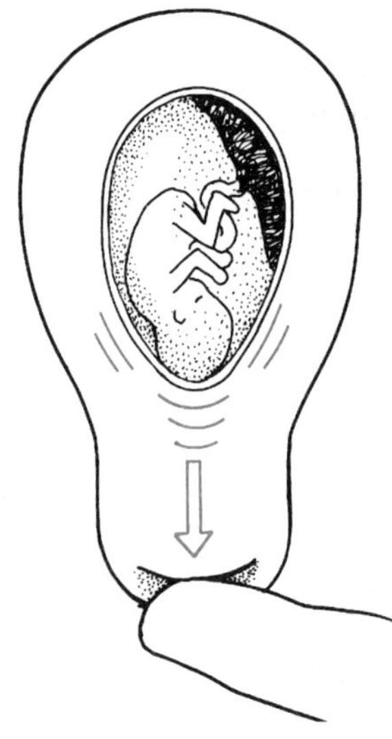

figure 7-1 *Ballottement. The principle of ballottement is that an object floating in fluid can be made to move upward by a tap and its rebound can be felt. The examiner gently taps the bottom of the cervix, causing the fetus to rise in the amniotic fluid sac. When the fetus sinks back to the bottom of the amniotic sac, a gentle tap can be felt on the examiner's finger. This response is a probable sign of pregnancy.*

table 7-2 causes of false readings of pregnancy tests

False–Negative Reading	*False–Positive Reading*
Performed to early or late in pregnancy	Protein or blood in the urine sample
Urine too dilute	Prolonged life of the corpus luteum
Urine stored at room temperature	Effects of certain medications
Effects of certain medications	Hydatitidform mole
Tubal pregnancy	Chorionic carcinoma
Missed abortion	

the test is not performed immediately). Table 7-2 lists reasons for inaccurate test results.

skin pigmentation changes

Skin pigmentation changes that occur during pregnancy include the following:

- *Linea nigra*: a dark brown line, seen particularly in brunettes, that extends from the umbilicus to the symphysis pubis
- *Chloasma*: "mask of pregnancy;" a blotchy tan or brown discoloration that appears on the face; may fade following delivery
- *Striae gravidarum*: stretch marks; stretching of the skin, which produces red or pink streaks, particularly on the abdomen but also on the breasts; following pregnancy fade to silver but never disappear entirely

Linea nigra and chloasma also may be caused by the use of birth control pills. Striae gravidarum can result from obesity.

positive signs

The *positive signs* of pregnancy are diagnostic and 100% accurate. They include fetal heart sounds, fetal movement felt by the examiner, and ultrasound imaging of the fetus.

fetal heart sounds

Once the heartbeat of the fetus can be heard by a clinician, pregnancy is confirmed. Using a Doppler device, the clinician can detect the fetal heartbeat as early as the 8th to 10th week (Fig. 7-2*A*). Using a standard fetoscope (less commonly used since the development of the Doppler device), the heartbeat can be heard at 18 to 20 weeks' gestation (see Fig. 7-2*B*). The woman and her family may enjoy listening with the Doppler device; this is their first experience of hearing their child. In addition to the fetal heartbeat, two other sounds may be heard: the *funic souffle* and the *uterine souffle*. The *funic souffle* is a soft whirling or whizzing sound heard as the fetal blood rushes through the umbilical cord; it matches the tempo of the fetal heartbeat (between 120 and 160 beats/min). The *funic souffle* is considered a positive sign of pregnancy; however, it is heard only in about one sixth of all clients. The *uterine souffle* is a soft whirling or whizzing sound heard as the maternal blood swishes through the large uterine vessels. This

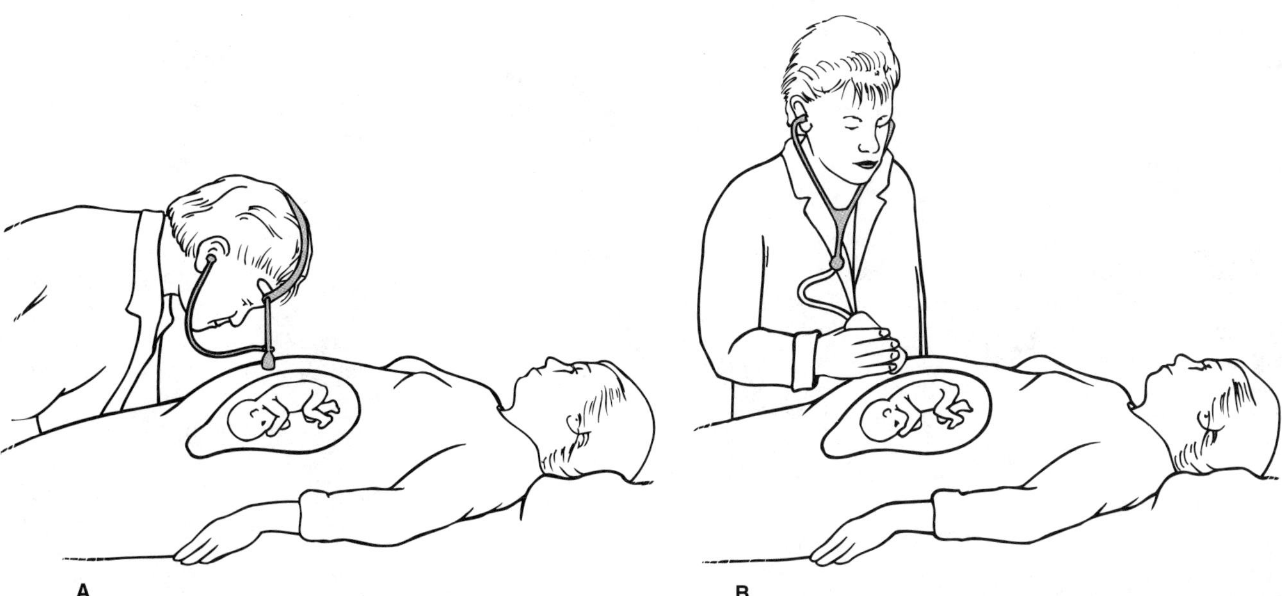

figure 7-2 *Auscultation of fetal heart tones.* ***(A)*** *Doppler ultrasound.* ***(B)*** *Fetoscope.*

sound matches the tempo of the mother's pulse (approximately 80 beats/min). Thus, it is simple to differentiate the uterine souffle from the funic souffle by counting the maternal pulse rate (approximately 80) and comparing it with the count made when listening to the fetal heartbeat through the maternal abdomen.

fetal movements felt by examiner

By the end of the fifth month of pregnancy, the fetus is of sufficient size and strength that its movements can be detected by an experienced examiner. This is a positive sign of pregnancy.

ultrasound

Ultrasound may be used to diagnose pregnancy as early as 5 to 6 weeks' gestation. It also may determine that the products of conception are located in the uterus, thus ruling out ectopic pregnancy (see Chap. 8). As early as 10 weeks' gestation, the parents may see their offspring's heart beating and some of the larger body parts. Ultrasound using a transvaginal approach (a probe is inserted into the vagina to provide a *sonogram* [ultrasonic image]) can detect pregnancy as early as 2½ to 3 weeks (see Fig. 7-2*C*). Fortunately, ultrasound has replaced x-ray to diagnose pregnancy, eliminating the danger to the fetus of radiation exposure. However, the long-term effects of ultrasound are not known; thus, routine ultrasound screening is not recommended.

physiologic changes during pregnancy

The body of the pregnant woman undergoes many and varied physical changes during the 9 months between conception and birth. Most of the changes occur in the reproductive system but also affect the other body systems. After childbirth, the body systems generally revert to their prepregnant state.

reproductive system

The external structures of the reproductive system, the labia majora, labia minora, and clitoris, enlarge during pregnancy due to increased vascularity caused by high levels of circulating estrogen and an accumulation of fat. Although these structures reduce in size following delivery, trauma from birth and loss of muscle tone may prevent them from returning to their prepregnant state.

The internal structures of the reproductive system change dramatically during pregnancy. Ovulation ceases, and the placenta becomes the major endocrine gland of the reproductive system. Remarkable changes occur in the uterus, vagina, perineum, and breasts.

uterus

The nonpregnant uterus is a pear-shaped organ measuring approximately 7.5 cm (3 in) × 5 cm (2 in) × 2.5 cm (1 in); it weighs about 70 g (2.5 oz) and has a volume of about 10 mL (2.5 tsp). During pregnancy, the uterus increases in size, weight, and volume to accommodate the growing fetus. At full term, the uterus weighs about 1100 g (2.5 lb), and its capacity has expanded to 5 L (5 quarts), more than 500 times its prepregnant capacity. Table 7-3 summarizes these changes.

table 7-3 uterine growth during pregnancy

	Before Pregnancy	*At Full Term*
Length	7.5 cm (3 in)	32 cm (13 in)
Width	5.0 cm (2 in)	24 cm (9 in)
Depth	2.5 cm (1 in)	22 cm (8 in)
Weight	70 g (2.5 oz)	1,100 g (2.5 lb)
Volume	10 mL (2.5 tsp)	51 mL (5 qt)

During pregnancy, uterine muscle fibers develop extra elastic tissue and become wider and longer. This allows them to stretch during pregnancy, contract during labor, and ultimately return to normal size following delivery.

The blood supply to the uterus is increased by as much as 80% during pregnancy, with more than 16% of the body's total blood supply circulating through the uterus at one time. The uterine blood vessels widen and develop many new branches to accommodate the increased volume. The new blood supply is necessary to nourish the growing muscle tissue, provide adequate circulation to the placenta, and support the decidual lining of the uterus. This greatly increased blood flow means that vaginal bleeding at any time during pregnancy or immediately following delivery can be life-threatening.

During pregnancy, the cervix becomes shorter and softer. Progesterone causes an increase in production of cervical mucus and a mucus plug is formed to block the cervical os. This mucus plug prevents bacteria and other foreign matter from invading the uterine cavity. The mucus plug is expelled when the cervix dilates in preparation for birth.

vagina

Estrogen causes the vagina to develop an increased blood supply and causes the mucosa and smooth muscles to thicken and the joints to relax. The vagina also increases in length. These changes allow it to stretch to accommodate the passage of the infant.

Vaginal secretions increase during pregnancy, but the pH level falls from 7 to less than 5. Secretions are normally clear, thick, and odorless. The change in the pH prevents bacterial infections but increases the likelihood of yeast infections (particularly *Candida albicans*). This condition causes itching, burning, and a cheesy vaginal discharge. Medications may be ordered by the physician to ease the symptoms and cure the infection. If untreated, the infant may contract the yeast infection as it passes through the

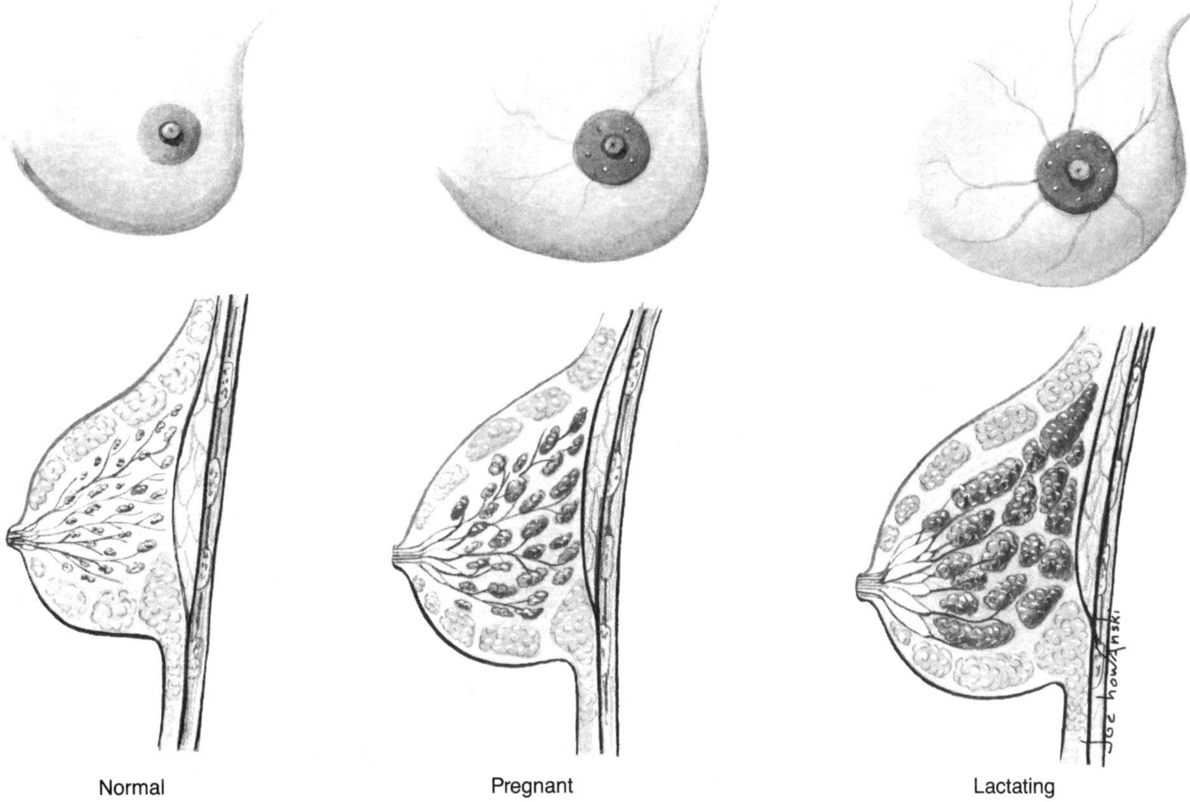

figure 7-3 *Breast changes during pregnancy.*

birth canal. This condition in the infant is known as *thrush*, a yeast infection of the mouth.

breasts

Early in pregnancy, rising levels of estrogen and progesterone cause the breast tissue to enlarge and feel tender. The breasts are preparing for milk production and nursing of the infant. The nipples become erect and enlarge (Fig. 7-3). The sebaceous glands on the areola enlarge and look like small bumps on the outer edges; these are called Montgomery's tubercles. These tubercles secrete oils to keep the nipples supple and to help prevent cracking when the infant nurses.

A few months into the pregnancy, the breasts will begin to secrete a thin yellowish fluid called *colostrum*. It contains protein, antibodies, and minerals but is low in sugar and fat. The breasts will continue to produce and secrete colostrum until 2 to 3 days after delivery when mature milk production begins.

respiratory system

Many changes occur in the respiratory system of the pregnant woman to improve or maintain adequate gas exchange. As pregnancy advances, the uterus pushes the diaphragm upward as much as 4 cm (1.5 in) to accommodate the growing fetus. This decreases expansion of the lungs. To compensate, progesterone relaxes the supporting ligaments of the rib cage, allowing the diameter of the ribs to expand. This change permits the lung capacity to remain the same.

As the abdomen enlarges, the woman shifts from abdominal breathing to thoracic breathing. Her respirations become deeper and faster, increasing by two breaths per minute, so she is taking in 30% to 40% more air to meet the added oxygen needs of the fetus. Crowding of the thoracic area and increased air intake may cause shortness of breath, especially during the last trimester.

Under the influence of estrogen, the upper respiratory tract becomes very vascular. This may cause nasal congestion, deepening of the voice, a sense of fullness in the eustachian tubes, and nose bleeds (*epistaxis*). Because of these symptoms, the woman may express concern that she has a "head cold."

nursing alert

Caution the mother that these upper respiratory symptoms are normal, and she should not take any over-the-counter drugs or other medications without consulting her physician.

cardiovascular system

The cardiovascular system changes significantly to meet the demands of pregnancy. These changes prepare the woman's body to meet the increasing needs of the fetus for oxygen and nutrition while meeting her own body requirements.

During pregnancy, the blood volume increases 30% to 50% to supply the increased vascular needs of the reproductive system, particularly the uterus and the placenta, which supplies the fetus with adequate oxygen and nutrition. It also builds a reserve blood supply for the anticipated blood loss during delivery. Maternal blood loss during a vaginal delivery is usually 200 to 300 mL; blood loss during a cesarean delivery is usually 400 mL or more.

As the blood volume increases, it temporarily dilutes the concentration of red blood cells and hemoglobin. This is called *physiologic anemia* and is a normal result of pregnancy. The woman's body continues to increase the number of red blood cells throughout pregnancy and by the last few weeks, has reached a normal range. Hemoglobin and hematocrit are monitored carefully; hemoglobin levels should never fall below 12 g, and the hematocrit should never fall below 35%. If levels decrease further, the woman is evaluated for true anemia. Generally, during the second trimester, iron supplements are prescribed for the woman to help build the hemoglobin essential for oxygen transport.

The expanded blood volume increases the workload of the heart, which, in turn, increases cardiac output. This can increase the normal pulse rate by 10 to 15 beats/min. Blood pressure decreases slightly during pregnancy. Systolic blood pressure decreases from about 12 to 26 weeks and then gradually returns to prepregnancy levels by about 36 weeks.

The increased workload presents no problems for a normal heart but may cause serious symptoms in a diseased heart.

gastrointestinal system

During the first trimester, the woman may experience nausea and vomiting due to hormonal changes and decreased carbohydrate metabolism. Throughout pregnancy, the sight and odors of certain foods may be disturbing. This may be particularly frustrating if they were previously favorite foods.

As the pregnancy advances, the woman may have increased salivation, heartburn, flatulence, and occasional constipation, all due to the decreased gastric motility caused by increased levels of progesterone. Hemorrhoids may develop from the pressure of the enlarging uterus on the veins lying directly beneath it.

urinary system

Urinary output increases 60% to 80% during pregnancy to excrete the fetal and maternal waste products. This causes a normal decrease in the specific gravity of the urine.

The kidneys and ureters dilate during pregnancy, and the muscle tone of the entire urinary system, including the bladder, decreases. These changes slow the flow of urine (*urinary stasis*) and predispose the woman to distention of the kidneys (*hydronephrosis*) and the ureters (*hydroureter*). Urinary stasis also increases the risk of urinary tract infections.

During pregnancy, the woman will retain water (as much as 6.5 L), which aids in increasing blood volume, hydrating the placenta, forming the amniotic fluid, and enlarging the breasts and uterus. In the past, diuretics were administered to decrease this water retention. Diuretics are contraindicated, however, because water is necessary for proper organ function and because diuretics endanger the woman and the fetus.

integumentary system

Skin and hair changes vary greatly during pregnancy. Women with blond hair, blue eyes, and fair skin generally have the fewest changes, whereas dark-eyed brunettes may experience the most significant changes. Some changes may be permanent; others will fade or diasappear after pregnancy. Changes include vascular markings, pigmentation changes, striae gravidarum, acne, and hair growth.

vascular markings

The woman may notice the formation of red spider-shaped markings (*nevi, angiomas*) particularly on her face, neck, chest, and extremities. Red patches may form on the palms of her hands (*palmar erythema*) and sometimes on her gums near the tooth line. These changes are caused by increased levels of estrogen. They usually fade after delivery, but they do not disappear completely.

pigmentation changes

Pregnancy may cause the areola, nipples, and perineal areas to deepen in color. The face may develop brown patchy areas (chloasma), and a dark line may appear from the umbilicus to the symphysis pubis (linea nigra; Fig. 7-4). These changes occur in response to the hormones and will fade or disappear completely.

striae gravidarum

Weight gain during pregnancy causes increased tension on the skin, which may produce stretch marks (striae gravidarum) on the breasts, abdomen, hips, and upper thighs (see Fig. 7-4). During pregnancy, they are pink or bright red; after delivery, they fade to silvery-white.

acne

Estrogen also causes increased oil production that can lead to the development of acne. Once the estrogen level falls, the excess oiliness disappears.

hair growth

High levels of estrogen also accelerate hair growth. The woman may experience the growth of facial hair. In addition, perspiration increases as estrogen levels rise. These changes normally resolve after pregnancy ends and hormone levels fall.

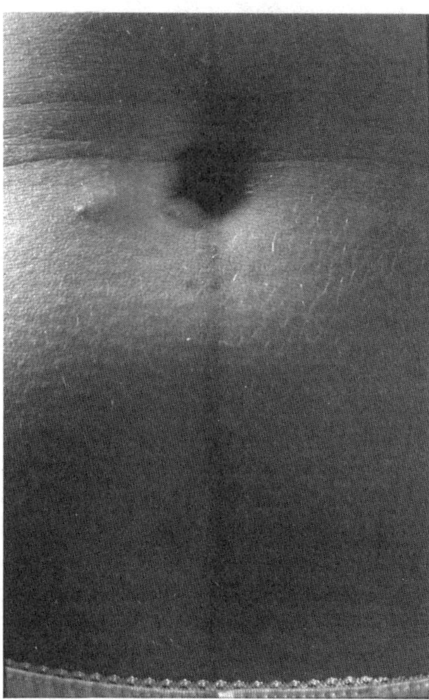

figure 7-4 *Linea nigra.*

musculoskeletal system

The musculoskeletal system responds to the many changes of pregnancy. The weight gain, change in posture from the protruding abdomen, and hormones secreted all play a role. The hormone *relaxin*, secreted by the corpus luteum, causes relaxation and increased mobility of the sacroiliac, sacrococcygeal, and pelvic joints. This contributes to the characteristic "waddling" gait the woman develops. As the uterus enlarges and increases in weight, the woman will lean backward, increasing the lumbar curve (*lordosis*) and shifting her center of gravity to keep her balance (Fig. 7-5). This change produces a strain on her lower back and can cause low back pain.

Relaxin also causes separation of the abdominal muscles to allow for growth of the uterus. Late in pregnancy, the woman's umbilicus becomes flattened or may protrude. The weight of the enlarging uterus pulls and stretches the broad ligament, and she may report sharp, stabbing pains when she attempts to change position rapidly.

metabolic changes

Metabolic function speeds up during pregnancy because of the increased oxygen consumption of the woman and the fetus and the demands of the woman's cardiovascular system. It may increase as much as 15% to 20% but returns to the normal prepregnancy levels following delivery.

endocrine system

The most striking change in the endocrine system during pregnancy is the development of a new temporary organ—the *placenta*. Ovulation stops, and the placenta begins to produce and release estrogen and progesterone.

Because estrogen and progesterone levels remain high throughout pregnancy, the pituitary gland ceases production of follicle-stimulating hormone and luteinizing hormone. Late in pregnancy, it begins secreting two very important "pregnancy hormones," *prolactin* and *oxytocin*. Prolactin is responsible for the production of breast milk (*lactation*). Oxytocin is responsible for the initiation and maintenance of labor contractions.

The cortex of the adrenal glands enlarges and increases production of the glucocorticoids, which increase the amount of circulating glucose in the blood. In response, the pancreas increases production of *insulin*, which is necessary for carbohydrate metabolism. Its effectiveness is hindered, however, by the increased levels of estrogen and progesterone, which inhibit the action of insulin. This makes control of diabetes during pregnancy a real challenge. It is also the reason why some prediabetic women develop high glucose levels and need to be placed on diabetic diets with daily insulin injections during pregnancy. This condition is called *gestational diabetes*. Usually, these women may follow a regular diet following delivery.

The adrenal glands increase production of aldosterone, which promotes sodium reabsorption. This is necessary to counteract the sodium-wasting effects of progesterone.

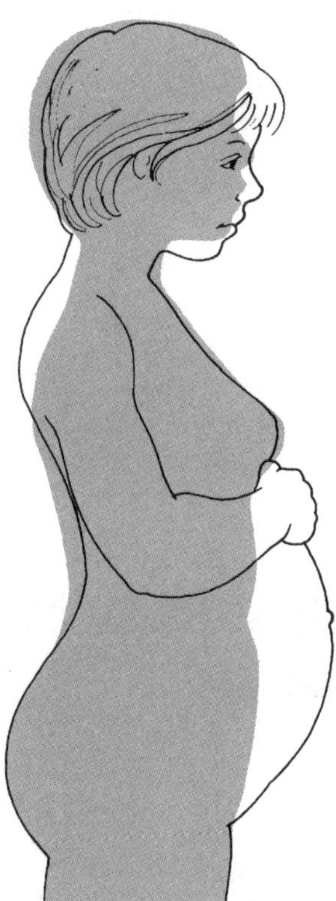

figure 7-5 *Postural changes during pregnancy. The pregnant woman's head assumes an exaggerated anterior flexion, and the shoulders slump anteriorly in an attempt to compensate for the body's gravity shift. The poor lumbosacral alignment that results from this compensation creates backache and unsure balance.*

psychosocial changes during pregnancy

All changes in life, whether positive or negative, produce stress. Pregnancy and its outcome represent a big change in the life of a woman and all other members of her family. How she and her family cope with the changes will depend on several factors:

* Their cultural beliefs
* Their spiritual beliefs
* Their support systems, such as family, friends, neighbors
* Their personal physical health
* Their ability to use positive coping mechanisms
* Their past experiences (positive or negative) with pregnancy and birth

In addition, the woman and her partner need to accomplish certain developmental tasks of pregnancy successfully to adapt to the pregnancy and future roles as parents. For ease of understanding, these tasks generally are discussed according to trimesters. These tasks may overlap and occur according to each parent's own timetable (Table 7-4).

Although the partner has fewer tasks to accomplish, he or she often provides the majority of the support for the woman. Being involved throughout the pregnancy can be very rewarding for the partner. In recent years, leaders in childbirth education have recognized the vital role the partner can play and now strive to include rather than exclude him or her. Depending on the couple, however, partners differ in their desired degree of involvement in the pregnancy and birth, and the nurse needs to respect the individual partner's preferences.

cultural considerations

Because pregnancy and birth are major life events, each culture has strong beliefs and customs about these events. However, individuals within each cultural group may not abide by the dictates of the culture; thus, the nurse should avoid stereotyping people from a particular culture.

table 7-4 maternal developmental tasks of pregnancy

FIRST TRIMESTER
Acceptance of the pregnancy and of the fetus
SECOND TRIMESTER
Development of a sense of physical and mental well-being
THIRD TRIMESTER
Transition to the role of parenthood

Many cultural groups view pregnancy and birth as a normal part of life that does not require medical intervention. Women from these groups may not seek prenatal care until late in pregnancy.

Cultural standards also can dictate how women behave during childbirth. For example, women from Southeast Asia tend to remain quiet when experiencing pain, believing that a display of emotion is shameful.

Cultural beliefs and customs also influence diet. For example, Filipino American women may avoid hot, spicy foods during pregnancy.

The role of the father also depends on cultural beliefs. Although the trend among affluent white Americans is to have the father present for prenatal classes, labor, and delivery, Mexican Americans often allow only women to be present for the birth.

first trimester

The first trimester is an adjustment phase. During this period, each person explores his or her own individual feelings about pregnancy, birth, and the potential task of parenting.

maternal tasks

The major goal for the woman during the first trimester is the acceptance of the pregnancy and the fetus. She may experience feelings of ambivalence and consider such questions as, "Is this the right time to be pregnant?" "Will I be a good mother?"

She may focus more on the physical discomforts and less on the fetus because it may not seem real to her. Depending on her relationship with her mother, she also may renew or strengthen that relationship as she examines her own identity as a woman and a potential mother. During this phase, she may develop fears or fantasies that the fetus is deformed or has a serious disease.

paternal tasks

Like the mother, the partner also must deal with the reality of the pregnancy during this time; however, he does not experience the same physical changes as the woman. He may worry about finances or his ability to be a good father and role model. He may be confused or experience guilt feelings because his partner is experiencing nausea, vomiting, and other discomforts associated with pregnancy. This problem is often compounded by the mother's frequent mood swings and tearfulness.

Some partners may develop *couvade* (a French term meaning "to hatch"). When this happens, the partner will experience many of the same symptoms as the woman, such as weight gain, morning sickness, and even abdominal pain when the woman goes into labor. Most often, these symptoms are seen in fathers who are very much involved with the pregnancy and concerned about the woman's physical condition.

second trimester

The second trimester is a plateau phase. The pregnancy begins to seem real for both parents. They develop a need to learn more about fetal growth and development, and this makes it an ideal time to provide prenatal education.

maternal tasks

The major goal for the woman during the second trimester is to develop a sense of physical and mental well-being. She has settled in with the idea that she is truly pregnant and begins to feel fairly comfortable with the progress. Her physical discomforts are somewhat relieved, and she may experience an increased energy level. She becomes less fearful about the well-being of the fetus if prenatal visits assure her that all is going well. She begins to see the fetus as separate from herself, having its own identity but still very dependent on her. As she explores her feelings, she may become introverted and self-centered. The nesting instinct may be apparent as she begins to plan the nursery, purchases or makes baby clothes, and day dreams about "what my baby will be like." She also may spend time watching other children with their mothers and imagining what type of mother she will be.

paternal tasks

The father may feel the baby move and experience joy with the idea of being a father. He also may experience some frustration as the mother becomes introverted, but as he contemplates fatherhood, he becomes somewhat self-centered also. The father may seek an active role in the pregnancy by watching the mother's diet, assisting with household chores, and talking frequently about the pregnancy. Some fathers may be less involved, taking on the role of an observer. These behaviors are largely determined by his personality and his past experiences, both cultural and social. During this trimester, he may focus on what type of provider and parent he will be.

third trimester

As the pregnancy enters its final stages, the mother and father are preparing for their roles of parenthood. They begin to anticipate the final event: labor and delivery.

maternal tasks

The major maternal goal during this phase of pregnancy is the transition to the role of motherhood. The woman may be forced to slow down her daily activities due to her increased size and returning fatigue. As she prepares herself for labor and birth, she may enroll in prenatal and childbirth classes. She may finalize birth plans along with her partner. They may decide to have their child at home, in a birthing center, or in a hospital setting. She may begin "nesting" activities, such as preparing the infant's room, purchasing or making clothes for the infant, and seriously considering names for the infant.

paternal tasks

This period also is a transition phase for the father. He may participate in planned classes, discuss possible names for the baby, and become more involved as the time draws near. Some fathers may draw back and become less involved with classes and so forth. Old fears about finances, ability as a support person, and ability as a father may resurface. If the couple has remained supportive of each other throughout the pregnancy, this can be a time of renewed closeness.

sibling involvement

Pregnancy can be a time of confusion for children in the immediate family. The age of a child will determine how he or she is prepared for the new arrival. The older the child, the more questions and involvement may be required. The child should be told of the expected baby in a positive, nonthreatening way and should be included in plans for this addition to the family. Parents should emphasize that the infant will be an addition to the family, not someone to take the child's place. Allowing children to participate in the plans can help make them feel more a part of the family. Taking children shopping and allowing them to assist in the selection of the items for the newborn, feeling the baby move in mother's abdomen, and reminiscing about their birth and early years are ways to ease the transition for the sibling.

✶ nursing considerations

During pregnancy, the pregnant woman and her partner will probably see the nurse more than any other member of the health care team. To provide effective, family-centered care, the nurse needs a solid background in maternity nursing. Much of the nurse's time will be spent educating the woman and her partner about the physical and psychological changes that occur during pregnancy.

The nurse will assume many roles while working with the couple: teacher, role model, counselor, and resource person. In addition, the nurse will perform routine clinical procedures. The nurse's listening skills are of utmost importance in determining the needs of the client. Verbal and nonverbal cues will help the nurse evaluate when interventions are needed. The couple may feel uncomfortable discussing important issues, such as sexuality, emotional stressors, or cultural beliefs. Listening with empathy and understanding can make them feel more comfortable and provide an open environment for them to explore their options and increase their understanding of the process of pregnancy.

what would you do?

Joan is a 25-year-old single woman. She has come to the clinic because she has missed two menstrual cycles, her breasts are tender, and she feels very fatigued. She has just been examined by the physician who has confirmed that she is pregnant. Joan is crying and visibly upset. She says to the nurse, "This can't be right. I did a home pregnancy test, and it was negative. I'm sure something is terribly wrong with me, and the doctor is not telling me. How can I be pregnant? I just don't believe it."

key points ✳

- ✳ Pregnancy is a normal physiologic process, not an illness.
- ✳ To calculate the estimated date for delivery using Nägele's rule, add 7 days to the first day of the last menstrual period and count back 3 months.
- ✳ The three major categories of the signs of pregnancy are presumptive, probable, and positive.
- ✳ Pregnancy affects every major body system.
- ✳ The internal structures of the reproductive system change dramatically during pregnancy, particularly the uterus.
- ✳ During pregnancy, the endocrine system develops a new temporary organ, the placenta, which is the lifeline between mother and fetus.
- ✳ The pregnant woman needs to accomplish several developmental tasks: acceptance of the pregnancy and the fetus; development of a sense of physical and mental well-being; and transition to the role of parenthood.

review questions ✳

1. The term used to describe the signs of pregnancy that appear early and are generally subjective is
   a. traditional.
   b. presumptive.
   c. probable.
   d. positive.
2. A soft, whirring sound that may be confused with the fetal heart beat is called
   a. fetal heart tones.
   b. funic souffle.
   c. uterine souffle.
   d. bruit.
3. Rita Nichols is 36 weeks pregnant. The nurse is listening to the fetal heart tones and questions whether the sound she is hearing belongs to the fetus or the mother. She could
   a. request an order for an ultrasound.
   b. report her problem to the charge nurse.
   c. check the mother's pulse and compare the two readings.
   d. change the mother's position and recheck.
4. Tiffany DiMento, who is 7 months pregnant, is concerned about the red "stretch marks" on her abdomen. She asks, "Will they always be there?" The nurse's best response would be,
   a. "Yes. They never go away."
   b. "Yes, but they will fade to a silver color."
   c. "No. They will disappear completely after delivery."
   d. "No. They will disappear shortly before you go into labor."
5. Allison Amundson will experience and accomplish several psychosocial tasks of pregnancy. The first task to be accomplished is
   a. the development of a sense of physical and mental well-being.
   b. the acceptance of the pregnancy and the fetus.
   c. the acceptance of her husband as a new father.
   d. the transition to the role of motherhood.

bibliography ✳

Cunningham, G., McDonald, P.C., Leveno, K.J., Gant, N.F., & Gilstrap, L.C. (1993). *Williams obstetrics* (19th ed.). Norwalk CT: Appleton & Lange.

Fortier, J., Carson, V., Will, S., & Shubkagel, B. (1991). Adjustment to a newborn: sibling preparation makes a difference. *Journal of Obstetric, Gynecologic and Neonatal Nursing, 20*(4), 73–78.

Kenner, C. A., & Mac Laren, A. (1993). *Essentials of maternal and neonatal nursing*. Springhouse, PA: Springhouse Corporation.

May, K. A., & Mahlmeister, L. R. (1994). *Maternal and neonatal nursing* (3rd ed.). Philadelphia: J.B. Lippincott.

Murphy, R. L. (1992) Couvade: The pregnant male. *The Journal of Perinatal Education, 1*(2), 13–17.

Olds, S. B., London, M. L., & Ladewig, P. W. (1992). *Maternal newborn nursing: A family-centered approach* (4th ed.). Redwood City: Addison-Wesley Nursing.

Pillitteri, A. (1995). *Maternal and child health nursing* (2nd ed.). Philadelphia: J.B. Lippincott.

Reeder, S. J., Martin, L. L., & Koniak, D. (1992). *Maternity nursing* (17th ed.). Philadelphia: J.B. Lippincott.

Sloan, E. (1993). *Biology of women* (3rd ed.). New York: Delmar.

needs and care of the expectant family

8

outline

objectives

After studying this chapter, the reader should be able to:

* Discuss measures that may be used to alleviate the discomforts of pregnancy.
* Discuss the information given and obtained during the first prenatal visit.
* List the danger signs that the pregnant woman should report during pregnancy.
* Using the nutritional pyramid, discuss nutritional needs during pregnancy.
* Discuss pain management techniques taught in prenatal classes.
* Describe the use of breathing techniques used during labor.

key terms

antepartum
contraction stress test
effleurage
focal point
Hoffman technique
hyperemesis gravidarum
Kegel exercises
kick count
leukorrhea
nipple stimulation test
nonstress test
oxytocin challenge test
pica
psychoprophylaxis
rapid plasma reagin (RPR)
Venereal Disease Research Laboratory (VDRL)

Neff C & Spray M. *Introduction to Maternal and Child Health Nursing,*

Pregnancy can be one of the most exciting events in the life of a woman and her partner. Whether the pregnancy is planned or unplanned, the woman receiving this diagnosis may experience a variety of feelings, both positive and negative. She may feel shock, pleasure, joy, and fear simultaneously. The family also may share some of these feelings. Caring for the expectant family can be exciting and challenging for the nurse.

A woman who receives adequate prenatal (*antepartum*) care is much more likely to have a healthy pregnancy that results in a healthy baby. Prenatal care includes regular physical examination by the physician or nurse practitioner, periodic diagnostic tests to assess maternal and fetal health, and health teaching about nutrition, hygiene, safety, and preparation for parenthood.

✷ nursing considerations

The nurse has a key role in prenatal care, in performing routine clinical procedures and in helping the woman and her partner learn more about the realities of pregnancy, birth, and becoming parents. As a health educator, the nurse teaches the woman self-care measures to cope with the common discomforts of pregnancy. The nurse also provides necessary information about lifestyle factors, such as diet, exercise, and safety, and directs the woman and her partner toward community resources that can help meet their needs.

discomforts of pregnancy

The discomforts of pregnancy are the result of the normal anatomic and physiologic changes taking place. Although these discomforts can be frustrating, they are temporary. Many can be alleviated with simple interventions.

nausea and vomiting

Nausea and vomiting usually occur during the first trimester as the result of hormonal changes and the slowing of peristalsis. Although often called "morning sickness," nausea and vomiting can occur at any time. Some women experience these symptoms throughout their pregnancy.

Nausea and vomiting are often relieved by eating dry crackers before arising in the morning. Other helpful measures include eating small, frequent meals; avoiding fatty, greasy, or fried foods; increasing fluid intake between meals; and avoiding liquids with the meal. Peppermint tea, soothing and comforting to the gastrointestinal tract, also may give some relief. Hot foods should be eaten while still very warm, and cold foods should be eaten very cold to increase their appeal.

Morning sickness should not be confused with severe nausea and vomiting (*hyperemesis gravidarum*), which can cause severe dehydration, putting the woman and fetus at risk and requiring hospitalization (see Chap. 9).

heartburn

Heartburn (indigestion or esophageal reflux) is not a "burning or pain in the heart" but primarily a result of the growing uterus pressing on the stomach, rising progesterone levels, and decreased gastric motility. These factors cause a burning sensation in the esophagus and may leave a sour taste in the mouth.

The measures suggested for relief of nausea and vomiting also will help relieve heartburn. Lying down after meals may increase the incidence. The physician may prescribe an antacid, for example, magnesium hydroxide (Maalox or Mylanta); however, baking soda and sodium bicarbonate (Alka-seltzer) should be avoided because these products will cause electrolyte imbalance.

constipation

Many women experience constipation during pregnancy, especially in the second and third trimesters due to the sluggishness of the intestines. Increased levels of progesterone relax the bowel, and the enlarging uterus displaces it. Iron supplements also can contribute to constipation.

Increasing intake of fresh fruits and vegetables, whole grain cereals, and fluids, especially water, may offer relief. Exercise, especially walking, may be beneficial. If constipation continues, the physician may prescribe a stool softener. Any self-medication is dangerous during pregnancy, and laxatives are no exception. Mineral oil interferes with the absorption of vitamins A, D, K, and E (the fat-soluble vitamins), which could cause deficiencies in the woman and fetus. Enemas are contraindicated because they can cause premature labor.

urinary frequency

This condition occurs during the first and third trimesters because the enlarging uterus is pressing on the bladder. During the second trimester, the uterus moves up into the abdominal cavity and provides temporary relief. If the woman coughs or sneezes during the third trimester, however, she may dribble small amounts of urine.

There is no special remedy for this problem. Perineal pads may be used to keep undergarments dry if dribbling becomes a problem. Fluids should not be limited. Instruct the woman to report any blood in the urine or burning with urination because urinary infections can develop frequently during pregnancy.

> **✷ nursing alert**
>
> *Encourage adequate fluid intake (8–10 8-oz glasses per day) to prevent dehydration.*

breast tenderness

Breasts, including the nipples, may become very tender. The woman may report fullness, tingling, and soreness, caused largely by increased levels of progesterone and estrogen. Wearing a well-fitted supportive bra with wide straps offers some relief.

ankle edema

Ankle edema is normal during pregnancy and results from normal sodium and water retention. As the enlarged uterus presses on the large veins in the pelvic region, it causes decreased venous return from the lower extremities, contributing to ankle edema.

Elevating the legs periodically helps relieve the edema; lying on the side also is helpful. Caution the woman to avoid knee high stockings and panty girdles, which constrict circulation.

dyspnea

As the uterus enlarges, it presses up against the diaphragm, causing shortness of breath. This problem occurs especially during the third trimester.

Maintaining good erect posture when sitting or standing helps relieve dyspnea by increasing oxygen intake. Pillows to elevate the upper torso may help when sleeping or resting in a reclining position.

vaginal discharge

It is normal for the pregnant woman to have increased vaginal discharge (*leukorrhea*), resulting from increased estrogen levels. Normally, it is white or yellowish; any itching, burning or odor indicates infection.

Irritation can be relieved by wearing loose cotton or cotton-lined underwear. Instruct the woman to keep the perineal area clean and dry.

> **nursing alert**
> *Instruct the woman to avoid the use of feminine hygiene deodorant sprays, tampons (even though she may have vaginal discharge), and vaginal douching unless ordered by the physician.*

varicose veins

Impaired venous return, mentioned previously, contributes to the formation of varicose veins. The legs may ache and feel "heavy" or tired.

Wearing support hose or elastic stockings may offer relief. For maximum benefit, the stockings should be put on before getting out of bed in the morning, before the veins become distended. The nurse cautions the woman to avoid crossing her legs because this can increase pressure on the lower extremity veins. Prolonged standing or sitting also should be avoided because this interferes with circulation.

> **nursing alert**
> *Instruct the woman to report any signs of thrombophlebitis: legs that are red, tender, swollen, or warm to the touch.*

muscle cramps

Many pregnant women suffer from painful leg cramps, especially during the night, interfering with their rest. These cramps result from decreased calcium levels in the blood, tension, and the normal stretching of the muscles and tendons.

Simple bed rest or elevation of the feet can offer some relief. Cramping can be immediately relieved by straightening the extremity and bending the foot toward the knee (dorsiflexion). Massaging the "muscle knot" may help; however, if there are any signs of thrombophlebitis (red, swollen, tender, or warm areas), the leg should not be massaged. If this continues to be a problem, the physician may order medications specific to the problem.

broad or round ligament pain

As the uterus increases in size and weight, it stretches and pulls on the broad and round ligaments that support it. Getting up from a sitting or reclining position or sudden twisting or jerking may cause a sharp pain in the lower outer aspect of the abdomen. It is more commonly experienced on one side but may occur on both sides at the same time.

Resting on the left side with the knees drawn up close to the abdomen can offer some relief. Sudden position changes, twisting, and jerking movements should be avoided. Localized heat may give temporary relief.

backache

The enlarging uterus causes the woman to change her posture to maintain her balance. The angle of the lumbar region increases (lordosis), straining the muscles and producing pain.

Wearing low-heeled shoes offers some relief, as does performing pelvic exercises. A firmer mattress may help by increasing support to the lower back. A bed board under the mattress also can achieve the necessary firmness.

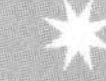

> **nursing alert**
> *Although backache is a common discomfort during pregnancy, it needs to be carefully assessed because it also could signal urinary tract infection or premature labor.*

hemorrhoids

Varicose veins occurring in the rectum are called *hemorrhoids* and result from the increasing weight of the uterus pressing on the rectal vessels. This causes them to enlarge or bulge and produces pain, itching, and generalized rectal discomfort. Constipation also can contribute to the formation of the hemorrhoids by making it necessary to strain during defecation.

Increasing fluids and fiber in the diet to prevent constipation offers some relief. Alternating use of ice packs and sitz baths also may bring temporary relief. If the hemorrhoids feel hard or cause rectal bleeding, the woman needs to notify the physician. He or she may order topical ointments or local anesthetics to relieve the pain. The woman should check with her physician before taking any over-the-counter medications.

orientation of parents to prenatal care

The first prenatal visit to the clinic or physician's office can be stressful for the client. She may come alone or with her partner. A warm and friendly attitude on the part of the nurse can allay many of her fears. By encouraging questions and giving clear, easy-to-understand explanations, the nurse helps make this initial visit a positive experience. The woman or couple should be made to feel welcome and encouraged to participate actively in the plan of care.

If the partner is present, the partner should be included in the orientation. If the partner is not present, the nurse extends a welcome for future visits. The partner may feel uncomfortable in a maternity setting, and a few words of encouragement may help alleviate this discomfort.

Orientation includes a description of the physical layout of the building, a tour of the facility, an explanation of the hours they are open, and telephone numbers to use in case of an emergency. A written copy of the information should be provided for later reference.

health history

At the first prenatal visit, the nurse needs to obtain the client's complete health history to assist in individualizing care. The history includes biographic data, obstetric history, information on the current pregnancy, and a medical history, including family history.

biographic data

The nurse needs to obtain the woman's name, address, phone number, age, and birth date. This is important because clients younger than 15 years or older than 35 years are at risk for prenatal complications (see Chap. 9). These women may need additional testing and monitoring throughout their pregnancy.

Information concerning the woman's marital status is helpful in determining her support systems. Family and friends can offer important emotional and physical support for the pregnant woman. This is a good time to determine whether the woman will need the assistance of social services for transportation, financial aid, housing, and so forth.

obstetric history

The obstetric history includes the number of past pregnancies and any pertinent subjective and objective information. Points to explore include the following:

- Number of past pregnancies
- Number of viable births
- Any abortions or stillbirths
- Any medical illnesses during the pregnancies
- Any spotting, bleeding, or edema during the pregnancies
- Whether the woman received prenatal care
- Length of gestation for each pregnancy
- Length of labor for each pregnancy
- Any problems during labor and birth (mother or infant)
- Any birth defects or congenital anomalies
- Type of deliveries
- Any problems with anesthetics
- Any excess bleeding or infections immediately following the births
- Any problems with postpartum depression

After obtaining this information, the nurse can use one of two methods (para + gravida or TPAL, discussed in Chap. 7) to record the number of pregnancies and their results.

history of current pregnancy

Information regarding the current pregnancy must be established during the first prenatal visit. At this time, the nurse needs to determine the estimated date of delivery (EDD) using Nägele's rule (see Chap. 7).

If the client cannot remember the date of her last menstrual period (this may happen, particularly if she has irregular menstrual cycles), the due date can be established by estimating uterine growth and using ultrasound.

The nurse also should assess the client's emotional status regarding this pregnancy. This would be an appropriate time to explore the need for information and referrals based on the client's responses.

medical history

A general medical history of the client and family is particularly helpful for establishing a baseline of information to develop a care plan for this pregnancy. It also alerts the health care team to potential complications that may arise during this pregnancy. The nurse should pay particular attention to a history of sexually transmitted diseases, tuberculosis, hereditary diseases, and any history of multiple births. A history of childhood diseases, medical diseases and their treatment, past surgeries, bleeding disorders, accidents, injuries, and emotional problems should be explored.

At this time the woman's blood type and Rh status should be determined and her weight and height obtained. A history of the use of medications (over-the-counter and prescription), allergies to medications or foods, menstrual problems, and the past use of contraception should be obtained. A current record of immunizations also should be obtained.

Information regarding the father's health history should be obtained. It should include a history of any health problems, exposure to industrial chemicals or hazards, blood type and Rh, a history of genetic or congenital disorders, and his attitude toward the present pregnancy.

physical examination

During the first prenatal visit, a complete physical examination will be performed, which includes the following:

* Vital signs should be recorded for use as baseline data for comparison with results later in the pregnancy.
* Height and weight are required to determine total weight gain.
* Examination of the breasts, including the nipples is necessary; special preparation for breast-feeding is required for a woman with inverted nipples.
* Palpation of the abdomen during the first trimester allows for examination of the liver, spleen, and bowel and auscultation of the fetal heart after 10 weeks' gestation. In the second and third trimesters, it allows for examination of fetal position and measurement of fundal height.
* Perineal examination allows infections, hemorrhoids, and varicosities of the vulva to be identified and treated.
* Pelvic examination is necessary to inspect the cervix visually and obtain laboratory specimens as needed (Display 8-1).

display 8-1
preparation of a woman for pelvic examination

1. Give thorough explanation to decrease fear and anxiety.
2. Have woman empty her bladder prior to examination to prevent discomfort and aid in exam.
3. Assist her in assuming a comfortable position on the table.
4. Instruct her to lie on her back with her hands at her sides.
5. Assist her in elevating her head slightly and flexing her knees to relax the abdominal muscles for easier examination.
6. Drape the woman so only the perineal area is exposed.

laboratory tests and screenings

Blood tests, urine tests, and screenings during pregnancy monitor the health and well-being of the mother and fetus.

blood type

Identifying the woman's blood type and Rh status is necessary to determine if any incompatibility exists, such as ABO or Rh, that might endanger the fetus (see Chap. 9). If the woman's blood type is Rh negative, the baby's father must be checked to determine his Rh factor. If his blood type is Rh negative, no other interventions are necessary. If his blood type is Rh positive, the woman must have antibody screenings to determine if her body is producing antibodies for Rh-positive blood. (This happens when the fetus has inherited the father's blood type.)

hemoglobin and hematocrit

The woman's hemoglobin and hematocrit are measured for signs of anemia. The hemoglobin should be 12 g and the hematocrit 35%. If the hemoglobin falls below 10.5 g or the hematocrit below 32%, the woman is anemic, probably due to a diet low in iron. Treatment usually consists of diet counseling and iron supplements.

serology

A serologic test, such as the Venereal Disease Research Laboratory (VDRL) test or the rapid plasma reagin (RPR), is performed to detect syphilis. If the test is positive, the woman is treated with antibiotics to eradicate the disease. If treated before 18 weeks' gestation, the fetus is not likely to be affected. If treated later, the newborn may need treatment after birth. Lack of treatment can cause prematurity, congenital syphilis, or intrauterine death. Sexual intercourse should be avoided for 1 month after treatment.

maternal serum alpha-fetoprotein

The developing fetus produces a protein called *alpha-fetoprotein* (AFP), and it is found in the amniotic fluid and maternal blood. The woman's blood may be tested for AFP between 16 and 18 weeks' gestation. Elevated levels of AFP may indicate neural tube defects, such as spina bifida. Abnormally low levels of AFP may indicate Down syndrome. Approximately 5 to 10 women out of every 100 screened will have abnormal test results (Cunningham, et al., 1993). This does not prove that the fetus has a defect but merely warrants further investigation. The test will be repeated, and if results are still abnormal, the doctor will order an ultrasound or amniocentesis for further clarification.

triple screen

Recent studies have shown that screening the AFP with two additional maternal serum hormones, unconjugated estriol and chorionic gonadotropin, increases the efficiency of screening for Down syndrome. This procedure is called the "triple screen." Women with a low AFP, low unconjugated estriol, and a high level of chorionic gonadotropin are more likely to have an infant with Down syndrome and are encouraged to follow these tests results with an amniocentesis to confirm the diagnosis.

hepatitis b

Hepatitis B virus (HBV) may be transmitted to the fetus in utero or during delivery. An estimated 18,000 to 22,000 infants are born each year to mothers who are positive for the hepatitis B antigen. Unless treated, approximately 4,000 to 6,000 of these infants will become carriers of the virus and may suffer from cirrhosis or other liver ailments later in life (Centers for Disease Control, 1990). The Centers for Disease Control and Prevention recommend that mothers who are at risk should be tested. Populations at risk include the following:

- Women of Asian, Pacific Island, and Alaskan Eskimo descent
- Women of Haitian descent
- Recipients of repeated blood transfusions
- Intravenous (IV) drug users or partners of IV drug users
- Women who have been exposed to hepatitis B
- Women who have had multiple sexual partners

Following delivery, the infant should receive immunization. Passive immunization with 0.5 mg of intramuscular hepatitis B immune globulin immediately following birth seems to be effective. This should be followed by injections of the hepatitis vaccine at 1 week, 1 month, and 6 months of age. Following these guidelines prevents 9 out of 10 cases of HBV infection and chronic carrier states (Centers for Disease Control, 1990).

urine tests

A variety of urine tests may be performed during pregnancy. Most commonly, the urine is checked for the presence of protein, which may indicate kidney disease or pregnancy-induced hypertension (PIH). The urine also is monitored for glucose, which if detected, necessitates further testing to rule out gestational diabetes. A urine culture and sensitivity test may be performed if the woman reports burning with urination.

screenings

Screenings are performed to rule out diseases or complications that can occur during pregnancy. The most common screenings performed are diabetic screenings and group B *Streptococcus* screenings.

diabetic screening Diabetic screening is performed at 24 to 28 weeks' gestation. The woman is given a sweet cola-flavored beverage to drink (Glucola). It contains 50 g of glucose. One hour later, a blood sample is drawn. If the blood sugar reading is higher than 135 mg, a more sensitive test (the 3-hour glucose tolerance test) is performed.

group b streptococcus Group B *Streptococcus* is present in approximately 20% of all pregnant women at the time of delivery. They are considered carriers because they do not actively have the disease but may pass it to their newborns during labor and delivery if the infant swallows or inhales the bacteria from the amniotic fluid. Only 1% to 2% of these newborns contract the disease, but if they are not treated, the disease can cause pneumonia, meningitis, lung and kidney damage, loss of vision, and hearing and developmental delays.

Screening for *Streptococcus* B requires periodic cultures of the cervix and pharynx at 26 to 28 weeks' gestation. If the cultures are positive, the woman is treated with antibiotics to decrease the risk of transmission to the infant.

other fetal–maternal evaluation tests

Many different tests to assess fetal well-being during late pregnancy have been advanced in the past few years. Some of these tests include maternal assessment of fetal movement, contraction stress tests (oxytocin challenge test, nipple stimulation test), and the nonstress test.

maternal assessment of fetal movement ("kick count")

Studies have shown that the movement of the fetus, "kick count," can provide information about the general well-being of the fetus. During the third trimester, the fetus should move a minimum of 10 times during a 2-hour period. If there is less movement, further diagnostic tests may be performed to rule out problems. The woman should be instructed to do kick counts twice a day, morning and afternoon, about 1 to 2 hours after eating. Lying on her left side, she counts the movements of the fetus until she reaches a total of 10. If the fetus does not move within ½ hour, she should eat or drink something containing sugar and recount. It she does not feel movement during the next 2 hours, she should contact her physician.

contraction stress tests

Contraction stress testing involves the use of an external fetal monitor (Fig. 8-1). The monitor is attached to two belts that are placed on the woman's abdomen. One belt contains a device to detect and record the fetal heart beat; the other belt contains a device that is placed over the fundus of the uterus to detect any uterine contractions. (See Chap. 12 for discussion of fetal monitoring and interpretation.)

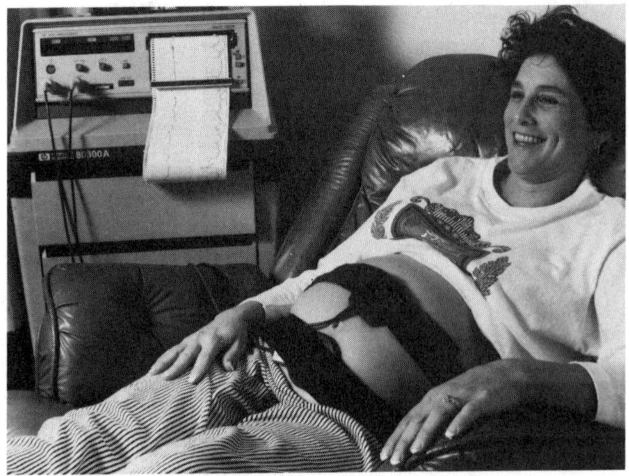

figure 8-1 *Electronic fetal monitoring.*

The two types of stress tests are the oxytocin challenge test and the nipple stimulation test.

oxytocin challenge test The oxytocin challenge test requires the use of a fetal monitor to record the uterine contractions and fetal heart beats. Oxytocin is administered intravenously in increasing dosages until the woman has three uterine contractions in a 10-minute period. The response of the fetal heart beat in relation to the contraction is then assessed. This test is usually performed after 30 weeks' gestation.

At the height of a normal uterine contraction, the blood supply to the fetus decreases, and the fetal heart rate drops briefly. If there is a normal placental reserve of oxygen, the heart rate immediately returns to normal. If there is placental insufficiency, however, the fetal heart rate may drop after the peak of the contraction and may not recover until after the contraction ends (late deceleration). This would indicate a positive test, and the physician should be notified. The placenta may be deteriorating, and delivery of the fetus should be considered. A negative test result indicates that the placenta is functioning normally and can withstand the ordeal of labor.

nipple stimulation test The nipple stimulation test is noninvasive and can deliver the same information as the oxytocin challenge test without the IV administration of oxytocin. This test is based on the fact that stimulation of the nipples causes the pituitary gland to secrete oxytocin. The woman is instructed to roll her nipples between the thumb and index finger in an attempt to develop three uterine contractions within a 10-minute period. If unsuccessful after 1 hour, an oxytocin challenge test is initiated. The results of the nipple stimulation test are interpreted the same way as the oxytocin challenge test.

nonstress test

The nonstress test measures the response of the fetal heart to fetal movement. If the fetus is healthy and the placenta is delivering adequate oxygen, the fetal heart rate will increase in response to fetal movement.

To perform the test, the nurse attaches a fetal monitor to the woman's abdomen. A monitor strip of approximately 40 minutes with at least two fetal movements and the corresponding fetal heart rate will then be interpreted.

A reactive reading indicates that the fetus had an increase of at least 15 beats/min lasting for 15 seconds or moved during a 20- to 30-minute period. A nonreactive test (unfavorable response) indicates fetal hypoxia.

biophysical profile

The *biophysical profile* uses ultrasonography to assess for the presence of fetal anomalies and fetal risks, including the potential for perinatal asphyxia. Five different variables are assessed: breathing movement, body movement, tone, amniotic fluid volume, and fetal heart rate. Each variable is assigned 2 points for a maximum total of 10 points. A score of 2 indicates normal; 1, questionable; and 0, abnormal. A score of 8 to 10 is considered normal. A fetus scoring 6 or less is at high risk for perinatal asphyxia or premature birth.

display 8-2
danger signs during pregnancy

1. Vaginal spotting or bleeding
2. Swelling of the face
3. Severe continuous headache
4. Blurred vision or other visual disturbances
5. Persistent vomiting
6. Abdominal pain
7. Painful urination
8. Lack of fetal movement
9. Sudden gush of fluid from the vagina
10. Fever above 100°F.

subsequent prenatal visits

The pregnant woman normally is scheduled for the following prenatal visits:

* Every four weeks until 28 weeks' gestation
* Every 2 weeks from 30 to 36 weeks' gestation
* Every week from 37 weeks' gestation to delivery

The woman will be seen more often if she develops an illness or one of the danger signs (Display 8-2). Otherwise, the routine visit will be a time for answering her questions and giving new information. A typical visit also includes the following:

* Blood pressure reading to assess for early signs of pregnancy-induced hypertension
* Measurement of weight to assess weight gain (normal versus abnormal)
* Urinalysis to check for elevated glucose (gestational diabetes) or protein (pregnancy-induced hypertension)
* Measurement of fundal height to assess for proper growth and development of the fetus

health promotion during pregnancy

Many women today realize that pregnancy is a normal physiologic event. However, many women and their partners are concerned about how pregnancy will affect their lifestyle. Although the old saying "all things in moderation" usually applies, the nurse needs to address the personal concerns of each woman or couple. This section includes a discussion of topics that concern many pregnant women: personal hygiene, breast care, sexual activity, exercise, employment, nutrition, and substances to avoid. See the Nursing Care Plan for the Pregnant Client: Health Promotion During Pregnancy.

personal hygiene and safety

Increased perspiration and vaginal discharge make daily baths or showers highly desirable. Usually tub baths may be continued throughout pregnancy unless dilation of the cervix has begun or the membranes are ruptured. Showers

nursing care plan
for the pregnant client: health promotion during pregnancy

NURSING DIAGNOSIS

Knowledge Deficit, related to diet, exercise, and breast care for first-time pregnant family

GOAL: expand and evaluate pregnant family's knowledge base on nutrition, exercise, and breast care during pregnancy

NURSING INTERVENTIONS	RATIONALE	EVALUATION
Evaluate client's knowledge base re: diet, exercise, and breast care.	To begin educating your client, you will need to realize the extent of teaching that will be necessary.	The nurse will have discovered the client knowledge base and teaching needs.
Educate the client regarding nutritional intake, specific caloric, nutrient, and vitamin needs, and normal weight gain.	Appropriate diet during pregnancy will make an important difference in the health of the mother and developing child. The mother will need to understand the basic 5 food groups, as well as recommended proportions. Vitamin requirements increase during pregnancy due to increase in metabolism, and a supplement will be necessary., Good sources for minerals such as calcium, phosphorus, and iron are vital to the developing fetus and for the mother. The pregnant client should gain 25–35 pounds.	The pregnant client and family will verbally express the importance of good nutrition and demonstrate an increase in their knowledge by review of a diet history. The client will gain 1 lb per week for the first trimester and 2–4 lbs per week for the remaining 2 trimesters.
Teach the client about the importance of physical fitness during pregnancy.	Exercise during pregnancy can promote good physical condition which, in turn, may lessen backstrain and muscle cramps and ease or shorten labor. It is especially important to strengthen abdominal, pelvic, and lower back muscles because of their use during pregnancy and delivery	Client will verbalize that she can continue most prepregnancy exercise after MD approval; however, she should avoid fatigue. Client will express when she should stop exercise (pain, nausea, vomiting). Client will demonstrate an understanding of the contraindications to exercise (vaginal bleeding, history of preterm labor)
Inform the client regarding supportive bras, avoidance of soap on nipples, and exercise to promote future breast-feeding for woman with flat or inverted nipples.	Supportive bras are helpful in providing comfort and preventing back strain. Soap can dry nipples, causing them to crack and bleed. Flat or inverted nipples can be prepared using the Hoffman technique to allow for breast-feeding.	The client will wear a supportive bra and explain proper breast care. If the client has inverted nipples and wishes to breast-feed, then she will demonstrate the Hoffman technique.

are fine; however, the woman should be cautioned to be especially careful in the later stages of pregnancy because her heavier body and shifting balance may make her awkward and prone to slipping and falling. Sitting on a stool during her shower can add to her safety and comfort.

Clothing should be loose and comfortable. Low-heeled shoes are more comfortable and provide better stability to help prevent falling. They also lessen back strain. The use of garters should be avoided because they increase pressure on the lower leg vessels, which contributes to development of varicose veins.

Dental check-ups should be performed early in pregnancy. Good dental hygiene is especially important during pregnancy because the gum tissue is soft and will allow pockets of food to adhere to the tooth near the gumline, increasing the likelihood of dental cavities. The woman needs to tell her dentist about the pregnancy to avoid the use of x-rays, which could harm the fetus. Daily flossing and the use of a fluoride toothpaste are recommended.

Generally, douching is contraindicated during pregnancy. In some cases, the physician may order medicated douches to combat vaginitis.

Car seat belts can continue to be used during pregnancy with some minor adjustments. The lap belt should be placed beneath the abdomen and across the upper thighs. The shoulder belt portion should be placed between the breasts and adjusted so it does not irritate the neck (Fig. 8-2).

Air travel is generally permissible but may require written permission from the physician in later pregnancy. It is a good idea for pregnant women to carry a copy of her medical records in case of an emergency.

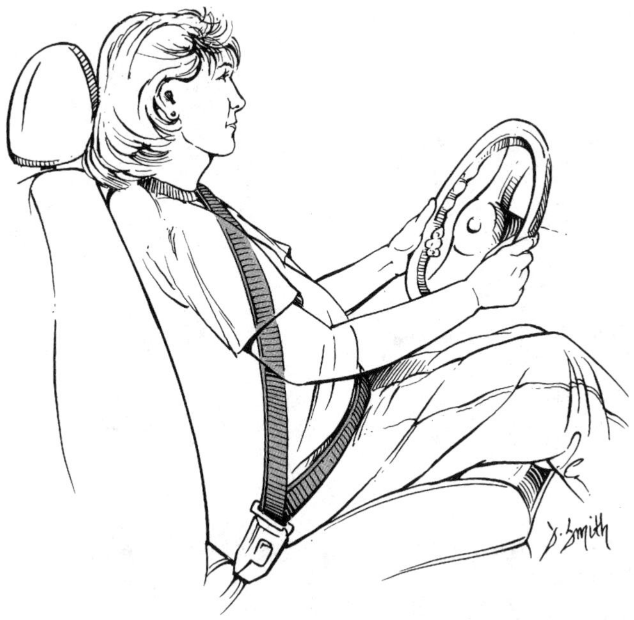

figure 8-2 *Pregnant women should wear seat belt with shoulder strap above the uterus and below the neck and lap belt low and under the abdomen.*

breast care

A proper fitting supportive bra is necessary for comfort and prevention of back strain. It may be necessary to obtain a larger bra as the pregnancy advances. The woman who plans to breast-feed may wish to purchase nursing bras because she can use them after the pregnancy. Breast pads or plastic liners in the bras should be avoided because they provide a dark, warm, moist environment, which promotes growth of bacteria. Soap should not be used on the nipples because it has a drying effect and may cause the nipples to crack and bleed.

Some women may have flat or inverted (resembling a slit or fold) nipples (Fig. 8-3). This condition does not prevent them from breast-feeding. During pregnancy, the nipples can be prepared by using the *Hoffman technique*. Twice daily the woman places her thumbs on either side of the nipple and pulls away from it. Next, she places her thumbs above and below the nipple and repeats the exercise. This will cause the nipple to become more erect and more easily grasped by the infant.

sexual activity

During the first trimester of pregnancy, the woman may experience a decrease in sexual drive. Frequent nausea and vomiting, breast tenderness, and the increase in estrogen levels all contribute to these feelings. The partner may be concerned that he will injure the fetus. During this time, he also may be adjusting to the fact that his partner will soon be a mother as well as his mate. This can temporarily decrease his interest in sexual activity. The need for closeness may still be met by hugging, kissing, and being together.

During the second trimester, the woman may experience an increase in sexual drive. Discomforts of the first trimester have usually decreased, and she begins to feel more physically fit. The vascular congestion of the pelvic organs may enhance enjoyment of sexual contact.

During the third trimester, the woman's abdomen has enlarged, and she tires easily. The couple may try alternate intercourse positions to relieve the discomfort. A side-lying position may produce physical satisfaction and be more comfortable for the woman.

Sexual intercourse during normal pregnancy will not harm the fetus. If the woman experiences vaginal bleeding or the membranes are ruptured, however, intercourse may be contraindicated because of the increased potential for infection. Women with a history of preterm labor may be instructed to abstain from intercourse during the last 8 weeks of pregnancy.

The woman or her partner may feel too embarrassed or uncomfortable to ask questions or express concerns about sexual activity. The nurse who has developed good rapport with his or her clients may introduce this topic during the routine prenatal visits. A good opening statement may be, "Many women worry about sexual contact during pregnancy. Do you have concerns that you would like to discuss?" Exploring sexual concerns may alleviate undue stress and guilt for the couple. Both partners must feel free to discuss their feelings and deal with what is happening and how it is affecting them.

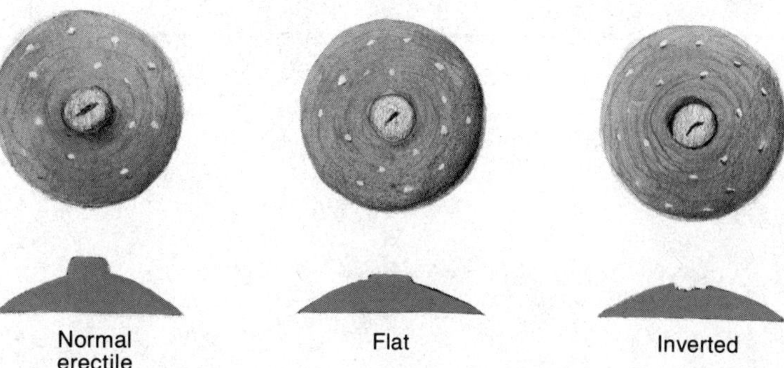

figure 8-3 *Variations of the nipple.*

exercise

Maintaining physical fitness is important throughout the life span. During pregnancy, it is particularly important because it strengthens the abdominal, pelvic, and lower back muscles and increases endurance and stamina. The woman who is in good physical condition may have a shorter labor and easier delivery because the muscles are toned and prepared to do their job. Exercising during pregnancy also can relieve some of the common discomforts of pregnancy, such as back strain and muscle cramps.

The amount of exercise tolerated by a pregnant woman depends on her age, stage of pregnancy, general physical condition, and any history of chronic disease. In general, the woman may participate in most of her usual types of exercise but should avoid exercising to the point of fatigue. She must stop any activity if she experiences pain, nausea, or dizziness. She also should avoid sports that could cause a blow to the abdomen. Pregnancy is not the time to engage in a new sport but a time to continue with most sports that the woman is conditioned to perform. Display 8-3 offers guidelines for exercise during pregnancy.

Exercise may be contraindicated or severely limited in the following circumstances:

- A history of preterm labor
- Extreme overweight or underweight
- A history of high blood pressure, heart, lung, or thyroid disease
- Vaginal bleeding
- Severe anemia

Walking is probably one of the most beneficial and inexpensive methods of exercise. The only special equipment needed is a sturdy, comfortable pair of shoes; the woman can pace herself according to her own condition. Walking also is an activity that may be initiated if the woman has not previously exercised. As the pregnancy advances, the woman may find that she tires more easily and becomes somewhat unstable on her feet. She may have to alter her exercise program to allow for these changes.

display 8-3
guidelines for exercise during pregnancy

1. Maintain adequate fluid intake.
2. Warm up slowly; use stretching exercises but avoid overstretching to prevent injury to ligaments.
3. Avoid jerking or bouncing exercises.
4. Be careful of loose throw rugs that could slip and cause injury.
5. Exercise on a regular basis (three times per week).
6. After the first trimester, avoid exercises that require supine position.

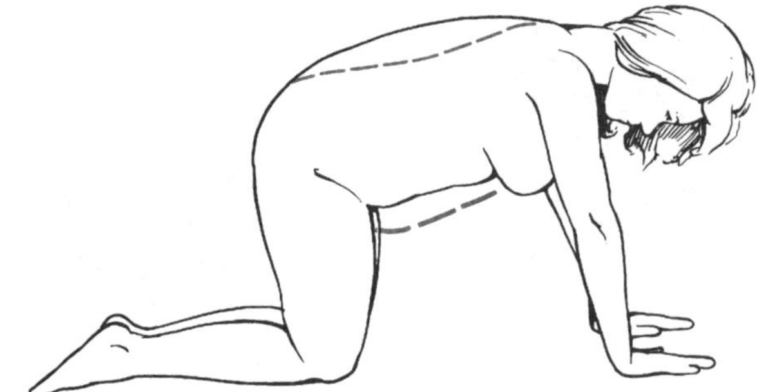

figure 8-4 *Pelvic rock.*

Prenatal classes usually introduce exercises to strengthen the abdominal muscles and limber specific body parts, such as the thigh muscles and perineal muscles. Three of the most commonly practiced exercises include the pelvic rock (tilt), tailor sitting, and Kegel exercises.

pelvic rock, tailor sitting, and Kegel exercises

The pelvic rock or tilt causes the lumbar spine to become more flexible and is helpful in decreasing back pain during pregnancy and labor (Fig. 8-4). Tailor sitting exercises stretch and tone the perineal and thigh muscles in preparation for labor and delivery (Fig. 8-5).

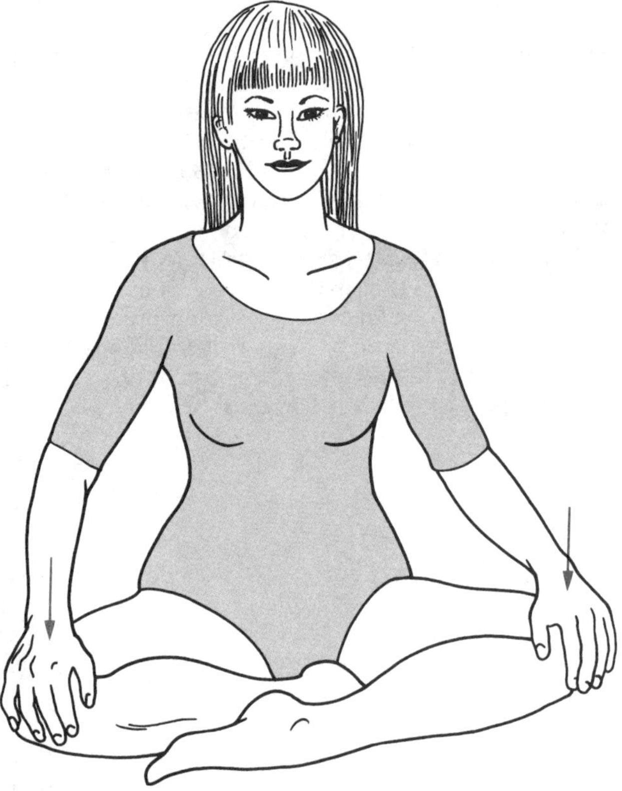

figure 8-5 *Tailor sitting. To perform correctly, place one foot in front of the other; gently push downward on the knees.*

Kegel exercises strengthen the muscles of the pelvic floor. To perform Kegel exercises, the woman should slowly contract and relax the pubococcygeal muscle. To do this, she might imagine that she is urinating and try to stop the flow midstream. Another way to practice is to imagine the perineum as an elevator. In relaxed position, the elevator is on the ground floor. Slowly contracting the perineal muscles takes the elevator to the top floor and then slowly returns to the ground floor as the muscles are relaxed. Practiced daily, Kegel exercises can provide the following benefits:

* Shortening the second stage or birth stage of labor
* Preventing urinary dribbling when the woman coughs, laughs, or sneezes (stress incontinence)
* Preventing a "dropped" bladder, rectum, or uterus (cystocele, rectocele, uterine prolapse) later in life
* Decreasing healing time for perineal sutures (episiotomy) and hemorrhoids

employment

In most instances, the pregnant woman can continue to work throughout her pregnancy. However, if her job requires her to stand longer that 3 hours, lift more than 15 lb, or to have a repeated exposure to vibration or extreme heat or cold, she needs to consider transferring or taking a leave of absence until the infant is born. She needs to avoid certain material or chemicals that may be harmful to the fetus (Display 8-4). If she develops problems, such as high blood pressure, vaginal bleeding, or extreme fatigue, the physician may require her to take a leave of absence. Federal law protects women who must take a leave of absence due to pregnancy. She is guaranteed a return to the same job with no loss of seniority. The nurse can be instrumental in acquiring the necessary forms and information for the client.

display 8-4
harmful materials and chemicals to avoid

1. Anesthetic gases
2. Mercury
3. Glycol ethers
4. Lead
5. Exposure to radiation
6. Carbon monoxide
7. Cell-killing agents
8. Hexachlorophene
9. Organic solvents
10. Pesticides and herbicides

substances to avoid

Many substances, including over-the-counter medications, can cause abnormalities in the developing fetus; such substances are called *teratogens*. Some substances may cause gross malformation of the fetus, while others may cause growth retardation, spontaneous abortion, or stillbirths. The nurse needs to educate the woman about these substances and their potential impact on the fetus. The most common substances that can harm the fetus are caffeine, alcohol, over-the-counter medications, cigarettes, and cocaine and other illegal drugs (controlled substances). Some women may develop a craving for nonfood substances (*pica*), which also may put them at risk.

The Food and Drug Administration (FDA) now requires drug labeling for teratogenicity. The drugs are divided into five categories based on their potential for causing harm to the fetus. The categories range from drugs that cause no harm to the fetus to drugs that are contraindicated for use during pregnancy due to severe harm or death to the fetus. To obtain the latest information on specific teratogens, nurses may call the California Teratogen Registry located at the University of California, San Diego Medical Center (1-800-532-3749).

caffeine

Caffeine is a central nervous system stimulant that is found in coffee, tea, colas, chocolate, and certain over-the-counter medications. The FDA has warned that substances containing caffeine should be limited during pregnancy to 300 mg or less per day. There is some controversy on the possible effects on the fetus but because there may be a link between low birth weight and premature rupture of the membranes, the nurse needs to counsel the woman to limit her use of substances containing caffeine to no more than the recommended amount (Table 8-1).

alcohol

Alcohol is a known teratogenic agent and should not be consumed during pregnancy. It can cause *fetal alcohol syndrome*, a cluster of irreversible birth defects, such as mental retardation, facial and cranial abnormalities, delayed motor function, and low birth weight. As the child matures, behavioral and psychosocial problems also may develop.

The pregnant woman should be counseled to abstain from alcohol consumption during pregnancy. Women with alcohol abuse problems should be referred to an alcohol rehabilitation program for help.

table 8-1 caffeine equivalents

Beverage or Item	*Caffeine*
Coffee (1 cup)	75 mg
Tea (1 cup)	50 mg
Cocoa (1 cup)	10 mg
Coca-Cola (12 oz.)	46 mg
Pepsi Cola	38 mg
Mountain Dew	54 mg

over-the-counter medications

No medications should be taken during pregnancy unless prescribed by the physician who is monitoring the pregnancy. Many women do not realize that aspirin, decongestants, ibuprofen, and many other over-the-counter drugs that are relatively harmless to most nonpregnant women can damage the fetus. For example, aspirin can cross the placental barrier and cause fetal bleeding or increased fetal heart rate; it also can prolong pregnancy or labor. Vitamin supplements also can harm the fetus and should be avoided unless prescribed by the woman's physician.

The nurse needs to emphasize the importance of avoiding the use of over-the-counter drugs. Some physicians will give their clients a list of drugs that may be used during pregnancy for routine discomforts, such as indigestion or mild aches and pains. When reviewing this list with the client, the nurse can impress on her the importance of adhering to the physician's orders.

cigarettes

Cigarette smoking is harmful not only to the mother, but to the unborn child. Nevertheless, about 20% of all pregnant women continue to smoke during their pregnancy (O'Connor, et al., 1992). The more the woman smokes, the more profound are the effects to her and her child. Cigarettes contain carbon monoxide, a toxic gas, that lowers the available oxygen for the woman and the fetus. They also contain nicotine, an addictive stimulant, that causes the blood vessels to constrict and decrease the blood flow. Other harmful toxins found in cigarettes are ammonia, arsenic, cyanide, and formaldehyde.

Smoking decreases maternal absorption and use of calcium, vitamin C, vitamin A, and some of the B vitamins. It has been linked to premature births, low–birth-weight infants, spontaneous abortions, and delayed mental and physical development of the child. In addition, it doubles the risk of sudden infant death syndrome (SIDS) after birth.

Pregnancy can be a strong motivator for cessation of smoking, making it an ideal time for the nurse to educate women about the effects of smoking on her and her child. If the woman is unable to quit, the nurse can urge her to limit her smoking as much as possible because any reduction in smoking can have profound positive effects for the fetus. The woman also should be instructed to avoid an environment in which others smoke because second-hand smoke (*passive smoking*) also can be harmful.

cocaine

Cocaine, a central nervous system stimulant, is an illegal drug that is available as a white powder or as white or colored chips (*crack*). As a powder, it can be inhaled or mixed with water and injected directly into a vein. Crack may be smoked and is more addictive than the powdered form. Because cocaine is addictive, the need for the drug may override the woman's concern for her unborn child. Cocaine addiction is one of the most serious drug problems affecting childbearing families. The numbers of drug-addicted mothers, including adolescents, is currently on the rise (Evans, 1991).

Pregnant women who use cocaine increase their risk of the following:

- Heart attack: An overdose can cause the heart to stop.
- Stroke: Cocaine raises blood pressure.
- Respiratory arrest: Cocaine can cause seizures, resulting in respiratory failure.
- Acquired immunodeficiency syndrome: This disease is transmitted from sharing needles with infected people.
- Spontaneous abortion: Miscarriage can be caused by vasoconstriction of the placenta, resulting in lack of oxygen to the fetus.
- Abruptio placentae: Miscarriage or hemorrhage can be caused by increased blood pressure.

The infant born to a cocaine-addicted mother is at high risk for the following:

- Growth retardation caused by vasoconstriction of the placenta
- Prematurity caused by vasoconstriction of the placenta
- General system failure (tremors, jitters, visual problems, poor tolerance to feeding, diarrhea, and increased startle response) caused by faulty organ development

Cocaine addiction is a serious problem affecting women in all walks of life. Most women are reluctant to admit to the use of cocaine because it is an illegal drug. The cocaine user is often difficult to identify because the drug is metabolized so quickly, disappearing from the urine within 24 to 48 hours after use. Identification of the signs of possible cocaine addiction requires keen assessment skills on the part of the nurse. These signs include mood swings, depression, changes in appetite, irritability, and lack of interest or motivation. The nurse needs to be supportive and nonjudgmental. Interesting the woman in a drug recovery program should be attempted; however, this is often a difficult task because the addiction is so strong.

Several states, including Texas, Wyoming, Connecticut, Indiana, South Carolina, and Kentucky, have prosecuted women for taking drugs during pregnancy. Although this trend shows concern for the unborn child, many health care professionals are concerned that addicted pregnant women will not seek prenatal care due to fear of prosecution. Cocaine abuse among pregnant women remains a national dilemma.

pica

Some pregnant women develop a craving for a nonfood substance, such as laundry starch, clay, coffee grounds, ice cubes, and a variety of other substances. Called *pica*, this condition is not limited to a particular ethnic or cultural group but is more common among lower socioeconomic groups. It is not unusual for these women to have iron-deficiency anemia, but it is not known whether this a cause of pica or a result. It is important to identify women with pica, to refer them for additional nutritional counseling, and to discuss the risks involved. Many women with

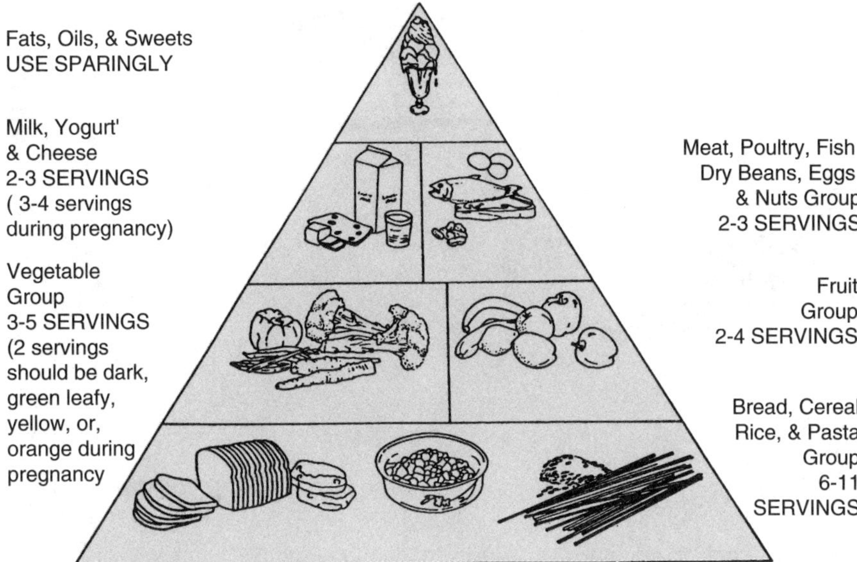

figure 8-6 *The food pyramid.*

pica will consume these substances to the extent that their daily nutritional requirements are not met.

nutrition

Adequate nutritional intake during pregnancy makes a profound difference in the health of the mother and her developing child. The nutritional status of the mother directly affects the growth and development of the fetus and can prevent the development of such maternal complications as anemia and pregnancy-induced hypertension. Adequate maternal nutrition helps prevent low birth weight and impaired organ development. Contrary to the popular myth that the growing fetus extracts needed nutritional requirements from the mother's body, the nutritional intake of the fetus depends on the mother's nutritional intake. In that sense, the pregnant woman really is "eating for two."

In 1992, the United States Department of Agriculture developed a pyramid (Fig. 8-6) to replace the basic four food groups. It emphasizes the importance of variety and proportions in the daily diet. The size of the block on the pyramid denotes the importance and proportion of the food group needed. The basic five food groups range from largest (greatest amount needed) to smallest, as follows: 1) grains, 2) vegetables, 3) fruits, 4) milk, and 5) meats. The very tip of the pyramid (the smallest section) contains fats, oils, and sweets (called "other group"); foods in this group have very little nutritional value. They may be eaten occasionally but should not replace any of the basic five.

The pyramid is an excellent teaching tool for the maternity nurse because it removes the mystique from nutritional counseling. The only change needed when instructing the pregnant woman on the use of the pyramid is to increase her calcium intake to the highest recommended number of servings (four).

During pregnancy, the need for most nutrients increases. The pregnant woman may need to learn how to make wise selections from the food groups to meet these needs. Food should always be discussed in terms of servings, not milligrams, calories, or percentages. The nurse should be sensitive to any cultural, economic, and psychosocial implications that diet changes may have for the client. Referrals should be made to a registered dietician as needed.

weight gain

The recommended weight gain during pregnancy is 25 to 35 lb. A woman who is underweight may need to gain as much as 40 lb. One who is obese may need to gain slightly less. Pregnancy is not the time for weight loss dieting because the woman may not receive enough nutrients. A woman who is carrying twins or triplets may need to gain more than one who is carrying a single fetus.

Typically, the majority of the weight is gained during the last two trimesters. The usual pattern of weight gain is 2 to 4 lb during the first trimester and an average of 1 lb/wk during the second and third trimesters (Display 8-5).

> **nursing alert**
>
> *Assess the pregnant woman for sudden weight changes. Sudden weight gain suggests fluid retention; sudden weight loss suggests medical illness.*

Most women lose approximately 10 lb at delivery (the combined weight of the baby and fluid loss) and 5 lb or more during the following month. The remainder of the weight gained during pregnancy is lost gradually during the next few months but may take 1 year or more if a great deal of weight was gained. Breast-feeding and exercise can hasten this process.

display 8-5
distribution of weight gain

Breasts: 1 to 3 lb
Uterus: 2 to 2.5 lb
Body fluid: 8 lb
Blood volume: 3.5 lb
Fetus: 7 to 7.5 lb
Placenta: 1.5 lb
Amniotic fluid: 2 to 2.5 lb

caloric intake

During normal pregnancy, the caloric intake should increase from 2,200 to 2,500 for the average woman, an increase of 300 calories. The added calories are needed because of the increased metabolic rate, the increased workload from the extra body weight that the woman is carrying, and the nutritional needs of the developing placenta and fetus. These calories should come from foods rich in essential nutrients. This means she should avoid foods from the tip of the food pyramid. Foods such as doughnuts, potato chips, and candy bars provide empty calories (low in nutritional content). The pregnant woman should be encouraged to make an additional choice from the calcium group and the protein group to supply the extra calories and additional nutrients.

nutrient needs

All foods are made of a combination of proteins, carbohydrates, and fats. Contained in these food substances are the vitamins (fat soluble and water soluble) and minerals necessary for a healthy body.

The National Academy of Science's Food and Nutrition Board establish the Recommended Dietary Allowances (RDAs) for the normal healthy adult. They also set RDAs for the pregnant woman (Display 8-6).

protein

Daily protein intake should increase to 60 g during pregnancy. This is an increase of approximately 20% above the prepregnancy recommended consumption and is needed for fetal growth and development and formation of the placenta and amniotic fluid. In the woman, this increase is necessary for growth of additional breast tissue, uterine tissue, and expansion of the blood volume. Excellent sources of protein include eggs, milk, yogurt, cheese, meat, poultry, and seafood.

carbohydrates

Complex carbohydrates should supply approximately 50% of the total calories in the nonpregnant woman. During the second and third trimesters, the intake should increase by 14%. Carbohydrates are necessary for the formation of red blood cells, digestion, growth of bones and tissues, and the formation of the digestive and nervous system. Excellent sources of complex carbohydrates include whole-grain breads, pasta, rice, and cereals.

fats

Fats are the most concentrated source of energy in the diet. Most body cells can directly oxidize fatty acids to produce energy. Two essential fatty acids, linoleic acid and linolenic acid, cannot be synthesized by the body and must come from the diet. These acids are necessary for the metabolism of cholesterol. The woman should use vegetable oils rather than animal fat (lard) to supply these essential fatty acids.

vitamins

Most vitamin requirements increase during pregnancy because of increased metabolism. The pregnant woman must eat a variety of foods to obtain the necessary vitamins. A vitamin supplement may be ordered by the physi-

display 8-6
recommended dietary allowance during pregnancy

PROTEIN (g)	60
FAT-SOLUBLE VITAMINS	
Vitamins	
Vitamin A (mcg)	800
Vitamin D (mcg)	10
Vitamin E (mg)	10
Vitamin K (mcg)	65
WATER-SOLUBLE VITAMINS	
Vitamin C (mg)	70
Thiamine (mg)	1.5
Niacin (mg)	17
Vitamin B_6 (mg)	2.2
Folate (mcg)	400
Vitamin B_{12}	2.2
MINERALS	
Calcium (mg)	1,200
Phosphorus (mg)	1,200
Magnesium (mg)	320
Iron (mg)	30
Zinc (mg)	15
Iodine (mcg)	175
Selenium (mcg)	65

Adapted from National Research Council (US) Subcommittee on the Tenth Edition of the RDAs: Recommended Dietary Allowances. Washington, DC: National Academy Press, 1989.

cian, but the woman needs to be careful about self-medication with vitamins to avoid serious complications. The two broad categories of vitamins are fat soluble and water soluble.

fat-soluble vitamins Fat-soluble vitamins (A, D, E, and K) are absorbed into the lymphatic system with fat. They cannot be excreted when consumed in excess but are stored in the liver and adipose tissue and can be toxic when consumed in large doses.

Vitamin A increases the body's resistance to infection and is necessary for cell, bone, and tooth formation. Good sources of vitamin A include dark green, leafy vegetables; yellow fruits and vegetables; and milk fortified with vitamin A.

Vitamin D helps the body use calcium and phosphorus in bone and tooth formation and in the absorption of iron. Good sources of vitamin D include liver, fish, fortified milk, cheese, and eggs. Vitamin D also is produced when the skin is exposed to sunlight.

Vitamin E is the most important antioxidant in the body. It also assists in maintaining the cell wall and protects red blood cells from breakdown. Good sources of vitamin E include vegetable oils; nuts; green, leafy vegetables; and grains.

Vitamin K is necessary for the formation of prothrombin, which promotes normal blood clotting. It is synthesized in the lower gastrointestinal tract but still relies on dietary intake to maintain adequate levels. Good sources of vitamin K include dark green, leafy vegetables and liver.

water-soluble vitamins The water-soluble vitamins include vitamin C and the B-complex vitamins (including folic acid). They are absorbed through the intestinal wall into the bloodstream. They are considered nontoxic because the excess amounts are filtered through the kidneys and excreted in the urine.

Vitamin C is responsible for the formation of teeth and strong bones, the formation of the blood vessels, and the production of the "glue" (*collagen*) that holds the body's tissues and cells together. Good sources of vitamin C include fresh fruits (especially citrus fruits), green and red peppers, greens, spinach, and broccoli.

b-complex vitamins The B-complex vitamins include folic acid, thiamine, riboflavin, niacin, and vitamin B_{12}. The B-vitamins are necessary for many of the metabolic functions of the body. Folic acid has received particular notice in recent years for its role in deoxyribunucleic acid (DNA) and ribonucleic acid synthesis (RNA), which is responsible for reproduction of cells and transmission of inherited characteristics. In 1992, the United States Public Health Service recommended that all women of child-bearing age consume 0.4 mg of folic acid per day. Research has documented that defects in the closure of the spinal column during embryonic development (neural tube defects) in newborns can be prevented if the woman ingests adequate levels of folic acid before and during pregnancy. Good sources of folic acid and the B vitamins include whole grains; eggs; dark green, leafy vegetables; beans; beef liver; and fresh fruits.

minerals

Minerals are essential to the structure and function of the body. They help to build cell structures, maintain acid–base balance, and transmit messages in the nervous system. The intake of calcium, phosphorus, iron, zinc, and sodium is particularly important during pregnancy.

calcium and phosphorus Calcium and phosphorus play a role in the formation of bones, teeth, cells, and tissues of the body. The woman's calcium requirements during pregnancy increase by 50% from 800 to 1,200 mg/d. The calcium is stored in the woman's bones for use by the fetus during the last trimester. Good sources of calcium and phosphorus include milk and dairy products, oatmeal, dry beans, and dark green, leafy vegetables.

iron Increased iron, the chief component of hemoglobin, is needed during pregnancy to manufacture maternal and fetal red blood cells. During pregnancy, the recommended amount of iron increases to 30 mg/d to meet these needs. In the third trimester, the fetal liver begins to store iron for use during the first 4 to 6 months after birth when breast milk or nonfortified formula fails to provide an adequate supply of iron. Because dietary iron is poorly absorbed, the physician will prescribe an iron supplement during pregnancy. The woman needs to know that iron supplements can cause her stool to be black and tarry and can contribute to constipation. She should increase her fluid and fiber intake to alleviate the problem. If constipation persists, the physician may order a stool softener. Good sources of iron include eggs, meat, and greens.

zinc During pregnancy, the woman should ingest 15 mg/d of zinc. Deficiencies of zinc may lead to congenital malformations, prolonged and difficult labor, and increased risk of bacterial infections in the amniotic fluid. Because zinc is found in most high-protein foods, adequate protein intake ensures adequate zinc. Good sources of zinc include fish, meats, egg yolks, and liver.

sodium Sodium is an electrolyte that is responsible for water and electrolyte balance. In the past, the pregnant woman was instructed to limit or restrict her salt (sodium) intake to prevent swelling (edema). We now know that the sodium requirement during pregnancy is actually increased to assist the kidneys with filtration. Because the American diet is rich in sodium, it is not necessary for her to increase the amount of salt. Two to three grams of sodium daily is sufficient to meet her needs. Because edema during pregnancy was formerly thought to be caused by sodium retention, the pregnant woman was often given diuretics. This practice has been discontinued, however, because the drugs can harm the woman and the fetus.

childbirth education and preparation

Many women expecting a child have a profound desire to learn about pregnancy and birth and want to be as well prepared as possible for this event; often, their partners share this wish to learn and prepare for birth. Many prenatal and childbirth programs are offered to meet this need in a variety of settings: prenatal clinics, the Red Cross, hospitals, and community colleges. Childbirth educators can become certified through ASPO/Lamaze (American Society for Psychoprophylaxis in Obstetrics) and other organizations to ensure that they have the professional skills and competence to meet the needs of expectant families.

While the program length and organization may differ among the various classes offered, all have certain content in common:

- Anatomy and physiology of the reproductive systems with emphasis on the changes that occur during pregnancy
- Fetal growth and development
- Proper nutrition during pregnancy and self-help techniques to cope with the minor discomforts of pregnancy
- Pain management, relaxation, and breathing techniques that can be used during labor and delivery
- The role of a support person during labor and delivery
- The possibility of high-risk birth, including cesarean delivery
- Preparation for parenting: breast-feeding and bottle feeding, infant growth and development, and well-baby care
- A tour of the maternal–newborn facility

Many other programs for family support also have become available, such as sibling support classes, which prepare the children of the family for the coming addition. Classes for grandparents discuss their role, encourage their support, and review current trends in infant care. Many facilities also offer breast-feeding classes. These classes include information on preparation of the breasts, techniques for breast-feeding, and advantages and disadvantages of breast-feeding.

teaching guidelines
assisting the woman with plans for prepared childbirth

- Select a support person that will act as your coach throughout the classes and the labor; be sure it is someone with whom you feel comfortable.
- It is important for you and your support person to attend all classes.
- Once classes have begun, be sure to practice the techniques daily; the more you practice, the more skilled you will become.
- Relax and enjoy learning; be sure to ask questions as needed.

family considerations

Today's family wants to make informed choices that are right for them and the developing child. Many questions are brought to mind when they hear terms like prepared childbirth, Lamaze, natural childbirth, and breathing patterns. The nurse can be instrumental in offering information that will allow the family to make the choices that are appropriate for them.

The nurse may assist the family in the following ways:

- Answering questions in easy to understand terminology
- Listening carefully for cues about cultural or religious beliefs that may affect the birth process
- Describing the various childbirth education classes available to the family, including names, times, and places
- Offering pamphlets, brochures, and other materials that the family may study at home

The Teaching Guidelines display also will help the woman with plans for prepared childbirth.

methods of pain management

Over the years, many methods have been developed to reduce the pain or discomfort of labor and birth. As early as the 1930s, women began to demand help and more control with this natural process. Three pioneers in this effort were Dr. Grantly Dick-Read, Dr. Robert Bradley, and Dr. Fernand Lamaze. Today, most programs are based on the Lamaze method or a combination of methods to meet the needs of the childbearing woman. Regardless of the approach, they are based on common principles:

- Providing information about the birth process diminishes fear and anxiety, which in turn diminishes pain.
- Physical preparation, such as relaxation and breathing techniques, diminishes the pain of labor.
- A coach or support person helps the woman maintain her focus, thus reducing her pain.

dick-read method

Dr. Grantly Dick-Read was one of the first physicians to show an interest in assisting the pregnant woman to a more rewarding labor and delivery. He believes that childbirth pain revolves in a vicious cycle: fear-pain-tension-fear. He believes that as the pain begins, the woman becomes fearful of the unknown. This increases the pain, resulting in increased tension. As labor progresses, the cycle continues to build, and the pain intensifies.

In his book, *Childbirth Without Fear*, he proposes the idea that this cycle can be broken by 1) educating the woman about her body and the birth process; 2) assisting her with relaxation; and 3) encouraging slow breathing during the contractions.

bradley method

In 1965, Dr. Robert Bradley published *Husband-Coached Childbirth*, in which he emphasizes the importance of the husband's role in childbirth. He believes that the husband should be with the woman throughout the labor process to coach and support her. This method uses breathing patterns and relaxation techniques similar to Dr. Dick-Read's method. He also emphasizes the importance of reduced environmental stimuli to promote comfort: dimming the lights and keeping the room as quiet as possible during labor. The Academy of Husband-Coached Childbirth prepares teachers to conduct prenatal classes on the Bradley method.

lamaze method

Dr. Fernand Lamaze, a French obstetrician, developed the method of prepared childbirth and pain management that bears his name. This method is based on his experiences in a Leningrad obstetric clinic in Russia. He uses the term *psychoprophylactic* (mental prevention) to describe his method for reducing childbirth pain. He studied Pavlov's works on *conditioned response* (a pleasurable response can be substituted for a painful response) and pain perception. Pavlov discovered that the mind can receive only one strong message at a time; all other messages become secondary and can be inhibited or greatly decreased, a phenomenon known as the *gate control theory*.

By bombarding the mind of the laboring woman with many messages, pain becomes a secondary message and may be eliminated or at least diminished. The Lamaze method uses a variety of techniques to accomplish this task, including relaxation, imagery, and breathing techniques. A support person, the woman's partner or a close friend, helps keep the woman focused on these techniques.

relaxation

Relaxation is the focused release of tension in all or part of the body. It is a learned behavior through which the woman recognizes the difference between tension and relaxation of various muscle groups. She also learns how to maintain conscious relaxation of the muscle groups by developing an awareness of her body, concentrating, and practicing this technique repeatedly. The more she practices, the more control she will learn to exert, even during intense labor contractions. Relaxation interferes with the normal tension that pain produces. This tension during labor can cause exhaustion, deplete the oxygen supply, increase the perception of pain, and even prolong the duration of labor.

imagery

Once the woman has learned to relax, she can begin to practice imagery. Imagery is a form of daydreaming, like taking a mental vacation to someplace serene. Some women may use a "focal point," such as a picture, card, or some memento that has special meaning. This focal point is placed in their line of vision, and they concentrate on it while forming mental images. Other women may choose to take a mental vacation to the beach, the mountains, or some other special place. For imagery to be successful, the woman must be totally relaxed. The more life she brings to the image, the more successful she will be in decreasing the painful stimuli. She should focus on special sounds, smells, tastes, sights, and feelings that the image or place brings to mind.

An example of imagery is to think of a sandy beach:

- It is quiet.
- There is a gentle breeze blowing through the palm trees.
- The sun is bright and warm.
- The sand is soft and warm as it sifts through your fingers.
- The surf can be heard as it gently rushes over the sand.
- There is a taste of salt in the air.

The more "real" the woman can make the image, the more relaxed and preoccupied she will become. The nurse or coach should not interrupt the woman during this time because it will break her concentration. The woman must select a place that is special for her. If she detests sand and surf, this scene would defeat the purpose because it would produce tension for her.

breathing techniques

Breathing techniques alone do not alter pain perception, but the concentration necessary to control the learned breathing patterns is linked to the ability to relax. To practice the breathing techniques, the woman should assume a comfortable, relaxed position. She should select her focal point or special image and begin and end each contraction with a slow, cleansing breath. This is important during practice and during labor. The cleansing breath oxygenates mother and fetus and is an indicator to maintain relaxation. Her coach may need to remind her to take the cleansing breaths. Most people prefer to breath in and out through the nose but mouth breathing or a combination of mouth and nose breathing also is fine. She may find her mouth gets dry; if so, she may use a lollipop, ice chips, or sips of water.

Years of research on breathing patterns has led to the four distinct patterns that are used today. These include *slow-paced breathing, modified-paced breathing, patterned-paced breathing, and expulsion breathing*. The woman may find that she uses one or all four of these patterns during her labor. The choice is up to her.

slow-paced breathing

Slow-paced breathing includes approximately 6 to 10 breaths per minute or about half the normal breathing rate. As she breathes in, the chest and abdomen should gently expand and then relax with exhalation. Some women may use a technique called *effleurage* during this type of breathing. Effleurage is the gentle, rhythmic stroking of the abdomen, thighs, or bed linens. This motion may help with relaxation. Corn starch applied lightly will decrease the friction or drag on her skin.

modified-paced breathing

As the contractions become more intense, the mother may find she cannot sustain her control with slow-paced breathing. Modified-paced breathing allows her to increase her rate to almost twice that of her normal respiratory rate. It is primarily chest breathing. The nurse needs to monitor the breathing rate and intensity because respirations that are too rapid and deep respirations can lead to excess loss of carbon dioxide (*hyperventilation*), which, in turn, leads to panic. If hyperventilation occurs, the nurse has the woman breath into cupped hands or a paper bag to restore normal respirations. These episodes, if they occur, are usually only temporary. Hyperventilation that lasts for a long time can cause loss of consciousness and a decrease in uterine blood flow, placing the fetus at risk.

patterned-paced breathing

This third type of breathing is a variation of the modified-paced breathing. This method is used when the contractions have reached such intensity that the woman has difficulty concentrating. By adding a soft blow every few breaths she increases her focus. This may be done every third or fourth breath, or she may create her own pattern. If she feels the urge to push and it is too early, she may find a ratio of 1:1 deep breaths to soft blows may be helpful.

expulsion breathing

When the cervix is fully dilated and the fetus is low in the birth canal, the woman may begin pushing to assist with the delivery. Two types of pushing are taught: 1) holding the breath and bearing down or 2) exhaling with a sound or groan coming from the throat while bearing down. There is some concern about holding the breath for long intervals (more than 5 seconds) because it could decrease the pressure in the chest cavity, reducing venous return to the heart. This would result in a decrease of cardiac output, lowering the amount of circulating blood to the uterus. Decreasing the blood supply to the uterus limits the available oxygen supply for the fetus, resulting in fetal distress. Proponents of the groaning push state that this type of expulsion breathing does not interfere with the woman's circulating blood but does cause the abdominal muscles to contract and push on the uterus, thus aiding in the expulsion of the fetus. Regardless of the method chosen, the woman must continue to take a cleansing breath before and after the contraction.

Relaxation is still the key to control. The nurse needs to remind the woman to relax as needed and to focus her pushing toward the perineal floor. It is important to praise and encourage the woman throughout this period.

what would you do? ✷

Amalia is expecting her first child in a few months. She and her husband speak Spanish and have been in this country for 6 months. She rides the bus to the clinic for her visits because she does not have a driver's license. She has expressed a desire to enroll in childbirth preparation classes. She has concerns that she has shared with the nurse: 1) She has a limited understanding of the English language and is afraid she will not understand the instructor. 2) Her husband does not want to participate in the birth experience because he feels that it is not appropriate for the man to be present.

key points ✷

- ✷ **The discomforts of pregnancy are the result of the normal anatomic and physiologic changes that occur during pregnancy. They disappear with delivery, and many can be alleviated with simple interventions.**
- ✷ **The first prenatal visit can be stressful for the woman and her partner. It is important to make them feel welcome and to encourage them to participate actively in the plan of care.**
- ✷ **Laboratory tests and screenings performed during prenatal visits include blood type and Rh status, hemoglobin and hematocrit, maternal serum alpha-fetoprotein, triple screen, RPR, hepatitis B, diabetic screenings, and group B *Streptococcus*.**
- ✷ **After the first prenatal visit, the woman is seen every 4 weeks until the 28th week, then every 2 weeks until the 36th week, then every week until delivery.**
- ✷ **During pregnancy, the woman should receive education regarding personal hygiene and safety, breast care, sexual activity, exercise, employment, and substances to avoid.**
- ✷ **Adequate nutritional intake during pregnancy can have a profound impact on the health of the woman and her unborn child. The food pyramid may be used for teaching the pregnant woman about her nutritional needs.**
- ✷ **Childbirth education classes include information on the birth process and teach relaxation and breathing techniques to reduce the perception of pain.**

review questions 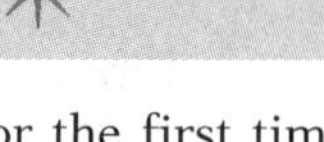

1. Tanya Moore is pregnant for the first time. Her last menstrual period began on January 12. She asks the nurse when her baby is due. The nurse uses Nägele's rule and calculates Tanya's due date as
   a. October 19.
   b. October 5.
   c. November 19.
   d. November 5.
2. Tanya is concerned because she has been very nauseated every morning for the last 2 weeks. Yesterday she

vomited after eating her breakfast. She is concerned that she may have the "flu." The nurse states,

a. "You are probably experiencing the beginning signs of the flu. Be sure and discuss this with the physician."
b. "You are probably just nervous about being here today, because it is your first visit."
c. "You are probably experiencing 'morning sickness.' Try eating some dry crackers or toast before getting out of bed."
d. "There are so many germs flying around; you need to discuss this with the physician because it could be something very serious."

3. Tanya is very concerned about gaining weight during her pregnancy. She wants to know if she could plan on gaining 7 or 8 lb because that is the weight of many newborns. The nurse tells her that the recommended weight gain during pregnancy is
   a. 10 to 15 lb.
   b. 10 to 20 lb.
   c. 25 to 35 lb.
   d. 35 to 50 lb.
4. The nurse has explaines to Tanya that she will have her urine checked during each prenatal visit. The urine will be checked for
   a. occult blood and white cells.
   b. glucose and protein.
   c. bilirubin and sedimentation.
   d. any signs of infection.
5. Tanya plans on breast-feeding but has inverted nipples. What may the nurse teach her to help with this problem?
   a. Using a breast binder for the remainder of pregnancy
   b. Exposing the nipples to air several times a day
   c. Kegel exercises
   d. Hoffman exercises

references

Centers for Disease Control (1990). Protection against viral hepatitis. Recommendations of the Immunization Practices Advisory Committee. *MMWR, 39*, 1.

Cunningham F. G., McDonald, P.C., Leveno, K.J., Gant, N.F., & Gilstrap, L.C. (1993). *Williams obstetrics* (19th ed.). Norwalk, CT: Appleton & Lange.

Driscoll, D. W. (1992). Perinatal transmission of hepatitis B. *RN*, 65.

Evans, A. (1991) Perinatal chemical use. In K. Niswander & A. Evans (Eds.), *Manual of obstetrics* (4th ed.) (p. 30). Boston: Little-Brown.

O'Connor, A., et al. (1992). Effectiveness of a pregnancy smoking cessation program. *JOGNN, 21*(5), 385–392.

bibliography

Amis, D., & Green, J. (1993). *Prepared childbirth—the family way* (5th ed.). Richardson, Texas: The Family Way, Inc.

Swinnerton, T. (1990). Alternate antenatal treatments. *Nursing Times, 86*(48), 68–69.

Campinha-Bacote, J., & Bragg, E. J. (1993) Chemical assessment in maternity care. *MCN, 18*, 24–28.

Corrine, L., Bailey, V., Valentin, M., Morantus, E., & Shirley, L. (1992). The unheard voices of women: Spiritual interventions in maternal-child health. *MCN, 17*, 141–145.

Dudek, S. G. (1993). *Nutrition handbook for nursing practice*. (2nd ed.). Philadelphia: J.B. Lippincott.

Evans, N. (1994). *The A to Z of pregnancy and childbirth.* Alameda CA: Hunter House.

Fishbein, E. G., & Phillips, M. (1990). How safe is exercise during pregnancy?. *JOGNN, 19*(1), 45–49.

MacLaren, A. (1992). *Maternity care.* Springhouse, PA: Springhouse Corporation.

Olds, S. B., London, M. L., & Ladewig, P. W. (1992). *Maternal-newborn nursing: A family-centered approach* (4th ed.). Redwood City, CA: Addison-Wesley Nursing.

Rhodes, A. M. (1992) Criminal penalties for maternal substance abuse. *MCN, 17*, 11.

Sherman, S. R. (1990). *Pregnancy—a special time for nutrition and good health*. Dairy Council: California.

Sullivan, J., Boudreaux, M., & Keller, P. (1993). Can we help the substance abusing mother and infant? *MCN, 18*, 153–157.

Sharts-Hopko, N. C. (1993). Folic acid in the prevention of neural tube defects. *MCN, 18*, 232.

nursing care during pregnancy at risk 9

outline

objectives

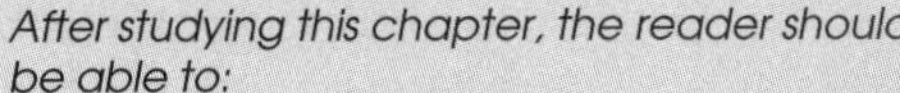

After studying this chapter, the reader should be able to:

* Define high-risk pregnancy.
* Discuss the signs, symptoms, and nursing care of a woman with a bleeding disorder.
* Describe the types of spontaneous abortion and the supportive nursing care.
* Discuss the events that occur with the formation of a hydatidiform mole and the importance of follow-up care.
* Explain the difference between placenta previa and abruptio placentae and the nursing care necessary for each condition.
* Define hyperemesis gravidarum and its possible effects on the maternal and fetal outcome.
* Explain the series of events involved in the development of hemolytic disease in the newborn due to blood incompatibility between the fetus and the mother.
* Describe the impact of cardiac disease and diabetes on the pregnant woman and fetus.
* Define toxoplasmosis and measures to prevent the disease.
* Discuss sexually transmitted diseases and their impact on the woman and fetus.
* Compare and contrast the goals of nursing care for pregnancy in the adolescent and older pregnant woman.

key terms

abortion
abruptio placentae
disseminated intravascular coagulation
ectopic pregnancy
gestational diabetes
HELLP syndrome
hemolytic disease
hydatidiform mole
hyperemesis gravidarum
placenta previa
pregnancy-induced hypertension
sexually transmitted disease
TORCH infections

Although most pregnancies proceed without serious health problems for mother or fetus and conclude with the birth of a healthy infant, complications can occur. These complications may be related to the age of the mother, pre-existing medical conditions, or a direct result of the pregnancy. When the health of the pregnant woman or the fetus is jeopardized, the pregnancy is referred to as pregnancy at risk or high-risk pregnancy. (Risk factors are listed in Display 9-1.) This chapter deals with nursing care of the woman with these complications. Early intervention and continuing assessment can increase the chances for a successful outcome.

✳ family considerations

During a pregnancy at risk, the woman and her family may experience anxiety due to the potential for complications. By developing rapport with the woman and her family as early as possible, the nurse can promote a healthy exchange of information about their anxiety and concerns. As the family gains trust, they will feel more comfortable sharing their concerns and their need for specific information.

All members of the health care team may be needed to address these concerns. Social services may be used for financial concerns, dieticians for dietary planning, and home health agencies for the home-bound client.

display 9-1
summary of high risk factors

AGE

* Adolescent
* Older than 35 years

ANATOMIC ABNORMALITIES

* Incompetent cervical os
* Cephalopelvic disproportion

CARDIOVASCULAR DISORDERS

* Pre-existing heart disease
* Development of hypertension during pregnancy
* Rh negative—sensitized

DRUG USE/ABUSE

* Alcohol
* Illegal drugs (eg, cocaine)
* Tobacco

METABOLIC DISORDERS

* Diabetes mellitus
* Thyroid disorder
* Adrenal disorder

SOCIOECONOMIC FACTORS

* Poverty
* Lack of prenatal care
* Lack of support group

conditions associated with bleeding

A bleeding disorder (*hemorrhage*) during pregnancy poses a threat to the woman and the fetus. The causes of bleeding disorders are usually associated with the trimester in which they occur (Table 9-1).

ectopic pregnancy

Ectopic pregnancy occurs when the zygote (fertilized ovum) implants outside the uterine cavity. The word ectopic means "away from the normal place." Ninety-eight percent of ectopic pregnancies implant in the fallopian tube and the remaining 2% in the abdominal cavity, ovaries, or cervix (Fig. 9-1). Ectopic pregnancies are the leading cause of maternal death in the first trimester and overall, the second leading cause of maternal death.

etiology and pathophysiology

Any condition that blocks passage of the fertilized ovum through the fallopian tube greatly increases the incidence of ectopic pregnancy. The most common factors are congenital or developmental anomalies, adhesions of the tubes, history of pelvic inflammatory disease, use of intrauterine devices, salpingitis (infection of the fallopian tube), multiple induced abortions, or a history of ectopic pregnancy.

Because the fallopian tube cannot accommodate the growing embryo, the tube ruptures, resulting in hemorrhage. The tube may tear and begin to bleed slowly or rupture spontaneously and bleed suddenly and severely. Any such bleeding requires immediate medical attention.

Symptoms of ectopic pregnancy include pain and rebound tenderness in the lower abdomen, vaginal bleeding, dizziness, shock, and possible peritonitis.

diagnostic tests

Blood is drawn for a complete blood count (CBC) to determine the effects of the bleeding. This may be indicated by a drop in the hemoglobin and hematocrit. A serum human chorionic gonadotropin (HCG) level may be drawn to confirm pregnancy. A needle may be inserted through the vagina for aspiration of fluid from the cul-de-sac (*culdocentesis*) to look for indications of bleeding. An endoscopic examination (*culdoscopy*) may be done to visualize the pelvic organs to observe for any abnormalities. Ultrasound also may be used to determine the presence and location of an ectopic pregnancy.

medical–surgical management

Treatment focuses on control of the bleeding and if necessary, surgical removal or repair of the fallopian tube. If the

table 9-1 summary of bleeding disorders

Condition	Cause	Symptoms	Occurrence
Ectopic pregnancy	Blockage of fallopian tube	Pain, rebound tenderness LLQ abdomen	First trimester
Spontaneous abortion	Possibly chromosomal	Vaginal bleeding	First trimester
Hydatidiform mole	Chorionic degeneration	Passage of grapelike vesicles	Second trimester
Placenta previa	Low implantation of placenta	Painless bleeding	Third trimester
Abruptio placentae	Unknown	Sharp abdominal pain with vaginal bleeding	Third trimester
Disseminated intravascular coagulation	Depletion of clotting factors	Hemorrhaging	First, second, or third trimester

fallopian tube has not ruptured, methotrexate, a chemotherapeutic agent, may be administered. Because methotrexate attacks rapidly growing cells, it attacks the fast-growing zygote, causing it to disintegrate, while leaving the tube intact.

If the tube has ruptured, a laparotomy is performed, and the tube is removed to control the bleeding. Blood is administered as indicated to prevent or alleviate signs of shock. To prevent problems with future pregnancies, patients who are Rh negative will receive Rh immunoglobulin (RhoGAM) to neutralize any Rh positive blood cells that may have entered the bloodstream.

nursing care

Nursing care includes monitoring vital signs for the development of hypovolemic shock or infection, observing for the presence and amount of vaginal bleeding, providing emotional support, and preparing the woman and her family for surgery if indicated. To document vaginal bleeding accurately, the nurse records the number of times the vaginal pad is changed, the amount of blood the pad contains, and the length of time the pad has been worn. This procedure is often referred to as a "pad count."

preoperative care Preoperatively, every effort is made to stabilize the patient. Intravenous (IV) solutions may be started as preliminary fluid replacement, bed rest is maintained, and the surgical consent form is signed. The nurse needs to be prepared to help the family deal with anxiety and fear during this crisis. Enlisting support from the hospital chaplain or family clergyman can sometimes be helpful.

postoperative care Postoperatively, care focuses on stabilizing the patient and preventing infection. Once the woman is stabilized, the nurse needs to focus on the loss the family has experienced and assist them with the grieving process. Referral to a local support group may be helpful. If the tube has been removed, explain that pregnancy can still occur, but the risk of tubal pregnancy in the remaining tube is increased. It is important to explain the need to recognize and report any signs or symptoms of another tubal pregnancy.

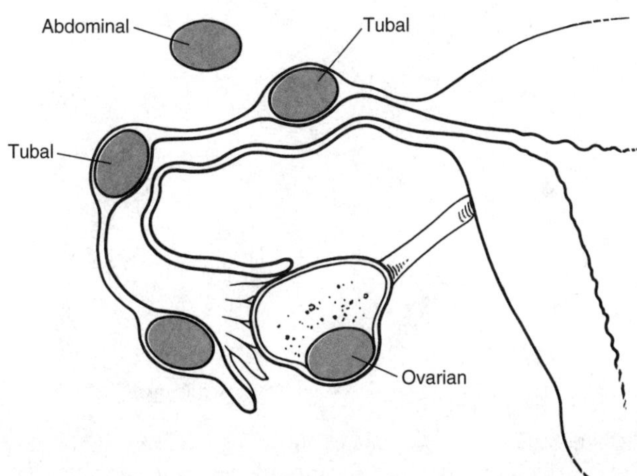

figure 9-1 *Sites of ectopic pregnancy.*

spontaneous abortion

Spontaneous abortion is the expulsion of the products of conception before the age of viability (capable of surviving outside the uterus). The age of viability is considered to be 20 weeks' gestation or fetal weight of more than 500 g. Because the term *abortion* can elicit a strong emotional response, the term *miscarriage* is used more commonly by lay people.

Approximately 15% to 20% of all pregnancies result in spontaneous abortion. About 10% of these patients are seen clinically; the rest lose the pregnancy in the first few days and are asymptomatic. The menstrual cycle may be delayed from a few days to 2 weeks and may seem heavier

table 9-2 types of spontaneous abortions

Classification	*Symptoms*	*Medical Management*
Threatened (may happen but may be averted with intervention)	Experiences vaginal bleeding and abdominal cramping	Bed rest Pad count
Inevitable (will happen; unable to sustain pregnancy)	Increase in vaginal bleeding Dilation of cervix Rupture of membranes	Allow uterus to evacuate Dilatation and curettage (D&C)
Habitual (unable to carry embryo or fetus)	Spontaneously aborts three or more pregnancies	D&C Purse-string suture for incompetent cervical os
Incomplete (aborts but retains products of conception)	Expulsion of fetus with retention of placental fragments	D&C
Missed (fetus dies but does not abort without intervention)	Retention of dead fetus in utero Maceration of fetuss	Oxytocin to initiate labor if it does not occur spontaneously

than usual. The body normally expels all gestational contents and heals itself without intervention.

There are five categories of spontaneous abortion, differentiated according to their symptoms (Table 9-2).

etiology and pathophysiology

Approximately 80% of spontaneous abortions occur during the first trimester, and often the cause is unknown. Causes of spontaneous abortion usually fall into one of two broad categories: defective development of embryonic or placental structures and maternal complications.

More than half of all spontaneous abortions result from chromosomal abnormalities that interfere with the development of the embryo, making it incompatible with life. The most common maternal complication leading to spontaneous abortion is *incompetent cervical os,* a mechanical defect of the cervix that makes it incapable of retaining the pregnancy. This condition usually occurs in the second trimester. The cervix dilates because it cannot support the weight of the embryo or fetus, the membranes rupture, and the products of conception are spontaneously aborted. Other causes of spontaneous abortion include infection, trauma, malnutrition, or substance abuse.

diagnostic tests

Routine laboratory tests, such as CBC and urinalysis, are usually done for baseline information. In addition, an ultrasound may be performed to evaluate the condition of the embryo.

medical–surgical management

The threat of spontaneous abortion demands bed rest and vaginal examination to confirm that the cervix is closed, and the membranes are intact. Close observation is maintained until the symptoms subside or the condition progresses to inevitable abortion.

If the diagnosis is *incompetent cervical os*, the physician may use a purse-string suture (*cerclage*) to support the cervix as long as the patient is not experiencing labor contractions (Fig. 9-2). This suture pulls the cervical os closed and is left in place until near term when the mother may go into labor normally or may be a candidate for a cesarean delivery. If the mother appears able to deliver vaginally, the doctor will clip the purse-string suture and allow labor to progress normally.

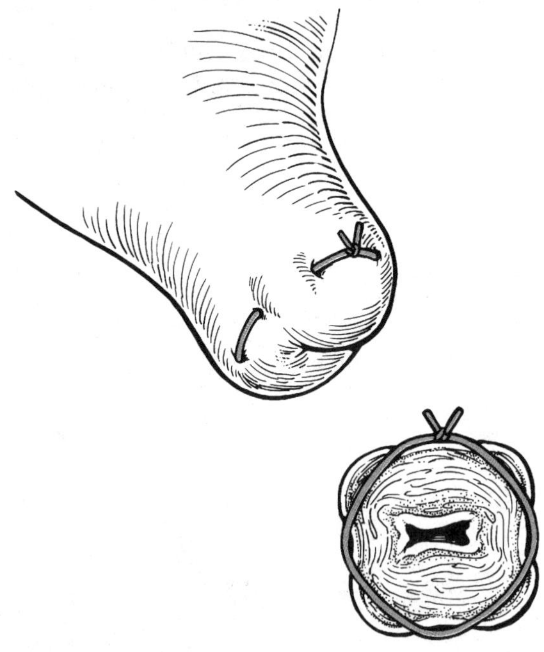

figure 9-2 *A cross-section of an incompetent cervix showing a purse-string suture in place. The suture is removed at term to allow cervical dilation and delivery.*

If spontaneous abortion does occur, fluid replacement is given as indicated, oxytocin is used to control bleeding, and a dilatation and curettage or vacuum aspiration is performed to clean the endometrium and control the bleeding. RhoGAM is given deep intramuscularly (IM) within 72 hours to prevent Rh sensitization as indicated.

nursing care

As soon as the patient is admitted and the diagnosis is made, the nurse begins monitoring vital signs, signs of vaginal bleeding, and any reports of pain. Emotional support is critical. The nurse explains all procedures and treatments to be performed and listens empathetically to concerns of the woman and her family. It is often helpful for the support person to remain with the patient as the situation permits. The hospital chaplain or the family's minister or other spiritual advisor may be notified to provide support.

If surgery is indicated, the preoperative consent form needs to be signed and witnessed. Whole blood or oral iron supplements may be administered as ordered to prevent anemia. Because the patient usually is discharged within 24 hours of surgery, referral to a grief process group is helpful. Many institutions follow up by telephone to assess the need for further intervention. Some communities have provisions for a follow-up home visit by a public health nurse to evaluate the woman's needs.

 **nursing alert**

Once the cervix has dilated and the membranes have ruptured, the loss of the fetus is inevitable, and emotional support is vital.

hydatidiform mole (gestational trophoblastic neoplasm)

Hydatidiform mole is a cystic degeneration of the chorionic membrane that results in a mass of clear vesicles (Fig. 9-3). The vesicles occur in grapelike structures within the uterine cavity. The embryo is absent but degenerating embryonic structures occasionally may be seen.

etiology and pathophysiology

There is no known cause for hydatidiform mole; it occurs once in every 2,000 pregnancies. Normal fertilization takes place, but when the placenta begins to form, the chorionic membrane breaks down. Usually there is rapid enlargement of the abdomen in relationship to the suspected gestational period. Signs and symptoms of a hydatidiform mole include a uterus larger than normal for expected gestational age, vaginal bleeding, anemia due to blood loss, excessive nausea and vomiting, abdominal cramping, and possibly *pregnancy-induced hypertension* (PIH) prior to 20 weeks' gestation.

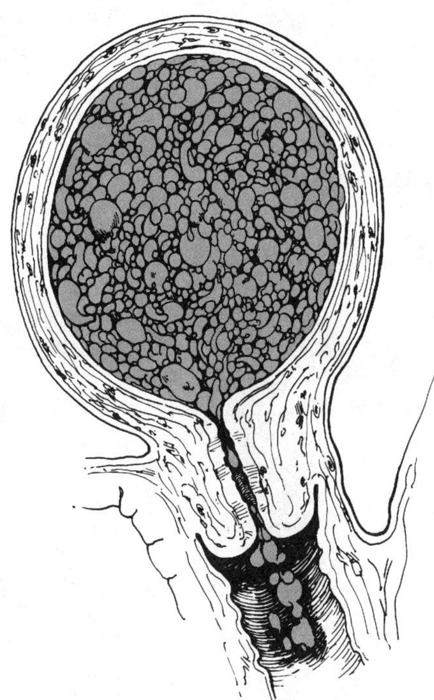

figure 9-3 *Hydatidiform mole.*

diagnostic tests

Auscultation for fetal heart sounds will prove negative. Ultrasound imaging reveals the absence of a fetus and the presence of a mole. A CBC is obtained to evaluate for signs of anemia.

medical–surgical management

Dilatation and curettage is performed to ensure complete removal of the mole. Levels of HCG are monitored for elevation, which indicates the development of chorionic carcinoma. A chest x-ray may be ordered to rule out metastatic carcinoma. Generally, prophylactic chemotherapy is not indicated. Pregnancy should be avoided to prevent the increase in HCG levels. If the HCG levels remain within normal limits for 1 year, the prognosis is good, and pregnancy may be attempted.

 **nursing alert**

Emphasize the importance of follow-up care to monitor for chorionic carcinoma.

nursing care

Preoperative nursing care includes accurate observation of vaginal drainage, observation for signs of hypertension, and preoperative teaching. Routine postoperative care is provided, including monitoring of vital signs and vaginal drainage, promotion of early ambulation, and prevention of postoperative complications. Patient and family teaching on the importance of follow-up care during the following year is critical. Empathetic listening and emotional support are essential to assist the woman and her family with the grieving process.

placenta previa

Normally, the placenta forms in the upper portion of the uterus, which allows for the normal changes that occur in the cervix during the latter term of pregnancy. With *placenta previa*, however, the placenta implants in the lower uterine segment near the internal cervical os. In severe cases, the placenta partially or totally covers the os.

Placenta previa is the most common cause of bleeding in the second and third trimesters of pregnancy. Normal changes in the lower uterine segment during the later stages of pregnancy cause the placenta to separate from the uterus, producing varying degrees of painless bleeding.

Three classifications of placenta previa have been named according to the relationship of the placenta to the internal cervical os (Fig. 9-4):

* *Marginal or low lying*: The placenta lies near the cervical os but does not cover any portion of it.
* *Partial*: The placenta covers only a portion of the cervical os.
* *Complete* or *total*: the placenta covers the entire cervical os.

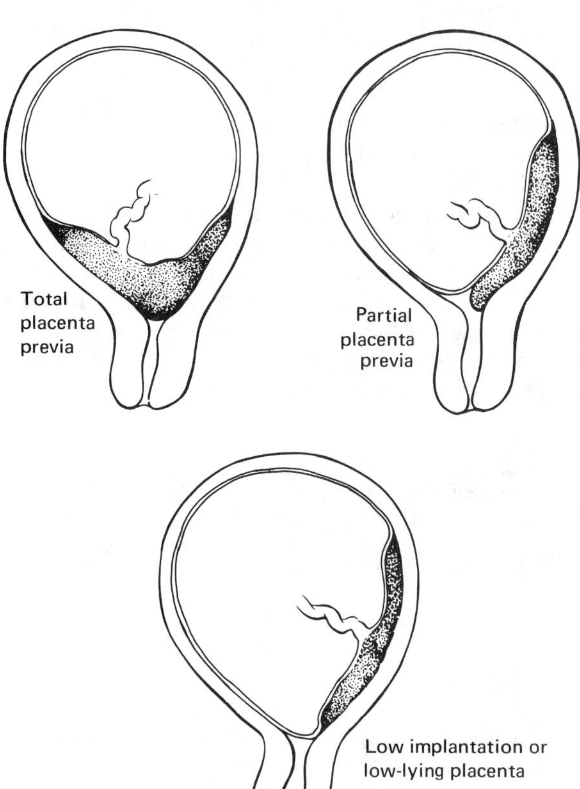

figure 9-4 *Variations of placenta previa.*

etiology and pathophysiology

There is no specific known cause for the development of placenta previa. It is seen in 1 of every 200 deliveries but rarely in a first pregnancy. The incidence seems to increase with a history of multiple pregnancies, advanced maternal age, or history of low cesarean delivery or other uterine incision. Each of these conditions lowers the vascularity of the uterine lining, forcing the placenta to thin out and cover a larger area to meet the needs of the developing fetus.

Sometime during the second or third trimester the patient with placenta previa develops the classic symptom, painless vaginal bleeding. The bleeding can vary from mere spotting to gross hemorrhage, depending on the degree to which the cervical os is covered. As the cervical os changes in preparation for labor, the placenta may tear loose from the uterine wall. Usually the first episode of bleeding is mere spotting. Each subsequent episode results in more severe bleeding until delivery. If the placenta totally occludes the cervix, the bleeding is more severe and may require a cesarean delivery to save the mother and infant.

The greatest threat to the fetus is the possibility of preterm delivery. Every effort is made to maintain the pregnancy as close to term as possible. Following are three reasons for early medical interruption of the pregnancy:

* Uncontrolled hemorrhage
* Fetal hypoxia due to excess detachment of placental tissue
* Fetal hypoxia due to hypovolemia in the mother

diagnostic tests

An ultrasound examination may be performed to locate the placenta. Research studies show that performing the ultrasound through the vagina (*transvaginal approach*) may give more conclusive data because it offers more accurate visualization of the internal os. Hemoglobin and hematocrit tests will be obtained to determine the necessity for blood replacement. Aspiration of amniotic fluid through the abdominal wall (*amniocentesis*) also may be performed to determine fetal maturity.

medical–surgical management

The treatment plan must take into account the gestational age of the fetus, the location of the placenta, and the actual amount of bleeding. If the mother is stable and bleeding is minimal, the physician may order bed rest and observation. An ultrasound is ordered to determine the location of the placenta for planning further intervention.

If the condition progresses and bleeding is more severe or if the ultrasound confirms total placenta previa, the physician may perform a cesarean delivery. Blood replacement is ordered as indicated, and prophylactic antibiotic therapy may be given to prevent infection because of lowered resistance.

nursing care

The mother will be placed on bed rest, preferably in a side-lying position to prevent pressure on the mother's vena cava, which could decrease the oxygen supplied to the fetus. The mother also may receive oxygen by mask to increase indirectly the level of oxygen to the fetus. The nurse monitors fetal and maternal vital signs. Any increase in pulse (*tachycardia*), decrease in blood pressure, or other signs of shock must be reported immediately. A perineal pad count must be maintained to keep accurate record of blood loss. The abdomen is palpated to assess for uterine contractions and the quality and duration of contractions noted. The nurse needs to prepare the family for the possibility of a cesarean birth and the care of a high-risk or premature infant. Answering questions and explaining treatments and procedures help reduce anxiety.

abruptio placentae

Abruptio placentae occurs when a normally implanted placenta separates prematurely from the uterine wall, resulting in bleeding that may be obvious or concealed. If the placenta separates at the edges, which occurs in 80% of cases, the bleeding is apparent. If the placenta separates at the center, the bleeding is concealed between the placenta and the uterine wall (Fig. 9-5).

etiology and pathophysiology

The exact cause of abruptio placentae is unknown; however, several risk factors have been identified. They include previous history of placenta previa, multiparity, history of PIH, essential hypertension, trauma to the abdomen, and history of alcohol or drug abuse.

Abruptio placentae generally occurs in the third trimester of pregnancy or when the woman goes into labor. It has occurred as early as the 20th week of pregnancy, however. The number of cases has recently declined, probably due to the decrease in multiparas and the increase in primigravidas. It is seen in about 1% of all pregnancies; incidence is higher among mothers who use crack cocaine.

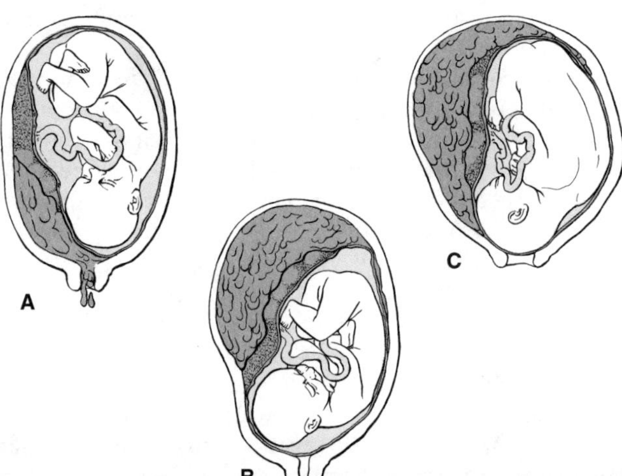

figure 9-5 *Abruptio placentae at various separation sites. **(A)** External hemorrhage. **(B)** Internal or concealed hemorrhage. **(C)** Complete separation.*

Signs and symptoms of abruptio placentae include a severely painful, rigid, boardlike uterus; dark red concealed or vaginal bleeding; signs of maternal shock; and signs of fetal distress, including the possible absence of fetal heart rate.

diagnostic tests

The symptoms of abruptio placentae are specific. Only an ultrasound is needed to confirm the medical diagnosis.

medical–surgical management

Medical treatment is based on the severity of the condition. If there is minimal separation, and maternal and fetal stability are confirmed, no specific intervention is needed. If the mother is hemorrhaging and there are signs of fetal distress, cesarean delivery is necessary. In addition, blood transfusions and prophylactic antibiotics are indicated.

nursing care

The nurse explains procedures and answers questions as indicated to help alleviate the patient's and family's fear. Because the potential for hemorrhage is high, vital signs and intake and output are monitored closely. Vaginal bleeding is observed for amount and frequency, and the pad count is documented. Comfort measures, such as back rubs and breathing techniques, can help calm the woman.

disseminated intravascular coagulation

Disseminated intravascular coagulation (DIC) encompasses a series of events, resulting in hemorrhage. Widespread clotting in the peripheral blood vessels leads to the depletion of the clotting factors, causing massive internal and external bleeding.

etiology and pathophysiology

The cause of DIC is not completely understood. Certain conditions are known to precipitate DIC, such as abruptio placentae, eclampsia, amniotic fluid embolism, and missed abortion.

Once the coagulation process begins, the fibrinogen, a protein necessary for clotting formation, is depleted. At this point, massive hemorrhaging occurs, and the woman's life is in jeopardy.

diagnostic tests

Blood studies are performed to check bleeding and clotting time, platelet count, and fibrinogen level. Typing and cross-matching of blood also are done in the event that transfusion is necessary.

medical management

The underlying cause of DIC must be corrected to halt the process. This is usually followed by administration of whole blood, plasma, fibrinogen, or cryoprecipitate (contains fibrinogen). Steps must be taken to prevent or manage shock and possible tissue necrosis that may have occurred because of blockage of peripheral capillaries, especially in the brain or kidneys.

nursing care

Vital signs and fetal heart tones need to be checked every 15 minutes and any changes reported. Urine and feces are monitored for signs of occult blood. A perineal pad count is made. The nurse monitors laboratory tests and reports any abnormal findings. A calm, quiet atmosphere is maintained for mother and family. The nurse explains procedures and answers questions as they arise.

✶ nursing process for the client with a bleeding disorder

assessment

Subjective data to be assessed include the following:

* Menstrual, obstetric, and medical history
* Abdominal pain
* Rebound tenderness in the lower abdomen
* Joint or bone pain indicating possible internal bleeding

Objective data to be assessed include the following:

* Presence, amount, and color of any vaginal bleeding
* Vital signs for indications of infection or shock
* Laboratory tests, including pregnancy test, urinalysis, CBC, bleeding and clotting times
* Ultrasound reports
* Decrease or absence of fetal heart rate indicating fetal distress
* Skin and mucous membranes for signs of bleeding
* Prolonged bleeding from IV or injection sites

nursing diagnosis

* Anxiety, related to threat to life of self or fetus
* Fluid Volume Deficit, related to blood loss
* Risk for Infection, related to peritonitis
* Anticipatory Grieving, related to possible loss of child

planning and implementation

Although the various conditions causing bleeding during pregnancy involve some specific nursing diagnoses, they all have certain nursing actions in common. The woman who experiences bleeding during pregnancy most often is extremely upset with the course of events and the potential threat to herself and her unborn child. The entire family is thrown into crisis. The nurse may best assist the mother and family by providing emotional support, evaluating their coping skills, intervening as necessary, and providing thorough explanations of all procedures.

Vital signs are monitored closely for signs of shock (pallor, clammy skin, drop in blood pressure, increase in pulse) and infection (increase in temperature). Any vaginal bleeding is observed for amount and color, and an accurate pad count must be kept. Laboratory data are collected, organized, and reported to the physician. See the Nursing Care Plan for the Pregnant Client with a Bleeding Disorder.

evaluation

* Client verbalizes a reduction of anxiety.
* Fluid volume will be within normal limits.
* No evidence of infection will be present.
* Client will demonstrate normal coping skills.

hypertensive disorders

pregnancy-induced hypertension

PIH, formerly called toxemia, is a multisystem disorder that is usually identified by symptoms of hypertension, proteinuria, and edema. Unless treated, PIH can lead to organ damage in the mother and impaired development in the fetus. Blood pressure elevation without other symptoms is usually called gestational hypertension. There is no increase in perinatal mortality associated with gestational hypertension. If the blood pressure is elevated along with edema and proteinuria, it is called *preeclampsia,* a potentially life-threatening condition. If the condition progresses to the point that the mother is experiencing convulsions, it is called *eclampsia* (Table 9-3). Eclampsia poses a very high risk for fetal and maternal death.

preeclampsia

Preeclampsia is most often seen in first time pregnancies, generally after 20 weeks' gestation. It is most common among adolescents, women older than 35 years, or women with a familial history of the disease. Incidence among African American women is twice that among white women. Low-income women also are at high risk for PIH, possibly because of poor nutrition or lack of prenatal care (Display 9-2).

Preeclampsia is divided into two stages: *mild* and *severe*. Mild preeclampsia may allow the pregnant woman to remain at home with frequent visits to her clinic or physician's office for assessment. As the symptoms become more severe, she may be hospitalized for close observation and aggressive treatment.

mild preeclampsia

Mild preeclampsia usually manifests with a blood pressure increase of 30 mm Hg systolic or 15 mm Hg diastolic, compared with the baseline blood pressure. In addition, proteinuria is present, usually measuring 1+ or 2+ on a urine reagent test strip. Edema is confirmed by a weight gain of 2 lb or more per week in the second trimester and 1 lb per week in the third trimester. The edema is usually noticed in the face, hands, and ankles, rather than just in the ankles as often experienced in pregnancy.

nursing care plan
for the pregnant client with a bleeding disorder

NURSING DIAGNOSIS
Fluid Volume Deficit, related to blood loss

GOAL: To detect and manage bleeding disorder while minimizing associated complications

NURSING INTERVENTIONS	RATIONALE	EVALUATION
Monitor vital signs	Drop in BP or increase in pulse indicate circulatory compromise with a compensatory response	Client will remain normotensive, with regular heart rate between 80–100 beats per minute
Assess skin for color, warmth, and sensation.	Pallor and cool, clammy skin and decreased sensation can signify initial shock state with decreased peripheral perfusion	Client will be well perfused with warm, dry skin, peripheral pulses and good color, sensation, and motion in extremities
Keep an accurate pad count, including color and amount	Objectively indicates the amount and type of bleeding (fresh/old bleeding; clotting or not clotting)	Lochia/bleeding will be less than 1 pad per hour
Evaluate laboratory data: CBC, PT, PTT, and platelets	Abnormal laboratory values low hemoglobin, elevated PT, PTT, and low platelets indicate a need for replacement therapy	Client will have laboratory values of bleeding and clotting indicators within normal limits

NURSING DIAGNOSIS
Anticipatory Grieving, related to potential loss of fetus

GOAL: Client and family will verbalize anxiety and fear over potential loss

NURSING INTERVENTIONS	RATIONALE	EVALUATION
Encourage client and family verbalization of feelings	Verbalization of feelings can promote anticipatory grieving, which may help the client and family incorporate the potential fetal death into their thoughts and better handle the anxiety related to it	Client and family will support each other and share their feelings with each other and the caregivers The client and family's anxiety level will be within expected and acceptable range for this type of crisis

The woman with mild preeclampsia may usually remain at home, but she will need weekly monitoring to assess for changes in her condition. Assessments may be performed by a physician, clinical nurse specialist, or nurse practitioner. The woman may be instructed to remain on bed rest in a side-lying position to increase blood flow to the fetus. Because she is losing protein in the urine, she also is advised to follow a high-protein, high-fiber diet with adequate fluid intake.

severe preeclampsia

Once the blood pressure increases to 160 mm Hg systolic and 110 mm Hg diastolic, with extensive edema and proteinuria measuring 3+ or 4+ on the urine test strip, the woman has progressed to severe preeclampsia. At this time, she may experience epigastric pain, nausea, and vomiting caused by liver distention. Pitting edema of legs, hyperreflexia, anxiety, and irritability may be present. Cerebral edema may cause visual disturbances, such as headaches, blurred vision, or seeing spots. Urine output may decrease to 400 to 600 mL per 24 hours due to retention of fluids.

Hospitalization is required, and medical care is directed toward preventing seizures, lowering the blood pressure, and delivering the fetus safely and as close to term as possible. Hydralazine (Apresoline) is the drug of

table 9-3 comparison of stages of pregnancy-induced hypertension

Mild Preeclampsia	*Severe Preeclampsia*	*Eclampsia*
Increase of systolic blood pressure by 30 mm Hg or increase of diastolic blood pressure by 15 mm Hg	Hypertension increases	Continues with hypertension
Edema in face, hands, and ankles, especially in the morning	Edema increases	Continues with edema
Weight gain of 2 lb in 1 week or 6 lb in 1 month	Weight gain continues or increases	Continues with weight gain
Proteinuria	Protein continues to spill into the urine (5 g/24 h or 3+ or 4+ protein on dipstick	Continues with protein in urine
	Blurred vision or other visual disturbances	Continues to have visual disturbances
	Oliguria (>400 mL/24 h)	Oliguria continues
	Headache	Headache may still be present
	Hyperreflexia, central nervous system irritability	Central nervous system irritability continues to increase
	Epigastric pain	Epigastric pain continues
		Convulsions, which may lead to death

choice for hypertension. It is usually given if the diastolic blood pressure is above 110 mm Hg. Hydralazine relaxes the blood vessels and increases cardiac output.

Magnesium sulfate ($MgSO_4$) is used to sedate the woman and control impending seizure activity. It causes vasodilation and depresses the central nervous system. It may be given IV or IM. If given IV, the loading dose is 3 to 4 g followed by hourly doses of 1 to 4 g. If given IM, it is given deep, using the Z-track method (to prevent leakage into the tissues); the usual dose is 5 g in each hip every 4 hours.

nursing alert

Calcium gluconate is the emergency antidote for magnesium sulfate. It should be readily available when administering magnesium sulfate.

display 9-2
contributing factors in development of pregnancy-induced hypertension

1. First pregnancy (increases with multiparity)
2. Poor nutrition
3. Lack of prenatal care
4. History of essential hypertension
5. History of diabetes
6. Age (younger than 16 years or older than 35 years)

eclampsia

The diagnosis of *eclampsia* indicates that in addition to hypertension, proteinuria, and edema, the woman has developed cerebral edema severe enough to cause seizures (convulsions). Left untreated, eclampsia may lead to coma and death. This life-threatening event demands emergency intervention to save the life of the woman and fetus.

Maternal mortality from eclampsia can be as high as 15% and fetal mortality as high as 25%. Seizure care and medications are continued, and every effort is made to deliver the fetus.

hellp syndrome

The initials HELLP signify *h*emolysis, *e*levated *l*iver enzymes, and *l*ow *p*latelets. This syndrome, a form of PIH, can occur with mild or severe preeclampsia late in pregnancy or immediately following delivery. Its effects mimic DIC, and it leads to postpartum hemorrhage. HELLP syndrome occurs in 1 of every 150 pregnancies with a maternal death rate as high as 20% (Sauer & Harvey, 1992). Laboratory tests show that hemolysis (a destruction of the red blood cells with the release of their hemoglobin into the surrounding tissues), elevation of liver enzymes (from hemorrhage and destruction of liver tissue), and low platelets (from widespread use in attempt to control the hemorrhage) has occurred.

The treatment and nursing care for HELLP syndrome are similar to those for preeclampsia and eclampsia with one exception: Once HELLP syndrome has been identified, delivery is encouraged regardless of the fetal gestational age.

etiology and pathophysiology

Although the cause of PIH is unknown, its effects are clear: The blood vessels constrict, causing the blood pressure to elevate. This increases the demands on the heart and reduces blood flow to the internal organs, which leads to possible necrosis (death of tissues) or thrombus (blood clot) formation; this can affect the brain, renal system, cardiovascular system, or hepatic portal system.

With PIH, the normal increase of blood volume (30%–40%) that occurs in normal pregnancy fails to occur. This can decrease circulation between the uterus and placenta, possibly resulting in chronic fetal hypoxia, retarded fetal growth, or fetal death.

diagnostic tests

The urine is monitored for protein. Blood tests include hemoglobin, hematocrit, blood urea nitrogen (BUN), creatinine, renal and liver function, and the coagulation time of the blood. If it becomes necessary to use magnesium sulfate for seizure activity, a serum magnesium level also may be needed.

medical management

Medical management is aimed at controlling the hypertension, improving the blood flow to the placenta to prevent fetal hypoxia, and preventing seizures and coma in the woman. The only known cure is delivery of the infant.

✳ nursing process for the client with pregnancy-induced hypertension

assessment

Subjective data to be assessed include the following:

* Blurred vision, headaches, or other visual disturbances
* Epigastric pain

Objective data to be assessed include the following:

* Any increase of systolic or diastolic blood pressure
* Edema in the face, hands, or ankles
* Weight gain exceeding 2 lb in 1 week
* Proteinuria
* Oliguria
* Hyperreflexia, central nervous system irritability, or seizure activity
* Fetal heart for signs of fetal distress
* Laboratory values for any deviations from normal

A woman with severe preeclampsia, eclampsia, or HELLP syndrome requires constant observation and assessment. The nurse needs to be vigilant in assessing and reporting any changes in the woman's status to prevent any further complications.

nursing diagnosis

* Risk for Injury to mother, related to possible seizure activity
* Risk for Injury to fetus, related to hypoxia
* Fear, related to inability to control the outcome of PIH
* Knowledge Deficit, related to the condition and its treatment

planning and intervention

Seizure precautions must be initiated to prevent injury. Side rails need to be padded and the room kept dark and quiet. Maximum rest with minimal stimulation should be enforced. A private room and no telephone also can help decrease stimulation. A padded tongue blade should *not* be used during a seizure to prevent biting of the tongue, because it is ineffective and may cause other injuries.

Deep tendon reflexes should be assessed every 4 hours for response to the medication (Table 9-4). Maternal vital signs and fetal heart tones are monitored every 4 hours. Face, hands, and ankles are assessed for signs of edema. The nurse weighs the patient daily and documents the weight. Urinary output is measured and assessed for possible protein content (*proteinuria*).

It is vital that the nurse explain carefully the importance of bed rest and a nonstressful environment. Explain to the family that one member may stay with the patient, but others should go to the waiting room. Enlisting the family's aid is helpful to the patient and the family. By offering emotional support, allowing family members to voice concerns, and answering questions, the nurse helps reduce stress and anxiety. Information should be relayed to the client and the family in a timely fashion to reduce stress.

> **nursing alert**
>
> *If the woman experiences a seizure, her head should be turned to her side to prevent aspiration. Support her gently to prevent her from injury, but do not hold her down because this increases the potential for injury.*

evaluation

* Patient remains free from injury.
* Fetus remains free from injury.
* Patient and family verbalize understanding of medical condition and its course of treatment.
* Patient and family verbalize fears.

chronic hypertension

The woman who becomes pregnant with preexisting hypertension (140/90 or more) or develops it before the 20th week of pregnancy, may experience a further increase in blood pressure. She also is inclined to develop proteinuria, edema, and sometimes superimposed PIH. The fetus is at high risk for intrauterine growth retardation (growth less than normal). During pregnancy, the woman is usually placed under the care of an internist and an obstetrician. She is monitored carefully throughout her pregnancy to prevent serious complications; her prenatal visits are

table 9-4 assessment of deep tendon reflexes

Type	Procedure	Scoring
Biceps reflex	Flex client's elbow, and place your thumb across the antecubital space. Strike your thumb with the reflex hammer.	0 = no response, abnormal 1+ = diminished, not abnormal 2+ = average response 3+ = brisk, but not abnormal 4+ = hyperactive, abnormal
Patellar reflex	Flex client's knee. Strike with reflex hammer just below the knee cap.	0 = no response, abnormal 1+ = diminished, not abnormal 2+ = average response 3+ = brisk, but not abnormal 4+ = hyperactive, abnormal
Ankle clonus	Use one hand to support client's leg with knee flexed. Sharply dorsiflex the foot.	Normal response = no rhythmic jerking of the foot after release (negative clonus) Abnormal response = rhythmic jerking of the foot after release (positive clonus)

scheduled every 2 weeks throughout the entire pregnancy. Care is similar to the woman experiencing PIH.

hyperemesis gravidarum

Hyperemesis gravidarum is a condition in which persistent, severe vomiting begins in early pregnancy and leads to weight loss, fluid and electrolyte imbalance, dehydration, and metabolic imbalance. If the condition is allowed to progress untreated, it can prove fatal.

etiology and pathophysiology

The exact cause of hyperemesis gravidarum is unknown, but stress and lifestyle are believed to play an important role. It is more common in the United States than in any other country. Some researchers believe that increased levels of hormones during pregnancy, particularly HCG, also may play a role.

Hyperemesis gravidarum results in dehydration, which decreases the uteroplacental circulation and the delivery of nutrients to the fetus. This can result in growth retardation of the fetus. Severe cases of hyperemesis gravidarum require hospitalization for IV therapy to correct the dehydration and resulting metabolic imbalance.

diagnostic tests

Blood tests are done to monitor electrolyte imbalance (decreased sodium, potassium, chloride), and urinalysis is done to assess for the presence of ketones, an indication the the woman's body is breaking down fat reserves to maintain cellular activity.

medical management

Home management consists of the use of antiemetics, high-carbohydrate meals, and reduction of stress. Hospitalization is necessary if the condition does not improve. Treatment consists of IV hydration, electrolyte replacement, and the continued use of antiemetics (promethazine [Phenergan] or hydroxyzine [Vistaril]). Psychiatric consultation for the development of coping and stress reduction skills also may be indicated.

✳ nursing process for the client with hyperemesis gravidarum

assessment

Subjective data to be assessed include the following:

* A 24-hour dietary recall
* History of nausea and vomiting

Objective data to be assessed include the following:

* Presence of continued vomiting
* Documented record of weight loss
* Pale, dry skin with poor turgor
* Vital signs to monitor increase or decrease in temperature and pulse
* Laboratory data for indications of electrolyte imbalance and starvation

nursing diagnosis

* Fluid Volume Deficit, related to vomiting
* Altered Nutrition: Less than body requirements, related to vomiting
* Ineffective Individual Coping, related to unidentified stressors

planning and intervention

By maintaining an empathetic, nonjudgmental attitude, the nurse encourages the woman to talk about possible stressors and assist her in developing coping mechanisms. Other health care team members, such as the social service worker or the family clergyman, can provide additional assistance. A calm, quiet atmosphere is important. In addition, the nurse monitors the woman's electrolyte status and keeps an accurate intake and output record. Antiemetics are given as needed. The emesis basin needs to be kept handy but out of sight to prevent unpleasant reminders. The woman takes nothing by mouth (NPO) until the nausea subsides, usually 24 hours to 48 hours. She is then given clear liquids and slowly advanced to a normal balanced diet.

evaluation

* Fluid volume will be within normal range
* Woman maintains adequate nutrition to meet needs of growing fetus
* Woman demonstrates use of effective coping skills

hemolytic disease

Hemolytic diseases cause jaundice and anemia in the newborn. These diseases result from incompatibility of maternal and fetal blood. Due to transplacental bleeding, blood from the fetus enters the maternal bloodstream, causing the formation of antibodies. Maternal blood then crosses to the fetus, usually during birth; however, it can occur anytime during the pregnancy. As little as 0.5 mL of Rh-positive fetal blood entering the Rh-negative mother may cause significant antibody formation. These antibodies then attack and destroy the fetal red blood cells. The two types of hemolytic diseases are Rh incompatibility and ABO incompatibility.

rh incompatibility

Rh is an antigen or blood factor that triggers the production of antibodies in people whose blood is Rh positive. Rh factor is present in 85% of white people and 90% of African Americans in the United States. Those missing the Rh factor (15% white, 10% African American) are Rh negative. When the mother is Rh negative and the father is Rh positive, the fetus may inherit the Rh factor, leading to *Rh incompatibility* in subsequent pregnancies. There is no physical harm to the pregnant woman, but in subsequent pregnancies, the fetus can suffer severe effects, including death. These events understandably have great emotional impact on the woman and her family.

etiology and pathophysiology

The Rh antigen (factor) is located on the surface of the red blood cell. Generally there is no transfer of fetal blood to the mother. However rupture of small vessels can occur during pregnancy, allowing some of the fetal blood to enter the maternal bloodstream. The woman then produces antibodies to the antigens. As maternal blood crosses the placenta to the fetus, the antibodies begin to destroy the fetal red blood cells. Large numbers of blood cells may be exchanged during delivery. When this happens, *Rh isoimmunization* occurs, producing anemia in the fetus during subsequent pregnancy. If severe, this anemia is called *erythroblastosis fetalis* and can prove fatal. As little as 0.25 to 0.5 mL of blood exchanged may set the mechanism in motion (Fig. 9-6).

Rh incompatibility can result from spontaneous abortions, induced abortions, ectopic pregnancies, and term pregnancies.

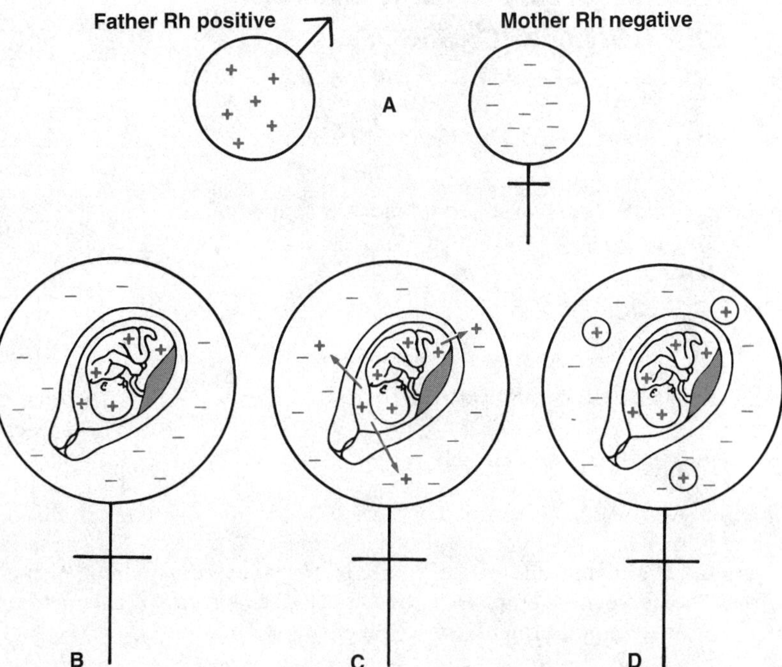

figure 9-6 *Rh isoimmunization. (**A**) Father Rh positive, mother Rh negative. (**B**) Mother Rh− pregnant with Rh+ fetus. (**C**) Transplacental bleeding transfers Rh+ blood to mother's bloodstream. (**D**) Mother forms Rh+ antibodies.*

diagnostic tests

At the first prenatal visit, blood is tested to determine type, Rh status, and antibody titer (indirect Coombs' test), which indicates the degree of maternal sensitization. An amniocentesis and amniotic fluid analysis may be done if the antibody titer has reached a critical level (1:16).

medical management

If prenatal antibody screening tests and blood typing identify potential problems, Rh immune globulin (RhoGAM) is administered within 72 hours of delivery to protect against Rh immunization for the next pregnancy. RhoGAM combines with and neutralizes any positive red blood cells that the mother may have received, thus protecting the next fetus.

Because RhoGAM does not cross the placental barrier, physicians have begun to administer it at 28 weeks' gestation to prevent Rh isoimmunization that can occur from bleeding during delivery. Immediately following delivery, the mother will have a repeat antibody titer and will receive another dose of RhoGAM if she is a candidate. If she has already produced antibodies, the medication will not be effective. No medication is available for protection against ABO incompatibility.

abo incompatibility

ABO incompatibility arises when the pregnant woman has type O blood and the fetus has inherited type A, B, or AB from the father. Occurring in 20% of pregnancies, this condition is usually much milder than Rh incompatibility, usually resulting in jaundice in the newborn. ABO incompatibility also occurs with transplacental bleeding but differs in that it can occur in a first-time pregnancy and does not have the potential to cause fetal death.

✳ nursing process for the client with hemolytic disease

assessment

Subjective data to be assessed include the following:

* History of past pregnancies or abortions

Objective data to be assessed include the following:

* Blood type for ABO and Rh factor

nursing diagnosis

* Fear, related to outcome of pregnancy
* Knowledge deficit, related to the tests and follow-up

planning and intervention

The nurse provides accurate and thorough information about all tests and the condition of fetus. He or she answers questions and allows the family to verbalize concerns. The nurse must emphasize the importance of keeping all prenatal appointments for follow-up care. This can be a good time to discuss the possibility of the use of RhoGAM at 28 weeks' gestation and postdelivery.

evaluation

* Family will verbalize concerns.
* Family will verbalize understanding of the condition.

pre-existing medical conditions

Pregnancy puts a tremendous workload on the body; however, the normal healthy female body is designed to withstand this strain. Some women have pre-existing medical conditions that add to the workload placed on the body. Two of the most common medical conditions are *cardiac disease* and *diabetes mellitus*.

cardiac disease

Cardiac disease is the leading nonobstetric cause of maternal death. The maternal cardiovascular system undergoes dramatic changes during pregnancy, with blood volume increasing 30% to 40%. Although this increased volume does not affect the healthy heart, it can have a major impact on a diseased cardiovascular system. The New York Heart Association has designed a Classification of Functional Capacity for the cardiac patient (Display 9-3). The pregnant woman with class I or II heart disease will likely be able to carry a fetus to term if she receives proper medical care. However, women with class III or IV disease are advised not to attempt pregnancy.

The most common cardiac conditions seen in the maternity patient are congenital heart disease and rheumatic heart disease. These conditions place a pregnant woman at risk for pulmonary edema and decreased cardiac output. They place the fetus at risk for low birth weight, prematurity, and intrauterine hypoxia.

etiology and pathophysiology

Increased blood volume, which peaks between 28 and 32 weeks' gestation, can overwhelm the maternal heart. Cardiac output is not sufficient to meet the body's needs and thus decreases oxygen and nutrition to the developing fetus.

diagnostic tests

An electrocardiogram, chest x-ray, and possibly vital lung capacity test may be performed to obtain baseline data. Any other tests (usually noninvasive) would be done based on reported symptoms.

medical management

The expectant woman with cardiac disease needs to be monitored closely throughout pregnancy. If the condition is severe, she usually is under the care of a cardiologist in addition to her obstetrician.

She is taught the signs and symptoms to observe and report: tachycardia, palpitations, dyspnea, edema, and chest pain. Strict adherence to proper diet, rest, and exercise is essential.

display 9-3
classification of heart disease

Class I: No cardiac symptoms; no limitation of physical activity
Class II: Symptoms felt with ordinary exertion; a slight limitation of physical activity
Class III: Symptoms felt even during limited activity; a more detailed limitation of physical activity
Class IV: Symptoms occur during any physical activity; a severe limitation of physical activity

If her heart condition is severe, the woman is placed on bed rest with supplemental oxygen. Medications may be ordered as indicated. Vaginal delivery is usually planned because the woman is not a good surgical risk.

✳ nursing process for the client with cardiac disease

assessment

Subjective data to be assessed include the following:

* Heart palpitations, dizziness, dyspnea, or chest pain
* Recent pattern of weight gain
* Tolerance of routine daily activity

Objective data to be assessed include the following:

* Breath sounds
* Vital signs
* Extremities, monitoring for signs of dependent or nondependent edema

nursing diagnoses

* Activity Intolerance, related to dyspnea and tachycardia
* Altered Tissue Perfusion to the placenta, related to inadequate circulation
* Fear, related to possible effects on pregnancy outcome

planning and intervention

If the symptoms do not warrant hospitalization, the patient is encouraged to have frequent rest periods during the day and a minimum of 10 hours sleep at night, to follow a nutritional low-salt diet, to take cardiac medications as directed, and to report for prenatal visits as indicated.

If hospitalization is indicated, bed rest will be mandatory. The nurse will administer oxygen at prescribed liter flow and administer cardiac drugs (such as digitalis) as ordered. The nurse needs to explain all procedures and treatments to the patient and family to allay anxiety and to help them verbalize fears and concerns.

display 9-4
maternal effect of diabetes

* Hydramnios (excess amniotic fluid)
* Hyperglycemia
* Increased incidence of PIH
* Urinary tract infections
* Possible birth trauma due to fetal size
* Increased incidence of postpartum hemorrhage

evaluation

* Patient demonstrates sufficient energy and strength to complete required activities.
* Patient identifies medical regimen, diet, medications activities that promote vasodilation.
* Patient reports increase in psychological and physiologic comfort.

diabetes mellitus

Diabetes mellitus is an endocrine disorder that results from the inability of beta cells in the pancreas to produce adequate insulin for metabolism of carbohydrates. Insulin is the endocrine hormone that enables glucose to enter the cells. Because synthetic insulin was produced in 1921, the lifespan of the diabetic patient has increased greatly. Before this time, many women with diabetes did not reach childbearing age. Those who did were sterile or subject to spontaneous abortion.

Approximately 1% to 5% of all pregnant women are diabetic, and an additional 2% to 3% develop *gestational diabetes*. Gestational diabetes occurs only during pregnancy and usually disappears after the birth of the child. However, women with gestational diabetes have an increased risk for developing diabetes mellitus later in life.

With better prenatal care, synthetic insulin, and more effective management of diabetes, women with diabetes now have the opportunity to have normal, healthy infants. The challenges to be met include careful monitoring of maternal glucose levels, promoting positive maternal feelings in meeting the demands of diabetes and pregnancy, and concluding the pregnancy with a healthy mother and newborn (see Displays 9-4 and 9-5 for maternal and fetal effects of diabetes).

display 9-5
fetal effects of diabetes

* Hypoglycemia
* Macrosomia (large size)
* Congenital anomalies
* Prematurity
* Respiratory distress syndrome

etiology and pathophysiology

Pregnancy causes changes in the glucose–insulin regulatory system of the woman with diabetes. The major problem throughout the pregnancy is control of the balance between insulin and blood glucose.

During the first trimester, the placenta produces a hormone (*human placental lactogen*) that counteracts the influence of insulin on glucose; estrogen and progesterone have a similar effect. In spite of this action, the maternal fasting blood sugar remains low, probably because the growing embryo uses the excess glucose.

Later in pregnancy, because the levels of these hormones continue to increase, the pregnant woman is prone to the development of *hyperglycemia* (elevated blood sugar). After the delivery and during the early postpartum period, the hormone levels drop and dramatically decrease the need for insulin.

diagnostic tests

A glucose screening test will be given to all pregnant women at 24 to 28 weeks' gestation and earlier if the mother has a history of diabetes. Later in pregnancy, oxytocin challenge tests may be used to assess placental viability. Ultrasound may be used to assess fetal age, growth, and development.

medical management

If the woman was diabetic prior to conception, her insulin and dietary needs will change with pregnancy due to the demands of the growing fetus. If she develops gestational diabetes, it will be apparent at 24 to 28 weeks and can probably be controlled with diet alone because gestational diabetes usually is a milder condition.

The woman with diabetes will be monitored closely throughout pregnancy with frequent prenatal visits. Blood glucose monitoring, diet and exercise instruction, insulin monitoring, and oxytocin challenge tests will be performed. If the blood glucose level remains high in spite of dietary management, the woman will be placed on insulin rather than oral hypoglycemic agents. These agents cross the placental barrier and can harm the fetus. The decision on vaginal versus cesarean delivery will be made late in the pregnancy and will depend on the severity of the disease and the eventfulness of the pregnancy. Infants born to diabetic mothers are usually large for gestational age and weigh 9 lb or more.

✳ nursing process for the client with diabetes mellitus

assessment

Subjective data to be assessed include the following:

* History of diabetes
* Previous delivery of a large infant (9 lb or more)
* History of excessive weight gain during the pregnancy
* Classic diabetes symptoms, such as excessive urination (*polyuria*), excessive thirst (*polydipsia*), or excessive ingestion of food (*polyphagia*).

Objective data to be assessed include the following:

* Elevated blood glucose in the urine (*glycosuria*)
* Elevated blood glucose level

nursing diagnoses

* Fear, related to the impact of diabetes on the pregnancy outcome
* Risk for Infection (urinary tract), related to diabetes
* Altered Nutrition: Potential for more than body requirements, related to possible nonadherence to dietary restrictions

planning and intervention

The nurse needs to discuss the basic pathophysiology of diabetes with the woman, answer her questions, and provide extra information about diet, exercise, and insulin management.

The woman needs to understand that glucose in the urine increases the risk of developing urinary tract infections and that increasing fluid intake can decrease the risk. The nurse encourages good handwashing habits and discusses signs and symptoms of infection. The nurse also reinforces the importance of reporting any abnormalities immediately. Having the patient do a 24-hour dietary recall can help identify potential problems in following the diabetic diet assigned. The woman also may be referred to a dietician for further counseling.

evaluation

* Patient will relate an increase in psychological and physiologic comfort.
* Patient will demonstrate knowledge of risk factors and practice appropriate precautions to prevent infection.
* Patient will demonstrate understanding of nutritional needs during pregnancy.

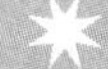

nursing alert

Emphasize the importance of home self-care and the need to adhere to diet, rest, and an exercise program for the best possible outcome.

infections

A woman of childbearing age can acquire numerous infections. The more common ones that can directly affect pregnancy or the outcome of the pregnancy are discussed here. These include urinary tract infections, sexually transmitted diseases (STDs), and a group of **teratogenic** infectious diseases associated with pregnancy, **formerly** identified by the acronym TORCH. The letters in TORCH represent the following:

T: toxoplasmosis

O: other (including hepatitis B, human immunodeficiency virus [HIV], syphilis, and chlamydial infection)

R: rubella
C: cytomegalovirus
H: herpes

Some teratogenic diseases are spread by sexual contact; others are spread by a variety of ways, but they all are capable of infecting the fetus.

urinary tract infections

Under the influence of hormones, especially progesterone, the urinary tract becomes especially susceptible to a variety of urinary tract infections (UTIs) during pregnancy because of the loss of muscle tone. The infections range from a minor case of bladder infection (cystitis) to a more serious kidney infection, such as pyelonephritis.

etiology and pathophysiology

During pregnancy, the lower ureter and renal pelvis narrow, and the upper ureter dilates. This leads to stasis of urine and delayed emptying of the bladder, which increases the potential for urinary infections; in addition, muscle tone is poor due to increased hormones, and there is mechanical pressure from the enlarging uterus.

diagnostic tests

Sterile or clean-catch urine specimens are obtained, and culture and sensitivity reports are used to identify the causative agent and the appropriate antibiotic.

medical management

Once the pregnant woman has been diagnosed with an infection, appropriate antibiotics are usually administered. Amoxicillin, ampicillin, and cephalosporins are the drugs of choice for UTIs because most bacteria causing these infections are sensitive to them, and their use during pregnancy is considered safe.

✳ nursing process for the client with a urinary tract infection

assessment

Subjective data to be assessed include the following:

* Pain in the lumbar region
* Malaise
* Dysuria, urgency, or frequency of urination

Objective data to be assessed include the following:

* Presence of bacteria noted on urinalysis
* Blood in urine (hematuria)
* Elevated temperature, chills
* Vomiting

nursing diagnosis

* Pain, related to inflammation and infection
* Altered Health Maintenance, related to knowledge deficit of prevention of recurrence

planning and intervention

Nursing care focuses on educating the woman on the proper use of antibiotics and the woman and her partner on practices to prevent further infections. The woman needs to be encouraged to drink 8 glasses of water daily, to wash the perineum from front to back to prevent fecal contamination, to avoid sexual practices that may irritate the meatus, and to void immediately when she feels the urge. In addition, she should be counseled to report immediately any recurrence of symptoms.

evaluation

* Patient will report relief of pain following medical and nursing intervention.
* Patient will verbalize understanding of practices needed to prevent recurrence of UTIs.

toxoplasmosis

Toxoplasmosis is caused by a protozoan called *Toxoplasma gondii*. It is transmitted by ingesting or handling raw meat or handling cat feces (generally from cleaning cat litter boxes).

The disease produces mild flulike symptoms in the woman but can produce devastating effects in the fetus. If the disease is acquired early in pregnancy, it may produce a spontaneous abortion. If acquired later, it may result in inflammation of the fetal brain (*encephalitis*), a small brain and head in relationship to the body (*microcephaly*), an abnormal collection of cerebrospinal fluid (*hydrocephaly*), convulsions, or mental retardation.

etiology and pathophysiology

Once the organism enters the woman's body, it travels throughout the body, crossing the placental barrier and entering the fetal tissue. Approximately 75% to 90% of exposed pregnant women have the potential for developing this disease.

diagnostic tests

Antibody titer blood tests are drawn to confirm diagnosis. To detect fetal involvement, an ultrasound and aspiration of amniotic fluid may be performed.

medical management

Toxoplasmosis can be prevented primarily through educational counseling. The person who prepares meals should be instructed to cook meat well and to wash hands thoroughly when handling raw meat. If cats are kept in the house, some family member other than the pregnant woman should empty the litter box.

If the pregnant woman has contracted toxoplasmosis, the drugs of choice are pyrimethamine or sulfadiazine. Studies show that these antimicrobials can limit or prevent damage to the fetus.

✳ nursing process for the client with toxoplasmosis

assessment

Subjective data to be assessed include the following:

* ✳ General malaise, listlessness, aching, and other vague flulike symptoms

Objective data to be assessed include the following:

* ✳ Elevated temperature and enlarged lymph glands

nursing diagnosis

* ✳ Fear, related to impact of disease on fetus
* ✳ Anxiety, related to lack of knowledge about disease process

planning and intervention

Prevention of toxoplasmosis includes educating the woman to avoid contact with raw meat and cat feces. Once the mother has been diagnosed with toxoplasmosis, the nurse explains all procedures and possible outcomes, emphasizing the importance of follow-up care. The woman must be able to verbalize her concerns. If spontaneous abortion occurs or if the newborn is disabled, the woman is referred for counseling. This may be done through local support groups, her minister or other spiritual advisor, or a mental health professional.

evaluation

* ✳ The woman reports an increase in psychological comfort.
* ✳ The woman demonstrates resolution of anxiety following education.

rubella

Rubella, commonly called 3-day measles or German measles, causes general flulike symptoms and a characteristic pink papular rash that appears first on the face, then the trunk, and finally the extremities. It lasts for 3 days and may cause minor itching. Side effects are rare, but in the fetus of an infected woman, the effects are devastating. If rubella is contracted during the first trimester of pregnancy, the fetus may develop congenital rubella syndrome (CRS). During the first month of pregnancy, the risk of developing CRS is 50%; during the second month, it drops to 25% and during the third month to 10%. During the second and third trimesters, the risk drops to less than 1% (Eisele, 1993). The major symptoms of CRS include blindness, deafness, heart defects, mental retardation, cleft lip, and cleft palate.

Infants born with CRS are infectious and must be isolated from other infants and from pregnant women. They may continue to shed the virus for several months following birth. Prevention of the disease is the best therapy. Women of childbearing age should be tested for immunity. A rubella antibody titer (blood test) of 1 : 8 or greater shows the individual has developed immunity to rubella. If the titer is less, immunization with live vaccine should be given, after which the woman should avoid pregnancy for 3 months to prevent transmission of the virus to the embryo. If the woman is pregnant, the immunization will need to be delayed until after delivery.

teaching guidelines ✳
prevention of sexually transmitted diseases

* ✳ Know your sexual partner; observe for signs of lesions or discharge.
* ✳ Use condoms; they can prevent most forms of sexually transmitted diseases (STDs).
* ✳ If you are sexually active, you need to have regular physical check-ups and report any lesions or discharges.
* ✳ Share your history of any STD infection with your sexual partner.
* ✳ Remember, there is no vaccination available to prevent STDs.

sexually transmitted diseases

STDs are diseases spread by any type of sexual contact: genital, oral-genital, or anogenital. As a group, STDs have reached epidemic proportions in the United States, affecting an estimated 30 to 40 million people. The Teaching Guidelines display provides guidelines to help reduce the risk or prevent the transmission of STDs. These diseases cause the greatest harm to women and infants, resulting in chronic infection, infertility, or spontaneous abortion. If the woman contracts the disease during pregnancy, the effect on the fetus is related to the trimester during which infection occurs. During pregnancy, the health care provider is challenged with eliminating the infection, preserving the future fertility of the woman, and preventing harm to the existing fetus.

The incidence of STDs is highest in young sexually active adults, ages 15 to 24, particularly in ethnic minority populations living in urban areas. Any sexually active person is at risk, however. Many people have more than one STD; for example, more than 20% of people infected with gonorrhea also have a chlamydial infection. Table 9-5 shows the various STDs, their effects on the woman and fetus, and the medical treatment of choice.

syphilis

Syphilis is caused by the spirochete *Treponema pallidum*. It is transmitted by sexual contact and can be fatal if untreated. Following an incubation period of 1 to 3 months,

table 9-5 sexually transmitted diseases seen in pregnancy

Disease and Causative Agent	*Maternal Effects*	*Newborn Effects*	*Medical Management*
Candidiasis (*Candida albicans*)	Erythema and pruritus of labia and vulva Thick white, curdlike vaginal discharge	Thrush	Maternal—Mycostatin vaginal tablets or cream during pregnancy Newborn—oral Mycostatin
Chlamydia (*Chlamydia trachomatis*)	Ectopic pregnancy Preterm labor	Sepsis Conjunctivitis Pneumonia	Maternal—Zithromax 1 g PO once or Vibramycin 100 mg PO b.i.d. for 7 d (including partner). *If pregnant*—erythromycin 250 mg PO q.i.d .for 14 d Newborn—erythromycin ointment in both eyes at birth
Gonorrhea (Neisseria gonorrhoeae)	Infection of the chorionic and amnionic membranes Preterm delivery	Sepsis Ophthalmic infections	Maternal—Rocephin 125 mg once with doxycycline, 100 mg PO b.i.d. for 7 d (including partner) *If pregnant*—Rocephin 125 mg IM for 1 d, then erythromycin 500 mg PO q.i.d. for 7 d Newborn—erythromycin ointment in both eyes at birth
Genital herpes (herpes types II)	Painful vesicles on genitalia	Local skin lesions on eyes, skin, and throat May become systemic; can result in fetal death, low birth weight, prematurity	Maternal—no known cure; to alleviate symptoms, may use acyclovir (not approved for use during pregnancy) Cesarean delivery may be necessary Newborn—no known cure; to alleviate symptoms, may use acyclovir
Syphilis (*Treponema pallidum*)	Chancre sores Ulcers on genitalia Rash CNS symptoms	May develop congenital syphilis	Maternal—penicillin. Newborn—penicillin
Trichomonas (*Trichomonas vaginalis*)	Foul, frothy, yellow-green vaginal discharge Vaginal pruritus	None	Maternal—Flagyl (including partner). If pregnant, Cleocin vaginal cream 2% during the first trimester
Condyloma, papilomavirus (genital warts)	Warts present on vulva Bleeding Vaginal discharge	Warts may be present on the larynx	Maternal—podophyllin drug of choice but contraindicated during pregnancy Cryosurgery (freezing of tissue) or laser surgery
Acquired immunodeficiency virus	AIDS-related complex (ARC) Kaposi's sarcoma *Pneumocystis carinii* Death	ARC Kaposi's sarcoma *P. carinii* Death	Maternal—no cure; AZT, antibiotics, and gamma globulin provide temporary relief Newborn—same treatment as maternal
Cytomegalovirus	Mild fever or asymptomatic	Mental retardation Deafness Death	Maternal—none Newborn—none

a painless lesion (chancre) appears where the organism entered the body, most often on the genitalia but does occur on the lips, mouth, or rectum (see Fig. 9-7*A* and *B*). If untreated, the lesion disappears, but the lymph glands may be enlarged. This is the *primary stage* of syphilis. As the individual reaches the *secondary stage*, 2 to 4 weeks after the initial lesion disappears, a generalized rash appears. An elevated temperature with sore throat, eye inflammation, and joint pain may occur during this time. These symptoms also will disappear after a few weeks. Within a few months, the individual reaches the latent phase of the infection. It may last several years and is no longer infectious to others except during pregnancy when it can be passed to the fetus. The *tertiary stage* (late stage) of syphilis is debilitating: The infected person experiences destruction of the heart and central nervous system. Congenital syphilis, transmission of the germ from the mother to the fetus, may appear any time during the infectious process. It may result in stillbirth, intrauterine growth retardation, or preterm labor. A blood test called VDRL (Venereal Disease Research Laboratory) test or RPR (rapid plasma reagin) is performed to detect syphilis. Penicillin is the drug of choice and may be used at any stage of the illness; however, any damage to the heart or central nervous system is permanent.

gonorrhea

Gonorrhea, caused by *Neisseria gonorrhoeae*, is one of the most commonly reported and easily transmitted STDs in the United States. Since 1986, approximately 1 million new cases have been reported each year. The rates are extremely high in teenagers and young adults, especially in the inner cities (Bowie, Hammerschlag, & Martin, 1994). The bacteria live in the mouth, throat, urethra, and cervix.

Four out of five woman with gonorrhea remain asymptomatic. Those with symptoms will experience pelvic pain, a yellow-green vaginal discharge, and vulvar irritation. Lack of treatment in the woman may result in the spread of the infection to the fallopian tubes. This may cause pelvic inflammatory disease (PID), resulting in scarring of the tube and sterility.

In 80% of men infected with gonorrhea, the symptoms include painful urination and a white, yellow, or yellow-green penal discharge. The remaining 20% of men remain asymptomatic. Lack of treatment may result in the spread of the infection the to testes, causing sterility.

Symptoms of gonorrhea may appear within 1 to 14 days after contact in the man and the woman. Diagnosis is made by culturing the penal or vaginal discharge. Because most woman remain asymptomatic, a cervical culture is part of routine prenatal care. An infant born to a mother with gonorrhea may develop *ophthalmia neonatorum* (gonorrheal conjunctivitis); most states require administration of prophylactic antibiotic eye ointment at birth.

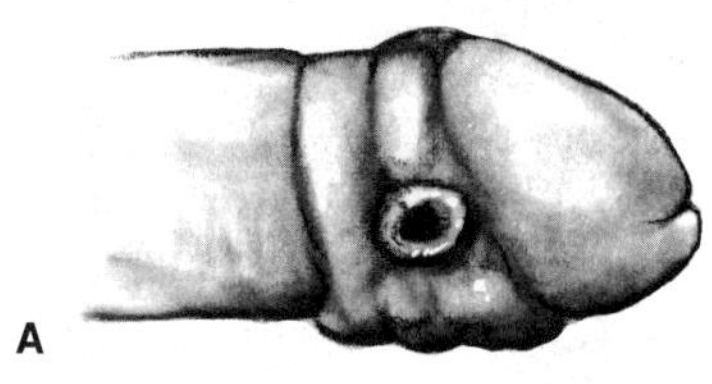

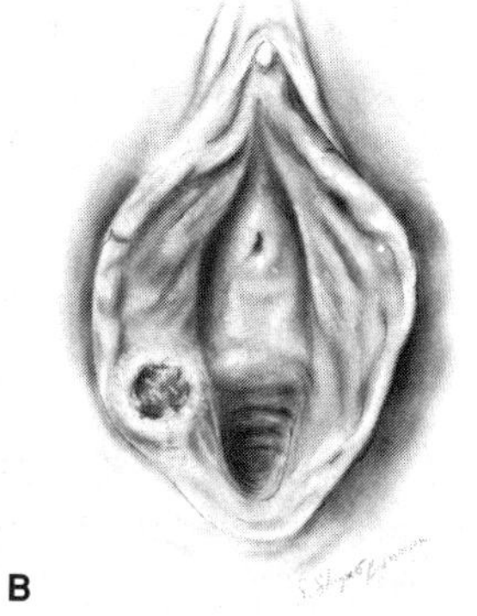

figure 9-7 *Common sites of syphilitic chancres. (**A**) Penis. (**B**) Vulva.*

hepatitis b

Hepatitis B is an inflammation of the liver caused by hepatitis B virus (HBV). The virus attacks cells of the liver, causing scarring (cirrhosis), liver failure, cancer, or death. It is spread by direct contact with infected blood or body fluids (including semen) through any of the following: blood transfusion, sharing needles, sexual intercourse, or passage through the birth canal of an infected woman. An individual's risk for acquiring HBV is increased if he or she lives in the same household with an HBV carrier or has a job that involving exposure to infected human blood.

Symptoms include nausea, vomiting, tenderness over the liver region, and later jaundice. Diagnosis is confirmed by a blood test detecting antigens in the blood, liver biopsy, palpation of tenderness over the liver, and late in the disease, the presence of jaundice. Treatment is supportive; there is no known cure. The woman is placed on bed rest and encouraged to eat a high-calorie diet.

Use of HBV vaccine can prevent perinatal transmission. The vaccine may be given to women during pregnancy if they test negative for the virus. It is given in a series of three shots, spread over 6 months. If the mother has HBV, the newborn can be protected from infection by receiving the first of three injections plus a dose of hepatitis B immune globulin within 12 hours after birth. The remaining two doses will be given with the other childhood immunizations at 1 and 6 months of age. The Centers for Disease Control and Prevention (CDC) recommend that all pregnant women be tested for HBV and that all infants receive the vaccine, regardless of the mother's HBV status (CDC, 1994).

trichomoniasis

In the woman, *Trichomonas vaginalis*, a protozoan infection, produces a frothy vaginal discharge, with intense itching and swelling of the vulva. *Dysuria* (pain with uri-

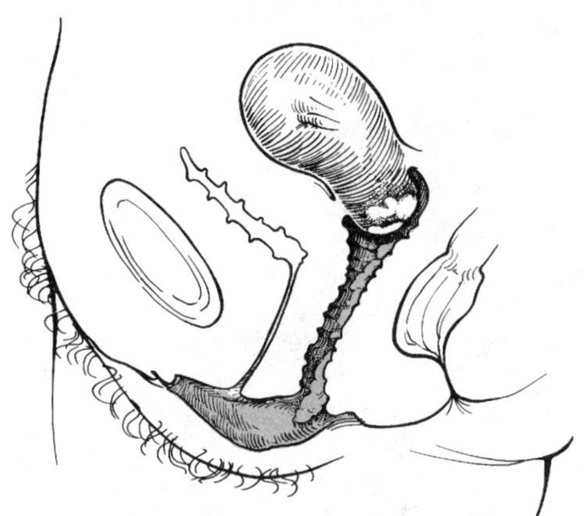

figure 9-8 *Candidiasis.*

nation) and *dyspareunia* (painful intercourse) also may develop. The infection often recurs.

An infected man is usually asymptomatic but occasionally develops prostatitis (infection of the prostate gland). Diagnosis is made by microscopic examination of vaginal secretions. Trichomoniasis does not spread to the uterus and fallopian tubes, so there is no risk of infertility, but the intense irritation to the vaginal tissues may cause atypical cells to show on the Pap smear.

Metronidazole (Flagyl) is the treatment of choice and may be used during the second and third trimesters but is contraindicated during the first trimester of pregnancy. The CDC guidelines recommend the use of clindamycin (Cleocin) 2% vaginal cream during the first trimester.

candidiasis (monilia)

Candida is a yeast (fungus) that is part of the normal flora of mucous membranes, including the vagina. It becomes a problem when it multiplies too rapidly (Fig. 9-8). It may be spread by sexual contact but also can be seen with an increase in estrogen levels (pregnancy, birth control pills) and with use of certain antibiotics that destroy the normal flora and changes the Ph. Certain hygienic practices also may contribute to the development of *Candida*. These include frequent douching, use of perfumed body sprays, and tight-fitting nylon underwear and pantyhose.

In the woman, the symptoms of *Candida* include a cheesy, white, vaginal discharge, intense vaginal itching, and red swollen vulva. An infected man may experience irritation of the penis. Miconazole nitrate (Monistat) vaginal creams or suppositories are ordered for insertion twice daily for 10 to 14 days. The nurse needs to instruct the woman on the insertion of the cream or suppositories. A vaginal pad can be worn to prevent staining of the underwear. Sexual intercourse should be avoided unless a condom is worn until drug therapy is completed.

cytomegalovirus

Cytomegalovirus (CMV) is a member of the herpes family and is spread by any close contact, such as kissing, sexual intercourse, or breast-feeding. More than 50% of all adults have antibodies for the virus. It is found in semen, cervical mucus, breast milk, saliva, and urine. If CMV is contracted during pregnancy, the mother may be asymptomatic, but the fetus can develop deafness or mental retardation or may die from severe tissue damage. There is no treatment for this disease.

genital herpes

Genital herpes (*herpes simplex virus type 2*) is a chronic STD that may be controlled but not cured. It produces small, red, painful blisters on the genital region around the vagina and rectum (Fig. 9-9). The blisters break and produce ulcerated areas that last up to 6 weeks. The herpes virus recurs throughout the life of the individual. If the woman develops herpes for the first time during the first trimester of pregnancy, it can be systemic, causing placental spread, resulting in spontaneous abortion. Genital herpes also is associated with prematurity and intrauterine growth retardation. If the woman has active herpes at the time of birth, cesarean delivery is recommended to reduce the risk of neonatal infection. Infants born vaginally

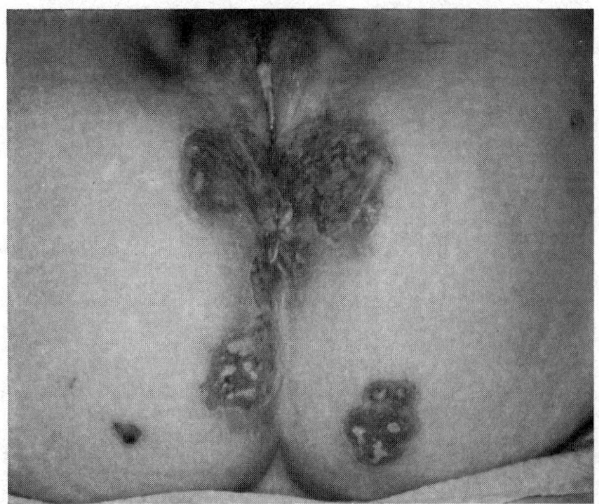

figure 9-9 *Herpes genitalis lesions are characterized by painful vesicles in the vulva and perineal areas.*

during active infections face a 50% chance of becoming infected, with a 60% death rate (Evans, 1994). The drug acyclovir can shorten the healing time but is not approved for use during pregnancy.

chlamydia

Chlamydia, caused by the bacterium *Chlamydia trachomatis*, produces a genitourinary infection. It is the most common STD seen in the United States, with 4 million new cases reported each year. Approximately 8% of all pregnant women in the United States are affected (Lott & Kenner, 1994). Single women with multiple sex partners who have unprotected intercourse are at highest risk. An estimated 15% to 20% of adolescents who use oral contraceptives are infected with *Chlamydia.*

Chlamydia is often considered the "silent STD" because its symptoms are generally mild and may mimic those of gonorrhea. Complications of chlamydia, however, can be serious, including PID and sterility. In the woman, chlamydia usually begins as an infection of the cervix. It can then spread to the uterus and fallopian tubes, producing scarring that can result in a high incidence of ectopic pregnancies or sterility. In the man, the first symptom of chlamydia is nongonococcal urethritis. If untreated, it leads to epididymitis, an inflammation of the testicles that results in sterility. A diagnosis is made by culturing epithelial cells from the cervix or penis. The pregnant woman may pass the infection to her unborn child, resulting in eye infection, conjunctivitis, or pneumonia.

condyloma acuminata (human papillomavirus, genital warts)

Genital warts are caused by human papillomavirus and are sexually transmitted. They appear as small pink or tan growths that itch and are spread by scratching. As they spread, they appear as cauliflower-like clusters. The warts appear on the vulva, vagina, cervix, and rectum of the woman. On the man, they occur on the penis and rectum (Fig. 9-10). Incubation time is from 1 to 3 months following contact. During pregnancy, the lesions increase in size, sometimes becoming so large that they interfere with vaginal delivery. Treatment of the nonpregnant individual consists of topical application of a 25% podophyllin. Podophyllin use during pregnancy is contraindicated because of its toxic effects on the fetus, but cryosurgery (freezing) or carbon dioxide laser surgery has been successful.

✳ nursing process for the client with a sexually transmitted disease

assessment

Assessment begins with the first prenatal visit. The nurse explores any vague reports of symptoms. Screening tests are usually performed during the first visit and later in the pregnancy as deemed necessary. It is important to educate the woman and her partner about STDs and precautions that should be taken.

Subjective data to be assessed include the following:

* Malaise or fatigue
* Abdominal discomfort or anorexia
* Pain with urination
* Vaginal irritation or itching

Objective data to be assessed include the following:

* Foul-smelling vaginal discharge
* Lesions of the vulva or labia
* Enlarged lymph nodes in the groin, axilla, or neck
* Rash
* Oral or genital lesions
* Elevated temperature

nursing diagnosis

* Fear, related to the consequence of condition on fetal outcome
* Knowledge Deficit, related to transmission, consequences, and prevention of STDs

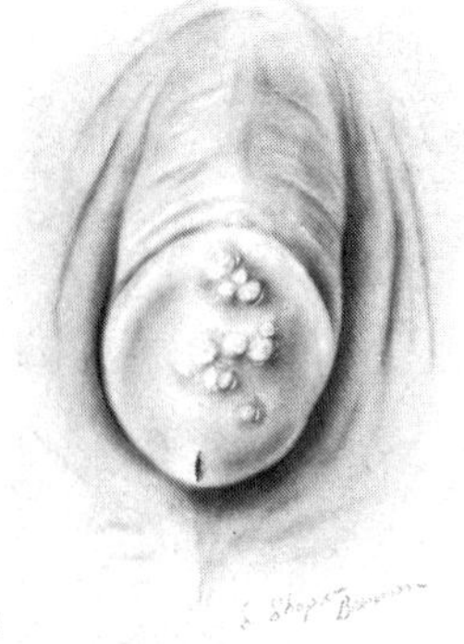

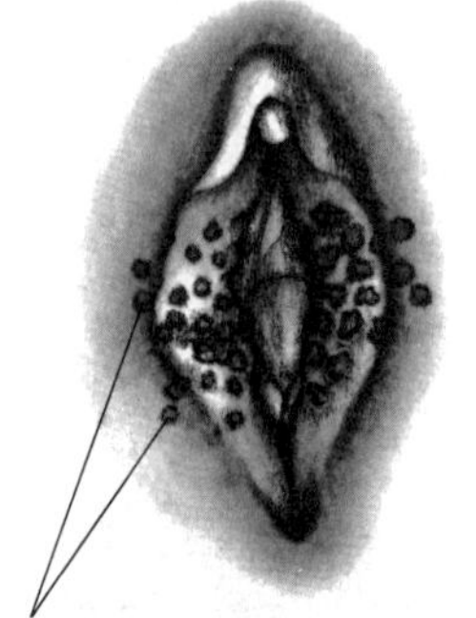

figure 9-10 *Venereal warts. **(A)** Venereal warts on penis. **(B)** Venereal warts on vulva.*

planning and implementation

When a woman has been diagnosed as having a STDs, she and her partner may experience a variety of emotions, especially fear for the fetus and the woman. By providing an open, nonjudgmental atmosphere, the nurse allows the couple to voice their concerns. Education and support are the two most important aspects of care. Education includes discussing the impact of the infection, the treatment ordered by the physician, and the importance of follow-up care and methods to prevent reinfection or recurrence.

evaluation

* Patient will report increased psychological comfort and coping skills.
* Patient is able to describe the route of transmission, consequences, and methods of prevention for STDs.

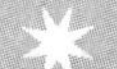
nursing alert
Remember the importance of universal precautions.

human immunodeficiency virus

The first case of acquired immunodeficiency syndrome (AIDS) was diagnosed in 1981. In 1983, the deadly virus believed to be responsible for this disease was isolated, and today it is called human immunodeficiency virus (HIV). It is the most deadly STD. The virus attacks and destroys the immune system, making the individual unable to fight infection. It attacks and changes the genetic makeup of the T lymphocytes responsible for immunity. The normal functioning T lymphocytes recognize foreign antigens and stimulate the B lymphocytes to produce antibodies. As the immune system becomes compromised, germs normally occurring in the environment invade and multiply, causing the individual to develop opportunistic infections that are life-threatening.

HIV is transmitted through blood and body fluids, including semen, breast milk, vaginal secretions, feces, and urine. See Display 9-6 for summary of HIV transmission. Women of childbearing age are the fastest growing group of HIV-infected people. Symptoms of HIV include fever, aches, pains, loss of appetite, night sweats, weight loss, swollen lymph glands, dry cough, diarrhea, and yeast infections. The individual is considered to have full-blown AIDS when he or she is diagnosed with one or more life-threatening opportunistic infections, such as *Pneumocystis carinii* pneumonia or toxoplasmosis of the brain.

Current research indicates there is no acceleration of HIV during pregnancy. Without treatment, however, 30% to 50% of infants born to HIV-positive women will be infected with HIV. The CDC currently recommends HIV testing for all pregnant women who are at risk for the development of the virus.

display 9-6
summary of transmission of human immunodeficiency virus

* **Sharing HIV-contaminated needles**
* **Oral, anal, or vaginal sex with an HIV-positive individual**
* **Receiving an HIV-contaminated blood transfusion**
* **Perinatally from mother to neonate**

diagnostic tests

The enzyme-linked immunosorbent assay (ELISA) antibody reaction blood test is used to diagnose HIV infection. If this test is positive, it is followed by the Western blot analysis for confirmation.

medical management

Once the woman has been identified as HIV positive, she is counseled to avoid pregnancy. If she is in the early stages of pregnancy, termination of the pregnancy is one option offered. High doses of antibiotics may be needed to fight infections that develop. If the woman has not been treated with antiviral drugs previous to the pregnancy, the risk of HIV transmission to the infant may be decreased by more than half with the administration of AZT (zidovudine) during pregnancy and for 6 weeks after delivery to the mother and the newborn.

✳ nursing process for the client with hiv infection

The symptoms of HIV infection are usually vague, and many can mimic the early signs of pregnancy. Women should be assessed carefully during prenatal visits.

assessment

Subjective data to be assessed include the following:

* Pain
* Loss of appetite
* Vaginal itching
* Reports of night sweats

Objective data to be assessed include the following:

* Elevated temperature
* Weight loss
* Swollen lymph glands
* Dry cough
* Diarrhea
* Yeast infections
* Positive test results for HIV
* Appearance of rashes or lesions
* Vaginal discharge
* Presence of opportunistic infections

nursing diagnosis

* Knowledge Deficit, related to disease process
* Fear, related to course of disease and possible transmission to the fetus

planning and implementation

Many HIV-positive women are not aware of their diagnosis until prenatal screening tests are performed. Emotional support and understanding are vital in assisting the woman and her family to accept the diagnosis and make plans for the uncertain future. The woman is instructed about the disease and the signs, symptoms, and changes to be reported. Medications are administered as needed. The nurse should explain medication use, schedule, and possible side effects for which to watch and report. Every attempt is made to prevent exposing the fetus to maternal blood. For example, during labor, internal fetal monitoring and scalp blood sampling are avoided.

nursing alert

During delivery, universal precautions require the use of gloves, gowns, and face shields or goggles due to the high risk of splashing of amniotic fluid and the presence of blood.

evaluation

* The woman will verbalize understanding of the disease process.
* The woman will demonstrate appropriate coping skills.

special pregnancy concerns related to maternal age

A woman's reproductive life extends from menarche to menopause, a period of 35 or 40 years. Childbearing at either end of this age continuum has special considerations and implications for the client and the nurse. Women younger than 16 years or older than 35 years face additional risks.

teenage pregnancy

Young people are becoming sexually active early in adolescence, and an epidemic of teenage pregnancy is the tragic result. Women between the ages of 15 and 19 are having in excess of 1/2 million babies per year in the United States (Harlap, Kost, & Forrest, 1991). The Guttmacher Institute, an institution that tracks sexual behavior patterns, reports that 9% of 12-year-olds, 30% of 15-year-olds, and 71% of 18-year-olds have had sex at least once.

Teenage mothers have unique and complex physical, emotional, and economic needs. They are "children having children," usually single parents with little financial security. Many try to complete their high school education while pregnant or while learning to be a mother; others drop out of school, impairing their economic future.

Physically, teenage pregnancy is considered high risk because of the increased incidence of PIH, iron deficiency anemia, preterm and low–birth-weight newborns, cephalopelvic disproportion, STDs, and stillbirths in women younger than 20 years of age. Compounding their problems is the fact that many receive no prenatal care.

Emotionally, the pregnant teenager is forced to deal with the developmental issues of adolescence and pregnancy at the same time. She may have low self-esteem, poor body image, or the inability to develop peer relationships. In addition, her parents may attempt to take over the decision-making or ask her to leave the family unit, totally abandoning her.

nursing considerations

The pregnant teenager needs patience, understanding, and empathy. The nurse may be her first contact with someone ready to listen and understand her needs and concerns. Time should be set aside during the first prenatal visit to explain fetal growth and development and the changes she can expect in her own body. Good basic nutrition should be emphasized because teenagers tend to have irregular dietary habits. Explaining the relationship between good nutrition, fetal development, and personal weight gain may assist in gaining the teenager's compliance.

The first prenatal visit is an excellent time to assess the teenager's level of psychological development and the level of family support and involvement. Financial concerns may be explored at this time. The nurse may need to call on social services for assistance for the teenager.

Care of the pregnant adolescent should focus on the following:

* Obtaining early prenatal care
* Determining the availability of adequate nutrition, housing, and continuance of education and financial assistance
* Enrollment in childbirth education classes
* Enrollment in parenting education classes as available

pregnancy in women older than 35 years

Although pregnancy after age 35 is still considered high risk, new research indicates there is "no relationship between pregnancy outcome and maternal age after coexisting maternal disease is excluded" (Catanzarite, Deutchman, Johnson, & Scherger, 1995). In today's society, most first-time pregnancies after the age of 35 are planned. Many women are waiting until their careers are established. These mothers are emotionally prepared, seek early prenatal care, and follow health care recommendations for pregnancy. They usually also seek and attend childbirth education classes.

Unfortunately, nearly 12% of pregnant women older than 35 years have chronic medical conditions, including hypertension, diabetes, cardiac disease, renal disease, thyroid disorders, and uterine malformations. As many as 50% of women older than 35 years also have infertility problems. Maternal age increases the chances for chromosomal abnormalities in the newborn, with Down syndrome being the most common.

A woman who is 35 years or older and considering pregnancy needs to understand the following:

* She is two to three times more likely to have a cesarean delivery.
* She is three times more likely to have twins.
* She has a slightly higher than average maternal mortality rate.
* She has an increased risk for the development of gestational diabetes.

nursing considerations

The pregnant woman older than 35 years should be encouraged to seek prenatal care early in her pregnancy. Tests such as the triple screen, chorionic villus sampling, or amniocentesis may be ordered to screen for fetal abnormalities. Thorough explanations need to be given. Care of the older pregnant woman is focused on the following:

* Careful monitoring of the mother and fetus
* Providing accurate information about the course of the pregnancy and the well-being of the fetus
* Teaching self-care and care of the newborn
* Offering emotional support, guidance, and appropriate referrals for social services as needed

key points

* **Spontaneous abortion occurs when the products of conception are expelled before the age of viability. It may be classified as threatened, inevitable, incomplete, missed, or habitual.**
* **Placenta previa results when the placenta implants in the lower segment of the uterus. The classic symptom is painless vaginal bleeding. It may be classified as total, partial, or low lying.**
* **Abruptio placentae is a condition in which a normally implanted placenta prematurely separates from the uterus. This produces hemorrhage and can result in the loss of mother and baby.**
* **PIH results in edema, hypertension, and proteinuria. The two stages of PIH are preeclampsia and eclampsia. HELLP syndrome, a variation of PIH, can occur with mild or severe preeclampsia.**
* **Hyperemesis gravidarum can occur during the first 16 weeks of pregnancy and may result in severe electrolyte imbalance. Hospitalization with the use of IV hydration may be necessary.**
* **Hemolytic disease may occur when the pregnant woman's and baby's blood are not compatible. Transplacental bleeding allows blood cells from the baby to enter the pregnant woman's bloodstream, and she in turn produces antibodies. These antibodies may mix with fetal blood in subsequent pregnancy, resulting in destruction of fetal red blood cells.**
* **The blood volume may increase 30% to 50% during pregnancy. Pregnant women with cardiac disease may not tolerate this physiologic change. Cardiac disease is the leading nonobstetric cause of maternal death.**
* **Some pregnant women may develop diabetes during pregnancy, which may disappear after the delivery of the child. This condition is called gestational diabetes. It requires careful monitoring of diet and medication during the pregnancy.**
* **STDs may be transmitted to the fetus in utero. Monitoring for the presence of STDs in the mother is an important prenatal assessment.**
* **Pregnant women should be monitored for the presence of UTIs during pregnancy due to their increased susceptibility.**
* **HIV, the AIDS virus, is the most deadly of the STDs; it is transmitted through blood and body fluids. The CDC recommends HIV testing for all pregnant women who are at risk for the development of the virus.**
* **Pregnancy occurring before 16 years or after 35 years places the woman at risk for complications during pregnancy.**

review questions

1. Mrs. Vasquez is in her sixth month of pregnancy and has developed bright red, painless vaginal bleeding. Her abdomen is soft and nontender. Fetal heart tones are within normal limits. The physician states that she has placenta previa and to monitor her carefully. The nurse would
   a. monitor vital signs, heart tones, and keep a pad count.
   b. encourage fluids and keep an accurate record of intake and output.
   c. encourage ambulation and keep her NPO.
   d. call the minister because she will need emotional support.
2. Mrs. Silverman is in her ninth month of pregnancy and has been admitted to the hospital with the diagnosis of abruptio placentae. A critical nursing intervention would be to
   a. give her a drink and assist her into a comfortable position.
   b. obtain blood pressure, pulse, and fetal heart tone readings.
   c. make her NPO and discuss the possibility of surgery.
   d. discuss the possible need for blood transfusions.
3. Mrs. Chang is in her 28th week of pregnancy and has developed hypertension and edema of the face, hands, and feet that does not disappear with rest. The physi-

cian has told her she has PIH and must return to the office next week. The nurse should tell her,
   a. "Don't worry. The baby will be perfectly fine."
   b. "The doctor will probably admit you to the hospital next week just to be safe."
   c. "It is important that you rest as much as possible."
   d. "You should begin checking your urine at home because you will probably develop gestational diabetes."
4. Pregnant women should avoid changing the cat litter during pregnancy to prevent
   a. *Chlamydia.*
   b. gonorrhea.
   c. toxoplasmosis.
   d. hyperemesis gravidarum.
5. Mrs. Garber is in her fourth month of pregnancy and has developed gestational diabetes. She can expect
   a. always to be a diabetic.
   b. to be placed on a diabetic diet with frequent monitoring of blood sugar.
   c. no special precautions because it will only last the length of the pregnancy.
   d. hospitalization for insulin injection technique.

references

Bowie, W. R., Hammerschlag, M. R., & Martin, D. H. (1994). STDs in '94: The new CDC guidelines. *Patient Care, 28*(7), 29.

Catanzarite, V., Deutchman, M., Johnson, C. A., & Scherger, J. (1995). Pregnancy after 35: What's the real risk. *Patient Care, 29*(1), 41–51.

Centers for Disease Control (1994). *Hepatitis B prevention and pregnancy.* Atlanta, GA: US Department of Health and Human Services.

Eisele, C. J. (1993). Rubella susceptibility in women of childbearing age. *Journal of Obstetric, Gynecologic, and Neonatal Nursing, 22*(3), 260–263.

Evans, N. (1994). *The A to Z of pregnancy and childbirth.* Alameda: Hunter House.

Harlap, S., Kost K., & Forrest, J. D. (1991). *Preventing pregnancy, protecting health: A new look at birth control choices in the United States.* New York: The Alan Guttmacher Institute.

Lott, J. W., & Kenner, C. (1994). Keeping up with neonatal infections: Designer bugs, Part I. *MCN, 19,* 207–213.

Sauer, P. M., & Harvey, C. J. (1992). Pregnancy-induced hypertension: Understanding severe preeclampsia and the HELLP syndrome. *Critical care nursing clinics of North America, 4,* 703.

bibliography

Burnhill, M. S. (1994). Adolescent pregnancy rates in the US. *Contemporary OB/GYN, 39*(2), 26–30.

Cordisco, M. E. (1994). Fighting DIC. *RN, August,* 37–40.

Flaskerud, J. H., & Ungvarski, P. J. (1992). *HIV/AIDS: A guide to nursing care* (2nd ed.). Philadelphia: W.B. Saunders.

Fleming, B. W., Munton, M. T., Clarke, B. A., & Strauss, S. S. (1993). Assessing and promoting positive parenting in adolescent mothers. *The American Journal of Maternal Child Nursing, 18,* 32–37.

Killion, C. (1993). Pregnancy: A critical time to target STDs. *MCN, 19,* 156–161.

(1992). *Lippincott's review series: Maternal-newborn.* Philadelphia: J.B. Lippincott.

MacLaren, A. (1992). *Nurse's clinical guide to maternity care.* Springhouse, PA: Springhouse Corp.

Martin, L. L., & Reeder, S. J. (1991). *Essentials of maternity nursing.* Philadelphia: J.B. Lippincott.

Olds, S. B., London, M. L., & Ladewig, P. W. (1992). *Maternal-newborn nursing* (4th ed.). Redwood City: Addison-Wesley.

Orellana, M. A., & Remington, J. S. (1990). Toxoplasmosis in pregnancy. *Hospital Medicine,* 26(9):09–111, 119–125.

Petrone, C., & Mandel, L. (1994). Hypertension: This patient is pregnant. *RN, February,* 50–55.

Pillitteri, A. (1995). *Maternal and child health nursing* (2nd ed.). Philadelphia: J.B. Lippincott.

Queenan, J. T. (1984). Rh and other blood immunizations. *Ortho Novum Publication,* 15–23.

Reeder, S. J., Martin, L. L., & Koniak, D. (1992). *Maternity nursing: Family, newborn, and women's health care* (17th ed.). Philadelphia: J.B. Lippincott.

Sipes, C. (1995). Guidelines for assessing HIV in women. *MCN, 20,* 29–33.

Tillman, J. (1992). Syphilis: An old disease, a contemporary perinatal problem. *Journal of Obstetric, Gynecologic, and Neonatal Nursing, 21*(3), 209–213.

Trustem, A. (1991). When to suspect ectopic pregnancy. *RN, August,* 22–25.

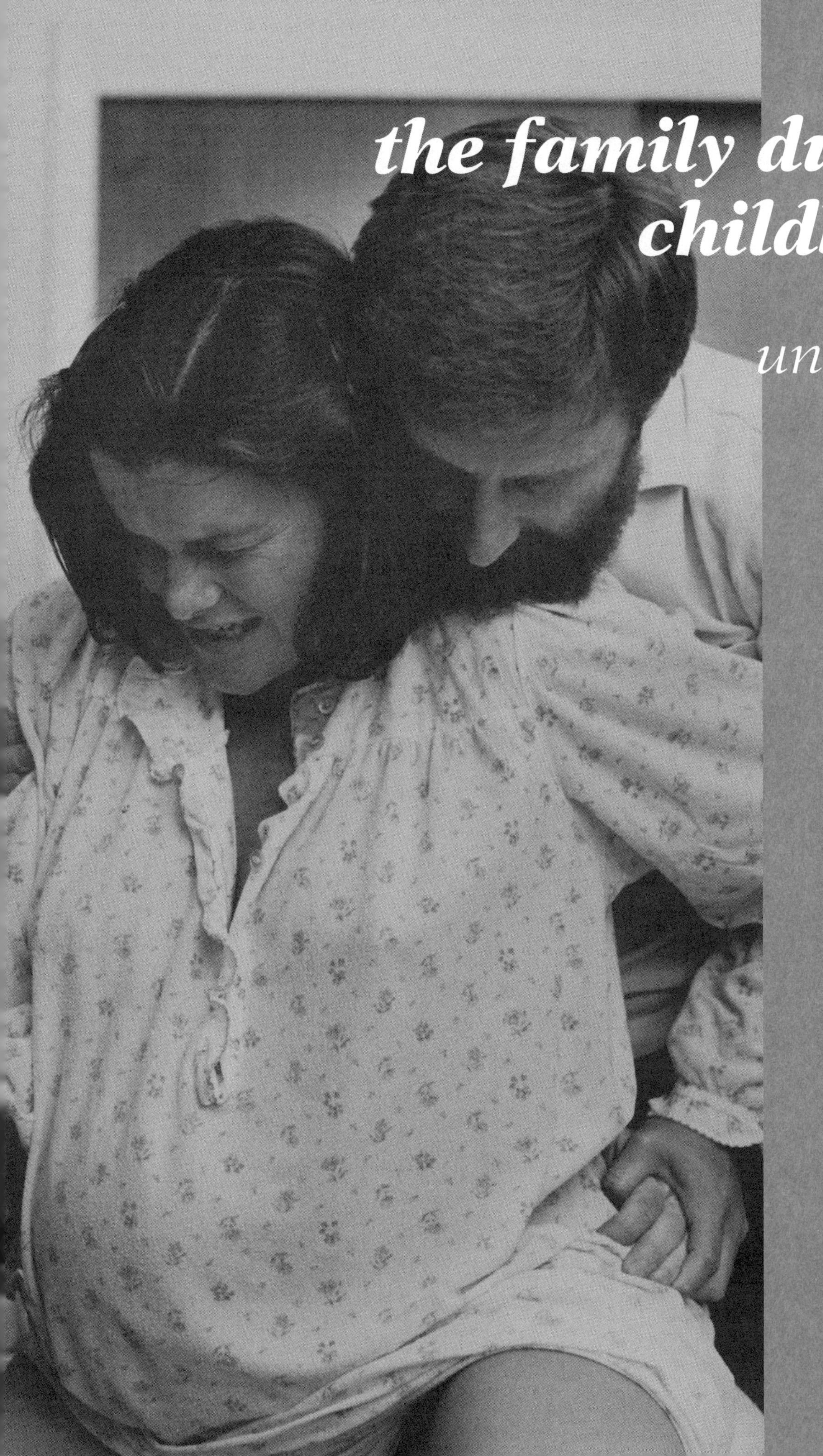

the family during childbirth

unit IV

the process of labor 10

outline

objectives

After studying this chapter, the reader should be able to:

* Define the preliminary signs of approaching labor.
* Define the differences between true and false labor.
* Discuss the four Ps that affect the course of success of labor.
* Describe the four types of fetal presentation.
* Define frank breech, complete breech, and footling breech.
* Define the six cardinal movements of the fetus during labor and birth.
* Discuss the terminology used to assess contractions.
* Discuss the impact of the woman's perception of labor and its outcome.
* Discuss the four stages of labor.
* Discuss the fetal and maternal physiologic effects of labor.

key terms

acme
attitude
cardinal movements
cephalopelvic disproportion
complete breech
crowning
decrement
diagonal conjugate
dilatation
duration
effacement
engagement
fontanels
footling breech
frank breech
frequency
increment
intensity
labor
lie
lightening
molding
mucus plug
oblique lie
occiput
restitution
retained placenta
ripening
station
transverse lie
vertex

Labor is the process of regular, involuntary uterine contractions leading to cervical *effacement* (thinning) and *dilatation* (dilation), resulting in the birth of the infant. It is a normal physiologic process that proceeds in a fairly predictable manner to the delivery of a healthy newborn. The course of labor is influenced by a variety of factors, making each birth unique and special (Table 10-1).

This chapter discusses the process of labor. Nursing care of the client and family during labor and delivery is discussed in Chapter 12, Nursing Care of the Family During Childbirth.

table 10-1 factors that impact the progress of labor

Element	*Impact*
Fetal position	* A well flexed vertex position is Ideal.
Gestational age	* Fetuses less than 37 weeks have a higher risk of malpresentation, which can lengthen labor.
	* Fetuses more than 42 weeks have a higher risk of large body size and birth complications, which can lengthen labor.
Birth weight	* Generally, the larger the fetus, the longer the labor.
Maternal age	* Young teenagers (younger than 16 years) have small immature pelvic structures, which can lengthen labor.
	* Older women (older than 35 years) have an increased incidence of twins and breech position, which can lengthen labor.
Maternal obesity	* Women who are obese generally have poor muscle tone, which can prolong labor.
Maternal position during labor	* A standing or upright position is more effective for dilation of the cervix.
	* A supine position can result in less effecient labor contractions because it works against gravity.
Maternal psychological status	* Stress and anxiety inhibit uterine activity.
Medications	* Narcotic analgesia can slow the progress of labor.
	* Epidural anesthetic may interfere with the mother's ability to push during the second stage of labor.
Parity	* First labors are usually longer than subsequent labors.
Status of membranes	* Rupture of membranes during labor brings the fetal head in close contact with the cervix for more efficient dilation.
	* Rupture of membranes also allows the uterus to remain partially contracted, causing more effective contractions.
Uterine contractions	* Contractions must be of sufficient quality to cause effacement and dilation.

preliminary signs of approaching labor

The pregnant woman often experiences preliminary signs alerting her that her body is preparing for labor and birth. These signs include *lightening,* Braxton Hicks contractions, the presence of bloody show, and spontaneous rupture of membranes (SROM).

lightening

Lightening is the phenomenon experienced when the fetus settles in the pelvic brim. This can occur 2 to 3 weeks before delivery in the primigravida and usually at the onset of labor in the multigravida. As the fetus and uterus "drop," the fundal pressure on the diaphragm is relieved, allowing the woman to breathe easier. This shift in position increases pressure in the lower abdomen, leading to urinary frequency, dependent edema in the lower extremities, leg cramps, development or exacerbation of varicose veins, hemorrhoids, and increased vaginal secretions due to congestion of the vaginal mucosa. Fetal movement at this time also may cause the woman to experience a feeling of pressure.

braxton hicks contractions

Braxton Hicks contractions are present throughout most of the pregnancy. They usually are painless, intermittent, and irregular but may increase in intensity during the last 6 to 8 weeks of pregnancy. If these contractions develop a fairly regular pattern, the woman may believe she is in labor. When this happens, it is called "false labor." This can be emotionally and physically exhausting for the woman. The nurse can alleviate some of the embarrassment by explaining that only by examination can true labor be differentiated from false labor.

bloody show (mucus plug)

The cervix becomes softer (also called *ripening*) and thinner and may begin to dilate in preparation for labor. The mucus plug, a collection of cervical secretions that seals the uterine opening, loosens and is expelled. This exposes small cervical capillaries that rupture, resulting in a pink or bloody vaginal discharge, referred to as *bloody show*. Bloody show signals that the beginning of true labor may occur within 24 hours.

spontaneous rupture of the membranes

Up to 12% of all women experience SROM prior to the beginning of labor. The amniotic fluid may gush suddenly or dribble slowly and continuously. In most cases, labor starts within 24 hours of the rupture. After 24 hours, there is an increased risk of intrauterine infection, and labor may be induced if the woman is near term. Some women may be concerned they will have a dry birth if the membranes are ruptured. The nurse can allay anxiety by explaining that amniotic fluid is continually produced until the birth of the child.

If the woman suspects that her membranes have ruptured, she should notify her care provider and proceed to the hospital or birthing center for examination. If she is slowly dribbling, it may be difficult to determine whether the membranes are still intact. Three methods may be used to confirm SROM: nitrazine paper, examination of fluid under the microscope, and vaginal examination with a speculum (Table 10-2).

other possible signs

A few days or hours before the beginning of labor, the woman may experience vague clues that something is about to happen. She may awake with a sudden burst of energy after feeling fatigued during the last month. She may experience an overwhelming desire to do heavy house cleaning, rearranging of furniture, or making changes in the general decor. This phenomenon is often called the nesting instinct. During the last week of pregnancy, she may actually lose 1 to 3 lb of weight after consistently gaining weight. Some women also may experience bouts of nausea, vomiting, or diarrhea preceding labor. Some of these events are due to the changes in hormonal levels prior to the onset of labor; others have no known cause.

characteristics of true labor and false labor

True labor contractions occur at regular intervals, increasing in intensity and duration, with a shortening of the intervals between each contraction. The contractions usually intensify with ambulation, and sedation or analgesic usually does not impede the progress. The woman may describe the contraction as starting in the lower back and circling to the front of the lower abdomen. The bloody show is usually present and increases in amount as the labor continues. Finally, and most important, the cervix dilates and effaces with true labor.

False labor contractions occur at irregular intervals that do not increase in intensity or duration. Ambulation does not intensify or otherwise affect the contraction, although sedation may slow or decrease the number of contractions. The discomfort is usually located in the lower abdomen, and usually there is an absence of bloody show. Most importantly, the cervix does not dilate or efface with false labor. For a comparison of true and false labor, see Table 10-3.

factors affecting labor

A successful labor depends on the "four Ps" (passage, passenger, powers, and psyche). The maternal pelvis must be large enough to allow *passage* of the fetus. The fetus (*passenger*) must be in an appropriate position and small enough to pass through the maternal pelvic cavity. The

table 10-2 tests for determination of the presence of amniotic fluid

Test	*Procedure*	*Results*
Nitrazine paper	With gloved hand, place a small piece of nitrazine paper in the vaginal orifice.	Amniotic fluid turns the yellow nitrazine paper blue because amniotic fluid is slightly alkaline (urine and vaginal secretions are both acidic).
Ferning or fern test	Using a sterile swab, obtain some of the suspected fluid from the vaginal orifice, and place on a glass slide to dry.	Dried amniotic fluid produces a fernlike pattern when examined under a microscope.
Examination with speculum	A sterile speculum is gently inserted into the vaginal canal; the woman is then instructed to bear down or cough.	If the membranes are ruptured, the examiner will see a pooling of amniotic fluid in the vaginal canal.

table 10-3 comparison of true versus false labor

Area of Consideration	*True Labor*	*False Labor*
Contractions	Regular intervals Increase in intensity Radiate from low back to lower abdomen Sedation does not stop the contractions Ambulation increases intensity	Irregular intervals Intensity remains the same Usually located in lower abdomen Sedation decreases or stops contractions No changes occur with ambulation
Cervix	Dilates and effaces	No changes occur
Bloody show	Present and increases as labor progresses	Not present

uterine contractions (*powers*) must be strong enough to cause effacement (thinning) and dilation (opening) of the cervix to allow for birth. Finally, the woman's psychological coping strategies (*psyche*) must be strong enough to support her throughout the process.

passage

For successful vaginal delivery, there must be sufficient room for the fetus to pass through the maternal pelvis. (See Chap. 4 for the types of pelves and their anatomy and physiology.) This trip through the true pelvis curves downward, forward, and upward. Measurements may be taken to determine safe passage. The *diagonal conjugate* is the most important measurement. It is the distance from the lower edge of the symphysis pubis to the sacral promontory (Fig. 10-1). This measurement must be a minimum of 10 cm for successful vaginal delivery. The transverse diameter, that is, the distance between the ischial spines, also must be at least 10 cm. Immobility of the coccyx, sharp raised ischial spines, or a narrowed pubic arch may interfere with the progress of labor. Imaging studies, such as computed tomography (CT) scans or sonograms, may be used to help assess pelvic measurements.

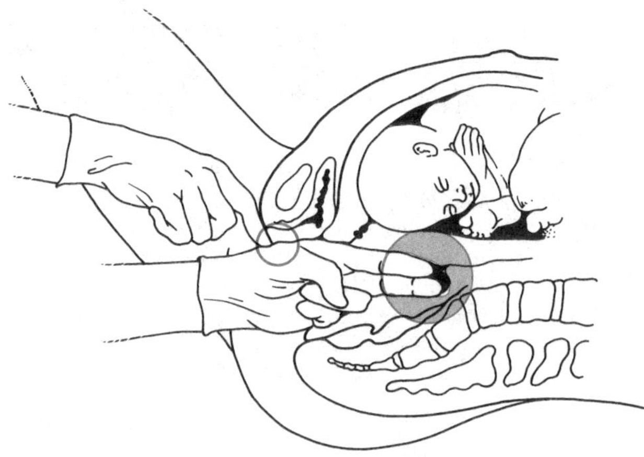

figure 10-1 *Diagonal conjugate. During the vaginal examination the examiner's middle finger touches the sacral prominence, and the index finger of the other hand marks the part of the examining hand that touches the symphysis pubis.*

If the fetus is too large, the pelvic anatomy too small, or the fetal position incompatible with a successful vaginal delivery, the condition is called *cephalopelvic disproportion* (CPD), and cesarean delivery is necessary.

passenger

Many factors affect the ability of the fetus to pass through the maternal pelvis. These include fetal head, *fetal lie, fetal attitude, fetal presentation* and position, and *cardinal movements*.

fetal head

The fetal head, the largest diameter of the body, is designed to withstand the pressure exerted on it as it pushes against the cervix. The bones of the head include the occipital bone, two temporal bones, two frontal bones, and two parietal bones. These bones are connected by strong connective tissue (*sutures*) that allows them to shift and overlap as the fetus passes through the birth canal. This process is called *molding*. The areas where the suture lines meet form two soft membranous areas called *fontanels*. The two most important fontanels are the anterior and posterior. The diamond-shaped *anterior fontanel* is the largest and is found just above the forehead. It remains open past the first birthday. The smaller, triangular *posterior fontanel* and the suture lines close shortly after birth.

fetal lie

Fetal lie refers to the relationship of the long axis (head to toe) of the fetus to the long axis (head to toe) of the woman. Approximately 99% of all fetuses assume a longitudinal lie; that is, the fetus' long axis is parallel with the woman's long axis. If the fetus' long axis is perpendicular to the woman's long axis, the position is called a *transverse lie.* The woman's spine and that of the fetus form a right angle. A transverse lie is usually the result of over-relaxation of the woman's abdominal wall caused by multiple pregnancies, an abnormal uterus, a contracted pelvis, or placenta previa. A transverse lie will always require ce-

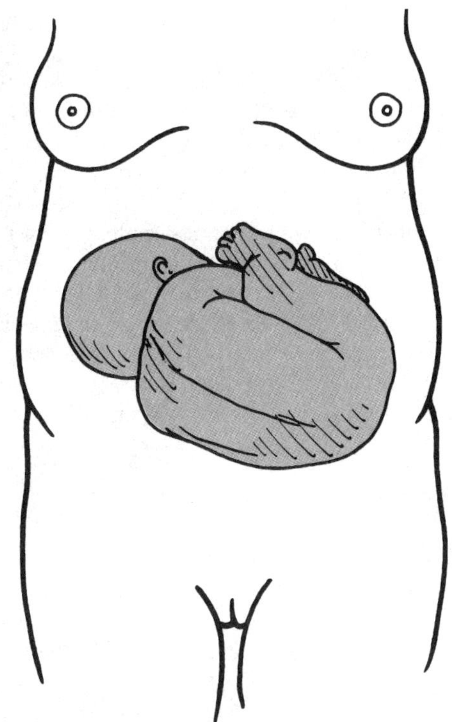

figure 10-2 *Transverse lie.*

sarean delivery because the head and the trunk of the fetus cannot enter the pelvis at the same time (Fig. 10-2). The fetus also may assume an *oblique lie* (the relationship of the spines forms less than a 45-degree angle); this position also will result in surgical intervention unless the fetus is able to assume a longitudinal lie before delivery.

fetal attitude

Fetal attitude refers to the relationship of the fetal parts to one another. Throughout pregnancy, the fetus may assume different positions in utero. In preparation for labor, most of the time, the fetus will assume a vertex (head first) position to allow for the smallest head diameter to enter the pelvis. In this position the fetus' head is flexed with its chin against its chest, the spinal column is curved forward, the upper extremities are folded against the chest, and the lower extremities are bent at the knees with the thighs on the abdomen. In this oval or egg-shaped position, the fetal body conforms best to the shape of the uterus.

fetal presentation and position

Fetal presentation (presenting part) refers to the part of the fetus that enters the birth canal first. Up to 97% of the time, the fetus presents head first (*cephalic*). If the head presents with the chin flexed toward the chest, it is called *vertex presentation.* This is the most common cephalic position and the easiest for the woman to deliver. More rarely, a *face presentation* occurs, the fetus's neck is hyperextended bringing the back of its head (occiput) in contact with its back. This causes the face to enter the birth canal first.

The remaining 3% of the presentations are called *breech presentations*. There are three basic types (Fig. 10-3):

* Frank breech: Buttocks are the presenting part, with the thighs flexed and the legs extended over the anterior surface of the body.
* Complete breech: Buttocks are the presenting part, with the thighs flexed on the abdomen and the legs positioned on the thighs.
* Footling breech: One or both feet are the presenting part or parts.

fetal position

Fetal position determines the relationship of a designated point of the presenting part in relation to the maternal pelvis. The designated points used for the various presenting parts of the fetus follow:

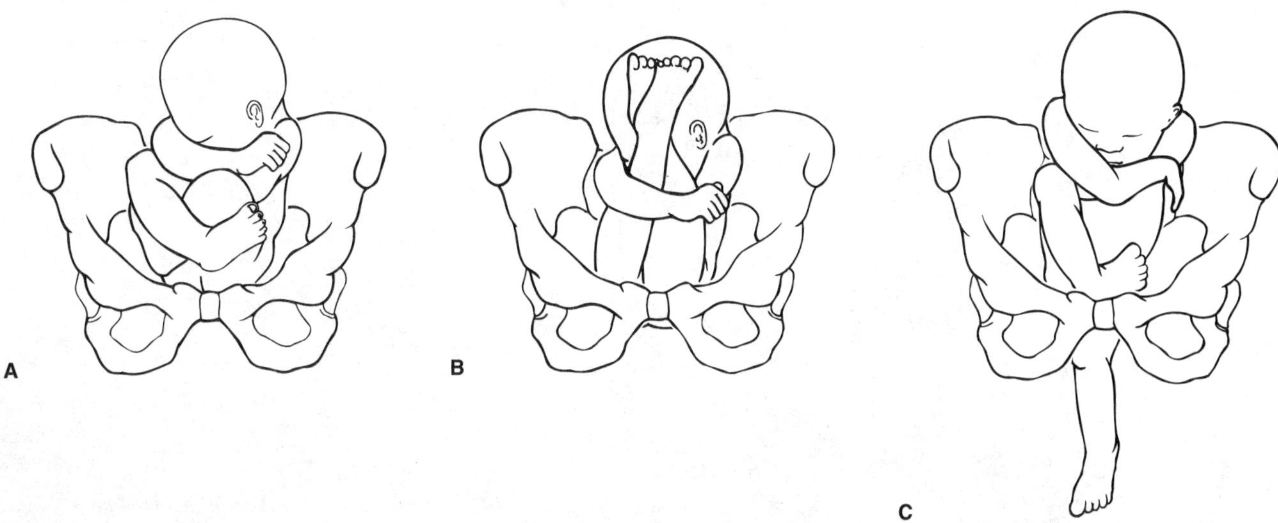

figure 10-3 *Breech presentation.* ***(A)*** *Complete breech.* ***(B)*** *Frank breech.* ***(C)*** *Footling breech.*

* Vertex presentation—occiput
* Face presentation—chin
* Breech presentation—sacrum
* Shoulder presentation—scapula

The designated points used for the maternal pelvis follow:

* Right side of the maternal pelvis (woman's right side)
* Left side of the maternal pelvis (woman's left side)
* Anterior (front of the woman's body)
* Posterior (back of the woman's body)

The various positions are usually expressed using the first initial of each defining word (Fig. 10-4). For example, LOA means the fetal head is presenting with the occiput directed toward the left side and anterior pelvis of the woman. This is the most common position and the easiest birthing position for the woman and the fetus.

One last indicator of position of the fetus in relation to the maternal pelvis is the *station*. Station refers to the relationship of the fetal presenting part to the maternal ischial spines (Fig. 10-5). When the presenting part is level with the maternal ischial spines (palpated by the physician or midwife during vaginal examination), the station is 0. This means the fetal presenting part has passed through the maternal inlet of the pelvis (engagement) and has begun descent through the birth canal. Station is measured in centimeters. If the fetus is above the ischial spines (floating), it is described as 1 to +4 cm. Below the ischial

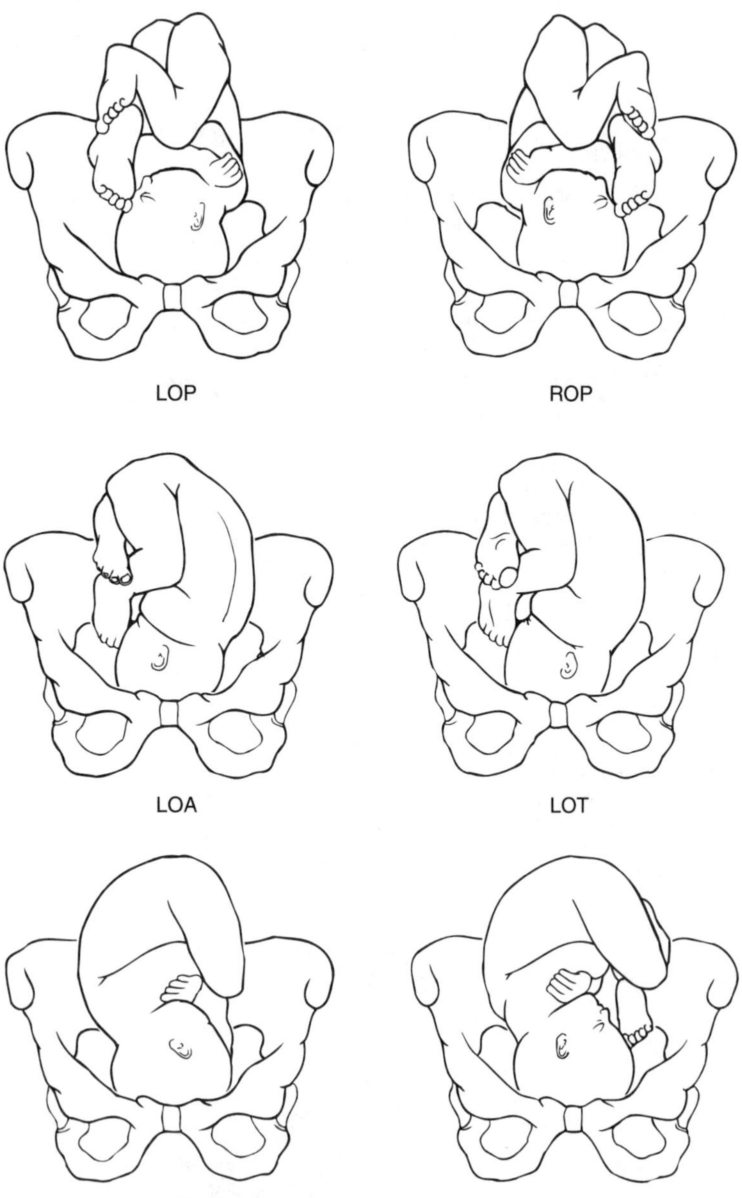

figure 10-4 *Vertex fetal positions include A = anterior; L = left; O = occiput; P = posterior; R = right; T = transverse.*

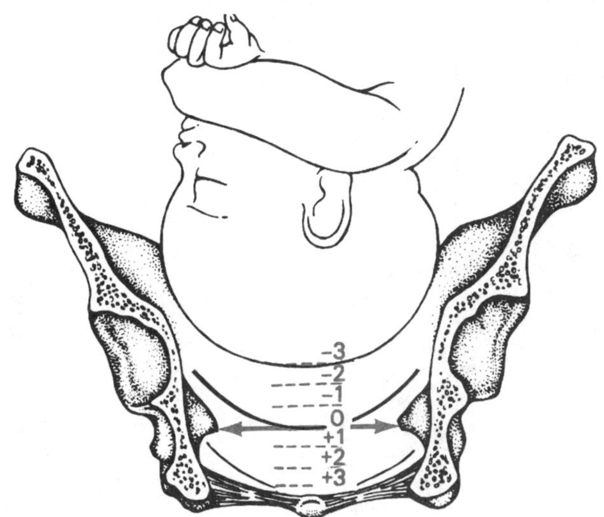

figure 10-5 *Stations of the fetal head:*
−3 station—vertex is 3 cm above the spines.
−2 station—vertex is 2 cm above the spines.
−1 station—vertex is 1 cm above the spines.
0 station—vertex is at the level of the spines.
+ 1 station—vertex is 1 cm below the spines.
+2 station—vertex is 2 cm below the spines.
+3 station—vertex is 3 cm below the spines.

spines, it is described as +1 to +4 cm. Once the fetus has reached +4 cm, the presenting part can be seen by spreading the labia. The appearance of the fetal head at the opening of the birth canal is called *crowning*.

cardinal movements of the fetus

The fetus assumes various positions as it passes through the birth canal to allow for ease of passage. Failure to progress through these various positions may result in complications with the progress of labor. These six positions are *descent, flexion, internal rotation, extension, external rotation,* and *expulsion* (Fig. 10-6).

descent Descent is the continuous downward movement of the fetus through the birth canal. The descent is aided by the pressure of the uterine fundus, the pressure of the amniotic fluid, and the bearing down of the woman during the final stage of labor.

flexion As the fetus descends, the pressure of the pelvic floor and the shape of the uterus cause the fetal neck to flex and the chin to rest on the chest. This allows the smallest diameter of the fetal head to enter the maternal pelvis.

internal rotation As the fetal head enters the maternal pelvis, it rotates from a diagonal or transverse position to an anteroposterior position. The occiput of the fetus rotates anteriorly, allowing the fetal head to pass beneath the pubic arch.

extension As the fetal head reaches the floor of the pelvis, it extends to allow for delivery of the occiput, face, and chin. Extension occurs in response to pressure of the uterine contractions and resistance to the shape of the pelvic floor.

external rotation Once the fetal head is delivered, it immediately rotates to the right or left (transverse) to assume the position it was in during engagement, the earlier part of labor. Rotation of the head at this point is called *restitution*. This mechanism brings the shoulders into an anteroposterior position for ease of delivery. The anterior shoulder, which appears beneath the symphysis pubis, is delivered first, followed by the posterior shoulder.

expulsion Once the shoulders are delivered, the rest of the infant literally slides out. The time of birth is recorded once the entire infant is born, not at the appearance of the head.

powers

The powerful force of the uterine contractions causes cervical effacement and dilatation. These contractions also assist with the cardinal movements of the fetus, leading to delivery of the newborn and later expulsion of the placenta.

As labor continues, cervical effacement progresses from 0% (no change, thick) to 100% (full effacement, almost paper thin). Cervical dilation progresses from 0 cm (closed) to 10 cm (fully dilated, ready for passage of the fetus; Fig. 10-7). Finally, the fundal pressure causes the fetus to descend and eventually to be expelled. Cervical effacement and dilatation are assessed throughout labor by gloved fingertip vaginal examinations, performed by the physician or nurse midwife. In some institutions, the registered nurse may perform vaginal examinations.

anatomy of a uterine contraction

Uterine contractions are intermittent and involuntary. The woman has no control other their length or interval. They usually begin about 5 minutes apart and last for 20 to 30 seconds. As labor progresses, contractions may be 1 to 2 minutes apart and last for 90 seconds. The rest period between each contraction is important because it allows the uterine muscle to relax, the woman to rest, and the fetus to become reoxygenated (for a brief interval at the height of the contraction, the oxygen supply to the fetus is blocked).

The following terminology is used to describe contractions:

Increment: the building of a contraction
Acme: the height or strongest segment of the contraction
Decrement: the declining or lessening of the intensity of the contraction
Duration: the time from the beginning to the end of one contraction
Frequency: the time from the beginning of one contraction to the beginning of the next contraction
Intensity: the strength at the acme of the contraction (Fig. 10-8)

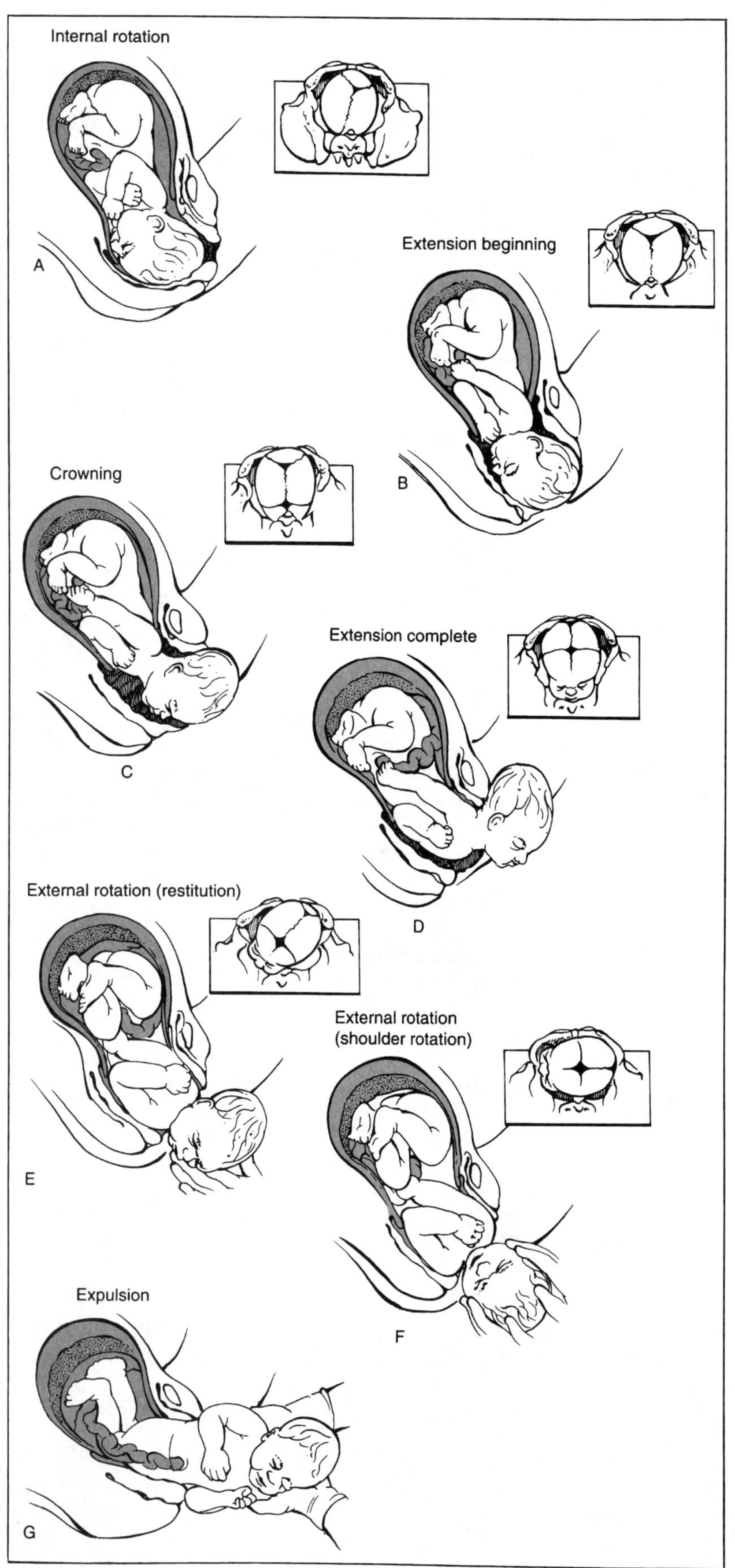

figure 10-6 *Mechanism of normal labor.*

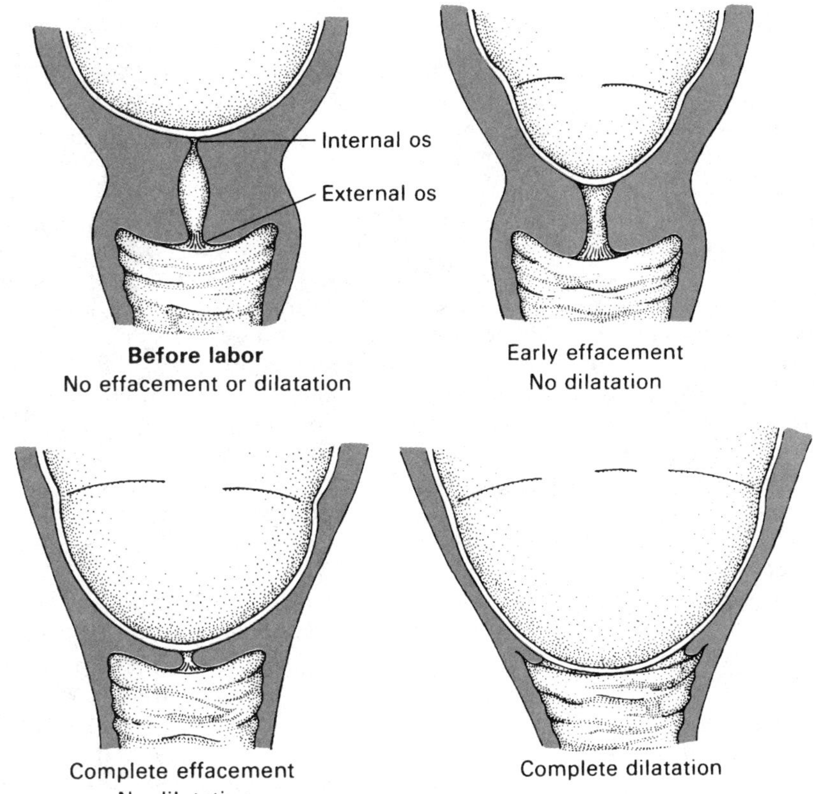

figure 10-7 *Stages in cervical effacement and dilatation.*

✳ nursing insight

To mimic the sensation of a contraction and to feel the three phases, increment, acme, and decrement, place the right hand over the deltoid muscle of the left arm. Slowly contract and relax the deltoid of the left arm. You can begin to feel the muscle contract (increment). Next you feel the muscle as it is totally contracted (acme). Finally, slowly release the contraction (decrement).

The uterine contractions are monitored for their intensity. This may be done by palpation, placing the hand over the fundus and feeling the degree of firmness at the height of the contraction. It is charted as mild, moderate, or firm. A mild contraction would allow the nurse to indent his or her hand easily into the fundal region at the height of the contraction. A firm contraction would prevent the indentation. A moderate contraction would fall somewhere between the two extremes.

Because this is a somewhat vague way to measure intensity, an intrauterine catheter may be used for more accurate monitoring. Once the membranes have ruptured, a small, sterile, water-filled catheter is inserted into the uterus. This catheter is connected to a strain gauge located on the electronic fetal monitor. It measures the intensity of the uterine contraction in millimeters of mercury (mm Hg). The normal resting measurement is about 10 mm Hg; at the height of a strong contraction it may measure 30 to 55 mm Hg.

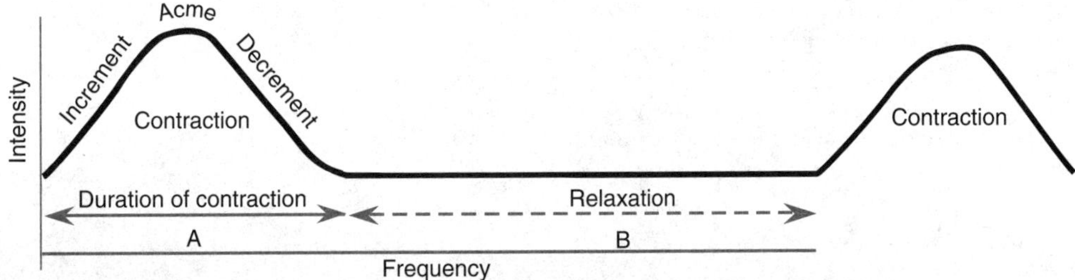

figure 10-8 *Assessment of uterine contraction: The interval and the duration of uterine contractions. The frequency of contractions is the interval timed from the beginning of one contraction to the beginning of the next contraction. The interval consists of two parts:* ***(A)*** *the duration of the contraction and* ***(B)*** *the period of relaxation. The broken line indicates an indeterminate period, because the time (B) is usually of longer duration than the actual contraction (A).*

psyche

The woman's perception of the birth process can impact the course of events during labor. High levels of anxiety can actually prolong the labor, decrease the length or intensity of the uterine contractions, and result in *dysfunctional labor*. The woman's ability to cope with the labor process depends on several factors, including her level of fatigue, cultural beliefs, patterns of coping, understanding of the process of labor, and personal response to pain.

Four major factors have been identified that increase the woman's belief that she can cope with labor (Lowe, 1991). These factors include previous successful coping with labor and childbirth; observing other women who have successfully coped with childbirth; discussions with others, including health care providers, that lead to confidence building; and physiologic arousal mechanisms in response to labor sensations.

Encouraging the woman to attend prenatal classes can increase her understanding of the process, thereby decreasing anxiety. Encouragement and praise by the health care team and her significant other also can increase her coping ability.

stages of labor

Labor is a continuous process. For ease of understanding, however, labor is divided into four stages beginning with the onset of contractions and ending with a critical observation period following the delivery of the placenta.

first stage of labor

The first stage of labor begins with the onset of contractions and ends with complete dilatation of the cervix. It is often called the dilatation stage. For the primipara, the first stage of labor lasts approximately 8 to 12 hours; for the multipara, the first stage lasts 6 to 8 hours. This stage is further broken down into three phases: *latent*, *active*, and *transition*.

latent phase

The latent phase begins with true labor contractions that are light in intensity, occur every 5 to 20 minutes, and last for 15 to 30 seconds. The cervix dilates to 3 to 4 cm. The woman is usually able to talk during a contraction, perform last-minute arrangements in preparation for the birth, and may begin to show excitement or apprehension. She may experience dull menstrual-like cramping, low back discomfort, the passage of the mucus plug (mucous secretions that form in the cervix during pregnancy), and light bloody show.

active phase

As the cervix dilates from 4 to 7 cm, the labor contractions become stronger, longer, and more frequent. Contractions are 50 mm Hg or stronger, lasting 45 to 60 seconds, and occurring every 3 to 5 minutes. The woman becomes more self-focused and may begin her learned breathing pattern or request pain medication during this time. As the contractions increase in intensity, she may find it difficult to ambulate, especially at the height of the contraction. There may be an increase in the amount of bloody show, and the membranes may rupture during this time.

transition phase

This is the most difficult phase for the woman. The cervix dilates from 7 to 10 cm. The contractions last 60 to 90 seconds and occur every 2 to 3 minutes. She may begin to experience nausea and vomiting, trembling of the legs, flushing, and irritability. She may become apprehensive that she is losing control. Rectal and vaginal pressure may cause her to want to bear down with contractions. The transition phase ends with full cervical dilatation and effacement.

second stage of labor

The second stage of labor, the expulsion stage, begins with full dilatation of the cervix and ends with the birth of the infant. The second stage is much shorter than the first, usually lasting 1 hour or less. The contractions are very strong, lasting 60 to 90 seconds, and occur every 2 to 3 minutes. The abdominal muscles begin to contract as the woman feels an overwhelming urge to push with her contractions. Her face may become flushed, and she may perspire from the exertion. All her energies are focused on expelling the infant. The perineum bulges, and the rectum may *evert* (turn outward) from the pressure of the presenting part (Fig. 10-9). The contractions may be rapid with little interval between. The presenting part becomes more visible with each contraction (*crowning*). As the head of the infant is expelled, the woman may feel burn-

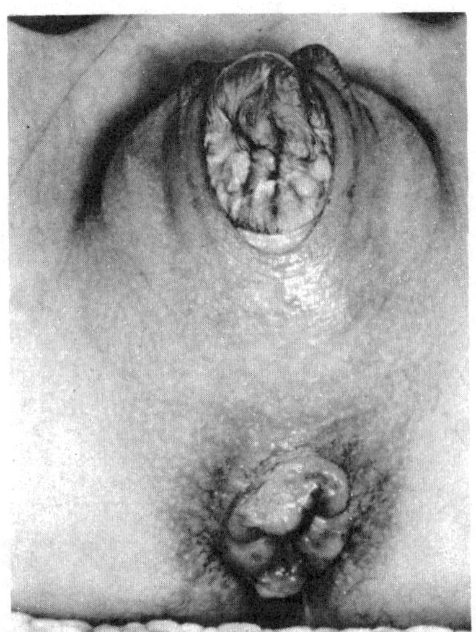

figure 10-9 *Perineum bulges; fetal head crowns and the rectum everts.*

ing, stretching, or a tearing sensation in the perineal region. The sensation of pain and pressure is relieved once the head is expelled; the remainder of the body usually follows with ease (Fig. 10-10).

third stage of labor

The third stage of labor, the placental separation and expulsion stage, begins immediately after expulsion of the infant and ends with the expulsion of the placenta. Following the delivery of the infant, the uterus contracts firmly; this empties the remaining amniotic fluid and allows the uterus to assume a smaller, globular shape. The shrinking of the uterus causes the placenta to begin to detach. This in turn causes bleeding at the site, leading to further separation. Placental separation usually occurs within 5 minutes after the birth. Signs indicating placental separation include a globular shaped uterus, a rise of the fundus in the abdomen, a lengthening of the cord, and increased vaginal bleeding (it may appear as a sudden gush). If the placenta has not separated within 30 minutes after delivery, it is considered a retained placenta, and surgical intervention may be necessary.

The placenta is expelled in one of two distinct ways: fetal side first or maternal side first. In 80% of cases, the placenta detaches from the center to the outer edges causing it to expel with the fetal side first. This is called the *Schultze maneuver*, commonly referred to as "shiny Schultze" because the fetal side of the placenta is smooth and shiny. In 20% of cases, the placenta separates from the edges inward, causing it to fold and deliver the maternal side first. This is called the *Duncan maneuver*, commonly referred to as "dirty Duncan" because the cotyledons on the maternal side give it a dull, bumpy, somewhat dirty appearance (Fig. 10-11).

Once the placenta is delivered, the uterus again contracts, which prevents uterine hemorrhage. Oxytoxic drugs (Pitocin) may be administered to keep the uterus contracted.

the fourth stage of labor

The fourth stage of labor, the immediate recovery stage, lasts from 1 to 4 hours after birth. It is a critical physiologic adjustment time for the mother. The uterus continues to contract to control bleeding. The mother may experience a trembling chill, which is thought to be a physiologic response to the end of labor. After all the work, she is usually tired, hungry, thirsty, and excited. Initial parental attachment usually occurs at this time.

physiologic effects of labor on the woman

During labor the focus is on the reproductive system, but labor also affects the other maternal systems. It includes a whole body adaptation and response.

nervous system

Endorphin levels increase during pregnancy. *Endorphins* are naturally occurring substances within the body that act as analgesics by binding with opiate receptors in the brain, thus increasing the pain threshold. Researchers are attempting to understand if this is the body's way of dealing with labor pain.

cardiovascular system

Because labor requires an intense amount of energy, the cardiovascular system responds by increasing cardiac output, blood pressure, and pulse rate. The systolic blood pressure may rise an average of 15 mm Hg during the height of the contraction, while the diastolic rises an average of 5 to 10 mm Hg. It returns to normal between contractions.

The pulse rate increases an average of 10 to 20 beats/min during the second stage of labor, especially in response to the woman's bearing down efforts. Between contractions, it returns to the normal resting pulse rate.

During the birth process, the woman may lose 300 to 400 mL or more of blood. This decrease in blood volume helps reduce the woman's blood volume to the prepregnancy levels.

urinary system

With the predictable decrease in fluid intake during labor and the increase in output of fluid from perspiration and hyperventilation, the kidneys begin to concentrate the urine. This helps the body conserve fluids and electrolytes. As the fetal head descends low in the birth canal, it puts pressure on the maternal bladder, and the woman may lose the sensation of "bladder filling." Requesting her to void every 2 hours will assist in maintaining bladder tone. It also prevents a full bladder from impeding the progress of labor.

gastrointestinal system

The gastrointestinal system becomes mostly inactive during the labor process. Any food ingested during this time will stay in the stomach and increase problems with nausea, vomiting, and the danger of aspiration. Fluids are encouraged to meet the demands of increased fluid loss and are readily absorbed.

respiratory system

Because of the anxiety, pain, and increased exertion associated with labor, the workload of the respiratory system increases. The respiratory rate increases to meet these increased demands (*hyperventilation*). If oxygen demands are not met (*hypoxia*), the woman can quickly slip into acidosis. Obesity or large amounts of narcotics can contribute to this problem. Prolonged hyperventilation can lead to a decrease in the normal levels of carbon dioxide.

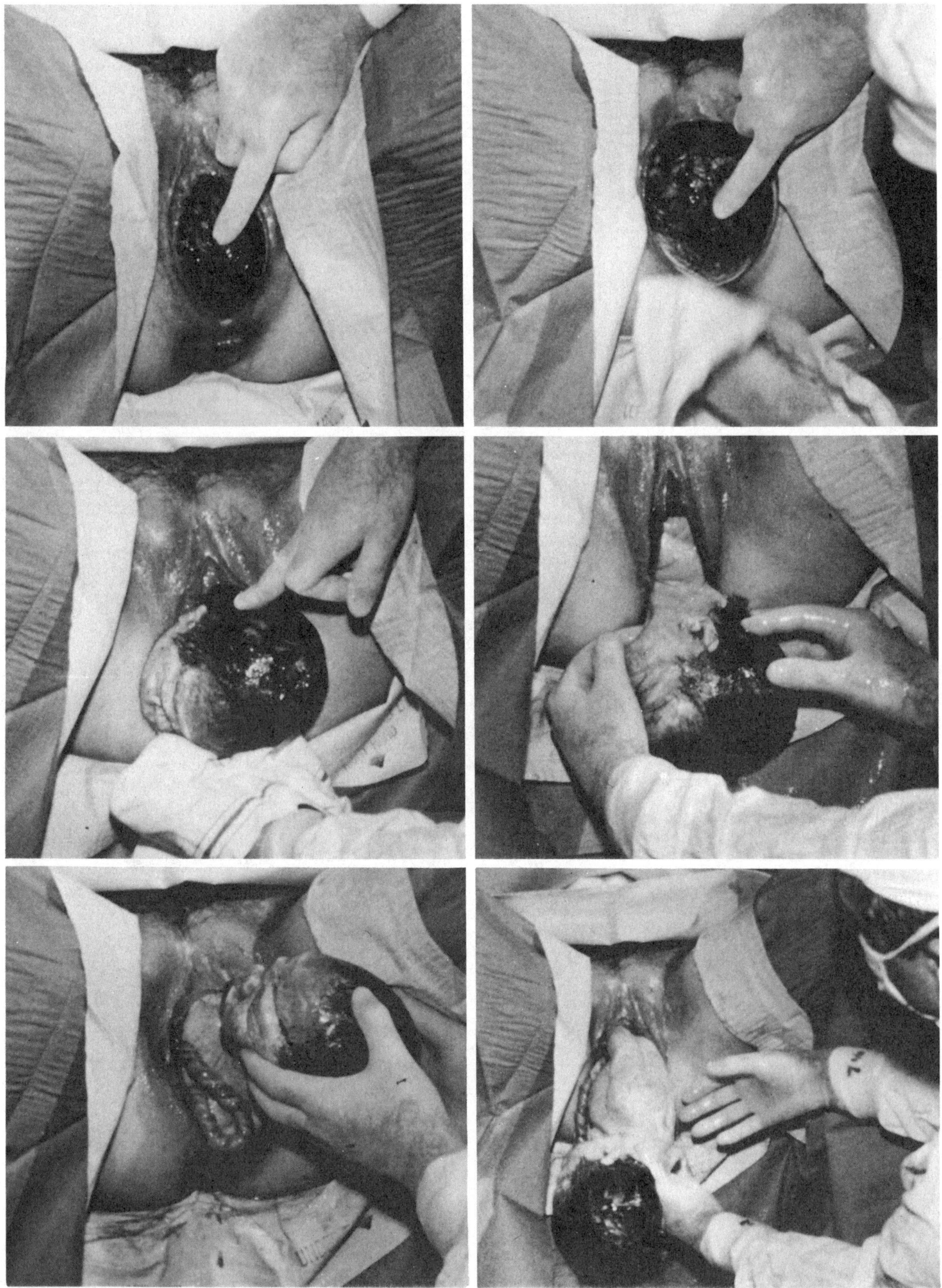

figure 10-10 *Birth sequence.*

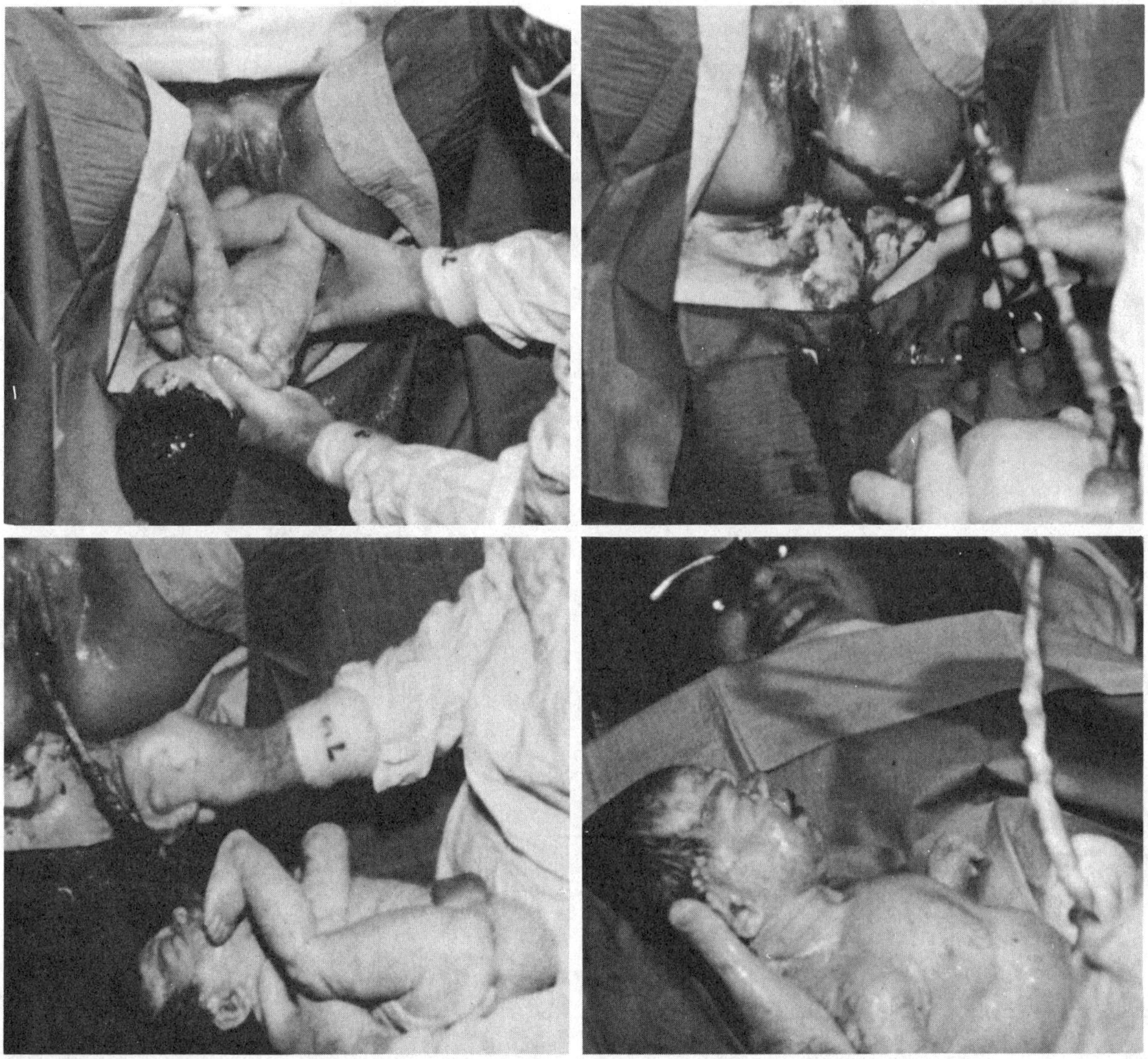

figure 10-10 (continued). *Birth sequence.*

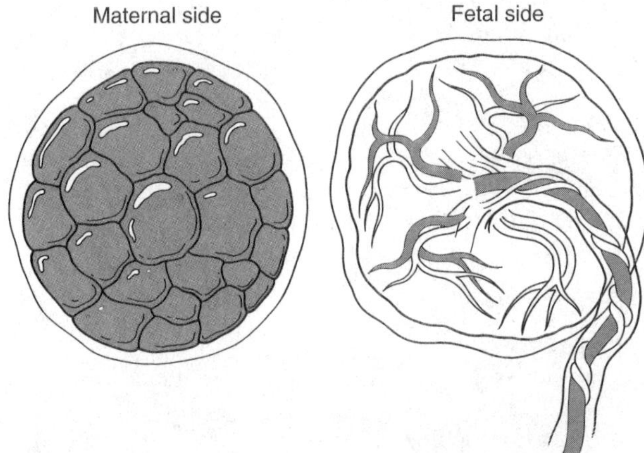

figure 10-11 *The placenta.*

This can interrupt the normal blood gas exchange at the placental site. Assisting the woman with breathing patterns during labor can alleviate these problems.

physiologic effects of labor on the fetus

Although the fetus is primarily a passenger during the labor process, labor has an indirect systemic effect on the fetus.

nervous system

The fetus with a normal functioning nervous system will have certain expected responses to the labor process. The pressure exerted on the fetal head during contractions produces vagal nerve stimulation. This causes the fetal heart rate to slow during the height of the contraction.

cardiovascular system

The normal pulse rate for a fetus is 120 to 160 beats/min. During the height of a contraction, the blood supply to the placenta is temporarily slowed due to constriction of the uterine arteries. The fetus responds with a slowing of the pulse rate during the height of the contraction. This does not interfere with normal fetal functioning because the fetal blood pressure elevates to meet circulatory demands.

respiratory system

During pregnancy, labor, and birth, the placenta is the respiratory organ of the fetus. As the fetus passes through the birth canal, the chest is compressed and amniotic fluid is expelled from the lungs to prepare for the first breath that inflates the lungs.

* nursing considerations

To assist the woman to meet the physical and emotional challenges of labor, the nurse must have an understanding of the process and its impact on the woman, the fetus, and the family. The nurse may play a vital role in preparing the expectant parents. Questions the nurse may encounter include the following: "How will I know when to come to the hospital?" "How will I know if my water breaks, and then what do I do?" "I plan to use Lamaze, but what if the pain is too strong and I can't continue?" The nurse must be prepared to answer these and similar questions to allay fear and anxiety. Labor and delivery call on all the coping strategies of the woman and her support person to meet the physical and psychological demands. The nurse needs to communicate to the family that he or she is there for them and will do everything to make this a positive and memorable time.

key points *

- **Preliminary signs of approaching labor may include lightening, Braxton Hicks contractions, bloody show, passage of the mucus plug, and SROM.**
- **The characteristics of true labor include regular contractions that increase in frequency and intensity, presence of bloody show, pain radiating from the lower back to the lower abdomen, and most important, cervical dilatation and effacement.**
- **A successful labor depends on the 4 Ps: adequate space for passage, appropriate position and size of the passenger, adequate contraction of the uterus (powers), and adequate maternal coping strategies (psyche).**
- **To ease the passage of the fetus through the birth canal, the bones in the fetal skull overlap. This process is called molding.**
- **The majority of the time, the fetus will assume a longitudinal lie and cephalic presentation.**
- **The most common fetal position for birth is left occipital anterior (LOA).**
- **Breech positions include frank, complete, and footling. These positions usually result in a cesarean birth.**
- **Engagement occurs when the presenting part of the fetus is level with the maternal ischial spines.**
- **For birth to occur, the cervix must be 100% effaced and dilated to 10 cm.**
- **The cardinal movements of the fetus include descent, flexion, internal rotation, extension, external rotation, and expulsion.**

review questions *

1. The nurse is aware that the most common birth position is
   a. LOA.
   b. LOP.
   c. ROA.
   d. ROP.
2. Ms. Champagne is a 39-week, para 0, gravida 1. She tells the nurse it feels like the baby has "dropped." She says she finds it easier to breathe but feels pressure in the perineal region, voids frequently, and has begun to have occasional leg cramps. The nurse understands that she has experienced
   a. beginning labor contractions.
   b. lightening.
   c. engagement.
   d. Braxton Hicks.
3. The nurse recognizes that the most important sign of true labor is
   a. frequent contractions.
   b. that walking eases the discomfort.
   c. that analgesics have no impact on the quality of the contraction.
   d. cervical dilatation and effacement.
4. For the fetus to pass through the birth canal successfully, a variety of pelvic measurements may be taken. One of the most important measurements is the diagonal conjugate. This measurement must be at least
   a. 6 cm.
   b. 8 cm.
   c. 10 cm.
   d. 12 cm.
5. The first stage of labor is called the dilatation stage. Full dilatation is
   a. 5 cm.
   b. 7 cm.
   c. 10 cm.
   d. 12 cm.

bibliography

Cunningham, F. G., McDonald, P. C., Leveno, K. J., Gant, N. F., & Gilstrap, L. (1993). *Williams obstetrics* (19th ed.). Norwalk, CT: Appleton and Lange.

Cassidy, J. (1993). A picture perfect birth. *RN, 56*, 45.

Chao, A., Herd, J., & Tabsh, K. (1990). The ferning test for detection of amniotic fluid contamination in umbilical blood samples. *American Journal of Obstetrics and Gynecology, 162*(5), 1207–1213.

Cosner, K. R., & DeJong, E. (1993). Physiologic second stage labor. *MCN, 18*, 38–43.

Kenner, C. A., & MacLaren, A. (1993). *Essentials of maternal and neonatal nursing*. Springhouse, PA: Springhouse Corporation.

Lieberman, A. B. (1991). Why labor hurts. *American Baby*, 66–70.

Lowe, N. (1991). Maternal confidence in coping with labor. *Journal of Obsterics, Gynecologic, and Neonatal Nursing, 20*(6), 457.

May, K. A., & Mahlmeister, L. R. (1994). *Maternal and neonatal nursing: Family-centered care* (3rd ed.). Philadelphia: J.B. Lippincott.

Olds, S. B., London, M. L., & Ladewig, P. W. (1992). *Maternal newborn nursing: A family-centered approach* (4th ed.). Redwood City, CA: Addison-Wesley Nursing.

Pernoll, M. L. (1991). *Current obstetric and gynecologic diagnosis and treatment* (7th ed.). Norwalk, CT: Appleton and Lange.

Pillitteri, A. (1995). *Maternal and child health nursing* (2nd ed.). Philadelphia: J.B. Lippincott.

Reeder, S. J., Martin, L. L., & Koniak, D. (1992). *Maternity nursing* (17th ed.). Philadelphia: J.B. Lippincott.

Scott, J. R., et al. (1994). *Danforth's obstetrics and gynecology* (7th ed.). Philadelphia: J.B. Lippincott.

analgesia and anesthesia 11

outline ✳

objectives 

After studying this chapter, the reader should be able to:

- ✳ List the labor nurse's goals for pain management.
- ✳ Describe the causes of labor pain.
- ✳ Explain the benefits of pain control in the laboring woman.
- ✳ Discuss the use and benefits of systemic analgesia in the laboring woman.
- ✳ Discuss the types and effects of regional anesthetics.
- ✳ List the teaching considerations for the woman undergoing epidural anesthesia.
- ✳ Compare and contrast the effects of regional and general anesthesia.

key terms 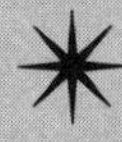

analgesia
anesthesia
antagonist
blood patch
epidural anesthesia
paracervical block
pudendal block
spinal block

Pain control during childbirth has been used in one form or another (pharmacologic or nonpharmacologic) since the Middle Ages. Chloroform, a gas anesthesia, was used by Queen Victoria in 1858 (Fields & Wall, 1993). Throughout history, objections have been raised about the use of analgesia and anesthetics for childbirth, sometimes for moral or ethical reasons and other times because of possible health risks.

Many people felt that because childbirth was a normal physiologic process, it would not cause pain; others believed that pain was to be expected. Still others believed that only women who were "emotional" experienced pain. Some people believed that any use of anesthesia was totally unsafe. Changing attitudes in today's society and newer and better medications have led to increased use of analgesia for pain control during labor and delivery (Fields & Wall, 1993).

Labor pain can range from mild discomfort, a feeling of pressure, to severe overwhelming, consuming pain. As nurses, one of the most rewarding tasks is helping the woman and her partner to experience the process of labor and delivery in as positive and comfortable a manner as possible; this can be through the use of nonpharmacologic methods, such as Lamaze techniques, walking, and changing positions, or through the use of medications. This chapter focuses on the use of analgesics and anesthetics to relieve the pain associated with labor. See Chapters 8 and 12 for discussions of nonpharmacologic comfort measures.

✳ family considerations

Most women express concern about the pain associated with the labor process. Questions such as the following are common, especially during the later stages of pregnancy: "How much will it hurt?" "How long will it last?" "I plan to use my Lamaze training, but what if I lose control?" The primigravida will have no personal experience on which to draw other than stories from her friends and family. The multigravida, realizing that each labor experience is different, may still be concerned about the pain, especially if she had a difficult delivery in the past.

The partner also may express concern about the discomfort the woman may experience. Many times partners are particularly upset because they feel responsible for the pregnancy. They may express a feeling of helplessness.

✳ nursing considerations

The nurse recognizes that labor proceeds in predictable stages, but the discomfort experienced depends on the woman's perception of a variety of factors (Display 11-1).

The following are goals of the labor nurse:

* Provide maximum comfort with minimal risk to the woman and fetus.
* Help make labor and delivery a positive experience for the woman and her family.

display 11-1
factors affecting pain response

1. **Knowledge or education of the birth process**
2. **Cultural beliefs about the expression of pain**
3. **Anxiety**
4. **Fatigue or sleep deprivation**
5. **Experiences with labor pain**
6. **Fetal size and position**
7. **Personal coping mechanisms**

The labor nurse must monitor the woman receiving analgesics or anesthesia closely to prevent complications, such as hypotension or aspiration of vomitus. The fetus must be monitored carefully to make sure adequate oxygenation is maintained because any disturbance in the woman's blood flow indirectly affects the fetus (Fig. 11-1).

causes of pain

During the first stage of labor, pain results from the dilatation and effacement of the cervix. Most of the pain is felt in the lower abdomen and lower back. During the second stage of labor, the pain results from pressure of the fetus on the vagina, bowel, bladder, and uterine ligaments and is felt primarily in the perineal region. Pain is usually most acute during this stage. During the third stage of labor, the pain results from hypoxia in the uterus caused by compression of the uterine blood vessels and by uterine

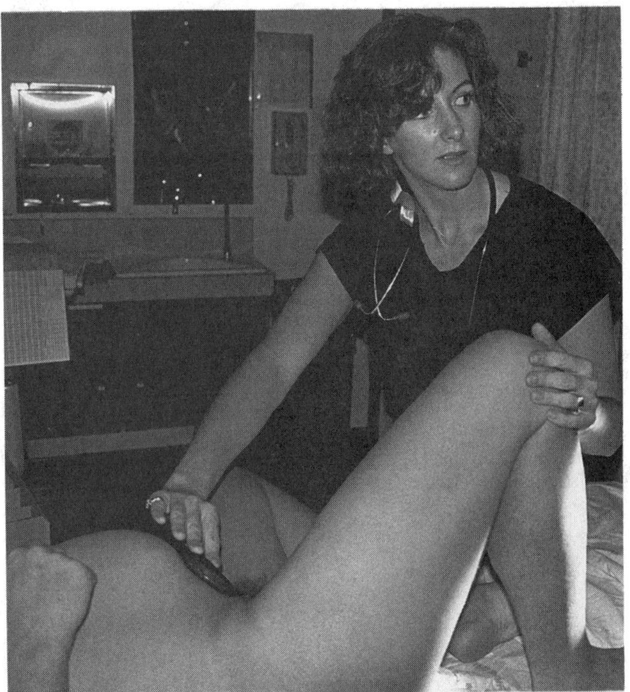

figure 11-1 *After administering analgesics or anesthesia, the labor nurse must monitor the woman and fetus closely. (Photo by Kathy Sloane.)*

contractions that expel the placenta. This pain is milder and somewhat like the pain felt early in the first stage of labor.

benefits of pain control

Appropriate pain management breaks the fear-tension-pain cycle (see Chap. 8), thus contributing to the woman's feelings of self-esteem. The woman who feels more in control of herself and her environment can become a more active participant in the birthing process. Effective pain control also decreases the fatigue associated with excess anxiety and fear. It allows the woman to rest and conserve her energy for the "pushing" phase. These positive feelings can actually prepare her for a more positive attachment with her newborn.

pharmacologic pain relief methods

Pain relief during labor and delivery may include the use of systemic analgesia, such as narcotic analgesics, sedatives, and tranquilizers. These medications are used to relieve pain and anxiety during the first stage of labor.

Anesthesia is used when analgesia alone does not offer adequate pain relief. Anesthesia is used to block the nerve pathways, resulting in partial or complete loss of feeling. Regional anesthesia relieves pain without loss of consciousness; general anesthesia renders the individual unconscious.

The choice about pain management is usually made during prenatal classes. The woman may decide to use pain medication, anesthesia, or Lamaze, Dick-Read, or a variety of other nonpharmacologic pain management methods. The woman who has chosen nonpharmacologic pain relief measures but finds she is losing control may find that analgesics will help her regain control. Then she can continue to use her breathing techniques and other nonpharmacologic pain relief methods (Borneman, 1995). The nurse needs to respect the woman's decision, praise her for her progress, and try to prevent her from feeling any guilt because of her choices.

nursing insight

The decision to use pain relief medications during labor and delivery should be left to the woman, without interference from the nursing staff, regardless of their own beliefs.

systemic analgesia

Once labor is well established, usually during the active phase or 4 to 5 cm dilatation, systemic medications may be administered without slowing or stopping the progress of labor or harming the fetus.

narcotic analgesics

Narcotic analgesics act on the brain to increase the pain threshold and produce mild euphoria. Narcotics are often given with a tranquilizer to relieve the labor pain and promote rest between contractions. Caution must be exercised in using narcotics. Administered too early, narcotics may impede the progress of labor. Administered during transition, narcotics can cause respiratory depression in the infant. Narcotics commonly used in labor and delivery include meperidine (Demerol), butorphanol (Stadol), and nalbuphine (Nubain; Table 11-1).

nursing alert

If analgesia is given too early, it will impede the progress of labor. If it is given too late, it will cause fetal respiratory depression.

table 11-1 common narcotics used during labor and delivery

Drug	*Dosage, Route*	*Maternal Side Effects*	*Fetal Side Effects*	*Nursing Considerations*
Meperidine (Demerol)	25 mg IV 500–100 mg IM q3–4 h	Respiratory depression, nausea and vomiting, urinary retention, orthostatic hypotension Impedes labor if given too early	Respiratory depression	Check for drug allergies Monitor vital signs Monitor stage of labor for administration
Nalbuphine (Nubain)	0.3 mg/kg over 10–15 min IV 10 mg IM q3–6 h	Induces withdrawal symptoms in narcotic-dependent client Respiratory depression, nausea and vomiting, drowsiness, orthostatic hypotension	CNS depression, respiratory depression	Check for drug allergies Monitor vital signs Monitor stage of labor for administration
Butorphanol Tartrate (Stadol)	1 mg IV q3–4 h 2 mg IV q3–4 h	Induces withdrawal symptoms in narcotic-dependent client	CNS depression, respiratory depression	Check for drug allergies Monitor vital signs

narcotic antagonist

Demerol and other narcotic analgesics may produce respiratory depression in the newborn. The narcotic antagonist naloxone hydrochloride (Narcan) is used to reverse the narcotic respiratory depressive effects, often in as little as 1 to 5 minutes. It is the drug of choice for newborn respiratory depression. Narcan replaces the narcotic drug at the neural receptor sites, thus inactivating the effects of the narcotic. The usual dosage for the newborn is 0.1 mg/kg, administered through the umbilical vein at birth (American Academy of Pediatrics and American College of Obstetricians and Gynecologists, 1992). If respiratory depression is suspected, Narcan can be administered to the woman shortly before birth because it crosses the placenta rapidly. The usual maternal dosage is 0.4 mg/kg, preferably given intravenously (IV). Resuscitation equipment should be readily available to assist in ventilation as needed. The newborn should be observed closely for 6 to 8 hours following the dosage, because once the drug wears off, respiratory depression may recur.

sedatives and barbiturates

These drugs cause maternal sedation and relaxation but offer no analgesic properties. They are reserved for the client experiencing false labor or who is in the latent phase of labor. Their use is contraindicated in active labor client because they rapidly cross the placenta, they have prolonged effects on the fetus, and no medication is available to reverse their effects. Side effects seen in the newborn include central nervous system depression, delayed sucking ability causing poor nutritional intake and impaired establishment of feeding pattern, and extreme drowsiness. This group of drugs includes secobarbital (Seconal), phenobarbital (Luminal), and pentobarbital sodium (Nembutal). They are usually administered orally (100 mg) but may be given intramuscularly (IM; 100 mg).

tranquilizers

Tranquilizers are used to decrease the anxiety and apprehension that occur during labor, to relieve the nausea that some pain medications produce, and to potentiate the effects of the narcotic analgesia, thus decreasing the amount of narcotic needed to produce the desired pain relief. Commonly used tranquilizers include promethazine (Phenergan) and hydroxyzine (Vistaril). The recommended dosage for both is 25 to 50 mg intramuscularly (IM) administered alone or with the appropriate narcotic. Maternal side effects include hypotension and a potentiation of respiratory depression when used with narcotics. Newborn side effects include lethargy and hypothermia.

> **nursing alert**
> *Monitor respirations when using tranquilizers with narcotics. Do not give medication if respirations fall below 12 breaths per minute. Also, monitor blood pressure, and hold medication if the woman becomes hypotensive.*

anesthesia

Anesthesia blocks sensory nerve transmission to produce a numbness or lack of feeling, with or without loss of consciousness, relieving pain and discomfort. A variety of anesthesia methods are used in obstetrics (Fig. 11-2). Regional anesthesia is generally used for pain management during labor, vaginal delivery, and repair of perineal tears and episiotomies. General anesthesia is reserved for cesarean deliveries.

regional anesthesia

Regional anesthesia refers to the injection of anesthetic agents to block the sensory nerve transmissions from a specific region of the body. Regional anesthesia may be

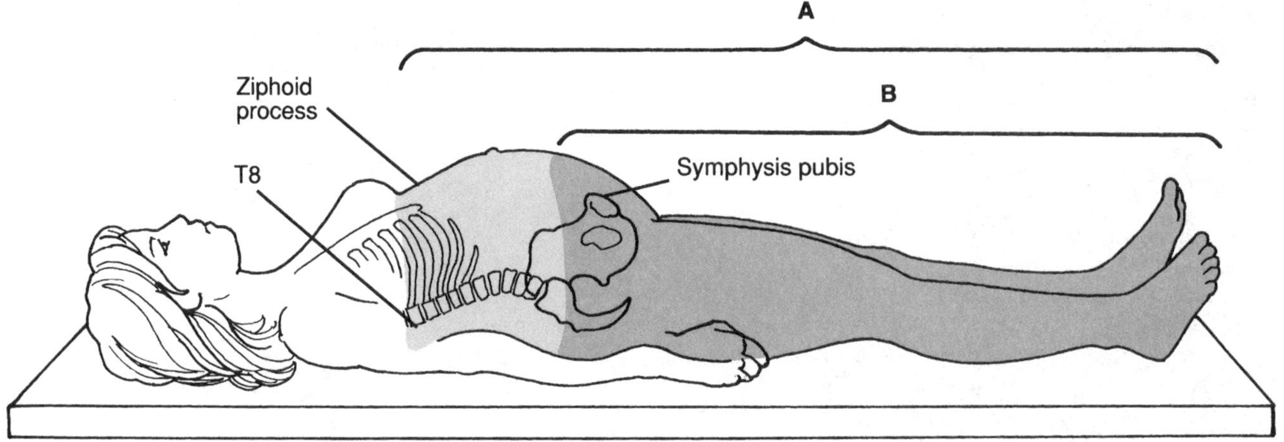

figure 11-2 *Levels of regional conduction anesthesia for obstetrics: Spinal (subarachnoid) block and lumbar epidural. **(A)** Anesthesia for cesarean section must extend from xiphoid process of sternum (near the level of T8) to provide analgesia of entire abdominal cavity. **(B)** Anesthesia for vaginal delivery extends from umbilicus or symphysis pubis to provide analgesia for delivery and repair of an episiotomy.*

table 11-2 effects of regional anesthetics

Advantages	*Disadvantages*
Area that is blocked is totally pain-free	May fail to take effect
Usually they have few depressive effects.	May only partially take effect
Client is awake and can be a participant in vaginal delivery.	May result in toxic reaction
	Can have rare severe side effects, such as respiratory or cardiac arrest in isolated cases
	Catheter placement can result in nerve damage in isolated cases
	Epidurals can result in hypotension

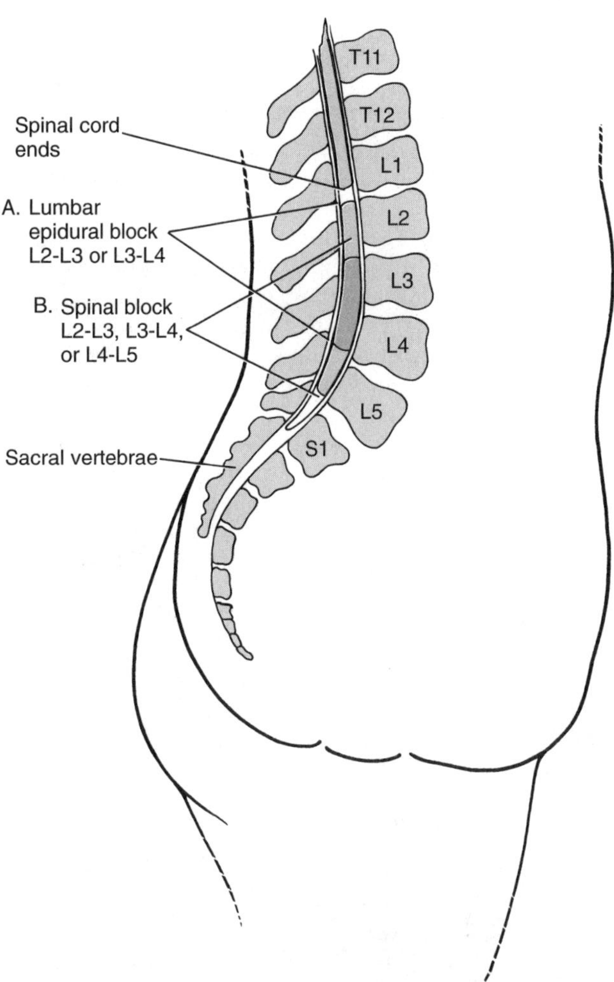

figure 11-3 *Sites for anesthetic administration during labor and delivery.* ***(A)*** *Site for lumbar epidural block. Lumbar epidural block is usually continuous and provides analgesia and anesthesia from active labor through delivery. Client may be sitting or in a lateral position for insertion. The catheter remains in place so additional doses of medication can be administered.* ***(B)*** *Site for spinal block, often called a saddle block. This block is administered just before delivery. A local anesthetic drug is injected directly into the spinal fluid in the spinal canal (subarachnoid space) with client in a sitting or lateral-recumbent position.*

administered as a single injection or as a continuous infusion through a catheter. Types of regional anesthesia include spinal block, lumbar epidural, pudendal block, paracervical block, and local infiltration. Advantages and disadvantages of regional anesthesia are summarized in Table 11-2.

spinal block

A spinal block is administered to relieve pain during a cesarean delivery. It is a rapid, reliable form of anesthesia with minimal fetal or maternal side effects. The nurse assists the woman into a sitting or side-lying position with her shoulders parallel, her chin resting on her chest, and her back arched forward to widen the intervertebral spaces. The nurse anesthetist or anesthesiologist cleanses the lower back with an antimicrobial scrub, numbs the area with a local anesthetic, and introduces a spinal needle into the subarachnoid space between L2 and L5 (Figs. 11-2 and 11-3). This produces total loss of feeling and motor paralysis from the abdomen to the toes for 1 to 2 hours. The woman is monitored carefully for signs of hypotension, which can result from sympathetic blockade. This is usually temporary and often can be avoided with IV hydration. The use of a vasopressor, ephedrine, may be necessary if the blood pressure becomes dangerously low or does not respond to IV hydration.

Some women develop a spinal headache. These headaches, appearing within 24 to 72 hours following delivery, are caused by leakage of cerebrospinal fluid into the epidural space, resulting in tension on the intracranial neural structures. These headaches can be severe and are positional, worsening when the woman is upright and subsiding when she is in a reclining position. The woman is usually placed on bed rest, given analgesics for the pain, and given increased IV fluids. If the headache does not respond, the physician may consider a "blood patch." This procedure consists of the physician obtaining 10 to 20 mL of the woman's own unclotted blood, usually from the arm, and injecting it into the original puncture site of the spinal anesthesia, thus sealing the dural puncture site. This technique has been successful, and most women experience relief within a few minutes of the procedure.

epidural anesthesia

Epidural anesthesia is fast becoming the most popular form of obstetric anesthesia (Taylor, 1993). It can be used for pain control during the first and second stages of labor and for surgical procedures, including cesarean delivery. The woman remains awake, alert, and cooperative and is usually able to respond to the urge to push during the second stage of labor. Occasionally, the woman may experience some nausea and vomiting and breakthrough pain. Hypotension is the most common maternal side effect; few if any side effects occur in the fetus.

Epidural anesthesia requires a small catheter to be threaded into the epidural space of the spinal column. This space lies between the vertebrae and the dura mater, the outermost membrane covering the spinal cord. This area is filled with veins, fatty tissue, and the nerve roots that exit the spinal cord. As the medication is injected into the catheter, it bathes these nerve roots, resulting in a block that provides pain relief. Because the medication does not penetrate the dura mater, there is no chance of spinal headache from leaking fluid.

Although epidural anesthesia can be administered at any time, it is usually administered to the primigravida when she is dilated 5 to 6 cm and to the multigravida when she is dilated 3 to 4 cm (Taylor, 1993). In preparation, the nurse obtains maternal baseline vital signs and fetal heart rate. Prior to the procedure, the woman is encouraged to void to prevent urinary retention due to diminished neural bladder sensations. At this time, she also is hydrated with 500 to 1,000 mL of IV fluid to prevent hypotension, the most common side effect; this results from the marked vasodilation produced by blocking the sympathetic neurons. For introduction of the catheter, the woman is positioned on her side with her shoulders parallel and her legs slightly flexed or in a sitting position with her head flexed, elbows on her knees, and feet flat on a stool. In either position, the woman's back should remain fairly straight to slightly flexed (Fig. 11-4). Severe flexion is avoided because it increases the chances of piercing the subarachnoid space, which would allow the medication to enter the cerebrospinal fluid much like a spinal anesthetic. The catheter is then secured with tape and aspirated to check for appropriate placement by making sure there is no blood or cerebral spinal fluid return. A test dose of medication is administered to rule out placement in the subarachnoid space or epidural vein. This is important because the amount of medication used in an epidural is five times the dosage used in a spinal block. The medication can be administered in intermittent bolus doses or as a continuous infusion with drip rate controlled by an infusion pump (Fig. 11-5).

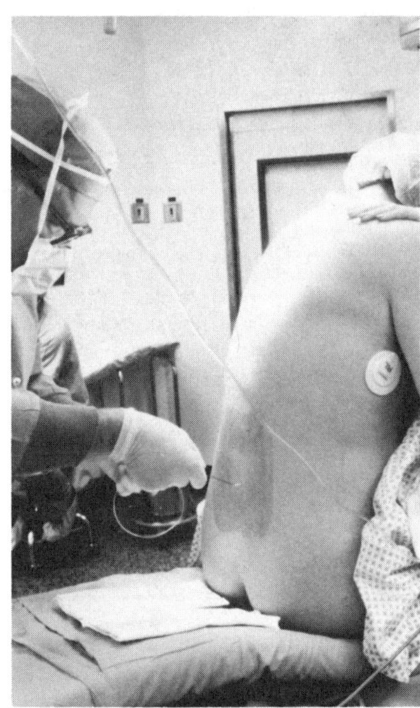

figure 11-4 *During the insertion of an epidural catheter, the woman should be seated with her head slightly flexed and back straight.*

teaching guidelines
lumbar epidural anesthesia

- ✶ Once you have decided to have the procedure and all your questions have been answered, you will be asked to sign a consent form.
- ✶ Your blood pressure, pulse, and respirations will be checked frequently before, during, and after the procedure.
- ✶ Your baby's heart rate also will be monitored frequently.
- ✶ You will be asked to assume a sitting or side-lying position for insertion of the catheter. This may be uncomfortable, but the nurse will assist you.
- ✶ You will be asked to void prior to starting the procedure, and you will be reminded to void at intervals following the procedure. If you are unable to void, you may need to be catheterized.
- ✶ A local numbing agent will be administered before insertion of the medication catheter. This will produce a momentary stinging or burning sensation.
- ✶ You will be asked to maintain a side-lying position to help prevent low blood pressure during your labor.
- ✶ When delivery is imminent, the nurse may need to remind you to push with your contractions.

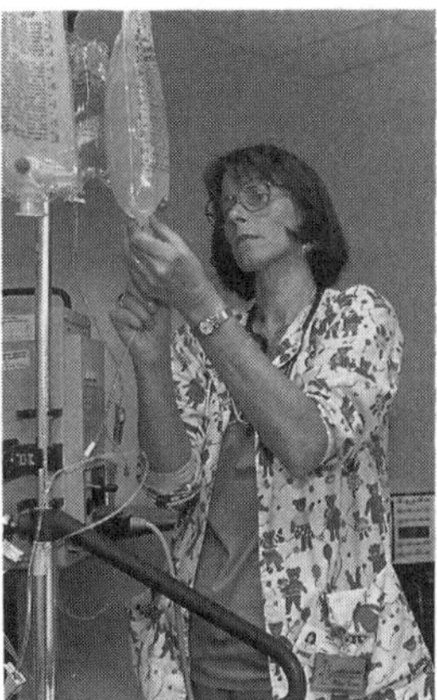

figure 11-5 *The nurse monitors the epidural infusion pump.*

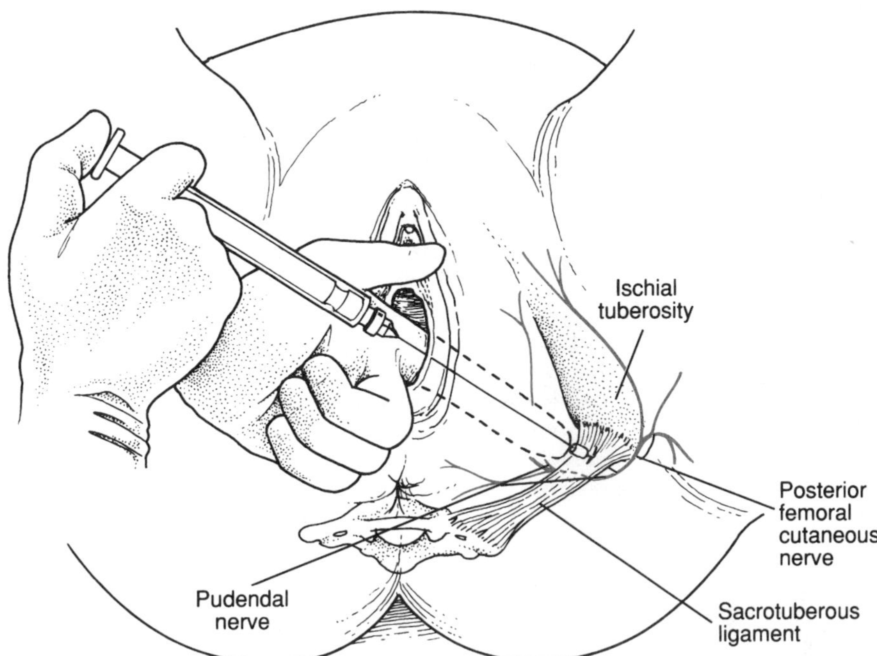

figure 11-6 *Pudendal block. Pudendal nerves are located lateral to tips of the ischial spine.*

pudendal block

A pudendal block is administered during the second stage of labor to numb the perineum for birth, repair an episiotomy or lacerations, or prepare the woman for a forceps delivery. The drug is injected by the physician into the pudendal nerve on either side of the sacrum (Fig. 11-6). The medication takes effect within 2 minutes and lasts up to 1 hour. Possible complications include hematoma formation, trauma to the sciatic nerve, accidental injection into a blood vessel, or perforation of the rectum.

paracervical block

A paracervical block is an injection of local anesthetic near the uterine fibers on either side of the cervix (Fig. 11-7). This relieves the pain of cervical dilatation during the active phase of labor. A paracervical block is usually administered when the woman's cervix is dilated 4 to 5 cm. Maternal complications are related primarily to systemic toxic reaction to the drug itself. Fetal reactions include bradycardia, fetal distress, or inadvertent intracranial injection. It is rarely used today because of the high incidence of fetal reactions.

local infiltration

Local infiltration is injection of an anesthetic into the superficial tissues and nerves of the perineum to numb the area for repair of lacerations and episiotomies. It is particularly useful for women who have chosen nonpharmacologic pain relief methods for the birth process. This procedure is safe for the woman and the fetus because it is practically free from side effects other than a momentary burning sensation during the injection.

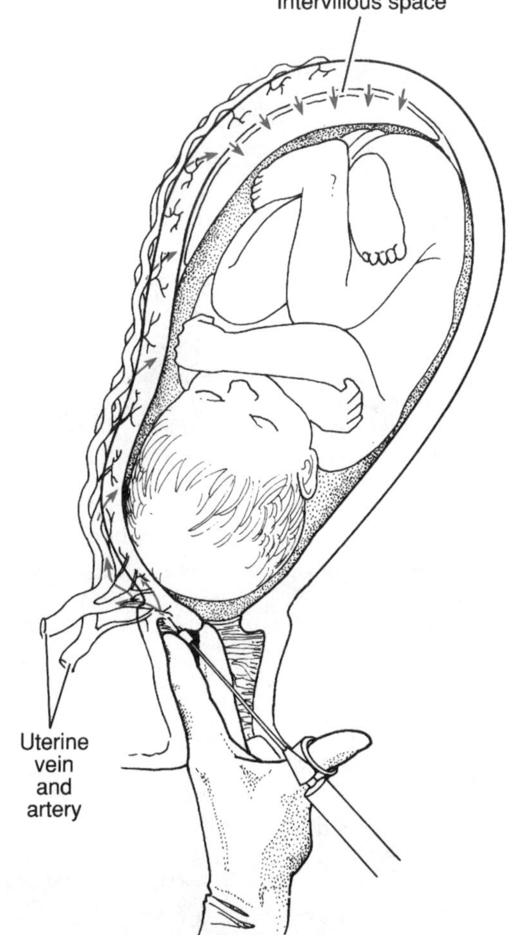

figure 11-7 *Paracervical block. Paracervical block is an effective and relatively simple method of relieving pain during labor.*

general anesthesia

General anesthesia renders the woman unconscious through the use of IV medication, inhalation of gases, or a combination of these agents. Because she is intubated, the woman is at risk for regurgitation and aspiration of the highly acidic gastric contents, which could result in chemical pneumonitis and possible death. Prior to anesthesia, the woman is given an antacid to neutralize stomach contents or a dose of cimetidine (Tagamet) to improve gastric motility (Fields & Wall, 1993). Other possible maternal complications include cardiac arrhythmias and uterine atony, which could lead to hemorrhage in the early postpartum period. General anesthesia also places the fetus at risk because the anesthetic rapidly crosses the placenta, resulting in respiratory depression or hypoxia. Today, this method of anesthesia is reserved for emergency cesarean delivery.

✳ nursing process for the woman receiving analgesia or anesthesia

assessment

There are two phases in the assessment of a woman receiving analgesia or anesthesia for pain during labor and delivery. First, the nurse makes an initial assessment to determine if the woman is a candidate for medication. Second, the nurse assesses the client after the administration of the medication to determine its effectiveness and impact on the well-being of the woman and the fetus.

premedication assessment

* Review the woman's medical history for any contraindications to medications (allergies, history of drug

nursing care plan for the pregnant woman receiving epidural analgesia/anesthesia

NURSING DIAGNOSIS

Pain, related to labor contractions

GOAL: Client's pain during labor and delivery will be bearable

NURSING INTERVENTIONS	RATIONALE	EVALUATION
Assess client's pain level objectively, using a numeric scale.	Use of a numeric scale to measure pain will assist the nurse in evaluating the effectiveness of the treatment.	The client will state an improved rating on the numeric scale after treatment. The client will subjectively be more comfortable as evidenced by her ability to respond to instructions and converse.
Discuss various treatment options regarding her pain, and ensure that the client understands the use of epidural anesthesia.	Pain relief during labor may include systemic analgesia, spinal blocks, pudendal block, etc. Optimally, the client will decide during her prenatal classes on her choice and at this time the discussion should be understood by her and the health care team.	The client and her family will state their readiness and understanding of epidural anesthesia during labor.
Encourage the client to void before the procedure.	Epidural anesthesia diminishes neural bladder sensations. The nurse will need to monitor for bladder distension.	The client will void before the procedure. The nurse will observe for bladder distension throughout the treatment.
Obtain baseline vital signs and hydrate the patient with IV fluid as ordered.	Hypotension is a side effect of epidural anesthesia and assuring client is adequately hydrated can prevent this complication. Prompt identification of hypotension is assisted by knowing the client's baseline vital signs.	The client will remain normotensive and adequately hydrated. Vital signs will remain stable.
Evaluate the ongoing effect of the epidural anesthesia.	The client may require more or less epidural anesthesia and an ongoing evaluation is necessary.	The client will receive adequate analgesia and continue to be comfortable.
Monitor for other complications of the epidural anesthesia	The second stage of labor may be prolonged with an epidural, and the client may need to be reminded to push.	The client's labor will progress normally, and the client will push when reminded.

dependence, medical diseases or disorders, malformations, injuries or disease processes affecting the spinal column).

* Obtain current information about any medications she has been taking, last food and fluid intake, her preferences in pain management, problems during this or any previous pregnancies, time labor started, intervals between contractions, and status of membranes.
* Determine fetal status for presentation, position, gestational age, fetal heart rate, and response to labor.

postmedication assessment

* Check for side effects or allergic reactions.
* Monitor fetal and maternal vital signs for stability.
* Assess maternal pain relief and response to medication.

nursing diagnosis

* Knowledge Deficit, related to expected pain level and procedures for medicating for pain
* Anxiety, related to fear-tension-pain cycle
* Situational Low Self Esteem, related to inability to manage labor pain effectively without intervention

planning and implementation

When planning care for the woman in labor, the nurse needs to consider the cultural beliefs of the woman and her family, the woman's perceptions of labor pain, her knowledge of the labor process, and plans for controlling pain. The goal of nursing care is to provide information about the labor process, causes of the pain, and interventions to relieve the pain. Comfort measures, such as positioning, ice chips, and breathing techniques, also can be introduced if the woman is receptive. Thorough explanations of all procedures are given to the woman and her partner, with emotional support and praise as appropriate. The nurse administers medications as ordered to relieve the pain while minimizing side effects to the fetus. The woman is monitored for any side effects, including hypotension, respiratory depression, and urinary retention, and the fetus is monitored for any signs of respiratory depression. See the Nursing Care Plan for the Pregnant Woman Receiving Epidural Analgesia/Anesthesia.

evaluation

* The woman and her partner will express a basic understanding of the causes of labor pain and the interventions available.
* The woman will express a relief of anxiety.
* The woman will be more in control and appear more self-assured.

key points

* **Pharmacologic or nonpharmacologic management of childbirth pain has been used since the Middle Ages.**
* **The goals of pain management for the nurse assisting the family with labor and delivery are to provide maximum comfort for the woman with minimal risk to her and the fetus and help make labor and delivery a positive experience for the entire family.**
* **Appropriate pain management allows the woman to become a more active participant in the birthing process.**
* **Systemic analgesia (narcotics, sedatives, and tranquilizers) may be administered during the first stage of labor to relieve pain and anxiety.**
* **Naloxone hydrochloride is a narcotic antagonist used in emergencies to reverse narcotic depressive effects in the newborn.**
* **Anesthesia blocks sensory nerve transmission, with or without consciousness, to relieve pain during labor and delivery.**
* **Regional anesthesia blocks sensory nerve transmission to a specific region or portion of the body, alleviating the woman's pain without loss of consciousness.**
* **General anesthesia renders the woman unconscious and is reserved for emergency cesarean delivery.**

review questions 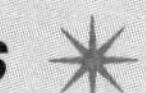

1. Felicia Evans, a primigravida, is in labor and dilated 5 cm. She has expressed a great deal of fear and anxiety and is requesting medication. Which of the following medications ordered by Felicia's physician would be most helpful?
   a. Seconal
   b. Narcan
   c. Vistaril
   d. Nembutal
2. Rita Froehlich is going to have a spinal anesthetic in preparation for a cesarean delivery. The nurse assists her into a sitting position with her back arched forward. This is done to
   a. make Rita more comfortable.
   b. shorten the time needed to do the procedure.
   c. widen the intervertebral spaces for needle insertion.
   d. allow the nurse to get a better hold on Rita to prevent her from moving.
3. Hannah Levy has just been admitted to the obstetric department. She plans to have an epidural anesthetic during her labor. The nurse explains to Hannah that her blood pressure will be checked frequently because
   a. it is institutional policy in most hospitals.
   b. hypotension is the most common side effect of epidural anesthesia.
   c. the blood pressure can give an indication of the stage of labor.
   d. taking frequent blood pressure readings allows the nurse to make other assessments while in the room.
4. The nurse recognizes that Demerol given late in labor can result in respiratory depression in the newborn.

The medication given to counteract this condition is called
   a. Vistaril.
   b. Seconal.
   c. Narcan.
   d. Phenergan.
5. Denise Williams has just delivered a healthy, 7-lb baby boy. She was able to control her labor pain with the use of Lamaze techniques but developed perineal lacerations during delivery. The physician has elected to use an anesthetic before suturing the area. The nurse recognizes that the physician most probably will use
   a. a spinal block.
   b. a lumbar epidural.
   c. a general anesthetic.
   d. a local infiltration.

references 

American Academy of Pediatrics and American College of Obstetricians and Gynecologists (1992). *Guidelines for Perinatal Care* (3rd ed.).

Borneman, T. (1995). Controlling pain, using non-drug interventions to relieve pain. *Nursing 95*, 21.

Fields, S. A., & Wall, E. M. (1993). Obstetric analgesia and anesthesia. *Primary Care*, *20*(3), 705–712.

Taylor, T. (1993). Epidural anesthesia in the maternity patient. *Maternal Child Health*, *18*, 86–93.

bibliography

American College of Obstetricians and Gynecologists (1992). Anesthesia for emergency deliveries. *ACOG Committee Opinion*, No. 104. March 1992.

Cunningham, F. G., McDonald, P. C., Leveno, K. J., Gant, N. F., & Gilstrap, L. (1993). *Williams obstetrics* (19th ed.). Norwalk, CT: Appleton and Lange.

Deglin, J. H., & Vallerand, A. H. (1993). *Davis's drug guide for nurses* (3rd ed.). Philadelphia: F.A. Davis.

Green, M. J. (1993). Expectations and experiences of pain in labor: Findings from a large prospective study. *Birth*, *20*, 65–72.

Kenner, C. A., & Mac Laren, A. (1993). *Essentials of maternal and neonatal nursing*. Springhouse, PA: Springhouse Corporation.

May, K. A., & Mahlmeister, L. R. (1994). *Maternal and neonatal nursing: Family-centered care* (3rd ed.). Philadelphia: J.B. Lippincott.

Olds. S. B., London, M. L., & Ladewig, P. W. (1992). *Maternal newborn nursing: A family-centered approach* (4th ed.). Redwood City, CA: Addison-Wesley Nursing.

Pappas, A. B. (1994). *NSNA review series—maternal newborn nursing.* New York: Delmar.

Pillitteri, A. (1995). *Maternal and child health nursing.* Philadelphia: J.B. Lippincott.

Reeder, S. J., et al (1992). *Maternity nursing* (17th ed.). Philadelphia: J.B. Lippincott.

Reiss B. S., & Evans, M. E. (1993). *Pharmacological aspects of nursing care* (4th ed.). Albany: Delmar.

Wild, L., & Coyne, C. (1992). The basics and beyond: Epidural analgesia. *American Journal of Nursing*, *90*(4), 26–34.

nursing care of the family during childbirth

12

outline

objectives

After studying this chapter, the reader should be able to:

* Discuss the guidelines for admission for labor and delivery.
* Describe the information gathered during the admission procedure.
* Discuss the use of Leopold's maneuvers in determining fetal lie, position, and presentation.
* Discuss the difference between internal and external fetal monitoring.
* Define the terms used to interpret fetal monitoring patterns.
* Describe the nursing care given during labor and delivery.
* Describe immediate care and assessment of the newborn.

key terms

accelerations
bulb syringe
deceleration
doula
early decelerations
electronic fetal monitoring
external electronic monitoring
fetal scalp blood sampling
internal electronic monitoring
late decelerations
Leopold's maneuvers
monitrice
radiant warmer
strain gauge
variability

The birth of a child remains one of life's most exciting, miraculous events. After months of waiting and anticipation, labor begins; this is a process as old as humanity itself, yet it is a unique experience for each woman and each family. For most healthy women, this normal physiologic process follows a predictable course, concluding as a new life enters the world. The nurse is a privileged participant in this process, carefully monitoring the health of the woman and her fetus and offering comfort and physical and emotional support to the woman and her partner. This chapter describes family-centered care of the woman at low risk for complications. Care of women at risk for complications during labor and delivery is discussed in Chapter 13.

✷ family considerations

Determining when to seek care for labor and delivery in the hospital, clinic, or at home is an important consideration for the family. This period of indecision can be both stressful and exciting. Ideally, plans for child care and functioning of the household will be in place, and only a few phone calls to finalize arrangements and notify others will be needed (see Teaching Guidelines). The initiation of labor marks a change in the family unit; roles will change as a new member or members are added.

Factors that effect the labor experience for the family include the following:

- Experiences with past labors
- Cultural beliefs about the labor experience
- Personal beliefs about the labor experience
- General physical health of the woman
- Maternal age
- Childbirth preparation classes
- Prenatal care
- Support system

teaching guidelines ✷
when to go to the hospital or birthing center

The following signs indicate that it is time to go:

- You experience a sudden gush of fluid from the vagina. This means your bag of waters has ruptured.
- Contractions are approximately 5 minutes apart. (Check with your physician for exact time; be sure he or she knows how long it will take you to reach the hospital.)
- If you have bright red vaginal bleeding, with or without contractions, you should immediately go to the hospital.

✷ nursing considerations

The nurse recognizes that admission to the labor department is a time of anxiety, heightened anticipation, and uncertainty for the woman and her support person. The goals of nursing care follow:

- Establish a warm, welcoming environment.
- Assess maternal and fetal well-being.
- Provide clear, concise explanations about the physical environment, procedures, expectations, and equipment used.

admission of the woman in labor

Once the woman has been introduced to the routine and is comfortable, the admission process should be quick and efficient. The earlier in labor the admission is accomplished, the easier it will be for her. Maternal assessment includes a history and physical examination, necessary laboratory tests, and evaluation of the woman's psychological status. Fetal assessment includes determination of fetal position and lie and fetal status.

✷ nursing process for the client in labor

maternal assessment

history

A history should be compiled as soon as possible. Many institutions receive a copy of the woman's prenatal information from the physician. This is mailed, brought in by the mother, or faxed to the obstetric unit. The nurse may review this information in preparation for the admission. Regardless of whether this information is available, history needs to include the items listed in Display 12-1.

physical information

A general head-to-toe assessment should be performed to determine the overall status of the woman. The nurse needs to listen to the patient and ask open-ended questions during this time to determine the woman's chief complaint. The nurse should not assume that the woman is in active labor. Her membranes may have ruptured, she may have a urinary tract infection, or various other concerns may have brought her to the hospital.

Vital signs are assessed at this time. Temperature should be within normal limits (97° to 99.6°F); any elevation may indicate infection or dehydration. The pulse normally will be between 70 to 80 beats/min but may run as high as 100 due to anxiety. A persistent elevated pulse may be due to dehydration or exhaustion. Respirations normally will fall between 16 and 24 breaths per minute. Elevated respiratory rate may been seen with hyperventilation due to anxiety, pain, or infection. Blood pressure is assessed between contractions with the woman lying on her left side to obtain the most accurate reading. If the blood pressure is elevated, the nurse should wait a few

display 12-1
essentials of maternal history

* Name
* Age
* Attending obstetrician or nurse-midwife
* Pediatrician
* Weight
* Allergies
* Blood type and Rh
* History of previous medical condition
* Prenatal problems
* Para and gravida
* Results of any testing during prenatal period
* Prenatal education
* Plans for breast-feeding or bottle feeding
* List of any medications taken during pregnancy
* Any foods or fluids ingested in the last 24 hours
* Onset of contractions
* Status of membranes
* Estimated date of confinement

minutes and reassess it to verify the elevation. If the reading remains high, the nurse should assess for signs of pregnancy-induced hypertension (see Chap. 9).

Once it has been determined that the woman is in labor, the nurse will assess the contractions for frequency, duration, and intensity. A vaginal examination may be performed by the registered nurse to assess cervical dilatation, station, effacement, and status of the membranes. If the status of the membranes is in question, nitrazine paper may be used to check for the presence of amniotic fluid in the vaginal canal. The fern test also may be used for confirmation (see Chap. 10). The status of the amniotic fluid is important:

* It is an indication of the beginning of labor if it has not already begun.
* Once the membranes are ruptured, there is an increased chance of intrauterine infection.
* There is a chance of umbilical cord prolapse if the fetal head is not engaged in the pelvis.

✷ nursing alert

Be alert for signs of potential clinical problems during the physical assessment, for example, genital lesions (STDs), edema (PIH), back pain, or history of fractured coccyx (difficulty with delivery of fetus).

laboratory tests

A urine specimen is obtained and immediately checked with a dipstick for protein and glucose. The remainder of the specimen may be sent for routine urinalysis, depending on the physician's preference.

A blood sample is drawn for syphilis screening (VDRL), hemoglobin, hematocrit, hepatitis B antibodies, and blood typing. Drug screening also may be done if the maternal history indicates the need.

psychological status

The psychological preparation of the woman and her support person is assessed by observing body language, posture, and verbal responses. Cultural considerations are discussed as indicated, and every attempt needs to be made to meet these considerations in the plan of care.

fetal assessment

Once it has been established that the woman is in active labor, the fetus is assessed for position, lie, and presentation, using Leopold's maneuvers. The fetal heart rate is assessed to determine if it is within normal limits. Fetal heart tones (FHT) are heard using a fetoscope or handheld electronic Doppler. An electronic fetal monitor may be applied, internally or externally, to provide continuous information for assessment of fetal well-being.

✷ nursing insight

Regardless of whether fetal heart tones are obtained by the manual method or by the electronic method, they are recorded every 30 minutes during the latent phase of labor, every 15 minutes during the active phase, and every 5 minutes during the second stage.

leopold's maneuvers

Leopold's maneuvers are a combination of four observations and palpations used to determine the fetal lie, position, and presentation (Fig. 12-1). The four maneuvers include the following:

1. Palpation of the fundal region. One hand is placed on either side of the fundus; generally the buttocks are palpated and feel soft, smooth, and move only with the entire torso. If the head is felt, it is smooth, firm, and more round and moves independently of the torso.
2. Palpation of the sides of the uterus. One hand is placed on either side of the body of the uterus and depressed to feel for the location of the back and extremities. The back feels firm and smooth, while the extremities feel nodular.
3. Palpation just above the symphysis pubis. This is accomplished by grasping with the dominant hand. The head is more firm and rounded than the buttocks. If the fetal head is not engaged, the fetal part will move freely.
4. Palpation for the cephalic prominence (the brow of the fetus). Both hands slide down toward the symphysis pubis. The fetal brow can be felt on the same side as the extremities.

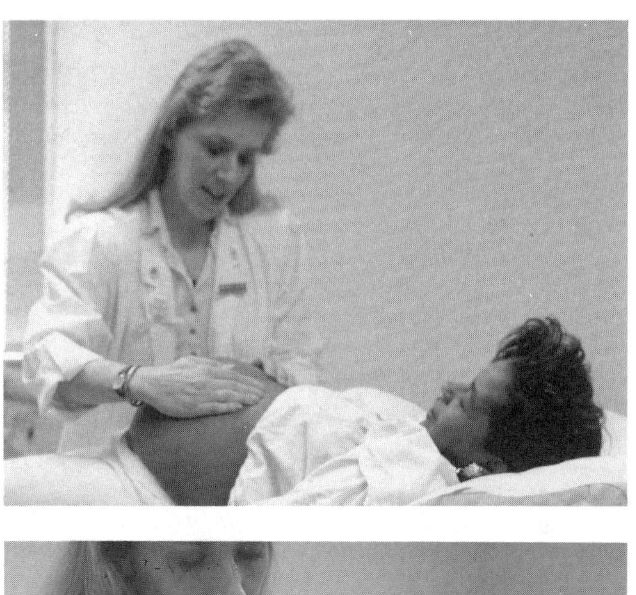
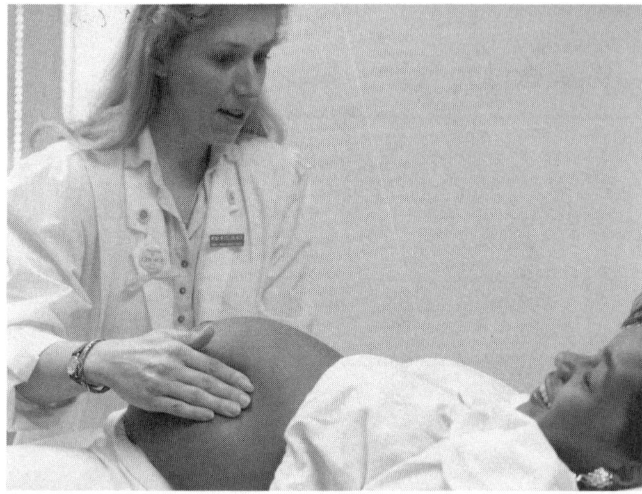
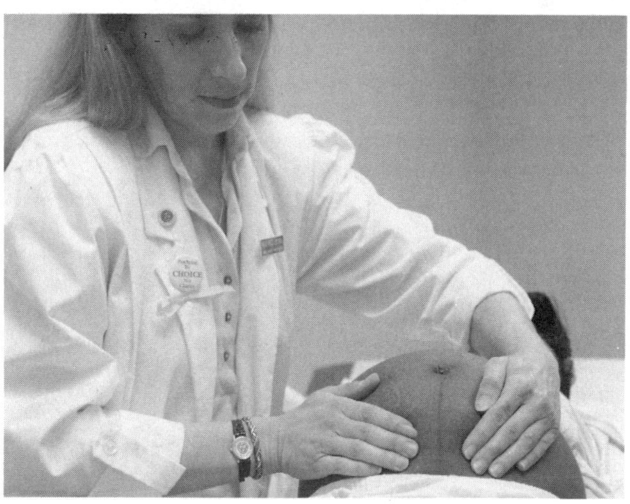
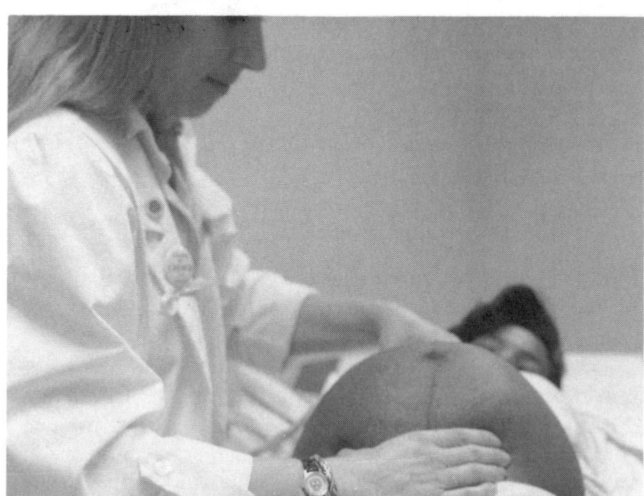

figure 12-1 *Leopold's maneuvers are used to assess fetal position and presentation.*

fetal heart tones

The fetal heart rate should range between 120 and 160 beats/min. Below 100 or above 180 can indicate fetal distress. After performing Leopold's maneuvers, the fetoscope or ultrasound Doppler is placed in the area where the heartbeat is loudest. Usually the fetal heart can be heard best through the fetal back. With a face presentation, FHTs are better heard through the fetal thorax. The majority of the time the fetus will be in a cephalic or vertex position, so the heart will be heard more clearly in the lower maternal abdomen. If the fetus is breech, the fetal heartbeat will be heard more clearly in the upper portion of the maternal abdomen. Because it is difficult to hear FHTs during a contraction, continuous electronic fetal monitoring may be used for a more complete picture.

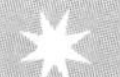 **nursing alert**

Always palpate the woman's radial pulse when assessing for the fetal heart rate. This will avoid confusing the maternal heart rate with the fetal heart rate because the fetal rate is much faster.

electronic fetal monitoring

Electronic fetal monitoring may be performed internally or externally. The monitor produces an audible sound of the FHTs plus a continuous tracing (Fig. 12-2). Using fetal monitoring provides a clearer picture of the fetal heart rate because it monitors continuously before, during, and after a uterine contraction. The monitor also provides a tracing pattern of uterine activity. Depending on the local protocol, fetal monitoring may not be used on a "low-risk labor" patient. (See Display 12-2 for indications for fetal monitoring.)

external electronic monitoring To monitor externally, a tocodynamometer transducer ("toco") is placed on the maternal abdomen over the fundus of the uterus and is strapped in place with Velcro or similar materials. This measures the pressure of the uterine fundus during a contraction and converts it to an electrical pattern that is recorded on graph paper.

An ultrasound transducer, similar to the ultrasound Doppler, is then strapped over the maternal abdomen where the FHTs are the loudest. A water-soluble lubricant is applied to the transducer to improve conduction of the

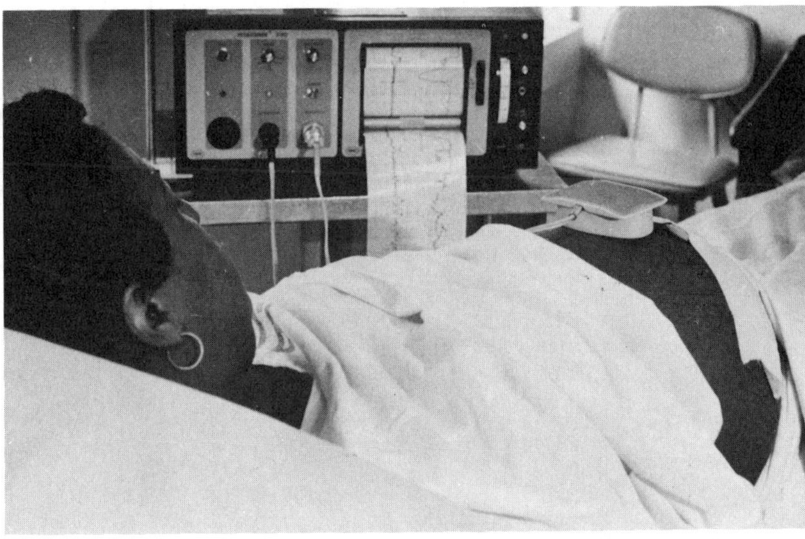

figure 12-2 *Client with external fetal monitor applied. Note that the monitor function can be observed and heard by the client.*

sound. The FHTs may be heard throughout the room, while being converted to an electrical pattern that is also recorded on the graph paper (Fig. 12-3). Initially hearing the fetal heartbeat can be encouraging and exciting for the parents. Later, when the labor becomes active, the nurse may elect to turn the sound off if it distracts the mother and her support person.

External fetal monitoring is noninvasive and easily applied. It gives a permanent record that may be stored along with the legal chart. A poor tracing of the pattern may occur if the maternal abdomen is obese, the fetus moves excessively, or the amniotic fluid is excessive. See Table 12-1 for interpretation of fetal heart pattern.

internal electronic monitoring To monitor the uterine contractions internally, the cervix must be dilated at least 2 cm and the membranes ruptured. Using sterile technique, the physician, midwife, or specially trained registered nurse inserts a soft water-filled catheter into the uterus, past the presenting part of the fetus. This catheter is connected to a *strain gauge* (a device or transducer that measures pressure) located on the fetal monitor. It converts the pressure measurement to an electrical pattern that is recorded on the fetal monitor graph paper.

To monitor FHTs internally, the cervix must be dilated 2 cm, the membranes ruptured, and the presenting part of the fetus identified and engaged. Using sterile technique, a sterile spiral electrode is attached to the fetal scalp. This electrode converts the reading to an electrical pattern that is recorded on the fetal monitor graph paper similar to the external monitor. The internal reading is much more accurate and is not interrupted by fetal or maternal movement.

interpretation of the data To interpret the data from the monitor tracings properly, the health care provider compares the tracings with the clinical events that occur. Special classes, in-services, and clinical experience help personnel to become adept at interpretation. This may take several years. Many terms are used in this interpretation.

Tachycardia and *bradycardia* refer to the fetal heart rate. The normal fetal heart rate is 120 to 160; this is called the normal baseline fetal heart rate. The baseline is obtained by monitoring the fetal heart rate for 10 minutes between contractions. When the fetal heart rate increases above 160, it is defined as *fetal tachycardia*. This condition may be seen with fetal immaturity, fetal distress, and fetal or maternal fever. *Marked bradycardia* occurs when the fetal heart rate falls below 100 beats/min. This condition may been seen with fetal acidosis, cord compression, postmaturity, maternal hypotension, or placental separation. It also may be seen following an epidural procedure (Miller, 1993).

Variability is an indication of the functioning of the autonomic nervous system of the fetus. The sympathetic nervous system response increases the fetal heart rate, and

display 12-2
indications for fetal monitoring

* Maternal hypertensive states
* Rh incompatibility
* History of stillbirth
* Premature labor
* Post-term labor
* Failure to progress
* Labor induction
* Multiple gestation
* Intrauterine growth retardation
* Meconium-stained amniotic fluid
* Placenta previa and abruptio placenta
* Diabetes
* Umbilical cord prolapse
* Prolonged or premature rupture of membranes
* Decreased fetal movement

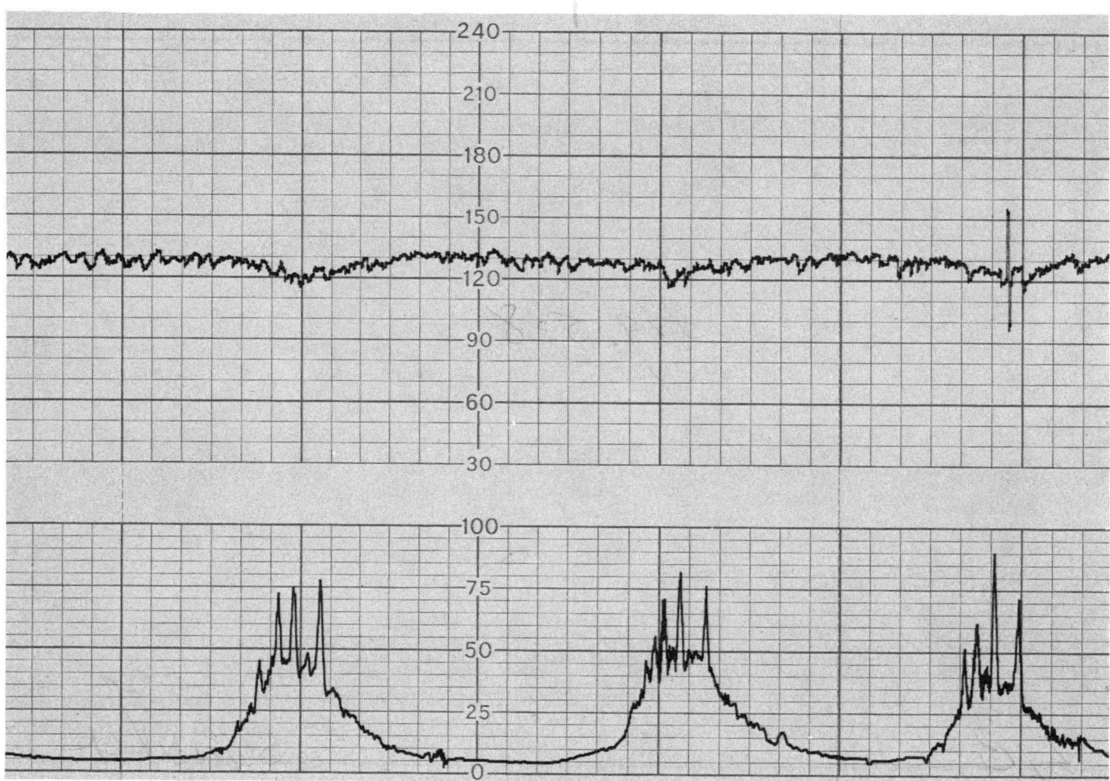

figure 12-3 *Monitor strip from internal monitor. Lower reading is the uterine pressure. Spikes during contractions indicate the mother was pushing down to assist with the descent of the baby. Slight dipping in the fetal heart rate (upper line) is normal during contractions.*

the parasympathetic nervous system decreases the fetal heart rate. Normal beat-to-beat variability using an internal monitor (for accuracy) is one of the most important indicators of fetal well-being. It is demonstrated by a range of 2 to 10 beats/min around the baseline. Absence of variability may be due to maternal narcotic or barbiturate medication, fetal immaturity, fetal hypoxia, or acidosis. The baseline variability is described as short term or long term. *Short-term variability* (beat-to-beat) refers to the fluctuations seen from one beat to the next. It is usually about 2 to 3 beats/min. *Long-term variability* refers to the wavelike fluctuations from the baseline that occur two to six times per minute with a normal range of 6 to 10 beats/min.

Accelerations are the temporary normal increases in fetal heart rate in response to fetal activity or compression of the cord during a contraction. They last for a short time and return to normal. Accelerations are an indication of fetal well-being (Fig. 12-4).

Decelerations are a periodic drop in the fetal heart rate. To evaluate a deceleration to determine if it is a normal or abnormal response, the health care provider looks at the relationship of the deceleration to the contraction and the severity of the drop.

Early decelerations occur late in labor and are a response to fetal head compression. They usually begin when the contraction begins and end with the end of the contraction. The fetal heart rate rarely falls below 100 beats/min. If decelerations occur early in labor before the fetus has descended, they may be an indication of cephalopelvic disproportion.

Late decelerations occur after the acme of the contraction and continue past the contraction. This is usually a serious sign. It could indicate uteroplacental insufficiency. An attempt to increase the blood flow should be made by placing the woman on her left side to increase blood flow to the uterus. Oxygen by mask also may be initiated. If the pattern does not correct itself, a cesarean delivery may be considered.

Variable decelerations should be considered a serious sign. These occur at varying unpredictable times during the contractions. Variable decelerations usually indicate cord compression. To relieve pressure on the cord, the mother may be placed in a Trendelenburg position. Oxygen also may be given by mask. If these interventions do not correct the problem, a cesarean delivery is performed.

fetal scalp blood sampling

When late decelerations or other signs of fetal distress occur, the physician may elect to obtain a specimen of fetal blood to check for acidosis. This sample (0.25 mL) may be obtained by piercing the scalp of the fetus and drawing the

table 12-1 interpretation of fetal heart pattern

Terminology	Definition	Nursing Consideration
Tachycardia	Fetal heart rate above 160 for more than 10 minutes (causes: maternal infection, drugs, fetal distress)	Continue to monitor fetal and maternal vital signs. Document findings. Report continued elevation.
Bradycardia	Fetal heart rate below 120 for more than 10 minutes (causes: fetal distress, maternal hypotension, severe contractions in response to oxytocin)	Continue to monitor fetal and maternal vital signs. Change maternal position. Give oxygen per mask. Slow or stop oxytocin drip. Document findings. Report continued decrease.
Variability	Indication of function of the fetal autonomic nervous system	An increase in variability does not require intervention. A decreased variability should be reported to physician for interpretation of cause. Document findings.
Baseline	2–10 beats around the baseline	
Short term	Fluctuations seen from one beat to the next	
Long term	Wavelike fluctuations that occur two to six times per minute with a normal range of 6 to 10 beats/min	
Accelerations	Temporary normal increases in FHR	No intervention is needed.
Decelerations	Periodic drop in FHR	No intervention is needed for early decelerations.
Early	Begin when the contraction begins and end with the end of the contraction (causes: cord compression)	For late decelerations, turn the mother to left side to increase blood flow to fetus; give oxygen per mask; document and report response; prepare for cesarean section if needed.
Late	Occur after the acme of the contraction and continue past it (causes: uteroplacental insufficiency)	
	Occur at varying unpredictable times during the contractions (causes: cord compression or cord around neck)	For variable decelerations, position on left side or knee chest to relieve cord compression; prepare for cesarean section if needed.

blood into a tiny glass capillary tube. If the pH of the sample is 7.20 or less, this indicates severe fetal acidosis, and the obstetric team should prepare for an immediate cesarean delivery.

nursing diagnosis

* Anxiety, related to birth process and foreign surroundings
* Knowledge Deficit, related to the birth process and techniques and procedures used
* Pain, related to labor contractions

planning and implementation

To individualize the nursing care and interventions during labor and delivery, planning and implementation are discussed according to the stages of labor. See the Nursing Care Plan on page 186.

first stage of labor

Care of the woman in the first stage of labor requires monitoring her and the fetus and providing comfort, support, and reassurance. For women who have not had prenatal care or childbirth preparation classes, the early stage of labor provides an opportunity for the nurse to offer information and special assistance (Display 12-3).

To understand specific nursing interventions throughout the first stage of labor, nursing care is described in terms of the needs during the three phases: latent, active, transition.

latent phase During the latent stage of labor, the cervix dilates to 3 to 4 cm. Contractions produce mild discomfort, occur every 5 to 30 minutes, and are 30 to 40 seconds apart. Most women will remain at home during this phase, making last minute arrangements for admission. If the woman has been admitted to the hospital, her blood pressure will be taken hourly. Pulse, respirations, and temper-

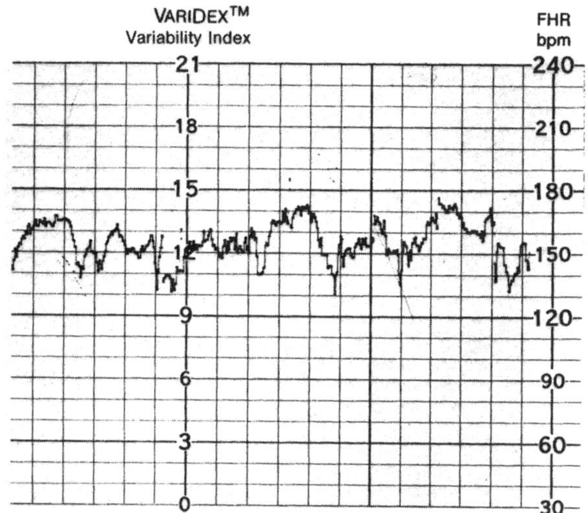

figure 12-4 *Transient accelerations of fetal heart rate.*

ature are taken every 4 hours. The fetal heart rate is checked every 30 minutes. Any deviations from normal are reported.

If the woman is to receive an enema and vaginal preparation (shaving of the vaginal area in preparation for delivery), this is the ideal time—before the contractions become stronger and closer together. In the past, the vaginal preparation consisted of shaving the mons pubis and entire perineal area, including the rectum. This procedure has been modified to include only the labial region or from the fourchette to the rectum, where lacerations or episiotomies are sutured. Some physicians no longer require this controversial procedure. It was originally thought that shaving decreased the chance of infection, but it might actually increase the possibility of infection due to small cuts or razor irritation.

The physician may order an enema to evacuate stool to prevent contamination of the sterile field, to prevent embarrassment due to expelling stool during bearing down efforts, and to stimulate uterine contractions. Types of enemas given include soap suds, tap water, and Fleets. Many physicians no longer order enemas if the woman has had a normal bowel movement in the past 24 hours. The enema is uncomfortable, and it may not produce the desired effect. Enemas are always contraindicated during premature labor, in the presence of vaginal bleeding, and if labor is progressing rapidly or birth is imminent. If these procedures are ordered, the nurse should explain the procedure, provide privacy, and use universal precautions.

As soon as all information is obtained, the admission and assessment are complete, and preliminary procedures are finished, the woman is encouraged to ambulate, and her support person is encouraged to accompany her. The nurse will continue to assess vital signs and fetal heart rate as necessary. The woman is encouraged to continue oral intake (125 mL/h) of ice chips, water, or clear liquids to prevent dehydration. No solid food is permitted because peristalsis is slowed during labor. The nurse also will encourage the woman to void frequently to prevent distention, which delays the progress of labor.

active phase As the active phase of labor begins, the contractions are 3 to 5 minutes apart and last 45 to 60 seconds. The cervix dilates from 4 to 7 cm. The woman becomes self-focused because the pains are progressively stronger and closer. If she has attended prenatal or Lamaze classes, she may begin her breathing patterns or request pain medication. The support person's participation is encouraged (Display 12-4). If the mother prefers to use analgesics or an epidural, they are usually administered during this phase (see Chap. 11).

Blood pressure is assessed every hour between contractions, preferably with the woman in a side-lying position. Fetal heart rate is assessed every 15 minutes during the active phase. Temperature is assessed every 4 hours unless the membranes have ruptured (which they often do during this phase), in which case it is assessed every hour. Contractions are assessed for frequency, duration, and intensity every 15 minutes. Cervical dilatation, effacement, station, and position of presenting part are assessed at appropriate intervals.

Once the membranes rupture, the nurse checks FHTs, checks for the presence of the cord in the vaginal orifice, and checks the fluid for amount, color, and odor. If the fetal head is not engaged, there is a risk of prolapsed cord

display 12-3
assisting the unprepared woman with labor

Some pregnant women may not have attended prenatal classes for a variety of reasons. The nurse may prepare these women early in labor with certain suggestions:

- **Attempt to relax your abdominal muscles as you feel your uterus tighten.**
- **Slow your breathing to one half the normal rate—about 6 to 10 breaths per minute.**
- **Use abdominal and chest muscles when breathing.**
- **Use this pattern of breathing throughout the entire contraction.**
- **At the beginning and end of each contraction, take a deep breath and release it slowly; this helps deliver oxygen to your baby.**
- **Concentrate on the nurse's face; he or she will assist you with pacing your breathing.**
- **As labor progresses, you may switch to rapid chest breathing, about 20 to 30 breaths per minute.**
- **Watch the nurse closely; he or she will help you pace your breathing.**
- **Try to rest and relax between each contraction; this will help you conserve your energy.**

display 12-4
measures that promote family or support person involvement

* Speak and to welcome family members or support person during the admission process.
* Assess the level of involvement the woman and family expect. This can range from periodic visits to continual presence and active coaching.
* Encourage their participation, and assist in making them comfortable in the environment.
* Encourage them to take breaks during the labor process to decrease their fatigue, stress, or tension.
* Explain procedures and equipment that is used.
* Relay updates to family members who choose to wait in the waiting room.

because the fluid can float the cord into the birth canal in front of the presenting part. As the fetus descends into the canal, pressure on the cord prevents the delivery of oxygen to the fetus. A drop in the fetal heart rate following rupture of the membranes may be the first sign of prolapsed cord (see Chap. 13). The time of rupture is documented on the chart. Fluid is normally odorless and clear. Greenish brown fluid indicates meconium staining, which may signal fetal distress because the anal sphincter relaxes. If the fetus is in breech position, meconium staining is a normal sign. As the fluid continues to leak, the nurse changes the absorbent bed pad to keep the mother more comfortable. Vaginal examinations are performed as needed to determine the woman's progress.

To provide comfort to the client, the nurse or support person may give backrubs or apply counterpressure to the woman's lower back, wipe her forehead with cool cloths, praise her efforts, and emphasize relaxation. The nurse needs to remind her to void at least every 2 hours to prevent bladder distention, which could impede the process of labor. It is important to assist her with mouth care to freshen and moisten the oral cavity, which can become dry, especially if she is using breathing techniques. The nurse encourages the support person to take breaks as needed and reassures the support person that the nurse will continue coaching and providing comfort measures for the woman during this time. Recently, a special type of support person has begun to attend the birth process, a professional labor assistant called a *doula* or a *monitrice*. Some couples engage the services of a doula or monitrice for additional support. A *doula* is an individual who provides physical and emotional support during the birth process. A *monitrice*, often a nurse-midwife, provides physical and emotional support and clinical assessment of the mother and fetus. Recent studies indicate the use of a doula or monitrice has shortened the length of labor and reduced the rate of cesarean deliveries, forceps deliveries, and epidural anesthesia (Perez, 1994).

No single position is ideal for all stages of labor, and a woman's ability to change her position is an important comfort measure. Encouraging the woman to change her position gives her a feeling of more control over the situation and can decrease anxiety. Ambulation may be continued if the woman is not connected to a fetal monitor and can tolerate the effort. Walking changes the pelvic dimensions and works with the force of gravity, improving rotation and descent of the fetus. Sitting in a chair also is useful. Sitting with the body angling forward straightens the path of the birth canal, and spreads the pelvis, making more room. A hand–knee position is helpful for the mother experiencing back labor from an occiput-posterior fetal position because it assists the fetus with rotation. The woman also may assume a squatting position for comfort during contractions. Squatting relieves back pain, widens the pelvic outlet, and takes advantage of gravity. A back-lying position should be avoided because it puts pressure on the vena cava, decreasing blood flow to the placenta, forces the woman to work against gravity, and can actually prolong labor by impeding the rotation of the fetus.

transition phase Transition is the most intense phase of the first stage of labor. During the transition phase, the cervix dilates from 7 to 10 cm; contractions are strong and long, occurring every 2 to 3 minutes and lasting 60 to 90 seconds. The woman may experience several physical cues that she is entering the transition phase. These include an increase in bloody show, shaking and chills, nausea and vomiting, perspiration, leg cramps, backache, and a sensation of pressure in the perineal region. The nurse continues to monitor maternal vital signs and FHTs just as during the active phase. Providing comfort, assisting the woman to maintain control, and preventing hyperventilation are the major goals during transition.

Some women may feel the urge to push even if the cervix is not fully dilated. To prevent the cervix from swelling and impeding the process, the nurse may assist the woman in changing the breathing pattern. Using the patterned pace breathing (adding a soft blow every few breaths) may assist the woman in regaining control. If the urge to push becomes overwhelming, a ratio of 1:1 is most helpful. This type of breathing resembles a puffing or panting type breathing. Because of the intense discomfort, fatigue, frequency, and length of the contractions, the woman is at risk for losing control. She may express fear of being alone but prefers little touching or interaction. She appears frustrated, restless, confused, and may seem to have difficulty understanding directions.

Nursing measures that may be helpful include the following:

* Change absorbent pad frequently to keep her clean and dry.
* Assist her into a position of comfort, avoiding the supine position.
* Decrease outside distractions.

nursing care plan
for the family during childbirth

NURSING DIAGNOSIS

Anxiety, related to labor and delivery experience and foreign surroundings

GOAL: *Client will tolerate stress of labor and verbalize anxiety*

NURSING INTERVENTIONS	RATIONALE	EVALUATION
Encourage the client and family to verbalize their fears and anxiety.	By eliciting the information causing the client's and family's fears the nurse can address each fear and provide accurate information.	The client and family feel comfortable in openly discussing their thoughts and sharing their feelings.
Support relaxation techniques and reinforce appropriate coping behaviors.	By showing approval of appropriate behavior, the nurse reinforces the behavior and the client continues to use measures to decrease anxiety.	The client shows objective signs of decreased anxiety (decreased heart rate) and states a decreased level of anxiety and a lessening of fear.

NURSING DIAGNOSIS

Powerlessness, related to the labor process

GOAL: *Increase the client's feelings of power by increasing the capability to make decisions*

NURSING INTERVENTIONS	RATIONALE	EVALUATION
Encourage the client to express her feelings any way she is comfortable with.	Encouraging expression of feelings gives credence to the client's feelings and increases her control over the situation.	The client will be comfortable in her expression of her feelings during labor.
Allow the client to make decisions regarding her comfort, such as position and what mode of analgesia she prefers.	Decision-making should be encouraged and shows respect to the client while giving her power and control during the labor process.	The client will make appropriate decisions and feel comfortable in asking questions. The client will state she feels some control in the labor process.

* Provide warm blankets for shaking and chills.
* Offer ice chips; fan or wipe her face with a cool cloth to relieve the perspiration that occurs, particularly on the face.
* Offer frequent praise and encouragement to alleviate feelings of apprehension and irritability.

To assist the woman in maintaining her focus, the nurse maintains eye contact, gives firm but gentle instructions, and breathes with her. To counteract fatigue, it is important to remind her when the contraction is over and to rest until the next one starts. Many women are able to doze and even fall asleep during these short periods. This is helpful in conserving her strength. Sacral pressure can relieve the back discomfort. If vomiting occurs, her head needs to be turned to the side, and her face cleansed with a cool cloth. The nurse reassures her that this is normal during this phase. She needs to be reminded that soon she will be completely dilated and ready to begin pushing.

second stage of labor

The second stage of labor begins with full dilatation and ends with the expulsion of the fetus. Contractions occur every 2 to 3 minutes and last 60 to 90 seconds. All energies are focused on delivery. Maternal pulse and blood pressure are monitored every 30 minutes; FHTs are monitored every 5 minutes. As the second stage of labor begins, the woman experiences an involuntary urge to push, bloody show increases, the fetal head crowns, the perineum bulges, and perspiration suddenly appears on her upper lip. She may make low grunting sounds and complain of perineal pressure; the membranes may rupture if they have not already done so.

A vaginal examination may be performed to confirm the woman's readiness for pushing. Comfort measures, such as mouth care, provision of dry bedding, and positioning for pushing, are provided (Fig. 12-5). Positions for pushing should ensure that the presenting part is in alignment with the axis of the pelvis. These positions include

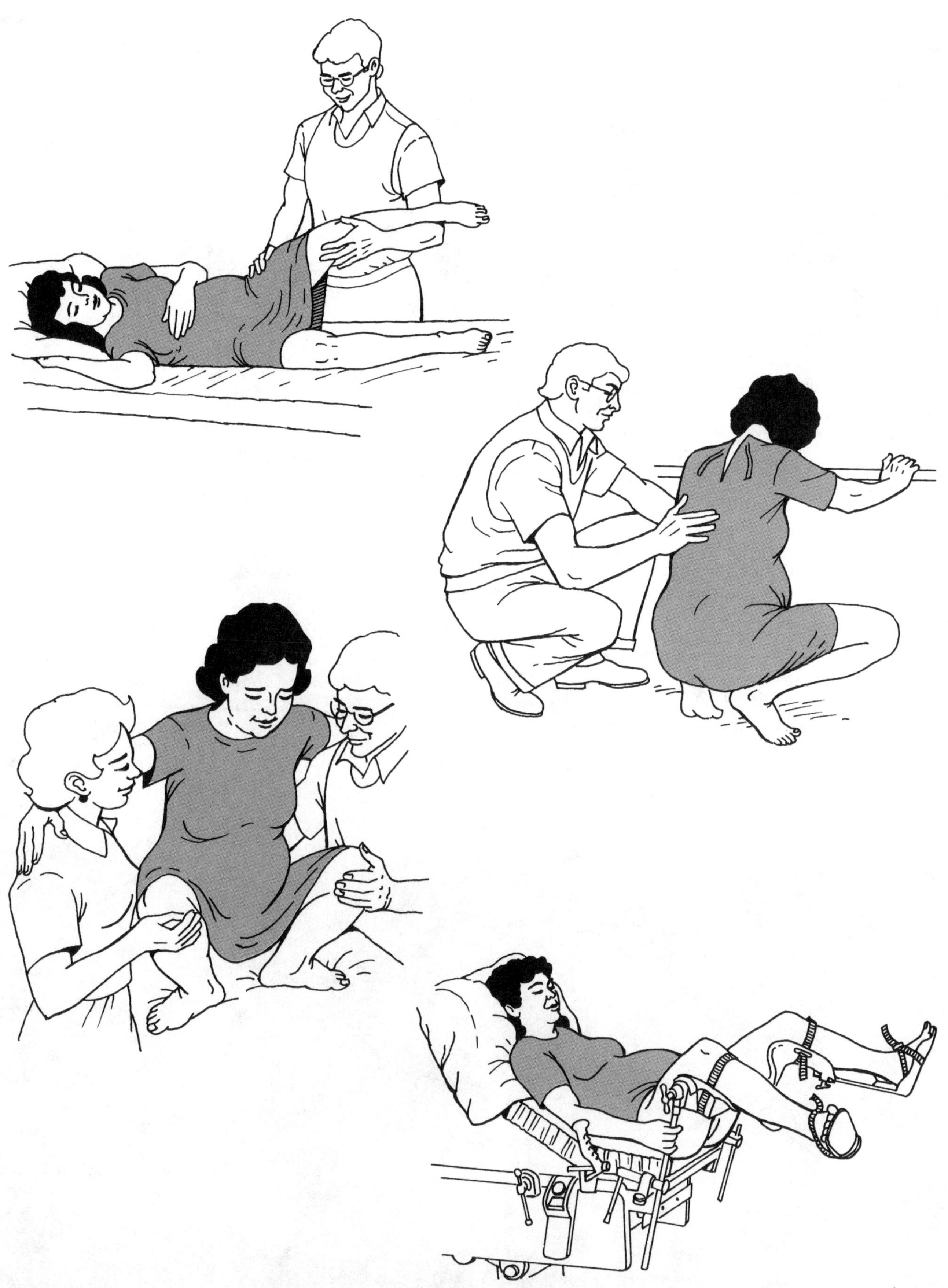

figure 12-5 *Some commonly used positions for pushing in the second stage of labor. Most of these positions take advantage of gravity to aid bearing-down efforts. Laboring women will naturally assume many of these positions for bearing down if position choices are not restricted.*

display 12-5
guidelines for assisting the woman to push in a semi-Fowler's position

* Assist to semi-Fowler's position.
* The support person or nurse may assist the mother in bringing her chin toward her chest. They also may place their arms beneath her shoulders for support.
* Instruct her to flex her thighs onto her abdomen and grasp her legs just below the knees at the beginning of the contraction,.
* As she maintains this position, she should be encouraged to bear down or push as if having a bowel movement.
* Remind her to take her cleansing breaths before and after the contraction.

semi-Fowler's, squatting, kneeling, or standing. In the hospital, the woman most often will assume a semi-Fowler's position. Guidelines for assisting the woman in pushing are summarized in Display 12-5. She needs to be supported in her desired position and instructed to push only when she has the urge; to use her abdominal muscles to assist with pushing; to use short pushes lasting no longer than 6 to 7 seconds; to hold her breath while pushing or to release it slowly, making a sound or groan from her throat; and finally to take a cleansing breath at the beginning and the end of the contraction (Fig. 12-6). Usually the woman experiences intense satisfaction when pushing, but she also is tired and sometimes experiences increased pain. The nurse continues to offer praise and encouragement. Frequently, the woman experiences leg cramps during this period. Cramps can be relieved by extending the leg and dorsiflexing the foot. The nurse explains that this is common and completely normal.

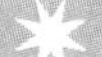 **nursing alert**

The cervix should be fully dilated (10 cm) before allowing the woman to push. Pushing before dilatation can result in the cervix becoming edematous, preventing further dilation, necessitating a cesarean delivery.

preparation for delivery Regardless of the type of delivery used (see Chap. 2), certain preparations are similar:

* Notifying the birth attendant that delivery is imminent
* Notifying the anesthesiologist or anesthetist if anesthesia is planned
* Cleansing and sterile draping of the perineal region to prevent the introduction of microorganisms into the uterus
* Preparing the supplies and area for delivery
* Ensuring the availability of equipment for the newborn (eg, sterile blankets, cord clamp, bulb syringe, radiant warmer)
* Ensuring the presence of emergency resuscitation equipment for the woman and newborn
* Preparation the support person for delivery (eg, scrub clothes, camera)

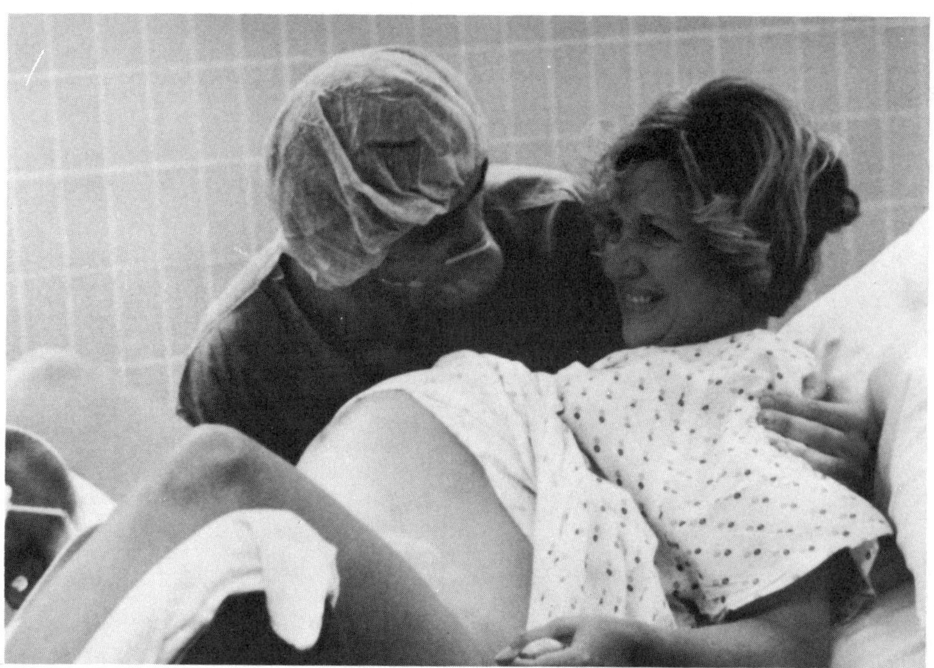

figure 12-6 *Bearing-down efforts in a conventional delivery room. The woman is supported in a semirecumbent position by pillows and by the support person. Her legs are supported by well-padded stirrups; handholds are in place to assist pushing efforts. (Photo by BABES, Inc.)*

> **nursing alert**
> *During delivery, universal precautions require that those at risk for splashing wear gowns, gloves, and goggles or face shields.*

If the woman plans to deliver in a traditional delivery room, she is transferred in time to prevent delivery on the way to the room. A primigravida is usually transferred when she is crowning, a multipara is transferred when she is dialated 7 to 8 cm. The side rails should be up for transfer. If the woman plans to deliver in a birthing room, extra absorbent pads may be placed under the perineum to absorb blood and amniotic fluid (see Chap. 2).

delivery During the delivery process, the nurse is actively involved in assisting the birthing attendant and encouraging and praising the woman and her support person. A small incision (*episiotomy*) may be performed midline or mediolaterally to prevent laceration of the perineum (see Chap. 13). As the head passes over the perineum, sterile gauze is used to wipe the face of the newborn, and a bulb syringe is used to suction secretions from the mouth. Often the physician or midwife will then show the infant to the mother and support person. When the umbilical cord stops pulsating, it is clamped and cut (Fig. 12-7). Sometimes the support person is permitted to cut the cord. The physician holds the newborn up for viewing by the mother or places it on the mother's abdomen to promote attachment. The mother and her support person are encouraged to look at and touch the newborn (Fig. 12-8).

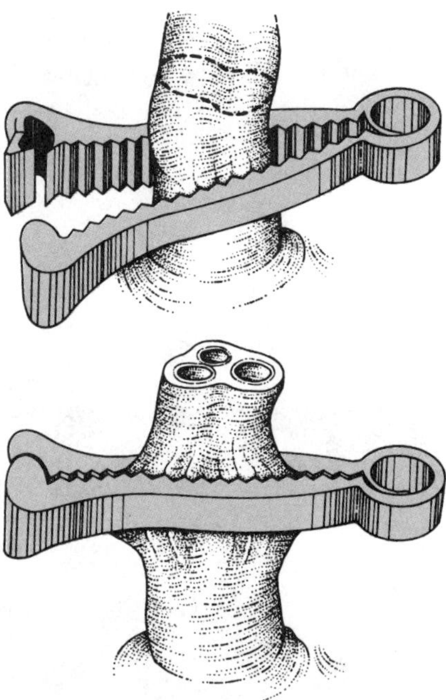

figure 12-7 *Umbilical clamp applied to cord.*

immediate care of the newborn Following initial contact with the parents and family, the newborn is then wrapped in sterile blankets and placed in the radiant warmer. He or she is wiped dry, and a small stockinet cap is placed on the head to prevent heat loss. The newborn's umbilical cord stump is assessed for two arteries and one vein. (Absence of one artery has been associated with heart and kidney anomalies.) Apgar scores are assessed at 1 and 5 minutes. The Apgar scoring system has five categories of evaluation: heart rate, respiratory effort, muscle tone, reflex irritability, and color. Each category is given a value of 0 to 2 points for a maximum score of 10. A score below 7 warrants intervention by the physician (Table 12-2). For identification purposes, the infant's footprints (fingerprints of the newborn are not developed adequately to be used for identification purposes) and the mother's index fingerprint are recorded. Identification bracelets with the mother's name, physician, newborn's date of birth, and sex are placed on the ankles of the newborn and wrist of the mother. Prophylactic antibiotic ointment (usually erythromycin) is inserted into the newborn's eyes to prevent gonococcal and chlamydial conjunctivitis (*ophthalmia neonatorum*). A recent study found that using povidone-iodine instead of the usual erythromycin eye ointment was effective not only for gonococcal and chlamydial infection but also against viruses, such as herpes simplex. In addition, povidone-iodine is less costly and easy to administer (Isenberg, Apt, & Wood, 1995).

Once the initial assessment and identification process is completed, the infant is wrapped in a warm blanket and placed with the mother to encourage further attachment. If she is breast-feeding, the newborn may be put to the breast for the first time.

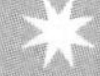

> **nursing alert**
> *The nurse follows universal precautions when handling the newborn because the newborn is covered with amniotic fluid and blood.*

third stage of labor

The third stage of labor begins immediately after the expulsion of the infant and ends with the expulsion of the placenta. The average length of this stage is 5 to 15 minutes but may last up to 30 minutes. The nurse observes for signs of placental separation. These include a sudden lengthening of the umbilical cord, a sudden gush of blood from the vagina, a globular shaped uterus, and a rise of the fundus in the abdomen. The nurse documents the time of delivery of the placenta and administers oxytocin (Pitocin) as ordered. This ensures the continued contraction of the uterus and reduces the potential for postpartum hemorrhage. Blood pressure and pulse are assessed. The per-

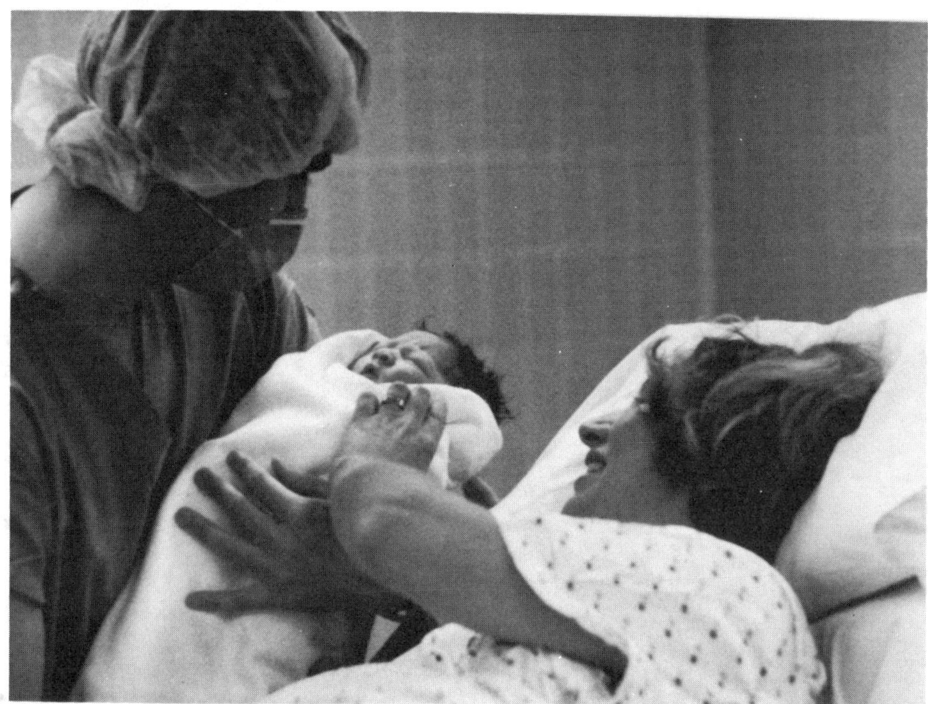

figure 12-8 *The happy couple greet their newborn. (Photo by BABES, Inc.)*

ineum is cleansed, and sterile perineal pads are applied. Ice bags also may be applied to the perineum to reduce swelling from trauma to the tissues. If the legs were in stirrups, they are removed from the stirrups simultaneously to prevent maternal hip injury. A clean gown and warm blankets are provided. Family members present for the birth may hold and visit with the newborn while the mother is comforted. If the mother has given birth in a traditional delivery room, she is now transferred to a recovery room.

fourth stage of labor

The fourth stage of labor lasts from 1 to 4 hours after birth (until the uterus remains contracted). This is usually a happy and peaceful period for the mother and her family. The mother is usually tired but hungry. She may eat a regular diet with juices and other fluids to replenish her system. In addition to monitoring the mother and newborn for physiologic adjustment, the nurse observes for attachment and interaction within the new family.

Maternal vital signs are monitored every 15 minutes for the first hour. The fundus is palpated to ensure continued contraction. The lochia (vaginal discharge) is observed for amount, color, and the presence of any clots. The bladder is assessed for distention. The mother is encouraged to void if able. Following labor and delivery, most mothers are excited, hungry, thirsty, and extremely tired. After visiting with the baby, eating and drinking, and visiting with her family, the mother is encouraged to rest to rebuild her strength (see Chap. 14).

table 12-2 *apgar rating system*

Sign	*Score*		
	0	*1*	*2*
Heart rate	Absent	Slow (less than 100)	More than 100
Respiratory effort	Absent	Slow, irregular	Good, crying
Muscle tone	Flaccid	Some flexion of extremities	Active motion
Reflex irritability	No response	Weak cry or grimace	Vigorous cry
Color	Blue, pale	Body pink; extremities blue	Completely pink

evaluation

* The mother verbalizes feelings of comfort and satisfaction.
* The mother verbalizes an understanding of the birth process and techniques and equipment used.
* The mother expresses relief from labor contractions following the birth process.

> **what would you do?**
>
> *Julie, age 15, para 0, gravida 1, has been admitted to the labor department in active labor with a term pregnancy. She is apprehensive, crying, and saying, "Please do something; I can't stand the pain.": She has had no prenatal care and does not understand what is happening to her. Her mother states, "Let her suffer; it's what she deserves. Maybe she'll listen to me the next time." What would you do?*

key points

* **Signs that admission for labor and delivery is necessary include a sudden gush of fluid from the vagina, contractions 5 minutes apart, or bright red vaginal bleeding.**
* **Goals for nursing care during the admission process include establishing a warm, welcoming environment; assessing maternal and fetal well-being; and providing a clear, concise explanation about the physical environment, procedures, expectations, and equipment used.**
* **Leopold's maneuvers are a combination of four observations and palpations to determine the fetal lie, position, and presentation.**
* **Electronic fetal monitoring may be internal or external and is used to give a continuous clear picture of the FHT in response to labor contractions.**
* **Encouraging the woman to change her position during labor is an important comfort measure. It gives her a feeling of control and can decrease feelings of anxiety.**
* **During transition, the nurse can assist the woman with maintaining her focus by maintaining eye contact, giving firm but gentle instructions, and breathing with her.**
* **During the second stage of labor, the nurse may assist the woman by supporting her in the desired position and instructing her to push only when she has the urge, to use her abdominal muscles to assist with pushing, to use short pushes that last no longer than 6 to 7 seconds, and to take a cleansing breath at the beginning and end of the contraction.**
* **To establish a patent airway in the newborn, the face is wiped with gauze as it passes over the perineum and then is suctioned with a bulb syringe.**
* **For identification purposes, the newborn's footprints and the mother's index fingerprint are recorded.**
* **Following delivery of the placenta, oxytocin is administered to keep the fundus firm. The blood pressure is assessed, the perineum cleansed, and perineal pads and a clean gown applied. Finally, the woman is covered with a warm blanket.**

review questions 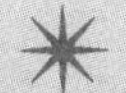

1. The nurse is admitting Dina Gemelos to the obstetric department. Dina, para 0 gravida I, is in active labor. What question is most pertinent at this time?
   a. "How long did it take you to get here?"
   b. "When did you first find out you were pregnant?"
   c. "Was this a planned pregnancy?"
   d. "When did your labor contractions start?"
2. The nurse recognizes that Dina's membranes have just ruptured. Her first action would be to
   a. call the physician.
   b. ask Dina to have a seat in the chair while she changes the linens.
   c. assess the fetal heart rate.
   d. tell Dina that things will progress quickly now.
3. The nurse encourages Dina to try a variety of positions for comfort but reminds her to avoid lying on her back to prevent
   a. infection.
   b. vaginal bleeding.
   c. slowing of the contractions.
   d. supine hypotension.
4. The nurse recognizes that Dina has entered the transition phase of labor. Dina's needs can best be met by
   a. giving her sips of water.
   b. breathing with her to help her maintain control.
   c. calling the physician.
   d. telling her support person to take a short break.
5. Dina's baby is born at 7 PM. The nurse's first priority in caring for the newborn is
   a. maintaining a patent airway.
   b. notifying the other family members of the birth.
   c. obtaining the footprints.
   d. assisting the father with obtaining pictures of the newborn.

references

Isenberg, S. J., Apt, L., & Wood, M. (1995). A controlled trial of povidone-iodine as prophylaxis against ophthalmia neonatorum. *New England Journal of Medicine, 332*(9), 562.

Miller, S. (1993). Continuous assessment. *Nursing Times, 89*(23), 48.

Perez, P. G. (1994). Another kind of labor partner. *Lamaze.*

bibliography

Biancuzzo, M. (1993). Six myths of maternal posture during labor. *Maternal Child Nursing, 18,* 264.

Biancuzzo, M. (1993). How to recognize and rotate an occiput posterior fetus. *American Journal of Nursing, 93,* 38.

Cassidy J. (1993). A picture-perfect birth. *RN, 56*(6), 45.

Cosner, K. R., & DeJong, E. (1993). Physiologic second-stage labor. *Maternal Child Nursing, 18*, 38.

Cunningham, G., MacDonald, P., Gant, N., Leveno, K., & Gilstrap, L. (1993) *Williams obstetrics* (19th ed.). Norwalk, CT: Appleton & Lange.

Guild, S. D. (1993). A comprehensive fetal monitoring program for nursing practice and education. *Journal of Obstetric, Gynecologic, and Neonatal Nursing, 23*(1), 34.

Kenner, C. A., & MacLaren, A. (1993). *Essentials of maternal and neonatal nursing*. Springhouse, PA: Springhouse Corporation.

Mackey M. C., & Stepans, M. E. (1994). Women's evaluations of their labor and delivery nurses. *Journal of Obstetric, Gynecologic, and Neonatal Nursing, 23*(5), 413.

May, K. A., & Mahlmeister, L. R. (1994). *Maternal and neonatal nursing: Family-centered care* (3rd ed.). Philadelphia: J.B. Lippincott.

Olds, S. B., London, M. L., & Ladewig, P. W. (1996). *Maternal newborn nursing: A family-centered approach*. (4th ed.). Redwood City, CA: Addison Wesley Nursing.

Pappas, A. B. (1994). *NSNA review series—Maternal-newborn nursing*. Albany, NY: Delmar Publishers.

Pernoll, M. L. (1991). *Current obstetric and gynecologic diagnosis and treatment* (7th ed.). Norwalk, CT: Appleton and Lange.

Pillitteri, A. (1995). *Maternal and child health nursing* (2nd ed.). Philadelphia: J.B. Lippincott.

Reeder, S. J., Martin, L. L., & Koniak, D. (1992). *Maternity nursing: Family, newborn, and women's health care* (17th ed.). Philadelphia: J.B. Lippincott.

Spence, A. (1992). Fast labors. *American Baby, 31*.

complications and emergencies during childbirth

13

outline

objectives

After studying this chapter, the reader should be able to:

* Define the term dystocia.
* Discuss abnormalities of the passage, passenger, powers, and psyche.
* List reasons for induction of labor.
* Discuss the nursing care of the woman undergoing induction.
* Discuss the nursing care of the client with premature rupture of the membranes.
* Describe nursing interventions for the client experiencing preterm labor.
* Describe the care of the client with an episiotomy or perineal laceration.
* Identify the differences between a forceps delivery and a vacuum extraction.
* List the most common reasons for a cesarean delivery.
* Discuss the nursing care of the client undergoing a cesarean delivery.

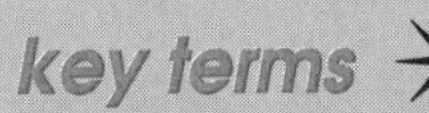
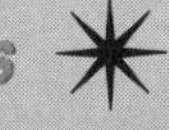

key terms

amniotomy
cephalopelvic disproportion
cervical ripening
dystocia
episiotomy
forceps
induction
laminaria
malposition
malpresentation
precipitous delivery
preterm labor
prolapsed cord
premature rupture of membranes
tocolytic agent
vacuum extraction
vaginal birth after cesarean

Childbirth is usually a joyous time for everyone involved. The waiting is over, and the woman and her family welcome a healthy newborn. Sometimes, however, complications and emergencies arise that threaten the health and well-being of mother or infant. In the event of a high-risk pregnancy, the woman and her physician may have anticipated and prepared for possible complications. When the pregnancy has proceeded normally, however, complications and emergencies can have physiologic and psychological implications for the woman and her family.

✶ family considerations

Complications arising during the birth process place an extra emotional burden on the family when they realize that even the best medical and nursing care does not guarantee a healthy mother and newborn. These problems may occur during any phase of labor and delivery and can have lifelong effects. Families whose infant is premature, for example, may face the initial life or death crisis of neonatal intensive care. This can be a long, expensive, exhausting ordeal for the family, and the newborn may still have multiple handicaps.

Women who prepare for a vaginal delivery but because of complications have a cesarean delivery may feel disappointed or guilty of having "failed."

✶ nursing considerations

When complications arise, the nurse needs to prepare the family with knowledge about the technical interventions and offer additional emotional support. Although these procedures are designed to provide the safest and most satisfying results—a healthy mother and newborn—they are not always successful.

dystocia

Dystocia means difficult labor, normally due to mechanical factors that result in prolonged, painful labor for the woman. The causes are usually abnormalities of the three Ps: the passage, passenger, or powers. The fourth "P" (psyche) cannot be overlooked because it affects the other three.

abnormalities of the passage

Abnormalities of the passage usually result in *cephalopelvic disproportion* (CPD). In CPD, the pelvic size is not adequate to allow passage of the fetus, or the pelvic shape is not favorable for the passage. This can lead to failure of the labor to progress, premature rupture of the membranes (PROM), or uterine rupture. If the fetal head cannot become engaged before the membranes rupture, cord prolapse can occur. Prolonged labor also can cause fracture of the fetal skull or fetal intracranial hemorrhage. To decrease these risks, abnormalities of the passage usually end in a cesarean delivery (discussed later in this chapter).

abnormalities of the passenger

Fetal dystocia, or abnormalities of the passenger, result from an abnormally large fetus, malpresentation, malposition, or multiple gestation. These abnormalities can prevent the fetus from passing through the birth canal and also usually require a cesarean delivery.

malpresentation

Breech presentations (frank, complete, or footling) can pose problems for the laboring woman and her fetus. Sometimes the physician is able to turn the fetus by external manipulation (external version) if the head is not engaged. If the physician elects to deliver the fetus vaginally, he or she encourages the woman to push, then delivers the breech and trunk and supports and lifts the trunk while manually delivering the posterior shoulder followed by the anterior shoulder. The physician then carefully delivers the head (Fig. 13-1). Vaginal breech deliveries are associated with a high risk for intracranial hemorrhage and prolapsed cord. Today, more than 90% of breech presentations are cesarean deliveries (Brown, Karrison, & Cibils, 1994).

malposition

In approximately 25% of all deliveries, the fetus assumes a malposition or posterior rather than anterior position, with the back of the fetal head in the maternal hind pelvis. This usually results in a prolonged or dysfunctional labor pattern because the fetal head must turn 135% (rather than the normal 90%) during internal rotation. The woman experiences back pain and pressure because the fetus must rotate against the sacrum, producing sacral nerve compression. About three fourths of the time, the fetus completes the rotation when it nears the pelvic floor and may be delivered vaginally; the newborn experiences an increase in caput formation and molding of the fetal head. In the remainder of cases, the fetus remains in the posterior position, and the physician may elect to perform a low forceps delivery to prevent maternal lacerations of the perineum.

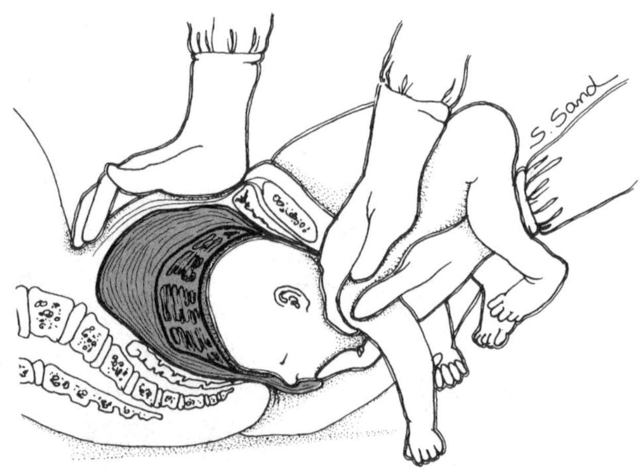

figure 13-1 *Breech delivery. Support of trunk while delivering head.*

nursing care Regardless of whether the infant rotates, posterior labor can be exhausting for the woman. The goal of nursing care is to assess carefully for signs of fetal or maternal distress and provide comfort and encouragement. Maternal vital signs and fetal heart rate (FHR) are monitored closely for signs of distress. Applying sacral pressure and warm packs, giving backrubs, and assisting with position changes help relieve back pain. A hands and knees position places the uterus in a "hanging position," relieves the back pain, and assists with rotation because gravity pulls the fetus' heaviest parts toward the anterior maternal abdomen. Support and reassurance are offered to alleviate feelings of frustration and exhaustion.

prolapsed cord

Prolapsed cord may be defined as the protrusion of the umbilical cord into the vagina before engagement of the fetal presenting part. This results in cord compression as the fetal presenting part descends into the maternal pelvis (Fig. 13-2). The risk for prolapsed cord increases with malpresentation or malposition. Emergency measures are instituted to keep the fetus from suffocating from lack of oxygen. The woman is placed in a knee-chest or Trendelenburg position. The physician, midwife, or registered nurse may insert a sterile gloved hand into the vagina to remove pressure from the umbilical cord and restore the oxygen supply to the fetus. Maternal vital signs and FHR are monitored closely until plans are instituted for an emergency cesarean delivery. To reduce anxiety, the nurse speaks calmly and quietly to the family, answering all questions and explaining all procedures.

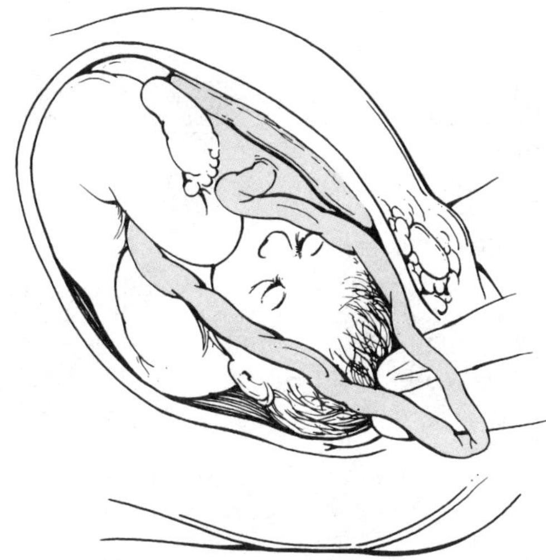

figure 13-2 *Prolapsed cord. Reduction of cord compression using gloved examiner's hand in vagina to elevate presenting part.*

multiple gestation

Multiple gestation can cause uterine dysfunction because of the extreme stretching of the uterus, the possibility of preterm labor, polyhydramnios, and fetal malpresentation (Fig. 13-3). This is considered a high-risk delivery, requiring the regular delivery attendants and a pediatrician and an extra nurse for each newborn.

The woman is instructed to report immediately to the hospital when the membranes rupture or when labor be-

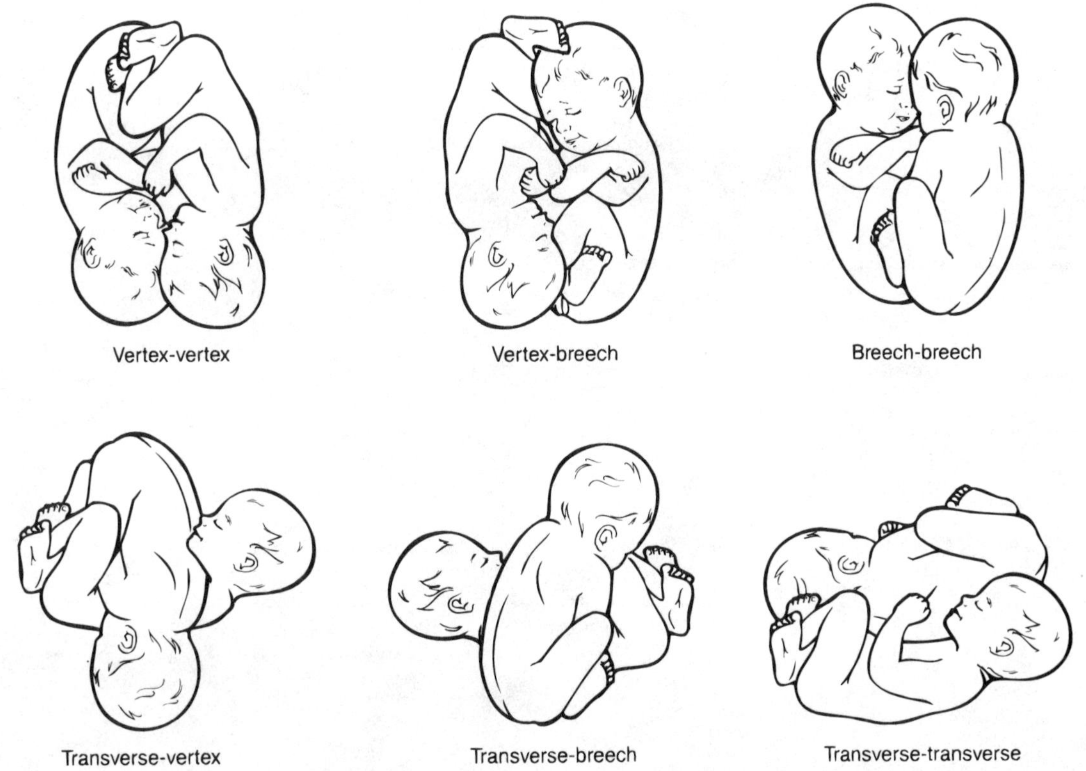

figure 13-3 *Variations of twin presentations.*

gins if a cesarean delivery is not already planned. Cesarean delivery is usually planned if there are three or more fetuses or if twins are not in the vertex position. If the fetuses weigh less than 3 lb, cesarean delivery also is indicated to decrease the chance of fetal hemorrhage.

> ✳ **nursing insight**
>
> *In addition to dealing with an emergency cesarean delivery, these parents may have just learned that they are about to have twins. Additional emotional support is vital for this couple.*

nursing care The nurse monitors the FHR and maternal vital signs continuously throughout labor and delivery. The woman is placed in a semi-Fowler's position to assist her breathing. The nurse explains preparations for the impending birth to the family. As the newborns are delivered, they must be identified appropriately. They are usually labelled "twin A" and "twin B" until names are selected by the parents.

Following delivery, the mother is monitored closely for signs of postpartum hemorrhage due to overstretching of the uterus. (See Chap. 15 for nursing care of postpartum hemorrhage.) The nurse may contact social services as needed to assist in home care planning and financial services.

abnormalities of the powers

Abnormalities of the powers or ineffective uterine contractions result from hypotonic labor, hypertonic labor, precipitous labor, or prolonged labor (Table 13-1).

abnormalities of the psyche

Fear and anxiety can affect the woman's ability to work with and through her contractions and can actually impede her progress. By offering moral support and providing comfort measures, a quiet environment, and explanations of procedures and events, the nurse can assist the woman and her family to cope with complications and emergencies that arise. See the Nursing Care Plan for the woman with dystocia.

induction

Induction is the intentional, artificial initiation of labor before the start of spontaneous labor contractions. Labor may be induced to protect fetal and maternal health. Post-

table 13-1 management of abnormalities of the powers

Term	*Definition*	*Causes*	*Medical Treatment*	*Nursing Intervention*
Hypotonic labor	Contractions that decrease in frequency and intensity	Medication in early labor, cephalopelvic disproportion (CPD), fetal malposition	Augmentation with pitocin, amniotomy; may result in cesarean delivery	Monitor intake and output; check for bladder distention; monitor vital signs, fetal heart rate (FHR), and contractions. Ambulate. Monitor pitocin infusion.
Hypertonic labor	Ineffective, intense, uncoordinated contractions	Muscle fibers not allowing for resting period; continuous stimulus. Extreme anxiety contributes	Bed rest, medication for pain, sedation	Darken room; provide quiet atmosphere, clean linens, mouth care. Administer medications as ordered. Provide reassurance and support.
Precipitous labor	Rapid labor that is completed in less than 3 h	Multiparity, pitocin, amniotomy, cocaine abuse	Monitor closely for impending birth	Assist with breathing techniques. Monitor contractions, vital signs, FHR for signs of distress.
Prolonged labor	Labor that lasts longer than 24 h	Ineffective contractions, CPD, fetal malposition, cervical swelling, or unripe cervix	Prostaglandin gel for cervical ripening, amniotomy, oxytocin (Pitocin), cesarean delivery if indicated	Provide comfort measures: clean linen, mouth care, position changes, assistance with breathing techniques. Administer medications as ordered; monitor maternal vital signs, contractions, FHR for signs of distress.

nursing care plan for the woman with dystocia

NURSING DIAGNOSIS

Fatigue, High Risk for, secondary to failure to progress in labor

GOAL: Client will rest during labor and maintain adequate energy

NURSING INTERVENTIONS	RATIONALE	EVALUATION
Encourage client to rest between contractions.	Fatigue can cloud a client's perceptions and make it more difficult to tolerate the labor process.	The client will rest in between contractions.
Assess client's level of pain and assist in appropriate treatment to allow rest without discomfort.	If the client is experiencing intolerable pain she will not be able to get the rest she needs.	The client will receive adequate analgesia to allow her to tolerate the pain and to rest.
Explain all procedures to client and family.	The labor experience is an intense process, and the client experiencing the complication of dystocia will have even more anxiety related to the process, which can be relieved by explaining all treatments and procedures.	The client will understand all treatments, exhibit decreased anxiety, and express confidence in the care she is receiving.
Monitor patient's glucose level and administer intravenous solution as ordered.	Glucose stores can become depleted quickly during labor, requiring prompt identification and correction of the abnormality.	The client will have normal glucose levels and have sufficient energy to continue with the labor process.
Advise client to lie on her side.	This will increase the blood supply to the uterus and prevent hypotension.	The client will be comfortable in a side-lying position. Labor will continue to progress.
Encourage client to void every 2 hours during labor.	A full bladder may hinder descent of the fetus and slow uterine contractions, further impeding the progress of labor.	The client will void every 2 hours during labor.

NURSING DIAGNOSIS

Fluid Volume Deficit, related to prolonged labor

GOAL: the client will maintain adequate fluid and electrolyte balance

NURSING INTERVENTION	RATIONALE	EVALUATION
Monitor the client's intake and output and electrolyte levels.	The client experiencing dystocia is at high risk for fluid volume deficit, especially if vomiting or diarrhea are present. Diaphoresis and hyperventilation further increase fluid and electrolyte losses via insensible loss during prolonged labor.	An accurate intake and output record will objectively record the client's fluid status.
Test the urine specific gravity.	This will provide the health care team with information regarding the client's level of hydration.	The specific gravity will be recorded and, if necessary, treatment will be started to maintain adequate hydration.
Administer intravenous fluid as prescribed.	Intravenous fluids can reestablish the client's hydration status and provide important electrolytes, thereby preventing intrapartal and postpartal complications.	The client will receive appropriate intravenous fluid to restore hydration and electrolyte levels.

date pregnancy is the most common reason for induction (Miller & Lorkovic, 1993). Other maternal reasons for induction include pregnancy-induced hypertension (PIH), diabetes, and PROM. Some fetal reasons for induction include postmaturity, hemolytic disease, or fetal demise. Labor may be induced by mechanical means (*amniotomy*) or by chemical means (*oxytocin, Laminaria, prostaglandin*).

amniotomy

In preparation for an amniotomy, the woman is placed in the dorsal recumbent position and the physician inserts a sterile *amnihook* (it looks like a long crochet hook) into the cervix and punctures the membranes. This procedure allows the presenting part to make close contact with the cervix. It also decreases the fluid volume in the uterus, providing better uterine contractions because a partially contracted muscle is always is more efficient. Immediately following the procedure, the nurse assesses the FHR and examines the perineum to confirm that the umbilical cord did not prolapse when the fluid exited. The fluid also is examined for color, amount, and odor.

An amniotomy is performed only after the cervix is soft, partially effaced, and slightly dilated. Ideally, the presenting part is engaged to prevent prolapsing of the cord.

cervical ripening

Cervical ripening is a technique used to cause the cervix to dilate, soften, and efface. Two therapies that produce this effect are *Laminaria* and prostaglandin E_2 (PGE_2). *Laminaria* is a special type of sterile, dried, compressed seaweed; when inserted into the cervical os, it absorbs moisture and swells to three to five times its insertion size. Within a few hours, *Laminaria* creates the desired effect on the cervix.

Prostaglandin E_2 may be applied intracervically or intravaginally to relax the smooth muscles of the cervix and to stimulate the musculature of the fundus. The Food and Drug Administration has approved the intracervical application, but the intravaginal application is still considered experimental (Miller & Lorkovic, 1993). After signing a consent form, the woman is placed in the supine position and the PGE_2 gel is inserted into the cervix or vagina. The woman is kept on bed rest for approximately 2 hours while her vital signs, uterine activity, and FHR are monitored. Following this period, if she is not in labor, she may be dismissed with instructions to return in the morning for induction with oxytocin (Pitocin) or to return if contractions begin before morning.

intravenous oxytocin

Oxytocin works on the myometrium, causing it to contract. Normally, oxytocin is released by the posterior pituitary gland to initiate labor contractions. Synthetic oxytocin may be administered to induce or augment (increase) weak or ineffective labor contractions. Because the drug is so powerful and even minute amounts can cause excessive contractions that could result in rupture of the uterus, oxytocin is always administered with an intravenous infusion pump to control the dosage administered. A fetal monitor is applied, and maternal vital signs, uterine activity, and FHR are monitored and documented every 15 to 30 minutes.

premature rupture of the membranes

Premature rupture is defined as rupture of the membranes 1 hour or more before the onset of true labor. In a term pregnancy, it is a concern if they have ruptured more than 24 hours before the onset of labor because of the risk of infection. If they rupture before the 37th week, prematurity of the newborn is a concern.

etiology and pathophysiology

Premature rupture occurs in approximately 10% of term pregnancies, and the cause is unknown. Some of the predisposing factors include malpresentation, weakened areas in the amnion and chorion, and incompetent cervical os. The woman usually reports a sudden gush or continuous trickle of fluid leaking from the vagina. Infection is the prime concern because ruptured membranes provide a portal of entry for microorganisms.

diagnostic tests

To confirm the presence of amniotic fluid, the fern test or nitrazine paper may be used (see Chap. 10). A complete blood count with differential is drawn to assess for infection. A catheterized urine specimen is collected for culture and sensitivity. An ultrasound examination is done to assess or confirm gestational age.

medical–surgical management

The physician may adopt a "wait and see" attitude, admitting the woman and watching her carefully until she goes into labor on her own. During this time, maternal vital signs are monitored, especially for signs of infection. The FHR is monitored for signs of fetal distress. Other medical interventions may include induction of labor or a cesarean delivery.

✳ nursing process for the client with premature rupture of the membranes

nursing assessment

Subjective data to be assessed include the following:

- Reports of leakage of fluid from the vagina
- Reports of any contractions

Objective data to be assessed include the following:

* Maternal vital signs for signs of infection
* Noticeable discharge with a foul odor
* Fetal tachycardia
* Positive results of tests for confirmation of amniotic fluid

nursing diagnosis

* Risk for Infection, related to rupture of membranes
* Anxiety, related to changes in anticipated course of events

planning and implementation

Monitor maternal vital signs every 2 hours; tachycardia could be an early sign of infection. Monitor FHR every 30 minutes. Tachycardia could indicate infection; bradycardia could indicate fetal cord compression (often seen if the presenting part is not engaged in the pelvis). If the presenting part is engaged, the woman may ambulate for comfort and to stimulate contractions; otherwise, bed rest is maintained. Change bed linens, and provide perineal care as needed, due to leaking amniotic fluid. Provide oral hygiene, and encourage adequate fluid intake, either orally or intravenously. Explain all procedures, and give updates on the progress of labor.

evaluation

* There is no evidence of fetal or maternal infection.
* Client demonstrates reduced anxiety and verbalizes an understanding of the course of events.

preterm labor

Premature labor may be defined as true labor that begins after the 20th week of gestation and before the 37th week of gestation. Premature births comprise 6% to 10% of all deliveries and are the leading cause of neonatal morbidity and mortality in the United States (Cowan, 1993).

etiology and pathophysiology

Conditions associated with the development of preterm labor include maternal infections, multiple gestation, placenta previa, abruptio placenta, drug abuse, smoking, teenage pregnancy, uterine structural anomalies, and trauma. Preterm labor also is associated with poor hygiene, poor nutrition, and poverty.

medical–surgical management

Some women may be candidates for tocolytic therapy to prevent premature birth. Tocolytic agents soothe and quiet uterine activity to prolong the pregnancy, allowing fetal lungs to mature. Examples of tocolytic agents include magnesium sulfate, terbutaline sulfate (Brethine), ritodrine (Yutopar), indomethacin (Indocin), and nifedipine (Procardia). Contraindications for use of tocolytic agents include PROM, cervical dilatation of 4 cm or more and effacement of more than 50%, maternal hemorrhage, severe PIH, and signs of fetal distress. In the United States, terbutaline sulfate is the drug of choice for home therapy. Once the initial preterm labor episode has been stabilized, the woman may be sent home on terbutaline sulfate orally or on a portable infusion pump (Cowan, 1993). If the physician chooses to use the infusion pump, hospitalization is prolonged by 2 to 3 days to teach the woman and her family about use of the medication and infusion pump. Home visits are then scheduled weekly or biweekly by a home health nurse (usually a registered nurse) for continued monitoring. The woman must remain on bed rest throughout the course of therapy.

If tocolytic therapy is not successful or the woman does not meet the criteria for therapy, she then proceeds to labor and delivery. The use of analgesics or anesthetics is avoided to prevent fetal respiratory complications because the fetal respiratory system is already compromised. (See Chap. 17 for care of the preterm infant.)

✳ nursing process for the preterm labor client

nursing assessment

Subjective data to be assessed include the following:

* Reports of backache, pelvic pressure, changes in vaginal discharge, diarrhea
* Reports of uterine contraction

Objective data to be assessed include the following:

* Frequency, duration, and length of rhythmic uterine contractions
* Cervical dilatation and effacement
* Presence of bloody show
* Status of membranes
* Maternal vital signs, FHR

nursing diagnosis

* Anxiety, related to possible risk to fetus
* Knowledge Deficit, related to plan of care

planning and implementation

The woman is placed on strict bed rest. An external fetal monitor and transducer are applied to observe FHR and uterine activity. A set of baseline vital signs is obtained. If a tocolytic drug is prescribed, the medication is administered orally or intravenously per the physician's order. The maternal vital signs are monitored every 15 minutes until the required maintenance dose of tocolytic therapy is achieved and the maternal and fetal vital signs are stable. The woman is instructed to report any signs of chest pain or discomfort, dyspnea, or coughing because tocolytic therapy can cause cardiopulmonary side effects.

If the decision to allow the woman to labor and deliver has been made, the nurse will monitor the labor just as with any other client, paying close attention to signs of fetal or maternal distress. (See Chap. 12 for care of the laboring woman.)

evaluation

* The client demonstrates effective coping skills.
* The client verbalizes an understanding of the plan of care.

operative procedures

episiotomy

An episiotomy is a surgical incision that extends from the fourchette downward through the perineal floor. Episiotomy is performed during the second stage of labor, based on the long-held belief that it facilitates the birth of the fetal head, shortens the second stage of labor, and prevents perineal tearing. Recent studies (Larsson, et al., 1991; Viktrup, et al., 1992) have questioned the value of episiotomy and have indicated that it should not be performed routinely but selectively (Cunningham, et al., 1993). Indications for episiotomy include preterm delivery, shoulder dystocia, breech delivery, forceps or vacuum extractor deliveries, and occiput posterior deliveries. This controversial procedure is performed because the physician believes that a surgical incision is less painful and heals more effectively than a perineal tear; however, some authorities question this belief (Larsson, et al., 1991). Nevertheless, the incidence of episiotomies among primigravidas may be as high as 90%. Nurse midwives usually rely on alternative procedures, such as perineal massage and alternative birthing positions to assist with the stretching of the perineum and birthing of the fetal head.

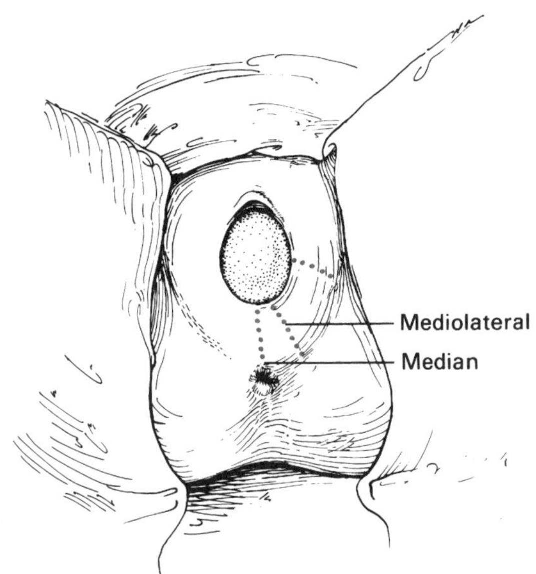

figure 13-4 *Types of episiotomies.*

The two major types of episiotomies performed are the midline and the mediolateral (Fig. 13-4). The midline is the most common procedure performed because it is less painful and causes less scarring. A disadvantage of the midline is that it may extend (tear further) than the incision line during the birth.

Because the intense pressure of the fetus on the perineum temporarily numbs the area, an anesthetic may not be necessary for the incision but will be necessary for the repair following the birth. A local anesthetic, such as lidocaine, provides perineal anesthetic and may be used for the incision (if necessary) and the repair following the birth.

If tearing does occur, with or without an episiotomy, it is classified as follows:

* First degree—extends from the fourchette through the perineal skin and mucous membrane
* Second degree—extends through the skin and mucous membrane and includes the perineal muscles
* Third degree—extends through the skin, mucous membrane, and perineal muscles and continues through the rectal sphincter
* Fourth degree—extends through the skin, mucous membrane, perineal muscles, and rectal sphincter and continues up the anterior wall of the rectum

✳ nursing considerations

Whether the mother has an episiotomy or laceration repair, the area will be tender and possibly edematous. The application of ice or cold compresses (20 minutes on, 20 minutes off) may soothe and comfort the area. The nurse observes the area daily for signs of infection or hematoma formation. The mother is instructed to cleanse the area from front to back with soap and water at least once or twice a day. A "peri" bottle filled with lukewarm tap water may be squirted over the area following each voiding and bowel movement. Sitz baths may be ordered two to four times per day to promote comfort and healing. The mother is instructed to apply her perineal pad from front to back and to avoid touching the part that goes next to the perineum. Enemas, laxatives, and suppositories are contraindicated with third- and fourth-degree lacerations. The mother is usually prescribed stool softeners and encouraged to increase fluid intake and to ambulate to avoid constipation.

forceps delivery

Forceps are sterile surgical instruments with two interlocking blades used during the second stage of labor to extract the fetus from the birth canal, assist with the rotation of the fetus, or shorten the second stage of labor. Today, only "low-forceps" deliveries are performed; that is, the fetus lies low in the perineum (Fig. 13-5). It is a relatively safe procedure with few complications; bruising of the fetal head, minor perineal lacerations, or vaginal trauma

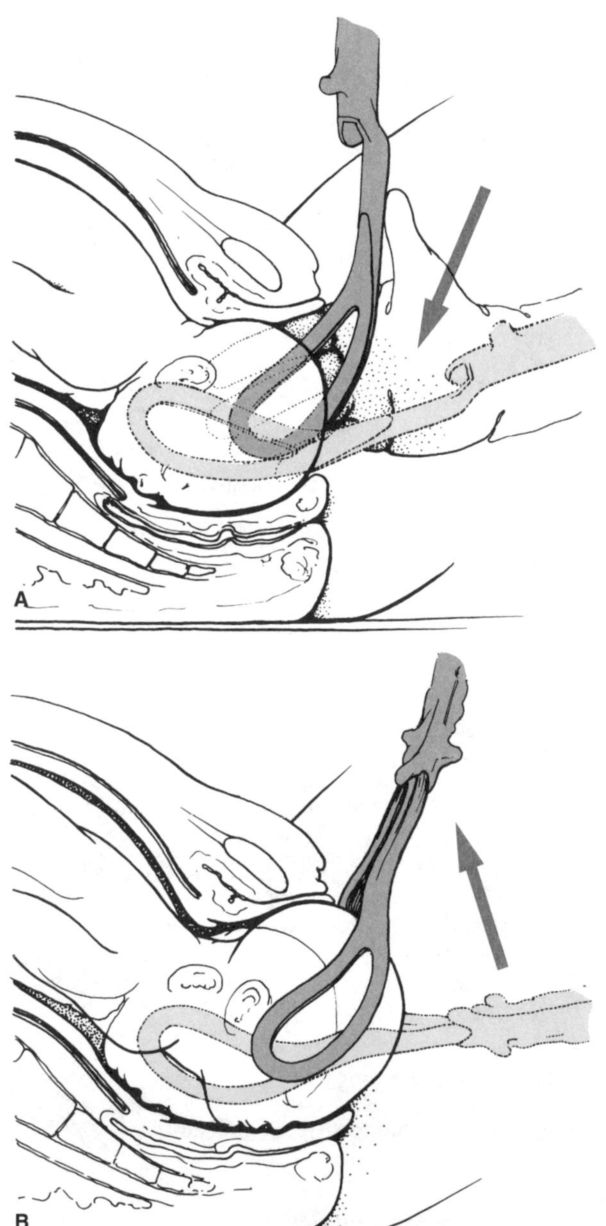

figure 13-5 *(A) Insertion of forceps blade and (B) applied forceps and direction of traction.*

may occur. The woman is usually given a pudendal block or a light anesthetic before the procedure. "High-forceps" or "midforceps" deliveries carry considerably more risk; these are no longer performed except in extreme emergencies when no other interventions, such as cesarean delivery, are available.

vacuum extraction

Vacuum extraction has largely replaced the use of forceps. A suction cup, called the ventouse, is placed over the posterior fontanel of the infant and connected to suction. The combination of suction and traction on the instrument results in delivery. The woman will feel a pulling sensation and discomfort from the birth process but not from the instrument itself. The nurse cautions the parents that the newborn will have caput succedaneum (soft tissue swelling of the head) but that the condition will disappear shortly after birth without lasting complications.

cesarean delivery

A cesarean delivery is a surgical procedure in which the physician makes an incision through the abdominal and uterine wall to deliver the newborn. Cesarean deliveries are performed because of maternal or fetal risk, not as an alternative to vaginal delivery. Some indications for cesarean deliveries include CPD, dysfunctional labor, fetal distress, abruptio placentae, or active genital herpes. A more complete listing is shown in Display 13-1.

A recent study indicates that cesarean deliveries may reduce by 50% the transmission of human immunodeficiency virus from infected mothers to their newborns. The current theory is that cesarean delivery prevents fetal contact with cervical and vaginal secretions, thereby protecting the infant from infection (Newell et al., 1994).

etiology and pathophysiology

Cesarean delivery is the most frequently performed surgical procedure in the United States, and the United States has the third highest cesarean rate among developed countries. Currently, 15% to 20% of all births in the United States are cesarean deliveries (Taffel, Placek, & Kosary, 1992).

A cesarean delivery may be scheduled and planned before labor begins. This is called an elective cesarean. It also can be an emergency procedure, arising from a life-threatening condition (see Display 13-1). The two most common types of cesarean deliveries performed are the lower segment transverse cesarean and the classic cesarean (Fig. 13-6). The lower segment transverse incision is preferred because the incision is made in the lower portion of the uterus, where the uterine wall is the thinnest and has the

display 13-1
indications for cesarean delivery

- Cephalopelvic disproportion
- Fetal distress
- Breech presentation
- Active herpes lesions
- Condylomata acuminata
- Repeat cesarean
- Multiple gestation
- Cord prolapse
- Prolonged labor
- Cervical swelling
- Dysfunctional labor patterns

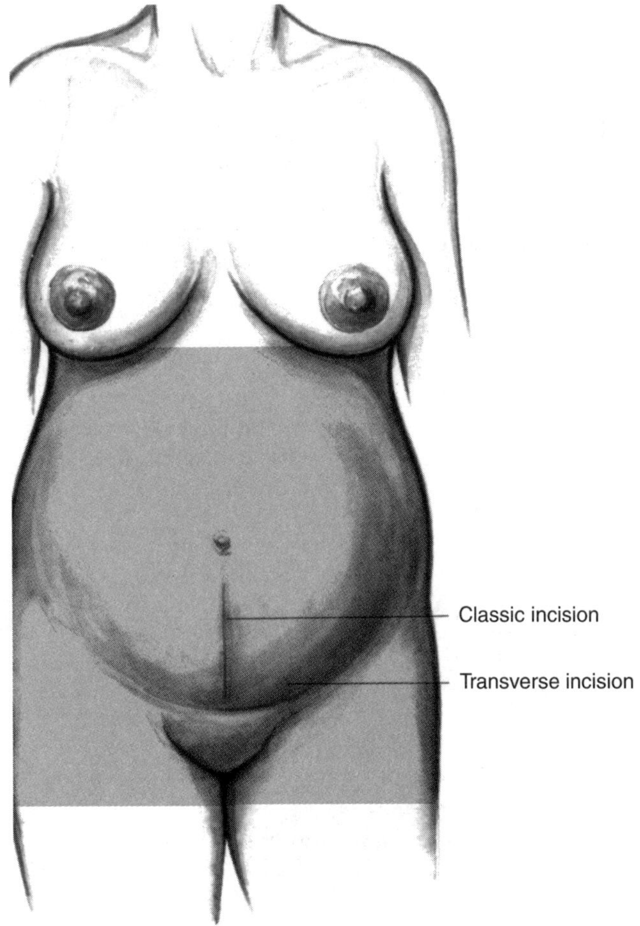

figure 13-6 *Colored area shows skin preparation area. Note classic incision versus transverse incision.*

least activity during contractions. This results in minimal blood loss and permits the woman to consider vaginal delivery for future deliveries. The classic cesarean incision consists of a vertical cut directly into the body of the uterus where the uterine muscle wall is the thickest and most active. This procedure requires cesarean deliveries for all future births because of the possibility that the uterus may rupture during labor contractions. The classic cesarean is generally reserved for emergency situations.

medical–surgical management

The procedure is explained to the client, and an informed consent is signed. The woman takes nothing by mouth for 6 to 8 hours prior to the procedure (unless it is an emergency). An intravenous line will be started to deliver needed fluids and medications. Generally, the woman is given a spinal or epidural anesthetic. In certain situations, especially emergencies, she may be given a general anesthetic. Prophylactic antibiotics may be administered as a precautionary measure.

✶ nursing process for the client undergoing a cesarean delivery

nursing assessment

Preoperative subjective data to be assessed include the following:

✶ The woman's and family's understanding of the procedure
✶ The woman's and family's psychological preparation for the procedure; feelings of fear or disappointment

Postoperative subjective data to be assessed include the following:

✶ Complaints of pain
✶ Maternal–infant attachment behaviors

Preoperative objective data to be assessed include the following:

✶ Maternal vital signs and FHR
✶ Maternal blood type and Rh
✶ Last time solid food or liquid was taken

Postoperative objective data to be assessed include the following:

✶ Fundal position and firmness
✶ Maternal vital signs at least every 15 minutes during the first hour
✶ Lochia (amount, color, and presence of any clots)
✶ Condition of dressing and incision
✶ Foley catheter for patency and color of urine
✶ Bowel sounds
✶ Breath sounds
✶ Intake and output

nursing diagnosis

✶ Acute Pain, related to surgical incision
✶ Risk for Infection

planning and implementation

In preparation for a cesarean delivery, the nurse obtains the signed operative consent form. The nurse prepares the woman and her family for the experience by explaining the procedure and answering any questions. They are reassured that the fetus is delivered within 5 to 10 minutes after the beginning of the surgery and that the mother's surgery will be completed in approximately 1 hour. She may feel pressure but no pain during the delivery. The family will be reunited as soon as possible after delivery. The father or support person is often allowed to stay with the woman during the surgery. The support person is given scrub clothing, shoe and hair covers, and instructions on the proper wearing of a mask. Drapes are positioned so that the support person may be near the head of the bed for maternal support but does not see the abdominal incision.

For safety reasons, the support person is brought into the surgical suite only after the room, staff, and patient are ready for the procedure. The maternal abdomen is prepped by shaving and scrubbing with an antimicrobial soap from the nipple line to upper thigh.

The nurse must be aware that following the procedure, the new mother is not only a maternity patient but also a surgical patient. Care includes monitoring the vital signs, intake and output, bowel and breath sounds, and the fundus and lochia. The mother is told that she will experience postoperative pain, but medications will be available to decrease the discomfort. She will need to turn, cough, and deep breathe, assisted by the nurse. She will have a Foley catheter for at least 24 hours and will not have to void during this time. Following removal of the catheter, the nurse will assist the woman to the bathroom for voiding. (See Chap. 14 for routine postpartum nursing care and assessments.)

The nurse needs to encourage the mother and her family to talk about the birth experience. Referring to it as a cesarean birth or cesarean delivery rather than a "surgery" or "section" may help the family put the experience into perspective.

evaluation

* The mother will experience a decrease in the initial postoperative pain.
* The mother and newborn will demonstrate an absence of infection.

vaginal birth after cesarean

Women who have previously had a low transverse incision for a cesarean delivery may successfully experience a vaginal birth after cesarean (VBAC). In the past, when classic cesarean deliveries were performed, VBAC was not an option because of the high risk of uterine rupture during labor. This risk existed because the incision for a classic cesarean cuts through the body of the uterus where the majority of contraction activity takes place.

The length of labor is not significantly different from a woman experiencing her first vaginal delivery (Clemeson, 1993). Not all women are candidates for VBAC, even with a low-segment transverse incision, because the original condition leading to the cesarean delivery may still be present, for example, CPD. Three major criteria are necessary for permitting the woman to labor:

* A previous lower segment transverse incision
* The woman's willingness and desire to attempt normal labor
* No history of medical conditions that prohibit VBAC

Many women eagerly anticipate VBAC because of decreased pain following the delivery, a quicker recovery phase, a shorter hospital stay, and a decrease in overall expense.

nursing care

The nurse encourages women who desire and plan a VBAC to attend childbirth education classes to prepare them for the experience. Some communities have specialized classes for the couple planning VBAC. During the labor, the woman may be fearful not only of the labor process, but of the possibility of uterine rupture. The nurse may need to offer additional encouragement and support. The nurse needs to explain to the woman that her labor will be monitored carefully for signs of failure to progress, fetal distress, or any other untoward signs and that a cesarean delivery will be performed if necessary.

key points ✳

* **Dystocia or difficult labor usually is a result of abnormalities of the passage, passenger, or powers. The fourth "P" also impacts the other three.**
* **CPD is the most common abnormality of the passage. It results in failure to progress because the fetus cannot pass through the birth canal.**
* **Abnormalities of the passenger include an abnormally large fetus, malpresentation, malposition, and multiple gestation. These conditions also can prevent the fetus from passing through the birth canal.**
* **Prolapsed cord is the protrusion of the umbilical cord into the vagina before the engagement of the fetal presenting part. This is an emergency condition that can result in suffocation of the fetus. The woman is placed in knee-chest or Trendelenburg position until arrangements for a cesarean delivery can be made.**
* **Fear and anxiety can impede the woman's progress during labor. The nurse can assist the woman by offering moral support and providing comfort measures and a quiet environment.**
* **Induction is the intentional, artificial initiation of labor before the start of spontaneous labor contractions. Induction can be accomplished by mechanical means (amniotomy) or by chemical means (oxytocin, *Laminaria*, or prostaglandin).**
* **The main concern with PROM in a term pregnancy is the possibility of infection. The main concern if membranes rupture before 37 weeks is prematurity.**
* **The two most common types of episiotomies are midline and mediolateral.**
* **Enemas, laxatives, and suppositories are avoided in women with third- or fourth-degree lacerations.**
* **A cesarean delivery is a surgical procedure in which an incision is made through the abdominal and uterine wall to deliver the newborn. The nurse must be aware that the new mother is not only a maternity patient but also a surgical patient.**

review questions

1. Charise, para 0, gravida 1, has been in labor for 8 hours. She states that her back hurts more than anything. To comfort Charise, the nurse would
   a. apply sacral pressure and give backrubs.
   b. tell her support person to continue to coach her; delivery will be soon.
   c. give her mouth care and sips of water.
   d. have her ambulate to increase the intensity of the contractions.
2. Maria, para 2, gravida 3, has ruptured membranes and is in the first stage of labor. Because the membranes have ruptured, the nurse knows it is important to
   a. monitor the urine for glucose.
   b. monitor the temperature and pulse for signs of infection.
   c. monitor the blood pressure for signs of elevation due to PIH.
   d. perform frequent vaginal examinations using clean gloves.
3. The physician has just inserted *Laminaria* into the cervix. The nurse explains to the patient,
   a. "this will cause your contractions to start."
   b. "this will soften and dilate your cervix."
   c. "this will cause your baby to turn to the appropriate position."
   d. "this is routinely done for all patients."
4. Nita has just given birth to a 7-lb boy. The physician used vacuum extraction during the second stage of labor, and the newborn has caput. The nurse explains,
   a. "this condition will require needle aspiration to remove the excess fluid."
   b. "this is normal following this procedure and will disappear without intervention."
   c. "I will need to call the physician and report it.
   d. "all newborns experience this condition."
5. Annette is concerned that she will be unable to get up to use the bathroom immediately following her cesarean delivery. The nurse explains
   a. that assistance will be available.
   b. that Annette will have a catheter for a least the first 24 hours.
   c. that she will have nothing by mouth so she will not need to void.
   d. that she will obtain a bedside commode so Annette will not have far to walk.

references

Brown, L., Karrison, T., & Cibils, L. A. (1994). Mode of delivery and perinatal results in breech presentation. *American Journal of Obstetrics and Gynecology, 171*(1), 28.

Clemeson, N. (1993). Promoting vaginal birth after cesarean section. *American Family Physician, 47*, 139.

Cowan, M. (1993). Home care of the pregnant woman using terbutaline. *MCN, 18*, 99.

Cunningham, F. G., McDonald, P. C., Leveno, K. J., Gant, N. F., & Gilstrap, L. (1993). *Williams obstetrics* (p. 389). Norwalk, CT: Appleton & Lange.

Larsson, P., et al. (1991). Advantage or disadvantage of episiotomy compared with spontaneous perineal laceration. *Gynecol Obstet Invest, 31*, 213.

Miller, A. M., & Lorkovic, M. (1993). Prostaglandin E_2 for cervical ripening. *MCN, September/October*, 23.

Newell, D. T., Dunn, C. S., et al. (1994). Cesarean section and risk of vertical transmission of HIV-1 infection. *Lancet, 343*(8911), 1464.

Taffel S., Placek, P. J., & Kosary, C. L. (1992). US cesarean section rates 1990: An update. *Birth, 19*(1), 21.

Viktrup, L., et al. (1992). The symptom of stress incontinence caused by pregnancy or delivery in primiparas. *Obstet Gynecol, 79*, 945.

bibliography

Brouillard-Pierce, C. (1993). Indications for induction of labor. *Maternal Child Nursing, September/October*, 14.

Eganhouse, D. J., & Burnside, S. M. (1992). Nursing assessment and responsibilities in monitoring the preterm pregnancy. *Journal of Obstetric, Gynecologic, and Neonatal Nursing, 21*(5), 355.

Goff, K. J. (1993). Initiation of Parturition. *MCN, September/October*, 7.

Griese, M. E., & Prickett, S. A. (1993). Nursing management of umbilical cord prolapse. *Journal of Obstetric, Gynecologic, and Neonatal Nursing, 22*(4), 311.

Miovech, S. M., Knapp, H., Borucki, L., Roncoli, M., Arnold, L., & Brooten, D. (1994). Major concerns of women after cesarean delivery. *Journal of Obstetric, Gynecologic, and Neonatal Nursing, 23*(1), 53.

Patterson, E. T., Douglas, A. B., Patterson, P. M., & Bradle, J. B. (1992). Symptoms of preterm labor and self-diagnostic confusion. *Nursing Research, 41*(6), 367.

Pernoll, M. L. (1991). *Current obstetric and gynecologic diagnosis and treatment* (7th ed). Norwalk, CT: Appleton and Lange.

Pillitteri, A. (1995). *Maternal and child health nursing* (2nd ed). Philadelphia: J.B. Lippincott.

Reichert, J. A., Baron, M., & Fawcett, J. (1993) Changes in attitudes toward cesarean birth. *Journal of Obstetric, Gynecologic, and Neonatal Nursing, 22*(2), 159.

Reeder, S. J., Martin L. L., & Koniak, D. (1992). *Maternity nursing: Family, Newborn, and Women's Health Care* (17th ed). Philadelphia: J.B. Lippincott.

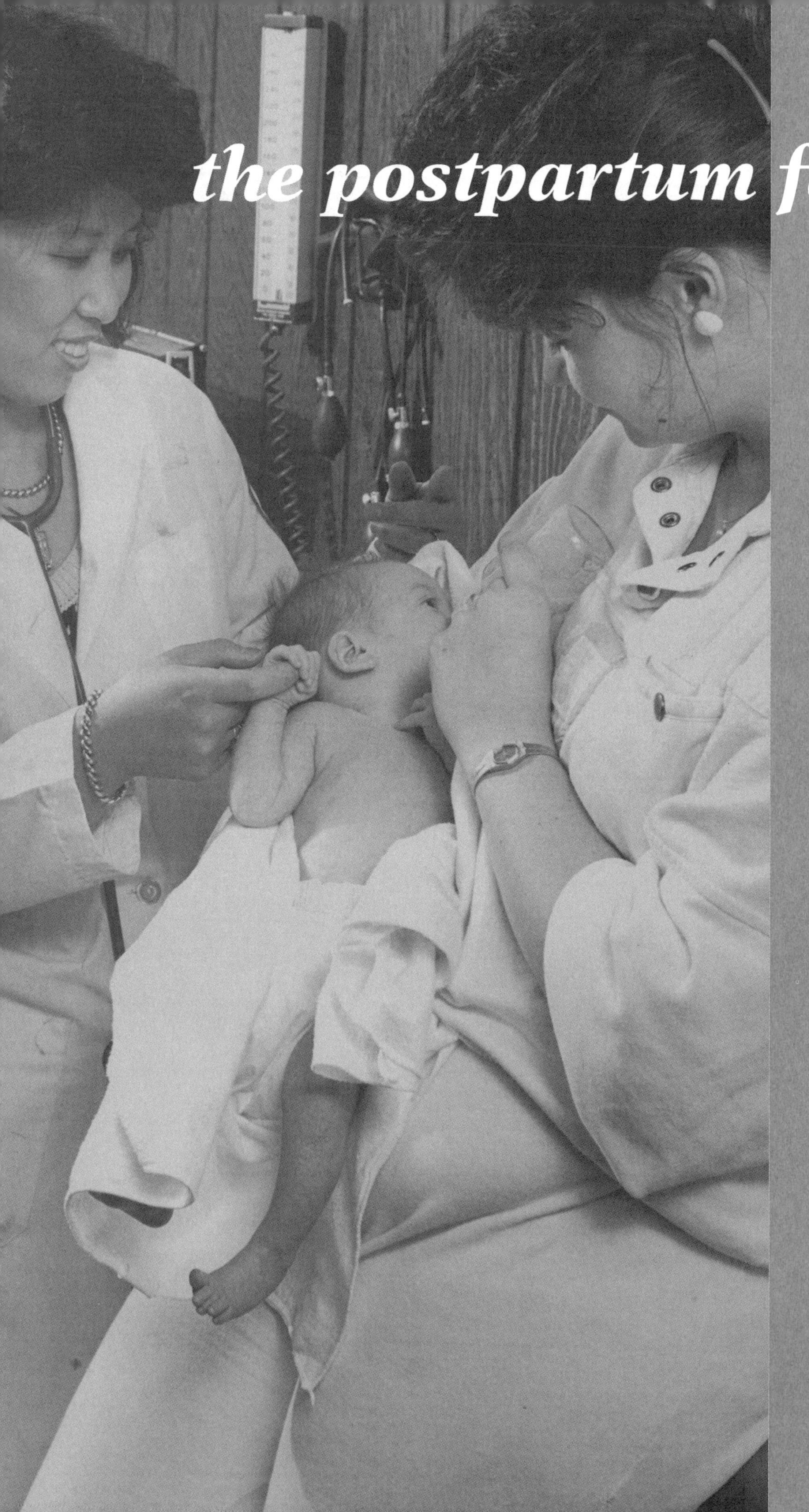

the postpartum family

unit V

nursing care of the postpartum family

14

outline

objectives 

After studying this chapter, the reader should be able to:

* Identify nursing goals during the postpartum period.
* Discuss the postpartum physiologic changes in the body systems.
* Describe the three psychological phases that the new mother experiences.
* Describe the three types of lochia.
* Discuss the psychological adaptations that the traditional father experiences.
* Describe the physical assessment the postpartum nurse performs.
* Discuss the psychosocial behaviors the postpartum nurse observes.
* Discuss nursing interventions used to relieve perineal discomfort.
* Discuss the instructions given to the breast-feeding or bottle-feeding mother.
* Discuss discharge instructions, including danger signs that the mother needs to report to her physician.

key terms 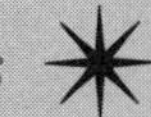

afterpains
attachment
diaphoresis
diastasis recti abdomini
engorgement
exfoliation
involution
La Leche League
let-down reflex
lochia alba
lochia rubra
lochia serosa
postpartum blues
postpartum chill
puerperium

Neff C & Spray M. *Introduction to Maternal and Child Health Nursing,*

The 6-week period immediately following childbirth is called the *puerperium* and is often considered the fourth trimester of pregnancy. This a period of major change for the woman and her family. During the puerperium, the woman's reproductive organs gradually return to the non-pregnant state (*involution*). Family members begin to restructure their roles to allow for acceptance of the newborn. This chapter discusses the physical and psychosocial changes that occur and the nursing interventions that will assist the family during this period.

✳ family considerations

The postpartum period is a time of readjustment for the family. The mother will begin to adapt to the "real infant" rather than the fantasy child she has imagined throughout the pregnancy. This can be very stressful for the mother, especially if the infant has a medical problem or is not the desired sex. Even selecting the appropriate name for the infant can be stressful.

The woman's partner may feel excluded because the main attention is on the mother and newborn. The partner may become frustrated in searching for his or her own role in the new atmosphere. This frustration may be displayed as irritability or total withdrawal.

Siblings also are affected by the birth of a new baby. Fortunately, many birthing centers realize the importance of including the siblings during the readjustment period. This helps the siblings see that their mother is alright and still loves them, and it gives them a "get acquainted" period to adjust to the newborn. The siblings' response will depend largely on their own stage of growth and development. Sibling visitations may decrease the initial problems with adjustment, such as feelings of jealousy or anger. They often can prevent or decrease regressive behavior that is common in siblings (Fig. 14-1).

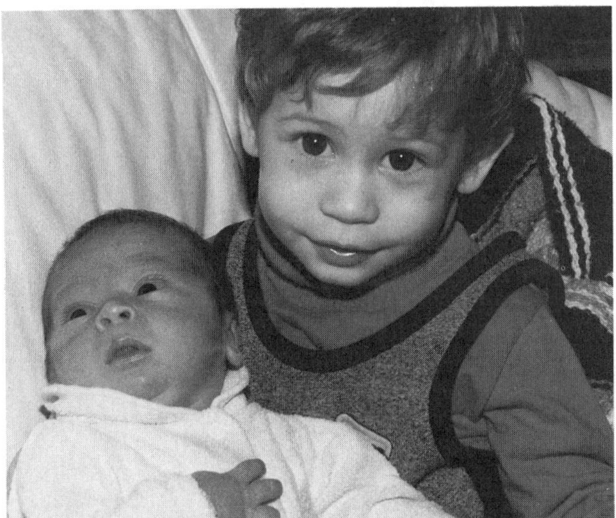

figure 14-1 *Toddler with new infant.*

✳ nursing considerations

Hospital stay following delivery ranges from 12 to 24 hours for vaginal birth to 3 days for cesarean birth. During this relatively short time, the nurse needs to assist the mother to become self-sufficient and to meet the emotional and physical needs of her newborn. The nurse also needs to help the family reorganize their roles to allow for acceptance of the newborn.

Nursing goals during this period include the following:

1. Preventing postpartum discomfort and complications
2. Teaching the mother to care for herself and her newborn
3. Offering educational and emotional support to the breast-feeding mother
4. Developing effective discharge planning, including follow-up care

In addition to teaching, the nurse needs to observe and assess the postpartum mother carefully. Hemorrhage and infections are the greatest threat to the woman. In addition, she needs to be monitored for signs of urinary retention, the development of blood clots in the lower extremities, and a variety of other conditions (see Chap. 15).

physiologic adaptation

Following the expulsion of the placenta and for the next 6 weeks, the woman's major body systems, particularly the reproductive system, are busy reverting to the prepregnant state.

Hormone levels are changing, producing physiologic and psychological effects, including the return of menstruation in women who are not breast-feeding.

reproductive system

uterus

The return of the uterus and other reproductive organs to the prepregnant state is called *involution*. The uterus must contract and remain firm to shrink to near its prepregnancy size and weight and to prevent bleeding at the placental attachment site.

Immediately following delivery, the uterus shrinks to approximately the size of a 20-week pregnancy (about the size of a grapefruit). The fundus should be firm and found near the umbilicus. The uterus continues to descend into the pelvic cavity at the rate of 1 cm (1 finger-breadth) per day. Usually by the 10th to the 14th day, the uterus is no longer palpable (Fig. 14-2).

The uterus also decreases in weight from 2.2 lb (1,000 g) at birth to 1.1 lb (500 g) during the first week. By the sixth week, as involution becomes complete, it will weigh less than 0.2 lb (100 g) and will be about the size of a pear. This reduction is due primarily to the decrease in size of the myometrial cells (they do not decrease in number, only in size).

Immediately following delivery, the placental attachment site on the uterine wall is open, jagged, and torn.

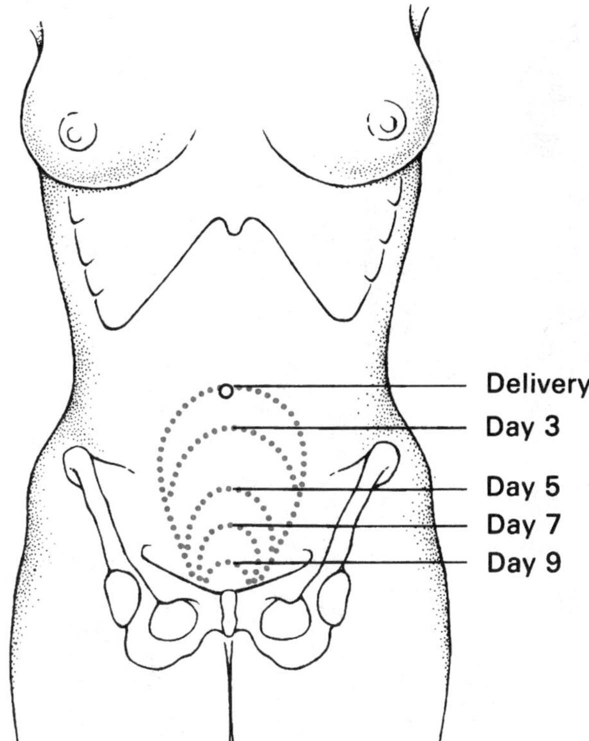

figure 14-2 *Involution of the uterus.*

Bleeding from the site is prevented because the blood vessels are occluded by the contracted myometrium of the uterus. As the blood clots over this area, it seals the raw, open areas. New endometrial tissue forms to cover the area, a process called *exfoliation*. This is important because it prevents scarring of the endometrium, which could prevent further pregnancies.

fundal firmness and position To check for fundal firmness and position, the nurse asks the woman to lie flat on her back. The nurse palpates the fundus of the uterus by placing the fingers of the dominant hand near the umbilicus and pushing downward on the abdomen (Fig. 14-3). He or she places the fingers of the nondominant hand slightly above the symphysis pubis and applies slight pressure. This pressure prevents the uterus from becoming inverted. If the woman has had a cesarean delivery, the nurse uses a slow, gentle motion to press on the abdomen toward the uterus, avoiding sutures or staples. If the fundus of the uterus is soft or "boggy" and higher than expected, the nurse massages the uterus to elicit a uterine contraction and thereby reduce the risk of uterine hemorrhage. If the uterus is slightly to the side of midline, usually to the right, the nurse asks the mother to void and then rechecks the fundus. This occurs because the uterine ligaments are still stretched, and the bladder can easily push the uterus to one side.

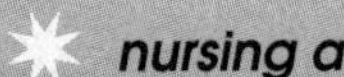
nursing alert

The fundus must remain firm to prevent postpartum hemorrhage. Massage if necessary.

afterpains The mother may experience "afterpains" for 2 to 3 days following delivery. These pains are caused by contractions of the uterus as it decreases in size. They are common in the multipara but also are seen in the primipara. These pains may be more severe for mothers of large infants, twins, or other multiple births or in women with hydramnios, because the more the uterus has been stretched, the more it needs to contract to regain its tone. If the mother is breast-feeding, the pains may be more severe, especially when the infant is nursing, because stimulation of the breast tissue causes the release of oxytocin from the pituitary gland. This causes the uterus to contract more vigorously. Frequently the physician will order analgesic medication to ease the discomfort.

lochia After delivery, the innermost lining of the uterus, the *decidua*, becomes necrotic and sloughs off. The sloughed decidua, combined with red blood cells, white blood cells, cervical mucus, and bacterial cells, forms the uterine flow called *lochia* (Table 14-1). For the first 2 to 3 days after delivery, the flow consists mainly of blood, is bright to dark red, and is called *lochia rubra*. The flow is usually heavy to moderate, saturating a perineal pad within 1 hour. The woman also may pass small clots. The flow has a characteristic musty odor, much like regular menstrual flow. The fundus should be checked for firmness at least once each shift and more often if the mother passes clots or the flow remains heavy.

Days 3 through 7, the lochia changes to pink or pink-brown and is called *lochia serosa*. The flow is much lighter (less than 4 inches on a pad in 1 hour or more), and the musty odor is not as apparent. No clots or fresh blood is seen during this time unless there is a complication.

Between days 7 and 21, the lochia has become light yellow or creamy yellow and is called *lochia alba*. The flow is scant and odorless. If the lochia remains red or changes

table 14-1 characteristics of lochia

Rubra	*Serosa*	*Alba*
Days 1–3	Days 3–7	Days 7–21
Dark red	Pink or pinkish-brown	Light yellow to creamy
May have small clots	No clots	No clots
Musty odor	Less odor	No odor
Heavy to moderate flow	Moderate to scant flow	Scant flow

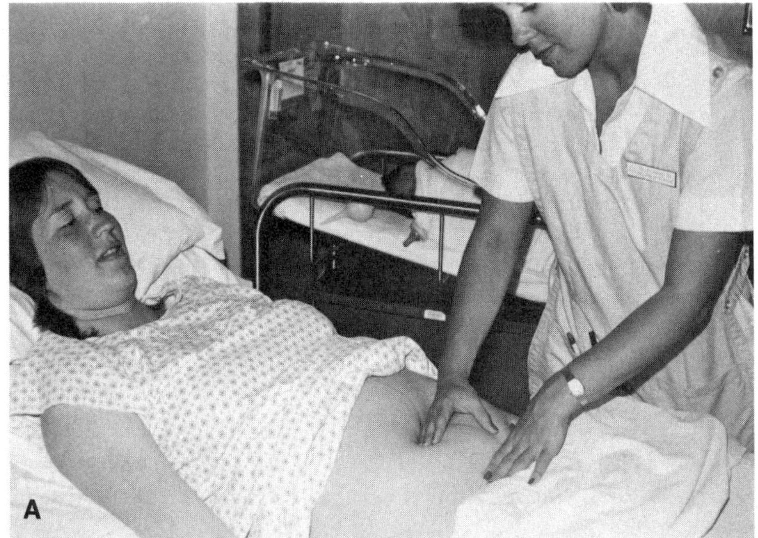

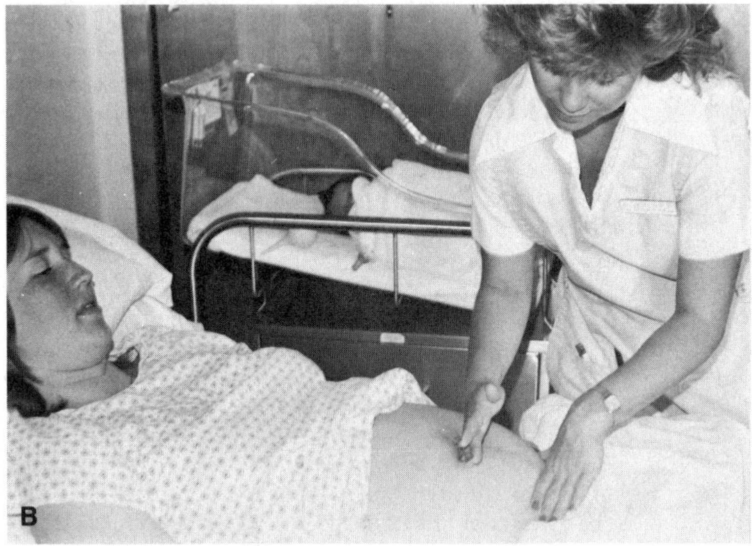

figure 14-3 *Assessing fundal position and height.* ***(A)*** *The nurse notes the position of the fundus.* ***(B)*** *The nurse assesses its height in centimeters from the umbilicus (Samuel Merritt College).*

back to red or if the mother is passing large clots, retained placental fragments may be preventing the uterus from contracting sufficiently. This should be reported to the physician. If the lochia develops a foul odor, an infection may be present and needs to be reported.

Following delivery, the cervix is very soft, usually lacerated, and dilated approximately 2 cm. By the end of the first week postpartum, the cervix has become firm and may be dilated only 1 cm. As it heals, the cervical opening takes on a characteristic transverse slit appearance, which distinguishes it from a nullipara's cervix, which has a round opening (Fig. 14-4). Following vaginal delivery, the walls of the vagina are dilated and smooth. They may be edematous and bruised. The hymen is permanently destroyed and heals as small taglike structures surrounding the vagina. As the vagina heals, the rugae reappear, and the walls become thicker. This process is usually complete within 6 weeks; however, the vagina, like the cervix, remains slightly larger in diameter than the prepregnant state.

abdomen and perineum

Following delivery, the abdomen is soft and flabby. The return of muscle tone may take several weeks; exercise will help in the return to normal. The mother may usually begin exercises to strengthen the muscles between 3 and 6 weeks postpartum but should consult her physician or health care provider about the timing based on her physi-

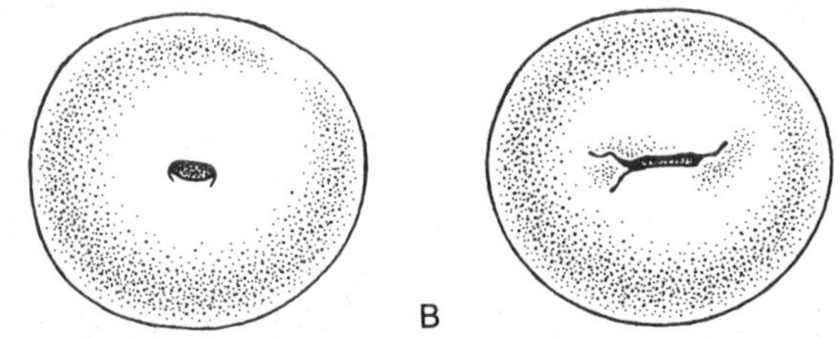

figure 14-4 *The perfectly round os of the nulliparous cervix becomes elongated after childbirth. The cervical os may gape if there have been significant lacerations during delivery.* ***(A)*** *Round os of nulliparous cervix.* ***(B)*** *Transverse slit of os in parous cervix.*

cal condition. The striae gravidarum fade from bright red to silver but never disappear. In the cesarean patient, the nurse inspects the incision site and evaluates for color, warmth, edema, discharge, degree of approximation (distance between the edges of the incision), and the condition of sutures, staples, or dressings.

The perineum is usually tender and swollen and may have bruises or sutures from an episiotomy. The mother also may have rectal hemorrhoids. The nurse assesses the perineal area for signs of bruising, tenderness, and redness. Perineal sutures should be checked for signs of separation, bleeding, or infection (redness, warmth, and tenderness).

breasts

As stated in Chapter 4, the breasts are prepared for lactation throughout pregnancy. During the last trimester, they begin to secrete *colostrum*, a thick yellow fluid rich in protein and minerals. Breast milk production begins about the third day postpartum (when the levels of estrogen and progesterone have decreased sufficiently). Breast milk is a thin, watery, liquid that resembles skim milk and supplies all the daily requirements for the newborn. As lactation begins, the breasts may become larger, firmer, and tender (*engorgement*). If the mother is breast-feeding, engorgement may be relieved by frequent nursing of the infant. If the mother is not breast-feeding, she is instructed to wear a tight-fitting bra or breast binder. Ice packs and analgesics also may relieve the discomfort. Breast engorgement usually subsides within 2 to 3 days using these measures. In the past, lactation-suppressing drugs were routinely administered to the non–breast-feeding mother to "dry up the milk." Today these drugs are rarely used, and the Food and Drug Administration no longer recognizes breast engorgement as an indication for their use.

endocrine system

Estrogen and progesterone levels drop to prepregnancy levels during the first 2 weeks postpartum. The level of human chorionic gonadotropin is negligible by the end of the first day. These rapid changes in hormonal levels are responsible for most of the physiologic changes seen in the other body systems and for the mild depression (postpartum blues or baby blues) that often occur in the early postpartum period.

Menstruation usually returns during the 3 months following delivery in the nonlactating mother. It may take up to 6 months to return in the lactating mother, with some mothers not menstruating for the entire time they breastfeed their infant. Remind the client that absence of menses does not prevent conception (see Chap. 4).

respiratory and cardiovascular systems

Following delivery, the rib cage gradually reverts to its normal diameter, and normal lung expansion returns. This relieves the shortness of breath and decreased activity tolerance associated with pregnancy.

The blood volume drops significantly following delivery and returns to the normal prepregnancy levels by the 4th week postpartum. As the heart adjusts to its decreased workload, the mother may experience temporary bradycardia with pulse rates of 50 to 70 beats/min. Blood pressure generally remains close to the predelivery reading but may drop slightly in response to decreased circulating blood volume. Any significant drop should be reported immediately because this could indicate postpartum hemorrhage.

During the first 72 hours postpartum, the hemoglobin, red cell count, and hematocrit levels may fluctuate but remain near normal levels despite rapid changes in body fluid content. This occurs postdelivery because the mother experiences hemoconcentration or packing of the cells despite fluid loss. These levels generally are within normal range by the end of the first week postpartum. The white cell count increases due to the stress and trauma of the birth process and may be as high as 25,000/mm.

Because of a decrease in plasma volume resulting in hypercoagulability, the mother is at risk for thrombophlebitis in the early postpartum period. With the delivery of the infant, pressure is decreased on the vessels in the lower extremities. This allows a gradual improving in hemorrhoids and varicose veins that may have occurred during pregnancy.

urinary system

The urinary system aids in the removal of excess fluid retained in body tissues during pregnancy, causing the mother to void as much as 3 L daily; however, it is not uncommon for the mother to experience urinary bladder distention after delivery due to trauma, bruising, and edema of the urethra. Increased bladder capacity due to the absence of the fetus and possible diminished sensations within the bladder also contribute to bladder distention. The nurse needs to monitor the mother carefully, because a distended bladder can lead to relaxation of the uterus, which can result in postpartum hemorrhage. Bladder distention also can lead to urinary retention and stasis, increasing the risk of urinary tract infection. Normally, the mother will void within 4 to 6 hours following delivery. Assisting her to ambulate to the bathroom may encourage voiding. Normal bladder function usually returns within a few days following delivery.

gastrointestinal system

Following a vaginal delivery, the mother is usually very hungry and thirsty. Peristalsis and digestive processes usually return to the prepregnant state within the first couple of days postpartum. Early ambulation and eating regular meals help to reestablish normal bowel patterns.

For a variety of reasons, constipation can be a problem following delivery. Hemorrhoids may be painful due to the pushing during the final stages of labor. Normal bowel function is just beginning to return. Perineal sutures, if present, may discourage bearing down. Many physicians prescribe stool softeners to assist the client. If the mother has not had a bowel movement by the third day postpartum, the physician usually prescribes a rectal suppository or small enema to initiate the return of normal bowel movements.

musculoskeletal system

For the first few days following delivery, the mother may experience muscle soreness and fatigue due to the intense work of labor. During the first couple of hours postpartum, she may experience a "postpartum chill"—trembling and feeling cold. This is probably due to the abrupt physiologic changes of childbirth rather than the temperature of the surroundings. The nurse should provide her with extra blankets and explain that this is a normal physical response following delivery.

In some women, the abdominal muscles may have separated during the later stages of pregnancy. This condition, called *diastasis recti abdomini*, will usually heal during the first few weeks postpartum. Once healing has occurred, the mother may begin her postpartum exercises to strengthen the abdominal muscles further. Joints, tendons, and ligaments tighten to their prepregnancy state.

integumentary system

Most of the pigmentation changes that occur during pregnancy (chloasma, linea nigra, and palmar erythema) fade but may not completely disappear (especially in dark-skinned individuals). Striae gravidarum will fade to silver. Hair and nail growth will slow to prepregnant growth rates.

The mother may experience periods of profuse sweating (*diaphoresis*) for the first few days postpartum. This is a normal physiologic response that aids the kidneys with the removal of excess fluids.

psychological adaptation

adaptation of the mother

The postpartum period is physically and psychologically stressful for the mother because of the many events that occur. This period has been described in three classic stages: the taking-in phase, the taking-hold phase, and the letting-go phase (Rubin, 1977).

the taking-in phase

During the *taking-in phase*, the mother is passive and dependent. It is a time of reflection during which the mother reviews, discusses, and relives her labor and delivery experience in an attempt to integrate the experience into her life. She may rely heavily on the nurse for basic care and instruction. She needs this time to recover from the sleep deprivation and extreme exertion of labor. In the past when most women received general anesthesia for childbirth, the taking-in phase lasted 2 to 4 days. Today when most women are awake for delivery, this period may last only a few hours.

the taking-hold phase

During the *taking-hold phase*, the woman begins to accept her new role eagerly and is excited and interested in assuming responsibility for herself and her newborn. She may express frustration with her lack of strength or any remaining soreness from the delivery because she is anxious to get on with her life as a new mother. At the same time, she may feel insecure and wonder if she will be a "good and capable mother." The nurse can help boost the woman's confidence by supporting and praising her progress in caring for the infant.

the letting-go phase

The *letting-go phase* usually occurs after the mother has been dismissed from the hospital and has settled into her home environment. It is a time when she finally accepts her role as a mother. She has separated fantasy from reality. She accepts her own labor and delivery experience and the fact that the infant is no longer part of her but a separate individual. If this is her first child, she accepts that her own role in the family has a different meaning. This may involve a grieving process and is normally the time that the mother may experience mild depression.

adaptation of the mother's partner

The postpartum adaptation of the woman's partner has been a neglected area of research. Some studies have been conducted on the response of the traditional father, but little is known about the response of the fathers in unmarried couples or of female partners in lesbian couples. The following is a description of responses of the traditional father.

integration of the birth process

Many new fathers have the same need to relive the birth process as the new mother. This may sometimes be difficult for the new father because the attention surrounds the new mother and infant. Many times he may feel frustrated in his attempts to be part of the group, particularly if complications have arisen during the birth process that may have prohibited his involvement. Time alone with the newborn can help ease the father as he begins to bond with the child and focus on his new caregiver role (Fig. 14-5).

physiologic responses of the father

Research by Ferketich and Mercer (1989) found that men may experience postpartum blues or mild depression similar to the mother's. Their research shows that many men report complaints of anxiety and depression as much as 8 months following the birth of the child. Many express financial concerns, irregular sleep patterns, and insecurity over their parenting abilities.

parental involvement of the father

Studies done by Fishbein (1990) show that the parental involvement by the father is most strongly influenced by the

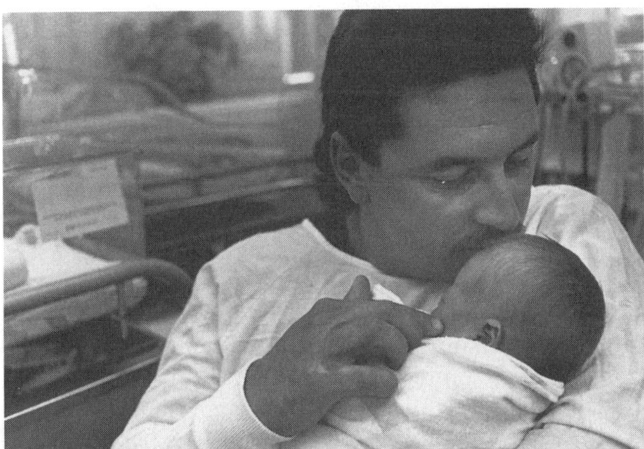

figure 14-5 *In the nursery, the father has an excellent opportunity to explore and interact with his new daughter. (Photo by Kathy Sloane.)*

mother. She is seen as the "gate-keeper" for his access to the infant. Society sends mixed messages to the father: On one hand, he is encouraged to be an active participant in the birth process; on the other hand, he is still perceived in the traditional role of supporter of the mother rather than participant in the actual care. Nurses and other health care professionals need to consider the father and the mother during this special time.

nursing care of the postpartum client

assessment

Observation of physical changes should include the following (Table 14-2):

- Vital signs: Elevated temperature could indicate infection; a decrease in blood pressure and an increase in pulse could indicate shock (usually from hemorrhage); an increase in blood pressure could indicate lingering signs of pregnancy-induced hypertension.
- Uterus: The uterine fundus (the top portion) may be palpated with the nurse's hand. The fundus should be firm and located at or near the umbilicus; it will descend (involution) from the umbilicus at the rate of 1 cm/d. Uterine discharge (lochia) should be assessed for the amount, color, and odor.
- Abdomen: Following delivery, the abdomen will be soft and flabby. If the mother has had a cesarean delivery, the nurse needs to assess the surgical wound for signs of healing. See Chapter 13 for care of cesarean clients.
- Perineum: The perineal area should be clean. A small amount of swelling due to the trauma of delivery is normal. The nurse observes for signs of tenderness, extreme swelling, bruising, or collection of blood beneath the skin *(hematoma)*. The nurse must check for the presence of any sutures and their condition and for the presence of hemorrhoids.
- Breasts: Immediately following delivery, the breasts are normally soft with the nipples intact, and they begin to secrete colostrum. On or about the third day postpartum, the breasts may become more firm and begin to secrete milk. The nurse assesses the breasts for signs of firmness, tenderness, warmth, or redness and assesses the nipples for tenderness, cracks, or bleeding.
- Lower extremities: The nurse assesses for signs of swelling or blood clot and vein inflammation *(thrombophlebitis)*. Dorsiflexion of the foot should not produce discomfort (negative Homans' sign).
- Elimination: The nurse observes urinary output. The mother normally will void within 4 to 6 hours following delivery. If she has not voided or is voiding frequent small amounts, she may need to be catheterized. Her bowels will probably not move until the second or third day postpartum.
- Nutritional status: The nurse assesses for adequate food and fluid intake. The mother will probably be extremely hungry and thirsty following delivery. Generally she may resume a regular diet.

Assessment of psychosocial changes should include observation of the following:

- Reaction to the childbirth process: The mother usually needs to discuss or relive the labor and birth process. The nurse observes for signs of low self-esteem, signs of embarrassment, or feelings of inadequacy.
- Attachment: The nurse observes for positive signs of maternal attachment, such as cuddling, holding, and talking to the infant. The nurse also observes other family members, including the father, for similar positive signs of attachment.

table 14-2 postpartum assessment (first 24 hours)

Area of Concern	*Expected Observation*
Vital signs	Within normal range
Breasts	Soft, nipples intact, bra on
Uterus	Fundus firm
Lochia	Rubra, moderate to heavy flow, may be small clots
Perineum	May be edematous; no sign of inflammation; any sutures present intact may have hemorrhoids
Lower extremities	No evidence of areas of redness, warmth, or tenderness
Elimination	Should void within 4 to 6 h of delivery
Bonding	Should show progressive signs of cuddling, holding, and talking to infant

* Postpartum blues: Many mothers experience a "let down" or short period of mild depression. This may be observed as periods of tearfulness, loss of appetite, withdrawal, poor concentration, irritability, and difficulty sleeping. The nurse needs to assess carefully to distinguish from true postpartum psychosis (withdrawal from reality), which may require hospitalization and intensive psychotherapy (see Chap. 15).

nursing diagnoses

The nursing diagnoses are based on the individual client. Even though most postpartal clients are healthy, the nurse needs to remember that the woman still has special needs. The following are some selected nursing diagnoses:

* Pain related to the trauma of the birth process
* Risk for Infection
* Fatigue related to labor process
* Ineffective Breastfeeding, related to inexperience
* Altered Urinary Elimination, related to decreased bladder tone
* Constipation, related to decreased gastric motility
* Impaired Skin Integrity, related to perineal laceration and trauma
* Knowledge Deficit, related to self-care and newborn care
* Conflict, related to changing parental role

planning and implementation

vital signs

During the first hour following delivery, the nurse or midwife is usually in attendance to detect or prevent immediate postpartum problems. Pulse, blood pressure, and respirations are monitored at least every 15 minutes until stable. During the next 24 hours, vital signs, including temperature, are assessed every 4 hours (see Table 14-2).

As stated previously, the pulse may remain slightly below normal due to the decreased circulating blood volume. Blood pressure will remain within normal limits. The temperature may be slightly increased during the first 24 hours due to dehydration but should be within normal limits following this period. Any significant changes should be reported immediately.

uterus

The fundus is checked for firmness, and the lochia is monitored for amount, color, odor, and the presence of clots. The fundus may need to be massaged to prevent hemorrhage if it becomes relaxed or boggy.

During the first hour after delivery, the fundus and lochia are checked at the same intervals as the vital signs (every 15 minutes). Once it is determined that the fundus is remaining firm, the nurse checks it and the lochia once per shift.

perineal care

The perineum should be observed for the presence of redness, edema, hematoma formation, lacerations, and hemorrhoids. If the mother has had any tears or lacerations that needed to be sutured or has had an episiotomy, the nurse must be sure that the sutures are intact and there is no evidence of infection (purulent discharge, redness, edema along the suture line). To prevent unnecessary discomfort to the mother while assessing the perineum, the nurse asks her to assume a side-lying position with the uppermost leg flexed (Fig. 14-6). With gloved hands, the nurse may gently lift the upper buttock to expose the area. Adequate lighting is important to ensure optimal visualization of the area.

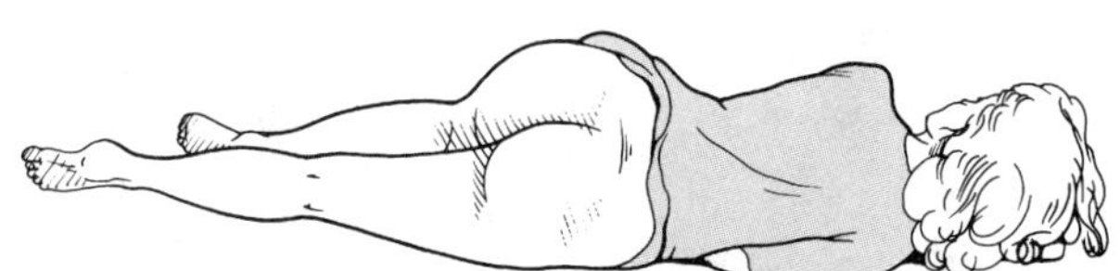

figure 14-6 *Positioning for perineal care.*

The mother is taught to cleanse the perineal area from front to back to prevent contamination. During the first 12 to 24 hours after delivery, an ice pack may be applied for relief of swelling and perineal discomfort. It should be used for no more than 20 minutes at any time, with ample intervals between applications. Care should be taken to prevent tissue damage from prolonged exposure to the cold.

Warm sitz baths may be used to provide cleansing, promote healing, and decrease discomfort (Fig. 14-7). Some facilities teach the mother's to use peri-bottles after each voiding or bowel movement. These are small plastic squirt bottles that may be filled with warm tap water. The mother is instructed to squirt the water gently from front to back to cleanse and relieve discomfort.

The mother is taught to wash her hands before and after perineal care and to apply her perineal pad from front to back by touching only the outside portion. This method keeps the part of the pad that touches her body clean and germ free.

The physician may order topical anesthetics to relieve perineal discomfort or pain from hemorrhoids. Those most commonly used are benzethonium (Americaine) and benzocaine (Dermoplast) sprays, Nupercainal ointment, and Tucks. The nurse needs to instruct the mother on proper application. Sitz baths also are soothing to the hemorrhoidal tissue.

nursing alert

Universal Precautions require the nurse to wear gloves to prevent contact with blood and body fluids. Postpartum care places the nurse at high risk for contamination, so he or she needs to be extremely diligent in following these guidelines.

elimination

Early ambulation is encouraged to promote the return of normal bowel and bladder function. The mother should be

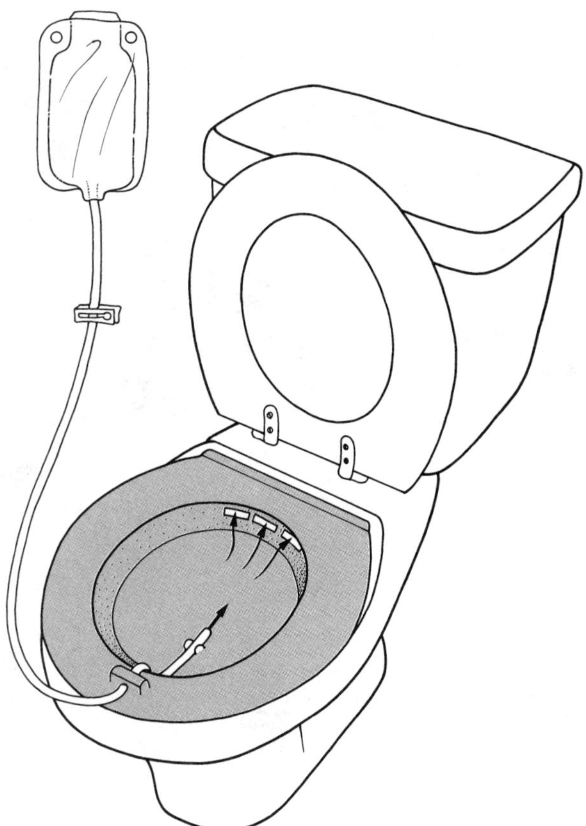

figure 14-7 *Sitz bath.*

encouraged to void within the first 4 hours following delivery. Assisting her to the bathroom and running the water in the sink or giving perineal care with a peri-bottle (according to institutional policy) may assist her. If the bladder becomes distended, she may need to be catheterized. Some physicians may require the insertion of a Foley catheter for 24 hours if the bladder has become distended.

To assist with the return of normal bowel pattern, the nurse should encourage liquids and fiber in the diet. Some physicians will administer stool softeners to ease the strain of the first bowel movement. Usually by the second or third day, the mother will have a bowel movement. Rectal suppositories or small-volume enemas may be ordered to assist the return to normal. See the Nursing Care Plan for the Women Adjusting to the Postpartum Period: Elimination.

nutritional status

The mother needs to continue the sound nutritional habits developed during pregnancy. If she plans to breast-feed her infant, the Food & Nutrition Board of the National Research Council recommends that she increase her food intake by 500 calories/d to meet the demands of milk production. Four or more servings of milk are needed to meet the calcium requirements. Extra servings of fruits and vegetables are good sources of vitamins and minerals. The mother should be encouraged to drink 2 to 3 quarts of fluids daily. She should avoid carbonated beverages, sweetened fruit drinks, and beverages that contain caffeine. Fluids to be encouraged are water, milk, and nonsweetened fruit juices. As an added precaution, the physician may require the breast-feeding mother to continue taking her prenatal vitamins.

reaction to the childbirth process

The mother needs to spend time discussing and relating her interpretation of the birth process. The nurse needs to listen carefully to determine if the woman perceives the birth process as a negative or positive event. Some mothers may express feelings of inadequacy or embarrassment over the series of events. Praising the mother for a job well done can be very supportive. It also is helpful for the nurses who were involved during the process to visit the mother and offer praise and congratulations. Answering questions and helping the mother to perceive the birth experience as positive can help her to integrate this experience in a positive manner.

Many families today are videotaping the birth process to keep with other family mementos. Studies by McKay and Barrows (1992) report that mothers viewing a video of their child's birth experience an intense emotional response. Many felt they even reexperienced the birth. McKay reports that many new mothers found that watching the videotape and discussing it with a nurse, midwife, or other professional birth attendant was helpful with "their emotional growth into motherhood." Mothers should wait to watch the tape until they feel ready (this may be several weeks after delivery) and that they should have a health care provider in attendance to discuss their feelings and perceptions following the viewing. This routine can help the mother better integrate the birth process into her life.

attachment

The formation of mother–child *attachment*, sometimes referred to as *bonding*, may be influenced by a variety of factors. These include religious beliefs, cultural patterns, social status, mother's level of energy, mother's psychological status, and mother's level of comfort. Positive attachment may be progressive in nature. The nurse should watch for signs of touching and cuddling, direct eye contact with the infant, and progressive involvement with infant care (Fig. 14-8). Additional positive cues could include comments about the resemblance of the infant to other family members, calling the infant by name, or talking to the infant.

The nurse may encourage the progress of attachment by assisting the mother to see the infant as a unique individual. This may be accomplished by encouraging the exploration of the newborn's body. Comments that may be offered may include the following:

- See how soft and small your baby's toes are?
- Look how your baby grasps your hand.
- Your baby has the same color hair as you.

nursing care plan
for the woman adjusting to the postpartum period

NURSING DIAGNOSIS

Constipation, related to decreased gastric motility

GOAL: The client will have a return of normal bowel pattern.

NURSING INTERVENTIONS	RATIONALE	EVALUATION
Encourage early ambulation.	Early ambulation can promote early return of bowel function.	The client will ambulate on postpartum day #1, increasing her mobility daily.
Provide and promote sufficient fluid and fiber in the client's diet.	Adequate fluid intake and a diet that includes roughage will help to prevent constipation.	The client will state an understanding of the importance of adequate fluid and fiber in her diet.
Administer stool softeners as prescribed.	Stool softeners work by increasing the water and fat entering the intestine and allowing for easier passage of stool.	The client will take the stool softeners as prescribed and understand their action.
Administer stool suppositories or small volume enemas as ordered after the 3rd day of postpartum.	Cathartics are avoided until the 3rd day since the increased intestinal mobility may lead to increased activity in the uterus and decrease the effectiveness of uterine contractions.	The client will inform the nurse of her bowel status and understand the potential need for a cathartic.

NURSING DIAGNOSIS

Altered Urinary Elimination, related to postpartum perineal swelling and decreased bladder tone

GOAL: The client will void within 4–6 hours following delivery

NURSING INTERVENTIONS	RATIONALE	EVALUATION
Offer the client a bedpan in the first hour postpartum.	The client may have residual effects of the epidural to prevent pain from voiding at this time.	The client will void early in the bedpan.
Assess the client's abdomen in the postpartum period.	A full bladder is felt as a hard area above the symphysis pubis and must be evaluated for frequently postpartum to prevent permanent damage from overdistension.	The client's bladder is frequently assessed for fullness and if unable to void, catheterization is prescribed to avoid complications.
Assist the client to void in the bathroom.	Walking to the bathroom may promote voiding.	The client is able to void within 4–6 hours postpartum.
The client is catheterized if no void after 4–6 hours.	Bladder infection from stasis of urine, decreased uterine contractions, and permanent bladder damage can occur if the client's bladder remains distended with no void after 4–6 hours postpartum.	The client is catheterized without difficulty, and the bladder is emptied.

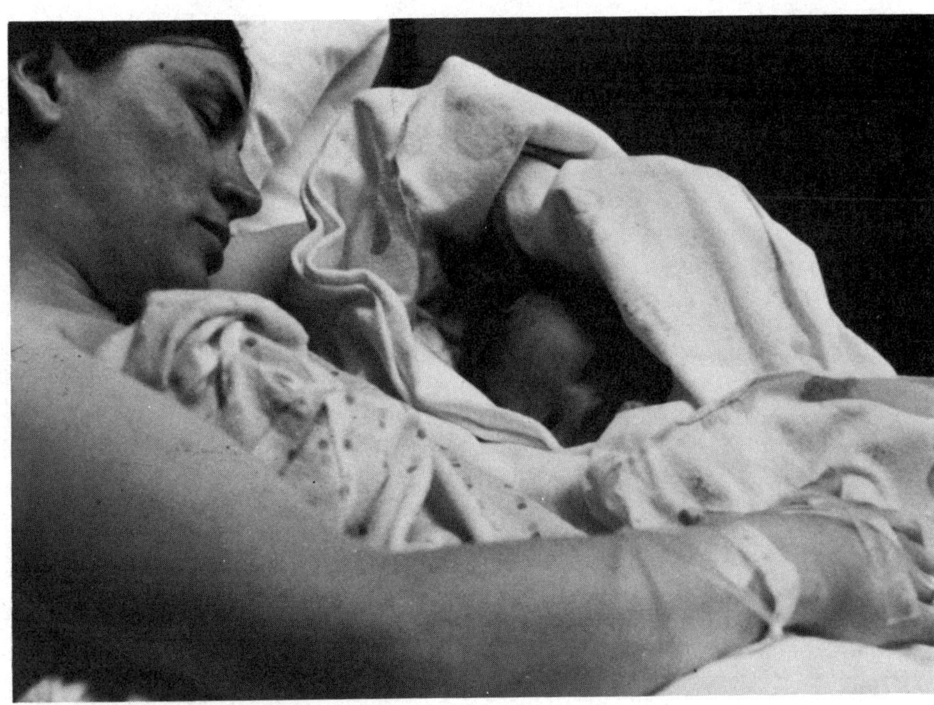

figure 14-8 *The mother snuggling with her resting newborn shows signs of mother–child bonding. (Photo by BABES, Inc.)*

The mother also may be encouraged to breast-feed early or to cuddle closely when bottle feeding. Assisting the mother to a comfortable position may enhance the feeding experience. The nurse also needs to provide time alone for the mother and infant (or couple and infant) to become acquainted.

postpartum blues

Hormonal fluctuations, lack of sleep, pain, stress of assuming the role of a new mother, and the fantasy of living "happily ever after" all contribute to the let down feeling or postpartum blues. It is normal for many women to experience these feelings.

The nurse needs to convey to the mother that these feelings are normal. The woman may feel tearful or inadequate as a mother; she may experience a decrease in appetite and difficulty sleeping. The basic nursing skill of "listening with a therapeutic ear" is extremely important. This allows the mother to verbalize her concerns and sort through what she is feeling. In addition to listening, the nurse needs to give the new mother plenty of tender loving care. It is helpful to provide adequate rest periods to allow the mother to regain her strength.

The nurse needs to explain to the family that postpartum blues are normal; this will help allay fears that the family is contributing to the problem or that there is something seriously wrong with the newborn that the mother has chosen to keep to herself. The family needs to know that they can help the mother most by being supportive and understanding of the situation.

evaluation

- The mother verbalizes relief from pain and displays relaxed body posture.
- Absence of infection is demonstrated by normal vital signs and involution.
- The mother denies feelings of fatigue.
- The mother demonstrates normal elimination patterns for voiding.
- The mother demonstrates normal bowel elimination by having at least one normal bowel movement.
- Perineal region is free from infection with apparent signs of healing.
- The mother demonstrates positive self-care and newborn care behaviors.
- The mother and her partner demonstrate positive parental behaviors.

wellness promotion during the postpartum period

Many concerns need to be addressed during the postpartum period. Because the postpartum nurse mostly deals with well clients, she spends much of her time educating the mother about care of herself and her newborn. Some of the topics that need to be discussed are postpartum hygiene, exercises, breast-feeding, bottle feeding, resumption of physical activity, and the need for rubella vaccine and RhoGam.

postpartum hygiene

Assisting the postpartum mother with her first bath or shower gives the nurse the opportunity to answer questions about self-care. It also provides the needed time for specific information about care of the breasts and the perineum.

The mother is instructed to wash the breasts first, using only clear water because soap may cause drying and cracking of the nipples. The nurse may need to remind the mother of the importance of wearing a supportive bra at this time.

As stated previously, the mother needs to do perineal care after each bowel movement or voiding. When cleansing the area during the bath or shower, she needs to remember to use a clean cloth and cleanse from front to back to avoid contamination of the vaginal area with stool.

breast-feeding

Breast-feeding provides a total, easily digestible diet for the newborn. Because breast-feeding is so beneficial to the newborn, the American Academy of Pediatrics, the American College of Obstetricians and Gynecologists, and the American Academy of Family Physicians recommend it as the preferred method of infant nutrition (Freed, 1993; Display 14-1). Breast-feeding seems to be most common among urban, white, college-educated women. The lowest rates of breast-feeding are seen among teenagers, high school dropouts, and African-Americans living in poor southern or rural areas (Freed, 1993).

In September 1990, the United Nations held the World Summit for Children. Many issues regarding child health were discussed. One of the priorities set was "the empowerment of all women to breast-feed their children." In 1991, the United Nation Children's Fund and the World Health Organization began the Baby-Friendly Hospital Initiative. The goal of the program is to make health care professionals around the world leaders in creating an environment that promotes and supports the practice of breast-feeding.

Most mothers make the decision to breast-feed or bottle feed during the second or third trimester of pregnancy. The nurse can be instrumental in assisting the mother to make the decision by offering education and support. Explaining early in the pregnancy the advantages of breast-feeding gives the mother ample time to make the decision that is best for her. Mothers who choose to breast-feed their newborn need education, support, and reassurance. Those who choose not to breast-feed or those who are unsuccessful in breast-feeding must not be made to feel guilty about their decision.

display 14-1
advantages of breast-feeding

1. It is a pleasurable, close time for the mother and newborn.
2. Breast milk is easily digested by the newborn.
3. No special preparation is needed prior to feeding.
4. It may decrease potential for newborn allergies or asthma.
5. Breast milk contains natural antibodies that may protect the newborn against certain infections.
6. Breast-feeding hastens the process of uterine involution.
7. Breast milk meets the nutritional needs of the newborn.
8. Breast-feeding promotes normal development of the teeth and jaws.
9. No additional costs or supplies are needed for breast-feeding.

composition of breast milk

Breast milk is considered the ideal nutrition for the newborn because it contains all the essential amino acids and is completely digestible by the newborn. Because the fat content is more digestible, absorption of vitamins A and D is increased. Breast milk also contains a higher level of lactose than cow's milk. Lactose is the easiest carbohydrate to digest, and it increases calcium absorption. Iron content of breast milk is low but much more easily absorbed; the infant also has stored iron in utero, creating reserves that last for 3 to 6 months following birth.

Breast milk contains antibodies that help to protect the infant against a variety of diseases and conditions. It alters the intestinal flora of the newborn, which decreases the potential for the development of diarrhea.

Certain drugs can affect the composition or quality of breast milk. The mother should check with her physician before taking any drugs while breast-feeding.

mechanism of lactation

The production of breast milk works on the theory of supply and demand: The more the infant suckles and ingests, the more the breasts produce. Milk production takes place in the milk glands of the breast under the influence of the hormones prolactin and oxytocin.

Prolactin, secreted by the anterior pituitary, stimulates milk production. Once the milk is produced, it must be carried through the ducts to the nipple. This occurs in response to the let-down reflex, which is initiated by the infant's suckling. This causes the posterior pituitary to release *oxytocin*, which causes the milk glands to contract and eject the milk.

assisting the mother with breast-feeding

Once the mother has made the choice to breast-feed, it should begin as soon as possible after delivery. This initial close contact helps begin the process of mother–infant attachment. It may be delayed if the mother is overly fatigued or the newborn needs immediate medical intervention. Breast-feeding is a learned skill. Many mothers may become nervous and frustrated during the first few feedings, especially when the newborn does not respond as expected. It is important to explain to the mother that these initial "trials" are important for the formation and release of the breast milk. The nurse also needs to alert the mother to watch for signs and symptoms of dehydration because it is difficult to assess how much milk the infant is receiving. Caution the mother to watch for signs of listlessness (this is not a sign of a good baby as thought), check the fontanels daily (they should be level with the scalp, not sunken), and check the urinary output (the infant should have at least six wet diapers per day).

After the mother has washed her hands, the nurse demonstrates how to hold the infant during breast-feeding. The mother and the infant must be comfortable; the mother can either sit or recline while nursing. If she chooses to recline, she can lie on her side with her arm raised. The infant can lie beside her, either flat on the bed or supported in a "football" hold with the feet toward her shoulder and her arm supporting the infant's head and back (Fig. 14-9).

The infant's mouth needs to cover the entire nipple and most of the areola. This decreases the potential for nipple soreness and promotes release of the milk. The mother may need to depress the breast tissue with her index finger to allow the infant breathing space. If this is necessary, she should be careful not to break the suction the infant has created.

Before removing the infant from the breast, the mother needs to break the suction to prevent injury to the breast tissue. She may accomplish this by gently inserting a clean finger into the side of the infant's mouth. The initial feedings should last about 3 to 5 minutes on each breast. Exposing the breasts to room air for 15 to 20 minutes following the feeding can help prevent nipple soreness (Display 14-2).

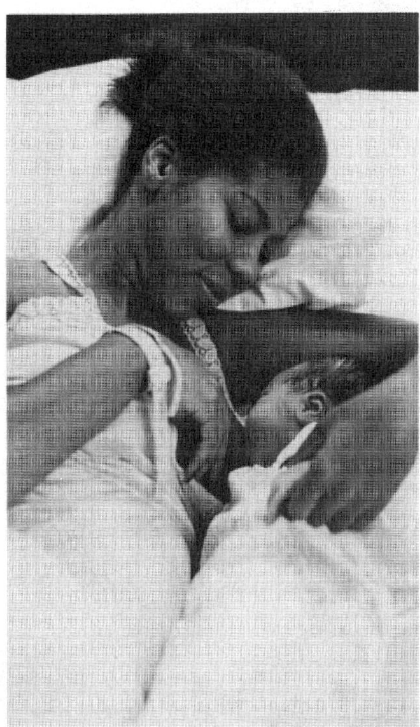

figure 14-9 *For comfort following delivery, the mother may assume a side-lying position to breast-feed her infant.*

display 14-2
teaching guidelines to prevent nipple soreness

Preventing nipple soreness can make breast-feeding more comfortable for both the mother and the infant:

- **Wash the breasts and nipples with clear water during bathing to prevent drying of the tissues.**
- **Wash the hands prior to breast-feeding to prevent the introduction of bacteria.**
- **Expose the nipples to air for 15 to 20 minutes after feeding to keep the nipples dry.**
- **Breast pads or a clean folded cloth may be inserted in the bra cup to keep the breasts dry.**
- **Change any breast pad liners as they become damp.**
- **Make sure the infant has the whole nipple and most of the aerola in the mouth during nursing.**
- **Feed the infant on demand to prevent breast engorgement and too vigorous suckling by the infant.**

Breast-fed babies usually require feedings every 2 to 3 hours around the clock. They receive most of the milk from the breast in about 5 to 10 minutes of feeding. Both breasts should be offered during the feeding period, and the mother should always start with the breast that was used last during the previous feeding. As the mother becomes more adept at feeding, she will begin to recognize the infant's cry that is associated with hunger.

The mother will need continued support after discharge. Many hospitals and clinics have lactation consultants available to the mother. The lactation consultant is a professional who has received specialized training and experience in breast-feeding and problems that can occur. La Leche League International, a group of nursing mothers, also can assist the breast-feeding mother.

breast milk expression

At times the breast-feeding mother may need to express her breast milk, for example, for bottle feeding the infant during her absence. She can express it manually or with the aid of a breast pump. If she plans to save the milk for feedings, the milk needs to be put in a sterile bottle, labeled with the date and time, and refrigerated immediately. It can be stored in sealed containers in the refrigerator for 1 to 2 days, in the refrigerator-freezer for 2 to 3 weeks, and up to 6 months in a deep freezer.

If she prefers to express the milk manually, she first washes her hands and then massages the breast to initiate the let-down reflex. Next she places her thumb on the top of the areola and her first two fingers on the bottom of the areola. Then she gently pushes toward the chest wall and squeezes toward the nipple. To prevent soreness and to better empty her breast, she should slightly rotate her fingers and thumb around the areola.

In using a breast pump, the woman needs to make sure the pump and her hands are clean before touching the breast. The breast pump exerts gentle suction to express the milk. She must read all directions to be sure she is using the pump properly. After pumping the breast, the pump should be washed and stored securely for the next use.

bottle feeding

If the mother has chosen to bottle feed the infant, the nurse educates and assists the mother as needed (Display 14-3). The methods for sterilization are taught (Display 14-4). In addition, the nurse emphasizes the following:

* The infant needs to be held close to the mother or other caregiver, much the same as when breast-feeding. This provides the cuddling, closeness, eye contact, and psychological nurturing that are as important as the physical nourishment.
* Bottles should never be propped; the infant could aspirate the milk or develop otitis media from blockage of the eustachian tube.
* The nipple should have a large enough hole to allow drops to flow (but not in a steady stream) when the bottle is inverted.
* The nipple should be well in the mouth, on top of the tongue, and full of liquid at all times during feeding. This prevents excess air from entering the infant's stomach.
* The infant should be bubbled (burped) midway through and at the end of each feeding; this empties excess air that may have accumulated in the stomach and prevents excess regurgitation.

display 14-4
bottle sterilization

TERMINAL METHOD

1. Assemble all equipment needed (bottles, formula, can opener, large pan).
2. Wash hands thoroughly.
3. Wash and rinse the bottles, caps, and nipples (also the can opener and lid of the formula).
4. Fill the bottles with the appropriate amount of prepared formula (bottles of water also may be filled and prepared at this time).
5. Place the prepared bottles in the pan with 2 to 3 in of water in the bottom.
6. Cover the pan and boil for 25 minutes; allow to cool.
7. When cool enough to handle, tighten the lids, and place in the refrigerator for later use.

ASEPTIC METHOD

1. Assemble all equipment.
2. Wash hands thoroughly.
3. Place all items needed for formula preparation in a large pan, and boil for 5 minutes.
4. In another pan, boil the amount of water needed for mixing the formula and for preparing fresh drinking water for the infant. Boil for 5 minutes.
5. Mix the formula with the sterile water in the sterile pitcher as ordered.
6. Use sterile tongs to remove the bottles; fill and place nipples and caps with the tongs.
7. Place in the refrigerator for later use.

This method made be adapted for use of bottles with sterile liners.

resumption of physical activity

Postpartum exercises may be individually ordered by the physician. The exercises are directed toward strengthening the abdominal and perineal muscles. Many of the exercises discussed in Chapter 8 may be used. Kegel exercises are particularly helpful for the perineal muscles and may be started as soon as the mother feels strong enough, usually within a few days after delivery. Mothers should avoid heavy exercise for at least 6 weeks to allow healing.

Some mothers return to work within 3 weeks of delivery, but many wait until the 6th week. Regardless of the mother's decision, she needs to avoid heavy lifting, excessive stair climbing, and strenuous activity for the first few weeks. She needs to get adequate rest, including naps, during the first week home to aid in the healing process.

Sexual intercourse may resume as soon as the lochia has ceased and the perineum has healed, generally in about 3 weeks. If she has had vaginal tearing or an episiotomy, she may need to wait an additional 2 or 3 weeks.

display 14-3
advantages of bottle feeding

1. Formulas are readily available in many stores.
2. Formulas are easy to mix; many are "ready to pour."
3. It may be easier to use for the mother who works outside the home.
4. It avoids possible embarrassment of breast-feeding infant in public.

rubella vaccine

During the early postpartum period, the mother needs to have a rubella titer drawn. If it registers less than 1:10, she should be given 0.5 mL of live rubella vaccine subcutaneously. This will prevent fetal anomalies due to exposure to rubella during future pregnancies. She must be instructed to avoid pregnancy for a minimum of 3 months following the administration of the vaccine.

rhogam (rho (d) immune globulin)

Mothers who are Rh negative and have given birth to an Rh positive infant are candidates for RhoGAM if they have not been previously sensitized. The infant's cord blood (direct Coombs' test) must be negative for antibodies and the mother must be negative for antibodies (indirect Coombs' test). This causes destruction of any fetal red blood cells that may have entered the mother's bloodstream before any antibodies have been produced that could cause problems for the next pregnancy. If the mother is a candidate, she is given RhoGam (1 mL deep IM) within 72 hours of birth.

display 14-6
sample discharge instructions

* Avoid heavy lifting or straining for at least 3 weeks.
* Limit stair climbing to 1 flight per day for at least 1 week.
* Begin or continue postpartum exercises as directed by the physician.
* May take tub baths or showers.
* No vaginal douching until directed by physician.
* No sexual intercourse for at least 3 weeks to allow for healing.
* Be sure to return to physician for postpartum check-up.
* If using or planning birth control, follow individual orders.

discharge instructions

Before the mother is discharged, her postpartum assessments must be within normal ranges. If there are any deviations, any special care needed is discussed. The physician or nurse midwife will perform an examination and give any individual instructions at this time. The nurse needs to be available to discuss these instructions and to assess for the mother's level of comprehension.

The nurse reviews all postpartum instructions on self-care and care of the newborn and on danger signs that are to be reported (Displays 14-5 and 14-6). The mother needs ample time to have all questions and concerns addressed. Follow-up care by a home health agency, La Leche league consultant, or other care provider should be arranged if desired or required. A copy of the specific care ordered by the physician will be given to the mother at discharge. A postpartum follow-up examination is usually scheduled for 3 to 6 weeks postpartum. The nurse may make this appointment, or the mother may schedule it if that is more convenient. Information on birth control can be given at this time (see Chap. 5).

display 14-5
postpartum danger signs that should be reported to physicians

1. Elevated temperature
2. Return of bright red vaginal bleeding
3. Foul-smelling vaginal discharge
4. Passage of clots with vaginal discharge
5. Prolonged perineal or abdominal pain
6. Pain in the calf of the leg, especially with redness, warmth, or tenderness
7. Difficult or burning urination; absence of urination

Discharge can be a happy but stressful time for the woman and her family. She is about to return to her home but may feel insecure about being on her own. The nurse needs to be supportive, praising her as much as possible to boost the woman's confidence, especially if this is her first baby. Many hospitals and clinics make follow-up phone calls to check on new mothers. They also give the mother their phone number so that she may call when she has questions. This can help ease the temporary insecurity that a new mother may have.

what would you do?

Shalleen, an 18-year-old homeless girl, was brought through the emergency department in labor. She delivered a full-term 5 lb 10 oz baby girl with Apgar scores of 8 and 9. Shalleen wants very much to keep her daughter but has no home or means of support. All that she owns are the clothes on her back and a tattered blue blanket that she uses to cover herself at night.

key points

* The nursing goals during the postpartum period are prevention of discomfort and complications, teaching the mother self-care and care of her newborn, assisting with breast-feeding, and developing effective discharge planning, including follow-up care.
* Involution is the regression of the uterus to the prepregnant state. The uterus must remain contracted and firm to prevent bleeding.
* Postpartum vaginal discharge, called lochia, changes color with time. Initially it is red (lochia rubra), then pink or pink-brown (lochia serosa), and finally light yellow or creamy yellow (lochia alba).

- ✶ According to Rubin, the mother goes through three phases of psychological adaptation following delivery: the taking-in phase, the taking-hold phase, and the letting-go phase.
- ✶ The nurse must observe for positive signs of mother–infant attachment. These include progressive cuddling, eye contact, and talking to and holding the infant.
- ✶ Perineal care following delivery is necessary to promote healing and to provide comfort. It includes the use of sitz baths, the proper application of the perineal pad, use of peri-bottles and topical anesthetics.
- ✶ Breast-feeding provides a nutritionally complete and easily digestible diet for the newborn. Mothers who choose to breast-feed need encouragement and instruction to make it a positive experience.
- ✶ Mothers who have a rubella titer of less than 1:10 should receive rubella vaccine to prevent fetal anomalies due to exposure to rubella during future pregnancies. If they receive the vaccine, it is important to explain that they should avoid pregnancy for a minimum of 3 months following vaccination.
- ✶ Mothers who are Rh negative, have given birth to an Rh positive infant, and have not been previously sensitized should receive RhoGAM within 72 hours following birth to protect future pregnancies.
- ✶ Before discharge of the postpartum mother, the nurse needs to review all postpartum instructions on self-care and care of the newborn.

review questions ✶

1. Lola, a gravida 1 para 1, is one day postpartum and has a moderate amount of red vaginal discharge. The nurse would record this as
   a. moderate amount of lochia rubra.
   b. moderate amount of lochia serosa.
   c. moderate amount of lochia alba.
   d. moderate amount of red vaginal discharge.
2. The nurse assesses Lola's fundus on the afternoon following the delivery of her infant and finds that it is firm but displaced to the right. What action, if any, should the nurse take?
   a. No action is necessary.
   b. Have Lola void, and recheck the fundus.
   c. Explain to Lola that it is normal for it to be displaced to the right.
   d. Notify the physician of the findings.
3. Lola has progressed well to her third day postpartum. When the nurse enters the room, she asks, "Why are my breasts beginning to feel firm on the sides?" The nurse would respond,
   a. "Maybe you are getting an infection; let me check."
   b. " It is normal for your breasts to feel a little more firm today; your milk is beginning to come in."
   c. "I don't know, but I will check with the doctor when she makes rounds."
   d. "Oh that sometimes happens; it's really nothing to worry about."
4. Ruth has never used a perineal pad before and wants to know how to put it on. The nurse would explain,
   a. "Just follow the instructions on the package; it's really simple."
   b. "It's important to make sure your hands are clean and you only touch the outside of the pad when applying it."
   c. "Oh don't worry about it; just place it against your vagina, and it will absorb the drainage."
   d. "It's not necessary to wear a pad; you can wear a tampon if you would like."
5. Jane, a gravida 1 para 1, wants to nurse her baby but is concerned about making sure he gets enough to eat. The nurse would explain,
   a. "You can pump your breast and measure it between feedings to see how much milk there really is."
   b. "The lactation nurse will explain all about it when she comes in."
   c. "The doctor will explain it when he makes his next visit."
   d. "Breast milk production is made on a supply and demand principle; the more the baby removes, the more the breast produces."

references ✶

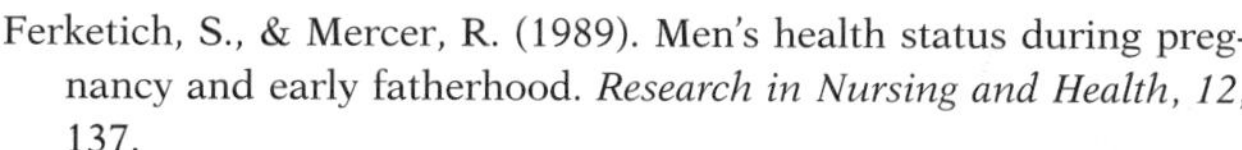

Ferketich, S., & Mercer, R. (1989). Men's health status during pregnancy and early fatherhood. *Research in Nursing and Health, 12,* 137.

Fishbein, E. (1990). Predicting paternal involvement with a newborn by attitude toward women's roles. *Health Care for Women International, 11,* 109.

Freed, G. L. (1993). Breast feeding—a time to teach what we preach. *Journal of the American Medical Association, 269,* 2, 243–245.

Mc Kay, S., & Barrows, T. L. (1992). Reliving birth: Maternal responses to viewing videotape of their second stage labors. *Image: Journal of Nursing Scholarship, 24,* 27–31.

Rubin, R. (1977). Binding-in in the postpartum period. *The American Journal of Maternal Child Nursing, 6,* 67.

bibliography ✶

Cunningham, F. G., McDonald, P. C., Leveno, K. J., Gant, N. F., & Gilstrap, L. (1993). *Williams obstetrics* (19th ed.). Norwalk, CT: Appleton and Lange

Kenner, C. A., & Mac Laren, A. (1993). *Essentials of maternal and neonatal nursing.* Springhouse, PA: Springhouse Corporation.

Kyenkya-Isabirye, M. (1992). UNICEF launches the baby-friendly hospital initiative. *The American Journal of Maternal Child Nursing, 17,* 177–179.

May, K. A., & Mahlmeister, L. R. (1994). *Maternal and neonatal nursing* (3rd ed.). Philadelphia: J.B. Lippincott.

Olds, S. B., London, M. L., & Ladewig, P. W. (1992). *Maternal newborn nursing* (4th ed.). Redwood City: Addison-Wesley Nursing.

Pernoll, M. L. (1991). *Current obstetric and gynecologic diagnosis and treatment* (7th ed.). Norwalk, CT: Appleton and Lange.

Pillitteri, A. (1995). *Maternal and child health nursing* (2nd ed.). Philadelphia: J.B. Lippincott.

Reeder, S. J., et al (1992). *Maternity nursing* (17th ed.). Philadelphia: J.B. Lippincott.

Sloan, E. (1993). *Biology of women* (3rd ed.). New York: Delmar.

complications and emergencies of the postpartum period

15

outline

objectives 

After studying this chapter, the reader should be able to:

* Discuss the causes of postpartum hemorrhage.
* Describe the nursing care of the mother experiencing postpartum hemorrhage.
* Describe the nursing care of a woman experiencing thrombophlebitis or emboli.
* List the teaching guidelines for prevention of venous stasis.
* Discuss the symptoms the mother may experience with puerperal infection, mastitis, and urinary tract infections.
* List the instructions for home care of the mother experiencing mastitis.
* Discuss the nursing care of the mother experiencing urinary retention.
* Discuss the difference between postpartum blues, depression, and psychosis.
* Describe the nursing care for the family experiencing a serious illness, deformity, or death of their infant.

key terms 

embolus
hematoma
mastitis
placenta accreta
postpartum blues
postpartum depression
postpartum psychosis
pyelonephritis
subinvolution
thrombophlebitis
uterine inversion

The 6-week period following delivery, the *puerperium*, is generally uneventful. The mother is stabilized, her body systems begin to revert to their prepregnant state, maternal–infant attachment continues, and the family begins to adjust to the new baby. Unfortunately, some mothers may develop complications. Continued, careful nursing assessment of the mother during this period can help alleviate or prevent these complications.

Physiologic complications of the postpartum period can include hemorrhage, infection, thrombophlebitis, and emboli. Occasionally, the mother may experience psychosocial complications, such as postpartum psychosis, dealing with the death of an infant, or coping with an infant with a serious illness or birth defect. This chapter discusses these conditions and the nursing interventions that are used to assist the mother.

✳ family considerations

When the mother experiences complications, she and the family face a crisis. Concerns develop not only about the physical well-being of the mother but also her ability to bond with and care for the infant. The mother's illness may interfere with her ability to meet the needs of the newborn. Her partner may suffer similar problems because concern about the mother may interfere with the attachment process. Illness also may prevent the mother from breast-feeding and cuddling the infant, resulting in feelings of inadequacy and adding to the mother's stress. Siblings may be concerned about the infant's condition but at the same time, feel neglected or slighted. They may express this through acting out behaviors, which may increase the family stress level.

✳ nursing considerations

The goals of nursing care of a mother with a postpartum complication include the following:

- Providing appropriate nursing care to minimize the risk of postpartum complications
- Providing comfort and pain relief measures to the mother
- Educating the mother and family about the mother's condition and the treatment that is needed
- Reducing mother-newborn separation and promoting bonding as the mother's condition permits
- Reducing the mother's and family's fear, anxiety, or grief

postpartum hemorrhage

Postpartum hemorrhage is defined as blood loss in excess of 500 mL following the birth of an infant. The bleeding may occur as a sudden gush or a continuous trickle. If the hemorrhage takes place any time during the first 24 hours, it is called *early* postpartum hemorrhage. *Late* postpartum hemorrhage develops most commonly during the following 2 weeks but may happen as late as 6 weeks postpartum.

table 15-1 postpartum hemorrhage

Source of Hemorrhage	*Definition*	*Cause*
Uterine atony	Muscles of the uterus do not contract.	Excessive manipulation of the uterus, some general anesthetic agents, prolonged labor, multiple pregnancies, overstretching of the uterus (twins, large fetus, hydramnios)
Lacerations	Tears occur during childbirth in the labia, perineum, uterus, cervix, or vagina.	Spontaneous delivery (precipitous) or operative delivery of a large infant
Retained placental fragments	The placenta or fragments of the placenta may adhere to the uterine wall, preventing the uterus from contracting.	Manual removal of the placenta, poor management of the second stage of labor, or growth of the placenta into the muscles of the uterus (placenta accreta)
Hematomas	A collection of blood trapped beneath the skin.	Injury to blood vessels in the perineum
Subinvolution	The uterus fails to return to its prepregnant size, remains larger and softer than normal, resulting in heavier bleeding.	Retained placental fragments, uterine tumors, or infection
Uterine inversion	The uterus turns inside out.	Application of pressure on the fundus when the uterus is not contracted, pulling on the umbilical cord to remove the placenta
Disseminated intravascular coagulation	The clotting ability is deficient.	Low level of fibrinogen

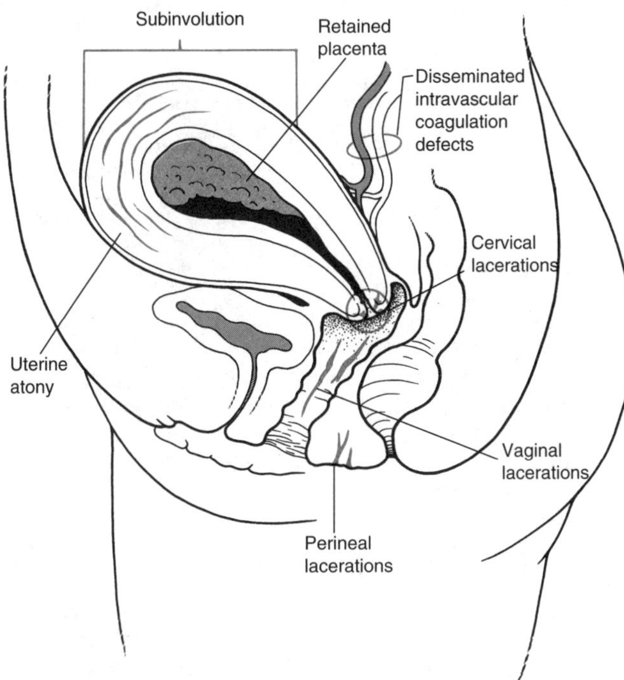

figure 15-1 *Common causes of postpartum hemorrhage.*

etiology and pathophysiology

Postpartum hemorrhage is the third leading cause of maternal mortality in the United States (Pernoll, 1991). The most common causes are uterine atony (responsible for up to 50% of deaths), lacerations, retained placental fragments, hematomas, subinvolution, or inversion of the uterus (Table 15-1 and Fig. 15-1). Postpartum hemorrhage also may be the result of disseminated intravascular coagulation (DIC). (See Chapter 9 for assessment and nursing care of the client with DIC.)

uterine atony Uterine atony occurs when the uterus fails to contract following the delivery. If the uterus is totally relaxed, hemorrhage will occur suddenly, and the mother will experience a continual gushing of blood from the vagina. Shock will follow quickly if the bleeding is not stopped. Sometimes the uterus may contract initially after delivery but begin to relax during the first hour. The uterus will feel boggy, and there will be a continual trickle of blood from the vagina. In this case, fundal massage will usually initiate uterine contraction and cause the bleeding to subside.

lacerations It is not uncommon for perineal tissues to be torn slightly during childbirth. Occasionally, the mother experiences significant tears that include blood vessels; such lacerations can result in serious bleeding. These tears usually result from vaginal delivery of a large infant, use of forceps, breech delivery, extension or tearing of an episiotomy, or a delivery that progresses too rapidly. If the tears are sutured, absorbable suture thread is used so that sutures will not need to be removed. If the tear is near the urinary meatus, a Foley catheter may be inserted to splint the area and prevent difficulty in voiding. It is usually removed within 24 hours or as soon as the swelling is decreased to allow for adequate voiding.

> **nursing alert**
> *If the mother is bleeding and the uterus is firm, the bleeding is probably from a laceration. Report this immediately!*

retained placental fragments Placental fragments left in the uterus prevent it from contracting, resulting in hemorrhage. Small fragments may adhere to the walls of the uterus, or one or more of the cotyledons may imbed in the muscular wall of the uterus (*placenta accreta*). To prevent this condition, the physician carefully examines the placenta and membranes to make sure that all placental tissue has been removed from the uterus.

hematomas Hematoma formation is the result of trauma to a blood vessel, with or without signs of trauma to the surface layers of the skin (Fig. 15-2). They most often occur in the vaginal or perineal areas. As much as 250 to 500 mL of blood may collect beneath the skin, causing severe pain and perineal pressure. It occurs most often when the second stage of labor has been prolonged, and the fetus has exerted pressure on the soft tissues of the birth canal.

subinvolution of the uterus Subinvolution of the uterus is usually discovered at the post-hospital check-up. The uterus is still soft and enlarged. It usually is the result of a small retained placental fragment. It also may be caused by an infection or uterine tumor. The mother may think she is just bleeding a little heavy. She may feel exhausted due to anemia.

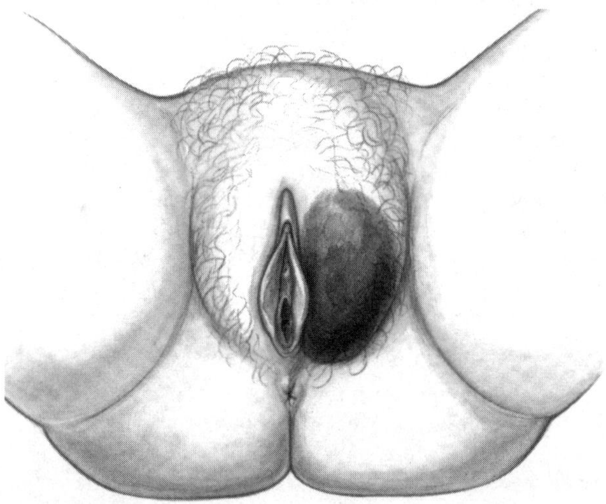

figure 15-2 *Appearance of a perineal hematoma from a bleeding subcutaneous vessel.*

uterine inversion Uterine inversion is the collapse of the myometrium, which results in the uterus turning inside out. In severe cases, the uterus may protrude from the vagina. The mother experiences acute pain and complains of a fullness in the vagina. The physician will place pressure on the inversion, causing it to revert back to the normal position. If the treatment is delayed, the cervix will swell, preventing the uterus from returning to normal position. If this happens, hysterectomy may be required.

medical–surgical intervention

Careful examination of the placenta (for missing pieces or parts of the membranes), cervix, vagina, and perineum following the third stage of labor is the best way to prevent hemorrhage.

If bleeding does occur, once the physician has established the cause, the following procedures may be used:

* Intravenous oxytocic agents, methylergonovine (Methergine), ergonovine (Ergotrate), or prostaglandins may be used to initiate contraction of the uterus (Table 15-2)
* Manual massage of the fundus to initiate contraction
* Transfusions as needed to replace blood loss
* Manual examination of the interior of the uterus for removal of retained placental fragments or suturing of lacerations
* Visual inspection of the cervix, vagina, and perineum for signs of lacerations; suturing as needed
* Hysterectomy if the body of the uterus is severely lacerated, inverted, or ruptured
* Ice packs applied to the perineum to reduce swelling and hematoma formation
* Incision and drainage of large hematomas with the use of analgesics for pain and antibiotics to prevent or cure infections

✱ nursing process for the woman with postpartum hemorrhage

assessment

To prevent or control postpartum hemorrhage, the nurse must be aware of conditions that place the mother at risk (Display 15-1). All mothers are closely observed because hemorrhage can occur early (first 24 hours) or late (after 24 hours up to 6 weeks) and can place the mother's life in jeopardy. Thorough and accurate assessment with immediate intervention can reduce or prevent serious consequences.

Subjective data to be assessed include the following:

* Vague statements from the mother, such as the following: "I feel all wet." "I feel like something just came out down there." "There is so much pressure; is that normal?"
* Complaints of perineal pain or pressure, especially with increasing severity

Objective data to be assessed include the following:

* Fundal firmness
* Amount and color of lochia
* Presence of clots
* Vital signs (for signs of shock or infection)
* Perineum swelling or discoloration
* Voiding pattern

nursing diagnosis

* Fluid Volume Deficit, related to a decrease in circulating blood volume
* Risk for Infection, related to prolonged rupture of the membranes, invasive procedures, or contamination of the perineal region
* Altered Parenting, related to the discomfort and fatigue caused by the postpartum complication

planning and implementation

If the bleeding has been caused by a boggy uterus, the nurse massages it to initiate contractions. Vital signs are monitored for signs of shock (rapid, thready pulse; decrease in blood pressure; pallor; excessive thirst; restlessness) or infection (increase in temperature and pulse rate). The bed is kept flat to encourage blood flow to the brain and kidneys. The mother is encouraged to void at least every 4 hours because a full bladder can contribute to uterine atony. If the mother is unable to void within 6 to 8 hours, she may need to be catheterized. The lochia is observed for amount, color, and presence of any clots. An accurate pad count should be kept (see Chap. 12). At least 2 U of blood are typed and crossmatched and held to be administered as ordered. Oxytocic drugs are administered as ordered to keep the uterus contracted. Oxygen may be given by mask to relieve respiratory distress caused by decreasing blood volume. Analgesics and ice packs may be used for perineal hematomas to relieve the pain and accompanying edema. Prophylactic antibiotics may be used to prevent infection. The nurse explains all procedures and answers any questions the mother and family may have to alleviate emotional stress. To facilitate bonding and attachment, contact with the infant is provided as the mother's condition permits.

evaluation

* The mother will return to normal fluid state as demonstrated by a normal blood count and flow of lochia.
* Absence of infection will be demonstrated by normal vital signs and involution.
* The mother will demonstrate effective parenting by cuddling, holding, and talking to the infant.

thrombophlebitis and emboli

Thrombophlebitis is the inflammation of a blood vessel accompanied by a clot formed from a grouping of cells, platelets, and fibrin. If the clot breaks loose from the ves-

table 15-2 common drugs used to control postpartum hemorrhage

Drug	Classification	Dosage/Route	Side Effects
Pitocin (oxytocin)	Hormone—oxytocic	10 U IV diluted in compatible IV solution	Water retention
Ergotrate (ergonovine maleate)	Oxytocic	PO 0.2–0.4 mg q6–12 h for 2–7 d IV 0.2 mg q2–4 h up to five doses; then PO	Headache, dizziness, chest pain, sweating, tinnitus
Methergine (Methylergonovine maleate)	Oxytocic	PO 0.2–0.4 mg q6–12 h for 2–7 d IV 0.2 mg q2–4 h up to five doses; then PO	Dizziness, headache, tinnitus, dyspnea, hypotension, nausea, vomiting, sweating
Prostin/15 m (prostaglandin)	Oxytocic, Prostaglandin	IM 0.25 mg q1½–3 h (total dose not to exceed 12 mg over 2 d)	Headache, wheezing, diarrhea, vomiting, flushing, fever, chills

sel wall and becomes free floating, it is called an *embolus* and can travel to the lungs, possibly resulting in death.

etiology and pathophysiology

Pregnancy predisposes a woman for clotting problems because the hormones circulating in the mother's body cause a loss of tone in the veins and make blood return from the lower extremities sluggish. The weight of the growing uterus places pressure on the veins, further impeding the return of the venous blood (*venous stasis*). Other predisposing factors include the following:

* History of thrombophlebitis
* Obesity
* Bed rest
* Previous cesarean deliveries
* History of recent infection
* History of varicose veins
* Older maternal age
* Forceps delivery
* Multiparity
* Lactation suppression with estrogens

By being aware of these factors and following the Teaching Guidelines display, the pregnant woman can take measures to prevent venous stasis.

medical–surgical intervention

Treatment of thrombophlebitis depends on whether the veins involved are superficial or deep. Superficial thrombophlebitis usually involves the saphenous venous system and causes calf pain, warmth, tenderness, and redness. Deep vein thrombosis produces the same symptoms plus swelling of the area. Conservative treatment requires complete bed rest with continuous warm, wet compresses. Anticoagulant therapy, such as heparin or coumadin, may be prescribed. Surgical intervention (thrombectomy) or thrombolytic therapy (streptokinase) may be used in severe cases.

diagnostic tests

A positive Homans' sign (pain in the calf with dorsiflexion of the foot) indicates thrombophlebitis. Vascular Doppler ultrasound may be used to visualize the venous structure of the extremities. Blood tests to determine bleeding and clotting time will be ordered to determine dosages of anticoagulant therapy. If an embolus has formed and traveled to the lungs (pulmonary embolus), a chest x-ray, arterial

display 15-1
maternal risk factors for postpartum hemorrhage

Placenta previa
Abruptio placentae
Prolonged or difficult labor
Precipitious delivery (rapid delivery)
Multiple fetuses
Hydramnios (excess amniotic fluid)
Forceps delivery
Induction of labor with oxytocic agent (Pitocin)
High parity

teaching guidelines
prevention of venous stasis

* Avoid prolonged sitting or standing.
* Elevate feet when sitting.
* Avoid crossing legs when sitting.
* Wear antiembolism hose if there is a history of thromboembolic disease.
* Ambulate early following delivery.

blood gases, and pulmonary angiogram may be performed to confirm the diagnosis.

✳ nursing process for the woman with thromboembolic disease

assessment

Subjective data to be assessed include the following:

- Tenderness or pain in the calf region, which indicates thrombophlebitis
- Severe dyspnea and chest pain, which indicate a pulmonary emboli

Objective data to be assessed include the following:

- Positive Homans' sign, redness at the site, swelling of the extremity, all of which indicate thrombophlebitis
- Rapid, shallow breathing; dyspnea; cough; rapid pulse; bloody sputum; chest pain; and elevated temperature, which indicate pulmonary emboli

nursing diagnosis

- Pain
- Impaired Physical Mobility
- Knowledge Deficit

planning and implementation

Vital signs are monitored every 4 hours. The extremities are measured once each shift and recorded. Laboratory studies are reviewed, and anticoagulants are given as ordered. If heparin is being administered, the antidote, protamine sulfate, should be readily available (usual dose is 1 mg/100 U of heparin). The nurse needs to watch for signs of bleeding, paying careful attention to the amount and color of the lochia, oozing of blood from injection sites, blood in the urine (hematuria), or bleeding from mucous membranes. Analgesics are given as ordered for complaints of pain. Bed rest is maintained. Warm compresses are changed frequently to maintain warmth and to assess the extremity for any changes. The nurse encourages contact with the infant and assists with positioning during feeding.

If the mother develops pulmonary emboli, it is an emergency situation. Oxygen by mask at 8 to 10 L/min is initiated. The head of the bed is elevated 30 to 45 degrees to relieve respiratory distress. Aminophylline, a bronchodilator, may be administered to relieve breathing discomfort. Heparin may be given intravenously to prevent further clot formation. Morphine is used to releive the pain. Many mothers need to be transferred to the intensive care unit for continuous cardiovascular and respiratory monitoring. Procedures are explained to the mother and family to relieve emotional distress.

evaluation

- The mother will express that she is free from pain.
- The mother will be able to resume her normal activities of daily living.
- The mother will express an understanding of her condition, its causes, and methods to prevent further complications.

postpartum infections

The trauma and stress to the body during labor and delivery reduce the body's resistance to and increase the chances for postpartum infection, especially in the pelvic region (puerperal infection). Other sites of potential infection include the breasts (mastitis) and the urinary system (urinary tract infections).

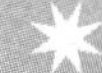
nursing alert

Good handwashing technique and adherence to strict aseptic techniques are vital in the prevention of infection.

puerperal infection

Puerperal infection is an infection of the reproductive tract that can occur any time during the postpartum period. The most common site is the uterine lining at the unhealed site of the previous placental attachment. If the mother's resistance is extremely low or the bacteria are particularly virulent, the infection may spread throughout the uterus, fallopian tubes, ovaries, and to the peritoneum (*peritonitis*). Perineal lacerations also can become infected as can the suture line of an episiotomy or a cesarean incision (Fig. 15-3).

etiology and pathophysiology

Once the fetal membranes rupture, a portal of entry for infection exists in the uterine cavity. After the placenta has been delivered, the site of placental attachment is open and vulnerable to infection. The most common infectious agent in puerperal infections is *beta-hemolytic Streptococcus*. *Staphylococcus* and *Escherichia coli* also may invade the area, however. A temperature elevation of 100.4°F (38°C) after the first postpartum day is usually the first indication of infection. A foul or purulent lochia accompanied by tenderness in the uterine area usually follows. The mother also may develop tachycardia ranging from 100 to 120 beats/min.

medical–surgical intervention

After culture samples of the suspicious drainage are obtained, antibiotic therapy is initiated. Antibiotics are usually started intravenously and later given orally. The mother will remain hospitalized. She may be given analgesics for discomfort and antipyretics for the elevated temperature.

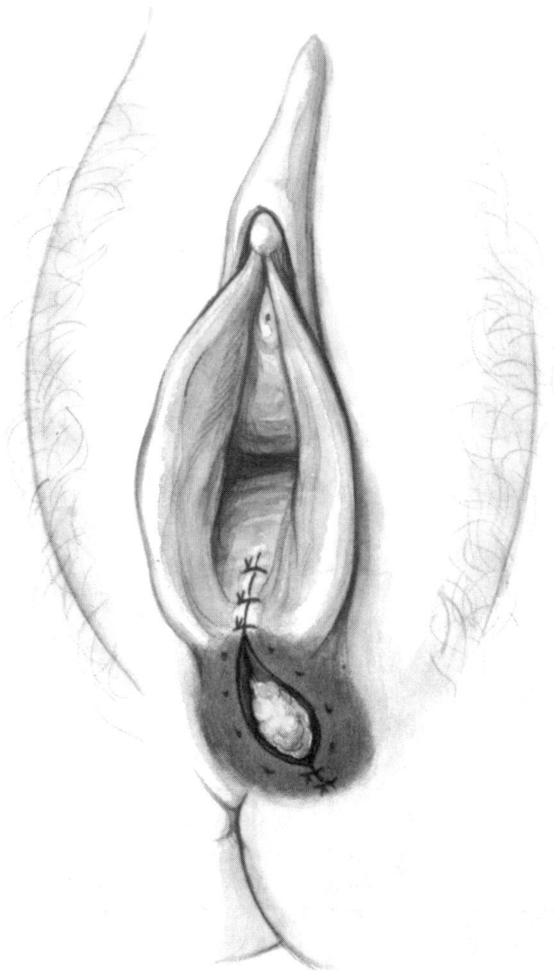

figure 15-3 *An infected suture line appears reddened, edematous, and often with infected secretions present.*

If infection occurs along a suture line (episiotomy, laceration repair, or cesarean incision), warm normal saline compresses may be ordered. If the area has abscessed, the physician may open the wound edges to allow drainage of the purulent material and necrotic tissue. Wet-to-dry dressings may then be used to promote secondary intention wound healing (wound edges remain separated, and the wound heals from the bottom upward and from the inside out).

diagnostic tests

A wound culture and sensitivity test is ordered to identify the causative bacteria and the antibiotic of choice. A complete blood count is ordered with special emphasis on the white blood cell count.

nursing care

Medications, such as antipyretics to lower the temperature, analgesics to relieve discomfort, and antibiotics to eliminate the infection, are administered as ordered. Vital signs and response to medication are carefully monitored. The nurse assists with bathing, turning, and positioning for comfort as needed. Adequate fluid and food intake is encouraged because of the loss of fluids with increased temperature, possible nausea, and general loss of appetite. Explanations of all procedures and treatments are given to decrease anxiety. In some hospitals, if the mother is unable to hold and care for her newborn, the nurse performs the newborn's care in the mother's room. If hospital policy or the virulence of the mother's infection makes this impossible, the nurse gives the mother frequent reports on her infant and acts as a vital link between the mother and her child.

mastitis

Mastitis is an infection of the breast tissue that can occur in the lactating mother during the second or third postpartum week. Because mastitis can interfere with breastfeeding, prevention is important for mother and infant.

etiology and pathophysiology

Mastitis occurs more often in primigravidas. *Staphylococcus aureus* is the most common cause, although other bacteria have been identified in mastitis. The breast usually becomes swollen and filled with milk (engorgement) just prior to the infectious process. The infection can range from mild inflammation to the formation of an abscess (Fig. 15-4). The breast may have purulent drainage in more severe cases. Usually only one breast or a part (*lobule*) of one breast is affected, although both breasts may be involved.

medical–surgical intervention

A sample of milk from the affected breast is obtained for culture and sensitivity. Appropriate antibiotic therapy is started immediately. If there is no purulent discharge, the infection usually is resolved within a couple of days. The mother is encouraged to continue breast-feeding unless there is an abscess. It is then advised that breast-feeding be discontinued until healing has occurred.

If an abscess has formed, it must be incised and drained. The area is then packed with sterile gauze, which is advanced slowly during daily dressing changes. This allows the area to heal from the inside out. When healing is complete, breast-feeding can be resumed.

nursing care

Prevention of mastitis can prevent pain, frustration, and emotional and physical discomfort for the mother (see Teaching Guidelines display). If mastitis does occur, it usually appears after the mother has been discharged from the hospital. Thus, the nurse needs to give complete and accurate instructions for home care:

* Directions for self-administration of antibiotics must be explained.
* Fluid intake should be increased to 8 to 10 glasses per day.
* If breast-feeding is to be continued, it needs to be done every 2 to 3 hours to prevent engorgement and to promote continued flow of the milk.

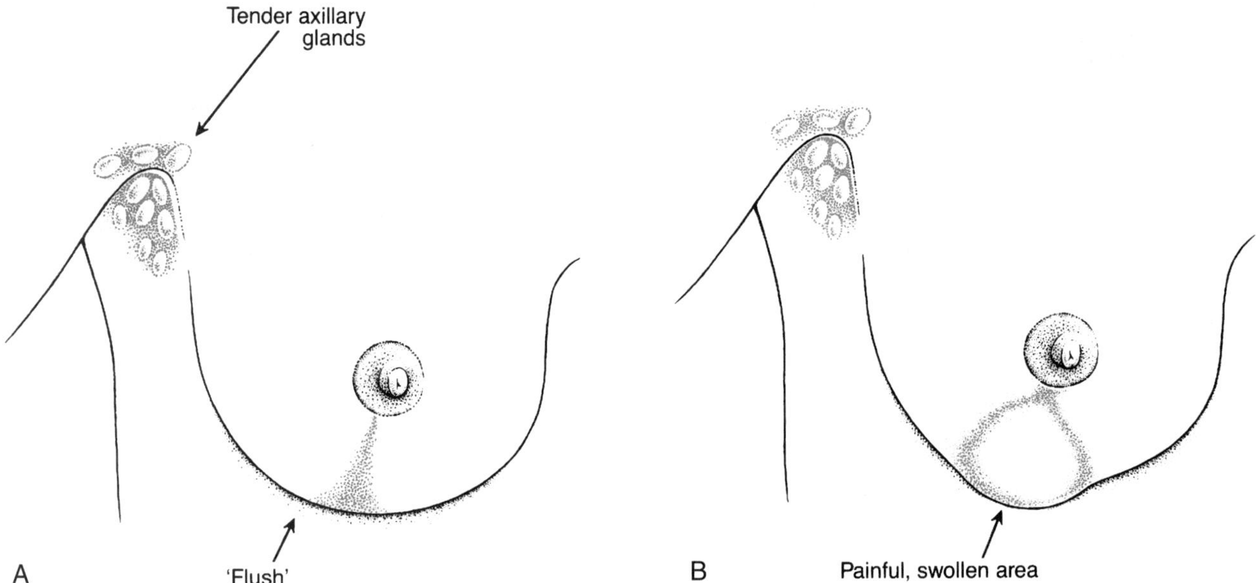

figure 15-4 *Mastitis. **(A)** Early mastitis. Fever is followed by a painful area on the breast and a "flush" that is red and tender but not fluctuant or swollen. **(B)** Overt inflammation in mastitis. A swollen, painful, red-to-brawny area develops. The purulent drainage gradually localizes into an abscess; when fluctuant, it must be incised and drained.*

✳ If breast-feeding is to be temporarily discontinued, the mother is instructed to pump her breasts to continue production of milk until breast-feeding can be resumed.

urinary tract infections

Urinary tract infections (UTIs) are a common postpartum complication. The infection may occur in the bladder (*cystitis*) or may travel up the ureters to the kidneys (*pyelonephritis*).

etiology and pathophysiology

The normal distention of the ureters and bladder, increased diuresis, and decreased sensitivity to the urge to void increase the risk of UTI. Birth trauma, catheterization, and repeated vaginal examinations expose the urinary tract to bacteria. These conditions cause 2% to 4% of all postpartum women to develop infection in the urinary tract. *Cystitis* produces complaints of burning or pain with urination, urinary frequency and urgency, and a low-grade fever. *Pyelonephritis* may cause fever, chills, malaise, flank or low abdominal pain, hematuria, and occasionally nausea and vomiting.

medical intervention

If a UTI is suspected, a routine urinalysis is performed to check for white blood cells, protein, or blood in the urine. A urine test for culture and sensitivity is then obtained by catheterization or the clean catch method to identify the bacteria causing the infection and determine the appropriate antibiotic. The drug of choice is usually a cephalosporin (most UTIs are resistant to ampicillin) given intravenously until the temperature is normal for 24 to 48 hours. The woman is then given the medication orally for 10 to 14 days.

nursing care

Applying ice to the perineum to decrease swelling, medicating for pain, and assisting the woman to void on the bedpan may help prevent retention of urine following delivery. However, if she is voiding small amounts frequently, she may be retaining urine. If there is suprapubic tenderness (an indication of bladder fullness) she may need to be catheterized. The physician needs to be notified and an order for catheterization obtained. If a UTI is suspected, a urine specimen may be obtained by catheterization or the clean catch method, depending on the physician's preference. If the mother needs to obtain a clean catch urine specimen, the nurse gives thorough, step-by-step instructions (see the Teaching Guidelines display).

teaching guidelines
prevention of mastitis

- ✳ Wash the hands before handling the breast to prevent contamination.
- ✳ Wash the nipples and breast with clear water; do not use soap because it could cause drying and cracking.
- ✳ Change breast pads when they are wet.
- ✳ Wear a clean bra daily.

teaching guidelines
clean catch specimen

* Oral fluid intake should be normal; it is not necessary to force fluids.
* Do not attempt to obtain the specimen until there is an urge to void.
* Cleanse the perineal area from front to back with povidone-iodine (Betadine) wipes or sterile wipes according to institutional policy.
* A sterile gauze pad or cotton ball may be placed over the vaginal opening to prevent lochia drainage from mixing with the urine specimen.
* The urine container is sterile; be careful to touch only the outside.
* Begin to urinate; once the stream has started, pass the sterile container under it to obtain a specimen. Remove the container carefully, and continue to urinate until the bladder feels empty.
* Carefully place the lid on the container to avoid contamination.
* The nurse will then label the container and send it to the laboratory for analysis.

✶ nursing process for the woman with postpartum infection

assessment

Subjective data to be assessed include the following:

* Pain or tenderness in the abdomen, breasts, perineal region, or flank region
* Pain or burning with urination
* Urinary frequency and urgency
* Loss of appetite
* General malaise
* Nausea

Objective data to be assessed include the following:

* Elevated temperature and pulse
* Redness and edema at site of infection
* Chills
* Hematuria
* Purulent drainage
* Foul odor of the lochia

nursing diagnosis

* Interrupted Breastfeeding, related to postpartum complications and possible antibiotic therapy
* Pain
* Risk for Injury, related to bladder distention, UTI

planning and implementation

The nurse continues to monitor the vital signs and observe for signs of changes in the infectious process. Specimens are obtained and sent to the laboratory as needed. The mother is taught good handwashing technique and care of her breasts and perineum to prevent reinfection. Dressings, perineal pads, and breast pads are changed frequently to monitor the areas and keep them clean and dry. Adequate fluid intake (2,000 mL/d) is encouraged. Antibiotics and pain medications are administered as ordered. If the mother is to continue the medications at home, the nurse instructs the mother on proper self-administration. Emotional support is given to the mother and her support person. See the Nursing Care Plan for the Woman with Puerperal Fever.

evaluation

* The mother will successfully reestablish breast-feeding.
* The mother will be pain free.
* The mother will void normally with no signs of infection.

postpartum blues, depression, or psychosis

Following delivery, the mother may experience varying degrees of mood alteration. These include (in order of severity) *postpartum blues, postpartum depression*, and *postpartum psychosis.* Other circumstances that can affect her emotional well-being are the birth of a child with a severe illness or deformity, stillbirth, or death of a newborn. These complications can affect the well-being of the mother, her partner, and the entire family unit.

Postpartum blues are experienced by more than half of all postpartum women. They begin about the third day after delivery and last less than 2 weeks. The woman may experience tearfulness, irritability, headaches, and anxiety. Postpartum blues result from decreased estrogen and progesterone levels, exhaustion from the labor and delivery, physical discomfort, and the sudden realization that she has the responsibility for another person. Postpartum blues usually resolve without medical intervention.

Postpartum depression may develop anytime during the first 3 months following delivery. In the United States, postpartum depression occurs in 10% to 26% of mothers (Beck, Reynolds, & Rutowski, 1992). The mother may experience prolonged tearfulness, withdrawal from family and friends, extreme fatigue, insecurity, loss of interest in daily activities, and the desire to harm herself or the newborn. The exact cause of postpartum depression is not known. Research indicates that the predisposing factors include a history of severe bouts of postpartum blues, marital dissatisfaction, depression during pregnancy, and lack of a support system (Beck, et al., 1992). Other research studies indicate that it may be caused by difficult birthing experiences (Ralph & Alexander, 1994). Medical treatment may include the use of antidepressant medica-

nursing care plan
for the postpartum client experiencing the complication of an infection

NURSING DIAGNOSIS

Risk for Infection (puerperal), related to rupture of membranes more than 24 hours before delivery

GOAL: The client will not encounter any signs of postpartum infection.

NURSING INTERVENTIONS	RATIONALE	EVALUATION
Assess for signs of postpartum infection.	The uterus is a closed space and anaerobic organisms may grow rapidly.	The client's temperature will be less than 38°C or 100.4°F, excluding the first day.
Evaluate lochia for smell and consistency.	Purulent, absent or foul-smelling lochia can indicate infection.	The lochia will be present, will not be purulent, and will not have a foul odor.
Monitor vital signs.	Sinus tachycardia is a compensatory response to fever.	The client's vital signs will remain stable.
Monitor fluid status and encourage adequate fluid intake.	Fever can cause an increase in insensible water loss.	The client will remain adequately hydrated, with balanced intake and output.
Administer antipyretics and antibiotics as prescribed.	Antipyretics will lower the temperature while antibiotics eliminate the infection.	The client will receive antibiotic-specific treatment and respond appropriately to the treatment without evidence of further infection.
Evaluate response to treatment.	The antibiotic may need to be reevaluated after specific cultures are obtained or if the client is not responding to therapy.	Persistent signs of infection will be reported and treatment adjusted promptly.

tion, individual psychotherapy, and group therapy, either outpatient or inpatient.

Postpartum psychosis is a relatively rare occurrence (only 1 or 2 cases per 1,000 births). Psychosis is a condition in which the individual loses contact with reality. These mothers may hallucinate and hear voices that tell them to kill themselves or their newborn. Hospitalization is always required. Intensive psychiatric treatment is necessary and may include individual and group therapy, antidepressants, antipsychotics, or lithium. With treatment, these mothers usually recover and are able to return home. Postpartum psychosis may recur in future pregnancies, however.

nursing care

The mother who experiences mood alterations, whether mild or severe, requires assistance in meeting her own daily needs and the needs of her newborn. The nurse needs to observe for positive signs of maternal–infant attachment. Lack of mother–infant attachment is often the first sign that intervention is needed. The nurse can assist the mother by being supportive and empathetic and encouraging the mother to express her concerns and feelings freely. Reporting signs of serious mood alterations is imperative for the safety of the mother and her newborn.

serious illness, deformity, or death of the infant

Assisting the family who experiences the birth of an infant with a serious illness, deformity, or death can be one of the most challenging tasks of the maternity nurse. For months, the parents have prepared and anticipated the birth of a beautiful, perfect, healthy newborn. If the child is born with a serious illness or deformity, the parents may be guilt ridden. Comments such as the following are not uncommon: "It's all my fault; I should have followed my diet more carefully." "I should have helped my wife more. She worked too hard. It's all my fault." "I knew smoking could harm my baby; I should have quit." The couple may experience a variety of emotions ranging from anger, denial, bargaining, depression, to acceptance. The nurse needs to remain supportive and nonjudgmental, allowing the family to express their grief in their own way.

nursing care plan
for family experiencing the death of the newborn

ASSESSMENT:

Janet Dailey is a 26-year-old gravida 1 para 0. Her husband, Doug, is a computer salesman at a local store. They have anxiously awaited the birth of their first child. Janet has had good prenatal care, and everything has been normal. She enters the hospital in active labor and gives birth to an 8-lb girl who does not breathe following delivery. Emergency intervention fails to resuscitate, and the infant is pronounced dead. Both Janet and Doug begin crying. Doug runs out of the room. Janet says, "This can't be happening. I want my baby. Where is Doug?" The nurse finds Doug just outside the room. He says, "How can I face Janet? I've let her down. We came here for a baby, and you have given us nothing. Why? Why?"

NURSING DIAGNOSIS:

Ineffective Individual Coping, related to the death of the newborn

NURSING INTERVENTIONS:

Spend time with each partner, allowing each to express feelings.
Rationale: This allows each partner to sort through individual feelings and builds rapport.
Contact their minister or hospital chaplin.
Rationale: This will provide additional support and counseling.

EVALUATION:

Janet and Doug will verbalize their individual feelings about the death of their newborn.
Each will begin to work through the grief process.

NURSING DIAGNOSIS:

Anticipatory Grieving, related to death of the newborn

INTERVENTIONS:

Discuss the death of the infant with the family.
Rationale: This assists the family in realizing the death has really occurred.
Express sorrow over their loss.
Rationale: Empathy helps to establish trust and rapport.
Allow family to express their grief openly.
Rationale: This supports the family in working through the stages of grief.
Prepare the infant for the parents' final visit, and provide privacy.
Rationale: This allows parents to say goodbye and aids in the grieving process.

EVALUATION:

Janet will be able to express her grief.
Doug will be able to express his grief.
Both partners will be able to share their grief with each other.

Parents of a seriously ill newborn may withdraw because of fear of injuring the infant further. Parents of the infant with a birth defect may be unable to look at the deformity. If the infant must be transported to a larger facility, physical distance may further complicate the situation. The nurse needs to help keep the lines of communication open, lend emotional support, and encourage attachment with the infant.

The death of an infant is one of the most tragic experiences a family can encounter. The excitement and expectations of the impending birth are brought to an abrupt, devastating end. The family is often in shock and may express denial of the death. The nurse can support the family by empathetic listening and caring. Preparing the infant for the last visit with the family is an important nursing task.

nursing care

When assisting the family to accept and care for an infant with a serious illness or deformity, the nurse strives to pro-

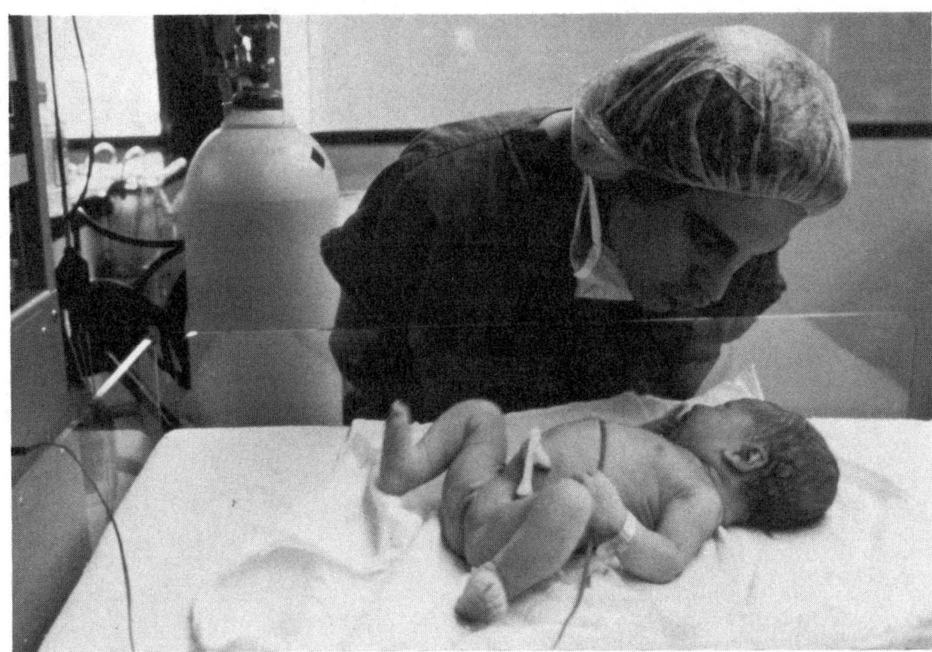

figure 15-5 *It is important that the family have an opportunity to interact and bond with an ill, isolated newborn.*

mote attachment by offering emotional support, providing accurate information about the infant's condition and proposed treatment, and teaching appropriate caregiving skills (Fig. 15-5). Referrals to local self-help groups, such as parents of Down syndrome infants, may help the family adjust. Social services may be helpful in assisting the family with the unexpected financial burden that can result from the infant's condition.

If the infant has died, the parents must have the opportunity to hold and say goodbye to their infant. Seeing the infant may help them to accept the reality of the death. It is a traumatic time for the grieving family, and the nurse needs to provide privacy for them. It is sometimes helpful for the nurse to offer to call other family members, call the funeral home of choice, and make arrangements for baptism of the infant if the family requests this. Many families find it helpful if the nurse notifies and requests the presence of the hospital chaplin or rabbi. The preparation of a memory packet also may be helpful. This could include a picture of the infant, a hospital identification bracelet for the infant, a lock of hair, footprints, and a copy of the birth certificate. Referrals to local support groups, such as Compassionate Friends, may assist the family with the grieving process.

key points ✳

- ✳ **The goals of nursing care of a mother with a postpartum complication are to minimize the risk of further complications, provide comfort and relief measures, educate her and the family about the condition and its treatment, promote maternal-infant bonding, and reduce the fear, anxiety, and grief associated with the condition.**
- ✳ **The most common causes of postpartum hemorrhage are uterine atony, lacerations, retained placental fragments, hematomas, subinvolution, or inversion of the uterus.**
- ✳ **Pregnancy predisposes the mother to clotting problems, such as thrombophlebitis and emboli, because the circulating hormones cause a loss of tone in the veins and make the return of blood to the heart sluggish.**
- ✳ **The most common site for infections in the pelvic region following delivery is the unhealed site of the previous placental attachment.**
- ✳ **Mastitis, an infection of the breast tissue, occurs most often during the second or third week postpartum and is usually caused by *S. aureus*.**
- ✳ **To prevent the development of mastitis, the mother must wash her hands before handling the breast, wash the nipples with clear water to prevent drying, change breast pads when they are wet, and wear a clean bra daily.**
- ✳ **Postpartum blues are experienced by more than half of of all mothers. Symptoms are tearfulness, irritability, headaches, and anxiety. They are transient and last less than 2 weeks.**
- ✳ **Postpartum depression can occur anytime during the first 3 weeks following delivery. Medical treatment is usually necessary.**
- ✳ **Postpartum psychosis is rare but causes the woman to lose contact with reality; she may be a threat to her own life or the life of her newborn.**

review questions

1. Juanita Lopez gave birth 1 hour ago to a healthy, 8-lb baby boy. When assessing her, the nurse finds that Juanita's fundus is firm, but she has a continuous trickle of blood coming from her vagina. The nurse would
   a. take no action because this is normal.
   b. report this immediately to the physician.
   c. change her peri-pad, and document it on the chart.
   d. massage Juanita's fundus.
2. Jane Norris is 2 days postpartum after a vaginal birth of a healthy, 7-lb girl. She tells the nurse, "My left calf hurts." Jane's leg is red, warm, and tender to the touch. The nurse would
   a. document this on Jane's chart.
   b. tell Jane to take a shower; the warm water may make it feel better.
   c. tell Jane to remain in bed, and notify the physician of the findings.
   d. take no action.
3. Lynne MacDonald is breast-feeding her baby. She complains of sore nipples. The nurse would
   a. tell her to stop nursing until the soreness is gone.
   b. check to see if the infant is attaching properly to the breast when nursing.
   c. tell her to cut the nursing time in half until the soreness is gone.
   d. tell her that this is normal when you are nursing an infant.
4. Brenda Zagarinski is 7 hours postpartum and has voided 75 mL, 100 mL, and 25 mL consecutively since the birth. The nurse would
   a. record these amounts on the intake and output sheet.
   b. force fluids to increase her output.
   c. notify the physician to obtain an order for catheterization for residual.
   d. take no action.
5. Danielle Munisteri is 3 days postpartum and has been crying and states she feel irritable and "out of sorts." She asks the nurse, "What is wrong with me? The baby is fine, and I am fine; why am I acting like this?" The nurse would tell her,
   a. "ask your physician when she visits."
   b. "I did the same thing when I had my last baby."
   c. "Many mothers experience these feelings after birth. It is probably due to all the hormonal and physical changes in your body. It will pass."
   d. "It is probably normal. I just hope you get over it before your husband brings your other children in to visit."

references 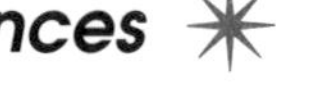

Beck, C. T., Reynolds, M. A., & Rutowski, P. (1992). Maternity blues and postpartum depression. *Journal of Obstetric, Gynecologic, and Neonatal Nursing, 21*(4), 287–292.

Pernoll, M. L. (1991). Current obstetric and gynecologic diagnosis and treatment (7th ed.). Norwalk, CT: Appleton and Lange.

Ralph, K., & Alexander, J. (1994). Borne under stress. *Nursing times, 90*(12), 28–29.

bibliography

Carpenito, L. J. (1995). *Nursing diagnosis application to clinical practice* (6th ed.). Philadelphia: J.B. Lippincott.

Cronin, R., Quansah, M., & Larson, E. (1993). Obstetric infection control in a developing country. *Journal of Obstetric, Gynecologic, and Neonatal Nursing, 22*(2), 137–143.

Cunningham, F. G., McDonald, P. C., Leveno, K. J., Gant, N.F., & Gilstrap, L. (1993). *Williams obstetrics* (19th ed.). Norwalk, CT: Appleton and Lange.

Gerbaso, F.R., Bottoms, S., Farag, A., & Mammen, E. (1990). Changes in hemostasis activity during delivery and the immediate postpartum period. *American Journal of Obstetrics and Gynecology, 162*(5), 1158–1163.

Goldaber, K. G., Wendel, P. J., McIntire, D. D., & Wendel, G. D. (1993). Postpartum perineal morbidity after fourth-degree perineal repair. *American Journal of Obstetrics and Gynecology, 168*(2), 489–492.

Harrigan, R., Haber, M. M., Hensen, K. A., Tse, A., & Perez, D. (1993) Perinatal grief: Response to the loss of an infant. *Neonatal network, 12*(5), 25–31.

Kenner, C. A., & Mac Laren, A. (1993). *Essentials of maternal and neonatal nursing.* Springhouse, PA: Springhouse Corporation.

May, K. A., & Mahlmeister, L. R. (1994). *Maternal and neonatal nursing: Family-centered care* (3rd ed.). Philadelphia: J.B. Lippincott.

Olds, S. B., London, M. L., & Ladewig, P. W. (1992). *Maternal-newborn nursing: A family-centered approach* (4th ed.). Redwood City, CA: Addison-Wesley Nursing.

Olsen, C. G., & Gordon, R. E. (1990). Breast disorders in nursing mothers. *American Family Physician, 41*(5), 1509–1515.

Pillitteri, A. (1995). *Maternal and child health nursing,* 2nd ed. Philadelphia: J.B. Lippincott.

Reeder, S. J., Martin, L. L., & Koniak, D. (1992). *Maternity nursing* (17th ed.). Philadelphia: J.B. Lippincott.

Schmidt, J. M., & Schimpeler, S. M. (1990). Obstetric and gynecologic abdominal wound infections:a comprehensive nurse-managed program. *The Journal of Perinatal and Neonatal Nursing, 4*(3), 25–43.

Trevelyan, J. (1994). Please tell mother. *Nursing times, 90*(9), 38–39.

Ugarroza. D. N. (1992). Postpartum affective disorders: Incidence and treatment. *Journal of Psychosocial Nursing, 30*(5), 29–32.

nursing care of the normal newborn

16

outline

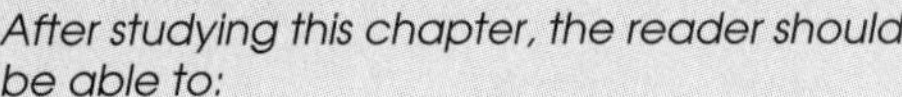

objectives

After studying this chapter, the reader should be able to:

* Name the seven immediate needs of the newborn.
* Discuss the benefits of breast-feeding.
* Evaluate the nutritional status of the newborn.
* Assess the physical characteristics of the newborn.
* Measure vital signs in the newborn.
* Discuss the physiologic transition from intrauterine to extrauterine life.
* Name 10 reflexes present in the newborn at birth.
* Describe three appropriate methods for holding a newborn.
* Perform a newborn bath.
* Describe the circumcision procedure and nursing care after circumcision.

key terms

acrocyanosis
caput succedaneum
cephalhematoma
cradle cap
Epstein's pearls
erythema toxicum
fontanel
hemangioma
icterus neonatorum
lanugo
milia
mongolian spots
neonate
nevus flammeus
phimosis
pathologic jaundice
physiologic jaundice
telangiectatic nevi
thermogenesis
vernix caseosa

During pregnancy, the fetus develops and matures until approximately 40 weeks' gestation, when he or she is fully prepared to separate from the warm, fluid intrauterine environment and enter extrauterine life. During development, the fetus depends on fetal circulation to meet basic physiologic needs of oxygen and nutrients. At birth, the neonate must adapt to extrauterine life by establishing and maintaining respirations, ingesting and digesting nutrients, eliminating waste material, and regulating body temperature.

nursing considerations

The first few hours in a newborn's life are the most critical. To be able to make and perform accurate nursing assessments and interventions, the nurse must have a thorough understanding of physiologic and behavioral changes that occur as the newborn adapts to extrauterine life. If the nurse observes deviations from normal at the initial assessment, serious complications in the newborn may be prevented. The nurse also must educate and support the family during this adjustment period.

Nursing goals include the following:

* Initiation and maintenance of a patent airway
* Prevention of hypothermia
* Prevention of infection
* Protection from injury
* Promotion of attachment
* Education of caregivers about newborn care and recognition of the need for medical intervention
* Provision of additional information and support for the teenage mother and the mother older than 35 years

family considerations

Becoming a parent is exciting and frightening. A demanding, totally dependent newborn requires attention, regardless of the needs of other family members. Family roles and positions change. Mothers, fathers, siblings, and grandparents are busy adjusting to their new roles based on personal attitudes, cultural practices, and belief systems. Most parents are eager to learn and embrace the challenge of parenthood.

Teenage mothers are faced with the challenge of becoming a mature adult who is responsible for a tiny, dependent individual. This requires knowledgeable, responsible parenting. Some continue to live at home and receive assistance and support from their parents, while others choose to live on their own and need financial assistance.

The first-time mother who is older than 35 years also may have adjustments to make. Many women older than 35 years have established careers and organized, scheduled lives. It can be a shock to find that the newborn sets its own schedule and will demand "loudly" that its needs be met.

Parents require compassion, patience, and support from the maternity nurse to meet new challenges that await them.

needs and care of the newborn

All newborns *must* be identified before leaving the delivery room. Several methods of identification may be used, such as bracelets or ankle bands. Identifying information should include the identification numbers of the infant and the mother. Newborn footprints and maternal fingerprints also are obtained shortly after birth.

When the newborn arrives in the nursery, the nurse confirms the presence of identification bracelets, places the infant under warming lights, and weighs and measures him or her. Temperature is assessed by placing the thermometer in the axilla and holding the arm gently against the chest. The thermometer must touch the skin to obtain an accurate axillary temperature. The nurse assesses physical characteristics, vital signs, gestational age, and body systems of the newborn.

The newborn has several needs that must be met to survive:

* Establishment of a patent airway
* Maintenance of respirations
* Maintenance of body temperature
* Nutrition
* Protection from infection and hemorrhage
* Sleep and rest
* Attachment

Nursing care is directed at meeting these needs and preparing the mother or other caregivers to continue care of the infant at home.

patent airway and maintenance of respirations

A patent airway must be established to maintain respirations in the newborn. The infant's airway may be filled with amniotic fluid, blood, or other fluids associated with the birthing process. The head is lowered to facilitate drainage of secretions. It may be necessary to suction gently the nose and mouth of the newborn using a soft bulb syringe.

nursing alert

When suctioning the newborn with a bulb syringe, always suction the mouth first and then the nose to prevent aspiration of mucous into the lungs.

Gentle manipulation of the newborn, such as rubbing the back, may stimulate crying. Lusty crying will cause the infant to draw in oxygen, causing full expansion of the lungs.

The respiratory rate of the newborn is usually 40 to 60 breaths per minute; however, a transitory tachypnea (with brief periods of apnea lasting less than 10 seconds) can occur in which the rate will range between 60 and 80 for the first day or two of life. Activity such as crying increases the respiratory rate.

maintenance of body temperature

Maintaining the newborn's body temperature in the immediate postpartum period is critical. In utero, the body temperature of the fetus is approximately 1 degree higher than that of the mother. At birth, the infant experiences an immediate drop in body temperature. Therefore, it is important to dry and wrap the infant in a blanket, place a cap on the head, and give the infant to the mother to hold. After the initial attachment period, the infant may be placed under a radiant warmer to maintain body temperature (Fig. 16-1).

The skin of the newborn is relatively thin, with little subcutaneous fat to insulate the internal organs. In addition, the nervous system, which controls heat production, is immature. This causes instability in the regulation of body temperature. The cardiovascular system is not yet fully functional, as seen by *acrocyanosis*, the transitory bluish discoloration of the hands and feet of the newborn, which lasts approximately 12 hours after birth. All of these factors place the newborn at risk for hypothermia.

The full-term newborn is born with brown fat, which helps to increase body temperature. Brown fat is located behind the sternum, in the neck, and between the scapulae of the newborn. Norepinephrine is released by the adrenal gland at the site of nerve endings in brown fat tissue, aiding in the metabolism of fats and resulting in *thermogenesis* (production of heat). Increased metabolism and oxygen consumption also cause thermogenesis. Even with these compensating factors, the newborn is at risk for loss of acceptable body temperature. The axillary temperature of the newborn should be between 97.6° and 98.6°F (36.5°–37°C).

Newborn infants do not shiver. If shivering is noted in the newborn, it indicates that the metabolic rate has doubled. The extra muscular activity created by shivering is of little help in raising the body temperature.

The newborn can lose body heat into the surrounding environment through evaporation, conduction, convection, and radiation. *Evaporation* can occur whenever the infant is wet. *Conduction* of body heat occurs when the infant's skin is touched by cold surfaces or objects. *Convection* of heat occurs through cold moving air, such as in a drafty room. *Radiation* heat loss occurs when the infant is placed near (but not touching) cold objects, such as walls or windows. Heat loss causes cold stress, which can result in hypoglycemia, hypoxia, metabolic acidosis, pulmonary vasoconstriction, and increased respiratory distress.

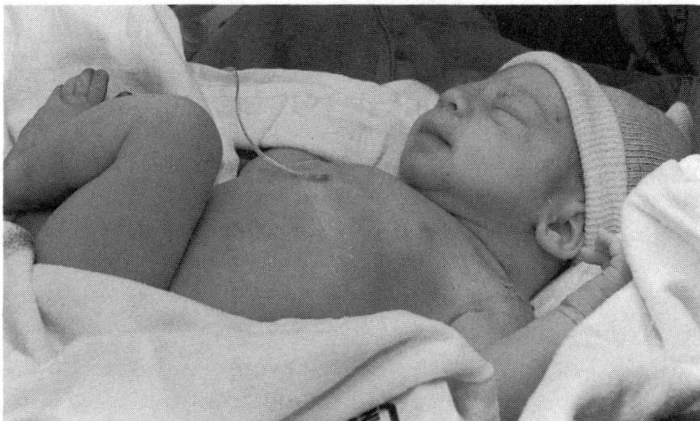

figure 16-1 *Newborn under radiant warmer.*

When assessing the newborn, the nurse does not evaluate body temperature based on the temperature of the hands and feet. Acrocyanosis will cause the fingers and feet to feel cool to the touch due to the immature cardiovascular system.

The nurse also monitors the newborn to make sure the body temperature is not too high. The *sudoriferous glands* (sweat glands) are not fully functional until approximately 4 weeks after birth. If the newborn becomes overheated, a red, pinpoint rash will appear, sometimes called *prickly heat.*

nutrition

The newborn may be "born hungry" or may fail to show interest in eating for a day or two after birth. The nurse needs to recognize signs of hunger in the newborn, which include restlessness, crying, rooting, and sucking. The newborn's need for nourishment can be met by breast-feeding and bottle feeding. Regardless of the method, feeding the infant can be an emotionally satisfying time for mother and newborn. If formula feeding is chosen, the father and other caregivers can participate in this experience as well.

breast-feeding

Breast-feeding is universally accepted and recommended as the ideal method of infant feeding. Breast-feeding provides the infant with immunity against certain diseases to which the mother has been exposed. In addition, breast-fed babies seem to have fewer respiratory infections and gastrointestinal disturbances than formula-fed infants.

If the mother has chosen to breast-feed, the newborn will often be placed at the breast immediately after birth, even before the placenta has separated from the uterine lining. The newborn is fed on demand, usually every 2 to 3 hours. The mother needs to know that it may take three or four days before her supply of breast milk is well established. Until that time, a thin, yellow, milky fluid called *colostrum* is secreted. Colostrum contains proteins, minerals, less fat, and fewer carbohydrates than breast milk and is easily digested by the newborn.

The mother and newborn should be comfortable during feeding. The cradle hold (Fig. 16-2*A*) is used most often. However, the mother may assume a side-lying position and use pillows to help support the infant.

The nursing mother needs to maintain a balanced diet. Caloric intake should be increased approximately 500 calories more per day than the prepregnancy diet. The diet needs to include at least 1 quart of milk daily, and the physician will probably recommend additional intake of vitamins A, B complex, and C. The physician should be consulted about any prescription or over-the-counter

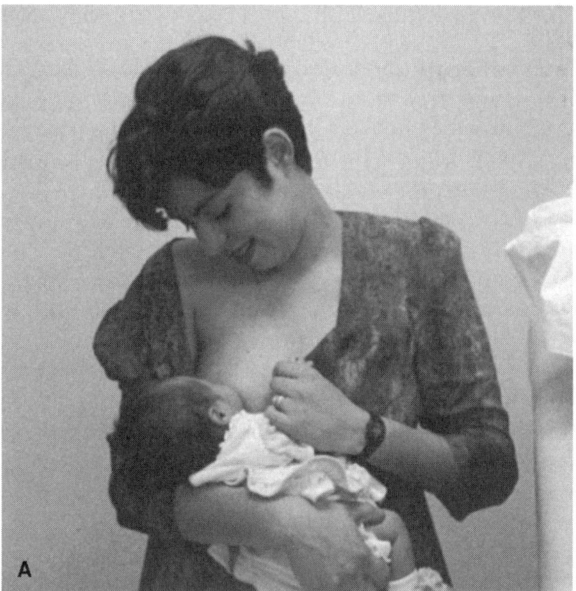

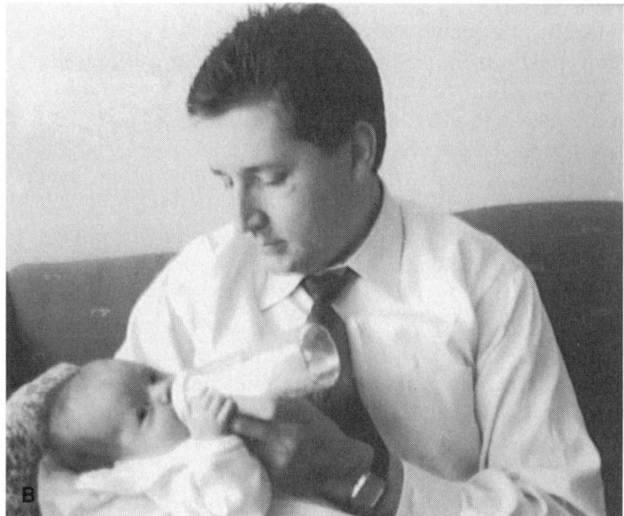

figure 16-2 *The cradle hold.* ***(A)*** *Breast-feeding.* ***(B)*** *Bottle feeding.*

medications taken by the mother because many of these are secreted in breast milk. (See Chap. 14 for more information.)

bottle feeding

Some mothers may choose not to breast-feed, or they may not be able to breast-feed. They should not be made to feel guilty or inadequate regarding their decision. Many kinds of infant formulas are available that meet the infant's nutritional needs.

The infant needs to be burped after each ounce of formula taken. This releases swallowed air that otherwise may cause colic.

The cradle hold is recommended when bottle feeding the infant (see Fig. 16-2*B*). Studies indicate that middle ear infections can result from feeding the infant in the supine position or from propping the bottle. Under no circumstances should the bottle be propped for feeding. (See Chap. 14 for more information.)

nutritional assessment

All newborns lose weight during the first few days after birth. This weight loss can be as much as 10% of the birth weight and can be alarming to the new mother. The nurse needs to reassure the caregiver that some weight loss is normal and expected during the first few days of life.

The nutritional status of the newborn may be evaluated by observing the following:

* Signs of dehydration. The newborn should have at least six wet diapers per day. Signs of dehydration include dry, hard stools; dark urine; dry mucous membranes; and sunken fontanels.
* Behavior. The newborn should appear content after feedings.
* Weight gain. Daily weight is monitored; normal weight gain is approximately 1 oz per day after the initial weight loss.

protection from infection and hemorrhage

The newborn has little resistance to infection. For this reason, each newborn is kept in a separate crib. Personnel with communicable infections (eg, sore throat, herpes simplex) are excluded from caring for mothers and newborns until the infection has cleared. Babies born outside the hospital are isolated until cultures demonstrate that they are free of infection. Caregivers and visitors need to be taught proper handwashing techniques and reminded to wash their hands thoroughly before holding or feeding the newborn.

While still in the delivery suite, the nurse follows universal precautions and uses a soft cloth to wipe amniotic fluid and blood gently from the face and scalp of the newborn. Some vernix may be removed during this process; however, vernix is considered a protectant and lubricant for newborn skin and is generally left in place. Bathing of the newborn is delayed until the newborn's temperature has stabilized.

Most states legally mandate the instillation of prophylactic antibiotic ointment (erythromycin 0.5% or tetracycline 1%) into the eyes of the newborn to prevent *ophthalmia neonatorum,* caused by maternal infection with *Neisseria gonorrhoeae.* Because this treatment temporarily interferes with newborn vision, it may be delayed for 1 hour after birth to allow time for the infant and mother to establish eye contact and initial attachment.

After cord pulsation has stopped, the cord is compressed using two compression clamps placed about 2 in from the abdomen. This delayed clamping supplies the newborn with approximately 100 mL of blood from the placenta, which provides extra iron. The cord is observed frequently for bleeding. An intramuscular injection of vitamin K (0.5–1 mg) is given in the anterior thigh to decrease the possibility of hemorrhage due to the naturally low prothrombin levels in the newborn.

cord care

Care of the umbilical cord stump consists of the application of Triple Dye or other antiseptic, such as alcohol 70%, which promotes drying of the stump. (Other solutions may be used, depending on hospital policy.) Triple Dye is applied at the base of the cord, skin margins, and tip of the cord. The antiseptic solution is applied at the time of bathing and at diaper changing. The stump is kept clean and dry and is observed for signs of infection, such as redness, malodor, moisture, or drainage from the site. Any of these signs should be reported immediately to the supervising nurse.

attachment (bonding)

The importance of attachment or bonding in establishing positive parent–child and caregiver–child relationships is being increasingly emphasized. The newborn needs to be nurtured and loved to survive. Nursing assessment needs to include observation of signs of attachment to plan effective intervention if a problem is apparent.

The newborn is more active and alert during the first hour after birth than during the hours that follow. No matter how long or difficult the labor has been, the new mother usually experiences a feeling of elation when she first sees her newborn. The mother usually places the newborn in a position facing her, establishes eye contact, and talks to the newborn in soft tones. She then inspects every part of the newborn (first counting the fingers and toes) and tells the newborn how beautiful he or she is. The mother relies on her sense of sight, touch, and hearing to get to know her newborn during this initial acquaintance phase of bonding.

The nurse should observe the attachment process with the following questions in mind:

* How does the mother interact with the newborn?
* Does she take part in daily infant care?
* Does she verbalize pleasure with the appearance and sex of the newborn?
* Does the mother seem to understand the needs of her newborn?

These same questions may be used when assessing the attachment of the father or other caregivers and the newborn.

sleep and rest

The newborn sleeps approximately 18 to 20 hours a day. The newborn may awaken occasionally in response to noise or other activity but easily settles back to sleep. Hunger will cause the newborn to awaken every 3 to 4 hours. Eventually, the hours of wakefulness increase.

assessment of physical characteristics

Assessment of the newborn begins with careful inspection and observation of the newborn's appearance. Working from head to toe, the nurse assesses general physical characteristics and measures weight, length, head and chest circumference, and vital signs (Table 16-1).

general physical characteristics

skin

The skin of a white newborn should be pink tinged and slightly warm. The African American newborn's skin will appear reddish black. Asian newborns will have skin the color of tea with a rose tinge. The ruddy color of newborn skin is attributed to the concentration of red blood cells in the blood vessels and limited subcutaneous fat. The turgor of normal newborn skin is elastic, although the skin of the hands and feet may be dry and peeling.

Vernix caseosa is a whitish yellow, greasy textured, cheeselike substance that covers the fetus in utero. It consists of epithelial cells and secretions of the sebaceous glands. Distribution of vernix over the body varies, but it is usually more pronounced in folds of skin and in the labia. Vernix is a skin protectant and lubricant. Although it is customary for the nurse to gently wipe off the vernix, some authorities now suggest that it be left in place to provide lubrication for the skin of the newborn. The amount of vernix decreases with the maturity of the newborn; thus, full-term and postterm newborns have less vernix caseosa than the preterm infant.

Milia appear as small, raised white spots on the face, especially across the bridge of the nose. They are easily recognized because they resemble what is commonly known as a pimple. Milia result from clogged sebaceous glands. The new mother may be concerned about the appearance of milia, but she should be reassured that they will disappear shortly. Milia should never be squeezed or pinched.

Lanugo is the soft, downlike growth of hair commonly seen on the shoulders and back of the normal newborn. Some infants may have lanugo on the forehead and face, especially on the sides of the cheeks, resembling sideburns. Like vernix caseosa, lanugo decreases with maturity of the newborn; thus, it is more evident in the preterm infant. It disappears in the first few days after birth.

Erythema toxicum, also known as "newborn rash," appears as firm white or whitish yellow papules or pustules varying in size from 1 to 3 mm. Erythema usually appears

table 16-1 summary of newborn physical assessment

Assessment Area	Usual Findings	Deviations
GENERAL OBSERVATIONS		
Muscle tone	Flexed position; good tone	"Floppy"; rigid or tense
Skin		
Color	Pink to ruddy when crying; appropriate to ethnic origin; acrocyanosis	Pallor; cyanosis; jaundice; ecchymosis; petechiae
Texture	Smooth; dryness with some peeling; lanugo on back; vernix	Excessive peeling or cracking; roughness
Rashes and pigmentation	Erythema toxicum; milia; mongolian spots	Impetigo; hemangiomas; nevus flammeus (port-wine stain)
Hydration	Skin pinch over abdomen immediately returns to original state	Skin maintains "tent" shape after pinch
Cry	Lusty	Shrill; weak; grunty
MEASUREMENTS		
Weight	2,700–4,000 g (6–9 lb)	
Length	48–53 cm (19–21 in)	
Head circumference	33–37 cm (13–14.5 in)	
Chest circumference	31–35 (12.5–14 in)	
VITAL SIGNS		
Temperature	Axillary (preferred method)—36.5–37°C (97.7–98.6°F) Rectal—36.5–37.2°C (97.7–99°F)	Hypothermia; fever
Respirations	40–60 respirations/min; quiet and shallow; diaphragmatic; occasional periods of rapid breathing, alternating with short periods of apnea	Prolonged rapid breathing; apnea lasting longer than 10 sec; grunting; retractions; persistent slow rate
Heart rate (apical pulse)	120–160 beats/min; faster when crying (up to 180 beats/min); slower when sleeping (down to 100 beats/min)	Tachycardia—greater than 160 beats/min at rest Bradycardia—less than 120 beats/min when awake
HEAD	Vaginal delivery—elongated (molding) Breech or cesarean birth—round, symmetrical Size within normal range	Caput succedaneum; cephalhematoma; hydrocephaly; microcephaly
Fontanels	Flat; soft; firm	Bulging; sunken
Anterior	Diamond shaped; 2–3 cm wide; 3–4 cm long; smaller at birth with molding	Small; almost closed; closed (craniostenosis); widened
Posterior	Triangular shape; small; almost closed	Enlarged
Face	Small; round; symmetrical; fat pads in cheeks; receding chin	Asymmetrical; distorted
Eyes	Edematous lids; usually closed; blue or slate-gray; no tears; red reflex present; pupils equal, round, react to light	Elevation or ptosis of lids; epicanthal folds; absence of red reflex; unequal, dilated, or constricted pupils
	Common variations—subconjunctival hemorrhages; chemical conjunctivitis; occasional slight nystagmus or convergent strabismus	Purulent discharge; frequent nystagmus; constant, divergent, or unilateral strabismus
Mouth	Intact lips, gums, palate; epithelial pearls; "sucking blisters" on lips; tongue midline, mobile, appropriate size for mouth; can extend to alveolar ridge	Cleft lip or palate; white, cheesy patches on tongue, gums, or mucous membrane; large or protruding tongue

(continued)

table 16-1 summary of newborn physical assessment (continued)

Assessment Area	*Usual Findings*	*Deviations*
Nose	In midline; even placement in relation to eyes and mouth; nares patent; septum intact, midline	Flattened or bruised; unusual placement or configuration; obstructed nares; deviated or perforated septum
Ears	Well-formed cartilage; appropriate size for head; upper attachment on line extended through inner and outer canthus of eye; external auditory canal patent	Floppy, large, and protruding; malformed; low set; obstruction of canal
NECK	Short; thick; full range of motion; no masses	Webbing; abnormal shortening; limitation of motion; torticollis; masses
CLAVICLES	Straight; smooth; intact	Knot or lump; decreased movement of extremity on one side
THORAX	Round; symmetrical; protruding xiphoid process	Asymmetrical; funnel chest
Breath sounds	Loud; bronchial; bilaterally equal	Decreased breath sounds; increased breath sounds; absent breath sounds
Heart sounds	Regular rate and rhythm; first and second sounds clear and distinct	Murmurs; arrhythmias
Breasts	Symmetrical; flat with erect nipples; engorgement 2nd or 3rd day not unusual	Redness and firmness around nipple
ABDOMEN	Symmetrical; slightly protuberant; no masses	Scaphoid or concave shape; distention; palpable masses; asymmetrical
Liver	Palpable 2–3 cm below right costal margin	Enlargement
Spleen	Tip may be palpable in left upper quadrant	Enlargement
Kidneys	May be palpable at level of umbilicus	Enlargement
Femoral pulses	Bilaterally equal	Unequal or absent
Umbilicus	No extensive protrusion or herniation; no signs of infection	Umbilical hernia; omphalocele; redness; induration; foul-smelling discharge
	Cord—bluish white, moist → black, dry; 3 vessels; no oozing or bleeding	Two vessels; bleeding or oozing from stump
GENITALIA	Appropriate for gender	Ambiguous genitalia
Female		
Labia	Edematous; labia majora cover labia minora; vernix in creases	Hematoma; lesions; fusion of labia
Vagina	Mucous discharge, possibly blood tinged	
Male		
Foreskin	Adherent to glans of penis	Opening below tip of penis (hydrospadias)
Urethra	Opening at tip of penis	Opening above tip of penis (epispadias)
Testes	Palpable in each scrotal sac	Palpable in inguinal canal; not palpable
POSTERIOR OF BODY		
Spinal column	Straight, flexible; intact, no masses	Exaggerated curves; spina bifida; any masses; pilonidal cyst
Anus	Patent	Imperforate anus; anal fissures
EXTREMITIES	Symmetrical in size, shape, and movement	Unequal or abnormal size or shape; asymmetrical or limited movement of one or more extremities
Digits	Five on each hand and foot; appropriate size and shape	Missing digits; syndactyly (webbing); polydactyly (extra digits)

(continued)

table 16-1 summary of newborn physical assessment (continued)

Assessment Area	*Usual Findings*	*Deviations*
Hips	Even leg length, knee height, gluteal folds; no resistance or limitation to abduction	Uneven leg length, knee height, or gluteal folds; uneven or limited abduction; hip "click" or "clunk" on abduction
Feet	Straight, or postural deviation easily corrected with gentle pressure	Structural deformities—talipes equinovarus (clubfoot; metatarsus abdductus)
REFLEXES		
Rooting and sucking	Turns toward object touching cheek, lips, or corner of mouth; opens mouth; begins sucking movements; strong suck, pulls object into mouth	No rooting; weak, ineffective, or absent suck
	May be diminished or absent after eating	
Grasp		
Palmar	Fingers grasp object when palm stimulated and hang on briefly	Weak or absent
Plantar	Toes curl downward when soles of feet are stimulated	Weak or absent
Moro	Symmetrical response to sudden stimulus—lateral extension of arms with opening of hands, followed by flexion and adduction	Asymmetrical; absent; incomplete
Stepping	Stepping movements when infant held upright with sole of foot touching surface	Asymmetrical or absent

within a day or two after birth. It is widespread over the body but does not appear on the palms of the hands or the soles of the feet. The rash usually disappears within a few hours or days after birth and does not require treatment. The cause is not known, and cultures from the lesions do not show bacterial growth.

Icterus neonatorum, also known as *physiologic jaundice,* appears in many newborns on the second or third day after birth, giving the skin a yellowish appearance. This is a normal manifestation of the breakdown of excessive red blood cells in the newborn, causing the yellowish skin color. During intrauterine life, when the oxygen needs of the fetus were met by the fetal circulation, more red blood cells were needed. With the establishment of external respirations, however, the need for red blood cells is greatly reduced. Breakdown of red cells also causes a rise in serum bilirubin levels to 12 mg/100 mL by the fifth day of life.

If yellowish discoloration of the skin appears within 24 hours of birth, the condition is called *pathologic jaundice.* This condition is characterized by serum bilirubin levels above 6 mg/100 mL within the first 24 hours of birth or jaundice that persists for more than 7 days. This condition most often results from Rh and ABO incompatibilities.

birthmarks

Several kinds of birthmarks may be noted on the skin of the newborn. Some of these are temporary and will fade with time. Others may be large and disfiguring, requiring surgical or other treatment to remove.

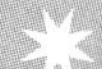

nursing alert

If the newborn develops jaundice within the first 24 hours of birth or if it persists longer than 7 days, it is pathologic and requires intervention.

Mongolian spots are slate-gray discolorations present at birth and most frequently noted on the buttocks or lower portion of the back of the newborn. They are seen more frequently in African American, Asian, or Mediterranean newborns. These spots do not require treatment and usually fade during the preschool years.

Nevus flammeus is a type of hemangioma, also known as "port wine stain." This is a capillary angioma located just below the epidermis. These birthmarks are not elevated, are red to purple, and generally appear on the face. They do not increase in size, nor do they fade with time. In the African American newborn, the nevus may be jet black. The port wine hemangioma may be treated with laser surgery or the injection of a sclerosing agent.

Telangiectatic nevi, commonly referred to as "stork bites" are temporary, superficial vascular lesions formed by the dilation of a group of small blood vessels. They may appear as a fine red line and are sometimes seen at the nape of the neck, upper eyelid or upper lip. They do not require treatment and usually disappear spontaneously within the first year. Other types of superficial hemangiomas, which include "strawberry" or "raspberry" marks, often disappear without treatment as the infant matures.

Stork bite redder when cries, disappears later

forceps marks and vacuum extraction marks

Forcep deliveries may produce bruised areas on the newborn. They resemble the shape of the forceps, fade within a few days, and produce no lasting effects.

Vacuum extraction of the newborn may produce caput swelling. The swelling usually subsides within a few days and produces no lasting effects.

head and neck

The head of the normal newborn is relatively large in proportion to the body and is approximately 70% of its adult size. During labor and delivery, the head is subjected to pressure in the birth canal and may initially appear misshapen, a condition referred to as *molding.*

The neck of the newborn is relatively short and creased. The normal newborn's head should be able to be turned freely from side to side. The neck cannot support the weight of the head, although when in the prone position, the newborn may be able to raise the head slightly. When the newborn is lifted, the head needs to be supported.

molding The flexibility of the cranial bones allows them to adapt to the shape of the birth canal, sometimes giving the newborn's head an asymmetric appearance. The degree of molding depends on the amount and duration of pressure exerted during labor and delivery. This can be alarming to the mother, who needs reassurance that the molding is temporary and should disappear within a week. With cesarean delivery, newborns typically have round, well-shaped heads.

fontanels The two spaces or "soft spots" where the cranial bones come together are called *fontanels.* The *anterior fontanel* is a diamond-shaped opening at the juncture of the two parietal and two frontal bones of the cranium. It is approximately 3 cm (1.2 in) long and 2 cm (0.75 in) wide, although the size varies considerably from one newborn to another. It may be possible to see pulsation at the anterior fontanel.

The triangular *posterior fontanel* is smaller than the anterior fontanel and appears almost closed. The posterior fontanel closes between 6 weeks and 2 months of age; the anterior closes within 9 to 18 months of age.

Occasionally *cradle cap* (seborrheic dermatitis), a build-up of thick, oily crust formations, occurs over the anterior fontanel. This condition most commonly occurs when the area is not cleansed properly, probably because of fear on the part of the mother or caregiver. The mother should be assured that both fontanels are protected by a thick, cartilaginous membrane and that normal shampooing of the head and scalp is not harmful. See Chapter 37.

As the nurse assesses the location and size of the fontanels, the head of the newborn is evaluated for soft-tissue edema or bruising. Depending on the duration and difficulty of labor, the bruising can range from minor to severe.

cephalhematoma When labor is unusually prolonged and the birth canal is small in relation to the size of the fetus, blood vessels are ruptured and blood collects between the periosteum and skull bone; this is called a *cephalhematoma.* The skin over the cephalhematoma may feel loose and slightly edematous. This condition usually resolves within a few weeks without treatment.

caput succedaneum Sustained pressure during labor or the use of a vacuum extractor to aid in delivery can cause *caput succedaneum,* an area of edema (and sometimes bleeding) between the scalp and the periosteum. Caput succedaneum is easily recognized by the nurse and can be differentiated from cephalhematoma because caput crosses suture lines and a cephalhematoma does not (Table 16-2). Caput succedaneum usually resolves without treatment during the first few hours or days after birth, depending on the size. When the condition is caused by a vacuum extractor, it usually takes longer to resolve than caput caused by pressure on the presenting part in the birth canal.

eyes

Most infants have dark blue or blue-gray irises and bluish sclera; however, dark-skinned infants have darker eyes. The true color of the infant's eyes is not apparent until 3 to 6 months of age. Strabismus (crossed eyes) may be present at birth due to poor neuromuscular control. The newborn can see and fixate on faces, shapes, and colors. Visual acuity is best within a range of 9 to 12 in.

The nurse should assess the newborn's eyes for pupillary size and equality, pupillary reaction to light, and presence of the blink reflex. Some newborns may have small subconjunctival hemorrhages resulting from changes in ocular pressure during birth. Parents need reassurance that these hemorrhages will resolve within a few days without treatment.

It is not uncommon for the eyelids to be swollen during the first few days after birth due to the trauma of delivery. Prophylactic administration of antibiotic drops or ointment may irritate the eye.

The lacrimal glands are not fully functional at birth and do not mature until approximately 2 months of age. Thus, the cries of the newborn are tearless.

ears

The ears of the newborn may be flattened and folded against the head, but the cartilage is normally well formed. The sometimes crumpled appearance is due to the position of the fetus in utero. In the normal newborn, the top of the ear is parallel with the outer canthus of the eye. Low-set ears may indicate chromosomal abnormalities, often resulting in kidney disorders.

The newborn is able to hear and responds to noise from birth. Hearing is usually evaluated by the infant's response to loud noise. Some states require hospitals to incorporate a hearing test as part of newborn screening. This test is performed within 24 to 48 hours or before the infant leaves the hospital. The infant must be in a quiet resting or sleep state to assess hearing ability accurately.

table 16-2 comparison of caput succedaneum and cephalhematoma

Caput Succedaneum	Cephalhematoma
Localized soft-tissue edema	Soft, fluctuant, localized swelling
Appears at birth	Appears several hours after birth
Does not increase in size	Increases in size for 2–3 days
Disappears several days after birth vague, poorly defined outline	Disappears approximately 6 wk after birth
Has crosses suture lines	Has well-defined outline
Caused by diffuse, edematous swelling involving the soft tissues of the scalp	Never crosses suture lines
Complications; rarely, anemia	Caused by subperiosteal hemorrhage
	Complications: jaundice, underlying skull fracture, intracranial bleeding, shock

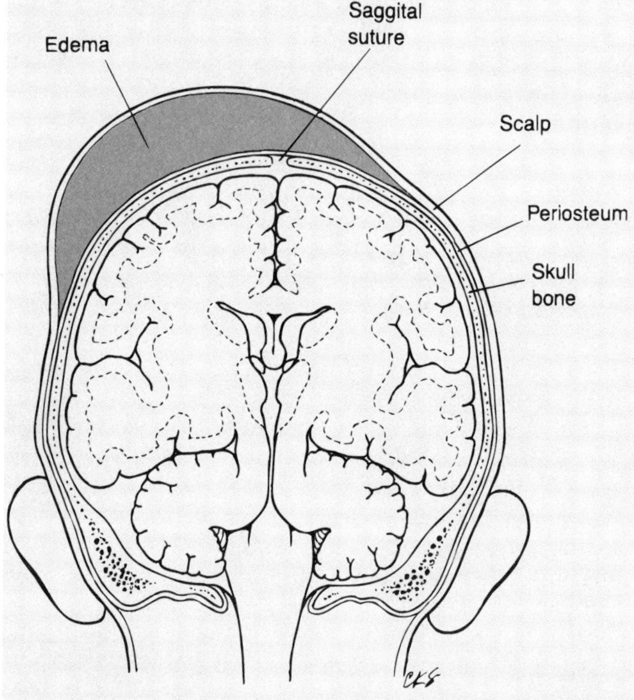

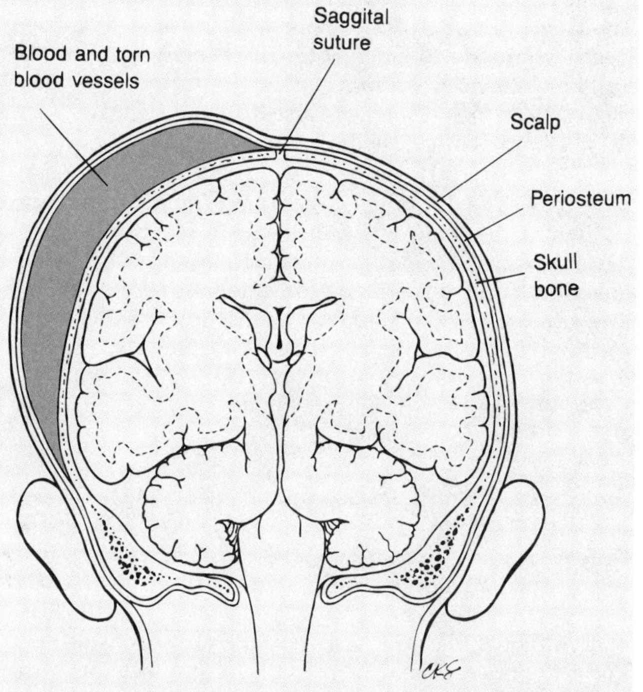

face

The newborn's face is designed for sucking. The chin is recessed, the nose small and flat, and the cheeks filled with fat pads to aid in sucking movements. The lips are normally pink and may have sucking calluses caused by strong sucking activity in utero. The sucking response is easily elicited by touching the lips.

The mouth of the newborn is easily observed if the infant is stimulated to cry by depressing the tongue with a clean, gloved finger. Crying causes the infant to open the mouth wide. *Epstein's pearls*, small, hard, shiny white specks on the hard palate and gum margins, are of no significance and disappear within a few days after birth. Oral mucous membranes in the newborn are normally moist and pink. Because the salivary glands are immature and produce little saliva, any heavy drooling or bubbling of oral mucus may indicate a tracheoesophageal fistula (see Chap. 17).

Monilia, commonly referred to as *thrush*, is a fungal infection caused by *Candida albicans* and is often transferred to the infant from the infected mother during birth. It appears as a white coating on the tongue and white patches on the cheeks and may be mistaken for milk curds. The white patches cannot be rinsed off with water and adhere to the mucous membranes. If the patches are scraped off, a reddened inflamed area can be observed, and bleeding may occur. Thrush is treated with nystatin instilled in the mouth and swabbed on oral lesions.

The newborn is a nose breather, making it essential to keep the narrow nasal passages open. Any mucus or swelling can lead to respiratory distress. Sneezing is the newborn's way of clearing the nasal passages.

The nurse assesses patency of nasal passages by closing the infant's mouth and holding one naris shut while checking the passage of air from the other naris. A mirror or a wisp of cotton can be placed at the open naris to check for movement of air.

abdomen

The abdomen of the normal newborn is cylindrical and slightly protruding. Initially, the umbilical cord is white and gelatinous; the two umbilical arteries and one umbilical vein are clearly visible. The nurse carefully observes the cord for signs of bleeding, especially for the first 24 hours after birth. The clamp applied at the time of birth needs to be checked and compression of the cord stump maintained. A bactericidal dye, such as Triple Dye or alcohol, is applied to the stump at bath time and with each diaper change to help prevent infection. Within 1 to 2 hours after birth, the cord begins to dry. Within a few days, it shrinks and becomes discolored, eventually turning dark. The nurse teaches the parents to check the cord for purulent discharge, swelling, and redness. Folding the diaper down away from the cord helps keep it dry. After about 10 days, the cord stump will slough off.

The abdomen is palpated to assess for masses or tenderness. The liver may be palpated approximately 1 cm below the right costal margin. Bowel sounds are present within 15 minutes after birth and may be heard as a tinkling sound in all four quadrants.

genitalia

female genitalia The genitalia of the newborn female may appear swollen due to maternal hormone activity. In the full-term infant, the labia majora completely cover the labia minora. In the preterm infant, the labia are underdeveloped, exposing the labia minora and the clitoris.

The nurse identifies the vaginal opening and the urinary meatus. A mucous discharge, possibly tinged with blood, may be apparent at the entry to the vagina. This is called *pseudomenstruation* and results from withdrawal of maternal estrogen at birth.

male genitalia The size of the penis and scrotum of the newborn boy will vary. The penis is assessed for correct placement of the urethra. The urethra is normally located at the center of the tip of the glans penis. The penis also is assessed for *phimosis*, a narrowing of the opening of the foreskin (prepuce) so that it cannot be retracted over the glans penis. The foreskin is not easily retracted at birth; however, true phimosis is rare. True phimosis will interfere with voiding; therefore, the adequacy of the urinary stream must be assessed. The full-term newborn boy urinates in a forceful stream that can project 6 to 8 inches upward in an arc. If parents choose to have the infant circumcised, the foreskin is surgically removed. See the Nursing Care Plan for the Family of the Male Newborn About to be Circumcised.

The scrotum of the full-term newborn boy is large and pendulous and the skin is rough. In the preterm boy, the scrotum is small and smooth, and the skin is shiny. The scrotum is gently palpated for the presence of both testicles. Normally the testicles will descend into the scrotal sac by the eighth month of intrauterine life. Cold temperature can cause the testicles to retract.

weight

The average newborn weighs between 6 and 8½ lb (2,700–3,850 g). The newborn boy weighs approximately ½ lb more than the average newborn girl. During the first few days after birth, it is not unusual for a newborn to lose up to 10% of the birth weight. The weight loss is attributed to elimination of urine and feces by the infant and to the initial decrease in fluid intake.

length

The average newborn measures between 19 and 21 in (47.5–53 cm). The average newborn boy is 20 in long, while the average newborn girl is 19.5 in long.

head circumference

The head of the newborn averages 13 to 14.5 in (33–37 cm) in circumference, approximately 2 cm larger than the chest circumference. The head is relatively large in proportion to the rest of the body, representing approximately one fourth of the total body size of the infant. In contrast, the head of the normal adult is approximately one eighth of total body size.

chest circumference

The circumference of the chest averages 12.5 to 14 in (31–35 cm), approximately 2 cm less than the head circumference. The chest is bell shaped, and the ribs are flexible. As previously mentioned, the breasts of the male or female newborn may be engorged due to maternal hormone levels. A pale, milky substance, commonly called "witches milk" may be expressed from the nipple. This condition usually occurs about the third day after birth and disappears within 2 to 4 weeks without treatment. The breasts of the infant should never be squeezed or massaged.

vital signs

respiratory rate

The respirations of the newborn are typically diaphragmatic or abdominal. The normal newborn respiratory rate is 30 to 60 respirations per minute but can increase with activity, such as crying. A quiet resting or sleeping respiratory rate of 45 or greater is considered abnormal. If respirations are costal in character or if sternal retraction or sucking in of the chest wall occurs, the charge nurse should be notified immediately because this is a sign of respiratory distress, which merits prompt attention.

The newborn usually breathes quietly. Newborns are nose breathers, so the nares should be kept free of dried mucus or other obstruction. Grunting type respirations on expiration or flaring of the nares during inspiration are signs of respiratory distress and should be brought to the attention of the supervising nurse.

nursing care plan
for the family of the male newborn about to be circumcised

NURSING DIAGNOSIS

Anxiety, Family, related to potential newborn pain with circumcision

GOAL: *Family will understand and be less anxious about the procedure, and the baby will not experience pain*

NURSING INTERVENTIONS	RATIONALE	EVALUATION
Educate parents on the importance of circumcision.	Circumcision is done for ease in hygiene, and potential for decrease in urinary tract infections. Uncircumcised males have a higher incidence of penile cancer.	The parents will state they understand the reason for the circumcision.
Inform parents of the procedure and the use of local anesthetic.	By informing the parents of the anesthetics used for this procedure the nurse can help to decrease their anxiety.	The parents will fell less anxious and ask appropriate questions related to the procedure.
Instruct the parents on the expected length of time the procedure will take.	The infant will be returned to the room within 1 hour and monitored for the following 4 hours.	The infant will be monitored hourly for signs of bleeding, and any complications will be reported immediately.

NURSING DIAGNOSIS

Knowledge Deficit, related to care of the newly circumcised male infant

GOAL: *Family will demonstrate the appropriate care and be able to verbalize signs that would warrant concern.*

NURSING INTERVENTIONS	RATIONALE	EVALUATION
Educate the parents on the appropriate care of the circumcised area.	This will give the parents the knowledge that will allow them to gain control of the new experience.	The parents will verbalize appropriate care of the newborn's circumcised area.
Teach the parents to clean the penis gently, using soap and water and, after rinsing well, to pat the area dry. Neosporin should then be applied to the site.	This will encourage adequate healing.	The parents will demonstate circumcision care prior to discharge from the hospital.
Inform the parents to notify the pediatrician if they see redness, purulent discharge, or if the babty cries in constant pain or has a fever >101°.	These are signs of infection and require prompt attention.	The parents will evaluate the healing process and state signs that indicate infection and require reporting.

pulse and blood pressure

The initial heart rate of the newborn immediately after birth is approximately 170 to 180 beats/min. Within 12 to 24 hours after birth, the rate will slow to approximately 120 to 150 beats/min during sleep and rise to 180 beats/min when the newborn is crying. The apical heart rate should be counted for 1 full minute, preferably while the newborn is sleeping or resting quietly because crying increases the heart rate. Peripheral pulses also should be monitored to ensure adequate circulation.

In the full-term newborn at rest, blood pressure is approximately 80/50. Crying may increase systolic and diastolic readings. A baseline blood pressure is measured during the initial assessment. The size of the blood pressure cuff depends on the size of the infant; blood pressure also should be assessed using Doppler for accuracy.

determination of gestational age

Determination of gestational age using scoring systems assists in determining the newborn's physical and neuromuscular maturity. Three commonly used tools include Dubowitz's maturity scale, Ballard's assessment tool, and Brazelton's neonatal assessment scale.

dubowitz's maturity scale

Dubowitz developed the first maturity rating scale. It was based on 21 criteria for evaluating physical and neuromuscular activity. The scale is highly accurate but time consuming to use and has largely been replaced by the modified form developed by Ballard.

ballard's assessment of gestational age

The Ballard assessment scale should be completed during the first 24 hours after birth because changes in the newborn's skin make it less reliable by the second day. Ideally, it is performed within the first 2 hours of life. The scoring takes approximately 5 minutes or less and is recommended by the Committee of Fetus and Newborn of American Academy of Pediatrics.

The Ballard scale assesses and scores physical characteristics (skin, lanugo, plantar creases, breast tissue, ears, and genitalia) and neuromuscular characteristics (posture, wrist flexion, arm recoil, popliteal angle, scarf sign, and heel-to-ear extension). The scores are added and compared with a column listing the gestational age. After determining the gestational age, the nurse then looks at birth weight, head circumference, and body length to determine if they are appropriate for gestational age.

brazelton's neonatal assessment scale

Terry Brazelton, a pediatrician, developed a scale to assess newborn behavior. Because it identifies normal versus abnormal behaviors in the newborn, the Brazelton assessment scale has been a valuable tool in assisting with parent–newborn attachment. The nurse must receive special training to perform the assessment. The newborn must be at least 3 days old, so the test is not usually performed in the hospital setting due to early discharge.

metabolic screening tests

phenylketonuria

Most states require screening for phenylketonuria, an autosomal recessive disorder that results in defective protein metabolism. If undetected, severe brain damage or mental retardation can result. The newborn should receive 2 to 3 days of breast milk or formula before the screening test is performed. The test requires using a heel stick to obtain three drops of blood that are placed on a card or special blotter paper. If the newborn is discharged before obtaining the sample, the parents are instructed to return after the appropriate amount of time for the sample collection. The results are usually mailed, and an appointment for follow-up can be made by the parents or caregivers.

blood sugar

Some infants are at risk for hypoglycemia (low blood sugar). Infants at risk include those larger than 9 lb, subjected to cold stress, or born to diabetic mothers. These infants have their blood sugar levels checked with a heel stick procedure. Some hospitals require all newborns to have a routine blood sugar test as part of the initial assessment. The normal newborn blood sugar is 40 to 80 mg/dL.

✱ nursing insight

To perform a heel stick properly on the newborn, the nurse does the following:

1. *Wears gloves*
2. *Washes and dries the heel*
3. *Wipes the heel with alcohol*
4. *Sticks the lateral side of the heel to obtain the specimen*

adaptation of body systems

As nurses assume more responsibility in the initial care and physical assessment of the newborn, it is essential to have a basic understanding of the neonate's physiologic transition from intrauterine to extrauterine life and how that transition affects all body systems. This enables the nurse to assess the newborn adequately, recognize deviations from the norm, and institute appropriate nursing interventions.

respiratory system

As if preparing for extrauterine life, the fetus "practices" respirations or breathing movements while in utero. However, because oxygen is supplied through the placenta and fetal circulation, these initial respiratory efforts serve no real purpose. During vaginal birth, the thorax is squeezed, and most of the fluid retained in the lungs during intrauterine life is forced out. The small amount of fluid remaining in the lungs is absorbed. When the chest wall expands after delivery, the first breath of air is inhaled. This causes an increase in alveolar PO_2 with subsequent relaxation of the pulmonary arteries. Pulmonary vascular resistance decreases, allowing increased pulmonary vascular flow. This results in oxygenation of newborn tissues.

Surfactant, a phospholipid, decreases the surface tension of the alveolar sacs. This allows them to fill with air and prevents them from collapsing with expiration, thereby maintaining functional residual capacity. Sufficient amounts of surfactant are usually not present in the fetus until the 36th week of gestation. Infants born before the 36th week usually require assisted ventilation.

cardiovascular system

Just as the expansion of the lungs with the first breath of the newborn decreases pulmonary vascular resistance, the clamping of the umbilical cord increases systemic vascular resistance with a subsequent rise in left atrial pressure. This physiologic change begins independent cardiovascular circulation in the newborn. It also initiates the closure of two fetal shunts, the *foramen ovale* and the *ductus arteriosus.* In utero, these shunts direct blood flow away from the lungs (see Chap. 6). When independent respiration is established, pressure in the left atrium increases due to decreased pulmonary resistance and increased pulmonary venous return to the left atrium. Pressure in the right atrium decreases due to the opening of the pulmonary circuit. These changes cause the closure of the foramen ovale, the opening between the right and left atria. Closure of the foramen ovale normally occurs within 1 to 2 hours after birth, and permanent closure occurs within several weeks.

Closure of the ductus arteriosus, the fetal vessel between the pulmonary artery and the aorta, usually occurs within 15 hours after birth. Closure is caused by increased systemic vascular pressure and increased pulmonary blood flow, reversing the blood flow across the ductus. Closure of the ductus allows the blood flow in the pulmonary artery to be directed entirely to the lungs. In addition, increased PO_2 levels cause constriction and subsequent fibrosis of the ductus arteriosus. Complete fibrosis of the ductus usually occurs within 21 days.

The exact mechanism for the closure of a third fetal shunt, called ductus venosus, is not fully understood. However, it appears that increased systemic vascular resistance causes decreased systemic venous return. This ends umbilical venous return, which in turn causes the ductus venosus to close. Closure of the ductus venosus allows perfusion of the liver. The transition from fetal to neonatal circulation is summarized in Figure 16-3.

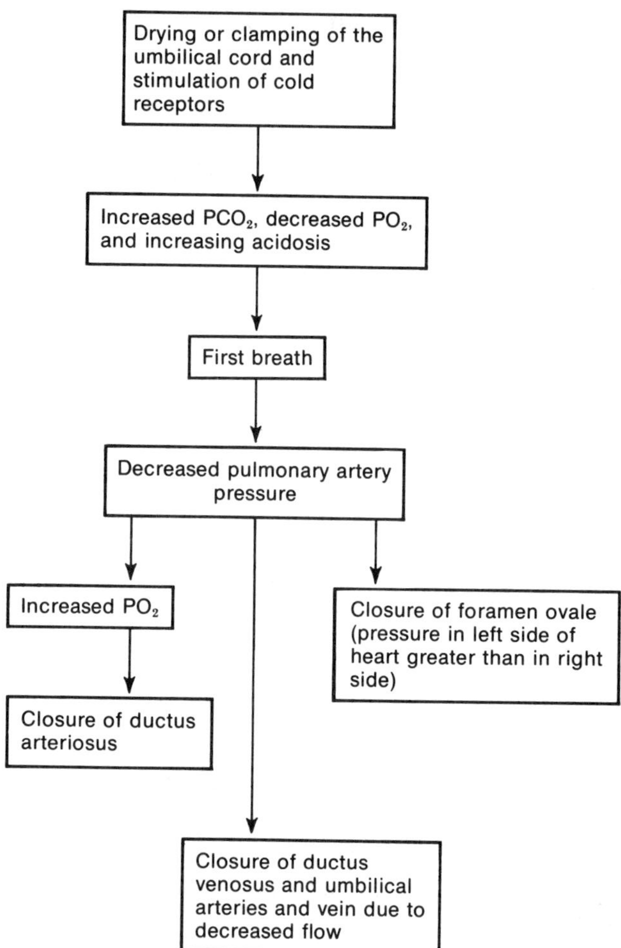

figure 16-3 *Circulatory events at birth.*

endocrine system

Luteal, lactogenic, and estrogenic maternal hormones cross the placental barrier and may cause temporary physical changes in the breasts of all newborns. These hormones can cause swelling and secretion of the newborn's breasts.

nervous system

The newborn's immature nervous system makes makes him or her unable to perform purposeful activity of any kind. Movements of the newborn are rapid and diffuse. Any response to stimulus is a reflex. Development of the peripheral nervous system and muscular control progresses from the head to the arms and then the legs, with control of the hands coming later.

Because the nervous system is immature at birth, the newborn is equipped with inborn reflexes to maintain life and provide protection until the nervous system matures. Inborn reflexes that are important to newborn nutrition include sucking, swallowing, and rooting. Other reflexes present at birth, such as sneezing, gagging, blinking, and Moro reflexes, are protective. These reflexes are present during the first 3 months of life but usually disappear during the first year. Nursing assessment includes determining the presence and function of these reflexes (Fig. 16-4).

sucking reflex

The sucking reflex is well established at birth. Newborns have been observed sucking their thumb at the time of birth. This reflex can be elicited by touching the lips or the skin near the infant's mouth.

swallowing reflex

The swallowing reflex is present before birth, as confirmed by the presence of amniotic fluid in the meconium. It is elicited by stimulation of the palate.

rooting reflex

The rooting reflex is present at birth and is elicited by touching the side of the cheek. The newborn will turn his or her head toward the object that touches the cheek in search of a nipple, either bottle or breast.

gag reflex

The gag reflex, also called the *pharyngeal reflex*, is present at birth and persists throughout life. It is elicited by touching the back of the tongue or the wall of the posterior pharynx.

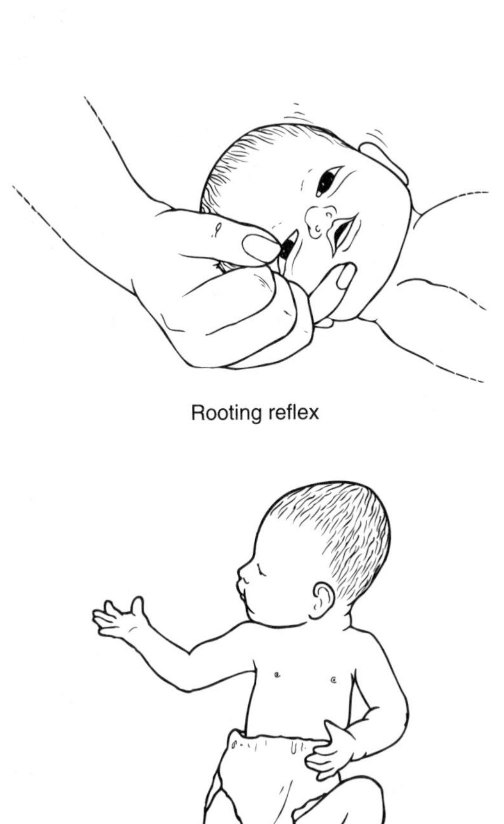

Rooting reflex

Tonic neck reflex

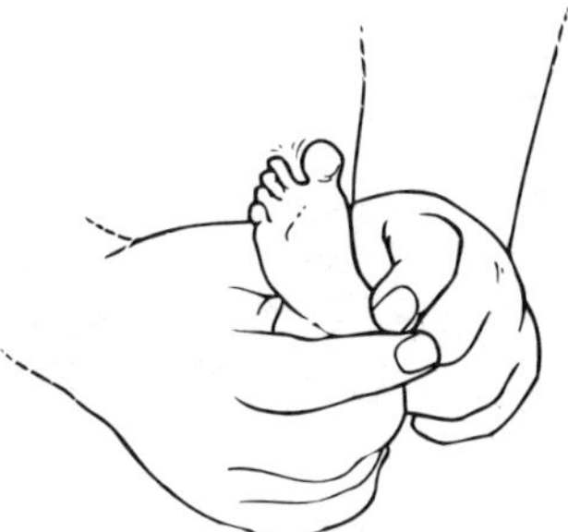

Babinski reflex

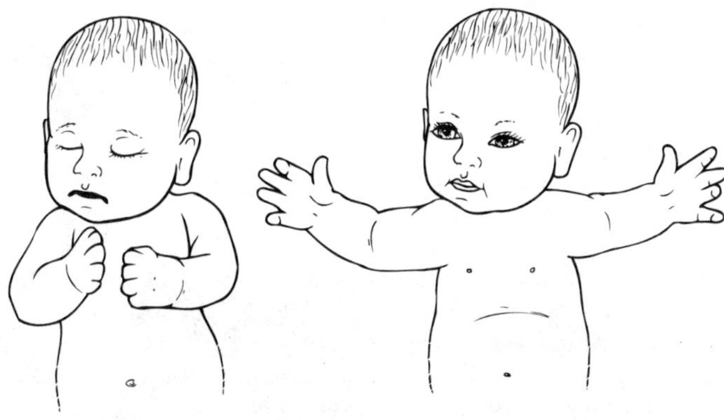

Startle reflex

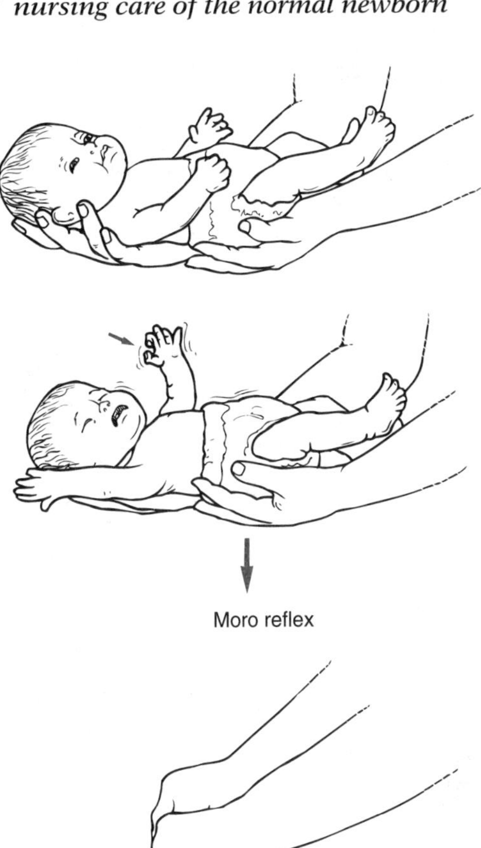

Moro reflex

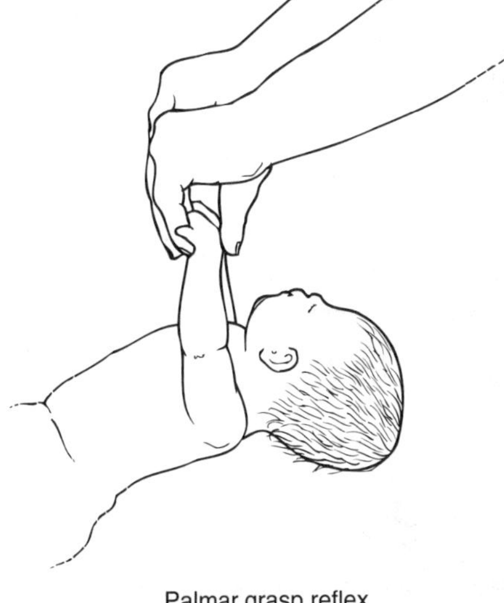

Palmar grasp reflex

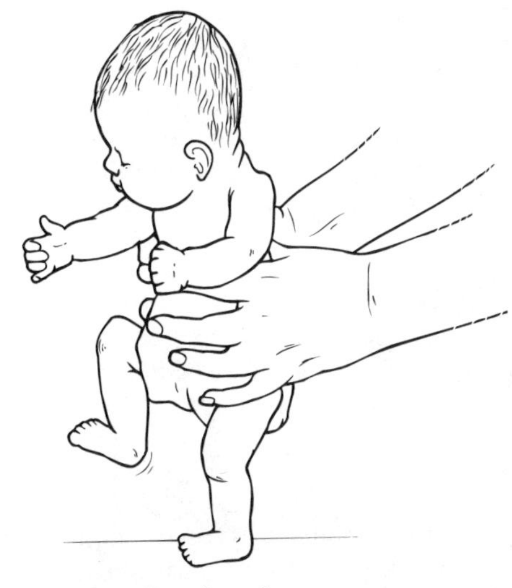

Stepping reflex

figure 16-4 *Neonatal reflexes.*

tonic neck reflex

The tonic neck reflex is elicited by placing the newborn in the supine position. It is characterized by the extension of the arm and leg on the side to which the head is turned and flexion of the opposite arm and leg. The newborn appears to assume the "fencing position." This reflex is usually present until about 4 months of age.

grasp reflex

The grasp reflex is present at birth. The infant clenches the fingers or toes when the palm of the hand or sole of the foot is stimulated. The grasp of the newborn is strong. This can be demonstrated by placing a finger on the palm of the hand of the newborn to elicit the grasp reflex and then gently lifting the newborn slightly off the examination table surface. The grasp reflex is present for approximately 3 months and then diminishes.

babinski reflex

The Babinski reflex is elicited by a firm stimulus, such as scraping on the sole of the foot, resulting in dorsiflexion of the great toe with an outward flaring of the smaller toes. It is present at birth and is normal during the first 12 to 18 months of life. After approximately 18 months of age, the presence of the Babinski reflex is considered abnormal, indicating a malfunction in motor control originating in the cerebral cortex.

moro reflex

The Moro reflex also is called the "embrace reflex." It is elicited by any sudden change in the equilibrium of the newborn, such as jarring. This reflex is characterized by flexion of the newborn's thighs and knees and fanning out of the fingers, followed by tight clenching of the fingers. The arms are first thrown away from the body and then rapidly drawn toward the trunk as though attempting to hold something closely.

The Moro reflex is the most commonly tested reflex of the newborn. Its absence usually indicates brain damage. It diminishes by 4 months and disappears by 6 months when the infant is able to roll.

startle reflex

The startle reflex is sometimes confused with the Moro reflex. This reflex is elicited by loud noise and is a good indication of the hearing ability of the newborn. The startle reflex is characterized by abduction of the arms and flexion of the elbows.

stepping reflex

The stepping or "dancing" reflex is elicited when the newborn is held upright so the soles of the feet touch a flat surface. The newborn will attempt walking or stepping movements until approximately 6 weeks of age.

urinary system

It is important to monitor the urinary output of the newborn and note the time of the first voiding. Normally the first voiding occurs within 4 to 6 hours of birth. If the newborn has not voided during the first 24 hours, medical intervention is required. Because urine is present in the bladder at the time of birth, it is not unusual for the neonate to void during delivery.

The renal system of the newborn is initially unable to concentrate urine due to the immaturity of the kidneys. For this reason, the newborn's urine will be dilute. Dehydration may occur rapidly because water is not reabsorbed freely by the nephrons in the kidneys. Large amounts of uric acid in the urine of the newborn can cause a rusty red stain on the diaper, which may be alarming to the mother. The nurse should explain that this is a normal, temporary condition caused by the crystallization of uric acid on the diaper.

gastrointestinal system

During intrauterine life, nutrients are supplied to the fetus through the placental circulation. Evidence that the fetus swallows in utero has been documented by the presence of lanugo in the meconium. This indicates that gastric emptying and intestinal peristalsis are present before birth. However, the digestive system does not begin to function until birth.

The stomach of the newborn has a capacity of approximately 60 mL (2 oz). Gastric emptying starts within a few minutes after feeding begins and takes 2 to 4 hours to be completed. It is not uncommon for newborns to swallow air. If the newborn is not burped properly and the swallowed air remains in the stomach, the infant may have difficulty finishing the feeding and may vomit. If the swallowed air enters the intestine, it will cause abdominal cramping (colic). Burping after each ounce of formula helps avoid this problem. Breast-fed newborns should be burped once or twice during the feeding.

The newborn may regurgitate a small amount of the feeding due to immature nervous system control of the cardiac sphincter. This is referred to as a "wet burp" or as "spitting up." Regurgitation during the first few feedings can be lessened by frequent burping and should subside with in a few months as the gastrointestinal and nervous systems mature.

The newborn should pass a meconium stool within 24 to 48 hours after birth. Meconium is formed in utero from swallowed amniotic fluid, cells shed from the gastrointestinal tract, and intestinal secretions. Meconium is thick, tarry, dark green, and odorless. If the newborn does not pass a stool within 24 to 48 hours of birth, it may indicate malformation of the gastrointestinal tract. The nurse notes whether the newborn had a stool at birth or meconium-stained amniotic fluid.

The passage of meconium is followed by *transitional stools*, which are a combination of meconium and fecal matter. Transitional stools are greenish brown and looser than meconium. Within 1 to 2 days after the appearance of transitional stools, fecal matter from the digestion of milk or formula will be passed. Stools of the breast-fed newborn are pale yellow or orange-yellow and more liquid than the stools of the formula-fed newborn. Stools of the formula-fed newborn are paler yellow than the breast-fed infant and somewhat curdlike in appearance. Breast-fed newborns may have more frequent stools than formula-fed newborns. The normal stool pattern for each newborn is individual and may vary from several stools a day to one a day.

immune system

The pregnant woman has active acquired immunity from antibodies developed in response to past illnesses or to immunization for certain illnesses. The fetus receives passive acquired immunity when immunoglobulin G is transferred across the placenta, primarily during the third trimester. Newborns therefore receive passive immunity to bacterial and viral infections to which the mother has formed specific antibodies, such as diphtheria, tetanus, measles, mumps, and polio. The period of immunity varies; immunity to some illness, such as measles, may last 4 to 6 months, whereas immunity to some bacteria may last only 4 to 6 weeks.

Immunization to begin the newborn's own active immunity begins within hours of birth when hepatitis B vaccine is administered. A series of other immunizations begins at 2 months of age (see Chap. 20).

procedures for newborn care

handling the newborn

The new mother or caregiver may be frightened at the prospect of lifting and holding a tiny newborn. The nurse has an important role in teaching the mother or caregiver that the baby will not break easily and that understanding certain principles of handling the newborn will help her feel more comfortable.

When the newborn is lifted, the neck, shoulders, and buttocks need to be supported. This is easily done if the newborn is in the side- or back-lying position. One hand can be slipped under the shoulders and neck and the other under the legs or buttocks. Using this method, the newborn can be lifted safely with support provided to the head.

Once the newborn has been lifted from the crib, the *cradle hold*, shoulder hold, or *football hold* will provide the necessary support. Any of these holds also will provide a feeling of comfort, closeness, and warmth for the newborn and the caregiver.

The *cradle hold* is frequently used during feeding. In this position, the head is cradled in the bed of the caregiver's elbow and the forearm provides support for the legs and buttocks. This position enables the caregiver and newborn to establish eye contact. The cradling effect provides a sense of security for the newborn and frees one of the caregiver's hands for other activities.

The *shoulder hold* also provides a sense of security and closeness. This upright position is recommended for burping. One hand is placed over the neck and shoulder region and the other used to support the buttocks.

The *football hold*, like the cradle hold, allows eye contact between newborn and caregiver and frees one hand for other activities. This hold is ideal for shampooing the newborn.

When the newborn is returned to the crib, the side-lying position is most frequently used. The infant's back is supported with a rolled receiving blanket or diaper. This position allows for drainage of secretions from the mouth. If the newborn is newly circumcised, the side-lying position will eliminate pressure on the penis and may be more comfortable. After feeding, the newborn should be placed on the right side to aid in digestion and prevent aspiration.

bathing and daily care

When the newborn's body temperature has stabilized, he or she may be bathed. Bath time provides the nurse an excellent opportunity for observation and assessment of the newborn. The procedure for bathing may vary from hospital to hospital, but the general principles remain the same. The following procedure is generally accepted in hospitals:

In preparation for bathing the newborn, the nurse thoroughly washes his or her hands and observes universal precautions. Before bathing, the following equipment and materials should be assembled:

1. Laundry hamper
2. Clean clothing: diaper, shirt, and receiving blanket
3. Sterile cotton balls
4. Applicators for cord care
5. Triple dye, Bacitracin, or alcohol for cord care, according to hospital protocol
6. Basin of warm water
7. Mild soap
8. Disposable washcloth or clean, soft cloth
9. Towels for drying

The newborn's temperature is taken following agency policy. The infant is undressed, weighed, and wrapped in a towel or blanket, exposing only the areas being bathed. This practice will prevent undue chilling during the bath. As a safety precaution, the newborn may remain in the bassinet during the bath.

The eyes are cleansed first, using a clean cotton ball moistened in warm water. The eyes are wiped beginning at the inner canthus and extending outward away from the lacrimal duct. A separate cotton ball is used for each eye. The external ear may be wiped with a cotton ball moistened in warm water, but nothing should be inserted into the canal. The face is cleansed with a soft cloth or disposable wash cloth, using plain water. Soap should not be used on the newborn's face.

After cleansing the face with warm water, the remaining parts of the newborn's body should be washed in the following order: head, neck, arms, front of body (omitting the cord area), back, legs, feet, lower back, and anus. The infant is patted dry. The water in the basin is changed and the genitalia cleansed last.

Special attention should be given to the areas around the scrotum and penis in the male and the vulva in the female. The genitalia should be cleansed using a cotton ball moistened in soap and warm water.

The prepuce (foreskin) of the penis is adherent to the glans during the neonatal period and needs to be retracted gently as far as it will go. It should *never* be forcibly retracted. The glans penis is gently and carefully cleansed using a cotton ball moistened in warm water, rinsed thoroughly, and patted dry. The foreskin is returned to the normal position after cleansing.

The vulva is cleansed gently using a cotton ball moistened in soap and warm water. It is important to cleanse the vulva from front to back (from the urethra toward the anus), using a clean cotton ball with each stroke. This helps reduce the possibility of transferring fecal organisms to the urethra and introducing a urinary tract infection.

Prior to discharge, the nurse must determine the mother's or caregiver's ability to bathe the newborn. Many hospitals use videotape demonstrations or return demonstrations by the mother or caregiver. This is an excellent time for the client to ask questions. The atmosphere should be relaxed to promote interaction. Instructions for home care should include the following:

- Newborns only need sponge baths until the cord falls off.
- Bath time should be an enjoyable experience for the caregiver and the newborn.
- Although baths do not need to be given daily, the face, creases, and perineal area should be cleansed daily.
- Avoid using strong or heavily perfumed soaps.
- Avoid using oils, powders, and creams; they clog the pores and cause skin irritation.
- Inspect the cord for signs of oozing or discharge; be sure to apply Triple Dye or alcohol as ordered by your physician.

care of circumcision

Based on cultural, social, and family traditions, parents may elect to have their newborn boy circumcised. Circumcision is a surgical procedure in which part of the prepuce (foreskin) is separated from the glans penis and removed. This procedure requires an informed surgical consent form signed by the mother. The infant is not fed for 1 to 2 hours prior to the procedure to prevent vomiting and aspiration. To prepare for the procedure, the nurse restrains the infant on a circumcision board (Fig. 16-5). The physician then uses a Gomco clamp or Plastibell to perform the procedure. Following the procedure, the nurse observes the site for bleeding, infection, or increased irritation. Yellowish drainage from the site is normal and lasts 1 or 2 days. Voidings are noted and recorded following the procedure because edema may interfere with urination. The penis of the circumcised newborn boy may be cleansed gently using soap and warm water, rinsed thoroughly, and gently patted dry. After cleansing, Neosporin or other antibiotic ointment is applied to the circumcision site. If a Plastibell has been used, a small plastic ring is left in place. It usually falls off within 1 week. Caregivers should be cautioned not to remove it manually.

discharge and home care instructions

Going home is an exciting time for the family, but it also can be a time of anxiety and concern for the new mother and father. The enormous responsibility of caring for a newborn can seem overwhelming. Thus, the nurse must provide written instructions and teaching materials so that the mother can review what she has learned in the hospital. This information should include sleep patterns, feeding and daily care, and when to call the physician if a problem arises. (See Teaching Guidelines: Circumstances that warrant calling the physician.) The nurse also emphasizes the importance of follow-up care, keeping appointments, phone numbers of the pediatrician and local hospital, and scheduled home visits.

Prior to discharge, the nurse verifies identification, assists with dressing the newborn, answers any last-minute

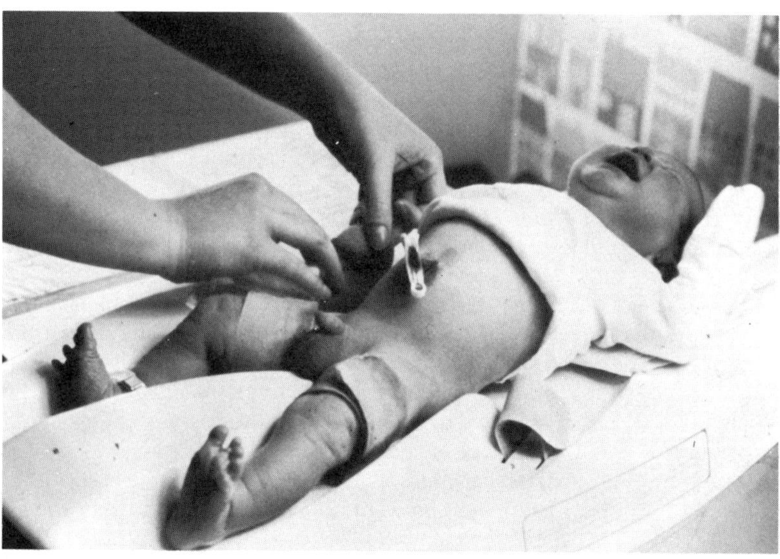

figure 16-5 *Infant in restraint for circumcision.*

teaching guidelines 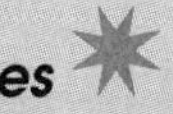
circumstances that warrant calling the physician

* Temperature above 100°F (37.7°C) axillary
* Difficult to arouse
* Signs of redness, puffiness, or drainage from the umbilical cord
* Projectile or persistent vomiting
* Diarrhea (green, liquid stools)
* Refusal of two consecutive feedings
* Difficulty breathing or fast, heavy breathing
* Blood in stool
* Abdominal swelling
* Excessive crying
* Pink or cloudy urine
* Less than 8 to 10 wet diapers per day
* Eye drainage
* Cough
* Runny nose

questions, and ensures the availability of an approved car seat for the ride home. Many hospitals supply a car seat for the parents.

nursing process for the normal newborn

assessment

Subjective data to be assessed include the following:

* Restlessness
* Crying pattern
* States of consciousness
* Attachment and bonding

Objective data to be assessed include the following:

* Airway patency
* Vital signs
* Intake and output
* Weight gain or loss
* General body systems responses

nursing diagnosis

* Risk for Ineffective Airway Clearance
* Risk for Fluid Volume Deficit
* Risk for Aspiration
* Risk for Hypothermia
* Risk for Injury, related to developmental status
* Risk for Altered Parent/Infant Attachment

planning and implementation

The newborn's breathing pattern is monitored closely. It is not unusual for the newborn to have a build-up of mucus that can alter the breathing pattern. The new parents should be taught to suction the mouth and nares of the newborn to assist with maintaining a patent airway.

Newborns should be monitored for adequate intake and output. Signs of dehydration include depressed fontanels and less than six wet diapers per day. To prevent aspiration, bottles should never be propped and the infant should be burped at intervals during feedings and positioned on the side when lying in bed. The newborn should be wrapped in a blanket, and a cap should be kept on the head to assist with maintaining body temperature. As much as 90% of body heat can be lost through the head. The infant should be placed in the crib or held securely to prevent injury. Parents should be encouraged to hold, rock, and talk with their newborns to promote attachment.

The nurse should complete a head-to-toe assessment during each shift to be alert to any subtle changes in the newborn that may require immediate intervention.

evaluation

* The newborn will demonstrate an effective breathing pattern.
* The newborn will demonstrate normal adequate hydration with normal elimination patterns.
* The newborn will maintain a body temperature within normal limits.
* The newborn will be free of injury.
* The newborn and family will demonstrate beginning normal parent–infant attachment.

key points

* **The seven immediate needs of the newborn include establishing a patent airway, maintaining respirations, maintaining body temperature, receiving nutrition, being protected from infection and hemorrhage, maintaining sleep and rest, and forming attachment.**
* **Breast-feeding is recommended as the ideal method of infant feeding. An infant who is breast-feeding is provided passive immunity against certain diseases to which the mother has been exposed. In addition, breast-fed babies seem to have fewer gastrointestinal disturbances and respiratory infections.**
* **A newborn's nutritional status may be evaluated by checking for signs of dehydration (less than six wet diapers per day; dry, hard stools; dark urine; dry mucous membranes; sunken fontanels), behavioral clues (the newborn should be content after feeding), and weight gain (normal gain is approximately 1 oz/d after intial weight loss).**
* **Assessing the physical characteristics of the newborn includes checking the skin (rashes, birthmarks, jaun-**

dice, forceps or vacuum marks), head and neck (molding, cephalhematoma, caput succedaneum), eyes (pupillary size, equality and reaction to light, presence of blink reflex), ears (position, response to noise), face and mouth (Epstein's pearls, thrush), abdomen (cord care), and genitalia (pseudomenstruation in girls, phimosis in boys). The newborn also is measured (length, head, and chest circumference) and weighed.

* The respiratory rate, pulse, and blood pressure are vital signs in the newborn that the nurse should measure. The normal newborn's respiratory rate is 30 to 60 respirations per minute, which increases with activity. The newborn's heart rate immediately following birth is 170 to 180 beats/min. Within 12 to 24 hours, this rate slows to 120 to 150 beats/min during sleep and 180 beats/min when the infant cries. A blood pressure of 80/50 is measured in the full-term newborn at rest.
* At birth, major physiologic changes occur in the infant. The respiratory, cardiovascular, endocrine, nervous, urinary, gastrointestinal, and immune systems undergo the most changes. The nurse needs to understand these physiologic transitions to assess the newborn adequately, recognize deviations for normal, and institute appropriate nursing interventions.
* Ten reflexes found in the newborn include sucking, swallowing, rooting, gag, tonic neck, grasp, Babinksi, Moro, startle, and stepping.
* The cradle, shoulder, and football holds are appropriate for handling the newborn. All three provide support for the neck, shoulders, and buttocks. These three holds also promote feelings of comfort, warmth, and closeness for the newborn and the caregiver.
* To perform an infant bath, the nurse or caregiver assembles the necessary equipment and materials. The anatomic order for bathing the infant is as follows: eyes, head, neck, arms, front of body (omitting the cord area), back, legs, feet, lower back, anus, and genitalia.
* Circumcision is an elective surgery for newborn boys. The surgical procedure includes separating and removing part of the foreskin from the penis. The male infant is restrained on a circumcision board, and a Gomco clamp or Plastibell is used to perform the procedure. Nursing care for the infant after surgery includes observing for bleeding, infection, or increased irritation. The penis is cleansed gently, rinsed thoroughly, and patted dry. Neosporin or another antibiotic ointment is applied to the circumcision site.

review questions

1. Tara Dennison wants to know why the nurse has placed a cap on her newborn. the nurse explains,
   a. "It is hospital policy."
   b. "It is to keep germs off the newborn's head."
   c. "It assists the newborn in maintaining an adequate temperature."
   d. "Local volunteers offer the caps to all newborns."
2. Sonya Connell is concerned about bathing her newborn while the cord is still present. The nurse explains that
   a. it is important to introduce the newborn to a tub bath as early as possible.
   b. a sponge bath will meet hygienic needs until the cord falls off.
   c. babies love water, so it is a great time for mother–baby interaction.
   d. she should probably ask her physician how he feels about it.
3. A mother questions the nurse about the white pimples on her newborn's face. The nurse recognizes that this is
   a. the start of an infectious rash.
   b. milia.
   c. lanugo.
   d. thrush.
4. When examining her newborn a mother notices a strawberry-shaped reddened area on her newborn's eyelid. The nurse explains,
   a. "The area can be removed with laser treatment."
   b. "These areas are common in newborns, and they disappear on their own."
   c. "This is a hereditary characteristic."
   d. "I will call the physician immediately."
5. Within a few hours of birth, the nurse scores an infant on the Ballard scoring system. This is to
   a. determine the average weight of the newborn.
   b. compare the newborn with other newborns.
   c. determine the newborn's gestational age.
   d. determine the need for additional nutritional supplement.

bibliography

Campinba-Bacote, J., & Bragg, E. J. (1993). Clinical assessment in maternity care. *Maternal Child Health, 18*(1), 24.

Gelbaum, I. (1993). Circumcision: Refining a traditional surgical technique. *Journal of Nurse Midwifery, 38*, 2.

May, K. A., & Mahlmeister, L. R. (1994). *Maternal and neonatal nursing: Family-centered care* (3rd ed.). Philadelphia: J.B. Lippincott.

NAACOG Committee on Practice (1991). *Physical assessment of the neonate*. Washington D.C.:

Olds, S. B., London, M. L., & Ladewig, P. W. (1992). *Maternal-newborn nursing: A family centered approach* (4th ed.). Menlo Park, CA: Addison-Wesley.

Pillitteri, A. (1995). *Maternal and child health nursing* (2nd ed.). Philadelphia: J.B. Lippincott.

Pontius, S., Kennedy, A. H., & Mittrucker, C. (1994). Accuracy and reliability of temperature measurement by instrument and site. *Journal of Pediatric Nursing, 9*(2), 114–123.

Reeder, S. J., Martin, L. L., & Koniak, D. (1992). *Maternity nursing: Family, newborn, and women's health care* (17th ed.). Philadelphia: J.B. Lippincott.

nursing care of the newborn at risk

17

outline

objectives

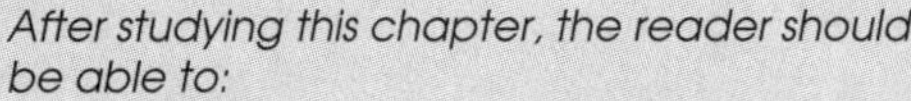

After studying this chapter, the reader should be able to:

* Use the nursing process to identify the high-risk newborn.
* Define small-for-gestational-age, large-for-gestational-age, term infant, postterm infant, preterm infant, and the associated health risks with each.
* Identify genetic disorders of the newborn and appropriate nursing care.
* Identify the four major cardiac defects and treatments for the newborn at risk.
* Describe hemolytic disease and differentiate the two categories of the disease.
* Identify the different types of birth trauma and appropriate nursing care.
* Define the various infections to which the newborn may be susceptible.
* Discuss the effects of maternal, prenatal substance abuse on the newborn.
* Explain how HIV/AIDS can be transmitted from the mother to the newborn and the effects of maternal antibodies on diagnostic tests.

key terms

apnea
asphyxia
atelectasis
birth trauma
brachial plexus
Candida albicans
cephalhematoma
caput succedaneum
congenital malformation
crepitus
Erb's paralysis syndrome
fetal alcohol syndrome
fetal alcohol effects
genetic abnormality
hyperbilirubinemia
hypoxia
kernicterus
large for gestational age
low birth weight
postterm or postmaturity
preterm or prematurity
purulent
respiratory distress syndrome
shoulder dystocia
Simian crease
small for gestational age
spina bifida
surfactant

Neff C & Spray M. *Introduction to Maternal and Child Health Nursing,*

The birth of an infant is usually an exciting, happy time. When an infant is identified before or at birth to be at risk, however, anxiety, fear, and sadness surround the birth experience. The family begins a grieving process, and the nurse helps them work through that process and provides care that can help minimize complications in the newborn.

Using the nursing process, this chapter provides the information necessary to help identify infants at risk and nursing care strategies to maximize neonatal health and minimize complications. It also discusses how the nurse can comfort and care for the family while teaching them how to care for their newborn.

✶ family considerations

Family members of the newborn at risk need to be included in the plan of care whenever feasible. Becoming active participants in the infant's care can help them meet their needs and the needs of the infant. The goal of nursing care is to help the family understand the infant care needed and to give them confidence by teaching them the necessary skills. To assist the family in becoming active participants, the nurse needs to provide information, teach the skills necessary for care of the newborn, and encourage parent–infant attachment and support systems. Parents of a newborn at risk may experience overwhelming anxiety about the chance that their child will not survive. As a result, they may experience anticipatory grief. This is evidenced by the following signs:

- Delay in naming the child
- Reluctance to visit the nursery
- Focusing on equipment and treatments when visiting the child
- Hesitancy to touch or hold the infant when possible

The nurse should provide the family with every opportunity to discuss their feelings and express their emotions. The nurse should encourage the parents to spend time with their infant. Information about the infant's medical status should be provided regularly.

alteration in size or gestational age

A newborn is classified using the criteria of gestational age and birth weight. Approximately one third of all infants who have a low birth weight are full term but small for gestational age (SGA; Pittard, 1993).

Gestation classification includes the following:

- Preterm—born before the end of the 37th week
- Term—born between 38 and 41 weeks
- Postterm—born after the completion of 41 weeks

Birth weight classification includes the following:

- SGA—birth weight at or less than the 10th percentile
- Appropriate for gestational age (AGA)—birth weight between the 10th and 90th percentile
- Large for gestational age (LGA)—birth weight at or greater than the 90th percentile

small for gestational age

etiology and pathophysiology

An SGA infant experiences intrauterine growth retardation (IUGR). The infant's birth weight will be at or below the 10th percentile on a growth curve. This occurs in 3% to 10% of all pregnancies, and affected infants have a four to eight times higher perinatal mortality rate than AGA infants (Gomella, 1992). Causes of IUGR include maternal malnutrition, smoking, diabetes mellitus, pregnancy-induced hypertension, heart disease, substance abuse, sickle cell anemia, placenta previa and infarction, and congenital infections, malformations, or multiple births. Complications of the SGA infant include perinatal asphyxia, meconium aspiration, hypoglycemia, increased heat loss, and congenital malformations (Table 17-1).

medical management

The focus of medical management is prevention and good prenatal care. Early detection may prevent further growth reduction, but when that is not possible, problems will be treated as they are assessed.

table 17-1 complications of small-for-gestational-age birth

Complication	*Cause*
Perinatal asphyxia	Decreased oxygen and nutrients leave little reserve to cope with labor and delivery
Meconium aspiration	Hypoxia causes relaxation of anal sphincter and passage of meconium, which fetus may swallow in utero or aspirate with first breath
Hypoglycemia	Increased metabolic rate in response to heat loss and increased use of glycogen stores cause hypoglycemia
Increased heat loss	Decreased brown fat (used to increase survival in utero) with inability to generate heat through nonshivering thermogenesis
Congenital malformations	Occurs 10 to 20 times more frequently due to insult to growth from various stressors

✳ nursing process for the small-for-gestational-age infant

assessment

The nurse assesses for the following objective signs of growth retardation throughout pregnancy:

- Lack of appropriate fundal height for gestation
- Less than optimum maternal weight gain
- Maternal malnutrition
- Maternal disease

After birth, the physical examination and appearance of the SGA infant will indicate the type of growth retardation sustained. Symmetric IUGR involves prolonged growth retardation because its onset is prior to 32 weeks' gestation, and it is caused by long-term maternal conditions or fetal genetic abnormalities. Infants with symmetric IUGR are SGA but usually vigorous and with normal body proportions. Asymmetric IUGR is associated with acute uteroplacental insufficiency and is not usually noticed before birth. Infants with asymmetric IUGR exhibit the following characteristics:

- Decreased weight
- Head and length within normal range (head appears large in relation to the body)
- Thin, emaciated appearance with loose skin folds
- Dry, peeling skin
- Thin umbilical cord, sometimes meconium stained due to intrauterine stress
- Vigorous with a wide-eyed appearance

nursing diagnoses

Depending on problems present at birth, nursing diagnoses may include the following:

- Risk for Injury and Hypoglycemia, related to increased needs and inadequate glycogen stores
- Altered Nutrition: Less than body requirements, related to increased metabolic rate, hypothermia, decreased subcutaneous fat
- Ineffective Thermoregulation, related to decreased subcutaneous fat
- Impaired Gas Exchange, related to intrauterine compromise and possible aspiration of meconium
- Altered Family Processes, related to the birth of a high-risk neonate

planning and implementation

Nursing care is directed toward preventing or minimizing complications. If oxygen is in use, careful monitoring of the flow rate is essential. Vital signs with auscultation of breath sounds are monitored every 4 hours. Skin and mucous membranes are assessed for cyanosis. Any negative changes are reported. A thermoneutral environment must be maintained. The infant needs to be in an isolette or wrapped in warm, dry blankets with a stocking cap on the head to maintain a normal axillary temperature between 97.7° and 99.7°F. Caloric intake is monitored and feedings often given every 3 hours. An intravenous line may be in place. Intake and output are recorded every 4 to 8 hours with 24-hour totals. Glucose testing is done per unit protocol based on the infant's status. Regular feedings or intravenous fluids plus glucose monitoring will help prevent hypoglycemia. Daily weights are important.

Care of the family also is essential. The nurse needs to explain procedures and treatments to the parents, allowing them access to their infant and encouraging them to assist in caring for the infant. Supportive care will help the family through this difficult, stressful time, including what may be an uncertain future.

evaluation

Interventions are successful in the following situations:

- The infant eats appropriately while maintaining normal glucose levels.
- The infant gains weight.
- The infant has pink, moist mucous membranes.
- The infant has vital signs within normal limits.
- The family understands the infant's status.
- The family feels comfortable assisting in the infant's care.
- The family asks appropriate questions to prepare for future care and monitoring of the infant.

large for gestational age

etiology and pathophysiology

An LGA infant's birth weight is at or above the 90th percentile on a growth curve. At one time, the large infant was considered a healthy infant. Now, however, it is known that accelerated growth can present a threat to the mother and the fetus during the birth process and to the infant during the neonatal period. Certain factors have been found to correlate with the LGA infant:

- Genetic predisposition: Large parents tend to have large infants.
- Multiparous women have larger infants than primigravidas.
- Newborn boys tend to be larger than girls.
- The leading cause of LGA infants is maternal diabetes.

The LGA infant is often born by cesarean delivery, or the mother is more likely to have a long, difficult labor and delivery. Birth trauma due to *cephalopelvic disproportion* is often associated with LGA infants. *Shoulder dystocia* (difficulty fitting through the pelvis) is common. Other complications include asphyxia, fractured clavicle, brachial plexus palsy, facial paralysis, skull fracture, and cephalhematomas. Large infants tend to be hard to arouse to a quiet, alert state and often have feeding difficulties (Pressler, 1991). They are predisposed to hypoglycemia, resulting from the long, difficult labor and the higher metabolic rate required for heat production in the larger body.

infant of a diabetic mother

Infants of diabetic mothers tend to have a larger body weight, but length and head circumference may be normal (Fig. 17-1). They appear polycythemic because of overproduction of red blood cells. Infants of diabetic mothers often have hypoglycemia because of increased fetal insulin in response to maternal hyperglycemia. After birth, the maternal source of glucose is lost. However, the increased fetal insulin remains and causes infant hypoglycemia. This persists until the infant's nutritional intake stabilizes the level of insulin.

The following complications are most often seen with an infant of a diabetic mother:

* Hypoglycemia
* Polycythemia
* Respiratory distress syndrome
* Hyperbilirubinemia

medical management

Medical management is directed at identification of the LGA infant prior to birth so that the appropriate delivery method can be anticipated and complications avoided. When identification is made, either before or after birth, care is directed at immediate assessment and treatment of common disorders.

✳ nursing process for lga infant

assessment

The LGA infant is usually easy to identify at birth by the large body size in relation to head and chest circumference. The infant's weight is plotted on a growth curve to identify those that may be borderline.

The nurse needs to assess the infant for objective signs of birth trauma:

* Clavicular fracture, often felt as a grinding when the shoulder is palpated
* Crying or wincing when moved or when a shoulder is touched
* Excessive skull molding because of a long, difficult vaginal delivery
* Brachial plexus palsy or facial paralysis, assessed by lack of facial symmetry or decreased or absent movement in one or both upper extremities

Signs of hypoglycemia are assessed:

* Jitteriness
* Irritability
* Lethargy
* Decreased muscle tone
* Apnea
* Cyanosis
* Blood glucose level less than 40 mg/dL (Hoskins, 1990)
* Hypothermia

The nurse assesses glucose levels and reports any abnormalities every 24 hours with decreasing or increasing frequency depending on the infant's condition. Feedings are initiated after bowel sounds can be heard (usually within 1 to 2 hours after birth) to help prevent hypoglycemia. When intravenous fluids are needed, monitoring of intake and output is essential.

Vital signs are assessed to detect signs of fetal asphyxia. The skull is assessed for signs of hematoma formation from the long, difficult birth (usually manifested within the first 12 hours after birth). When red blood cells in the hematoma break down, there is an increase in the total red blood cell mass of the blood. This increase in red blood cell mass, called polycythemia, predisposes the infant to jaundice. Polycythemia also causes decreased blood flow to all organs because it causes the blood to be excessively resistant to flow (hyperviscosity).

nursing diagnoses

Nursing diagnoses for the LGA infant may include the following:

* Risk for Injury, related to hypoglycemia, macrosomia (large body size)
* Impaired Physical Mobility, related to fractured clavicle, brachial plexus palsy, facial paralysis

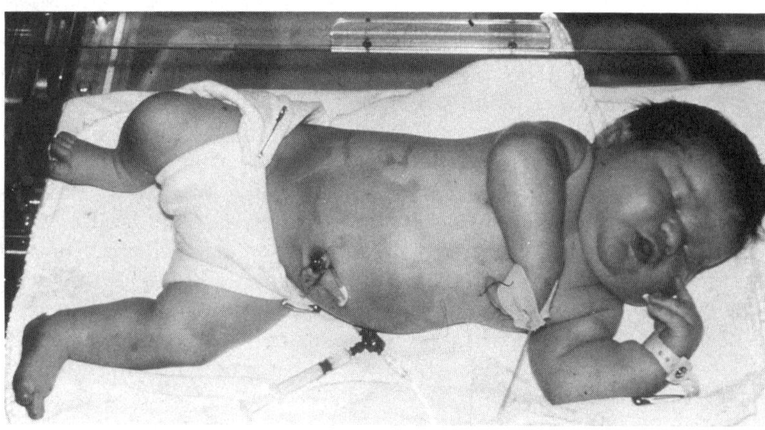

figure 17-1 *A macrosomic infant of a diabetic mother (IDM) has head circumference and length that are at the 90th percentile; the IDM's body weight greatly exceeds the 90th percentile. The IDM has considerable fat deposition in the shoulder and intrascapular area.*

* Altered Tissue Perfusion, related to polycythemia
* Ineffective Feeding Pattern, related to difficulty arousing
* Altered Nutrition: Less than body requirements, related to hypoglycemia, difficulty arousing

planning and implementation

Care of the LGA infant is centered around assessed needs. The plan of care follows these basic principles:

* Immediate assessment for signs of birth trauma
* Blood glucose assessment every 2 to 4 hours with decreasing or increasing frequency based on condition of infant (blood glucose level less than 40 mg/dL considered hypoglycemic)
* Feedings initiated after bowel sounds are present if respiratory rate is less than 60 per minute (if respirations are >60, it uses all the infant's energy to breathe and they are too exhausted to suck or ingest oral intake)
* No signs of cardiac compromise
* Maintenance of weight within normal limits for size and age
* Appropriate intake and output

the preterm (premature) infant

etiology and pathophysiology

Preterm infants are born before the beginning of the 38th gestational week. Technology has resulted in survival of infants that are smaller and more premature than ever before. More than 90% of infants weighing 750 g (1.65 lb) at birth now survive (Kliegman, 1990). Preterm infants may have long-term health problems (Display 17-1). Mild problems in development occur in 10% to 25% of preterm infants, and 5% to 10% have severe problems (Kleigman, 1990). Preterm birth is costly not only in financial terms, but in terms of the suffering of infants and families.

The exact cause of preterm birth is not known. The incidence in the United States ranges from 7% to 15%. One of the major factors associated with preterm birth is lack of prenatal care, especially among women who are single, young, and of lower socioeconomic status. These women are more likely to be malnourished, involved in substance abuse, have little education, have limited access to prenatal care, and have an inadequate support system.

The major problem of preterm infants is immaturity of all organ systems. There is a direct relationship between the length of gestation and the degree of organ maturity. An infant of 30 weeks' gestation will have a less mature system than an infant of 36 weeks' gestation.

medical management

Medical management is aimed at preventing preterm birth. When preterm birth is inevitable, it is essential to prepare for gestation-appropriate care to minimize complications. Care is directed primarily at assessment and management of circulatory and respiratory status and nutritional support.

display 17-1
long-term health problems of preterm infants

Damage to lungs
Damage to intestines
Blindness
Mental retardation
Developmental delays

* nursing process for the preterm infant

assessment

Preterm infants appear small, weak, and fragile (Fig. 17-2). Their underdeveloped muscle tone makes them limp with extension of their extremities. Their skin appears transparent, with little subcutaneous fat; blood vessels can be clearly seen. The body is covered with lanugo and vernix, and sole creases are minimal or absent. The labia majora of the female infant does not cover the labia minora. The male infant has undescended testes. Preterm infants are easily tired and have minimal energy for even simple body functions. Their cry is weak and feeble. Other areas of assessment are based on common problems seen with preterm infants. These include respiratory, circulatory, metabolic, neurologic, visual, auditory, and infectious problems (Table 17-2).

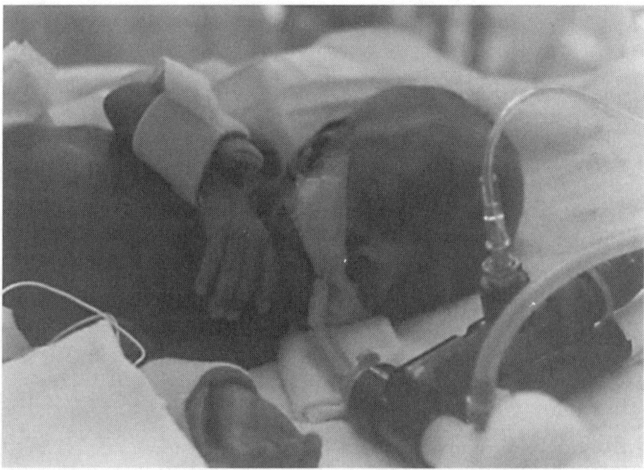

figure 17-2 *Preterm infant on ventilator appears to be so fragile.*

table 17-2 common problems of the preterm infant

System	Condition
Respiratory	Respiratory distress syndrome, apnea, bronchopulmonary dysplasia
Circulatory	Patent ductus arteriosus, intraventricular hemorrhage
Metabolic	Hypocalcemia, hypoglycemia, gastrointestinal dysfunction, hyperbilirubinemia, necrotizing enterocolitis
Neurologic	Ineffective thermoregulation
Infection	Inability to produce antibodies
Visual/auditory	Retinopathy, sensory overload

nursing diagnoses

Nursing diagnoses that may apply to the preterm infant include the following:

* Impaired Gas Exchange, related to immature pulmonary system
* Altered Nutrition: Less than body requirements, related to difficulty in feeding
* Fluid Volume Deficit, related to insensible water loss
* Ineffective Breathing Pattern, related to apnea and immature central nervous system
* Ineffective Thermoregulation, related to immature central nervous system, decreased brown fat
* Ineffective Airway Clearance, related to weak cough

planning and implementation

The nurse maintains respiratory function by assessing changes in vital signs, maintaining a patent airway, and observing for signs of respiratory distress, including the following:

* Nasal flaring
* Increased respiratory rate
* Apnea
* Cyanosis
* Tachypnea greater than 60 breaths per minute
* Tachycardia
* Chest retractions
* Stridor
* Expiratory grunting

Any alterations that suggest decreased respiratory function need to be reported to the registered nurse or physician. If oxygen is in use, the flow rate is monitored. Cardiac and respiratory monitors are maintained with alarms functioning. The infant is placed in a prone position or with the head slightly elevated if in a supine position for maximum air entry and oxygenation.

To minimize oxygen consumption and heat loss, the infant must be maintained in a thermoneutral environment. Warm oxygen and an isolette or heat shield are used. The infant should not be placed on cold surfaces, in drafts, or near cold walls or windows. The infant's skin is kept dry, and warm blankets and a cap are used if he or she is not in an isolette or under a heat shield. See the Nursing Care Plan for the Preterm Infant.

Hydration and nutritional status are determined by accurate intake and output along with daily weights. Preterm infants fatigue easily, so minimal handling is suggested. However, appropriate tactile and vocal stimulation is encouraged.

While the preterm infant is still in the hospital, parents are taught techniques on how to care for the infant and to observe for danger signs. The nurse should offer the parents the opportunity to learn infant cardiopulmonary resuscitation and should stress the necessity of follow-up medical care. Major danger signs of neonatal morbidity are summarized in Display 17-2.

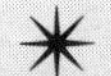
nursing insight

If oral feedings are taking place, avoid letting the infant suck for longer than 20 minutes to prevent increased energy demand and potential weight loss.

evaluation

Outcomes of nursing care are successful if the preterm infant does the following:

* Establishes effective respiratory function
* Consumes adequate nutrition and gains weight appropriately
* Shows no signs of heat loss
* Experiences minimal sequelae related to prematurity

the postterm (postmature) infant

etiology and pathophysiology

Approximately 10% of all deliveries are considered postterm, occurring after 41 weeks' gestation. The cause of postterm birth is not clearly understood; however, it occurs more frequently with primiparity, high multiparity, and a history of postterm pregnancy. It is believed that many are due to an inaccurate menstrual history, which results in an inaccurate estimate of the due date.

medical management

Medical interventions are aimed at preventing or minimizing the following problems associated with postterm birth:

* Asphyxiation, resulting in hypoxia and meconium aspiration syndrome
* Placental insufficiency, with effects ranging from mal-

nursing care plan for the preterm infant

NURSING DIAGNOSIS

Impaired Gas Exchange, related to immature pulmonary system and decreased surfactant production

GOAL: improve respiratory function

NURSING INTERVENTIONS	RATIONALE	EVALUATION
Monitor the infant's respiratory rate and observe respiratory pattern.	Measuring rate, recognizing periods of apnea and signs of increasing respiratory work, such as retractions, can assist in evaluating current treatment and indicate need for a change in treatment.	The infant's respiratory pattern and rate will be regular. The infant does not use accessory muscles for breathing.
Assess lung sounds every 2–4 hours.	Decreased breath sounds can indicate a worsening state of respiratory distress.	The infant's breath sounds will be evaluated every 2–4 hours, as indicated.
Use isolettes with oxygen inlets and humidifiers, as needed.	To establish adequate oxygen concentrations in the infant, while the moisture helps liquefy secretions for ease in mobilization.	The infant will have a pulse oximetry level higher than 94%. Pulmonary secretions are easily removed, as needed.
Place the infant in a prone position or with head slightly elevated.	This position will allow for maximum air entry and oxygenation.	The infant will be properly positioned, to promote adequate ventilation and perfusion.

NURSING DIAGNOSIS

Risk for Infection, related to immature immune system

GOAL: The infant will remain free of infection.

NURSING INTERVENTIONS	RATIONALE	EVALUATION
Ensure that all persons in contact with the infant wash their hands.	The most important prevention of infection remains effective hand washing.	The primary nurse will use proper hand-washing technique and ensure that all contacts with the infant also use proper hand washing.
Any personnel from other departments will wear protective scrub suits.	This will help to reduce the spread of infection from other departments to the infant.	The infant will remain afebrile and without signs of a nosocomial infection.
Change humidified water, IV tubing, suction equipment, respiratory equipment, and monitoring equipment on a regular basis.	All of these are measures to ensure cleanliness and prevent infection.	All equipment will be changed on a regular basis and documentation of this will be done.

nourished appearance to meconium staining of the skin and nails

* Polycythemia due to hypoxia
* Cold stress from decreased brown fat
* Hypoglycemia from depleted glycogen stores caused by nutritional deprivation

Management begins before delivery with tests of placental functioning, such as a nonstress test, contraction challenge test, or biophysical profile, if postterm dates are suspected. Labor is induced or a cesarean delivery performed if placental deterioration is found. With meconium aspiration, management will be more complex, usually in an intensive care unit. Most of the effort is directed at thermoregulation and nutritional support.

✳ nursing process for the postterm infant

assessment

On examination, the nurse will note the following signs of postmaturity:

display 17-2
major danger signs of neonatal morbidity

CENTRAL NERVOUS SYSTEM SIGNS
- Lethargy
- High-pitched cry
- Jitteriness
- Abnormal eye movement
- Seizure activity
- Abnormal fontanel size or bulging fontanels

RESPIRATORY SIGNS
- Apnea
- Tachypnea
- Nasal flaring
- Chest retractions
- Persistent rales and rhonchi
- Asynchronous breathing movements
- Expiratory grunting

CARDIOVASCULAR SIGNS
- Abnormal rate and rhythm
- Murmurs
- Changes in blood pressure
- Alterations and differentials in pulses
- Changes in perfusion and skin color

GASTROINTESTINAL SIGNS
- Refusal of two or more feedings
- Absent or uncoordinated feeding reflexes
- Vomiting
- Abdominal distention
- Changes in stool patterns

GENITOURINARY SIGNS
- Hematuria
- Absence of urine production
- Failure to pass urine

METABOLIC ALTERATIONS
- Hypoglycemia
- Hypocalcemia
- Hyperbilirubinemia and jaundice

TEMPERATURE INSTABILITY

- Meconium staining of the cord, skin, and nails
- Wide-eyed appearance, indicating hypoxia
- Hematocrit above 65%
- Loose skin with little subcutaneous fat
- Minimal or absent lanugo and vernix
- Dry, cracked, peeling skin
- Thick hair
- Nails extending over the end of the fingertips

nursing diagnoses

Nursing diagnoses common to the postterm infant include the following:

- Impaired Gas Exchange, related to decreasing efficiency of the placenta
- Altered Nutrition: Less than body requirements, related to intrauterine deprivation
- Ineffective Thermoregulation, related to parchment-like, desquamating skin and depletion of subcutaneous fat
- Risk for Aspiration, related to meconium aspiration syndrome
- Ineffective Airway Clearance, related to meconium aspiration syndrome
- Risk for Infection, related to meconium aspiration syndrome

planning and implementation

The role of the licensed practical nurse (LPN) in the care of the postterm infant is supportive, focused on prevention and symptomatic treatment of the identified problems (Table 17-3).

evaluation

Evaluation criteria include the following:

- Blood glucose level within normal limits
- Clear breath sounds
- Steady weight gain
- Maintenance of body temperature within normal range in open crib while dressed in a shirt, diaper, and wrapped in one or two blankets
- No signs of infection

genetic disorders

down syndrome

The presence of an extra chromosome 21 (trisomy 21) results in an infant with the distinctive clinical features of Down syndrome. Down syndrome (previously called mongolism) is the most common trisomy abnormality seen in newborns and is a major cause of mental retardation. The most distinctive features seen at birth include abnormally decreased tension or strength (*hypotonia*), slanted eyes, protruding tongue, and a transverse crease, called a simian crease, on the palm of the hand (Fig. 17-3). A complete cardiac assessment will usually show congenital heart problems. Medical technology is

table 17-3 postterm care plan

Diagnosis	*Outcomes*	*Interventions*
Altered Nutrition: Less than body requirements, related to increased use of glucose	Infant will ingest the amount of nutrition needed to: * Gain 1 oz/d * Maintain blood glucose above 45 mg/dL	* Initiate feedings within 2 h of birth if respiratory rate is within normal limits and bowel sounds are present. * Feed q2–4 h as tolerated. * Maintain IV if required for nutrition or glucose support. * Assess blood glucose per unit protocol, reporting levels less than 40 mg/dL. * Weigh nude daily on same scale and at same time.
Ineffective Thermoregulation, related to decreased glycogen and brown fat stores	Infant will display the following: * Maintain temperature within normal limits in open crib wearing shirt, diaper, and wrapped in 1–2 blankets * Maintain other vital signs within normal limits * Exhibit good skin perfusion assessed by capillary refill of less than 3 seconds and skin that is pink and that is warm to touch	* Initially after birth, place infant in isolette or under radiant warmer. * Place in open crib when physiologic status is within normal limits. * Assess vital signs q1–2h until within normal limits ×2 then assess q4–8h. * Assess capillary refill and skin perfusion q2–4h until within normal limits then once, 4–8 hours * Feed per unit protocol.

helping these children to live longer, often into their 50s and 60s. Educational support with technical training allows some mildly retarded children to live independently with minimal supervision and to perform simple job skills.

spina bifida

When the vertebral column fails to close during intrauterine development, the condition is called *spina bifida.* There are several forms of this condition:

* *Spina bifida occulta*—failure of the vertebral arch to close. A dimple occurs on the sacral area that may be covered by a tuft of hair.
* *Meningocele*—protrusion of the meninges (dura mater, arachnoid, and pia mater) usually covered by a thin membrane (Fig. 17-4*B*). There is no paralysis because the spinal cord is not involved.
* *Myelomeningocele*—protrusion of the meninges and spinal cord, covered by a thin membrane (see Fig. 17-4*C*). The extent of paralysis depends on the location of the defect. Hydrocephalus also may result with this defect.

> **nursing alert**
>
> *The primary intervention when an infant is born with a meningocele or myelomeningocele is to cover the defect with a sterile, saline-soaked dressing to maintain moisture and decrease risk of infection.*

Surgery is often performed the day of birth to correct the defect, minimize complications, and prevent infection. The nurse encourages the parents to become involved with care of the infant as soon as they are able. They need to learn techniques of feeding, range of motion exercises, positioning, catheterization (if prescribed), and skin care. The nurse must alert the family to potential problems and complications that accompany spina bifida.

congenital disorders

respiratory distress syndrome

Respiratory distress syndrome is caused by insufficient production of *surfactant* in the lungs. Surfactant is a phospholipid mixture produced by alveolar cells. It reduces surface tension of pulmonary fluids and promotes elasticity in pulmonary tissues. When surfactant is lacking, respiratory distress syndrome develops, and the lung alveoli collapse. Surfactant probably becomes sufficient to prevent alveolar collapse around 34 to 35 weeks' gestation. Each year, this disease affects approximately 40,000 infants in the United States, most of them preterm (Nugent, 1991).

Collapse of the lung alveoli (*atelectasis*) causes hypoxia and acidosis. Anaerobic metabolism (conversion of food into energy in the absence of oxygen) produces lactic acid. This impairs the ability of the heart to contract, decreasing cardiac output and blood pressure. Tissue perfusion in the organs is impaired, and respiratory failure occurs.

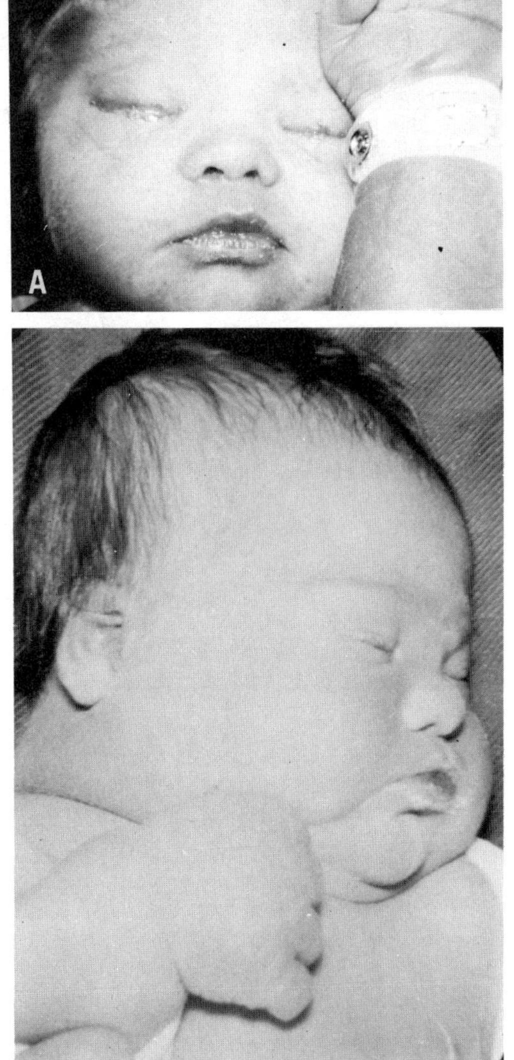

figure 17-3 *(A, B) Down syndrome.*

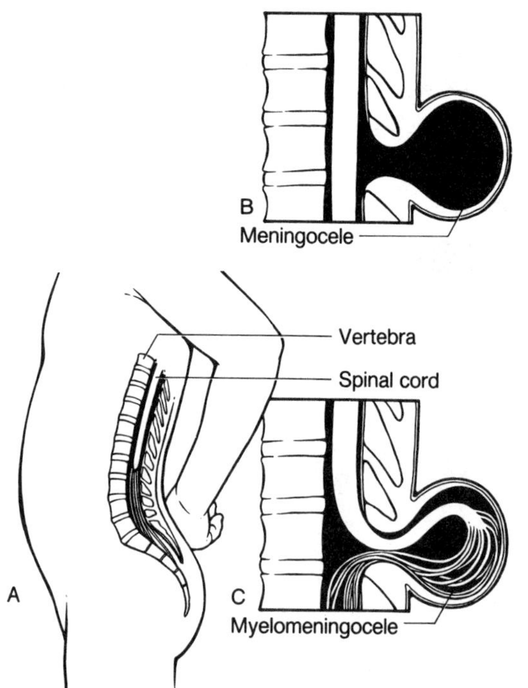

figure 17-4 *Cross-section of a normal spine **(A)** compared to a meningocele **(B)** and a myelomeningocele **(C)**.*

Nursing support at the LPN level usually includes monitoring of vital signs, oxygen and ventilatory supplementation, and noting signs of cyanosis and increasing respiratory distress, such as nasal flaring, grunting, or retracting. It is essential to report any negative change (see Chap. 30).

congenital heart disorders

patent ductus arteriosus

During fetal life, a vascular connection exists that is necessary to shunt oxygenated blood from the pulmonary artery out to the systemic circulation through the aorta. Blood in the fetal circulation is oxygenated through the placental circulation and not in the fetal lungs. This ductus usually closes spontaneously after birth. When it remains patent, the acyanotic condition is called patent ductus arteriosus, the most common congenital heart defect. This defect results in a harsh systolic murmur, eventually leading to right heart failure and pulmonary congestion. This defect is sometimes correctable by use of indomethacin, which causes vasoconstriction, or through surgical ligation of the ductus (see Fig. 17-5*A*).

coarctation of the aorta

This congenital defect is characterized by a narrowed aortic lumen, producing an obstruction of flow through the aorta. This in turn causes an increase in left ventricular pressure and results in congestive heart failure if surgical resection of the narrowing is not performed. Surgical interventions include enlargement of the constricted section using a prosthetic graft or a piece of the left subclavian artery or resecting the constricted portion using an end-to-end anastomosis of the aorta. A nonsurgical treatment is balloon angioplasty; however, tests are being conducted to determine its safety and effectiveness in infants (Fig. 17-5*B*).

septal defects

Septal defects are acyanotic heart defects. When an opening exists between the right and left sides of the heart, blood will flow from the greater pressure (left side) to the lesser pressure (right side). This does not produce

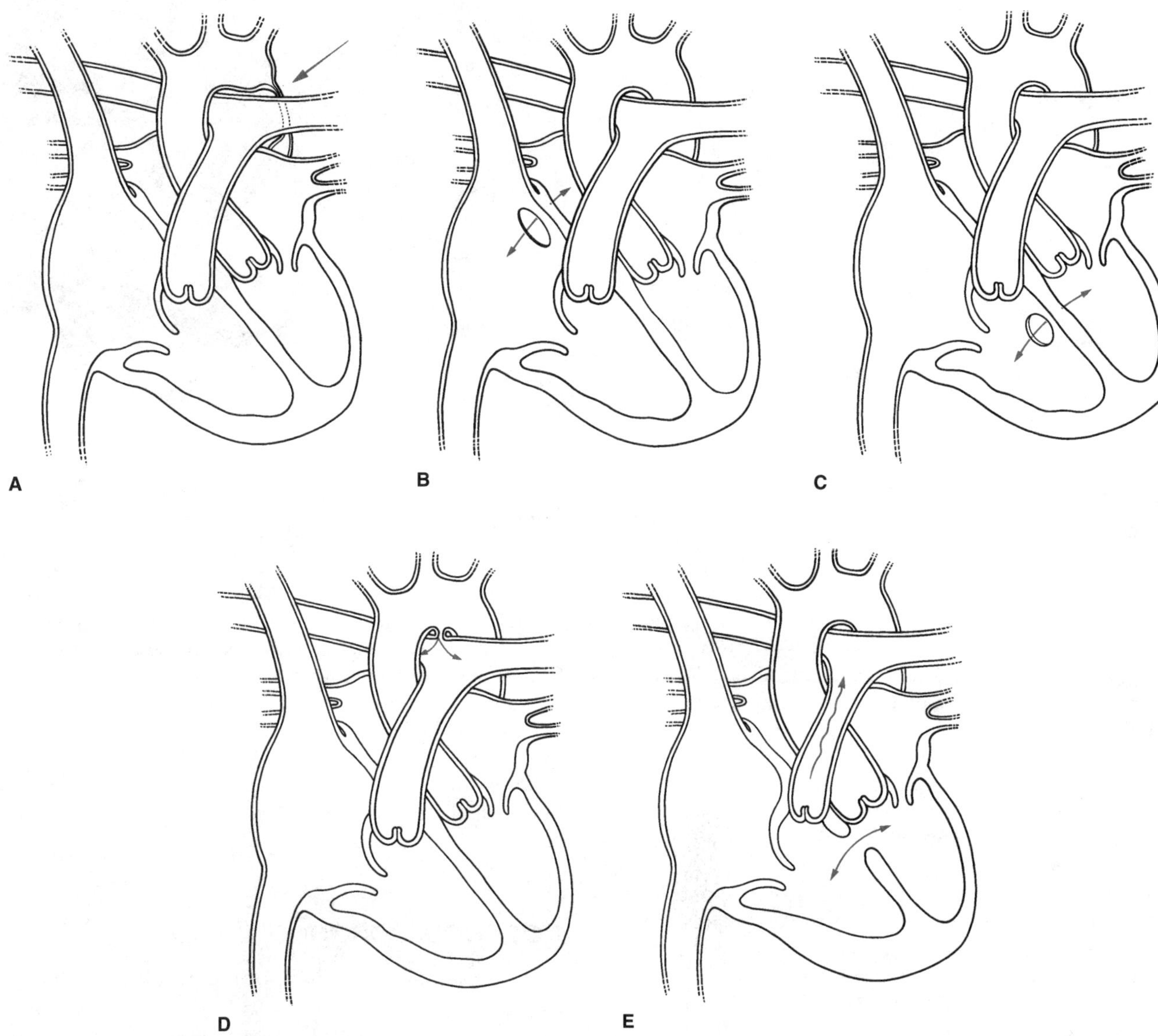

figure 17-5 *Major congenital anomalies that result in acyanotic heart disease.* ***(A)*** *Atrial septal defect is an abnormal opening between the left and right atria that leads to left-to-right shunting of blood.* ***(B)*** *Ventricular septal defect is a condition in which abnormal openings occur between the right and left ventricles.* ***(C)*** *Patent ductus arteriosus is the abnormal persistence of a vascular connection that, during fetal life, short circuits the pulmonary vascular bed and directs blood from the pulmonary artery to the aorta.* ***(D)*** *In coarctation of the aorta, an abnormal narrowing of the lumen of the aorta causes an increased left ventricular pressure and workload (Ross Laboratories). Major congenital anomalies resulting in cyanotic heart disease.* ***(E)*** *Tetralogy of Fallot is characterized by the combination of four defects: pulmonary stenosis, ventricular septal defect, an overriding aorta, and hypertrophy of the right ventricle.*

cyanosis because oxygenated blood is still being pumped to the systemic circulation. An abnormal opening between the right and left atria is called atrial septal defect (ASD). An abnormal opening between the right and left ventricles is called ventricular septal defect (VSD). A VSD will sometimes close spontaneously. A VSD and an ASD are correctable by surgery (see Fig. 17-5*C* and *D*).

tetralogy of fallot

The most common cyanotic heart defect is tetralogy of Fallot. This anomaly consists of four cardiac defects: pulmonary stenosis, ventricular septal defect, overriding aorta (aorta is displaced to the right, appears to arise from both ventricles, and straddles the VSD), and right ventricular hypertrophy (enlargement). The severity of symptoms depends on the severity of the individual defects. Symptoms in the newborn include cyanosis, characteristic murmur, hypoxia, and anoxic spells.

Corrective surgery involves resection of the pulmonary stenosis and closure of the VSD (see Fig. 17-5*E*).

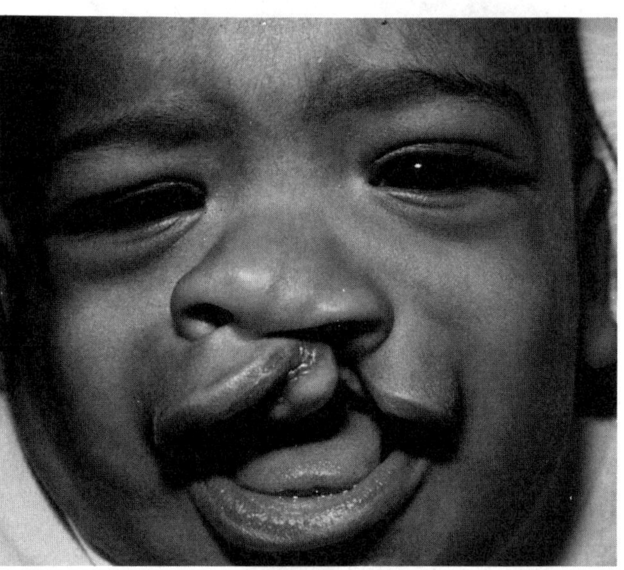

figure 17-6 *Unilateral cleft lip and palate. (Krause, C. J. et al. [1991].* Aesthetic facial surgery. *Philadelphia: J. B. Lippincott.)*

cleft lip and cleft palate

Among the most common congenital anomalies are cleft lip and cleft palate (CL/CP). These can occur separately or together and can be unilateral or bilateral. The degree of cleft may be from minor (notch at the lip or only the soft palate) to major (the entire lip and into the base of the nose or the entire hard and soft palates; Fig. 17-6). The cause could be genetic or environmental. Treatment includes prevention of aspiration and infection with emphasis on long-term care, including surgical correction and possibly speech therapy. Feeding the infant with a CL/CP presents a special problem to the nurse and parents. These infants have a decreased sucking ability, so liquid tends to escape out of the cleft palate through the nose. The nurse explains to the parents that the best way to feed an infant with CL/CP is to place the infant in an upright position and use specially designed nipples. The nurse should advise the parents that infants with CL/CP need to be burped frequently because of their tendency to swallow increased amounts of air.

clubfoot (talipes)

The most common congenital musculoskeletal anomaly is clubfoot (talipes; Fig. 17-7). This involves a deformity of the talus and metatarsals with a shortened Achilles tendon. It can affect one or both feet. In the most common form, the heel turns inward and the foot is plantarflexed. Sometimes position in utero may make the foot appear clublike. If the foot reverts to a natural position with full range of motion, true clubfoot is not suspected.

Clubfoot may be corrected with special shoes, casts, or braces. If these measures are not successful, surgical correction is indicated.

tracheoesophageal fistula

Tracheoesophageal malformations result from incomplete separation of the trachea and esophagus during intrauterine development. *Tracheoesophageal fistula* is char-

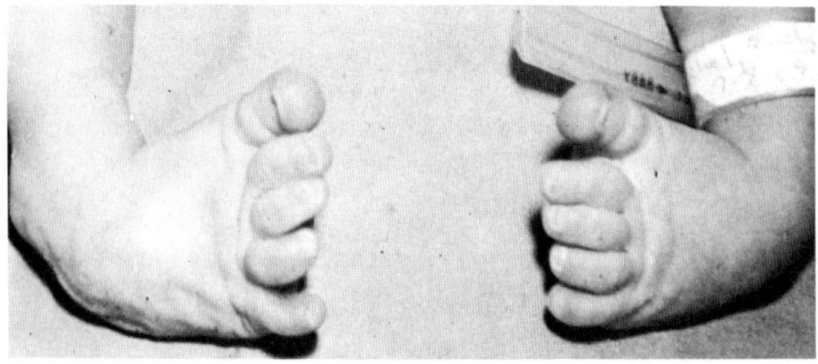

figure 17-7 *Talipes equinocavovarus foot (ie, clubfoot).*

acterized by an intact esophagus with a connection to the trachea. It is often associated with polyhydramnios (accumulation of more than 2,000 mL of amniotic fluid), thought to occur because of the inability of the fetus to swallow amniotic fluid. Symptoms after birth include excessive drooling and spitting up of feedings; increased need for suctioning; coughing, choking, or cyanosis with feedings; distended stomach; and inability to pass a nasal catheter into the stomach.

These malformations require immediate surgical correction, which consists of a thoracotomy with division and ligation of the fistula and an end-to-end anastomosis of the esophagus. The nurse monitors the infant's respiratory status, nutritional needs, fluid and electrolyte balance, and temperature regulation.

pyloric stenosis

This is a functional anomaly seen soon after birth with the symptom of progressive vomiting. It occurs because of hypertrophy of the pylorus muscle, causing obstruction at the pyloric sphincter. Projectile vomiting usually develops during the first week of life and leads to complete obstruction within 4 to 6 weeks. These infants appear dehydrated, malnourished, and lethargic. Surgery is the standard treatment for pyloric stenosis. Nursing interventions include monitoring vital signs, providing intravenous fluids, and recording intake and output. The nurse also looks for signs of stress or pain from surgery.

imperforate anus

Imperforate anus is an abnormal closure of the anus. It may be seen as a dimple where the anal opening should be, or it may manifest in a blind pouch in the lower or upper portion of the rectum. The defect is often noted first when attempting to take a rectal temperature. If the defect is high, imperforate anus must be considered if the newborn does not pass meconium within 24 hours after birth. The nurse needs to document passage of meconium and note abdominal distention or lack of bowel sounds to assist in the diagnosis. Surgical treatment is indicated in the infant with a midlevel or high malformation. Primary nursing interventions include keeping the perineal area clean and irritation free.

cryptorchidism

Cryptorchidism is failure of one or both testes to descend through the inguinal canal into the scrotum. As the child gets older, the heat of the body will damage his ability to produce sperm and may cause sterility. In an older child, administration of human gonadotropin may help the testes descend. Surgical treatment is called *orchiopexy*. (See Chapter 33.)

epispadias and hypospadias

Epispadias is a disorder in which the meatal opening of the urethra is located on the dorsal (upper) surface of the penis. In *hypospadias*, the meatal opening is found on the ventral (lower) surface of the penis. Surgical correction is possible for both defects and is usually performed when the child is 3 or 4 years old. Correction will improve the ability to direct the urine stream, the physical appearance of the genitalia, and the potential for normal sexual activity. For a full discussion, see Chapter 33.

phenylketonuria

Phenylketonuria (PKU) is an inborn error of metabolism. It is hereditary through autosomal recessive genes. The most common amino acid disorder, PKU is detected through mandatory newborn screening programs. The test involves laboratory analysis of a blood sample obtained through a heel stick.

Phenylalanine is needed by the body for growth. The newborn with PKU lacks the ability to convert excess phenylalanine to tyrosine. The accumulation of phenylalanine in the brain tissue leads to progressive mental retardation.

Nursing responsibility includes ensuring that the heel stick is performed before discharge and that the specimen is properly recorded and sent for analysis. Once the diagnosis of PKU is made, the nurse will assist with parent education for appropriate dietary management. A diet low in phenylalanine, if begun before 3 months of age, can limit damage to the central nervous system (see Display 17-3 for examples of foods low and high in phenylalanine). Blood phenylalanine levels should be kept below 15 to 20 mg/dL for life because brain myelination continues actively into adulthood.

display 17-3
foods high and low in phenylalanine

HIGH

- Meat or meat products
- Dairy products
- Sweetener (aspartame, NutraSweet, Equal)

LOW

- Vegetables
- Fruits
- Some cereals
- Breads
- Starches

*These foods should be measured to provide prescribed amount of phenylalanine.

hemolytic disease

Hemolytic disease of the newborn is a progressive disorder of the fetal blood characterized by *hyperbilirubinemia*. There are two categories of disease: Rh incompatibility and ABO incompatibility. Rh incompatibility occurs when an Rh-negative woman and an Rh-positive man produce an Rh-positive fetus. The Rh-positive cells of the fetus sensitize the mother to produce Rh-positive antibodies. In future pregnancies, an Rh-positive fetus will cause these antibodies to cross the placenta, resulting in *hemolysis* (destruction of red cells) of fetal blood. This causes fetal jaundice and anemia and will worsen progressively in future pregnancies with an Rh-positive fetus.

Nursing care as a preventive measure involves assessing mother and infant blood types and ensuring that the Rh-negative mother receives RhoGAM if she produces an Rh-positive infant. On a clinical level, once sensitized (by not receiving RhoGAM), the mother maintains a positive antibody screen but is otherwise asymptomatic.

The newborn will become jaundiced, usually requiring phototherapy. The nurse needs to maintain effective phototherapy through the use of an isolette with an ultraviolet light or phototherapy blanket. The infant's eyes must be properly shielded to prevent retinal damage. The infant is usually naked or has only a small covering over the genitals for stooling and voiding. Vital signs are taken every 4 hours and adequate fluid intake provided and recorded to prevent dehydration and promote elimination. Bilirubin is excreted in the stools and urine. Sometimes Rh sensitization causes such severe destruction of fetal red blood cells that the infant will require an exchange transfusion to minimize the chance of *kernicterus* (brain damage) from elevated bilirubin levels.

ABO incompatibility is usually less severe than Rh sensitization. It most often involves a mother with blood type O and an infant with type A, B, or AB blood. Type O blood contains anti-A and anti-B antibodies, which will destroy the infant's red blood cells, causing jaundice. This can occur, but less frequently, if the mother is type A (anti-B antibodies), and the infant is type B or vice versa. Phototherapy is the treatment of choice and is successful with this type of jaundice. All precautions, as stated previously, should be used with any type of phototherapy.

hydrocephalus

Hydrocephalus is the accumulation of excess cerebrospinal fluid in the ventricles of the fetal brain. The infant's head is shiny, with wide, bulging fontanels; prominent scalp veins; and separated suture lines. Increased intracranial pressure causes a downward cast of the eyes. If enlargement of the head continues untreated, brain damage occurs, and the infant will die. If hydrocephalus is identified early, surgery to insert a shunt to drain the excess fluid can help minimize brain damage (Fig. 17-8). Family support is a vital part of the nursing care. Comfort, nutrition, and support are important needs of the infant.

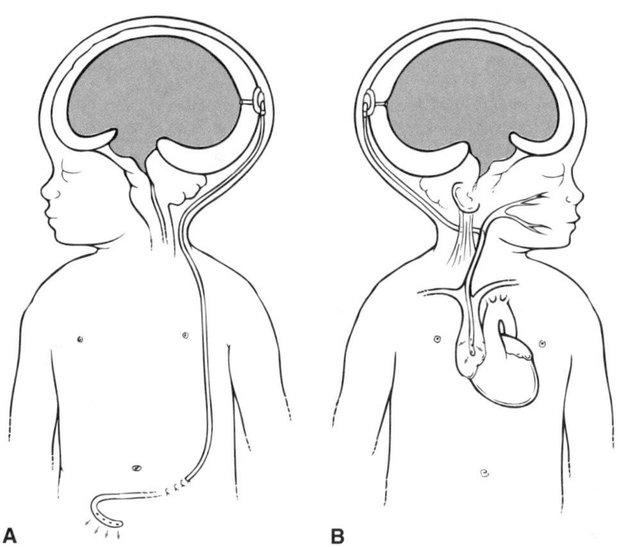

figure 17-8 *(A) Ventriculoperitoneal shunt. (B) Ventriculoatrial shunt. (From Milhorat TH. [1972].* Hydrocephalus and the cerebrospinal fluid. *Baltimore: Williams & Wilkins.* [p. 197])

Because placement of a shunt requires threading a drainage catheter into the peritoneum through an abdominal incision, most infants are fed using a nasogastric tube. After bowel sounds return postoperatively, fluids can be gradually introduced. Infants with hydrocephalus should be held when fed. Observe for vomiting, which is a sign of increased intracranial pressure, and constipation, which may increase intracranial pressure.

birth trauma

meconium aspiration

Meconium in the amniotic fluid results from fetal asphyxia in utero. The fetus responds to the asphyxia with increased peristalsis, anal sphincter relaxation, and passage of meconium. If meconium is aspirated into the tracheobronchial tree in utero or with the first breaths at birth, it produces a ball-valve effect in the lungs: Air is inhaled but cannot be exhaled. The alveoli become distended and create pneumothorax, bacterial pneumonia, or pulmonary hypertension.

Medical treatment involves immediate suctioning while the fetal head is on the perineum, before the infant's first breath. The infant will most likely be treated with ventilatory support in a neonatal intensive care unit.

Nursing care involves prevention through early identification and suctioning before the infant's first breath. If aspiration has occurred, oxygen must not be administered before the infant has been intubated and suctioned because the pressure of the oxygen may force bits of meconium further down into the lungs. Gas exchange is maintained through oxygenation and ventilatory support; vital signs are monitored, and intravenous fluid is maintained. If any specks of meconium remain in the lungs, the nurse may perform postural drainage with clapping and vibration to remove them.

asphyxia

Asphyxia is defined as insufficient oxygen in the blood (*hypoxemia*), excessive carbon dioxide in the blood, and decreased blood Ph. Initial assessment findings include rapid respirations, followed by apnea (absence of respirations), and then a decreasing heart rate. The infant then begins to gasp, the heart rate continues to fall, and the blood pressure drops. Respirations will continue to weaken until they stop altogether. Resuscitation is indicated to prevent cerebral hypoxia, metabolic imbalances, intraventricular hemorrhage, and necrotizing enterocolitis.

Apneic episodes, cessation of breathing for more than 15 seconds, is common among preterm neonates. These episodes are often preventable through nursing care that identifies and corrects their cause:

* Maintain appropriate blood oxygen levels to prevent acidosis.
* Provide adequate nutrition to prevent anemia and hypoglycemia or hyperglycemia.
* Provide a thermoneutral environment to prevent hypothermia.
* Maintain safety measures to prevent abdominal distention, regurgitation, and sepsis.

Central apnea, caused by insufficient neural impulses from the respiratory center, requires more intensive therapy.

retinopathy of prematurity (retrolental fibroplasia)

Retinopathy of prematurity (ROP) is primarily seen in preterm and very low–birth-weight infants who have been treated with oxygen therapy associated with respiratory conditions. The immature blood vessels in the retina may be damaged if arterial blood oxygen levels are too high. Other causes of ROP are being investigated because this condition also has developed in infants who have not received oxygen therapy.

Nursing care is preventive. Oxygen concentration and arterial blood oxygen levels must be monitored closely using such monitoring equipment as a pulse oximeter. This will allow the minimal amount of oxygen necessary for survival to be used and may decrease the incidence of ROP. Because other causes of ROP are uncertain, preventive measures in all aspects must be used. Protection of infant eyes from ultraviolet lights, such as bilirubin lights, is essential; dim but adequate lighting is maintained in the nursery. Administering the antioxidant vitamin E may prevent the occurrence of ROP because it minimizes tissue response to the effects of oxygen.

intraventricular hemorrhage

Intraventricular hemorrhage (IVH) most often occurs during the first 2 days of life in 20% to 30% of infants born at less than 32 weeks' gestation and weighing less than 1,500 g (5.5 lb; Minarcik & Beachy, 1993). Respiratory problems and hypoxia that increase blood pressure, vasodilation, and rupture of blood vessels are most often associated with IVH.

Observing and reporting signs of IVH are a part of the assessment routine. Signs of IVH include full or bulging fontanels, poor muscle tone, lethargy, irritability, forceful vomiting, and negative changes in vital signs.

fractures and brachial plexus injury

The clavicle is the bone most often broken during birth. Other fractures may occur but with less frequency. Assessment for fractures should be performed, especially when shoulder dystocia was present during delivery. The normal clavicle is straight. If a fracture occurred, a grating sensation called *crepitus* may be felt during movement. Eliciting the Moro reflex (seen only on the unaffected side) to evaluate symmetry of movement may help in the diagnosis. Treatment includes splinting the affected side against the chest and careful handling to prevent pain and further injury.

With a clavicular fracture or a fracture of any bone in the arm, damage to the brachial plexus may cause paralysis on the affected side. It occurs most often when traction is applied to the head of the newborn during a difficult delivery. The most common type of injury involves the upper arm, called *Erb's paralysis* (Erb's palsy at the fifth and sixth cervical nerves). The newborn's arm is limp, with the elbow in extension. The newborn is unable to elevate the affected arm, and the Moro reflex cannot be elicited on the affected side. Treatment involves passive range of motion exercises to prevent contractures and to restore function. Occasional splinting is necessary. With minimal injury, complete recovery is expected within a few months. Orthopedic follow-up is recommended to evaluate problems associated with the growth plate that may be seen later.

infections

Newborns are particularly susceptible to infectious agents due to the immaturity of their immune systems. Prompt diagnosis and treatment are important to prevent neonatal death.

diarrhea

Diarrhea in infants can be serious. Dehydration can occur quickly. Watery stools that leave little or no solid material on the diaper indicate diarrhea. The nurse assesses the infant's diaper for a "water ring," which shows where liquid has been absorbed. Infants with diarrhea must be evaluated by a registered nurse or physician for treatment.

Symptoms associated with moderate to severe diarrhea include increased frequency of stools, weight loss, irritability, vomiting, fever, stools containing mucus or blood, dehydration, and weakness. If left untreated, lethargy and coma may result. The nurse's role in caring for the infant with diarrhea includes daily calculations of intake, output, and weight; administering ointment to soothe the perirectal area; and noting the physical characteristics of the stool. The nurse should not take rectal temperatures, which could stimulate and traumatize the area.

conjunctivitis

Conjunctivitis may be chemical or infectious. Ophthalmic drops or ointment (erythromycin or tetracycline) instilled to prevent birth-related eye injury can cause the lid to swell. This chemical conjunctivitis, often seen with a clear discharge, appears a few hours after instillation and disappears in 1 to 2 days.

Infectious conjunctivitis may be caused by gram-negative bacteria, such as staphylococci, and requires treatment with ophthalmic antibiotics. A purulent exudate is present, and edema of the eyelids may be seen. The gonococcal and chlamydial organisms also may cause conjunctivitis. Newborns in the United States receive erythromycin or tetracycline ointment drops to prevent conjunctivitis.

The nurse should assess the infant's eyes routinely and remove any drainage with a clean, moist cloth; the eyes should be wiped from the inner to the outer canthus using a clean portion of the cloth for each wipe. If a purulent discharge is seen, the nurse reports this and administers treatment as ordered. Noting any maternal history of *Gonorrhea* or *Chlamydia* will aid in diagnosing the source.

thrush

If *Candida albicans* is present in the birth canal during delivery, the newborn may become infected. This condition, known as *thrush,* appears as white patches resembling milk curds on the tongue and cheeks. The patches may bleed if they are wiped. The infant is treated with a preparation of nystatin (Mycostatin).

impetigo

Impetigo contagiosa is caused by *Staphylococcus* and is common in the toddler and preschooler. The newborn also is susceptible to this infection because skin resistance to bacteria is low. It appears on the skin as a reddish macule, becoming vesicular and rupturing easily, leaving a moist exudate. The exudate dries to form a thick, honey-colored crust. Itching is common, and the infection is easily spread. Treatment includes the topical ointment mupirocin (Bactroban) or systemic antibiotics. Parents should be instructed to wash the lesions three to four times a day to remove any crusts. Nursing care is primarily preventive. This includes educating the parents about the necessity of prompt treatment of minor cuts and bites common in children. These skin openings tend to allow entrance of the *Staphylococcus* organism. The nurse also should state the importance of compliance with the treatment regimen to prevent the spread of infection.

streptococcal infection

One of the most common infections in the newborn is group B beta-hemolytic *Streptococcus,* which is transmitted to the infant during the birth process. The well infant develops a sudden onset of respiratory distress a few hours after birth. Respiratory assessment may reveal grunting, flaring, and retraction. The infant may be cyanotic or apneic or may exhibit signs of shock. Early assessment and reporting of clinical signs are essential. Assistance with cultures and monitoring support is needed. After cultures are obtained, immediate administration of antibiotics, such as a combination of ampicillin and gentamicin, is crucial to survival. The nurse should practice effective and frequent handwashing to prevent the spread of infection.

substance abuse

Substance abuse is epidemic in the United States and reaches every socioeconomic group. Substance abuse not only includes illegal drugs, such as heroin and cocaine, but legal substances, such as alcohol, tobacco, and caffeine. Almost all substances cross the placenta and enter fetal circulation. An infant born to a drug- or alcohol-dependent mother also will be drug or alcohol dependent. Some substances ingested by the mother may be teratogenic and result in congenital anomalies. It is not uncommon for a client to abuse more than one substance.

infant born to a drug-dependent mother

Because most drugs cross the placenta, the infant may develop problems in utero or shortly after birth. Complications include growth retardation, respiratory distress, prematurity, withdrawal symptoms. Symptoms of withdrawal usually occur within 24 to 72 hours after birth (Display 17-4). A significant number of newborns require treatment of their withdrawal symptoms with phenobarbital or paregoric. These medications are gradually tapered off and discontinued after several days. Nursing care primarily includes promotion of physical well-being, including monitoring of vital signs, adequate nutrition, holding, increased touch, a quiet and dimly lit environment, and medication. Family support includes counseling regarding available resources and ongoing evaluation to detect long-term problems. Hepatitis and acquired immunodeficiency syndrome (AIDS) are long-term problems frequently seen in infants of heroin-addicted mothers. Cocaine addiction has been known to increase the infant's risk to the following long-term disorders: sudden infant death syndrome, renal defects, cardiac anomalies, mild facial dysmorphic features, cerebral infarcts, necrotizing enterocolitis, low birth weight and length, and decreased head circumference.

display 17-4
infant drug withdrawal

SYMPTOMS OF DRUG WITHDRAWAL

* Hyperactivity
* Hyperirritability
* Tremors
* Sneezing
* Tachypnea
* Diarrhea
* Abdominal cramping
* Stuffy nose
* Sweating
* Excoriated buttocks, knees

fetal alcohol syndrome

Fetal alcohol syndrome (FAS) is characterized by prenatal and newborn growth retardation, mental retardation, delayed motor development, irritability, microcephaly, flat midface, and a thin upper lip. An infant with less severe effects of maternal alcohol use during pregnancy is said to have *fetal alcohol effects*.

The ideal treatment for FAS is prevention, advising pregnant women to avoid alcohol because it is not known how much alcohol is necessary to cause serious problems. Once FAS has occurred, assessment and documentation of withdrawal symptoms are important. Tremors, inconsolable crying, hyperactive rooting reflex, seizures, and sleeplessness often occur within 6 to 12 hours after birth. The nurse needs to monitor vital signs closely to detect signs of distress, prevent heat loss, protect the infant from injury, reduce environmental stimuli, encourage feedings, and administer any medication. As with drug dependency, family support is essential.

infant born with human immunodeficiency virus or acquired immunodeficiency syndrome

Human immunodeficiency virus (HIV) or AIDS can be transmitted through placental transfer, breast-feeding, or contaminated blood (Nair, 1992). Infants born to a mother infected with HIV carry the mother's HIV antibodies. This means that an infant who tests positive at birth may not actually be infected. Seroconversion may take up to 15 months.

Nursing care of the newborn with HIV or AIDS must include universal precautions, as is recommended with most patient care (gown, gloves, and handwashing), but with special emphasis on blood-borne transmission. The goals of care involve protection from opportunistic infections, keeping the newborn well nourished because failure to thrive is common, and facilitating growth and development. Disposable diapers are recommended, with disposal in special sealed plastic bags. Separate towels and washcloths are necessary, but clothing and linens can be washed with others unless visibly soiled with blood or body fluid.

key points

* **Using the nursing process will provide information to identify high-risk infants.**
* **Infants with alterations in size and gestational age are at risk for complications, which, when managed appropriately, can be minimized or prevented if recognized early.**
* **The four major cardiac defects (patent ductus arteriosus, coarctation of the aorta, septal defects, tetralogy of Fallot) are life-threatening but may be corrected successfully with medication or surgery.**
* **Hemolytic disease can cause kernicterus (brain damage from bilirubin) if not managed or treated.**
* **Infections in newborns are serious and must be treated medically to prevent systemic complications and possibly death.**
* **Maternal substance abuse produces serious withdrawal symptoms in the newborn.**
* **Care of infants born with HIV or AIDS requires emphasis on blood-borne pathogen transmission.**

review questions

1. The bone most commonly fractured during delivery is the
   a. femur.
   b. clavicle.
   c. sternum.
   d. ulna.
2. Which of the following soft-tissue injuries may contribute to hyperbilirubinemia?
   a. Caput succedaneum
   b. Petechiae
   c. IVH
   d. Cephalhematoma
3. Which of the following is a complication associated with high arterial blood oxygen levels in a preterm infant?
   a. IVH
   b. ROP
   c. Necrotizing enterocolitis
   d. Bronchopulmonary dysplasia
4. Newborns with substance-abusing mothers exhibit which behaviors?
   a. Cyanosis, constipation
   b. Strong suck, hypothermia
   c. Hyperirritability, difficulty feeding
   d. Fatigue, weak cry

5. Which is true about LGA infants?
   a. They are prone to hypoglycemia.
   b. They weigh more than 3,500 g.
   c. Fractured clavicles are common.
   d. Their weight is above the 80th percentile.

references

Gomella, T. L. (Ed.) (1992). *Neonatology: Management, procedures, on-call problems, diseases, drugs* (2nd ed.). Norwalk, CT: Appleton & Lange.

Hoskins, S. K. (1990). Nursing care of the infant of a diabetic mother: An antenatal, intrapartal and neonatal challenge. *Neonatal Network*, *9*(4), 39.

Kliegman, R. M. (1990). Fetal and Neonatal Medicine. In R. E. Behrman (Ed.), *Nelson essentials of pediatrics.* Philadelphia: W.B. Saunders.

Minarcik, C. J., & Beachy, P. (1993). Neurologic disorders. In G. B. Merenstein & S. L. Gardner (Eds.), *Handbook of neonatal intensive care* (2nd ed.). St. Louis: C.V. Mosby.

Nair, P. (1992). Early identification of HIV infection in children. *Pediatric AIDS and HIV Infection*, *3*(1), 40.

Nugent, J. (1991). *Acute respiratory care of the neonate*. Petaluma, CA: Neonatal Network.

Pittard, III, W. B. (1993). Classification of the low-birth-weight infant. In M. H. Kaus & A. A. Fanaroff (Eds.), *Care of the high-risk neonate.* Philadelphia: W.B. Saunders.

Pressler, J. L. (1991). Strategies useful in caring for macrosomic newborn. *Journal of Pediatric Nursing*, *6*(3), 149.

bibliography

Bobak, I. M., & Jensen, M. D. (1993). *Maternity and gynecologic care* (5th ed.). St. Louis: Mosby–Year Book.

Carpenito, L. (1995). *Nursing Diagnosis application to clinical practice* (6th ed.). Philadelphia: J.B. Lippincott.

Gorrie, T. M., McKinney, E. S., & Murray, S. S. (1994). *Foundations of maternal newborn nursing.* Philadelphia: W.B. Saunders.

Gulanick, M., Puzas, M. K., & Wilson, C. R. (1992). *Nursing care plans for newborns and children.* St. Louis: Mosby–Year Book.

Kenner, C. A. (1992). *Neonatal care—Nurse's clinical guide.* Springhouse, PA: Springhouse Corp.

Kenner, C. A., & MacLaren, A. (1993). *Essentials of maternal and neonatal nursing.* Springhouse, PA: Springhouse Corp.

Ladewig, P. W., London, M., & Olds, S. B. (1994). *Essentials of maternal-newborn nursing* (3rd ed.). Redwood City, CA: Addison-Wesley Nursing.

Mayers, M., & Jacobson, A. (1995). *Perinatal/neonatal nursing clinical care plans.* New York: McGraw-Hill.

Wong, D. L. (1993). *Essentials of pediatric nursing* (4th ed.). St. Louis: Mosby–Year Book.

growth and development

unit VI

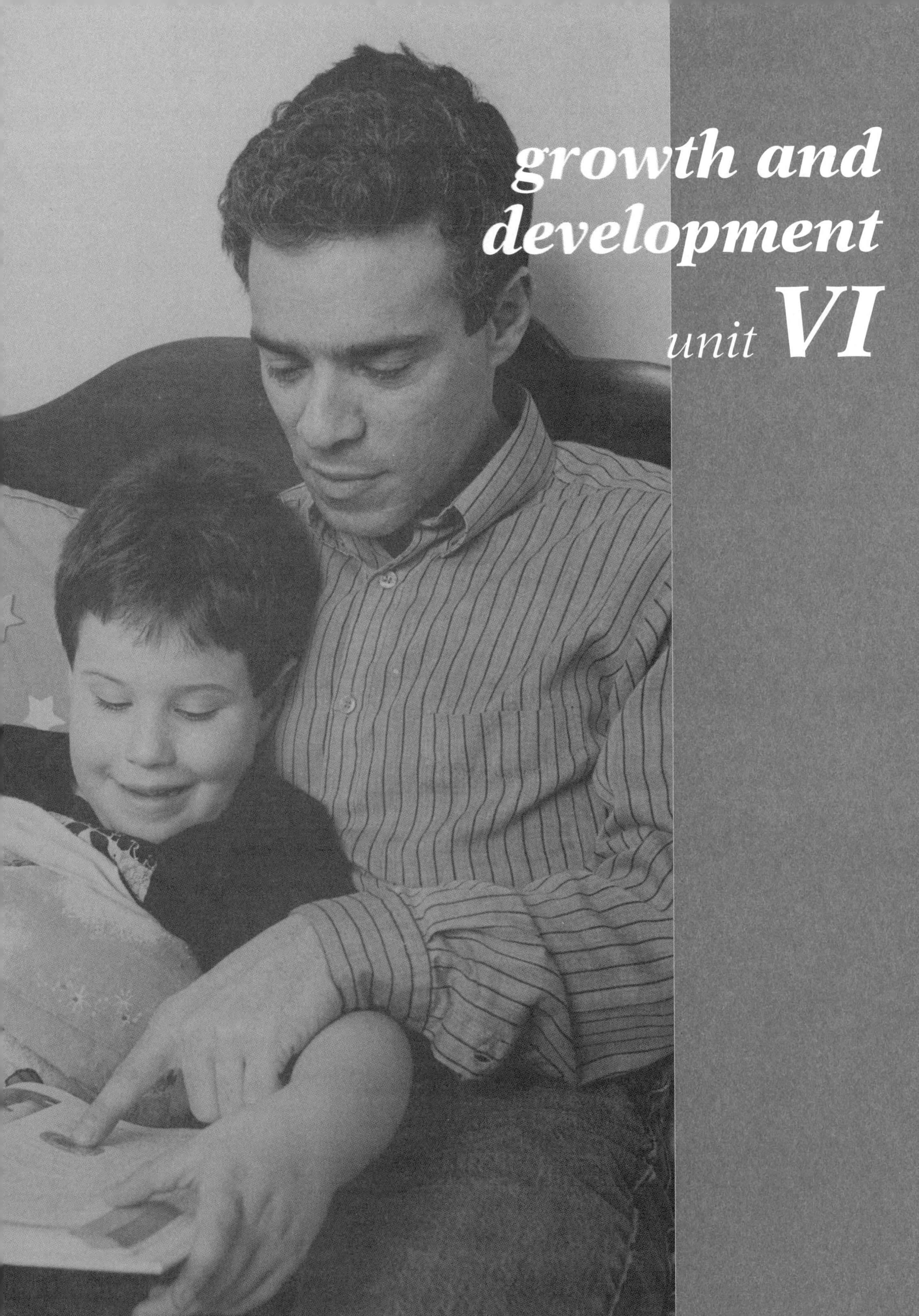

theories of growth and development

18

outline

objectives 

After studying this chapter, the reader should be able to:

* *Discuss why growth and development theories are important for nurses and parents to understand.*
* *Define growth, development, cephalocaudal, proximodistal, and developmental sequence.*
* *Compare Maslow's basic needs theory with Erikson's psychosocial theory.*
* *Describe the relationship between self-concept development and the theories of Maslow, Erikson, Skinner, and Bandura.*
* *Compare Bandura's observational learning theory with Skinner's Behaviorist theory in relation to violence.*
* *Compare Piaget's moral developmental theory with that of Kohlberg and Gilligan.*
* *List at least three influences on moral development.*
* *List two nursing interventions appropriate for altered growth and development.*

key terms 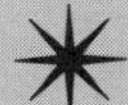

behavior modification
"catch-up growth"
cephalocaudal
conditioning
critical periods
developmental sequence
extinction
observational learning
personality
positive reinforcement
proximodistal
socialization
stimulus
reinforcement
response

Neff C & Spray M. *Introduction to Maternal and Child Health Nursing,*

Every field of study has developed theories to explain things that have not been proven as facts, and pediatrics is no exception. A *theory* is a set of assumptions based on observations of behavior or other phenomena; these assumptions attempt to explain or describe what happens.

Theories concerning growth and development help to identify specific milestones in a child's life, describe the current status of the child, and predict what will happen in the future as that child grows and learns.

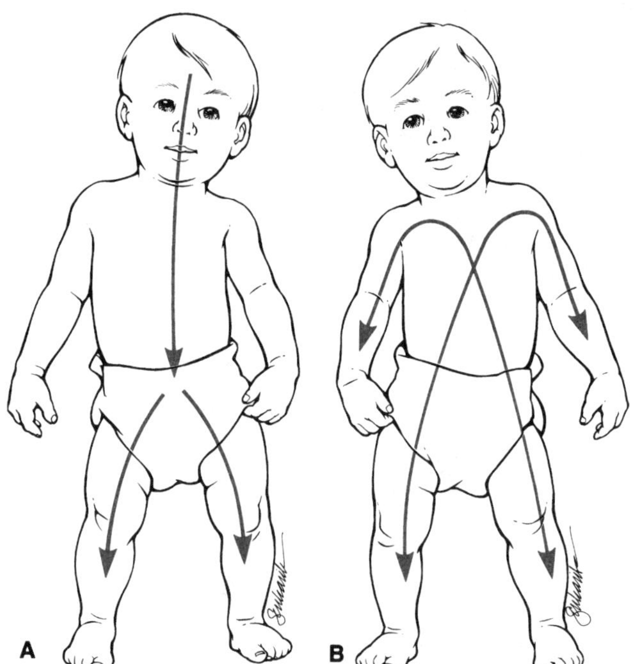

figure 18-1 *Principles of growth.* ***(A)*** *Cephalocaudal. Growth proceeds from the head to toe or tail.* ***(B)*** *Proximodistal. Growth proceeds from the center outward.*

importance of growth and development theories

Throughout the 20th century, theories concerning infant and child behaviors, development, and reasoning abilities have provided parents and other adults working with children with important information about personal learning concepts. Theories provide the building blocks necessary for understanding behavior.

Assessing the growth and development of children is an important nursing function. Competent pediatric nursing skills include the ability to recognize normal or delayed growth and development in children. Early intervention for delays in growth and development can often result in early correction that will enable the child to obtain or maintain optimum health functioning. Child development theories are significant to nursing because of the following:

* They explain and organize growth and development patterns in a sequential and logical order from birth until death.
* They provide an understanding of how children are alike and yet different.
* They offer explanations of behavior according to age categories.

growth and development

The terms *growth* and *development* are often used interchangeably; however, they have different meanings. *Growth* is the physical increase in height, weight, and body organ size caused by an increase in the number of cells. These characteristics can be measured in inches or centimeters and pounds or kilograms. *Development* is the increase in the complexity of function. For example, growth makes a child taller, whereas development makes it possible for a child to progress from crawling to walking. Development is a continuous process that takes time.

All growth, whether physical or mental, indicates organization. The body grows in a patterned, predictable way, just as the mind grows.

> **✳ nursing insight**
>
> *The pattern of growth is the most important thing to study and understand, not the exact time at which any single behavior occurs.*

patterns of growth and development

Growth and development follow a progression from head to tail, known as a *cephalocaudal* pattern, and from midline to the periphery of the body, known as a *proximodistal* pattern (Fig. 18-1). The cephalocaudal and proximodistal progression of growth and development are typically used to describe physical growth and motor development. For example, it explains the child's ability to gain control first over the head, then the torso, and finally the legs. However, the same general directional patterns can be seen in other aspects of development, such as the psychosocial development of children from being self-centered as toddlers to being more socially concerned as adolescents (Display 18-1).

sequence of growth and development

Development of children includes changes in physical function, such as sensorimotor skills, and changes in behavior, intelligence, and understanding. These changes occur in an orderly, predictable sequence known as *developmental sequence*. For example, between the ages of 6 and 10 months, an infant says "mama" or "dada" indiscriminately. Between 10 and 14 months, however, the child says "mama" or "dada" to specific individuals.

The development of new characteristics, skills, and behaviors is identified by periods in which the child is ready

display 18-1
principles of growth and development

* Growth and development of children are progressive, systematic, and sequential.
* Growth and development are not always consistent in pace; "spurts" of growth followed by "lags" are normal.
* Development evolves from general to specific and simple to more complex.
* Emotional development begins with feelings of trust in infancy and progresses to intense attachments in childhood.
* *Cephalocaudal* refers to the head-to-toe progression of growth and development.
* Cephalocaudal growth and development of the nervous system permit infants to progress from controlling their head movements to sitting, crawling, and walking.
* *Proximodistal* refers to growth and development that proceed from the center outward, allowing infants to first master rolling over, then to control their arms and legs, and finally to control their fingers and toes.

for certain activities. These periods are referred to as *critical periods* because a delay in the opportunity for development of new characteristics, skills, and behaviors can jeopardize future growth and development. For example, preschoolers need exposure to other children to help develop interaction skills. If the opportunity for interaction is not provided, children may have difficulty with social adaptation necessary during the school years. Although childhood development occurs in a predictable sequence, the pace of development and the timing of critical periods vary widely among individual children.

Assessing a normal pace of growth and development for children is based on continual, consistent growth patterns. The use of screening tools to plot the progression of children's growth and development helps nurses and other caregivers assess the child in comparison to normal ranges and thereby detect any delays and provide intervention. Growth charts or grids are used to plot the child's weight and height (Appendix).

One of the most commonly used screening tools for overall development is the Denver Developmental Screening Test (DDST). The Denver Developmental Screening Test evaluates four aspects of child development: gross motor skills, fine motor adaptive skills, language skills, and personal-social skills in children between the ages of 2 months and 6 1/2 years. The assessment tool consists of 125 items and can be administered in approximately 15 to 20 minutes. Test results do not reflect the child's intelligence ability but are used to assess developmental function expected at a given age.

influences on growth and development

Heredity and environment play a role in all growth and development. Basic growth and development potential is primarily established by genetics. How children use their potential, however, is influenced by environmental factors, such as nutrition. For example, a child of two parents who are short in stature may grow to be taller than either parent if the child's nutrition is better than the parents' nutrition during their childhood.

Environmental influences have a major effect on the child before and after birth. Prenatal exposure to drugs, such as alcohol, crack cocaine, or nicotine, and diseases, such as acquired immunodeficiency syndrome, rubella, and syphilis, can limit the child's physical and mental growth.

Birth order and socioeconomic status also affect growth and development. Caregivers may need reassurance that just because two siblings are different, there is no reason for concern as long as each falls within normal growth and development limits. Poverty contributes to poor nutrition, inadequate health supervision, and potential for limited stimulation, predisposing the child to altered growth and development.

Children with deficits, especially nutritional deficits, will grow more quickly when the deficits are corrected; this is the body's effort to catch up to the growth phase. Catch-up growth is noticeable in premature infants. Premature children without significant health problems can be expected to reach normal growth curves by the time they are in the preschool years.

sex differences

There are little scientific data on why the growth and development of boys differ from that of girls. However the differences are apparent from the time of conception. Some experts believe the sex differences occur because expectations for the sexes differ. However, it is generally accepted that boys are physically less strong than girls before birth and in the childhood years that follow.

Boys tend to develop more slowly, walking and talking later than girls and mastering toilet training later than girls. Nursery school studies reveal that boys and girls as young as 2 years display different play patterns. Girls usually are satisfied to engage in quiet play longer than boys, who tend to enjoy more active play.

The subject of gender involves many related ideas that are easy to confuse. Gender-related concepts include gender stereotypes, gender roles, and sexual orientation. Gender terms and descriptions are provided in Table 18-1.

studying child development

The most common method for studying children is called the *age-stage approach*. The age-stage approach relates landmarks in the developmental process (stages) to the

table 18-1 gender terminology

Term	Description
Gender	Classification of the biologic sex of a person into male, female, or intersexual
Gender identity	The child's awareness or perception of knowing which sex he or she is
Gender role	The expression of a child's gender identity, the image that the child presents to self and others; often involves culturally defined expectations about appropriate boy and girl behaviors
Gender stereotypes	Widely held, often inaccurate, beliefs about male or female abilities, personality traits, and social actions
Sex	A classification of male, female, or intersex determined at birth based on anatomic and chromosomal characteristics
Sexual orientation	A preference for certain sex partners: Heterosexuals, partners of the opposite sex; homosexuals, partners of the same sex; and bisexuals, partners of either sex
Intersex	Children with anatomic characteristics of both sexes or whose external genitalia are ambiguous, such as seen in hermaphrodites

various life periods (ages) in which they occur. The life periods or ages used are *prenatal, neonatal, infancy, toddlerhood, preschool, school-age,* and *adolescence* (Table 18-2). Researchers have studied various aspects of child development, including psychosocial, intellectual-cognitive, moral, and spiritual development.

table 18-2 age-stage framework for growth and development

Developmental Stage	*Age Range or Time Period*
Prenatal stage	Conception to birth
Neonatal stage	Birth to 1 mo
Infancy	First year
Toddlerhood	1–3 y
Preschool stage	3–5 y
School-age stage	6–11 y
Adolescence	12–18 y

✳ nursing insight

Age norms are not absolute standards. They are points of reference against which a child can be measured.

✳ family considerations

- ✳ Understanding normal age changes helps to determine which things about the child's behavior, good or bad, have been caused by outside influences and which are simply expected behaviors associated with growth.
- ✳ Celebrating birthdays as a cultural custom reflects significant progression toward maturity.
- ✳ Understanding undesirable behaviors that are typical (and usually temporary) for a particular age or stage reduces undue anxiety of caregivers and helps them to remain more calm and guilt free.
- ✳ Understanding growth and development theories provides guidelines for appropriate discipline of children, rather than discouraging discipline.

psychosocial development

Many theorists have studied and tried to explain human behavior, how each person develops. Psychosocial development refers to the evolution of *personality,* which includes who people are inwardly and how they present who they are to others. Personality includes temperament, emotions, self-esteem, self-concept, social behavior, and much more. The psychosocial theorists discussed in this section include Maslow, Freud, Erikson, Skinner, and Bandura.

maslow's basic needs theory

In the 1940s, Abraham Maslow (1908–1970) developed the theory that human behavior is shaped by an individual's attempts to meet basic human needs. Maslow grouped these needs in a hierarchy, sometimes shown as a pyramid, to illustrate that certain needs are more basic than others. The five levels of needs are described as *physiologic, safety and security, love and belonging, self-esteem,* and *self-actualization* needs. Normal growth and development parallel the upward progression from fulfillment of physiologic or survival needs, such as the need for food and water, to the need for psychological and emotional fulfillment in a career, vocation, or profession (Fig. 18-2).

Maslow's hierarchy of needs can be used as a tool to prioritize care of children. Children whose basic survival needs are not adequately met will be unconcerned about higher level needs. Children living in poverty or in an abusive family may be more concerned about food and safety than about education.

UNMET NEEDS CREATE:

5. LACK OF SELF-ACTUALIZATION

4. LACK OF SELF-WORTH
Feelings of insecurity and inferiority. Anxiety about personal worth.

3. UNLOVED-ISOLATED
Feelings of loneliness, rejection, and alienation.

2. LACK OF STABILITY
Feelings of fear due to chaos and disorganization.

1. LACK OF BASIC NEEDS
Preoccupation with survival. Physical suffering.

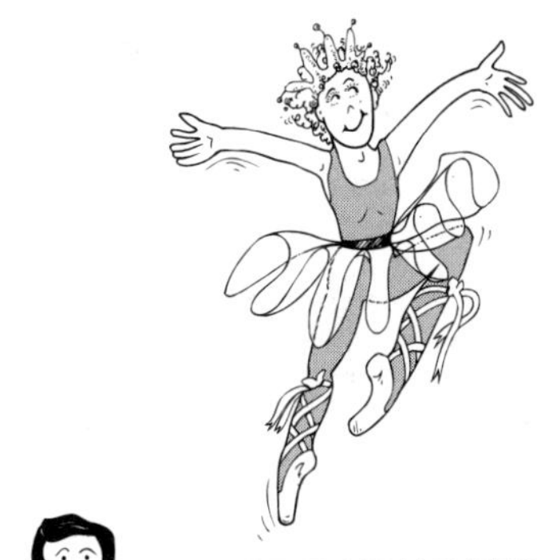

SELF-ACTUALIZED
Full use of talents.
5

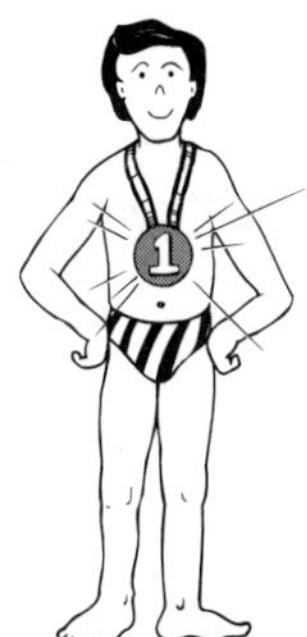

SELF-WORTH
Confidence in oneself to master one's world. Need for achievement and competence. Recognition of status from others.
4

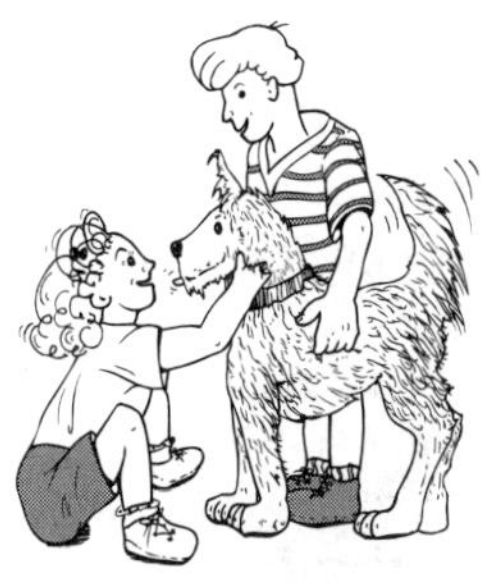

BELONGING-LOVE
Risk reaching out for affection, friends, and acceptance.
3

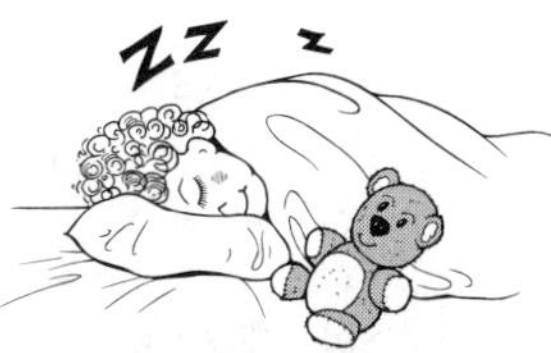

SAFETY & SECURITY
Order, structure, limits. A stable, routine, predictable environment from which to reach out.
2

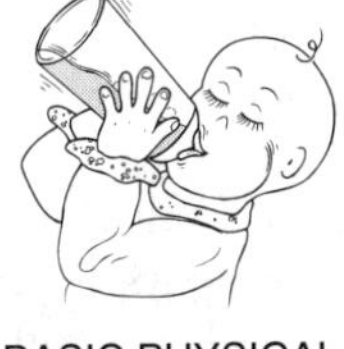
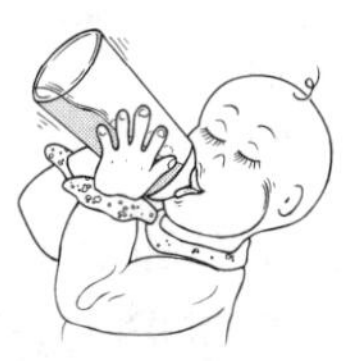

BASIC PHYSICAL NEEDS
Food, shelter, air, and sleep.
1

figure 18-2 *Maslow's hierarchy of needs.*

freud's theory of psychosexual development

In the 1930s, Sigmund Freud (1856–1939) described three components of the human personality as (1) the *id*, present at birth and made up of all the natural biologic urges or instincts to seek pleasure on an unconscious level; (2) the *ego*, based on conscious and rational thought determining what is possible within the limits of the child's world; and (3) the *superego*, encompassing all the internalized values and rules of behavior that are formed through the child's interaction with parents and others, creating feelings of guilt and pride (Fig. 18-3). According to Freud, socially acceptable behaviors develop when a healthy balance exists among the id, ego, and superego.

psychosexual development

Openly criticized by many modern theorists, Freud's theory describes personality development in relation to psychological features of sexual development. It includes the following stages: *oral, anal, phallic, latent,* and *genital*. The time periods include the following:

1. *Oral stage* from birth through 1 year when the child's gratification comes orally
2. *Anal stage* from 2 to 3 years when the child's attention is focused on the anal area
3. Phallic or *oedipal stage* from 3 to 4 years when the child's attention is on the genital areas
4. *Latency stage* from 5 to 15 years when the child's sexual and aggressive fantasies are dormant
5. *Mature genital stage* from 12 to 18 years when the adolescent begins to experience freedom from parents and the older teen leaves home

Freud's approach offends many individuals because his ideas of sexual repression and male dominance reflect a sexist bias.

Modern researchers attribute the differences between male and female behavior to physiologic differences found in the brains of boys and girls. These differences may result from the influence of male and female hormones. The anatomy and physiology of our brains affect how we think, learn, see, smell, feel, communicate, love, and fight. Considering hormonal effects on gender identity, social conditioning alone cannot determine sexual mindset.

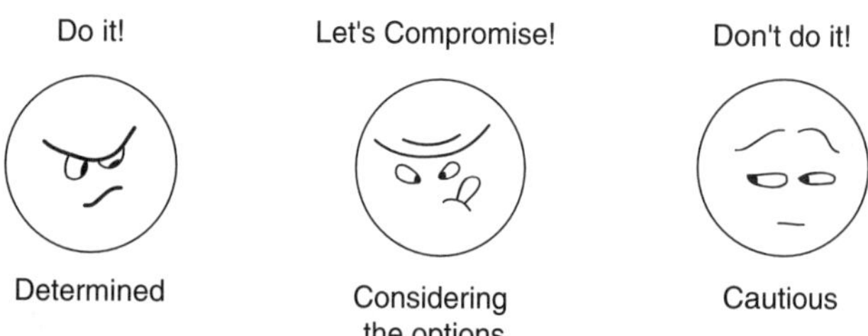

figure 18-3 *Freud's concept concerning id, ego, and superego.*

erikson's theory

A student of Sigmund Freud, Erik Erikson (1902–1994) proposed a theory emphasizing development of the individual's identity throughout the life span and in the context of parents, family, peers, neighbors, and culture. He describes five qualitative stages in psychosocial development of a child (Table 18-3). These stages represent the child's conflict between biologic needs and social demands.

The five stages described by Erikson follow:

1. *Trust versus mistrust*, from birth to 18 months, concerned with consistently meeting the needs of the infant
2. *Autonomy versus shame and doubt,* from 18 months to 3 years, concerned with the toddler's desire to become more independent and take control over personal actions and body functions, such as toilet training
3. *Initiative versus guilt*, from 3 to 5 years, concerned with the preschooler's need to initiate and experience a sense of purposefulness and accomplishment
4. *Industry versus inferiority,* from 5 to 11 years, concerned with the school-age child's need to learn and be accepted, a major influence on the child's feelings of self-esteem
5. *Identity versus role confusion,* from 12 to 18 years, concerned with the adolescent's search for role identity and peer acceptance

Each of these stages is discussed in more detail in subsequent age-specific chapters.

According to Erikson, a child must resolve the conflict encountered in each stage before progressing to the next. Failure to resolve the conflict can result in problems with self-concept and self-esteem.

self-concept and self-esteem

The terms self-concept and self-esteem are related but not synonymous. *Self-concept* is how a person sees himself or herself. *Self-esteem* is how a person feels about himself or herself. Obviously, if an individual sees himself as an attractive, valuable person (self-concept), he or she will feel good about himself or herself (self-esteem), and the reverse is also true.

The first step in the development of a child's self-concept is the recognition of being a separate being who can control and initiate actions. Self-concept includes the child's perceptions of his or her body and feelings. Children also use language to express and display a sense of self.

As a child develops a sense of self-concept, he or she begins to connect actions with outcomes. According to Erikson's theory, for example, a child who trusts is more likely to feel safe in exploring the environment and establishing a sense of self by separating from the mother.

As children grow, their concept of self becomes more complex. They begin to evaluate their strengths, weaknesses, accomplishments, and failures in comparison with

table 18-3 comparison of Erikson, Piaget, and Kohlberg's theories and age-related considerations

Age Group	*Erikson's Theory*	*Piaget's Theory*	*Kohlberg's Theory*	*Age-Related Considerations*
Infancy 1–12 mo	Trust versus mistrust	Sensorimotor period	No moral development	Trust formed when basic needs met Responds to being held Requires stimulation of senses Communicates by crying
Toddler 1–3 y	Autonomy versus shame and doubt	Preconceptual thought	—	Needs firm and consistent guidance Self-centered; asks many questions; responds to praise Has difficulty making choices
Preschool 3–6 y	Initiative versus guilt	Preoperational thought	Preconventional level	Tries to please Guilt is common when the child disobeys Enjoys repeating words; may count to 10 Acting out behaviors and masturbation common Morality is a matter of good or bad, based on a system of punishments
School-age 6–12 y	Industry versus inferiority	Concrete operations	Conventional level	IQ stable; enjoys stories and unusual situations Learning disabilities often identified Morality seen as following the rules of society Tries to be "good"
Adolescent 12–18 y	Identity vesus role confusion	Formal operations	Postconventional level	Peer group more important than family Has the ability to use logic and reason Teen is at risk for drug and alcohol abuse, social misconduct, antiestablishment behaviors, pregnancy, and sexually transmitted diseases Morality consists of standards beyond specific group or authority figure

others, especially their peers. They internalize adults' criticism and praise, especially that received from authority figures. Self-esteem emerges as the value that an individual places on his or her own identity and worth.

Children with high self-esteem tend to expect that they will be well received, successful, trusted, and respected for making sound decisions. Children with low self-esteem tend to experience lack of trust in themselves, apprehension about expressing unpopular ideas, and self-consciousness and preoccupation with personal problems.

skinner's behaviorist theory

During the 1940s, B. F. Skinner (1904–1990) developed a theory based on changing behavior through positive reinforcement or reward. The concepts of reward psychology promote positive reinforcement, rather than punishment, as an effective way to handle undesirable behavior in children. The emphasis in Skinner's work is on behavior response. Skinner suggests behavior is best changed or controlled by frequently using positive reinforcement, especially during toddlerhood; not giving reinforcements from time to time; and disregarding undesirable behaviors.

Skinner's concepts are often used in education. For example, students are rewarded or given positive reinforcement for giving correct responses to questions by receiving either a high class score or teacher or peer recognition. The questions act as a *stimulus,* an event that produces a physical or mental *response,* which is a reaction to the stimulus. *Conditioning* occurs when the child's responses result in new ways of learning. When the child stops getting high scores or recognition for correct responses, he or she may stop answering the questions, resulting in *extinction* of the response. Extinction is defined as the disappearance of a response as a result of the removal of the reinforcer.

✶ family considerations

Skinner's theory influences behavior by using a positive approach. Behaviors that promote positive recognition are emphasized, while negative behaviors are ignored. Caregivers practicing Skinner's theory will do the following:

* Reinforce every desired response of the child in the early stages of training.
* Omit reinforcements from time to time, once the child's learning is progressing. The ultimate goal is to achieve the desired behaviors without reinforcements.
* Avoid the use of punishment to foster learning because it is ineffective and can cause undesirable behavior patterns.
* Ignore undesirable behavior, and avoid negative reinforcement of undesirable behavior.

Using Skinner's approach to changing behavior is called *behavior modification* and applies the principles of *conditioning* (Table 18-4). Advocates of behavior modification assume that behavior is a product of learning, conditioning, and environmental control and consider that what is learned can be unlearned. Behavior modification techniques tend to be popular with people working with troubled school-age children and adolescents.

bandura's observational learning theory

Albert Bandura (1925–) proposed a theory of learning that expands on Skinner's reinforcement theory, describing learning as a response influenced by the observation of others, referred to as *models.* Observational learning involves being influenced indirectly by observing another person's reactions to specific situations. For example, 5-year-old Johnny observes his older brother behaving assertively with another child to avoid a fight. Johnny's brother benefits directly from the encounter (avoiding the fight); however, Johnny benefits indirectly because he is now aware of an appropriate way to respond to aggression.

Observational theory is useful for nurses:

* It identifies caregivers who experienced abuse as children as being at risk for becoming abusive caregivers.
* It reinforces the need for early intervention through education for at-risk caregivers.
* It offers helpful explanations for complex human behaviors.
* It explains why physical punishment can increase aggressive behavior in children when it is intended to do just the opposite.
* It explains how children are vulnerable to the power of television violence.
* It identifies the importance of positive role models in shaping behavior patterns.

table 18-4 behavior modification process and advantages

Behavior Modification Process	*Advantages*
Behaviors that are considered undesirable and in need of change are targeted	Behavior modification deals with specific undesirable behaviors, decreasing confusion often seen when behaviors are addressed in generality.
A reinforcer that offers positive reinforcement is selected.	Communication is encouraged between caregiver and child, helping to determine what value each one places on changing the behavior.
Reinforcement possibilities are selected and used to describe the exact behavior goals that need to be met and reinforced	Behavior control is encouraged, enabling the child to reach goals in a specified time.
The child's behavior goals and positive reinforcements are continually evaluated to monitor success or failure of the plan.	The evaluation process provides caregivers and children with an opportunity to evaluate the plan's success and celebrate behavior changes.

intellectual (cognitive) development

Intellectual or *cognitive* development is the way in which children learn to think, incorporate learning from experiences, solve problems, and communicate through language skills. It includes intelligence, perceptual ability, and the ability to process information. Cognitive development enables the child to acquire and retain knowledge of number systems, concepts of space and time, and laws of logic. Acquiring knowledge equips children to evaluate their world by understanding how objects, experiences, and events are connected and to respond to new situations. Cognitive development is measured by intelligence tests and an ability to function in the environment.

piaget's theory of cognitive development

Many researchers have studied cognitive development in children; the best known of these is Jean Piaget (1896–1980), a Swiss child psychologist. Piaget describes cognitive development as a sequential process, changing and adapting to biologic and environmental influences. He theorizes that the process consists of four phases: *sensorimotor activity, preoperational thought, concrete operations,* and *formal operations* (see Table 18-3). In each phase, the child uses *adaptation* to cope with a changing environment. Piaget describes adaptation as including two processes: assimilation and accommodation. *Assimilation* is the process of incorporating new experiences, impressions, and sensations into existing knowledge. *Accommodation* results when children replace their current way of thinking, believing, and behaving to adapt to new situations.

All children progress through these same phases but not at the same speed. The ages specified for each phase are estimated and differ for individual children.

sensorimotor activity (birth–2 years)

In the sensorimotor stage, infants come to know their world by reflexes, such as sucking and grasping, rather than "thinking" processes. They use their sense of taste, touch, sight, and sound to become acquainted with the world (Fig. 18-4).

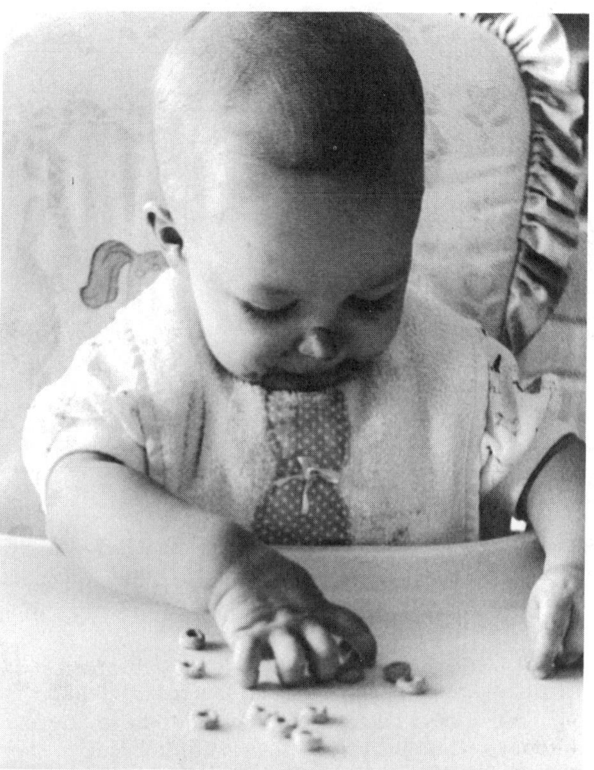

figure 18-4 *An infant learning to feed herself is often a messy affair.*

preoperational thought (2–7 years)

Between 2 and 4 years of age, a child sees the world in *egocentric* terms, that is, in terms of "me," and understands only what is seen. Ability to use language develops rapidly, and the child learns to associate words with objects.

As a child reaches preschool age, the egocentric thinking process changes to one that includes others. The child is able to focus on one idea at a time and to express thoughts in words (Fig. 18-5). Preoperational children tend to act as though everything has a purpose. This thinking is reflected in the child's constant asking "Why?" Nurses working with this age group need to be aware that simple explanations are more appropriate to the many questions asked. The answer may not be as important to the child as the ability to ask why.

concrete operations (7–11 years)

The *concrete operations* phase reflects thinking that is more internalized, logical, reversible, and used to solve problems. In this stage, Piaget refers to *concrete* to mean problems that involve recognized objects that are either perceived or imagined by the child. During this phase, the child has expanded social abilities, increased language skills, and an ability to understand other's views (Fig. 18-6).

formal operations (11–15 years)

During the *formal operations* stage, the adolescent becomes increasingly capable of understanding complex language and hypothetical situations. Adolescents have the ability to reason logically, which contributes to a tendency to be argumentative and idealistic. Adolescents engage in thinking about global or world issues. Peer influence is strong during adolescence, often leading to group conformity and adoption of faddish behavior (Fig. 18-7).

Nursing care of adolescents includes preparing them for normal developmental changes by offering thorough explanations to questions and concerns. Adolescents need to know what is considered normal. They have a natural

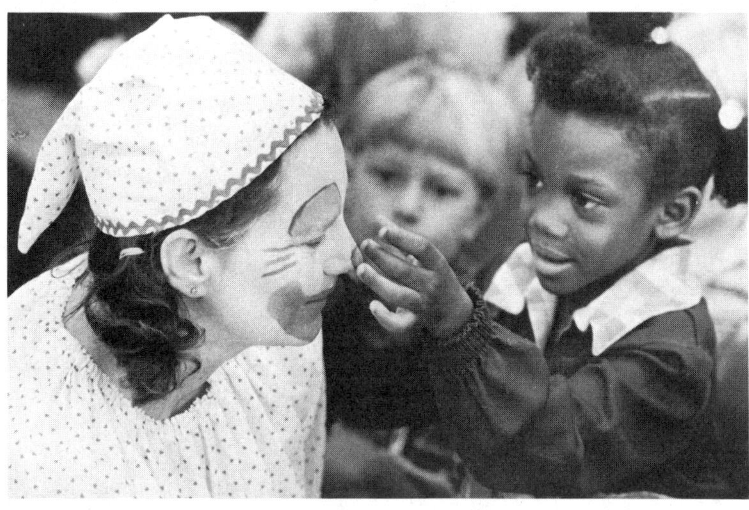

figure 18-5 *Young children possess a remarkable curiosity that observes and searches for causes.*

curiosity in the psychology of human behavior. A sharpened awareness of basic behavior traits that mark the stages of growing up can result in better self-understanding.

Piaget's theory is used in many nursing programs as a practical and applicable way to explain intellectual development. Critics of Piaget's theory point out that many children today reach the various phases of intellectual development earlier than theorized by Piaget. This accelerated development may result from training, education, and exposure to modern technology, such as television and computers, influences that were not considered in Piaget's theory.

moral development

Developing moral judgment is a gradual learning process that distinguishes behaviors as being acceptable or not acceptable, "right" or "wrong." Moral development is an important part of the child's socialization process. The process of socialization begins at birth and is the accumulation of behaviors, experiences, and ideas that enable the child to maintain interpersonal relationships appropriate for familial, cultural, and societal expectations.

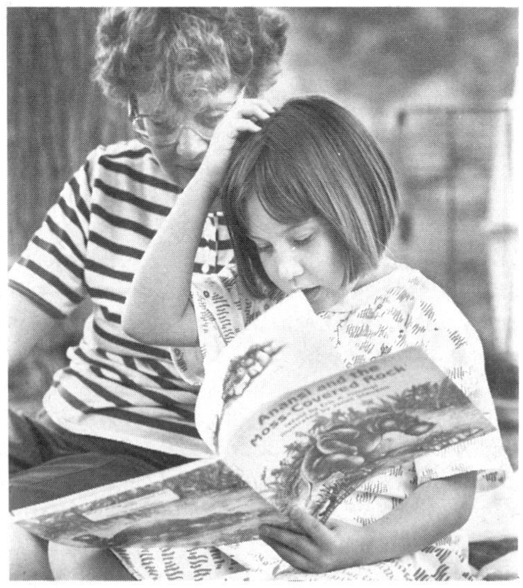

figure 18-6 *School-age child reflects on more complex issues, rationalizes, and resolves problems.*

piaget's theory of moral development

Jean Piaget proposed that a person's moral judgment depends on intellectual or cognitive understanding of various situations. His theory of moral development describes how reasoning about moral situations changes as children develop. His research ideas came from observing children playing marbles. Piaget discovered that children younger than 2 years would manipulate the marbles but could not play a game of marbles because they did not grasp the concept of game rules.

According to Piaget, children between 6 and 10 years attempt to follow rules but may perceive game rules differently, depending on their personal experiences. Children at this age regard rules as being unchangeable because they come from an adult authority. The combination of individual ideas of rules along with beliefs that rules are sacred helps explain why young school-age children often accuse one another of cheating.

At approximately 10 to 12 years, children understand that game rules provide a method for playing the game fairly and can be changed if everyone agrees. When game rules are broken, the players consider the child's reasons for breaking the rules and assign consequences accordingly.

morality of constraint

Piaget distinguishes two stages of moral development: morality of constraint and morality of cooperation. *Morality of constraint* is seen in children from 4 to 7 years and refers to the child's opinion that rules are absolute and unquestionable. Bad deeds are punished by an authority figure, and the punishment involves experiencing physical accident or misfortune. This type of thinking also is called "magical thinking."

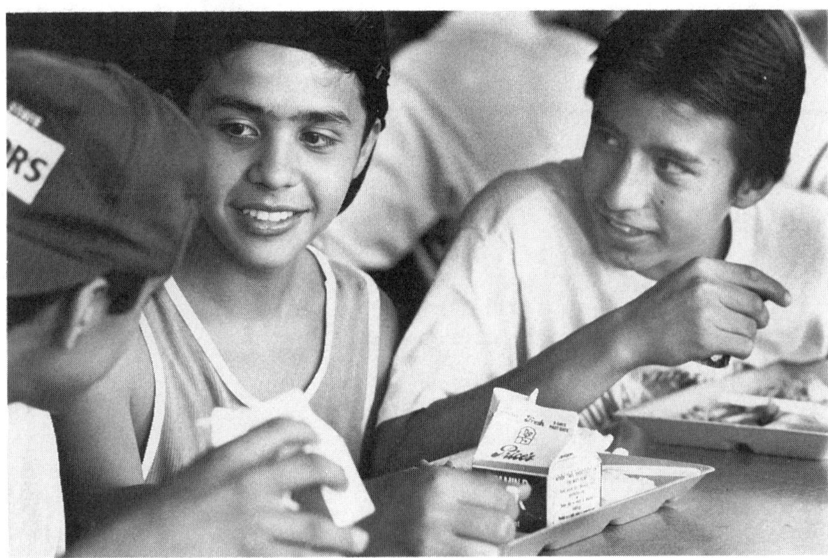

figure 18-7 *In early adolescence, the peer group is a major influence.*

✶ nursing considerations

Older preschoolers and young school-age children may believe they have suffered an injury because of lying to their parents. The child's notion that he or she is responsible for illness or injury because of bad deeds leads to feelings of guilt and depression. Reassuring the child that thoughts differ from actions and that "bad thoughts" cannot make "bad things" happen helps alleviate some of the child's self-blaming tendencies.

✶ family considerations

Siblings of sick children may feel responsible for the illness and display behavior changes as a result of guilt and depression.

> ✶ **nursing insight**
>
> *Siblings of sick children may feel responsible for the illness and display behavior changes as a result of guilt and depression.*

morality of cooperation

The second stage of moral development described by Piaget is called *morality of cooperation* and is seen in children 10 years and older. Morality of cooperation is described as an understanding that rules are arbitrary agreements that can be questioned and changed with compromise. Children at this age tend to question authority rules and attempt to compromise regulations.

✶ nursing considerations

Nurses caring for children older than 10 years can take advantage of compromise when seeking compliance to prescribed care. For example, the 10-year-old child who is reluctant to bathe during the morning may be more compliant if permitted to bathe in the evening. Choices or compromises should be offered only when they can be honored. Many nursing procedures or tasks need to be done on schedule, and offering a false compromise will only increase the child's frustration. For example, the child's medications must be administered on schedule; therefore, no compromise is possible.

✶ family considerations

Positive behaviors can be influenced by the use of compromise with this age group. For example, a child assigned to take out the trash has the understanding that prompt compliance in completing the task will result in a privilege, such as an extra phone use.

kohlberg's theory of moral development

Lawrence Kohlberg's theory of moral development relates closely to Piaget's theory and focuses on the reasons for making a judgment or decision, rather than on the morality of the judgment itself. According to Kohlberg, there are three levels of moral development: preconventional, conventional, and postconventional (see Table 18-3).

At the *preconventional* level, ages 4 to 10 years, the child learns to conform to rules imposed by authority figures and interprets right and wrong in terms of actions and their consequences. The child operates within and responds to physical consequences of actions. Good and bad are based on the rewards they bring and are encouraged by satisfaction of needs. An action is not considered bad if it produces no punishment.

Disciplining a child in the preconventional level includes explaining why certain behaviors are unacceptable, praising acceptable behaviors, and ignoring certain inappropriate behaviors to distract the child from seeking the attention gained by the behavior. Physical punishment and withholding privileges tend to give the child a negative view of morals.

In the *conventional* level, 10 to 13 years, the child makes decisions about right and wrong based on expectations of the family or of society. Behavior is directed at gaining family and peer approval. The child is impressed with "good boy" or "nice girl" conduct.

At the *postconventional level,* 13 years and older, the person tries to define personal moral values and standards independent of outside authority. Decisions about right and wrong consider the universal human rights of others.

✳ nursing considerations

Nurses need to be conscious of actions and words that express genuine concern and respect for children. Respect for children includes respect and acceptance of the child's value system and cultural orientation. Nurses must be willing to understand issues, morals, and value systems other than those they encourage for convenience, such as obedience.

✳ family considerations

Children need to have opportunities to interact with peers, children of different age groups, and adults to help them move to higher levels of moral functioning. Caregivers can promote moral development by providing opportunities for the child to make age- appropriate decisions and discuss the results of the decision.

gilligan's theory of moral development

After more than 10 years of research with female subjects, Carol Gilligan (1982) set forth a new theory on gender-related moral development. She proposed that moral judgment is learned differently by females. When Kohlberg's stages of moral development are used to measure girls, their responses to the dilemmas presented are often categorized incorrectly as reflecting a lower level of moral development. According to Gilligan, girls traditionally have been taught to equate goodness with helping others.

Gilligan's theory promotes the idea that from an early age, girls and boys have different perceptions of the world that influence their moral development. Boys associate morality with obligations, rights, and justice, while girls associate morality with addressing the needs of others within relationship settings.

Gilligan refers to the moral orientation of girls as the ethic of care and describes the orientation in three levels: caring for self, caring for others, and caring for self and others.

influences on moral development

Moral development is a complex process influenced by many sources. A child's morals are determined by family structure and parenting styles, peers, school, teachers, media, culture, and spiritual orientation.

family influence

Family structure and parenting styles have a great influence on a child's moral development. Parents and siblings begin influencing children's right and wrong behaviors at an early age. Disciplinary measures affect the child's perceptions of self and others.

Children exposed to a pattern of family interactions based on force, negative behaviors, and inconsistent discipline are more likely to develop antisocial behaviors obstructing moral development. Aggressive discipline or punishment through physical force or harsh words tells the child that aggression is a useful method to reach a goal. When parents reason with children, however, pointing out acceptable behaviors versus unacceptable behaviors along with behavior consequences, children are more likely to be generous, sympathetic, and compassionate with others. Childrearing practices that nourish warmth, positive behaviors, and cooperation enhance moral development.

Caregivers need encouragement regarding their parenting skills. Parenting is one of the most challenging tasks confronting an adult. Parenting is rewarding yet frustrating; it requires energy, courage, commitment, and a good sense of humor. The knowledge that your child is behaving within the normal limits of expected behavior is a great relief.

school influence

Family influences on the child's moral conscience tend to diminish as children get older and are exposed to babysitters, day care centers, school, media, and peers. Teachers and classmates influence a child's moral development by creating an atmosphere for modeling responses. Students often reflect teachers' demonstrations of compassion, honesty, altruism, and justice with behaviors to peers, parents, and school officials. Group discussions concerning moral issues can raise the level of moral reasoning among school-age children.

media influence

Research on how the media (television, movies, magazines, and newspapers) influence moral development has primarily studied the effects of television violence on aggression in children. Studies have shown that children exposed to a live or filmed model are likely to imitate the model shortly afterward, regardless of whether the model behaved socially or antisocially (Comstock & Paik, 1991). Because young children consider the consequences of behavior rather than the reasons for behavior, they tend to get the idea that it is all right to do bad things as long as you can get away with them.

cultural influences

Cultural expectations involve feelings, reasoning, and behaving and arise from the necessity for people to get along with one another and obey society's rules for daily living. The child's early introduction to cultural morality is in the home, where ideas of right and wrong are taught.

Different cultures emphasize different viewpoints on morality. For example, urbanized cultures tend to place more emphasis on the individual right for fairness and justice. Some cultures promote aggressive behaviors, while others believe in establishing a sense of self-control.

spiritual influence

Spirituality includes the child's beliefs about the purpose or meaning of life, a religious spirit, and the "natural" decency of people. James Fowler describes the spiritual dimension of life as *faith.* Basing his work on the theories of Piaget, Kohlberg, and Erikson, Fowler believes that faith develops as an interactive process between the individual and the environment.

Spirituality is closely linked with religious beliefs. Organized religion influences children by teaching them church-related beliefs. Rituals, prayers, and religious stories taught through church programs strengthen the child's moral convictions.

✶ nursing process related to growth and development

assessment

A child's growth is assessed through obtaining an accurate weight and length measurement and comparing the results with normal standards. Growth is considered altered when the weight falls behind height by 2 standard deviations and when the pattern of height and weight percentiles indicates a decrease. Development is considered to be altered when the child is unable to perform or has difficulty performing skills or behaviors typical of the age group.

Subjective data to be assessed include the following:

* Height and weight at birth
* Diet history
* Allergies
* Food intolerance
* Nausea, vomiting, and dysphagia
* Parental attitudes
* Child's behavior with parents, siblings, peers, and nurse

Objective data to be assessed include the following:

* General appearance
* Response to stimulation
* Interaction with parents and siblings
* Response to procedures and strangers
* Nutritional status
* Type of illness, treatments

nursing diagnosis

* Altered Growth and Development
* Knowledge Deficit

intervention

* Teach parents age-related developmental tasks.
* Differentiate between behaviors common to the age versus behaviors not appropriate for the specific age group.
* Carefully assess child's level of development in all areas of functioning by using specific assessment tools, such as the Denver Developmental Assessment Tool.
* Encourage the child to eat a balanced diet at mealtime and snack time, and teach caregivers basic nutrition facts.
* Provide play time with other children if possible.
* Provide a variety of age-appropriate toys.
* Allow hospital routine to be altered to suit child's schedule.
* Encourage safety by using specific safety devices, such as outlet plugs and door locks.
* Recognize speech and hearing impairments, and provide early intervention to prevent major delays in development.
* Evaluate fine and gross motor skills, and provide intervention before the child enters school.
* Encourage caregiver compliance with follow-up clinic or doctor's office visits.
* Encourage age-appropriate guidance and discipline measures.

evaluation

* Child will demonstrate behaviors in personal or social language, intellect, and motor activities appropriate to the age group.
* Height and weight measurements will be within normal ranges for child's age.
* Caregivers and child will verbalize an understanding of expected growth and development indicators.
* Child and caregivers will comply with recommended treatment plan for correcting any growth and development delays.

key points ✶

* **Theories concerning child development help explain current behavior and physical characteristics and predict physical, intellectual, social, emotional, and behavioral changes that will occur as children grow and learn.**
* **Growth refers to increases in height, weight, and body organ sizes (characteristics that can be measured in inches or centimeters and pounds or kilograms) and follows a head-to-tail (cephalocaudal) and midline-to-periphery (proximodistal) pattern.**

* Development refers to an increase in the complexity of function, a series of changes that occur in developmental sequence, such as the progression from crawling to walking.
* Abraham Maslow proposed that human behavior is shaped by the attempt to meet five levels of basic needs and grouped these needs in a hierarchy, beginning with physiologic needs.
* Freud's theory views personality development as a psychosexual process, divided into the following stages: oral, anal, phallic, latent, and genital.
* According to Kohlberg, moral judgment is influenced by cultural influences within interpersonal relationships and includes preconventional, conventional, and postconventional levels.
* Erik Erikson's theory views human development as occurring throughout the lifespan and within the context of parents, family, peers, neighbors, and culture. The first five stages of development, from birth to 18 years are trust versus mistrust, autonomy versus shame and doubt, initiative versus guilt, industry versus inferiority, and identity versus role confusion.
* B. F. Skinner developed a reward theory promoting behavior control through positive reinforcement as an effective way to change undesirable behavior in children without using punishment.
* Albert Bandura studied how children learn and proposed a theory of observational learning, a response influenced by observing others and imitating their behavior. This theory may help explain aggressive behavior in children after watching violence on television.
* Jean Piaget depicted four phases of cognitive development: sensorimotor activity, preoperational thought, concrete operations, and formal operations.
* Influences on moral development include the family, school, the media, and the culture in which a child is raised.
* Moral development theories include Piaget's ideas on cognitive understanding of various siutations and their prospective rules; Kohlberg's focus on the reasons for making a decision rather than the morality of the act; and Gilligan's gender-related moral development.
* Carol Gilligan proposes that boys and girls have different perceptions of the world and that these differences influence moral development. Girls' moral judgment includes an ethic of care.

review questions

1. Select the most appropriate statment concerning growth and development theories.
   a. They provide information about growth standards, child behaviors, fine and gross motor development, and reasoning abilities.
   b. They help professionals measure a child's intelligence.
   c. They set firm guidelines for normal growth and development.
   d. They deal primarily with behavior observed in children reared in poverty.
2. Mrs. Pompey is concerned that Francis, 6 months, is not walking. The nurse learns that Francis has just started sitting alone without support. Select the principle of growth and development that addresses this particular progression of Francis' development.
   a. Proximodistal
   b. General to specific
   c. Cephalocaudal
   d. Genetics
3. Mrs. Muñoz complains to the nurse that her 4-year-old son uses aggressive behavior after watching television. The theory that best describes how children are influenced through observational learning is
   a. Erikson's.
   b. Maslow's.
   c. Skinner's.
   d. Bandura's.
4. Brittany is a 5-year-old admitted to the hospital with diarrhea. She confides in the nurse that she was "bad" because she wished her brother would get sick, and her illness is a form of punishment. Another name for this type of thinking is
   a. cooperation thinking.
   b. magical thinking.
   c. preconventional thinking.
   d. gender-related thinking.
5. Chantal, age 3, is able to use language skills and has learned to associate words with objects. In what level of Piaget's cognitive learning is Chantal?
   a. Concrete operations
   b. Sensorimotor
   c. Formal operations
   d. Preoperational thought

references

Comstock, G., & Paik, H. (1991). *Television and the American child.* San Diego: Academic Press.

Gilligan, C. (1982). *In a different voice: Psychological theory and women's development.* Cambridge, MA: Harvard University Press.

bibliography

Berns, R. (1994). *Typical child development.* Albany, NY: Delmar Publishers.

Carpenito, L. (1995) *Nursing diagnosis: Application to Clinical Practice* (6th ed.). Philadelphia: J.B. Lippincott.

Castiglia, P., & Harbin, R. (1992). *Child health care.* Philadelphia: J.B. Lippincott.

Charlesworth, R. (Eds.) (1992). *Understanding child development.* Albany, NY: Delmar Publishers.

Jackson, D., & Saunders, R. (1993). *Child development.* Philadelphia, J.B. Lippincott.

Hoffman, M. L., & Saltzstein, H. D. (1967). Parent discipline and the child's moral development. *Journal of Personality and Social Psychology, 5,* 45–47.

Marhoefer, P., & Vadnais, L. (Eds.) (1992). *Caring for the developing child*. Albany, NY: Delmar Publishers.

Moir, A., & Jessel, D. (1991). *Brain sex, the real difference between men and women.* New York, NY: Carol Publishing Group.

Morrison, S. (1990). *The world of child development.* Albany, NY: Delmar Publishers.

Pillitteri, A. (1995). *Maternal and child health nursing* (2nd ed.). Philadelphia: J.B. Lippincott.

Schuster, C., & Ashburn, S. (1992). *The process of human development: A holistic life-span approach.* Philadelphia: J.B. Lippincott.

Weiten, W., & Lloyd, M. (1994). *Psychology applied to modern life: Adjustment in the 90's.* Belmont, CA: Brooks/Cole Publishing.

health maintenance and health promotion

19

outline ✳

objectives ✳

After studying this chapter, the reader should be able to:

- ✳ List the five national health care concerns for health maintenance and health promotion.
- ✳ Discuss the building blocks of health, including heredity, family size, culture, economics, nutrition, society, and environment, and their impact on children.
- ✳ Discuss the impact of poverty on the welfare of children.
- ✳ Discuss the impact of alcoholism and domestic violence on children.
- ✳ Compare child abuse with child neglect, and discuss legal implications to nursing.
- ✳ Compare nutritional needs of children with required nutritional intake for adults using the food pyramid.
- ✳ Define the term pesticide, and give at least three examples.
- ✳ Discuss the importance of cleanliness, proper storage, and food preparation as a means of reducing the risk of food-borne illness.
- ✳ Compare an infant's vital sign measurements with an adolescent's.
- ✳ State expected weight gains and length increases for a 5-month-old, 12-month-old, 3-year-old, and 5-year-old.

key terms ✳

Alateen
amblyopia
audiometer
caries
clostridium botulinum
cultural diversity
cultural bias
domestic violence
environment
Munchausen syndrome by proxy
pesticides
poverty
prejudice
Salmonella
scoliosis
shaken baby syndrome

Child health practices increasingly focus on the prevention of illness and the maintenance and promotion of health. Preventive practices implemented on a national scale include immunization programs, fluoridation of water, and regulation of chemical wastes.

National health care concerns include the growing number of families who are living in poverty,* uninsured and without access to medical care, distressed by drug and alcohol abuse, experiencing child abuse and neglect, and exposed to food, air, and water polluted with pesticides, chemical additives, and other toxins.

Parents and caregivers can help children understand the importance of maintaining physical, mental, and social well-being by acting as role models and teachers. This chapter deals with the building blocks of health, identified as heredity, family, culture, economics, nutrition, society, and the environment. Physical health assessment factors and the effects of violence on children and families are included.

building blocks of health

The health status of children depends on many factors, collectively called the *building blocks of health*. These factors include heredity, family size, culture, economics, nutrition, society, and environment. Each of these building blocks is dependent on the others to maintain the overall health of an individual. For example, weakness of economics threatens the integrity of the family, the environment in which family members live, and their nutrition.

Personal health behaviors of parents can have a positive or negative impact on children's health status. Proper nutrition, exercise, and safe play are positive influences on health. Poverty, illness, and violent lifestyles are negative influences, impairing physical and psychosocial well-being.

heredity

Heredity, the total genetic inheritance a child receives from parents, forms one of the essential building blocks for health. Heredity determines the boundaries for growth and development and health potential. Health problems such as heart disease, cancer, diabetes, allergies, blood dyscrasia, and mental health conditions may be linked to hereditary tendencies. Screening programs and genetic counseling promote early detection of hereditary disorders and can help minimize long-term effects on the child's life.

family

The family system in which a child lives and grows is a second building block of health. Family relationships, rules, values, and communication patterns help children learn and test skills needed to relate to the larger society. Family interactions teach children how to socialize with others.

Traditional family structure is changing. Half of all marriages end in divorce, nearly one third of all children are born outside of marriages, and one fourth of children live in fatherless homes.

Intellectual and psychosocial development is thought to be influenced by a child's family birth order. However, research findings conflict on exactly how this influence affects children. For example, in early studies, first-born children were described as high achievers with higher intelligence abilities; middle children were depicted as diplomatic with a tendency toward insecure personalities; and last-born children were viewed as affectionate and overly pampered. Current studies suggest birth order does not affect the child unless parents make birth order a significant issue. Parents who believe first-born children are more capable and deserving may treat them differently, enhancing the child's motivation and school success.

Family size and the number of siblings can affect a child's achievements and academic enthusiasm. Promoting or discouraging sibling rivalry colors a child's perceptions of self. Family energy used to promote child development and academic success sometimes is more apparent in small families than in larger families. However, in larger families, older siblings can help motivate younger family members.

divorce

Divorce is the leading disrupter of the traditional family unit, and it happens in half of all new marriages. Divorce creates changes in family member roles and a major reorganization of the family system. When the mother is awarded custody of children after divorce, the family income and standard of living often may be reduced dramatically, because women's salaries are generally less than men's salaries. Older children may need to assume more responsibility in helping to care for younger children and running the household. Children typically experience a great deal of stress at the time of divorce, displaying behavior problems and disruption in functioning.

domestic violence

Domestic violence is the ongoing, debilitating experience of physical, psychological, or sexual abuse in the home. It is often associated with the abuser's desire for control and involves increased isolation from the outside world and limited personal freedom and accessibility to resources. Domestic violence affects all communities, families, and children. It cuts across all age groups and social classes, but the victims are most often women and children.

Domestic violence can be direct and intentional, carried out with the intent of injury, or it can be indirect and accidental, causing harm to someone who is not the target of the violence. Domestic violence often is repeated regularly, increasing the risk of injury or death.

Factors contributing to domestic violence include parental consumption of excessive alcohol or other drugs, unemployment, or inability to pay bills. Domestic violence tends to follow a cycle of three phases: 1) increased tension, escalation of anger, blaming, and arguing; 2) battering and sometimes sexual abuse, verbal threats, and use of weapons; and 3) denial or making excuses for behavior, apologies, and promises to not be violent again.

Physical abuse is typically recurrent and escalates in frequency and severity. It often includes the following:

* Pushing, shoving, slapping, punching, kicking, choking, holding, tying down
* Assault with a weapon
* Leaving a child in a dangerous place
* Refusing to help a child when sick or injured

Emotional or psychological abuse may precede or accompany physical violence as a means of controlling through fear and degradation by using the following:

* Threats of harm
* Physical or social isolation
* Depriving, ignoring, or ridiculing needs
* Intimidation
* False accusations, blaming, and belittling

Family intervention is generally contraindicated in the presence of acute domestic violence until the immediate threat of harm has passed. Attempts to implement family therapy in the presence of ongoing violence may increase the risk of serious harm. The main concern must be for the safety of the abused parent and the children. Removing victims of domestic violence from the home is an emergency measure that saves lives.

child abuse *Child abuse* is defined as any situation or environment in which the child is not considered safe. The situation may involve intentional physical or sexual abuse of a child by parent, caregiver, or sibling or inadequate protection, exposing the child to hazardous conditions. Child neglect is defned as a failure of the caregiver to provide physical, social, and emotional needs.

The increase in child abuse and neglect is a national tragedy. Preschool and early grade school children are most frequently affected by abuse.

The causes of child abuse and neglect are complex and varied. Children who are born prematurely, have disabilities, are chronically ill, or demonstrate developmental abilities that are inconsistent with parental expectations appear to be at greater risk for abuse.

Physical abuse often begins as a means of punishment that escalates into severe and violent beatings. The *shaken baby syndrome* is commonly seen in infants who have been shaken vigorously, causing bleeding or bruising of the brain.

Emotional or verbal abuse is common in families in which adult demands and expectations are unrealistic for the child's age and developmental abilities. It is difficult to detect verbal abuse. Children subjected to verbal assault tend to be timid about trying new experiences, and they exhibit anxiety and behavioral outbursts.

Sexual abuse includes any sexual involvement between an adult and a child. Fondling, exhibitionism, rape, incest, child pornography, and prostitution are considered acts of abuse, regardless of whether the child consented to participate (Table 19-1).

Physical neglect is failure of a parent or legal guardian to provide for a child's basic needs. Basic needs include adequate food, shelter, clothing, personal cleanliness, and medical and dental care. Some states consider parents neglectful when children are not toilet trained before entering first grade or are not sent to school on a regular basis. Lack of appropriate well child care, including immuniza-

table 19-1 *physical examination for physical and sexual abuse in children*

Type of Abuse	*Assessment*	*Nursing Considerations*
Physical	Bruises; welts often resembling the article used; burns on soles, palms, back, or buttocks Immersion burns; splash burns on legs and buttocks; lacerations or abrasions, such as rope burns on wrist, ankles, neck, mouth, external genitalia Fractures of skull, ribs, long bones Abdominal injuries, retinal hemorrhage Symptoms of suffocation.	Assess the child's immediate needs; obtain medical and social history. Assess the likelihood of the injury with the parent's or caregiver's information. Determine the level of risk to the child if returned home.
Neglect	Undernutrition, poor hygiene, developmental delays, untreated medical conditions, large number of dental caries, discipline problems, lack of supervision	Assess family's priorities regarding child care and lack of resources.
Sexual	Display sexually provocative behaviors and distorted body image revealed through drawings Sexual promiscuity, pregnancy, test positive for sexually transmitted diseases Reports or signs of rectal or genital pain, rectal or genital bleeding	Children who are sexually abused are often mainpulated into secrecy. When abuse is admitted, confidentiality is very important.

tions; absence of necessary health aids, such as eyeglasses or hearing aids; undernutrition; and poor hygiene are considered signs of neglect.

Child abuse is often reported in families in which adult domestic violence occurs. Coordinated communication between advocates for victims of domestic violence and child protective service agencies are used to ensure the safety of the abused parent and the children. Children of battered women report a variety of worries about their mothers. Frequent concerns involve fears of abandonment, serious harm to themselves and their abused parent, and anxieties associated with intense anger and unpredictable behaviors. These children need compassion, tender interest, and concern for their experiences and feelings.

Children must be reassured that they are not the cause of domestic violence and that they have no way of controlling it. Breaking the cycle of domestic violence is not always easy but is possible with professional intervention. Even though they are not responsible for domestic violence, school-age children can be taught to recognize the signs of increased family tension and how to avoid displaying irritating behaviors (Display 19-1).

munchausen syndrome by proxy Munchausen syndrome by proxy is described as a particular syndrome of hospital addiction. The name comes from the fictitious Baron von Munchausen, who traveled widely and told false stories. The condition involves one person persistently inventing symptoms for another, often a mother inventing symptoms and faking signs of illness in the child. Evaluating the false symptoms can cause the child to undergo painful and unnecessary physical examinations and treatments. Terms such as *imaginary illness* and *somatization disorder* are used to describe this phenomenon.

display 19-1
suggestions for children living with domestic violence

Domestic violence can seriously affect children. Parents and caregivers can help children by communicating openly and constructively. Children, depending on age, can learn to lessen the violent experiences by the following:

* Learning when the cycle of violence is most likely to occur
* Understanding the clues that suggest the parent is starting to get upset
* Watching for signs of parental drinking or drug use
* Avoiding behaviors that may add to parental stress
* Staying away from parts of the house where the violence usually occurs
* Leaving the house when domestic violence begins
* Arranging to stay with a friend or relative and be honest about what is happening

A mother involved with Munchausen syndrome by proxy is often described as a woman with low self-esteem. The mother needs the hospital environment to provide her with a sense of competence and worth. The mother typically adopts the role of being dedicated, cooperative, and supportive of the medical staff. She displays intense worry over the sick child while adjusting well to hospital routine.

✳ nursing considerations

In every state, it is mandatory for nurses to report any suspected incidence of abuse or neglect. Suspicions of abuse and neglect do not have to be proven before they are reported. The law does not require that the family or adult be notified when a report is filed. The nurse must be knowledgeable concerning the health care agency's policy regarding child abuse.

Common symptoms of child abuse are bruises noted on the face, arms, legs, back, and abdomen in various stages of healing (Fig. 19-1). Burns on the legs and buttocks from scalding water and fractures at different stages of healing strongly suggest abuse. Repeated urinary tract infections with negative urine cultures, genital discharge, itching, or perineal bruises or bleeding indicate sexual abuse. Munchausen syndrome by proxy needs to be considered when children suffer from poisoning or repeated hospital admissions with vague symptoms.

alcoholism and substance abuse

It is estimated that more than 10 million Americans are addicted to alcohol (Gasbarro, 1992). Alcoholism is considered a family disease because of the harmful effect it has on all family members, even though only one parent abuses alcohol.

Children from alcoholic families often experience an unhappy childhood, distrusting authority and fearing the outside world. They live in a state of fear, turmoil, shame, guilt, and humiliation. Violence, incest, and other forms of sexual abuse are more common in alcoholic families than in the general population.

Children living in an alcoholic family often find it difficult to form close peer relationships. They tend to suppress feelings of anger and are more prone to emotional and behavioral problems and stress-related diseases.

Children are less likely to suffer long-lasting effects when the alcohol abuse is brief rather than chronic, financial stability is present, and supportive relationships within the family contribute to the child's emotional stability. Alateen is a support group for children from alcoholic families sponsored by Alcoholics Anonymous (AA). Alateen provides counseling and information for children living in an alcoholic family. Alatot provides support to children from 1 to 6 years of age. Information about Alateen and Alatot is provided by local chapters of AA.

Substance abuse may be used to rationalize violent behavior. Illegal drug use increases the risk of criminal behaviors, such as theft or prostitution, to support the drug habit. Parents focus on supporting their drug addiction rather than the needs of the child. Money needed for food,

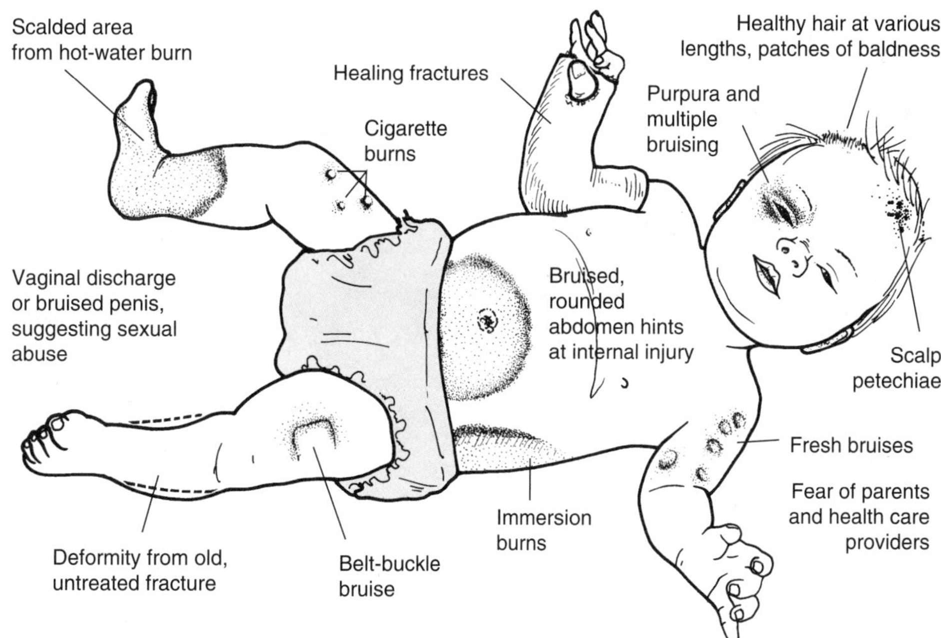

figure 19-1 *Signs and symptoms of child abuse.*

shelter, clothing, and so forth is used to buy drugs, forcing children to live in poverty and homelessness. Often children are the target for sexual abuse, increasing their risk of sexually transmitted diseases and emotional trauma.

Evidence indicates that while substance abuse and violent behavior frequently coexist, the violent behavior will not end unless interventions address the violence and the addiction (Ohio State Medical Association, 1992). Drug abuse clinics offer interventions aimed at treating the addiction; however, other problems associated with drug use require social service agencies and mental health counseling.

culture

Culture is defined as a set of values, beliefs, attitudes, and traditions that are held by a specific social group and handed down from one generation to another. Culture is a third building block of health that influences the way children view themselves, their health, nutrition, communication patterns, and language.

cultural diversity

Cultural diversity refers to the many differences that make each person unique. Some of the differences include race, education patterns, country of origin, socioeconomic class, language, and age.

As discussed in Chapter 1, North America has become a multicultural continent. In the United States, the number of nonwhite people is predicted to exceed the number of white people in the 21st century. Today, one American in four describes himself or herself as Hispanic or nonwhite. Current trends in immigration and birth rates reflect a growth in Hispanic, Asian, and African American populations.

Unfortunately, cultural diversity does not always equal cultural harmony. Conflicts already exist in some culturally diverse neighborhoods. Cultural bias and prejudice (an uninformed negative opinion about something or someone) can develop when children learn stereotypes based on race, gender, and ethnicity. Children of all ages are fascinated with similarities and differences between themselves and others. Prejudice often grows from a young child's limited experiences and immature ways of interpreting experiences provided through family encounters. As children gain a sense of respect for their personal lifestyles, they are more prone to accept the differences noted in others (see the Teaching Guidelines display).

Most Americans do not learn a second language, resulting in communication problems with children and parents who do not speak English as a primary language. Certain dialects or word meanings can cause differences in understanding. Nurses working in an area that has a large population of citizens speaking a language other than English need to learn pertinent words and phrases in that language or rely on an interpreter.

teaching guidelines
cultural differences

Families can help children cope with cultural differences by providing age-appropriate information about the following:

* Why people have different skin colors
* The importance of family values, religious and cultural rituals, and the significance of food customs
* Respect for others, regardless of race, culture, or creed

table 19-2 effects of poverty on health status

Characteristics of Living Conditions in Poverty	*Typical Health Problems*
Crowded living conditions Poor sanitation Inadequate nutrition Sharing utensils and personal hygiene articles Poor health habits Limited access to health care Lack of heat and electricity	Increased risk of infection and disease; more severe complications; longer recovery time Knowledge deficit concerning cause, treatment, and outcome of illness High incidence of noncompliance with treatment plan Feelings of worthlessness Loss of identity

economics

Economics is a key building block of health. The amount of money a family has affects the ability to meet basic needs and maintain health. More than 20% of American children (more than 44% of African American children) live in poverty, and this number is predicted to increase. Children living in poverty struggle for the necessities of food and shelter.

Poverty denies women proper prenatal care and increases the potential for neonatal difficulties. The mortality rate is substantially higher for infants born to mothers of low socioeconomic status. Poverty produces its own stressors: unsafe and undesirable neighborhoods, inadequate housing, chronic financial stress, and the dehumanization that often accompanies welfare dependency (Table 19-2).

In some families, poverty is passed from generation to generation. The United States tends to view poverty as an individual and local problem rather than relating it to such underlying causes as unemployment, inadequate wages, changing labor markets, and neglected and deteriorating local communities.

A growing number of young adults living in poverty are starting families in communities where health resources are scarce. Many poor families are headed by young, single women who frequently experience the breakdown of institutional and social support systems, increased interpersonal violence, and drug abuse.

Young, single parents who have been hurt and discouraged in previous relationships may try to provoke and recreate similar patterns in relationships involving the nurse. Single-parent attitudes communicated to nurses include apprehension, anger, hopelessness, and despair.

The nurse must build trust with families, particularly those who are poor and discouraged. Some young parents require nurturing before they can learn to trust. The nurse's behavior can show them how to develop effective parenting skills and provide care for their own children.

society

The society in which a child lives is the fifth building block of health. A primary concern in today's society is the increasing frequency of violent crimes and crime-related injuries and deaths. Rape, armed robbery, drive-by shootings and other murders, and drug-related crimes are in the news and on the minds of many citizens (Sharp, 1992). Fear of violent crime restricts the freedom of young and old alike, limiting many opportunities for play and other social activities.

nutrition

Nutrition, defined as the process used to take in and use nutrients (food) for body functioning and maintaining health, is the sixth building block of health. Food is essential for life, providing the energy needed for growth and development, tissue repair, and resistance to illness and infection.

Well-nourished children are less likely to become ill, and they tend to recover more quickly if they do become ill. Well-nourished children are more alert and attentive, whereas poorly nourished children display short attention spans and hyperactive and disruptive behaviors.

Good food habits are taught by parents and other caregivers. Children model behaviors seen in people they love and admire. Young children are surprisingly skilled at

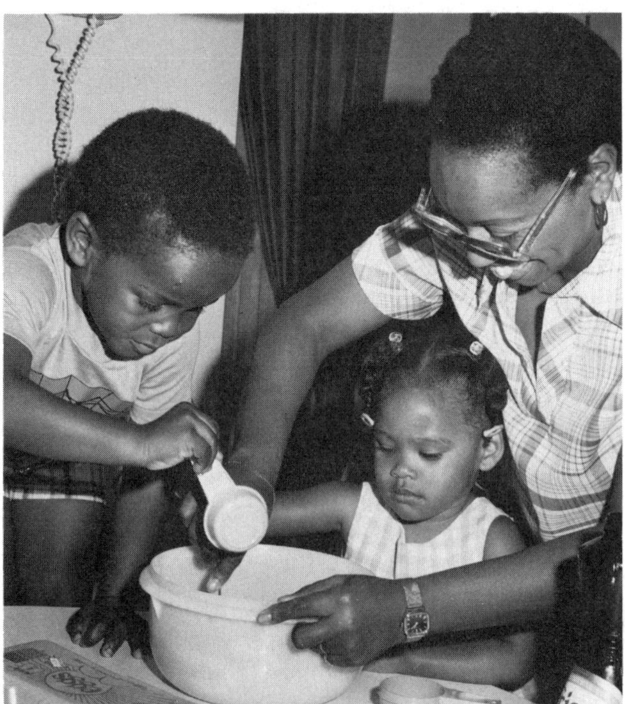

figure 19-2 *First-hand experience helps the child to build a repertoire of knowledge that serves as a foundation for healthy food choices.*

table 19-3 recommended pediatric daily allowances based on the food guide pyramid

Food Groups	Adult Allowances	Pediatric Allowances
Milk, milk products	2 cups daily	3 cups daily
Meat and meat alternates	Two or more servings with serving size 2–3 oz	Small children: 1 to 1½ oz
Fruit and vegetables	4 or more servings with serving size equal to ½ cup	Four or more servings with serving size half of adult portion
Bread and cereal	4 or more servings with serving size equal to ½ cup	Four or more servings with serving size half of adult portion
Fats, oils, and sweets	Small amount recommended due to high fat content	Same as adult

working out a balanced diet that includes essential nutrients for growth and development (Fig.19-2).

Parents are often concerned about their young child's food preferences and fluctuation in appetite. Parents need to be encouraged to evaluate a young child's food intake for several days rather than just at one meal to gain a more appropriate nutritional assessment. Nutritional recommendations are shown in Table 19-3.

The American Academy of Pediatrics recommends that children get approximately 30% of their calories from fat. Of that 30%, only one third should come from saturated fats and the other two thirds from polyunsaturated and monounsaturated fats. Fats are an important calorie source, and children need them for normal development. However, parents and children need to examine dietary practices and fat consumption because it is easy for children eating fast foods to exceed the 30% fat intake allowance. Dietary cholesterol should be below 300 mg daily. High fat and cholesterol intake contributes to obesity and heart disease.

✳ nursing considerations

Proper nutrition affects the health of all body systems. Knowledge about nutrition and diet therapy is necessary for all nurses but especially for those working with pediatric clients. When nutritional needs are not adequately met, gastrointestinal function is impaired, interfering with the child's normal growth and development.

communication with caregiver and child

Although some caregivers are familiar with the four basic food groups and the importance of a balanced diet, others may not be as well informed. They may have little or no understanding of food ingredients or special diet considerations (eg, liquid or high-protein diet; Fig. 19-3).

Cultural customs and beliefs about food must be considered when discussing a child's nutritional needs. Child and caregiver compliance to proposed changes in the diet is much greater when the nurse respects existing food customs and ideas in communicating with clients.

The nurse establishes rapport with children and caregivers by listening to their views on proper nutrition and health. Based on these views, the nurse can then provide factual nutritional information in a stimulating but nonthreatening way. For example, some families consider a chubby milk-fed baby a healthy baby. Information about milk-fed infants being at increased risk for obesity, heart disease, and anemia may not seem important to caregivers who perceive their child as being healthy. However, facts about nutrition may interest the caregiver who wishes to keep his or her baby healthy.

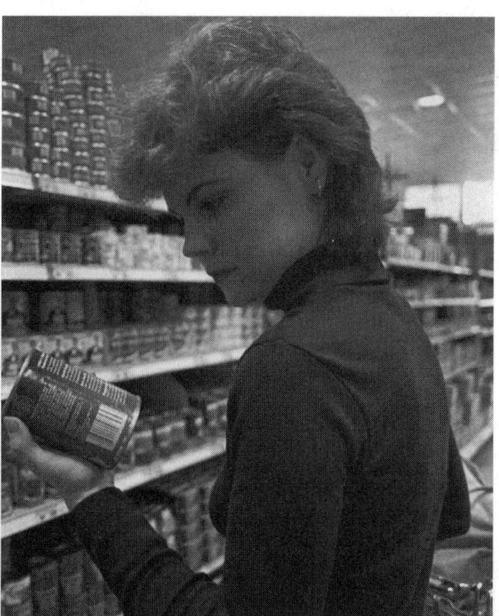

figure 19-3 *Nutrition labeling is a vital education tool. Caregivers can prepare well-balanced meals by learning what nutrients to look for on food labels. (Courtesy USDA Photo Lab)*

food safety

Food safety is of great concern because food-borne illnesses are disagreeable and can be dangerous, even fatal, to young children. Personal cleanliness, proper handling of food, and sanitation of food preparation, equipment, and serving areas reduce the risk of food-related illnesses (see the Teaching Guidelines display).

The most common cause of illness related to food consumption is contamination by disease-causing organisms. These organisms can enter food by hands soiled with urine or feces, coughing or sneezing over food, using contaminated equipment, or eating spoiled or undercooked meat.

Symptoms of food-borne illnesses include vomiting and diarrhea after eating. Young children are at risk for dehydration and electrolyte imbalance. *Clostridium botulinum* causes botulism, with symptoms involving the nervous system. The infected child will experience double vision, droopy eyelids, and difficult speech, progressing to difficult respirations and possible death.

pesticides in food

The popular news media have focused attention on concerns about the safety of the food supply in the United States. Much of the concern centers on the use of pesticides, food additives, and other chemicals and their potential for causing birth defects and cancer in children. Increasing research shows justification for concern. The federal government is beginning to take steps to reduce the use of chemicals in the production of the nation's food as a priority to protect the health of children and the environment. Providing children with safe food is a concern for all people (Display 19-2).

Pesticides are poisons used to kill or control pests. They include *insecticides* used to control insects; *fungicides* used to control fungi, such as mold and mildew; *herbicides* used to control weeds; and *rodenticides* used to control rodents. Widespread use of pesticides poses the threat of water, food, and air contamination.

The Natural Resources Defense Council (NRDC) has identified fruits and vegetables as common sources of pesticide contamination. Foods most likely to be exposed to pesticides are apples and apple products, strawberries, peaches, bananas, potatoes, celery, carrots, and food such as peanut butter and processed cherries.

Pesticides in foods are particularly disturbing for several reasons. Many foods contain the residue of multiple pesticides, which may interact with each other. Children

teaching guidelines ✱
food safety

Proper handling of food reduces the risk of food contaminated by bacteria and the serious consequences of food-borne illnesses.

FOOD HANDLING

Careful handwashing with soap and water:

✱ Before handling food
✱ After using the bathroom, playing with toys and pets, coughing, sneezing, or nose blowing

FOOD PREPARATION

✱ Clean all dishes, utensils, and work surfaces with soap and water after each use. (A solution of 1 tbsp chlorine laundry bleach in 1 quart of cold water destroys bacteria.)
✱ Serve foods immediately after cooking, or refrigerate.
✱ Keep hot foods above 140°F and cold foods below 40°F.
✱ Thaw frozen meat in the refrigerator.
✱ Use separate utensils for preparing and serving food.
✱ Microwave cooking does not always cook food evenly; observe microwave cooking instructions concerning standing time allowing heat to spread through the food.

FOOD STORAGE

✱ Never store cleaning supplies, pesticides, and drugs with food.
✱ Refrigerate perishable foods at 40°F or below or freeze at 0°F. (A cold environment will slow the growth of bacteria.)

FOOD CONTAMINATION

Bacterial Infections

✱ *Salmonella* comes from infected meat, poultry, eggs, unpasteurized milk, or uncooked eggs.
✱ *Staphylococcus* begins in food contaminated from skin pustules, such as boils or pimples, and throat infections. Susceptible foods are cheese, potato salad, cream-filled desserts. Cooking does not destroy the bacteria.
✱ *Clostridium botulinum* is common in foods that are home canned.
✱ *Escherichia coli* is found in stool and transmitted to food products by contaminated hands. Can be a way to transmit viral hepatitis.
✱ *Campylobacter jejuni* occurs from drinking untreated water, coming in contact with an infected pet, or eating undercooked meat.

Molds

✱ *Aflatoxin* develops in peanuts, peanut butter, grains, and animal products. Avoid eating moldy foods. Mold-ripened cheese is safe.

Parasites

✱ *Trichinosis* is found in raw or undercooked pork or game meats.

display 19-2
food safety information

The following information concerns food safety issues:

* Food ingredients and nutritional content are printed on food products to help educate the consumer.
* Foods containing high fat and sugar content are not recommended in large quantities, regardless of the child's age.
* Microbiologic contamination of food sources, such as meat, eggs, and canned foods, can be a major, even life-threatening, health risk.
* The healthy body has an efficient detoxification system, destroying low doses of harmful substances.
* Fresh fruits and vegetables must be washed thoroughly before they are eaten to remove chemicals used in harvest; it is safest to use only organically grown produce, even though it is more expensive.

consume more calories per unit of body weight, eat fewer types of food, and eat proportionally larger amounts of fruits and vegetables than do adults.

adolescent eating patterns

Teenagers often prefer "fast food" and "junk food," empty calories containing large amounts of carbohydrates and fat but little protein, vitamins, or minerals. When these teenagers are also parents, such a diet affects the entire family, contributing to weight gain without adequate nourishment. More than 20% of American children are obese. Lack of vegetables and protein in the diet increases the child's risk of developing iron-deficiency anemia and other disorders related to an unhealthy immune system.

Fad dieting also is common among adolescents. While such eating patterns may be harmless temporarily, they can impair health if extended for a long time. Older children may need counseling to help maintain self-esteem and learn diet requirements.

For several years, the fashion industry has promoted the idea that being thin is attractive. In an attempt to become thin or maintain a thin appearance, some children, especially girls, develop serious eating disorders. The two most common are *anorexia nervosa* (compulsive dieting to the point of starvation) and *bulimia* (a destructive cycle of binge eating followed by self-induced vomiting to prevent weight gain). The psychodynamics of both conditions are complicated and tend to involve severe family dysfunction. See Chapter 25 for more information on anorexia and bulimia.

environment

Environment provides the seventh essential building block for health. *Environment* is defined as the many circumstances and conditions, physical, psychological, and spiritual, that surround and influence the life and survival of a child.

Fetal environment consists of the uterus, placenta, and amniotic fluid. When this environment is altered by the mother's health habits, the child is at risk for congenital health problems. Maternal health habits linked with negative consequences on health include increased risk of low birth weight babies related to cigarette smoking, risk of fetal alcohol syndrome and drug addiction from maternal use of alcohol and illegal drugs, and increased risk of syphilis and acquired immunodeficiency syndrome as a result of unsafe sexual practices.

A child's environment is influenced by physical, social, economic, and cultural factors. Environmental factors, such as good dietary habits, physical exercise, adequate rest, medical and dental care, safety, cleanliness, limited stress, and promotion of interpersonal relationships, influence the manner in which a child's inherited abilities are strengthened.

Environmental influences putting children at risk for alterations in health, growth, and development include exposure to chemicals and pollution, abuse, illness, obesity, sedentary lifestyle, stress, poverty, poor diet, and inadequate medical and dental care.

assessment of vital signs

The nurse uses age-appropriate examination techniques when assessing vital signs and physical health of a child (Table 19-4). The normal range of vital signs in the child differs from that of the adult; younger children have lower blood pressure readings and higher pulse and respiration rates. Pulse, respiration, and blood pressure readings become similar to the adult as the child reaches adolescence (Appendix). Temperature values are similar to adult readings.

Vital sign values change more rapidly in children than in adults. Temperature ranges are often more extreme in children and more varied. Nurses need to be aware of the wide fluctuations and quick changes from normal to abnormal readings. Vital signs must be taken as often as the nurse thinks necessary, based on other assessment factors, such as warm skin, fussiness, difficult breathing, and cyanotic skin. A delay in obtaining a set of vital signs until the next scheduled time can have serious consequences if a temperature elevation results in fever convulsions.

temperature

Assessing a child's temperature can include rectal, oral, axillary, or tympanic methods. The manner in which the temperature is assessed depends on age, the child's cooperation, and existing medical or surgical problems that make one method more appropriate than another. Glass

table 19-4 age-appropriate physical examination techniques

Age	Procedure and Nursing Considerations
Newborn	Undress only the body part being examined (conserve body heat); encourage parent's help. Listen to apical pulse and breath sounds first before infant cries. Use the examination time to talk with parent. Examine throat and ears last.
Infant	Allow parent to hold infant. Talk to infant in a calm soothing manner. If the child is shy with strangers, avoid staring directly at the child's eyes because this can be perceived as threatening. Water bottles or pacifiers can be used to quiet a crying infant.
Toddler	Allow toddler to sit on parent's lap, and encourage parents help in undressing child. Allow toddler to handle equipment when possible. Pretend taking parent's blood pressure to help alleviate child's fears.
Preschool	Encourage undressing self. Allow child to wear underwear. Allow child to handle equipment and engage in "pretend" play using stuffed animals. Encourage parent(s) to stay during examination. Stickers can be used as a reward for bravery during the examination.
School-age	Allow child to decide if parent(s) will stay during examination. Provide child with simple explanations. Explain equipment and procedures.
Adolescent	Comment on body parts as they are examined (e.g. "Your skin is clear."). Examine genitalia last. Include health teaching about breast and testicular self-examination.

mercury thermometers take longer to record a temperature reading, while the electronic devices are much quicker.

rectal temperatures

Rectal temperatures are recommended for infants and for children who are unable to have an oral temperature reading because of an inability to follow directions. Temperatures also are taken rectally when the child is at high risk for seizure activity, making an oral reading dangerous; is experiencing breathing difficulties and is unable to keep the mouth closed; or has had oral surgery.

Normal rectal temperature ranges from 36.2° to 37.8°C (97°–100°F). The temperature reading may be obtained in a matter of seconds if an electronic thermometer is being used or in 3 to 5 minutes if using a glass thermometer. A more accurate reading is obtained when the infant is quiet. Gloves must be worn when taking a rectal temperature.

Disadvantages of a rectal temperature include alteration of temperature readings because of the presence of stool or potential for damage to rectal mucosa if the thermometer is inserted too deeply or if the child has had rectal surgery or is experiencing diarrhea.

oral temperature

Oral temperature readings are more acceptable to toddlers and older children. An oral temperature reading is obtained by using a glass mercury thermometer or an electronic thermometer. The normal range for oral temperature readings is 36.4° to 37.4°C (97.6°–99.3°F). It takes 6 to 9 minutes if using a mercury thermometer and only a few seconds for an electronic thermometer.

The child must keep the mouth closed and must not bite the thermometer. Oral temperatures respond more quickly and regularly to changes in arterial temperature than do readings taken rectally.

The child must not be left alone when taking an oral temperature. For security, safety, and accuracy, keep one hand on the thermometer when it is in place. Oral temperatures are contraindicated in a child who has had oral injuries or oral surgery.

axillary temperature

Axillary temperatures are often recommended for infants younger than 1 year. Normal axillary temperature values range from 35.9° to 36.7°C (96.6°–98°F). They are safe and easily accessible, taking 9 to 11 minutes to obtain the reading with a mercury thermometer.

Axillary temperature readings are recommended for children with diarrhea or who are at risk for rectal or colon perforation. Axillary temperatures are influenced by environmental temperature and airflow around the child that may alter the accuracy of the reading.

tympanic temperature

Tympanic membrane sensors provide a means for taking a child's temperature through the ear. The thermometer records the temperature rapidly with minimal distraction to the child. A disposable speculum is used for each child. Hospital policy and manufacturer's directions must be followed when using a tympanic thermometer. It is advisable to recheck temperature readings by using electronic or glass thermometers when tympanic readings are several degrees below normal. This is especially true if the child's skin is hot to the touch.

pulse

The pulse rate of an infant is taken apically (at the apex of the heart between left nipple and sternum) for 1 full minute. An infant's heart rate slows from 120 to 160 beats/min to 100 to 120 beats/min by 1 year of age and continues to decrease as the child grows (see Appendix).

The rate and rhythm, strength of beat, and activity of the child at the time the pulse is taken are noted and recorded. The pulse rate of an older child may be obtained at the radial, temporal, or carotid locations for 30 seconds. Changes in the pulse rate reflected by an increase or decrease of 10 beats/min must be reported to the registered nurse immediately. An increase in pulse rate often corresponds to an elevation in temperature; a decrease in pulse rate often corresponds to lowered temperature.

nursing insight

- *The pulse rate and respiratory rate must be assessed before taking a rectal temperature because small children tend to cry during a rectal temperature procedure.*
- *Crying increases the pulse rate and makes it difficult to hear an apical beat.*

respirations

An infant's respiratory rate averages 20 to 40 breaths per minute and is influenced by sleep, wakefulness, and feedings. This rate decreases as the infant ages until the rate is equivalent to the adult range of 12 to 22 (see Appendix). Infant respirations are counted for 1 full minute. Respirations may be counted for 30 seconds and multiplied by 2 in older children. Respirations are assessed for rate, rhythm, and depth.

Abdominal breathing is prevalent in infants and continues until school age, when an adult thoracic breathing pattern is established. Exposure of the infant's chest and abdomen is helpful when observing the respiratory pattern. When school-age children use abdominal breathing, they may be experiencing dyspnea.

Listening to the infant's chest with a stethoscope (auscultation) is necessary in assessing breath sounds. Unusual noises, such as expiratory grunts, crowing noises, wheezing, or inspiratory stridor, must be documented and reported to the registered nurse for further evaluation. Careful observation and reporting of signs of dyspnea, including restlessness, nasal flaring, cyanosis, and sternal or intercostal retractions, also are important (see Fig. 28-3).

blood pressure

An accurate blood pressure reading is difficult to obtain in an infant. An average blood pressure during the first year of life is 90/60, with differences noted according to activity level and weight. Blood pressure values increase as the child grows, reaching adult ranges in older children and adolescents (see Appendix).

The size of the blood pressure cuff is important for an accurate blood pressure reading. The recommended cuff size for an infant is 6 to 8 cm in width and 12 to 13.5 cm in length. The width of the cuff should not be less than one half nor greater than two thirds of the length of the upper arm or leg. A cuff that is too narrow will produce an increased reading, while a cuff that is too wide will produce a decreased reading. If the child is excited, restless, or uncomfortable, the systolic pressure may rise.

Preschoolers tend to be more cooperative if they are allowed to handle the equipment, pump the cuff, and so forth. Taking a parent's blood pressure before taking the child's can help relieve some anxieties. Preschool and young school-age children benefit from using the equipment on a doll.

physical health assessment and client and family education

Physical growth is assessed periodically by measuring the infant's weight, height, and head and chest circumference (Table 19-5). The data are plotted on growth charts and compared with previous measurements. Parental size and ancestry must be considered when comparing children with growth standards.

Risk factors for altered growth and development include prematurity, small for gestation age weight at birth, maternal use of alcohol or illicit drugs, maternal neglect or abuse, genetic disorders, and malnutrition. Growth delays or sudden slowing may mean illness or social or psychological problems requiring extra examination and care.

weight

Infants double their birth weight by age 6 months and triple their birth weight by 12 months. They gain approximately 5 to 7 oz (125–175 g) per week and up to 1½ lb (more than 453 g) per month.

Irregular increases are seen in a toddler's weight. By 3 years, the average child weighs about 14 to 15 kg (31–33 lb). Parents and other caregivers need to look at the physical, social, and emotional growth of the child as a gradual and continuous process.

table 19-5 recommended ages for health maintenance assessment

Age	*Time Interval*
1 mo–1½ y	Every month for the first 2 months, then every 2 to 3 months until the child reaches 1½ years
1½–2½ y	Every 6 months
2½–6 y	Every 12 months
6–18 y	Every 24 months

✱ nursing insight

If the toddler is too big to weigh on an infant scale and unable to stand on adult scales, weigh yourself on an adult scale, then hold the toddler, weigh yourself again, and subtract the difference between the two weights.

The preschool child experiences slow growth from 3 to 5 years. Genetic influences on body measurements are often apparent by the end of the preschool period. Normal weight gains are 3 to 5 lb (1.8–2.3 kg) per year. A 5-year-old can be expected to double the weight noted at 1 year of age.

During the school-age years, girls often grow faster than boys. Normal weight changes include a weight gain of 4½ to 6½ lb (2–2.9 kg) per year between 6 and 12 years.

During adolescence, hormonal activity causes secondary sex characteristics to appear and body mass to reach adult size. Boys tend to catch up to and exceed girls in weight with gains of 15 to 65 lb (6.8–29.5 kg) over a 4-year period. Girls gain 15 to 55 lb (6.8–25 kg) over a 3-year period.

height

Normal growth patterns for height include an increase of approximately 1 in (2.6 cm) per month, with a total increase of 50% over the birth length by 12 months. Most of an infant's growth occurs in the trunk of the body.

 **nursing insight**

Weight and height assessment tends to be more accurate if the infant is nude.

The child's height increases begin to taper off after the first year. Toddlers are expected to reach about half of their adult height by age 2.

Three-year-old toddlers can be measured by standing them against a growth chart or against a flat wall, marking the height and then using a yardstick or measuring tape to obtain the correct size. Taking a height measurement on a weight scale is difficult and usually not as accurate.

By 5 years, birth length is nearly doubled. As a result of greater increases in height compared with weight, preschoolers take on a thinner, taller appearance compared to chubby, pot-bellied toddlers.

School-age children grow in height about 2 in (5.2 cm) per year. Normal height changes during adolescence includes a gain of 2 to 8 in (5.1–20.5 cm) for girls and 4 to 12 in (10.2–30.8 cm) for boys.

laboratory values

The normal laboratory values for children vary, depending on the child's age. For example, the hemoglobin (oxygen-carrying protein) for a 1-month-old ranges from 10.7 to 13.9, whereas at 6 months, the hemoglobin ranges from 11.1 to 12.6. Hemoglobin reaches adult levels of 12 to 16 after 6 months. Decreases in hemoglobin caused by an inadequate supply of iron necessary for normal red blood cell formation occur most commonly in children between 6 months and 3 years. Called iron-deficiency anemia, this condition occurs when the diet includes too much milk and not enough solid, iron-rich food. Milk is a poor source of iron.

Laboratory tests are ordered by the physician as a screening measure for infants who manifest signs of altered growth and development or disease process. Specific laboratory tests are ordered when a child is considered at risk for certain conditions, such as exposure to lead-based paint.

Lead poisoning affects 4% of children 6 months to 5 years, with a high incidence noted at 2 to 3 years. Lead poisoning occurs six times more often in African Americans than in white people. Increased serum lead levels confirm the diagnosis (Appendix). Normal serum lead level value is less than 1 μg/dL.

vision

Assessment of vision in infants involves a description of the baby's activities. Eye movements that indicate the infant is following an individual with the eyes and smiling back at the caregiver reflect visual abilities. Infant vision is typically checked by the ability to follow a moving object to midline.

Toddlers and preschoolers are observed for behaviors indicating visual problems, such as rubbing the eyes frequently, squinting, frowning, or holding books or toys extremely close or far away from the face. Young children may wish to sit close to the television set or movie screen because they prefer seeing action up close. This habit is not necessarily associated with visual impairment; however, it needs to be discouraged because the exposure to electromagnetic fields from the television increases the closer the child sits to it.

Preschoolers are routinely screened for *amblyopia,* often referred to as "lazy eye." Because one eye focuses more quickly than the other, the child comes to depend only on the easily focused eye, which leads to deteriorating vision in the other eye. The Worth 4-Dot Test is used specifically to test for amblyopia. The test involves wearing special colored glasses and looking at a series of dots. The child will see four dots if both eyes are functioning properly.

Amblyopia is easily corrected during the preschool years by covering the child's easily focused eye with a patch, forcing the use and development of the other eye. If treatment is delayed after 6 years, chance of correction is decreased.

An "E" chart and Allen cards are used to check visual acuity in children who are unfamiliar with the letters of the alphabet. The procedure for using the "E" chart is similar to the Snellen chart except the child is asked to identify the position of the letter E. Normal vision for the preschool child is 20/50 using the E chart (Fig. 19-4*A*).

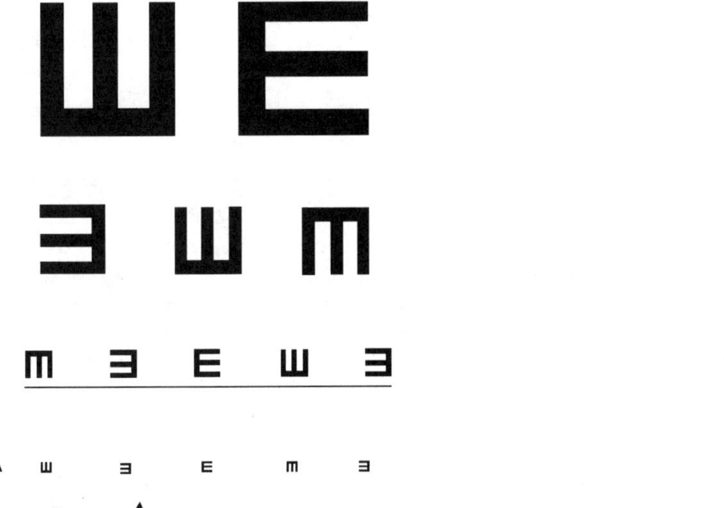

A

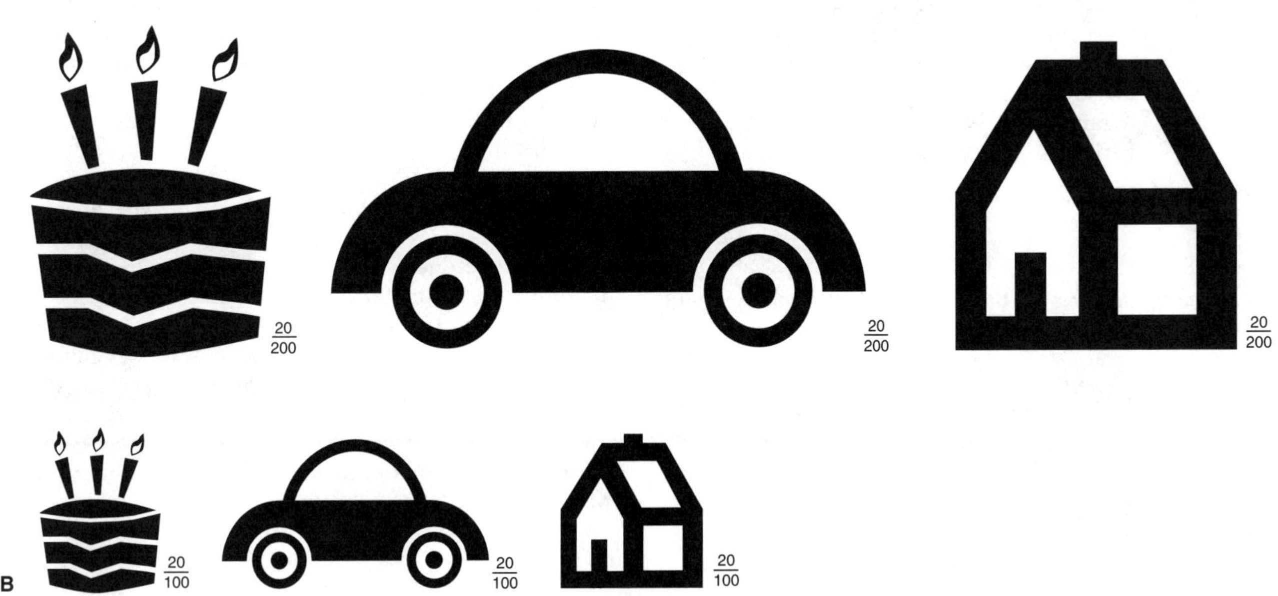

B

figure 19-4 *(A) E chart. (B) Allen cards.*

Allen cards have pictures of common objects, such as a car, house, and birthday cake. The cards are shown to the child at a distance of 15 ft, and visual acuity is determined by how well the pictures are seen (see Fig. 19-4*B*).

School-age children and adolescents may complain of frequent headaches when experiencing a vision problem. Poor academic performance, difficulty reading, and blurred or double vision indicate the need for an eye examination. The Snellen chart is used to check visual acuity in an older child. Normal visual acuity is considered 20/20.

hearing

Learning and the development of speech patterns depends on a child's ability to hear. Hearing impairment can affect the child's cognitive, social, and emotional development. Children should have their hearing tested at least once during the preschool years and more often if indicated.

Inappropriate responses and behavior may be the first clue that a child is not hearing accurately. Common behavioral signs of hearing loss include delays in developing language skills, difficulty in following directions, and using gestures instead of words to communicate needs. Hearing tests used for screening in preschool children use an audiometer. This nonmedical technique tests for normal range of tones used in everyday conversation (Fig. 19-5).

Hearing assessment includes a thorough history concerning familial hearing problems. An infant's hearing can be evaluated from the time of birth by checking responses to sound. These responses include blinking, turning the head toward the sound, and demonstrating the startle reflex in response to a loud noise. Infants at increased risk for hearing alterations include those born to mothers experiencing perinatal infections, such as rubella, herpes, cytomegalovirus, and syphilis; those whose birth weight was less than 1500 g; those with Apgar scores between 0 and 3; and those who have deafness in the family.

Many types of hearing problems can be effectively treated if they are identified early. Once a hearing problem is identified, the underlying cause may require drug ther-

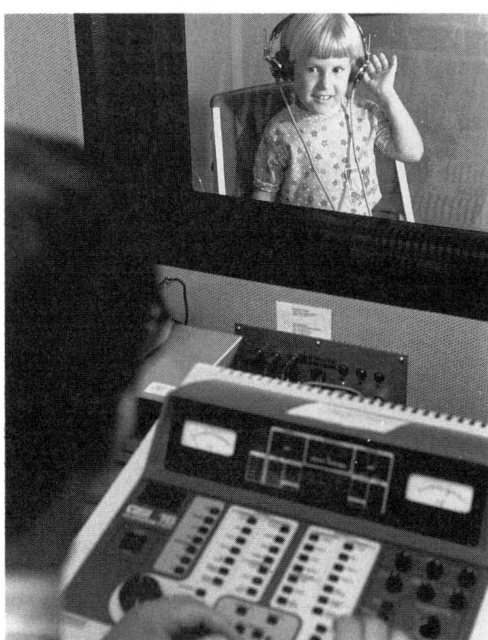

figure 19-5 *School-age child undergoing hearing screening assessment.*

apy, surgery, hearing aid placement, or teaching the child sign language.

speech and language

Speech and language development are influenced by many factors. Young children get many of their early language skills by copying speech heard at home. Language development increases as the child matures.

Most 2-year-old children speak in simple phrases, such as "go bye bye." By the time a child reaches preschool age, the vocabulary has expanded to include about 1,500 words, with the child using more complex sentences, such as "I want to play with Jane."

Normal speech and language development varies greatly according to culture and ethnic backgrounds. It may be difficult to determine speech impairment problems. The guidelines often used to screen children include an absence of speech by 2 years of age, stuttering, notably fast or slow speech, monotone voice, inability to understand the child's speech at 3 years of age, and no improvement in speech development. Early detection and treatment of speech difficulties is important for the young child to overcome speech impairments successfully.

scoliosis screening

Scoliosis screening is typically done on school-age children. The condition is characterized by curvature of the spine. The growth spurt common during adolescence can aggravate the condition, making early detection important.

The screening is done by having the child stand with the feet together and the back exposed. The back is observed for differences in the level of the hips and shoulders and balance of scapulae. The child is asked to bend forward and backward while the spine is observed for normal horizontal curvature (see Figure 36-5).

dental health

Proper dental health begins at birth and continues throughout the child's life cycle. Special attention must be given to diet, dental hygiene practices, regular dental examinations, and treatment of dental problems. Unfortunately, preventive dental care can be expensive and is often neglected by families experiencing economic problems.

Widespread education programs emphasizing the importance of brushing and flossing plus the addition of fluoride to public water supplies have helped decrease the number of dental caries (cavities) and reported gum disease problems in children during the last decade. Parental knowledge promoting early intervention for dental problems has made a significant improvement in children's dental health.

Many parents still have mistaken ideas about deciduous teeth ("baby teeth") being unimportant because they eventually fall out and are replaced by permanent teeth. However, deciduous teeth are necessary for chewing, maintaining spacing for permanent teeth, and speech development (Fig. 19-6).

A daily routine of good oral hygiene is important for the promotion of dental health. An infant's teeth can be wiped with a small, wet cloth to remove pieces of food. Toddlers can begin learning how to brush their teeth. A dental check-up is recommended for children between 2 and 2 1/2 years.

Dental caries are painful at any age, and infected teeth increase the child's risk for ear infections and more seri-

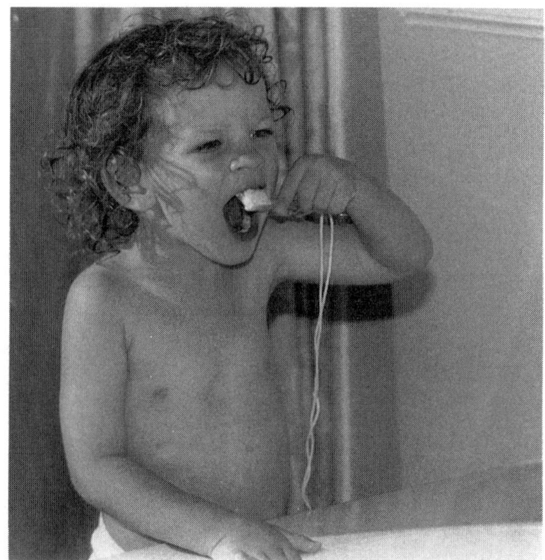

figure 19-6 *It is important for the young child to maintain healthy "baby teeth" and establish long-lasting brushing habits.*

ous infections, such as meningitis. Proper nutrition and good dental hygiene reduce the risk of dental caries.

health education

Primary responsibility for a child's health care belongs to parents and other caregivers. Parents are often the first to sense that their child has a physical, emotional, or cognitive developmetnal problem. Unfortunately, some parents delay seeking professional intervention. They may deny the seriousness or potential seriousness of the developmental delay and hope the child outgrows the problem.

Referral may be necessary to determine the meaning and cause of growth disturbances. Lack of growth or sudden delay may indicate illness or social or psychological problems that require treatment. Lack of motor development may indicate neurologic defects.

Parents often express concerns about their child's growing independence and may not understand the normal expectations related to the child's age. Abuse sometimes stems from a child's inability to perform according to parental expectations.

✳ nursing process in health maintenance

Periodic health assessment is necessary for young children (Table 19-5). The child's weight and height measurements are taken and compared with normal standards. Vision and hearing screenings are used to determine if the child has any impairments needing professional intervention. Dental health assessment involves screening children for the presence of caries.

nursing assessment

Subjective assessment is based on information obtained primarily from the child's parents or caregver. Parents must be asked how they feel the child is developing because family expectations and beliefs affect the child's development. Family history provides the nurse with information about genetic tendencies that may affect the child's growth and development.

Objective assessment of the child includes physical growth and development, including gross and fine motor development. Delays in growth and development requiring investigation include the following:

- Inability to hold head erect by 3 months
- No response to voices or common noises by 2 months
- Absence of teeth after 10 months
- No babbling by 10 months
- Inability to walk alone by 18 months
- Inability to kick when standing by 21 months
- Absence of toilet training by 5 years
- Significant weight loss or weight gain
- Loss of interest in friends, school, personal appearance, and so forth

nursing diagnoses

Nursing diagnoses are general because health maintenance spans many years of development.

- Risk for Altered Growth and Development, related to prematurity, maternal alcohol and drug abuse, malnutrition, genetic disorders, neglect or abuse, and poverty
- Risk for Knowledge Deficit of caregiver concerning expected growth and developmental needs of the child

nursing interventions

Nursing interventions concerning altered growth and development follow:

- Measure the child's weight, height, and head and chest circumference at every visit. Plot the data on growth charts and compare with previous measurements. Child will need to be referred if height and weight fall outside the 5th to 95th percentile. Observe for loss of deciduous teeth and eruption of permanent teeth. Take the child's blood pressure, pulse, respirations, and temperature. Observe whether the child moves all limbs with equal ease and range of motion. Ask about the child's favorite play activities, peer relationships, and hygiene habits.

Nursing interventions concerning risk for parental knowledge deficit concerning expected growth and development follow:

- Observe interaction between child and caregivers. Discuss with caregivers their expectations for the child now and in the near future. Demonstrate age-appropriate interactions. Examine the caregiver's concerns about sexual development, recreational drug and alcohol use, school and home responsibilities, and discipline.

evaluation

- Child's weight and height will fall between the 5th and 95th percentiles on a standardized graph. Child will demonstrate age-appropriate milestones for motor control, language development, and social, emotional, and cognitive development.
- Primary caregivers will describe expected developmental events for child's age.

home visiting programs

Home visiting programs in various forms have become increasingly popular to deliver health, welfare, and education services to children and families. Observing family interactions in the home provides people involved with the health and welfare of children an opportunity to identify specific family needs. Early detection and intervention are crucial in homes at risk for domestic violence, child abuse, and neglect.

key points

* National health care concerns include the increasing numbers of families that are living in poverty, uninsured and without access to medical care, distressed by drug and alcohol abuse, experiencing child abuse and neglect, and exposed to food, air, and water polluted with pesticides, chemical additives, and other toxins.
* Health status of children depends on many factors, including heredity, family size, culture, economics, nutrition, society, and environment.
* Genetic screening programs promote early detection of hereditary disorders, helping to minimize long-term effects.
* The family system is an important link to health because family interactions teach children values and communication patterns and how to socialize with others, follow rules, and learn and test skills needed to relate to the larger society.
* Culture is a set of values, beliefs, and traditions that are held by a specific social group and handed down from one generation to another, influencing the way children view themselves, their behavioral responses to others, family food preferences, communication patterns, and language.
* Cultural bias develops when children learn stereotypes based on race, gender, and ethnicity from the world around them; prejudice often grows out of a young child's limited experiences and immature ways of interpreting experiences provided through family encounters.
* American children raised in poverty lack the resources to meet basic needs, struggle for the necessities of food and shelter, live in unsafe and undesirable neighborhood environments with inadequate housing, experience the dehumanization that often accompanies welfare dependency, and have an increase in mortality rate because prenatal care is not adequate and health maintenance issues are neglected.
* A current concern is the increasing frequency of violent crimes and crime-related injuries and deaths associated with domestic violence as an ongoing, debilitating experience of physical, psychological, or sexual abuse involving children.
* Health maintenance assessment of children includes nutritional status; physical examination, including vital signs, weight, and height; normal laboratory values; and specific screening for vision, hearing, speech, and scoliosis.
* Health education issues affecting children include parental knowledge concerning developmental delays and the importance of early intervention; intervention for parents prone to violence, neglect, and sexual abuse; and factual information concerning nutrition and an awareness about pesticides in food.

review questions 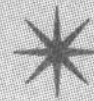

1. Select the most correct statement about the focus of national preventive health care concerns.
   a. Maintenance of physical, mental, and social well-being is affected by living in poverty, using and abusing drugs and alcohol, and experiencing potential dangers related to pesticide exposure.
   b. Maintenance of physical health centers on normal vital signs, normal weight and length increases, and family size.
   c. Maintenance of health and promotion of health care practices are influenced by birth order, heredity, and economic success.
   d. Maintenance of psychological health is only altered by domestic violence when actual abuse is experienced by the child.
2. A child's birth order affects intellectual ability when
   a. family size includes older and younger siblings.
   b. parents place much emphasis on the child's accomplishments relative to birth order.
   c. parents divorce immediately following birth of the child.
   d. the child is encouraged by younger siblings.
3. Select the most accurate statement providing a definition of culture. Culture includes
   a. stereotypes based on race, gender, and ethnicity.
   b. the many differences that make children unique.
   c. a set of values, beliefs, and traditions passed down through generations and specific to a social group.
   d. a limited experience and immaturity of interpreting experiences provided through family encounters.
4. Domestic violence tends to follow a cycle that includes
   a. decrease of hostility followed by an increase in sexual demands.
   b. decrease of physical abuse when verbal abuse increases.
   c. child neglect escalating to physical or sexual abuse involving mostly teenagers.
   d. increased tension and anger, followed by actual abuse then denial or excuses.
5. The American Academy of Pediatrics recommends that children receive approximately 30% of their calories from
   a. carbohydrates.
   b. proteins.
   c. fats.
   d. complex carbohydrates.

references 

Gasbarro, R. (1992). *Children of alcoholics growing up amid pain.* Waco, TX: Health Edco.

Ohio State Medical Association, Department of Human Services (1992). *Ohio physicians' domestic violence prevention project* (pp. 1–32), Columbus, OH: Ohio State Medical Association.

Sharp, R. (1992). *Effects of domestic violence on children.* York, PA: William Gladden Foundation.

bibliography

Devlin, B., & Reynolds, E. (1994). Child abuse. *American Journal of Nursing, March*, 27–31.

Donner, C. (1993). Recognizing child abuse. *American Journal of Nursing, March*, 58.

Gulanic, M., Gradishar, D., & Puzas, M. (1994). Ambulatory pediatric nursing. *RN*, .

Halpern, R. (1993). The societal context of home visiting and related services for families in poverty. *Home Visiting, 3*(3), 158–171.

Henry III, W. (1990). Beyond the melting pot. *Time, April 9*, 28–31.

Humphreys, J. (1991). Children of battered women: Worries about their mothers. *Pediatric Nursing, 17*(4), 342–345.

Kohn, A. (1990). The birth-order myth. *Health, January*, 34–35.

Marks, M. (1994). *Broadribb's Introductory pediatric nursing*. Philadelphia: J.B. Lippincott.

Marotz, L., Cross, M., & Rush, J. (1993). *Health, safety and nutrition for the young child* (3rd ed.). Albany, NY: Delmar Publishers.

Merina, A. (1994). Fighting school violence means taking on guns. *National Education Association Today, March*, 4–5.

McGehee, L. (1991). Coming to terms with the multiculturalists. *The Education Digest, December*, 4–5.

National Research Council (1993). *Changes needed to protect children from pesticides in diet.* Washington, DC: National Academy of Sciences.

Parlapiano, E. (1994). United against violence. *Futures, 1*, 22–26.

Ramey, C., & Ramey, S. (1993). Home visiting programs and the health and development of young children. *Home Visiting, 3*(3), 129–139.

Residue Monitoring (1991). Food and Drug Administration Pesticide Program, *9*, 1-3.

Rhodes, A. (l993). Family violence. *MCN, March/April*, 73.

Slaughter-Defoe, D. (1993). Home visiting with families in poverty: Introducing the concept of culture. *Home Visiting, 3*(3), 172–183.

Taylor, C., Lillis, C., & LeMone, P. (1993). *Fundamentals of nursing: The art and science of nursing care* (2nd. ed.). Philadelphia: J.B. Lippincott.

health protection and safety 20

outline

objectives

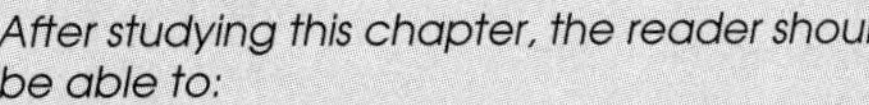

After studying this chapter, the reader should be able to:

* List two principal factors that protect the health of children.
* Define safety.
* Discuss at least six safety concerns when caring for young children.
* List the four types of poisons, and give an example of each.
* Discuss at least two issues concerning shooting accidents among children.
* Describe relevant car safety for infants, preschoolers, school-age children, and adolescents.
* List the four pathogens responsible for infectious diseases.
* List the immunizations available for nine infectious diseases.
* Discuss the causes for common childhood allergies.
* Discuss pediatric emergency care, including treatment of anaphylactic shock, respiratory distress, and cardiac arrest.

key terms

anaphylactic shock
angioedema
aspiration
caustic
convalescent
"doll's eyes"
electrocution
Heimlich maneuver
hypovolemic shock
immune deficient
immunizations
incubation stage
methane
plumbism
poison
prodromal stage
safety
urticaria

Protecting the health and safety of children includes preventing accidental injuries and protecting against communicable diseases. Accidental injuries are the leading cause of childhood mortality in the United States (Sewell & Gaines, 1993).

Parental knowledge of age-appropriate growth and development also promotes child safety and reinforces healthy family lifestyle patterns. Understanding and awareness of susceptibility to childhood illnesses increases compliance with immunization programs.

Immunization is aimed at reducing the child's risk of contracting and spreading communicable diseases. Communicable diseases in children can produce serious, sometimes fatal complications. Many children do not receive proper immunization even though clinics and public health care agencies provide immunization at little or no cost.

This chapter includes parental guidelines for child safety, general immunization information, and interventions for common childhood problems and life-threatening emergencies. Specific age-related immunizations are discussed in the appropriate growth and development chapters.

safety

Actions and practices that reduce the risk of disease, injury, or death are known as *safety*. Accidents are responsible for a large percentage of deaths in children between the ages of 1 and 14 years (Marotz, 1993). Childhood injury is the principal public health problem in America today, causing more deaths and disability than all childhood diseases combined. For example, accident-related deaths in 1994 were estimated at 3,400 in children up to 4 years old, 3,600 in children 5 to 14 years, and 13,900 in people 15 to 24 years (National Safety Council, l994).

Enforceable, age-appropriate safety rules help ensure safe environments for children. Developmental tasks that include motor skills and cognitive and psychosocial development affect a child's ability to play and understand danger and harm. For example, toddlers require constant supervision even though they can walk, talk, and appear to comprehend simple instructions. School-age children can be trusted to follow simple safety rules because of their ability to comprehend the fundamentals of danger, such as getting hit by a car while crossing the street. A child's progress in motor control, language development, and physical age may not be enough to guarantee a knowledge of health and safety. Age-appropriate guidelines are discussed in Table 20-1. Refer to Table 20-2 for a breakdown of accidental deaths according to age.

anatomic and physiologic considerations

Anatomic and physiologic differences between children and adults have important implications for health protection and safety. One of the most important anatomic differences between a child and an adult is the size of the airway. Children have smaller airways that can easily be obstructed by a slightly enlarged tongue, a small amount of mucus or blood, or a slight amount of swelling, or aspiration of food, toys, coins, and other foreign objects.

A child's head is larger in relation to the body than that of an adult. This contributes to falls, resulting in head and facial injuries.

There is less muscle in the thorax, increasing the risk of rib fractures. Fractured ribs can easily puncture a lung, causing *pneumothorax*, a collapsed lung resulting from penetration of the pleural covering of the lung.

Blood loss considered minor in an adult can quickly lead to hypovolemic shock in a child. A loss of l00 mL could amount to as much as 20% of a child's total volume. Signs and symptoms of shock are more subtle in children. Tachycardia is one of the first signs as the body attempts to raise cardiac output. A drop in blood pressure is a late sign of shock in a child. A child's body can compensate for a loss of up to 30% of total blood volume before the blood pressure drops.

home safety

Nurses have many opportunities to provide education about home safety. Caregiver education includes safe care of young children, emphasizing the importance of constant supervision; crib safety; safe toys; safeguarding from falls, burns, and poisons; appropriate first aid measures; and accessible emergency phone numbers.

All items within reach of the young child must be carefully inspected; items such as medicines, household cleaners, liquor, and sharp objects must be secured out of the reach of the child. Parental or caregiver supervision includes anticipation of hazards in the child's environment and protection by using precautionary measures, such as safety locks, guard rails, electric outlet covers, sturdy outdoor play equipment, age-appropriate toys, and education.

crib safety

Suffocation is defined as obstruction of air passages and is the leading cause of accidental death among children younger than 1 year old. Infants can suffocate in their cribs by getting their faces wedged between the sides of the crib and the mattress or by burying their faces under blankets. Waterbeds, soft mattresses, and bean-bag pillows are dangerous because infants can suffocate in the depressions made by their bodies.

Crib safety begins with the purchase of a crib that has met the requirements of the Consumer Product Safety Commission. Ornate crib headboards with cut-out designs are not recommended because the infant's head could get caught in large cut-out designs. Accordion-style baby playpens used in place of cribs are not recommended because they have wide openings that can entrap an infant's head and cause strangulation.

Cribs must be placed away from windows with blinds or draperies to reduce the risk of infants wrapping a dan-

table 20-1 age-related hazards and safety measures for children

Age	*Growth Features*	*Dangers*	*Safety Measures*
Infant 1–12 mo	Vulnerable to injury because head size is larger than the rest of body proportions Total dependence Puts objects in mouth	Burns, falls, choking, sharp objects, smothering, toys, bath water, poisoning	Provide constant supervision. Support head when holding. Lower hot water temperature to 130°F. Protect infant from rolling off flat surface or falling down steps. Select age-appropriate toys; keep infant away from faucets, hot drinks.
Toddler and preschool 1–4 y	Concrete thinking symbolized by fantasy and a belief that inanimate objects are capable of human feelings Use magical thinking Gains an unreal perception from television cartoons Trusts cars to not cause harm. Fascinated by fire	Windows, doors, water, poisons, burns, traffic, playing, animal bites	Ideal time to teach desirable health habits through short stories, puppet shows, song sessions, coloring activities, and role playing. Parental restrictions must be firm. Give child explanations about necessary restrictions. Avoid streets for play, matches, play with older children. Oversee play close to bodies of water. Teach swimming. Keep medications, cleaning products, matches locked.
5–9 y	Spends large part of day away from home at school or with peers May attempt dangerous activities to impress peers, such as reckless bike riding Participates in active sports	Traffic, firearms, sports, drowning	Teach specific safety rules; involve child as an active partner in learning about safety by providing concrete reasons for preventive actions. Teaching must gradually replace supervision.
10–14 y	Begins to develop abstract thinking abilities, enjoys reading Peer competition and approval important	Traffic, bicycle, skateboard, roller skating accidents, sports trauma, drug and alcohol abuse, sexually transmitted diseases (STDs), pregnancy, violence	Teach pedestrian and bicycle safety. Supervise competitive activities. Do not allow play in the streets or alleys. Provide sex education
15–19 y	Abstract thinking Strong urge for independence High degree of peer influence A sense of personal immortality	Automobile accidents, drug and alcohol abuse, violence, sports injuries, STDs, pregnancy, suicide	Teach scientific reasons for actions. Present statistics and case studies; encourage discussion and debate. Teach legal implications for drug and alcohol use, for example up to 0.10% is considered legal blood alcohol content.

gling cord around their neck. Pacifiers must not be tied around the infant's neck. Avoid using plastic bags to cover a mattress or pillow because infants can crawl into large plastic bags or pull smaller bags over their heads, causing suffocation.

As early as 2 months of age, an infant can roll from back to front and fall from a crib if the sides are down. To avoid burn injuries, cribs must not be placed near radiators or heating units.

falls

Children between the ages of 1 and 6 years are the most susceptible to falls because their coordination and judgment are not fully developed. Falling from open windows and down staircases can cause serious injuries or death.

Children are at risk for falling out of open windows, especially if window guards are not used on windows above ground level. Sitting or climbing against window screens is a safety risk because most window screens are not sturdy enough to support a child's weight.

Children love to run and climb, play on staircases, and rough-house around furniture. Staircases and furniture with sharp edges are potential dangers; placing them off limits can help reduce the risk of accidental injuries.

Holding handrails while climbing up and down stairs can reduce the child's risk of falling. When children are too young to use a handrail, "scooting" up and down the steps can be a fun way to travel and a safer way to get to

table 20-2 deaths reported in 1993 to unintentional injuries

Causes	*0–4 y*	*5–14 y*	*15–24 y*
Motor vehicle	1,000	2,000	10,600
Falls	90	80	230
Poisoning from solids (includes drugs, medicines)	40	30	280
Drowning	700	500	900
Fires, burns	850	350	200
Suffocation	140	30	30
Firearms	40	180	550
Poisoning from vapors (carbon monoxide)	40	30	110
Other (includes medical complications, machinery, mechanical suffocation, excessive cold)	500	400	1,000

Accident Facts (1994). National Safety Council.

the top and bottom. Young children with an unsteady gait can easily trip when attempting to walk on area rugs that are not secure to the floor.

When children are placed in feeding chairs, infant seats, and swings, safety precautions include the use of a harness or belt restraint and close supervision. The use of restraints does not lessen the need for constant supervision. Children can be spontaneous and creative in ways that contribute to falling out of chairs or being strangled from safety belts. See the Teaching Guidelines for safe climbing.

head trauma

Young children tend to fall on their heads, increasing the potential for brain trauma. When the brain is bruised, lacerated, or punctured, blood from ruptured vessels can flow between the brain and its protective coverings, causing pressure on the brain. When signs and symptoms indicate injury to the skull or brain, the child also may have a cervical spine injury. Care must be taken to immobilize the child and reduce the risk of permanent spinal cord damage.

Symptoms of serious head injury include the following:

- Decreased level of consciousness or personality changes
- Deep laceration or severe bruising on the scalp or forehead
- Elevated blood pressure, pulse, and respirations initially, then decrease
- Pain or swelling at site of the head injury
- Deformity of the skull, such as depression or large swellings (goose eggs)
- Altered appearance of the eyes, such as unequal pupils, "black" or sunken eyes, and "doll's eyes" (staying in midline position when the head moves)
- Altered vision and hearing
- Blood or clear fluid drainage from the ears or nose, suggesting cerebrospinal fluid loss

nursing care

When caring for children with head injuries, it is essential to secure an open airway, immobilize the neck and spine, and provide resuscitative measures if needed. To reduce the risk of intracranial pressure build-up, the entire upper body needs to be elevated or the entire body slanted to a head-elevated position. Oxygen administration is important if brain damage is a possibility. A pediatric trauma patient typically needs supplemental oxygen because a child's metabolic rate is about twice a fast as that of an adult.

Neurologic checks are done every 15 minutes and include assessment of alertness and orientation; pupil size, equality, and reaction to light; and ability to move all extremities on command (Table 20-3). Noting subtle differences and reporting and recording the findings can make the difference between a successful or an unsuccessful recovery. See the Teaching Guidelines for home care of head injuries.

teaching guidelines
safe climbing

Climbing is important to the child's motor development. When young children get the urge to climb, clear an area on the floor, and make a pile of sofa cushions and pillows. Throw a blanket over the top to give the appearance of a mountain and keep the pillows together, and then suggest that the child go mountain climbing.

table 20-3 neurologic checks

Acronym (PERL MAE)	*Explanation*
P	Pupils
E	Equal
R	Reactive to
L	Light
M	Moving
A	All
E	Extremities to command

Reproduced with permission from Rayfield, S. (1995). *Nursing made easy.* Shreveport, LA: I CAN Publishing.

teaching guidelines
home care of head injuries

When a child falls and hits his or her head, a common dilemma is whether to seek medical intervention or observe the child at home. The following information concerns both home care and tips on when to call the doctor.

HOME CARE

- ✳ Wake an infant every 4 hours for feeding.
- ✳ Wake an older child every 4 hours to assess his or her condition; check level of consciousness by asking name, place, and year.
- ✳ Give only sips of clear fluids, such as water, fruit juices, or ice pops, for the first 8 hours after the injury.

CALL THE DOCTOR WHEN

- ✳ Infant or child is difficult to arouse or becomes unconscious.
- ✳ Vomiting is noted about 8 hours after the injury.
- ✳ Infant or child becomes fussy, and ordinary calming methods do not work.
- ✳ Convulsions (seizures) occur.
- ✳ Child complains of headache and exhibits confused behaviors.

choking

Young children are well known for putting anything and everything into their mouths. Toys with small, removable parts; coins; marbles; pen caps; or other small round objects are unsafe for young children.

Infants are at risk for aspirating and choking on foods such as nuts, popcorn, or small candies. Boneless meats, fish, and chicken are given to children younger than 3 years as a safety precaution, reducing the risk of choking on small bones.

Crying children pose an increased risk of choking on food or medicines, resulting in vomiting and aspiration. Vomitus containing oily medicines can cause respiratory illness, such as pneumonia. Hydrochloric acid found in stomach contents can cause permanent damage to lung tissue.

When an infant vomits, he or she should be positioned head down with the hips lifted slightly to permit the liquid vomitus to flow out of the mouth. An older child can be positioned with the head bent forward.

Balloons pose a serious threat to young children because they can get sucked down the windpipe, where they are difficult to remove. Any condition that blocks a child's airway creates an emergency situation that must be resolved as quickly as possible. Emergency care for choking is discussed on page 327.

electrical injuries

Young children are natural explorers and will poke and probe light sockets with their fingers, increasing the risk of being electrocuted. Covers placed on wall outlets help keep adventuresome children from harm (Display 20-1).

burns

Smoke inhalation and burns are the third leading cause of death among children. Extra care must be taken when children are around stoves or other heating appliances. Many burn accidents occur in the kitchen from children pulling hot liquids or food off stoves and tables.

display 20-1
safety tips for childproofing the house

The greatest threat to a child's health is accidental injury. Because it is not possible to watch a child every minute of the day, surroundings need to be as safe as possible. The following safety tips will help.

- ✳ Use locks for cabinets containing medicines, cleaning supplies, guns, knives, gasolines, and other poisons, such as rat poison or insecticides.
- ✳ Use gates at the top and bottom of stairways and carpet stairways. Remove furniture with low, sharp corners. Test the sturdiness of window screens. Use unbreakable glass or Plexiglass on windows and storm doors that are in high-contact areas, such as family rooms, and *do not* use infant walkers unless child is closely supervised.
- ✳ Lower the temperature of your hot water heater to 120°F.
- ✳ Install antiscald devices in the bathtub and shower fixtures.
- ✳ Use smoke detectors and carbon monoxide detectors. Keep matches out of child's reach.
- ✳ Cover electrical outlets with safety plugs. Replace worn-out electrical cords. Keep electrical cords away from child.
- ✳ Use back burners on the stove. Turn pot handles toward back of stove; keep hot liquids away from child.
- ✳ Install window guards and stairway safety gates to prevent falls.
- ✳ Post emergency numbers next to the phone.
- ✳ Place irons, toaster, and other small appliances out of reach.
- ✳ Keep child away from wood-burning stoves, radiators, electric heaters, kerosene heaters, and fireplaces.
- ✳ Do not allow the child to play with toys with sharp edges or small parts that could be swallowed. Be alert to toys that are age and ability appropriate, and keep child from play with plastic bags.

Bathrooms are another area where children can receive burns. Scalding injuries can occur when bath water is too hot or children are unsupervised and accidentally turn on hot water. Temperature settings on hot water heaters can be lowered to reduce the risk of contact with scalding water. Curling irons and brushes left on by older siblings can burn younger children whose curious nature prompts them to explore the appliance. Burns are painful and can leave scars. Additional information on burns is found in Chapter 37.

Fire extinguishers must be readily accessible in case of fire. School-age children can be taught how to activate and use a fire extinguisher and call the local fire department.

Children between 3 and 8 years have a natural curiosity about matches and lighters. More than one third of the burns to children result from playing with matches. Young children can be taught that matches and lighters are tools for adults, not toys. However, the most effective measure is keeping matches and lighters out of a child's reach. See Teaching Guidelines for fire safety.

Family fire safety programs are effective in planning actions necessary in case of a house fire. Each family member participates and is knowledgeable about the program. Steps of the fire safety plan are practiced periodically. Most family fire safety programs are centered around the following:

* The safest and quickest escape route out of the house
* Keeping a bedroom or hall door closed to keep out fire long enough to escape through the escape route
* Agreeing on a way to sound a family fire alarm, such as pounding on walls and yelling, because fire may prevent walking to other areas in the house
* Not wasting time getting dressed or gathering valuables because precious seconds count
* Crawling on the floor if the house is full of smoke
* The importance of staying out of the house
* The significance of meeting parents and siblings in a preplanned location

Outdoor play on a sunny day may overexpose the child's skin to sun. Research links sunburn during childhood to increased risk of skin cancer later in life. Children can be spared some of the sun's intensity if they avoid outdoor activities between 10:00 AM and 3:00 PM. It is important to use a water-resistant sunscreen with a sun-protection factor of 15 or higher as an added safety precaution.

teaching guidelines
fire safety

Instruct parents to distinguish bedrooms of infants, small children, and invalids during a fire by placing a symbol, sticker, or sign on the windows, enabling firefighters to identify the room quickly.

teaching guidelines
clothing fires

Some children believe that their clothes will protect them from fire. If they are 3 years or older, teach them what to do in case their clothing catches on fire emphasizing stop, drop, and roll.

* Stop. Do not run because the fire burns faster.
* Shout for help. Do not run.
* Drop to the floor, and cover your face.
* Roll back and forth to put out the flames.
* Cool a burn with cool water.

drowning

Children are at increased risk for drowning because they lack the ability to judge water depth, and many have not learned to swim. Most children enjoy playing in water regardless of their swimming abilities.

Drowning can occur in swimming pools, ponds, lakes, bathtubs, commodes, and large liquid containers. Water only 2 inches deep can kill a young child in minutes. Large buckets (especially the 5-gallon size) pose a threat to the curious toddler who can fall into the bucket head first, be unable to get out, and drown, even in only 2 inches of liquid. It only takes enough water to cover the child's nose and mouth for drowning to occur.

Children require close supervision when swimming in a pool or lake. Younger children's lack of fear about water puts them at risk, while school-age children may be tempted to swim beyond their limits to impress their peers.

Swimming lessons are a way to provide children with the skills to enjoy water safely. Swimming with a friend is much safer than swimming alone. Swimming in authorized pools with lifeguard supervision contributes to water safety.

poisoning

Accidental poisoning ranks highest as a cause of death in children 1 to 5 years old. A poison is any substance that can harm the body. Poisons can be classified as ingested, inhaled, absorbed, and injected. Emergency care in poisoning cases presents special problems because signs and symptoms can vary greatly. A network of poison control centers has been established throughout the country with 24-hour service, providing information about all types of poisoning.

ingested poisons

Of deaths caused by accidental poisoning, 75% involve common household products, such as medicines (especially aspirin and birth control pills), cleansers, lawn fer-

teaching guidelines ✳ poisoning alert

Instruct the family to post the Poison Control Center number and other emergency phone numbers (especially 911) by all telephones.

tilizers, cosmetics, and pesticides (Fig. 20-1). Some products that appear to be harmless can be fatal; for example, vitamin overdose can cause liver damage and possible death. Mouthwash containing alcohol can cause an alcohol-induced coma when ingested by young children. Certain types of baby powder contain talc or asbestos fibers that can cause cancer.

Manufacturers have placed child-proof caps on many substances known to be dangerous to children. However, the most effective safety precaution in decreasing the risk of poisoning is to make the substances unavailable; they should be kept in a locked cabinet or other areas inaccessible to children. Children have been known to ingest poisonous substances while having a pretend tea party.

Household plants can be poisonous when ingested. Young children are often attracted to plant leaves, berries, and flowers. Common poisonous plants in the United States and Canada include the yellow and orange mushroom and the poinsettia.

Children can be attracted to the red leaves of the poinsettia plant. When the flower is ingested, the child's mouth and stomach become irritated. Poisoning related to plant materials requires immediate transport to the emergency room because antidotes for plant poisons are not available.

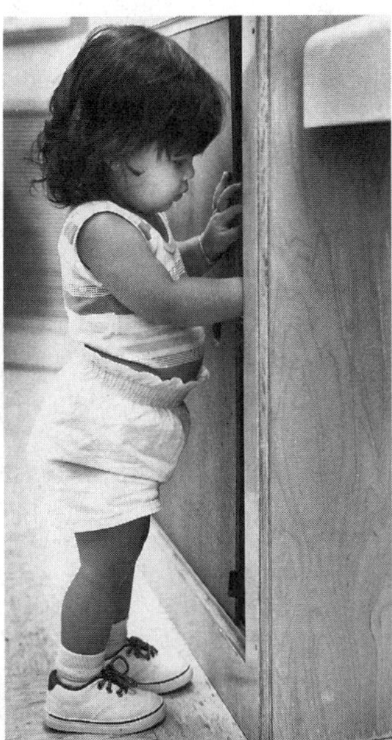

figure 20-1 *Toddler opening a cupboard. (Courtesy Child Care Center, University of Texas at El Paso.)*

lead poisoning

Many houses built before 1950 have lead plumbing and contain lead-based paint. The use of lead in older homes increases the risk of lead poisoning in children between 1 and 5 years. Lead poisoning also is called *plumbism*.

Lead poisoning is caused by eating, chewing, or sucking on objects that are covered with lead-based paint or other substances containing lead. Young children who are teething are at increased risk for lead exposure from chewing on toys, crib slats, windowsills, furniture, and pottery with lead glazes. Dust from deteriorating paint or water passing through lead pipes or lead joints can cause lead poisoning in young children.

Lead poisoning can cause serious health problems for the child. Testing blood levels of lead and analyzing bones or teeth, especially baby teeth that have fallen out, are two ways to detect lead poisoning. Lead will migrate to the bones a few months after invading the bloodstream and reenter the bloodstream when the child is experiencing stress from illness or emotional upheaval.

A balanced diet can help protect children from lead poisoning. When children do not eat enough iron, they tend to get lead poisoning more easily when exposed or have a more difficult time recovering from it. Foods rich in iron, meat protein, and vitamin C are especially important.

✳ nursing process for poison ingestion

assessment

Objective assessment of children suspected of ingesting poisons consists of noting any containers that might have contained the poisonous substance and examining the color, consistency, amount, and odor of vomitus. The child's mouth should be observed for burns or stains, and any unusual breath odors, body odors, or clothing odors should be noted. Abnormal breathing patterns and pulse rate also should be noted.

Subjective assessment includes questioning parents and older children about what type of poison was ingested. Determining the approximate time of ingestion and the child's behaviors following ingestion are important.

nursing diagnoses

- ✳ Risk for Injury, related to aspiration of vomitus
- ✳ Fear, related to invasive nature of treatments, such as gastric lavage
- ✳ Parental Anxiety, related to uncertainty of situation and feelings of guilt

planning and implementation

In most cases when poisons are ingested, emergency care consists of diluting the poison in the patients's stomach using one or two glasses of water or milk. The child is *not* given anything by mouth if he or she is unconscious. Vomiting should *not* be induced with syrup of ipecac or by any other means except on professional advice and never if the child is not fully conscious (Table 20-4).

When oily or caustic substances have been ingested, vomiting should not be induced. The increased risk of aspiration pneumonia or burning the throat as the caustic substance is vomited is too great. If the child is unconscious or having a convulsion, it is best to call 911 for emergency transport to the hospital.

Child and parental fears often center around the following ideas:

* Someone is to blame.
* The child will die.
* Parents may lose custody of the child.
* The child will be separated from the parents as punishment for their perceived "wrongdoing."

The nurse can help alleviate some of the fear if she or he speaks slowly, in a calm voice, and with a nonjudgmental attitude. Accepting the child's fear and providing an age-appropriate explanation is important, as is encouraging the child and parents to express feelings of helplessness or anger. The nurse needs to provide caregivers with information concerning the child's status and involve them in the care of the child.

evaluation

* Child will not aspirate vomitus.
* Fear about special procedures and treatments is decreased.
* Parental fear and anxiety are reduced.

table 20-4 *first-aid chart for caregivers*

Problem	*First-Aid Home Care*
Stings	Apply cool water and baking soda to site. Don't squeeze a bee-sting site. Keep emergency epinephrine kit handy.
Animal bites	Wash bite with soap and water. Identify the animal, and if possible, check animal's immunization against rabies.
Burns	Hold burned area under cool tap water for 5–10 min or until the pain is relieved. Apply antiseptic ointment and nonstick bandage. Do not break any blister.
Choking	If cough is present, do nothing. If child cannot talk, immediate action is necessary. Apply back blows for infant, Heimlich for older children. Refer to pg. 327 for choking information.
Cuts and scrapes	Apply direct pressure to stop bleeding. Wash cut with mild soap and water. Apply first-aid cream and nonstick bandage.
Head injuries	Apply pressure to stop bleeding. Do not move the child if there is a chance of neck injury.
Poison	Provide basic life support as needed (page 326). Save remainder of poison for identification purposes. Call local Poison Control Center. Do not induce vomiting with syrup ipecac or other means except on professional advice. Never induce vomiting if child is not fully conscious.
Fevers and convulsions	Be alert to signs of fever, such as listlessness, glassy eyes, and flushed, hot skin. Check child's temperature; if over 102.8°F, administer medications ordered by the doctor, such as Tylenol. Encourage fluids; remove excess clothing. Fever convulsions are frightening but last only a few seconds and are not dangerous. The important thing is to protect the child from injury.
Near drowning	Do not leave child alone while in a bathtub or near a body of water. Remove the child from the water. Check the mouth for any visible foreign matter or vomitus. If breathing is absent, begin rescue breathing. Stabilize the neck if there is any chance of neck injury.
Foreign objects in the eyes	Keep children from areas with a large amount of dust, sawdust, splinters. Teach children not to throw dirt or sand in a playmate's face. Examine the eyes. If an eyelash is seen in the corner of the eye, use a cotton swab to gently remove. Never apply pressure to an injured eye. If chemicals splash into the eye, rinse eye with large amounts of water for about 15 min. Keep child from rubbing eyes. Gently bandage a painful eye until seen by the doctor. Encourage crying because tears help wash dirt and sand out of the eye.
Twists and breaks	Provide playground supervision. Caution children about bicycle safety. Splint an arm or leg if a broken bone is suspected. If neck or back injury is suspected, do not move the child until medical help arrives. Call 911.

inhaled poisons

Inhaled poisons are present in the air and many can be absorbed through the skin. Carbon monoxide is a common inhaled poison. It is an odorless and tasteless gas that prevents normal red blood cell transport of oxygen to cells. Death can occur from hypoxia. This type of poison is often associated with motor vehicle exhaust.

Carbon monoxide can accumulate from the use of improperly vented wood-burning stoves, charcoal heaters, and indoor grills that are not vented. Malfunctioning oil, gasoline, coal-burning furnaces, and stoves also can be a source of carbon monoxide poisoning.

Other forms of inhaled poisons include chlorine gas, ammonia, agricultural chemical sprays or powders, and pesticides. Inhaled poisoning can occur from methane associated with vegetation decay, industrial solvents, and spray cans.

The Environmental Protection Agency proposes that more than 8 million homes contain radioactivity (known as *radon gas*) above federal safety standards. Radon comes from the natural breakdown of uranium in soil, rock, and water. It can get into any type of building and can build up to high levels in homes, schools, and so forth. Well water can be contaminated with high levels of radon.

Radon gas has been linked with lung cancer and poses a serious threat to young children. Testing is the only way to detect the gas and is inexpensive, easy, and quick. Test kits are available through state radon offices.

Gas fixtures must be checked periodically for leaks. In cold weather when the furnace is on, a small window should be opened to provide ventilation. A window must be opened when using cleaning fluids or paints that produce strong vapors.

✳ nursing process for inhaled poisons

assessment

Subjective assessment includes careful questioning of parents and children regarding exposure to gases, sprays, or powders. Carbon monoxide victims often have complaints of headache, dizziness, breathing difficulties, and nausea. Objective assessment of a child suspected of inhaling poisons includes noting broken containers holding toxic substances and being aware of distinctive odors, signs of fire or smoke, poor ventilation, cyanosis, and unconsciousness.

planning and implementation

The child must be removed from the toxic area. If he or she is conscious, deep breathing is encouraged. Cardiopulmonary resuscitation may be necessary if the child is unconscious.

> **✳ nursing alert**
> *Cherry-red skin color associated with carbon monoxide poisoning is a rare, late sign preceding death.*

absorbed poisons

Absorbed poisons typically irritate the skin. Chemicals and plants are the major sources of absorbed poisons.

✳ nursing process for absorbed poisons

assessment

Subjective assessment includes history of the child's activities and possible exposure to chemicals and plants and complaints of headache and difficulty breathing. Objective assessment includes observing the skin for signs of irritation, itching, abnormal pulse or respiration rates, generalized edema with hives, and unconsciousness.

intervention

Intervention includes bathing the exposed areas with clean water. Removal of all contaminated clothing is essential, followed by a call to the Poison Control Center. If symptoms of anaphylactic shock are present, call 911 for immediate transport to an emergency department.

injected poisons

Insect stings, spider bites, scorpion stings, and snake bites are common sources of injected poisons. Insect stings and bites are seldom dangerous; however, approximately 5% of the population is hypersensitive to insect venom and reacts with severe, life-threatening anaphylactic shock (see page 326).

All spiders are poisonous; however, most species cannot get their fangs through the skin, with the exception of the black widow and brown recluse spiders. Bites from these two species can produce medical emergencies.

Scorpion stings are common in the Southwest but do not ordinarily cause death. The *Centruroides exilcauda* scorpion is considered dangerous because the sting can cause respiratory failure in children.

Snake bite venom does not result in immediate death. It may take several hours for the symptoms to develop. It is safe to consider all snake bites poisonous because identifying the species may be impossible.

In the United States, there are two types of poisonous snakes: pit vipers, including rattlesnakes, copperheads, and water moccasins, and coral snakes.

✱ nursing process for injected poisons

assessment

Subjective assessment includes a history of events surrounding the incident. Parents and children are encouraged to tell what they saw and heard and describe the animal or insect responsible for the bite. Data include the child's complaints of blurred vision, nausea, and vomiting. Objective assessment of injected poison victims includes noting a bite on the skin, pain and swelling in the area of the bite, seizures, rapid pulse, labored breathing, and unconsciousness.

intervention

Appropriate intervention includes staying calm and keeping the child calm. Clean the bite mark with soap and water. Remove any constrictive clothing or jewelry from the affected extremity. Keep a bitten extremity immobilized and at heart level or below. Apply a light constricting band above and below the wound (never on both sides of a joint), and transport the child to the nearest emergency department.

nursing alert

Do not apply ice, cut the skin, or suck the venom from a snake bite.

poisoning from marine life

Marine life forms that produce sting injuries include the jellyfish, sea nettle, the Portuguese man-of-war, coral, sea anemone, and the hydra. Most children will experience pain but few complications from the sting. Applying alcohol to the sting site helps reduce the pain. If the child is allergic to the sting, anaphylactic shock can occur, resulting in death.

Puncture wounds from stepping on stingray, sea urchins, spiny catfish, or other forms of spiny marine life can produce painful and allergic reactions. Puncture wounds require medical attention and information concerning the date of the most recent tetanus shot.

animal and nonpoisonous insect bites

Children living in unsanitary conditions, particularly in low-income urban areas, are frequent victims of rat, flea, and bedbug bites. Infant beds must be placed high above the floor to reduce the risk of assault by rats.

Mosquitoes are most prevalent in warm, moist climates. They are most noticed in early morning and around dusk. Light spraying with an insect repellent safe for skin and clothing, such as Off, helps prevent bites. It is important to note safety warnings and contraindications provided by the manufacturer because some repellents have a toxic effect when absorbed through the skin, causing skin reactions such as blisters or hives, behavior changes, seizures, and coma; these are unsuitable for use on children.

Children playing in wooded areas are at risk for contracting Lyme disease. Lyme disease is caused by the bite of a pinhead-sized deer tick. Symptoms of the disease are red, circular rash; flulike symptoms; fever; chills; nausea; headache; stiff neck; and joint and muscle pains.

Children need to wear long-sleeved shirts and long pants when playing in wooded areas. Parents and children need to inspect the skin, hair, and clothing periodically for the presence of ticks. Ticks are removed gently with tweezers.

playing safe

Play facilitates learning and is often referred to as the "work" of a child. A child's approach to play corresponds to the ability to interact with siblings or peers. Infants typically engage in solitary play, while the preschooler enjoys cooperative play. Play enables the child to learn about the environment through the sense of touch, taste, hearing, smell, and sight.

Young children do not understand the concept of safe or unsafe play. They have a limited understanding of danger and a natural curiosity to explore, putting them at increased risk for injury. Adult supervision is always necessary for younger children at play (Fig. 20-2, Display 20-2).

Preschoolers are often fascinated by boxes or other items large enough to crawl into and hide, such as chests or abandoned refrigerators. The child can suffocate when doors are closed, trapping the child inside without adequate oxygen. It is now illegal to abandon chests or refrigerators without removing the doors.

Older children are interested in making things. Teaching children the proper use and storage of equipment,

display 20-2
safety at play

Playing safe involves more action than words on the part of parents and children.

- **Help the child form the habit of wearing a bike helmet when cycling, in-line skating, and skateboarding.**
- **Cross streets hundreds of times with children before letting them cross alone.**
- **Set a good example by using safety belts and child safety seats.**
- **Supervise children in and around water.**
- **Take a first aid and cardiopulmonary resuscitation course.**

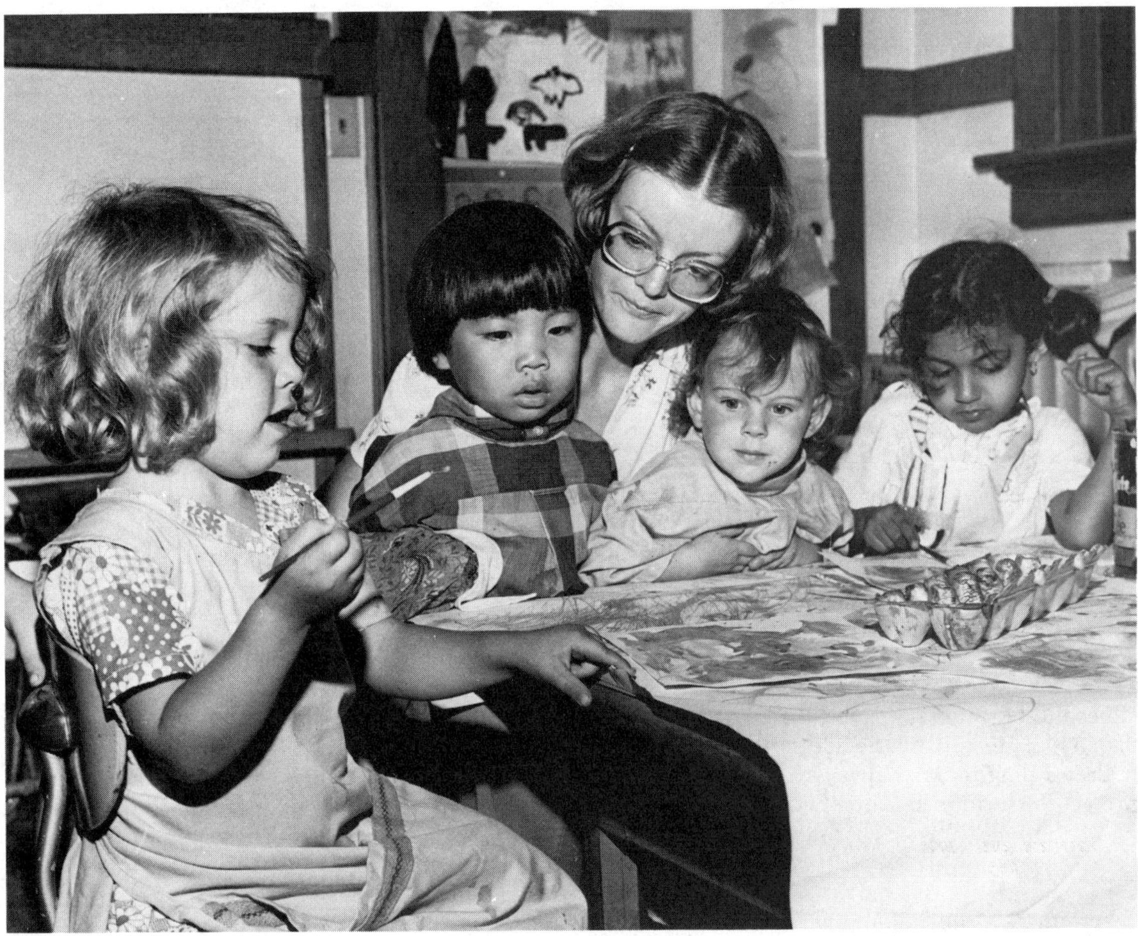

figure 20-2 *Adult supervision is necessary to ensure the safety of curious preschoolers.*

such as saws, nails, hammers, sewing machines, and gas and electric appliances, reduces the risk of injury. Children take pride in responsible behaviors, especially if given praise.

Young children are at risk for abuse and injury while playing with older children if the play is too aggressive (Fig. 20-3). A young child may be hit by a bicycle, swing seat, hard ball, or bat while playing with a crowd of mixed age groups.

Young children may be at risk for physical or sexual abuse by older children or disturbed adults. It is important to teach a young child his or her phone number, address, and what to do if he or she is fearful of another person (refer to page 375).

Preschoolers may voice their understanding of a safety rule but may just as quickly forget the rule while absorbed in play. Their expanding vocabulary enables them to learn simple safety rules. However, parents need to be cautious about giving them too much responsibility for their own safety.

With an increase in height and walking stability, preschoolers are able to travel further and faster than toddlers. Their interest in playing with others may take them away from home to play with friends where supervision is lacking.

Older children enjoy attending parties, carnivals, school dances, and sports events, making it difficult for parental supervision. Children need to keep parents informed of where they are at all times.

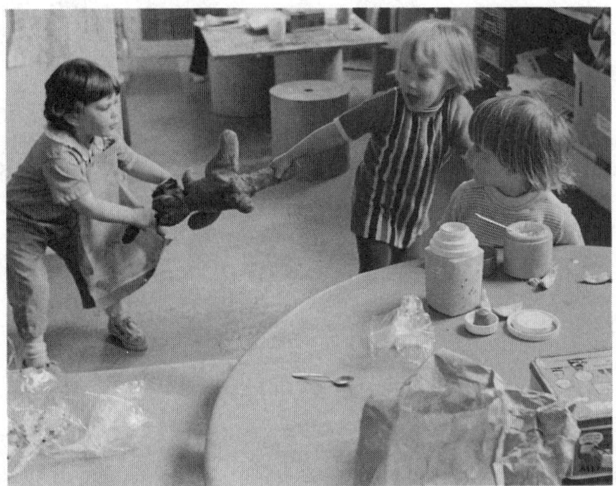

figure 20-3 *Aggressive and unsupervised play places the toddler in danger (© Elizabeth Hamlin/Stock Boston).*

toy safety

Manipulation of toys helps the infant develop motor skills in an unstructured, voluntary way. Toys can be categorized as language, muscular activity, imaginative, and sensory stimulators. The following guidelines are helpful when selecting toys for a child:

* Select toys appropriate for the child's stage of development.
* Toys must be free from sharp edges or loose parts.
* Toys must be safe for young children to place in their mouth and chew and free from toxic or chipping paint and splinters.
* Toys must be easy to clean.

bicycle safety

Gross motor development during the preschool years enables children to learn to ride tricycles or use toys with wheels. Their desire for adventure tends to make them reckless. Going fast on riding toys and not paying attention to other children and traffic put them at risk for serious injury.

A tricycle or bicycle is usually the child's first vehicle. Children need to be taught to regard the bike as a vehicle rather than a toy. Most bicycle accidents involve falls, not cars. Children riding bicycles always need to wear a helmet to protect the head in case of a fall.

sports safety

The number of American children participating in youth sports within and outside of school has increased in recent years, increasing the number of sports-related injuries. Sports injury can be a sudden acute injury from a collision or a fall involving bone fractures, contusions, sprains of joint ligaments, and strains of muscle tendons. Sports injuries also can involve chronic repetitive injury to tissue over an extended time, such as bursitis, tendinitis, or stress fractures (refer to Chapter 36). Contact sports, such as football and soccer, have the highest injury rate. In-line skating and skateboarding can be dangerous if the child fails to use proper safety equipment, such as helmets and knee and elbow pads. Physical fitness and experience play a key role in reducing the risk of injuries (Fig. 20-4).

teaching guidelines
bicycle safety

Bicycle safety includes the following:

* Ride the correct size bike; this involves having the feet touch the ground when sitting on the bicycle seat.
* Wear a helmet when riding your bike.
* Do not ride bicycles that do not have good brakes.
* Learn how the bicycle brakes work.
* Ride with traffic.
* Stop and look both ways before entering the street.
* Stop at all intersections. Obey all traffic signals.
* Use hand signals, and look all ways before turning.
* Do not ride a bike at dusk or in the dark.

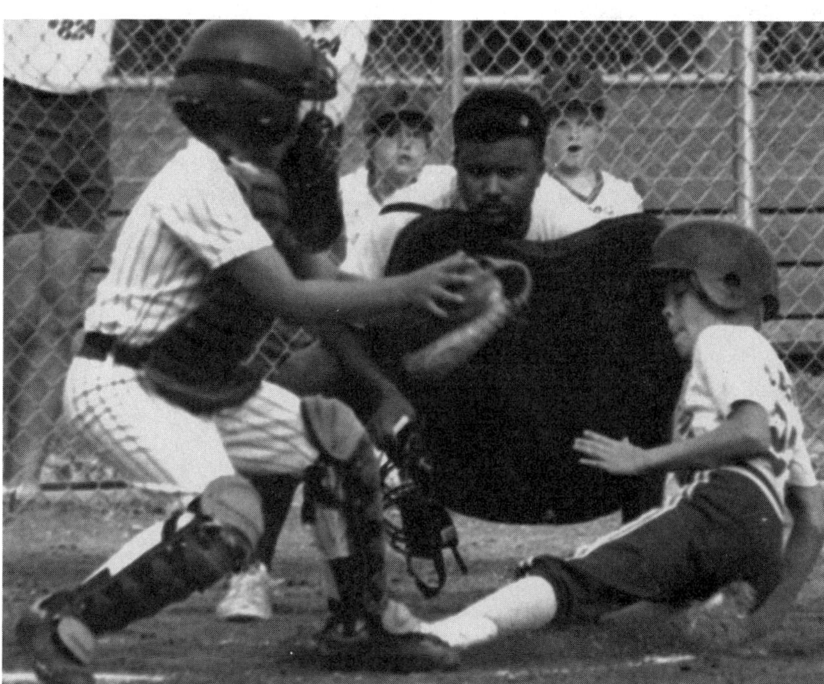

figure 20-4 *The risk of sports-related injury is greatly reduced when the child is protected with proper equipment and the knowledge of how to play safe.*

gun safety

If guns are kept in the home, they must be secured in areas inaccessible to children. Guns need bullets to kill or maim; consequently, safety precautions must be taken to ensure guns are unloaded and bullets kept in a separate locked area. Every day, 1.2 million "latch key" children return to homes in which there are guns.

The National Safety Council lists accidental shootings as the fifth leading cause of death for children younger than 5 years. Toddlers are not capable of understanding the difference between a play gun and a real gun. Some guns can be discharged by a child as young as 2 years.

violence

Teenagers are the most victimized by crime in the United States. They are victims in 3 of every 10 violent crimes (Bureau of Justice Statistics, 1994). African American youths between 15 and 19 years are approximately 50% more likely to be victims of murder than white youths (Merina, 1994).

Peer rivalry and gang activity increase the risk for violence and serious or fatal injuries from fighting, shootings, and knifings. Drive-by shootings have become too common in some areas. Children do not always understand the implications of using a weapon to settle disputes. They may have preconceived ideas from media exposure concerning violence.

Every day, 100,000 students carry guns to school in the United States; another 160,000 miss classes due to fear of physical harm. Thirty children are injured by gun violence each day, and every 2 days, 25 children are killed by guns (National Education Association, 1994).

Parents and caregivers need to set limits, provide guidance, and enforce consequences when rules are broken. Formal and informal instructions are helpful in the areas of appropriate social interactions.

teaching guidelines
dealing with school violence

Children and parents are urged to help reduce school violence by the following:

* Learning about violence prevention programs
* Reporting suspicious people or activities in the school to school authorities
* Calling 1-800-78-CRIME to report crimes or get advice and assistance for quitting a gang
* Calling 1-800-ATF-GUNS to report drug or gun activities

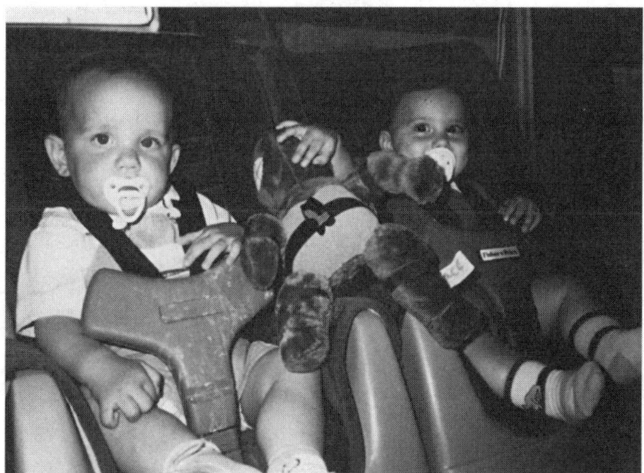

figure 20-5 *Children younger than 4 years and weighing less than 40 lb should always ride in car seats meeting vehicle safety standards of the Department of Transportation.*

car safety

Motor vehicle safety for an infant involves a safety seat. Safety car seats are most effective when they are installed according to the manufacturer's instructions. The safest position for any car safety seat is in the middle of the back seat. Convertible car seats can be used from birth until the child is older than 4 years and weighs approximately 40 lb. The car safety seat faces the rear of the car until an infant is 7 to 9 months old and weighs 17 to 20 lb. Seat belts and shoulder harnesses are used after the child has outgrown safety seats.

The car seat must meet the vehicle safety standards of the Department of Transportation. These include an anchoring device to the seat of the vehicle with a standard lap safety belt, a harness to keep the infant contained within the seat, and a head support to minimize the risk of whiplash injury (Fig. 20-5).

Car accidents are the most common cause of accidental injury in older children. Driver education and safety programs are offered at most schools and are beneficial to the young driver. The risk of automobile accidents is high in this age group, partly because they lack the maturity required to make safe driving decisions.

Adolescents often have a sense of immortality, increasing risky behaviors, such as drinking alcohol and driving. Many teenage deaths are associated with driving cars while blood alcohol levels are over the legal limit of 0.10%. Parents and caregivers are encouraged to teach adolescents to appoint a "designated driver," who refrains from alcohol consumption when traveling by car.

Young children need supervision while crossing busy streets. A toddler's hand is held securely when crossing streets or walking in areas of traffic. Playing or riding a tricycle in a heavy traffic area requires close supervision.

protection against infectious diseases

Infectious diseases are a leading cause of mortality in children. Many infectious diseases in children can be prevented with proper immunizations.

Infectious diseases are caused by *pathogens*. Pathogens are infectious organisms classified into five categories: viruses, bacteria, rickettsiae, helminths (worms), and fungi.

Infectious diseases progress through stages. The first stage is known as an *incubation* stage. This is the period between the invasion of an organism and the onset of symptoms of infection. With most childhood diseases, the incubation period ranges from 7 to 21 days.

The next stage is a *prodromal* period and involves a relatively short time span ranging from hours to a few days. This is the time between the nonspecific symptoms and specific symptoms. Nonspecific symptoms often include low-grade fever, fatigue, and low energy level. During this stage, children are capable of spreading disease to others.

The *illness* stage is characterized by specific symptoms of the illness. Many childhood diseases produce fever, increased white blood cell count, headache, and rash. The last stage in the course of an infectious disease is the *convalescent* period.

immunizations

Declines in the worldwide incidence (*morbidity*) and number of deaths (*mortality*) from infectious disease are a result of routine immunizations. The purpose of administering vaccines is to prevent disease. Until recently, infectious diseases and their complications were major cripplers and killers of children in the United States.

Vaccines contain antigens that stimulate immune responses. The different types of vaccine antigens include dead or weakened pathogens, parts of a pathogen, and inactivated bacterial toxins called *toxoids*. Live vaccines produce long-lasting immunity but are not recommended for children who are immunosuppressed from disease, radiation treatments, steroid therapy, or cancer drugs or for healthy children who have an immunodeficient family member, because of increased risk for getting the disease from a live vaccine.

Measles, mumps, and rubella vaccines are among the immunizations that contain live virus. Polio immunization is given in a live oral vaccine (OPV) or an inactive vaccine that is injected under the skin (subcutaneously). Oral polio vaccine causes live virus to be cast off in the stool and is not given to an immunosuppressed child. Infants suffering from gastroenteritis may not properly absorb OPV from the intestine and are not given it until the gastroenteritis is treated.

Vaccines do not cause disease (there may be a few rare exceptions). Vaccines take the place of the child's first exposure to the pathogen and stimulate production of antibodies and memory cells.

Routine childhood immunizations protect against nine diseases: measles, mumps, and rubella (usually given as one vaccine called the MMR); diphtheria tetanus, and pertussis (combined and called the DTP); poliomyelitis; *Haemophilus influenzae-B* (HiB); and hepatitis B (HBV). All of these diseases are contagious with the exception of tetanus. The maximal response is attained when all vaccines scheduled for the child are administered at the recommended time.

Children with human immunodeficiency virus or acquired immunodeficiency syndrome (AIDS), sickle cell anemia, or Hodgkin's disease receive pneumococcal vaccine to boost their resistance to *Streptococcus* pneumonia. The pneumococcal pneumonia vaccine is recommended for infants at age 6 months who are symptomatic with AIDS.

The HBV vaccine is a routine vaccination for infants. Universal infant HBV immunization is designed to reduce morbidity and mortality due to hepatitis B. Hepatitis B is an acute infection of the liver caused by HBV. The vaccine is given in three doses. The first dose is given within the first 12 hours after birth. The second dose is administered

teaching guidelines
immunizations against childhood diseases

The immunization that is given to your child may result in certain side effects that are not life-threatening but tend to make him or her somewhat irritable. The value of immunizations in preventing disease is important.

EXPECTED EFFECTS

- Low-grade fever (<102°F) within 24–48 h following DTP and *Haemophilus* B vaccine
- Fever within 7–10 d following MMR
- Measle rash approximately 2–4 days following administration of MMR
- Soreness, redness, and swelling at the injection site; mild rash

RECOMMENDED TREATMENT

- Give acetaminophen 10–15 mg/kg of body weight per dose. Do not give aspirin.
- Apply warm compresses to the injection site.
- Offer comfort measures, such as rocking, holding.

MORE SERIOUS EFFECTS REQUIRING MEDICAL CONSULTATION

- Fever >104°F
- Crying inspite of comfort measures for more than 3 h
- Unusual high-pitched crying
- Excessive sleepiness
- Limpness, paleness
- Convulsions

at 1 or 2 months, and third dose is given when the child is 6 to 18 months old. Children not immunized at birth will need to receive three doses by 18 months of age. Hepatitis B immune globulin also is given as a prophylactic measure to newborns of mothers who have a positive screen for hepatitis.

Diphtheria, typhoid, pertussis, and HiB are all inactive vaccines. The immunization schedule is shown in Table 20-5. When the recommended schedule is interrupted, it is not necessary to restart the complete schedule. Vaccinations may be delayed if an infant has a fever.

Parents may express concern about administration of the pertussis vaccine because of media attention to parental claims of severe side effects involving the central nervous system. It is important to emphasize the extremely rare chance of a severe reaction, which is outweighed by the benefits of immunization. Whooping cough can be deadly in infants younger than 6 months.

table 20-5 *recommended schedule of childhood immunizations*

Disease	*Description*	*Complications*	*States Mandating Vaccine*	*Schedule*
Diphtheria	Caused by a bacterium. Germ is passed through coughing or sneezing. Causes sore throat, fever, and chills.	Septicemia, heart failure, or paralysis	50	DTP 2,4,6,15 mo—4–6 y
Tetanus (lockjaw)	Caused by a bacterium found in soil, dust, manure. Enters body through a wound. Toxins cause headache, irritability, stiffness in jaw and neck.	Pneumonia, broken bones, exhaustion from muscle spasms	47	DTP 2,4,6,15 mo, 4–6, 14–16 y. Booster q10y
Pertussis (whooping cough)	Caused by a bacterium spread through coughing or sneezing. Severe spells of coughing often resulting in vomiting.	Pneumonia, convulsions, encephalitis	41	DTP 2,4,6,15 mo, 4–6 y
Polio	Caused by a virus. Fever, sore throat, headache, muscle pain.	Paralysis	50	OPV (live but weakened virus) 2,4,15 mo, 4–6 y Booster dose during an epidemic or for travel
Measles	Caused by a virus. Rash, high fever, cough, runny nose, and watery eyes last 1–2 wk.	Ear infection, pneumonia, encephalitis, convulsions, deafness, mental retardation Miscarriage	50	MMR 15 mo, 4–6 y College students and adults born after 1957
Mumps	Virus. Fever, headache, inflammation of salivary glands.	Meningitis, encephalitis, deafness, after puberty Males, orchitis; females, mastitis	39	MMR 15 mo, 4–6 y
Rubella (German measles)	Viral, infection. Fever, rash for 2–3 d, swollen glands, painful joints.	Birth defects, such as deafness, blindness, heart damage, small brains, mental retardation	50	MMR 15 mo, 4–6 y
Haemophilus influenza	Viral infection, meningitis	Permanent brain damage	None	2,4,6,15 mo
Hepatitis (HBV)	Acute phase mild or no symptoms; may become chronic.	Cirrhosis, hepatic cancer	None	0–2 wk

From Immunization Practices Advisory Committee (ACIP) Centers for Disease Control and Prevention (1994). MMWR, 43(RR-1), 10.

Vaccine not given to a child that is immunosuppresed

✱ nursing considerations

Injections cause discomfort and can be traumatic to the child who is not prepared. Reassure the child ahead of time that he or she may get a shot to help him or her stay healthy. Tell the child that the shot may hurt like a bee sting and will last as long as it takes to count to three. Do not discourage the child from crying, but comfort him or her and praise his or her bravery when the crying stops. Distraction can be used at the time of the injection to keep the child's fears from escalating.

allergies

Common childhood allergies include sensitivity to certain foods, tobacco smoke, animals, everyday lint, molds, and dust mites. Allergic reactions include mild to severe symptoms, depending on the child's contact with the allergen.

Hives (*urticaria*) are associated with allergic responses and are visible on the skin. Urticaria involves the upper dermis and results from localized edema caused by dilatation of the capillaries with the development of wheals. The wheals are usually flat, red, and intensely pruritic (itchy). Hives may occur close together or as isolated lesions.

Angioedema is edema of the skin and subcutaneous tissue resulting from the body's response to an allergen. Angioedema usually occurs with urticaria and is often seen on the eyelids, hands, feet, genitalia, and lips. Angioedema also can affect the larynx, causing asphyxiation and death. Allergens that usually cause urticaria and angioedema are drugs, foods, and insect stings.

✱ nursing considerations

Treatment for urticaria or angioedema is subcutaneous epinephrine or an oral antihistamine. Immediate intervention is essential for such an allergic response. After the response is treated, education about allergies needs to be provided to the child and caregiver.

Education programs for parents and children include the following:

- How to reduce the child's contact with a known allergen, especially in the home
- The value of administering small doses of an allergen subcutaneously to increase the child's tolerance to the allergen (allergy injections are usually given for 2–3 years)
- How to control the child's response to the allergen with medication, such as antihistamines or corticosteroids
- The importance of applying ice to an insect sting
- An awareness of the symptoms, serious consequences of anaphylactic shock, and importance of having an emergency kit available (emergency kits include two measured doses of epinephrine and an antihistamine)

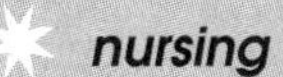
nursing alert

Children testing positive for egg allergy are given vaccines subcutaneously with increasing increments of 0.05 mL every 15 to 20 minutes to the full dose. Resuscitation equipment must be available during vaccine administration.

anaphylactic shock

Anaphylactic shock is an immediate hypersensitive reaction, an emergency that demands fast, effective intervention. Anaphylaxis is characterized by nausea, vomiting, diarrhea, bronchospasm, and a drop in blood pressure and pulse rate. Convulsions and death can occur as quickly as 10 minutes after exposure to an allergen. Children typically lose consciousness and cannot be aroused.

emergency measures for anaphylactic shock

Parents and older children can provide quick intervention by being taught to give a subcutaneous injection of aqueous epinephrine (Adrenalin) 1:100 at a dosage of 0.01 mL/kg of body weight up to 0.5 mL. Injecting aqueous epinephrine relieves laryngeal edema and bronchospasm. The child is positioned with the head even with the body, and 911 is called for emergency transportation to a health care facility. Emergency cardiopulmonary resuscitation may be necessary if the child's breathing and pulse are absent (refer to pediatric emergency care).

Oxygen by mask or prong is given in the presence of cyanosis. The child is at increased risk for respiratory and cardiac arrest. Emergency equipment used in respiratory and cardiac code situations must be readily available.

pediatric emergency care

Emergency care begins with airway, breathing, and circulation (ABC). Cervical spine alignment and immobilization are maintained while making sure the airway is patent, using the head tilt–chin lift or jaw thrust maneuver. The jaw thrust maneuver is used to open the airway while the cervical spine is completely immobilized. The head tilt–chin lift is avoided if neck injury is suspected.

Assess breathing by looking for the rise and fall of the chest and abdomen, listening for exhaled air, or feeling for exhaled air flow at the mouth. If spontaneous breathing is absent, provide two slow breaths by placing your mouth over the infant's mouth and nose. With a large infant or a child between 1 and 8 years old, the nurse makes a mouth-to-mouth seal and pinches the victim's nose tightly with the thumb and forefingers, using the hand to maintain head tilt.

If a pulse is present but spontaneous breathing is absent, *rescue breathing* is administered. Rescue breathing is a type of respiratory resuscitation given to a child who has an obstructed airway that is altering air exchange. Rescue breathing involves one breath every 3 seconds for infants, providing a rate of 20 breaths per minute until spontaneous breathing resumes. Rescue breathing performed rapidly may cause gastric distention and a decrease in lung volume.

Assessment of circulation involves palpating the brachial pulse in children younger than 1 year because the neck is typically short and chubby, making the carotid artery difficult to locate. However, in children older than 1 year, the carotid artery pulsation is the most accessible.

After the primary assessment, the nurse does a head-to-toe assessment, being alert for hidden injuries. A child must always be moved carefully. If trauma is suspected, the cervical spine must be completely immobilized and neck extension, flexion, and rotation prevented.

cardiopulmonary resuscitation

Cardiopulmonary resuscitation is accomplished by chest compressions, which are rhythmic compressions of the chest that circulate blood to the vital organs. Effective compressions are achieved on a hard, flat surface. The compression rate for infants and children is 100 times per minute (Fig. 20-6A–H).

cardiopulmonary resuscitation in an infant

The hand or forearm of the nurse or rescuer can provide the hard surface for infant resuscitation. The area of compression for infants is the lower third of the sternum. The index finger is placed on the sternum just below the intermammary line located between the nipples and over the breastbone. The middle and ring fingers are placed on the sternum, near the index finger. Using two or three fingers, the nurse compresses the sternum approximately one third to one half of the depth of the chest. This will correspond to a depth of about ½ to 1 in. The compression rate will be at least 100 times per minute.

cardiopulmonary resuscitation in the 1- to 8-year-old child

Any child between 1 and 8 years is considered a child for the purposes of administering cardiopulmonary resuscitation. The rescuer assesses proper hand position by tracing the lower margin of the child's rib cage to the notch where the ribs and sternum meet. With the middle finger on this notch, the index finger is placed next to the middle finger. The heel of the same hand is placed parallel to the sternum. The fingers are held up off the ribs while the heel of the hand remains in contact with the sternum. The chest is compressed to approximately one third to one half of the total depth of the chest (about 1 to 1½ in). The compression rate is 100 times per minute. With pauses for ventilation, the ultimate number of compressions will actually be at least 80 per minute. Basic life support maneuvers are summarized in Table 20-6.

External chest compressions require rescue breathing. At the end of every fifth compression, a pause of 1 to 1½ seconds is allowed for ventilation. In the infant and child, a 5 : 1 compression-ventilation ratio is maintained for one or two rescuers. The infant or child victim requires reassessing after 20 cycles of compressions and ventilation (approximately 1 minute) and every few minutes thereafter for any sign of spontaneous breathing or pulse.

emergency interventions for choking

Approximately 90% of deaths from foreign body aspiration occur in children younger than 5 years; 65% of the victims are infants (JAMA, 1992). Interventions to clear the airway are necessary when foreign body aspiration is witnessed or strongly suspected or when the airway remains obstructed during attempts to provide rescue breathing to an unconscious infant or child. The conscious infant or child needs encouragement to cough as a means of removing an aspirated object. Additional measures are required when the child's cough is ineffective or loses sound, an increase in respiratory distress is noted, or the child loses consciousness.

interventions for the choking infant

Back blows and chest thrusts are recommended when an infant is choking. Back blows are delivered while the infant is supported in a prone position. Chest thrusts are delivered while the infant is supine.

While holding the infant prone, support the head by firmly holding the jaw, allowing the infant's head to be lower than the trunk. Deliver up to five back blows forcefully between the infant's shoulder blades, using the heel of the hand.

After delivering the back blows, turn the infant over while carefully supporting the head and neck. Keep the head lower than the trunk. Provide up to five quick downward chest thrusts with one finger below the intermammary line. (Chest thrusts are done in the same location as chest compressions: the lower third of the sternum, one finger's breadth below the intermammary line.) Remove the foreign body if it can be seen. Open the airway, and attempt rescue breathing. If the airway remains obstructed, repeat back blows and chest thrusts until the object is removed and rescue breathing is successful.

heimlich maneuver for children

Emergency intervention for children who are choking but are conscious includes abdominal thrusts and can be done with the child standing or sitting. Standing behind the child, the thumb side of one fist is placed against the victim's abdomen in the midline, slightly above the navel and well below the tip of the xiphoid process. The other hand grabs the fist and exerts up to five quick upward thrusts. Each thrust must be a separate, distinct movement, delivered with the intent to relieve the obstruction.

A series of five thrusts is continued until the foreign body is expelled or the child loses consciousness. Abdominal thrusts are delivered to an unconscious child with the heel of one hand placed on the midline of the abdomen, slightly above the navel and well below the xiphoid process. The free hand is placed over the positioned hand. The thrusts are delivered by pressing the hands inward and up-

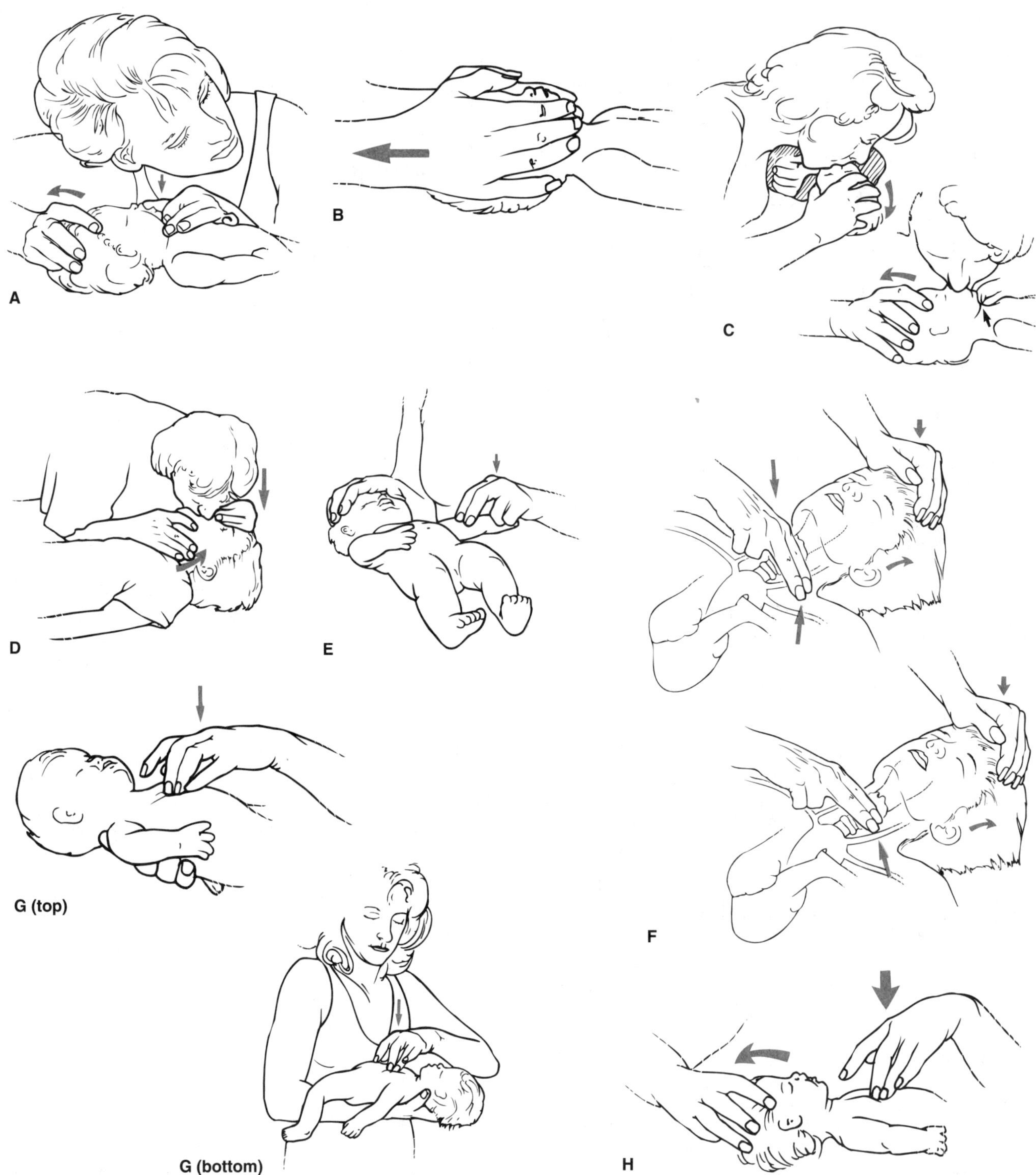

figure 20-6 *Cardiopulmonary resuscitation.* ***(A)*** *Opening the airway with the head tilt-chin lift maneuver. One hand is used to tilt the head, extending the neck. The index finger of the rescuer's other hand lifts the mandible outward by lifting on the chin. Head tilt should not be performed if cervical spine injury is suspected.* ***(B)*** *Opening the airway with the jaw-thrust maneuver. The airway is opened by lifting the angle of the mandible. The rescuer uses two or three fingers of each hand to lift the jaw while other fingers guide the jaw upward and outward.* ***(C)*** *Rescue breathing in an infant. The rescuer's mouth covers the infants nose and mouth, creating a seal. One hand performs head tilt while the other hand lifts the infant's jaw. Avoid head tilt if the infant has sustained head or neck trauma.* ***(D)*** *Rescue breathing in a child. The rescuer's covers the mouth of the child, creating a mouth-to-mouth seal. One hand maintains the head tilt; the thumb and forefinger of the same hand are used to pinch the child's nose.* ***(E)*** *Palpating the brachial artery pulse.* ***(F)*** *Locating and palpating the carotid artery pulse in the child.* ***(G)*** *Cardiac compressions.* ***Top:*** *Infant supine on palm of the rescuer's hand.* ***Bottom:*** *Preforming CPR while carrying the infant or small child. Note that the head in kept level with the torso. (Compare with H.)* ***(H)*** *Locating proper finger position for chest compression in infant. Note that the rescuer's other hand is used to maintain head position to facilitate ventilation. (From Pediatric Basic Life Support. JAMA 268[16]:268, Fig. 11-6.)*

table 20-6 cardiopulmonary resuscitation techniques for the infant, child, and adult

Actions	*Infant 0–1 Y*	*Child 1–8 Y*	*Adult Over 8 Y*
Shake and shout	Shake only	Yes	Yes
Call for help	Yes	Yes	Yes
Position victim	Flat surface or over forearm	Supine on flat hard surface	Supine on flat hard surface
Open airway	Use head tilt–chin lift if no trauma Keep neck immobile if trauma; use jaw thrust	Same as infant.	Same as infant.
Look, listen, feel for breath	Yes	Yes	Yes
Two breaths	Cover mouth and nose. Give 20 breaths per minute.	Cover mouth; pinch nose. Give 20 breaths per minute.	Same as child.
Check pulse	Brachial or femoral	Carotid	Carotid
Compression area, compression width	Lower third of sternum using two to three fingers	Lower third of sternum using heel of one hand	Lower half of sternum using heel of two hands
Compression depth	½–1 in	1–1½ in	1½–2 in
Compressions per minute	At least 100	80–100	80–100
Compression to ventilation ratio	5:1	5:1	15:2 (one rescuer) 5:1 (two rescuer)
Ventilations only	1 every 3 sec = 20/min	1 every 3 sec = 20/min	1 every 5 sec. = 12/min
Foreign body airway obstruction	Back blows/chest thrusts	Heimlich maneuver	Heimlich maneuver

ward toward the patient's diaphragm. If the child loses consciousness, the airway must be opened and rescue breathing attempted (Fig. 20-7).

finger sweeps

A finger sweep is an attempt to manually remove an airway obstruction. Gloves are worn to protect the rescuer from infectious agents. A gloved finger is positioned like a hook placed in the child's mouth and moved from one side to the other. A finger sweep is most effective if the foreign object responsible for the child's choking is visible. Care must be taken to avoid forcing the object further down the throat. Finger sweeps are not recommended on children who are conscious because stimulation of the gag reflex can induce vomiting, increasing the child's risk of aspirating vomitus into the lungs.

✶ nursing process for care of the child with a traumatic injury

Emergency care of children following accidental injury involves dealing with extreme parental and child anxiety and guilt. Parents may display defensive attitudes stemming from guilt and responsibility for the accident. They may be unable to use familiar coping strategies because of their overwhelming fear for their child's life. Some parents worry that they will be criticized as being neglectful or abusive parents.

Traumatized children feel pain. The pain is often enhanced by feelings of fear and guilt. Children may be frightened from the pain, the circumstances of the injury, and potential parental discipline for actions leading to the accident.

assessment

Subjective assessment is based primarily on a brief history of the accident obtained from the child's parents or other caregiver. The following questions provide valuable information.

- What happened?
- How long ago did the accident happen?
- What has already been done about the injury?
- If the child fell, how far was the fall, and on what body part did the child land?
- What do the parents feel is the most serious injury?
- What is the child's major complaint?
- Did the child cry immediately; has the crying been continuous or gotten weaker?
- Was the child unconscious at any time, and has the child been alert or confused since the accident?

Objective assessment of the child involves a quick assessment of apparent injuries, such as altered skin integrity as seen in cuts and burns, distorted extremities suggesting fractures, level of consciousness, and vital sign readings relevant to shock.

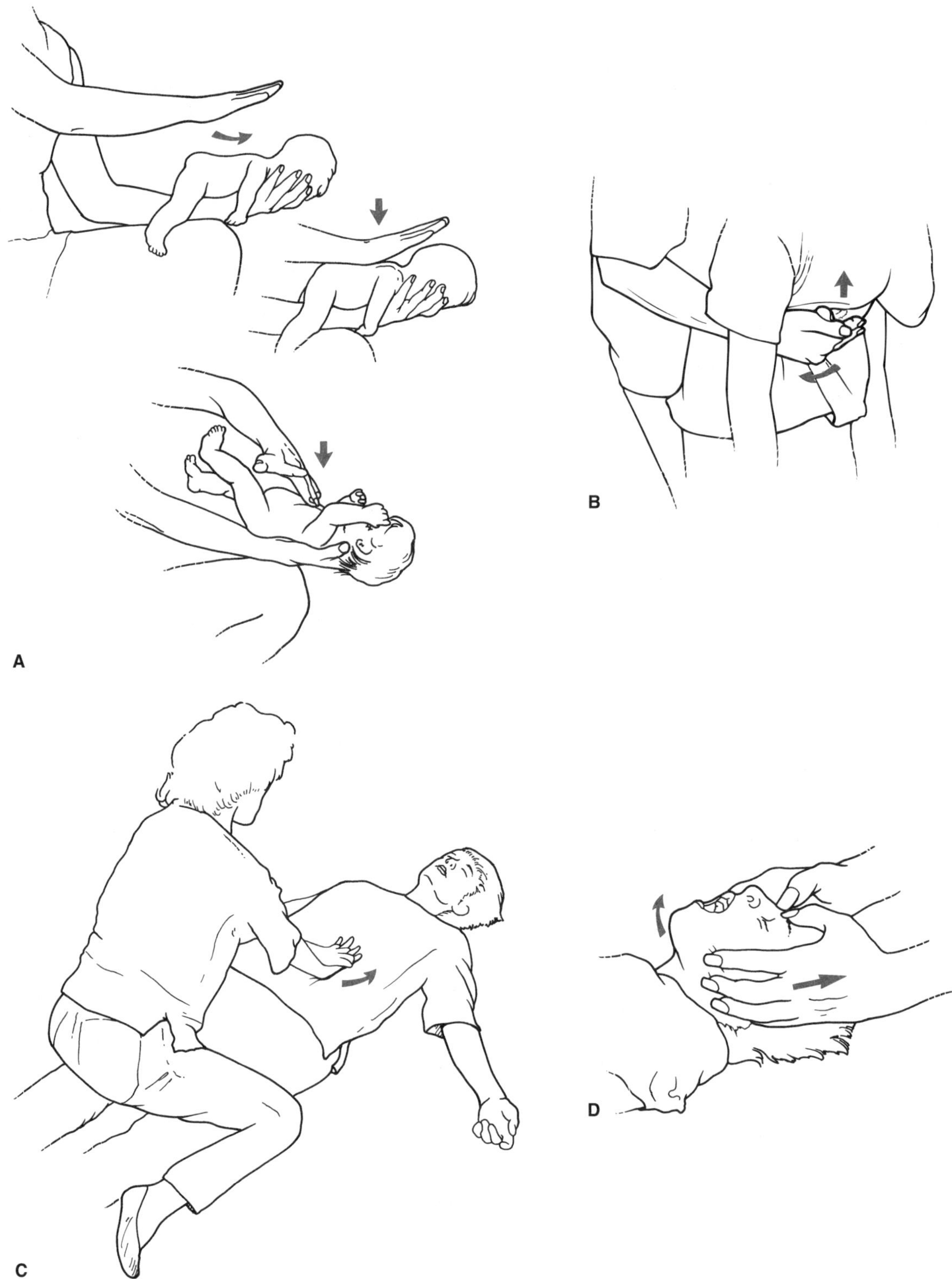

figure 20-7 *(A)* Back blows (top) and chest thrusts (bottom) to relieve foreign-body airway obstruction in infant. Hold infant over arm as illustrated, supporting head by firmly holding jaw. Deliver up to 5 back blows. Turn infant over while supporting head, neck, jaw, and chest with one hand and back with other hand. Keep head lower than trunk. Give 5 quick chest thrusts with one finger below intermammary line. If foreign body not removed and airway remains obstructed, attempt rescue breathing. Repeat these 2 steps until successful. ***(B)*** *Abdominal thrusts with child standing or sitting can be performed when child is conscious. Standing behind child, place thumb side of one fist against child's abdomen in midline slightly above navel and well below xiphoid process. Grab fist with other hand and deliver 5 quick upward thrusts. Continue until successful or child loses consciousness.* ***(C)*** *Abdominal thrusts with child lying can be performed on a conscious or unconscious child. Place heel of hand on child's abdomen slightly above the navel and below the xiphoid process and rib cage. Place other hand on top of first hand. Deliver 5 separate, distinct thrusts. Open airway and attempt rescue breathing if object not removed. Repeat until successful.* ***(D)*** *Combined jaw thrust-spine stabilization maneuver for a child trauma victim with possible head or neck injury. To protect from damage to cervical spine the neck is maintained in a neutral position and traction on or movement of neck is avoided. (From Pediatric Basic Life Support. JAMA 268[16]:266, Fig. 11-5, 1992.)*

nursing diagnoses

The most frequently used nursing diagnosis with injured children is Pain, related to the injury. Additional nursing diagnoses follow:

* Risk for Aspiration in children with loss of consciousness, as seen in head injuries, alcohol and drug use, and during vomiting in response to poison ingestion; impaired swallowing reflexes, as seen in premature infants; and decreased muscle tone of inferior esophageal sphincter
* Ineffective Airway Clearance, related to scarred esophageal tissue from ingestion of caustic poisons or foreign body obstruction
* Risk for Post-Trauma Response, related to accidental injury
* Risk for Injury, related to perceptual or physiologic deficit, a lack of awareness of hazards, or maturational age risks, such as suffocation from improper crib mattress, crib pillows, plastic bags, or unsupervised water activity; ingestion of environmental poisons, including plants, cleaning agents, and medications; burns from matches, fireplaces, or stoves; falls; careless operation of automobiles, bicycles, skateboards, and in-line skates
* Knowledge Deficit, related to child's age or parents' lack of understanding safety needs based on child growth and development expectations
* Self Esteem Disturbance, related to change in physical appearance if major features are altered, such as face, gait, speech
* Parental Fear, related to outcome after serious head, bone, and skin injuries
* Altered Family Processes, related to child's accident

planning and implementation

Nursing care is based on the extent of the injury, the body part injured, and the physiologic and psychological distress of the child. Criteria for hospital admission are typically based on life-threatening injuries. Children may be admitted to the hospital for a 24-hour observation period. Usually children are dismissed to the home with parents or other caregivers administering the necessary care.

Children and their parents must be provided with home care instructions; however, they are often too emotional to comprehend or remember what is being said. Thus, it is essential to provide written instructions that explain necessary care in a step by step way using simple terminology.

* Interventions reducing the risk of aspiration include maintain a side-lying position if not contraindicated by injury. Keep the head of the bed elevated unless contraindicated. Clear secretions from the mouth and throat with a tissue or gentle suction.
* Interventions promoting effective airway clearance include monitoring skin color, respiration rate and effort, voice or cry strength, and presence of crowing or stridor sounds with respirations. Maintain adequate hydration unless contraindicated. Feed child in a sitting position unless contraindicated. Plan rest periods before meals. Keep small objects away from young children. Evaluate toy safety according to level of growth and development.
* Interventions promoting resolution of stress associated with post-traumatic response include determining if the child has experienced a traumatic event. Evaluate the severity of the response and the effect on current level of functioning. Provide a safe environment where the child can regain control. Offer the child and parents support during episodes of high anxiety. Assist the child in talking about the experience and expressing feelings through play therapy sessions.
* Interventions promoting injury prevention include educating parents and children about maintaining safety at home, at school, and in the car (see Displays 20-1 and 20-2).
* Interventions to promote child's self-esteem include establishing a trusting nurse–client relationship by encouraging the child to express feelings, especially about self-views. Encourage the child to ask questions about health problems, treatment, progress, and prognosis. Provide reliable information; clarify any misconceptions the child has about self, care, or caregivers, and avoid negative criticism.
* Interventions to promote parental understanding and coping skills associated with child's injury include assessing parenting behaviors and determining the level of impairment. Provide parents with information regarding age-related development needs and problematic behaviors. Observe parent–child interactions. Support parental strengths, and encourage parental participation in child's care. Explain all procedures and potential patient reactions. Discuss resources available for counseling and financial assistance.

evaluation

* The child will not experience aspiration or respiratory distress.
* Child and parents will identify factors that increase the potential for injury, verbalize an intent to use safety measures to prevent injury, and describe safety practices applicable to home, environment, and automobile safety.
* Child will identify positive aspects of self, express a positive outlook for the future, and analyze his or her own behavior and its consequences.
* Parents will share feelings regarding parenting, identify factors that interfere with effective parenting, and identify resources available for assistance.

key points

* **Safety of children includes prevention of accidental injuries (the leading cause of childhood mortality in the United States) and protection against communicable diseases.**

* Actions and practices that protect children from risk of disease, injury, or death are known as *safety* and involve enforceable, age-appropriate safety rules based on a child's motor skills and cognitive and psychosocial development.
* Young children experience accidents that can be life-threatening, ranging from suffocation in cribs, falls resulting in head injuries, choking and aspiration of small pieces of food and other objects, drowning, burns, ingestion of poisons, and car accidents. School-age children also experience accidents involving bicycles, sports, drug and alcohol abuse, and peer violence.
* Poisons are any substances that can harm the body. A network of poison control centers has been established throughout the country with 24-hour service providing information about all types of poisoning, including ingested, inhaled, absorbed, and injected poisons.
* The National Safety Council lists accidental shootings as the fifth leading cause of death for children younger than 5 years, with reported cases of guns being discharged by children as young as 2 years. Teenagers (especially African Americans) are victims in 3 of every 10 violent crimes involving intentional shootings resulting from peer rivalry, gang activity, and illegal drug activity.
* Car safety for infants involves the use of safety seats installed according to the manufacturer's instructions and used from birth until the child is older than 4 years and weighs approximately 40 lb. For preschool and school-age children, car safety involves the use of seat belts and shoulder harnesses. Teenage car safety involves more than seat belts because most teens are interested in driving. Driver education and safety programs are a benefit to the young driver who may be at increased risk of car accidents because of the lack of maturity and risky behaviors, such as consuming alcohol and driving.
* Infectious diseases are a leading cause of mortality in children and result from exposure to pathogens, such as viruses, bacteria, rickettsiae, helminths (worms) and, fungi. Many childhood infectious diseases can be prevented with proper immunizations.
* Routine childhood immunizations protect against nine diseases: measles, mumps, and rubella; diphtheria, tetanus, and pertussis; poliomyelitis, HiB, and HBV.
* Common childhood allergies include sensitivity to certain foods, tobacco smoke, animals (especially hair and dander), everyday lint, molds, and dust mites; allergic reactions range from mild to severe symptoms depending on the child's contact with the allergen. Hives, pruritus, and angioedema are common; however, more serious reactions may result in anaphylactic shock and death.
* Pediatric emergency care involves the ABCs of cardiopulmonary resuscitation, including airway, breathing, and circulation. In addition, it is important to maintain cervical spine alignment and immobilization while making sure the airway is patent because many pediatric injuries include head and spine trauma.

review questions 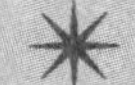

1. Select the most pertinent crib safety consideration.
   a. Use a soft mattress or water mattress to promote a sense of safety, trust, and warmth.
   b. Protect the crib mattress by covering it in plastic to reduce the risk of urine and stool contamination.
   c. Pacifiers can be tied around an infant's neck after the age of 1 month using a slip knot and satin ribbon for safety measures.
   d. Crib sides must be kept up at all times regardless of the infant's age.
2. Shawna is 2 years old and loves to climb. Shawna's mother is concerned about her risk of falling. Select the most appropriate nursing response to this concern.
   a. Children between 1 and 6 years are the least susceptible to falls because they have strong coordination skills.
   b. All children love to run and climb.
   c. Pile cushions and pillows in an area on the floor, and encourage Shawna to play with the pillows to promote growth and development.
   d. Shawna is at risk for head trauma if she falls and hits her head. You may need to administer a harsh punishment if she insists on climbing.
3. Select the most appropriate measure to prevent poisoning in toddlers.
   a. Teach the toddler how to get his or her own vitamins from the container with careful instructions on the importance of taking only one vitamin a day.
   b. Keep household products, such as vitamins, medicines, cleansers, lawn fertilizers, cosmetics, pesticides, and mouth wash, locked in a cupboard and out of the toddler's reach.
   c. Teach the toddler that household plants are not to be handled and involve the child in planting a small garden.
   d. Discourage toddlers from chewing on wood crib sides or window sills because of an increase risk of exposure to toxins from bacteria.
4. Select the most accurate statement concerning gun safety.
   a. Studies have shown that a child must be at least 5 years old before they have the ability to discharge a gun.
   b. Accidental shootings have decreased in the United States in the last 5 years.
   c. Teenagers (especially African Americans) are at increased risk for being victims of shootings resulting from peer rivalry, gang activity, and illegal drug activity.
   d. The National Safety Council lists children younger than 5 years as being a low risk for accidental shootings.

5. Infant immunizations include measles, mumps, rubella, diphtheria, tetanus, pertussis, polio, HiB, and
   a. varicella.
   b. HBV.
   c. herpes simplex.
   d. plumbism.

references

Bureau of Census, Economics, & Statistics Administration. (1994). *Statistical abstracts of the United States.* Washington, DC: U.S. Department of Commerce.

(1992). Guidelines for cardiopulmonary resuscitation and emergency cardiac care. *Journal of the American Medical Association, 268*(16), 2251–2301.

Marotz, L., Cross, M., & Rush, J. (1993). *Health, safety and nutrition for the young* (3rd ed.). Albany, NY: Delmar.

Merina, A. (1994). Fighting school violence means taking on guns. *National Education Association Today*, March, 4–5.

National Safety Council (1994). *Accident facts*. Itaska, IL: Author.

Sewell, K., & Gaines, S. (1993). A developmental approach to childhood safety education. *Pediatric Nursing, 19*(5), 464–466.

bibliography

Biehler, B. (1992). Impact of role-sets on implementing self-care theory with children. *Pediatric Nursing, 18*(1), 30–34.

Campbell, L., & Thomas, D. (1991) Pediatric trauma: When kids get hurt. *RN, August*, 32–39.

Children's Safety Network (1991). *A data book of child and adolescent injury.* Washington, DC: National Center for Education in Maternal and Child Health.

Environmental Protection Agency (1992). *The guide to protecting yourself and your family from radon*. Washington, DC: U.S. Government Printing Office.

Gulanick, M., Gradishar, D., & Puzas, M. (1994). *Ambulatory pediatric nursing*. Albany, NY: Delmar.

Igoe, J., & Giordano, B. (1992). Health Promotion and disease prevention: Secrets of success. *Pediatric Nursing, 18*(1), 61–62.

Levine, B., & Lavi, S. (1991). Perils of childhood immunization against measles, mumps, and rubella. *Pediatric Nursing, 17*(2), 159–161.

Marks, M. (1994). *Broadribb's introductory pediatric nursing* (4th ed.). Philadelphia: J.B. Lippincott.

McEwen, M. (1993). Should there be universal childhood vaccination against hepatitis B? *Pediatric Nursing, 19*(5), 447–451.

Metcalf, J., & Roberts, S. (1993). Strength training and the immature athlete. *Pediatric Nursing, 19*(4), 325–332.

Ostrum, G. (1993). Sports-related injuries in youths: Prevention is the key-and nurses can help! *Pediatric Nursing, 19*(4), 333–342.

Partners Active in Learning and Sharing (PALS). Pals (1994). *Instructions on safety.* Dayton, OH: The Children's Medical Center.

Pittman, K. (1992). Awakening child consumerism in health care. *Pediatric Nursing, 18*(2), 132–136.

Rollins, J. (1993). Nurses as gangbusters: A response to gang violence in America. *Pediatric Nursing, 19*(6), 559–567.

Schuster, C., & Ashburn, S. (1992). *The process of human development* (3rd ed.). Philadelphia: J.B. Lippincott.

Sweeney-Patterson K., & Stevens, J. (1992). Educating child care providers in child health. *Pediatric Nursing, 18*(1), 37–40.

Vessey, J., & Ritchie, S. (1993). The who, what, and when of pediatric immunization. *RN, September*, 42–48.

Wilson, P., & Dufour, L. (1993). Bicycle safety programs: Targeting injury prevention through education. *Pediatric Nursing, 19*(4), 343–346.

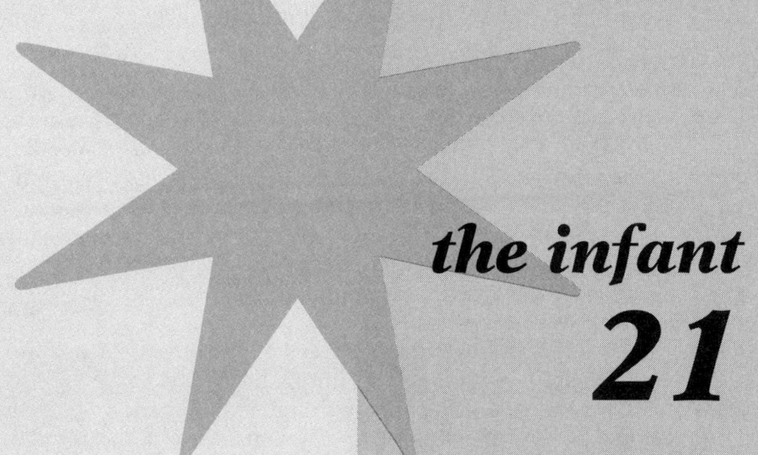

the infant 21

outline

objectives 

After studying this chapter, the reader should be able to:

* Describe three influences on infant growth and development.
* List the steps for accurately assessing an infant's temperature, pulse, respirations, and blood pressure.
* Discuss weight, height, and head circumference increases for an infant at 6 and 12 months of age.
* Describe at least five ways in which the sensory system enhances exploratory play in an infant.
* Describe developmental milestones at 3, 6, and 10 months.
* Compare breast-fed infants' and bottle-fed infants' stools, stating at least two differences.
* State the number of deciduous teeth and the age at which they erupt.
* Describe the infant's gross and fine motor development and the orderly progression that enables the infant to walk.
* Discuss the role of the parent or caregiver in the psychosocial development of the infant that focuses on trust versus mistrust.
* Discuss sensorimotor stage of cognitive development.

key terms 

retraction
hyperthermia
bottle caries
pincer reflex
gross motor development
fine motor development
colic
weaning
febrile convulsions

The infant is 1 month to 1 year old. The first year of life is a period of rapid, specific, progressive, and orderly growth and development. Each child grows and develops at an individual pace influenced by inherited genes, intrauterine environment, and extrauterine environment. A steady increase in height, weight, and head and chest circumference is a good indication of health in an infant. Any interruption in this steady growth and development should be cause for concern.

The infant and family accomplish tremendous physiologic, psychological, and social tasks during the first year. Parental understanding of infant growth and development is important; lack of understanding of infant needs can lead to child neglect and abuse. The infant is totally dependent on adults for meeting basic needs, which include the need for love and security.

This chapter addresses normal infant growth and development. Family issues, such as parental and sibling bonding, are included. Nurses must understand infant growth and development to fulfill their role as caregivers and teachers of children and families.

physical growth assessment factors

Infant growth is measured in terms of height, weight, and head and chest circumference and by assessment of vital signs and body systems. Infants are not only much smaller than adults, but their body systems are less mature. This immaturity can have important consequences in relation to health and illness (Fig. 21-1).

weight

Infants double their birth weight by 6 months and triple it by 12 months. They gain approximately 125 to 175 g (5–7 oz) per week and more than 453 g (up to 1½ lb) per month (see Appendix).

height

Infants normally increase in height approximately 2.6 cm (1 in) per month, with a total increase of 50% over their birth length by their first birthday. The average height for a 6-month-old infant is 68 cm (26 in). Standardized growth charts are used to plot an infant's height and weight and should demonstrate a pattern of normal growth curves. Most of an infant's growth occurs in the trunk of the body.

head

An infant's head is approximately 70% of adult size, and by 1 year, it will increase 10%, reaching 80% of its adult size. At birth, normal head circumference is about 35 cm (13.7 in). It increases approximately 1.3 cm (½ in) per month between 1 and 6 months and approximately 0.64 cm (1/4 in) per month between 7 and 12 months. Head circumference by 1 year is about 52 cm (20 in).

An infant's head size is influenced by genetics. Deviation from the standard growth parameters does not mean the infant has an abnormality; however, head size measurements that do not fall within the expected normal range (between the 10th and 90th percentiles on standard growth chart) need to be investigated.

 **nursing insight**

The anterior fontanel often becomes tense and appears to bulge when the infant cries, making accurate assessment of head circumference difficult until the infant has stopped crying.

chest

The chest of a newborn is smaller than the head circumference; however, an infant's chest at 1 year will equal the head circumference. The size of the chest will continue to increase after 1 year of age and will exceed the head size as the child matures.

vital signs

Vital signs are discussed in more detail in Chapter 19. Basic age-related information is included here for continuity of learning.

pulse

The heart rate of an infant slows from 120 to 160 beats/min to 100 to 120 beats/min by 1 year of age (see Fig. 21-1). The pulse rate of an infant is assessed apically (at the apex of the heart between left nipple and sternum) for 1 full minute. The rate and rhythm of the apical pulse are noted and recorded.

respirations

Respirations are assessed for rate, rhythm, and presence of retractions (the act of drawing back the sternum). An infant's respiration rate averages 20 to 40 breaths per minute and tends to have an irregular rhythm, ranging from deep to shallow respirations. Listening to the infant's chest using a stethoscope (auscultation) is another way to assess respirations and provides the nurse with information about breath sounds. Respiration rate is influenced by sleep, wakefulness, and feedings.

temperature

An infant's temperature is usually taken rectally; however, axillary and tympanic methods also can be used. Normal rectal temperature is 37.6°C (99.6°F). The temperature reading may be obtained in a matter of seconds if an electronic thermometer is being used or within 3 minutes if using a glass thermometer. Elevated temperature (hyperthermia) in infants can cause convulsions called *febrile convulsions*.

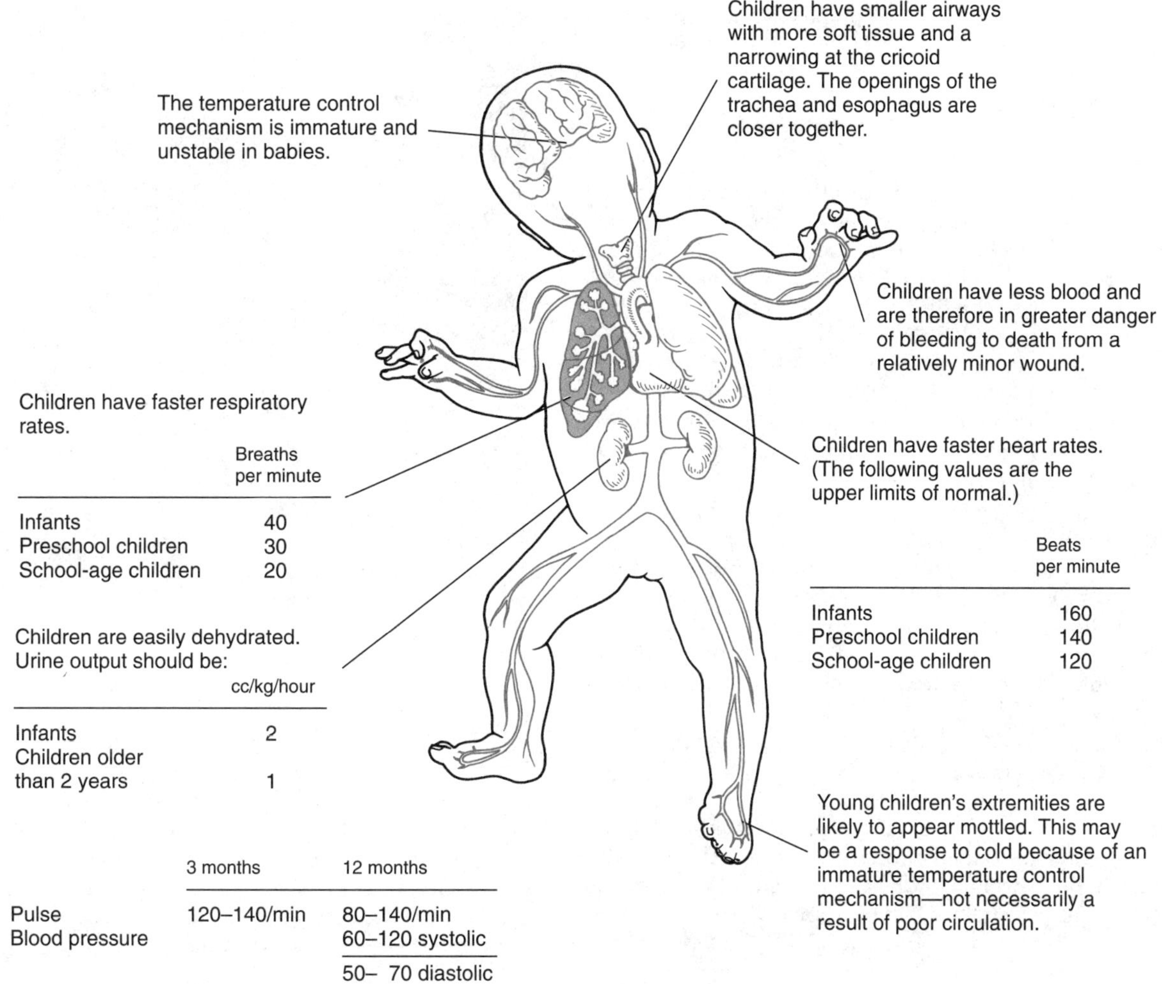

figure 21-1 *Children vs. adults: Important differences at a glance.*

blood pressure

An accurate blood pressure is difficult to obtain on an infant. An average blood pressure during the first year of life is 90/60, with differences noted according to activity level and weight (see Fig. 21-1). Electronic monitoring equipment is often used to obtain blood pressure readings.

developmental milestones

Development during infancy follows general principles reflected by specific events, such as holding the head up, rolling over, sitting, crawling, and walking. Typical patterns of development help describe skills considered normal at an approximate age.

Typical patterns are referred to as "norms." Norms are valuable for comparing and predicting normal development, but individual children can vary greatly and still fall within a normal range. Some important developmental milestones are summarized in Display 21-1.

Growth and development charts indicate average physiologic limits, but individual children must be evaluated in terms of health, race, gender, and genetic and environmental factors. An infant who lags behind the norm alerts pediatricians to look for possible problems, such as cerebral palsy or mental retardation.

Infants differ in appearance, personality, and the rate of growth and development. Body, hand, speech, and social development seem to change overnight. The 1-month-old infant differs when compared with a 3-month-old. Infant

display 21-1
developmental milestones

Infant assessment for developmental milestones includes the following:

- **Ability to head hold erect by 3 months**
- **Ability to sit without support on firm surface by 6 months**
- **Ability to bear a majority of weight on the legs by 10 months**

growth and development are compared and contrasted in Table 21-1.

1 to 3 months

body development

Infants at 1 to 3 months can turn their heads from side to side and use their eyes to follow a slowly moving object held overhead. When positioned on the stomach, the infant can lift the head to look around. A landmark for development starts with lifting the head (Fig. 21-2). This action will continue until the child is able to lift the upper trunk. Infants do not proceed to another activity without having accomplished the activity in the previous stage. Muscle development is accomplished by simple movement exercises, mobiles, and soft toys and by encouraging infants to reach, turn, and lift.

elimination

Breast-fed infants tend to have soft, unformed, bright mustard-yellow stools with little odor. Bottle-fed infants have yellow to yellowish-green stools that are more formed and have more odor. By 1 month of age, breast-fed infants have more frequent stools than bottle-fed infants.

3 to 6 months

Between 3 and 6 months, infants gain weight and appear to have grown into their skin. By 5 to 6 months, they double their birth weight and have gained additional body control. For example, a 7-lb newborn will weigh approximately 14 lb by 5 or 6 months, and when propped up, he or she can keep the head steady, looking around in various directions (see Fig. 21-2). He or she can roll from stomach to back, and from back to stomach, making it unsafe to leave the infant unattended if crib sides are down.

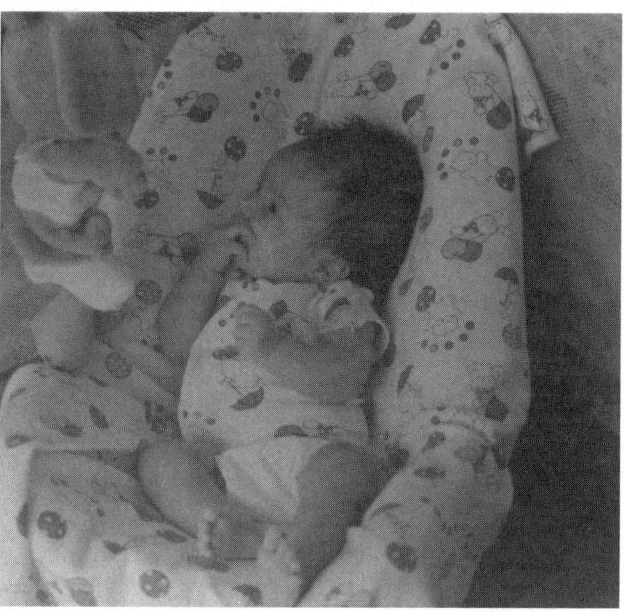

figure 21-2 *The month-old begins to explore her environment. (Photo by Elise Dinerman.)*

6 to 9 months

body development

By 6 months, infants can sit up without support for short periods of time. By 9 months, they can creep around on the floor, pulling themselves forward by moving their arms together and dragging their legs and torso. Some infants get up on their hands and knees and crawl around and may even pull themselves up to stand by 9 months.

teething

The process by which the crown of the tooth pushes through the area around the tooth (periodontal membrane) is known as "teething." The infant experiences red,

table 21-1 gross and fine motor growth and development

Growth	*1 Mo*	*3 Mo*	*4 Mo*	*7 Mo*	*10 Mo*	*12 Mo*
Gross motor	Turns and lifts head	Lifts head 90 degrees	Lifts head and chest with arm support May roll front to back	Sits; leans forward on hands; bears weight on legs	Sits with back straight; pulls to standing position; creeps or crawls	Walks holding onto hands, furniture
Fine motor	Uses eyes to follow for several feet Holds hands fisted, may try to reach overhead objects	Grasps rattle Eye–hand balance Shakes, waves, and throws toys	Hands open, reaches for objects Turns head when name called	Reaches and grasps large objects; transfers from hand to hand Palmer grasp	Pincer grasp; uncovers hidden toy	Pincer grasp improved; grasps a cup Releases objects on request

swollen, painful gums with increased drooling and irritability.

Teething does not cause infection, but because it begins at a time when the infant's maternal antibodies are low (around the seventh month), teething can make the infant less resistant to infections. Fever with temperature above 38.4°C (101.0°F), cold symptoms, diarrhea, and rashes need to be reported to the physician.

Teething discomfort can be relieved by offering a cold cloth, frozen teething ring, or a hard rubber teething ring for the infant to chew. Oral hygiene with a soft toothbrush is recommended as soon as the first tooth erupts. Infants are taught to brush their tongues to reduce the amount of bacteria in their mouths.

There are 20 deciduous teeth, often called "baby teeth" or "primary teeth." They are a guide for the proper positioning of permanent teeth. Deciduous teeth are a stimulus for growth of the jaws and aid in the development of speech.

The two lower central incisors usually appear by 6 to 7 months. By the first birthday, six deciduous teeth are in place (Fig. 21-3). There can be a familial tendency toward early or late tooth eruption without other signs of early or late development. Nutritional deficiency or prolonged illness also can interfere with tooth eruption.

dental caries or bottle caries

Dental erosion is frequently seen in infants who nurse or bottle feed at will during naps or at night. The sugar from the milk or juice collects around the teeth, causing cavities (dental caries). Another cause of dental erosion is repeated exposure to gastric acids seen in infants experiencing the return of stomach contents into the esophagus (*gastroesophageal reflux*).

biting

Biting often occurs after the first teeth erupt. The infant is quick to use the teeth to bite whatever is available (eg, nipples, siblings, pets, and even himself or herself).

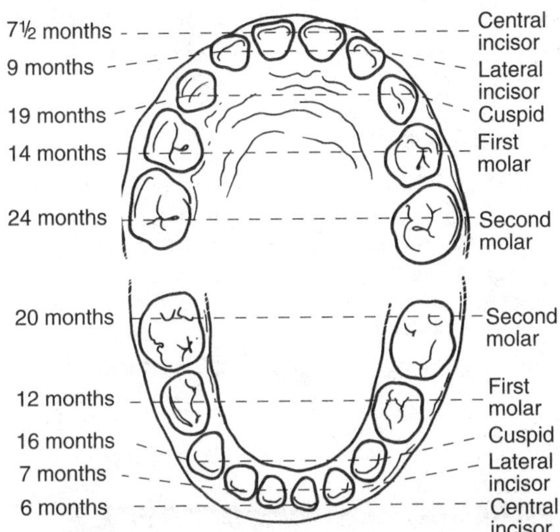

figure 21-3 *Approximate ages for the eruption of deciduous teeth.*

9 to 12 months

The 10- to 12-month-old continues to get around by crawling but may experiment with holding onto furniture and pulling up to a standing position. This ability to get around enables the infant to explore a larger environment, climbing up steps and onto chairs and furniture. Although the infant has little difficulty climbing up onto steps or furniture, help in getting down is usually necessary to avoid injury.

The infant will have tripled his or her birth weight by 12 months. For example, the 7-lb newborn will weigh approximately 21 lb by the first birthday.

sensory development

Infants experience the world through the five senses: touch, taste, smell, hearing, and sight. Development of these senses is unique to each infant; however, certain norms have been established to use in assessment.

touch

Touch is the first language that infants and parents use to communicate and includes active and passive touch. Active touch involves the infant's grasping clothes, toys, rattles, and bottles. Passive touch involves caregivers stroking and massaging the baby. Infants need to be touched and handled gently. Caressing and fondling are expressions of caring, essential to normal growth and development. Touching is a form of stimulation for the infant and is a way in which the infant learns about the environment.

Clothing that touches the infant's skin should be soft and comfortable. Infants have individual preferences as to whether they are bundled tightly or want skin-to-skin contact. Attentive caregivers become skillful at reading these preferences.

taste

Infants react to sour and sweet tastes much like an adult. Long before they have teeth, infants have what is called a "sweet tooth." Research studies have shown infants tend to suck faster when taking a sweet liquid.

smell

Infants learn early in life to identify the familiar smell of breast milk and associate this smell with their mothers. They also respond to irritating odors by drawing back from them.

hearing

An infant can distinguish its mother's voice from the voices of strangers. Infants prefer sounds that pulsate or are rhythmic and tend to pay attention to music on the radio but sleep through the noise of a vacuum cleaner. The development of hearing progresses as follows:

* A 1-month-old quiets momentarily at an unusual sound, such as a bell.
* A 2-month-old listens or stops an activity at the sound of spoken words.
* A 3-month-old turns the head in an attempt to locate a sound.
* A 5-month-old localizes a sound downward and to the side by turning the head and looking down.
* A 6-month-old locates a sound made from above the head.
* A 10-month-old recognizes his own name and listens when addressed.
* A 12 month-old easily locates and turns to a sound made in any direction.

sight

Eye contact is considered one of the infant's first social contacts. Infants can see and discriminate patterns. Infants will drop toys and become excited when they see them reappear. Bold colors tend to capture an infant's visual attention, and eye movement activity stimulates development of the brain's auditory cortex. Development of sight progresses as follows:

* A 1-month-old looks at objects that are approximately 46 cm (18 in) away. This is approximately the distance between a baby being held and the caregiver's face, which enables the infant to stare at the caregiver's face. Holding the infant is especially important during feeding to promote caregiver recognition and trust.
* A 2-month-old focuses well and follows objects with the eyes.
* A 3-month-old holds hands in front of the face as if studying them. He can follow an object or light across the midline or follow a light into all six positions of gaze.
* From 1 to 3 months, infants respond to a human face but show little or no fear of a stranger.
* From 3 to 6 months, infants smile at familiar faces but stare solemnly at strangers. Between 2 and 5 months, infant depth perception begins to mature, making the world three dimensional.
* From 7 to 12 months, the infant uses sight and greater mobility to explore, finding small obscure items and placing them in the mouth.

Eye color is usually gray-blue in light-skinned infants and brown in dark-skinned infants. African American infants often have a slight yellowing and small black spots on the sclera. Eye color stabilizes by 6 to 12 months.

> **nursing insight**
> *Blind children demonstrate the phenomenon of smiling at familiar faces and staring solemnly at strangers, indicating a cognitive or exploratory task of development rather than a test of vision.*

motor development

Infant motor development progresses from reflex activity to gross motor skills to fine motor skills. The process of development is orderly, beginning with control of the head, proceeding to the trunk, and advancing to the lower extremities. Motor development impacts the infant's ability to move in the environment to touch, explore, interact, and learn. Motor skills reflect neuromuscular development along with perceptual and cognitive development.

reflex activity

A 1-month-old infant demonstrates efficient reflexes even though arm and leg movements are still involuntary. By 2 months, the infant will have much smoother arm and leg movements. A startle reaction to sudden loud noise or loss of support (Moro reflex) is demonstrated by stiffening of the infant's body with arms and legs pulled into a clutch position as if to prevent falling (see Figure 35-5.).

At 3 months, the infant's body control changes from reflex to voluntary activity. The infant loses the stepping reflex and tonic neck reflex. The grasping reflex is weak, and voluntary grasping is still immature. The pincer grasp is a major milestone at 10 months, enabling the infant to bring the thumb and first finger together. This allows the infant to pick up small objects (see Figure 35-5.).

> **nursing alert**
> *Great care must be taken to provide the infant with a safe environment, free from small objects that can be picked up, put into the mouth or nose, and aspirated.*

gross motor development

At 1 month, the infant needs head support while being held (Fig. 21-4*A*). Between 1 and 4 months, the infant gains the ability to raise the head, roll from back to side, and attempt precrawling. At 6 to 9 months, infants demonstrate a *parachute reaction*, demonstrated by extending the arms similar to a response of protecting oneself from falling. Children with cerebral palsy do not have this response because they have maximum flexion activity. From 4 to 8 months, infants hold their heads erect continuously and sit with support for short intervals (see Fig. 21-4*B*). From 8 to 12 months, the infant sits without support, crawls, walks alone or with help, and feeds himself or herself (see Fig. 21-4*C* and *D*).

fine motor development

Between 1 and 4 months, fine motor development is characterized by purposeful attempts to grab objects but sometimes missing them and grasping objects with both hands momentarily. From 4 to 8 months, infants use their thumb and fingers to grasp objects (pincer reflex) and are able to hold objects in both hands simultaneously. From 8 to 12 months, infants can put objects in containers, feed themselves crackers or toast, and hold crayons to make marks on a paper.

psychosocial development

According to Erikson, the psychosocial development of the infant focuses on *trust versus mistrust*. Development of a sense of trust depends largely on caregivers and the child's

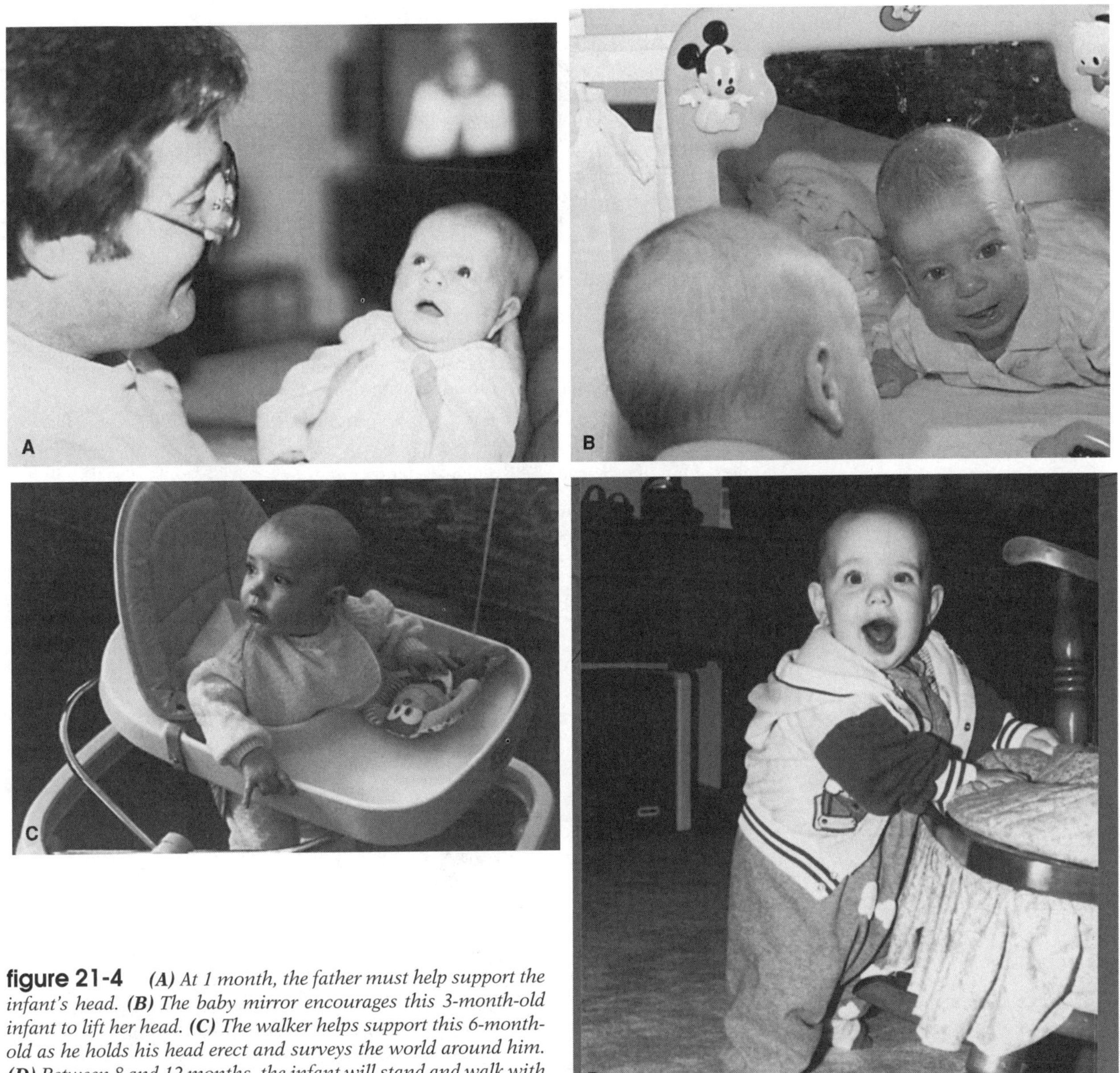

figure 21-4 *(A) At 1 month, the father must help support the infant's head. (B) The baby mirror encourages this 3-month-old infant to lift her head. (C) The walker helps support this 6-month-old as he holds his head erect and surveys the world around him. (D) Between 8 and 12 months, the infant will stand and walk with support.*

environment. The quality of the caregiver–child relationship and consistency of care are important factors in developing infant trust. The infant learns that certain sounds and touches indicate feeding, while other touches indicate bathing and so forth. These sounds, sights, and touches fall into patterns that the infant can recognize and trust. Infants like the same stories read over and over because they come to "trust" the pattern and outcome (Table 21-2).

Infant care that is attentive and timely teaches the infant that life is predictable. When care is inconsistent and the infant experiences a delay in the gratification of needs, uncertainty and mistrust can develop. Infants can become unresponsive if left alone most of the waking hours without stimulation from other people. A growing infant learns that people give care that provides enjoyment; consequently, they learn to trust people to meet their basic needs and reduce tensions.

Self-trust begins to develop when the infant learns to roll over, crawl, creep, and finally walk. Even falling and bumping the head is all part of "learning" to trust.

During the second 6 months of life, infants become capable of recognizing and responding to others. Infants respond to parents, siblings, and relatives by smiling and gesturing to be held. They display affection toward family members by kissing and following them around. They become attached to a particular toy and want to keep it close to them. They become upset when around strangers (Fig. 21-5).

As infants develop, they become more aware of themselves as separate beings. Infants during this time are less dependent on their mothers and more capable of being alone. The infant's success in adjusting to a change in his or her mother's attention depends less on the amount of time spent together than on the quality of the relationship.

table 21-2 psychosocial development of the infant

Age in Months	*Physical Development*	*Emotional Development*	*Intellectual Development*	*Social Development*
Up to 3	Head wobbly; whole body twitches when crying Kicks legs in air Tear ducts not fully developed—no tear production	Responds to human face, content when fed Develops sense of trust when basic needs are met	Crying communicates needs Learns to bring hand to mouth	Interest centered on caregiver Responds to being held Stops crying when sees parent
3–6	Holds head erect Cannot sit alone Can roll from one side to the other Plays with fingers and hands Enjoys touching Doubles birth weight	Smiles, laughs, coos, cries, kicks, and waves arms when distressed Enjoys playing peek-a-boo Smiles at familiar people	Each new activity result of mental growth Voluntary actions brain cell maturity Recognizes mother and father	Begins to interact with others Laughs, smiles at familiar people; enjoys attention; plays alone; learns that parents will return after they have left; begins learning love
6–9	Can pull up to sitting position and remain unsupported for a short time Can roll from stomach to back Likes to crawl Transfers objects from one hand to another Discovers feet Uses thumb and forefinger as a "pincer" movement to pick up small objects Likes to drag things First tooth	Responsive to other person's moods Enjoys imitation Reacts with shyness or aggression to fear	Talks to self in mirror; able to change facial expressions; enjoys pounding, banging, and throwing Mimics simple adult sounds Recognizes own name Crawls Perceives depth	"Stranger anxiety" common Highly responsive to caregiver's moods and emotions Enjoys imitating caregivers Enjoys "riding" on caregiver's knees
9–12	Can sit alone Crawls well Stands without holding on Enjoys playing with blocks Can grasp a cup by the handle May have 2–8 teeth	Shows affection by hugging Enjoys feeling, grabbing, and pulling hair Anger is directed at a specific thing Learns behaviors that are positive or negative	Mimics sounds; adds facial expression; can say simple words, wave "bye bye" Enjoys pointing games, "Where is your nose?" Learns by trial and error	Cooperates when being dressed Loves being "chased" by siblings Enjoys applause Enjoys rhymes; expresses jealousy, affection, and sympathy.

It is suggested that mothers need to be available often in 10- and 20-second intervals to give an added dimension to what the baby is already doing.

psychosexual development

Psychosexual development follows biologic growth in infants. The quality of physical intimacy between caregivers and infants during feeding, bathing, and other contacts reflects individual feelings about intimacy. Each contact represents an opportunity for the infant to experience pleasure with intimacy. If close contact with the infant is avoided by the caregiver because of fear associated with physical closeness, the infant will sense the fear and may feel it as rejection.

cognitive development

Piaget describes infancy as a sensorimotor stage that involves gaining knowledge and intellect of the environment through the senses. This stage represents developmental progression from involuntary activity to purposeful acts (see Table 21-2). The four sensorimotor stages include the following:

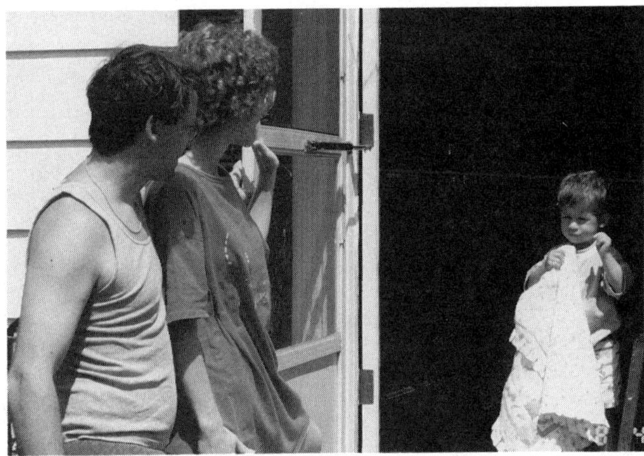

figure 21-5 *Child holding security blanket as parents leave.*

* Birth to 1 month: Inborn and predictable survival reflexes are seen. There is no concept of self or others. Infant is totally dependent.
* 1 to 4 months: Stereotyped repetition focuses on one's body as the center of attention. Infant is unable to differentiate self from others. Trial and error behavior is seen.
* 4 to 8 months: Attention shifts to objects and the environment. Infant displays more purposeful repetition of actions with goal-directed behavior and demonstrates an awareness that he or she is separate from others. A deliberate act elicits a certain response.
* 8 to 12 months: Infant moves toward independence from the mother figure. Infant demonstrates an awareness of events as being pleasant or unpleasant and associates gestures and behaviors with symbols.

language development

Infants understand the meaning of many words long before they speak them. They learn words by being exposed to them through books and conversations. By 1 month of age, an infant coos with vowel-like sounds. Infants learn language by imitating the speech they hear. If parents use only "baby talk," enunciation of words is likely to be poor as the infant begins to repeat words. Between 1 and 4 months of age, infants babble and make vowel sounds. Between 4 and 8 months, they use two-syllable words and form two-vowel sounds. By 8 to 12 months, they imitate word sounds and speak in syllables, respond to their own name, and demonstrate a three-word vocabulary.

Piaget suggests that infants are born with the ability to learn language but do not have definite language competence. He proposes that infants confront language skills according to their temperament. For example, early babblers may talk more quickly than quiet infants. He suggests that parents who talk to and maintain eye contact with their infants encourage early communication skills.

Exposing infants to names of people, objects, and animals helps promote speech. Infants are likely to repeat a word if given encouragement by the caregiver. Several factors influence speech development:

* Intellectual ability
* Relationship with parents
* Desire to talk
* Discovering that talking is rewarding
* Developing the muscles that control the mouth and larynx movements
* The range of opportunities that caregivers provide for the infant to listen and practice imitating speech

The first words spoken are usually nouns, such as "Mama" and "da-da." Action verbs, such as "run," "take," and "give" are learned as infants and toddlers gain an understanding of the activities of the words. Learning is enhanced when caregivers provide the infant with simple commands accompanied by physical gestures, for example, asking the infant to give a kiss while you are pursing your lips.

social development

The infant is a social being. As young as 1 month of age, infants demonstrate excitement and smile when a person or toy appears in their line of vision. They may hold still when gazing at a face and show contentment when being fed. Infant temperament is described as quiet, average, or active.

Between 4 and 8 months, infants begin to play with toys. They smile and laugh aloud when happy. They become easily frustrated and fearful of strangers. During this time, the infant may turn away from strangers and cry. Infants at 8 to 12 months make simple requests with gestures and play simple games, such as peek-a-boo. They show affection by hugging and may respond when asked for a kiss. They cry when disciplined and demonstrate anxiety when separated from their parents.

✳ nursing insight

Poor or missing language development may indicate neurologic disorder or hearing deficit. Language delays that need to be referred to a specialist include the following:

* *Lack of response to voices or common noises by 2 months*
* *Lack head posturing in the direction of sound by 6 months*
* *Lack of "jabber" by 10 months*

family relationships

Parental understanding of normal growth and development is important to infant–parent interactions. Parenting skills are learned, not inborn. Parent–infant attachment centers on the parent's interest in the infant and physical contact.

Mother–infant attachment is the main influence on an infant's sense of well-being; however, father–infant attachment also is important. Father attachment increases the father's willingness to take part in infant care and creates a stronger bond with the infant. Attachment is enhanced when parental expectations are reinforced by appropriate infant responses.

Infants tend to reflect the emotional state of the person providing care. Their basic attitudes toward life stem from early experiences with parents and siblings. The warm and loving way parents hold and communicate with infants gives them a secure feeling that the world is "okay."

crying

Parenting an infant can be an anxiety-producing experience. Because infants communicate by crying, parents can feel helpless and overwhelmed in meeting their infant's needs (Table 21-3).

The most difficult part is deciding what has caused the crying and what can be done to stop it. If the infant cries around the clock, it is time to make an appointment with the pediatrician. It is recommended that parents time the infant's crying episodes, because 5 minutes of lusty crying can seem like 60 minutes when trying to console the infant. Crying or fussing may stem from the following causes:

- Illness and immunizations. A DTP injection can cause crankiness for several hours.
- Infant immaturity. Infants mature at different rates. Some infants have immature nervous and digestive systems that make them more irritable when tired or hungry.
- Reactions to formula or breast milk. An infant may be sensitive to milk-based formulas or may be reacting to dairy products.
- Hypersensitive infants. Some infants have sensitive nervous systems, which cause them to overreact to noises, lights, sounds, and other stimulation. Infants differ in how easily they are soothed once a crying cycle begins.

colic

Colic is crying and irritability from a variety of causes, affecting more than 20% of all infants. Common symptoms of colic include continuous crying for extended periods each day. Colic is characterized by loud cries and screaming. The infant tends to draw the legs up tight against the abdomen. Colic usually lasts at least 3 weeks. Researchers think colic is caused by an immature nervous system. A predictable daily routine can provide comfort to a baby with colic.

Parents need reassurance and support in dealing with their colicky infant. Because the cause of irritability is not clear and the approach to managing colic is not well fo-

table 21-3 *infant cry assessment, possible cause, and suggested interventions*

Cry and Behavior	*Possible Cause*	*Suggested Interventions*
Loud, piercing, intense May hold breath; draws hands and feet up; squirms; strains; may pull at painful part (eg, ear)	Pain; diaper pin undone; hair wrapped around a finger, toe, or penis, altering blood flow	Check body and diaper for open pins, constricting hairs, and so forth. Call the pediatrician if irritability continues regardless of relief measures.
Cries after play Lack of tears Quiets when held or stimulated Crying quickly replaced by smiling	Loneliness or boredom after 3 mo	Hold; offer a toy or change of scenery; talk softly; stay relaxed.
Brief, rhythmic cries more intense at feeding time Attempts to suck fingers and fists May quiet briefly when given a pacifier, but resumes crying when no food is given	Hunger	Allow the infant to establish a feeding schedule.
Fussy crying after eating Spits up after eating	Overfeeding and gas bubbles	Keep in sitting position during feedings; offer small, frequent feedings; bubble during and after feeding.
Crying similar to hunger Feeding does not satisfy Refuses formula, or takes formula and does not swallow but allows it to drool from the mouth	Thirst, primarily in bottle-fed infants	Offer extra water either in a bottle or cup.
Irritable Eyes seem glazed, red, and swollen Turns away from adults	Tired or overstimulated	Offer quiet environment with security object. Wrap firmly with blanket. Rock gently. Allow infant to "cry it out" as an outlet for frustration.

cused, a family's stress is often increased as they try to cope. It is important to be sure that the baby is not crying due to lack of feeding or poor quality breast milk.

Behaviors that are common in mothers of colicky infants include crying, fatigue, depression, and resentment of the infant. A mother's feelings of frustration can have a negative effect on siblings in the family. The family needs reassurance that the colic is not long lasting. Family members need to support each other and take turns giving each other time for rest. A good sense of humor is helpful.

Massage can relieve infant stress by soothing, calming, and relaxing the infant. Massage relays love through touch, relaxes muscles, increases circulation, and may aid in relieving gas pain. If the infant is not enjoying the massage, it may be due to overstimulation. The massage can be saved for a more agreeable time.

setting limits

An infant learns to trust by encountering the world of "no-no's" or verbal discipline. "No-no's" give an infant's life dimension. They provide limits, similar to fences, beyond which the infant should not venture. The infant's internal constraints are not developed to control unacceptable behavior, so he or she must rely on external constraints, such as verbal discipline, to learn socially acceptable behavior. Security objects, such as blankets and toys, are often used by infants to provide comfort, especially during times of stress.

Setting limits begins in infancy and can include the use of negative voice and stern eye contact. Sensitive infants may be overly aggressive or overly timid, while quiet infants may be congenial. Infants grow to learn that negative behavior promotes disciplinary measures, while positive behavior wins parental approval.

Infants are encouraged to explore their environment by a natural curiosity. Their strong drive to taste, feel, and hold almost anything within reach encourages them to explore beyond acceptable limits of behavior. When the infant engages in unacceptable behavior, others (especially siblings) come back at them with anger and confrontation. This power struggle is the beginning of discipline concerns. The infant must learn that there are limits to behavior and that some behaviors are allowable while others are not.

It is difficult to spoil an infant with too much attention. Parents need to know that an infant must have needs met promptly because an infant does not understand delayed gratification. Care that is given with consistency and love during infancy influences the infant's feelings of trust. Meeting the infant's needs must take precedence over promoting discipline. Discussing an infant's needs with older siblings helps reduce the negative feelings generated by the infant's demands.

sleep

Infant sleep patterns can have tremendous influence on a young family. Sleep deficit affects everyone if the infant disturbs the household's normal sleep behaviors. Infants differ in the amount of sleep required and will satisfy their own requirements. Consequently, when the infant is tired, he or she will sleep (Fig. 21-6).

The typical sleep pattern during the first few months of life is one of frequent, short periods of sleep interrupted by crying and fussing. The infant makes peculiar but normal sounds during these nap periods, such as grunting, wheezing, gurgling, and sucking. This light, restless sleep is typical for the first 6 to 8 months. At about 8 months, infants begin to sleep more in the manner of an adult.

It is suggested that parents learn their infant's sleep patterns and adjust accordingly. Parents have little control over the infant's sleep pattern even though many try to gain control. For example, parents may decide to introduce solid foods early or give cereal-thickened milk before bedtime. However, these practices probably do little in helping the infant sleep through the night.

infant nutrition

Food is essential to the physical and psychological health of the infant. Feeding time gives the caregiver an opportunity to hold the infant securely, talk to him or her, and strengthen the attachment. Breast milk or formula provides complete nutrition during the first 4 months of life because a healthy, full-term infant has stored an adequate supply of iron in the tissues. After 4 months, however, an iron supplement is recommended. Commercial formulas are enriched with vitamins and minerals and contain 48% to 50% of their calories as fat, providing 20 Kcal/oz. Lactose is the main carbohydrate in formulas. Fluoride supplementation is recommended when using infant formulas. See the Teaching Guidelines for infant feeding.

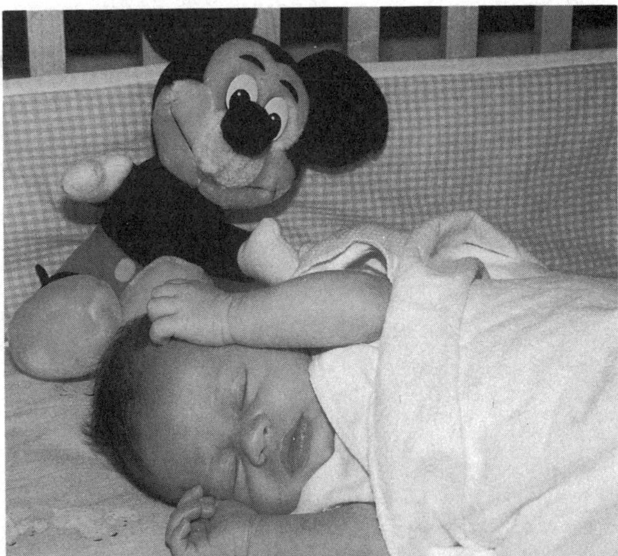

figure 21-6 *A sleeping infant is an endearing sight to exhausted new parents.*

teaching guidelines
infant feeding

- ✳ Feeding time is a good time to share your love. This is best accomplished by holding your baby, and supporting the head. Never prop the bottle.
- ✳ Burp the baby at least once during the feeding and again at the end.
- ✳ Position baby on the side after feeding.
- ✳ Feed the baby when hungry, demonstrated by rooting for a nipple, sucking hands, fussing, and crying. Breast-fed babies usually eat 8–14 times in 24 hours. Formula-fed babies may eat less often but at least six times per 24 hours.

controversial milk sources

Goat's milk is not recommended for infant feeding during the first year because it is deficient in iron, vitamin D, and vitamin C. Infants fed only goat's milk are at risk for megaloblastic anemia.

Unmodified cow's milk is not appropriate for young infants because it is deficient in iron, fluoride, and vitamins A, C, and D. Low-fat cow's milk, such as 2% or skim milk, is not recommended during infancy because of the low fat and caloric content. Whole milk is acceptable for infants older than 6 months of age, along with supplemental foods that make up at least one third of the caloric needs.

introduction of solid food

The suggested age for adding solid foods is between 4 and 6 months, depending on the pediatrician's guidance and developmental readiness based on fine and gross motor skills. Feeding actions are the consequence of motor development.

Before the age of 5 months, the infant will thrust the tongue out when food is put in the mouth. This is called the *extrusion reflex* and will disappear between the fifth and sixth month, about the time the infant demonstrates an ability to swallow semisolid foods. The process of moving food from the front of the mouth to the throat is a complex skill that must be learned.

A hungry baby is likely to become upset and cry when first offered solid foods. Parents need to know when infants thrust their tongues out, this does not necessarily indicate rejection of the food but merely represents a normal infant reflex. Providing the breast or a portion of formula before feeding solid food, along with a good measure of patience, can make the new experience more pleasant for infant and parent.

Dry cereal fortified with iron is a suitable starter food because it is easy to digest. Cereal is usually followed by fruits, vegetables, and then meat. New foods should be introduced one at a time, with 4 to 7 days between the introduction of foods. Solid food is offered in small amounts (1–2 teaspoons daily). This practice makes it easier to discover particular infant food intolerances or allergies.

When a particular food is refused, it can be excluded temporarily and reintroduced later. The infant may dislike certain foods. There are plenty of nutritious foods available to achieve a balanced diet. See the Teaching Guidelines for providing extra nutrition.

New foods should not be introduced when the infant is ill. Potentially allergenic foods, such as egg whites, fish, strawberries, oranges, soy, rice, beef, pork, chicken, and chocolate, should be offered in small quantities. Cow's milk is a common food allergy in infants.

Finger foods, such as dry toast, teething biscuits, small pieces of fruit, and cheese sticks, can be introduced when teeth begin to erupt. A spouted plastic cup is helpful when giving an infant liquids to drink. Fruit juices are diluted when first introduced.

Baby foods can be commercially prepared or fixed at home by using a food grinder, electric blender, food mill, or food processor. When solid foods are introduced, it is important to monitor the infant's height and weight and note progressive increases. If increases are not noted, the pediatrician should be informed.

teaching guidelines
providing extra nutrition

If your baby is growing slowly or is only taking small amounts of food, the following list provides ideas for giving "extra nutrition." The ideas are for babies who are eating cereal, fruits, vegetables, and meats. Ask your pediatrician before giving extra nourishment.

- ✳ Mix vanilla yogurt with strained fruits.
- ✳ Add cereal to strained fruits and vegetables
- ✳ Add 1–2 teaspoons of the baby's powdered formula to strained foods.
- ✳ Read baby food labels, and compare nutrition information.

weaning

Infants associate sucking with pleasure and satisfaction; therefore, weaning from the breast or bottle is best accomplished gradually. Introducing infants to cup drinking is suggested at of 5 to 6 months. Most infants are not ready to completely give up the breast or bottle at this age. Even though they are content to drink from a cup during the day, they often insist on a bottle or nursing during bedtime.

Some infants are reluctant to give up the breast or bottle, resulting in delayed weaning. Delayed weaning is considered a problem when it causes one or more of the following effects:

- ✳ Refusal to eat solid foods after 6 months of age
- ✳ Anemia confirmed in a routine screening at 12 months
- ✳ Tooth decay from overexposure to milk sugar

* Obesity caused from overeating on a predominately milk diet
* Lack of interest in play due to attention directed at nursing or taking a bottle
* Infant's refusal to take a bottle or cup when breast-fed

safety and hygiene

Most accidents during infancy can be prevented. Suffocation is the leading cause of accidental death among children younger than 1 year old. Infants are well known for putting anything and everything into their mouths. Choking can occur when small objects get caught in throats and windpipes.

Motor vehicle safety for the infant's first year of life involves primarily a safety seat. The safest position for any car safety seat is in the middle of the back seat. Convertible car seats can be used from birth until the child weighs approximately 40 lb. The car safety seat should face the rear of the car until an infant is 7 to 9 months old and weighs 17 to 20 lb. All car safety seats should be used according to the manufacturer's instructions. Refer to Chapter 20 for additional information about infant safety.

play

Play is the way babies learn and is often called the "work" of an infant. Caregivers are the most important teachers for their baby. During play, babies learn about talking and listening, how to follow objects with their eyes, and about the shape and feel of different objects. See the Teaching Guidelines for infant play.

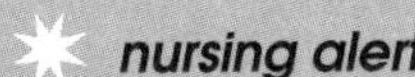

nursing alert

Infant carriers are different from car safety seats and should not be used as car safety seats.

teaching guidelines
infant play

Games will help develop your baby's senses.

* Repeat sounds made by the baby while looking into his or her eyes.
* Hold the baby facing you while singing songs.
* Position baby on his or her back, sit out of sight. Hold a noise-making toy about 12 in above the baby's face, and move the toy slowly in a circle; watch the baby's eyes follow the object.
* Collect objects of different shapes and sizes from around the house that are safe (eg, a plastic block, ball, plastic cup, toothbrush). Give the items one at a time to the baby, and allow him or her to explore them.

An infant's play is basically noninteractive with peers (solitary) and enables the infant to learn about the environment through touch, taste, hearing, smell, and sight. The manipulation of toys helps the infant develop motor skills in an unstructured, voluntary way. When selecting toys for an infant, it is important to choose the following types of toys:

* Appropriate for the infant's stage of development
* Safe for infants to handle; too large to swallow; free from sharp edges or loose parts
* Safe for infants to place in their mouth and chew; free from toxic or chipping paint and splinters
* Washable or easy to clean

infant bathing

Infant baths are needed only two to three times a week but may be done more often during hot weather. Regular tub baths are not given until 1 to 2 weeks after delivery when the cord has fallen off. Doors and windows are closed to prevent drafts and chilling during the bath.

Before starting the bath, necessary supplies are gathered. It is important not to leave the infant unattended (Fig. 21-7). Typical supplies needed for a bath include the following:

* Mild soap and baby shampoo
* Washcloth, towel, clean clothes, diapers, cotton balls, comb and brush
* Tub, dish pan, or clean sink

Tub bath procedure includes the following:

* Caregiver handwashing before starting the baby's bath
* Removing the infant's clothing
* Cleansing the baby's diaper area well before placing him or her in the water
* Washing the infant's face with a clean, wet washcloth; avoiding the use of soap
* Cleansing the eyes by wetting a cotton ball and wiping gently, starting close to the nose and wiping across the eye and using a clean cotton ball for each eye

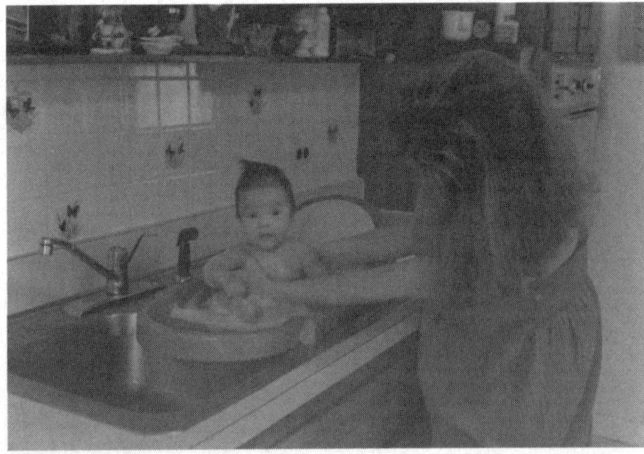

figure 21-7 *Bath time can be fun for infants and parents. (Photo by Elise Dinerman.)*

- Cleaning the ears and nose using a washcloth held snugly over the index finger (Cotton swabs are not used because the swab could be placed too deeply into the ear canal or push earwax in, causing trauma to the ear drum.)
- Shampooing the scalp by holding the infant's head over the water, supporting the back and head, rinsing off all the soap, and drying
- Placing the infant's body in the water slowly and carefully washing all folds of the skin, such as under the chin and behind the ears
- Removing the infant from the water and drying, taking care to prevent the infant from chilling

health maintenance

Parents often feel an overwhelming responsibility during the infant's first year to protect the infant from harm and maintain the infant's health. Health maintenance for the infant includes routine check-ups to assess growth and development, vision and hearing screening, and immunization schedules. Some common concerns and recommendations are summarized in Table 21-4.

screening tests for growth and development

The Denver Developmental Screening Test (DDST) is a systematic means of assessing infant skills in gross motor, language, fine motor adaptive, and personal or social areas (see Chap. 18 and Appendix). The DDST is helpful in giving nonthreatening socialization opportunities for infants and nurses.

The Carey Infant Temperament Scale (CITS) is designed to provide a profile of an infant's temperament. It is a questionnaire completed by parents on infant feeding, sleep, elimination, and play patterns. Used with infants 4 to 8 months of age, CITS provides helpful information for planning well child care and parental guidance. The Brazelton Neonatal Behavioral Assessment Scale helps caregivers "tune in" to their infant by learning more about infant personality and how caregiver responses affect the infant.

immunizations

Immunizations stimulate the infant's immunologic defenses to produce antibodies against the organism that causes a specific disease. Immunization against hepatitis is given at birth; diphtheria, tetanus, pertussis and oral polio vaccine are started at 2 months of age and repeated at 4 and 6 months (Table 21-5). Additional immunization information is found in Chapter 20.

> **nursing alert**
> *Children who get only one or two doses of a vaccine that requires four or five doses for immunity may be just as likely to get the disease as children who have had no doses.*

fever and other health concerns

Caregivers are often concerned about when to call their pediatrician about their infant's health. The nurse advises caregivers that because they know what is normal for their baby, they should not hesitate to call the doctor when they feel something is wrong. The following list can be used as a guideline. It is appropriate to call the pediatrician in the following circumstances:

- Fever (body temperature exceeding 38.4°C or 101.1°F)
- Not eating
- Vomiting more than once a day

table 21-4 common caregiver concerns and recommendations

Concern	*Recommendations*
Safe sleep	Place on back or sides in an approved crib with a firm, flat mattress. Do not use foam pads, foam sofa pillows, or water beds. Do not use fluffy bedding.
Effects of adult cigarette smoking on an infant's health	Infants can be burned or even blinded by a lighted cigarette or cigarette ash. Cigarette smoking during breast-feeding may decrease milk supply. Infants can develop vomiting, diarrhea, restlessness, and shock from nicotine in breast milk. Breathing cigarette smoke can increase the infant's risk of sudden infant death syndrome, colds, ear infection, and allergies.
Clothing needs	Dress the infant according to the weather and similar to what the caregiver is wearing. It is wise to cover the infant's head to provide warmth and protection from the sun and wind. Secure all buttons and snaps on baby's clothing.
Toy safety	Infants enjoy human faces and toys of bright and contrasting colors and textures. Toys with small parts and removable parts are considered unsafe because infants put things in their mouths.
Pacifier safety	Infants need to suck, and they get great pleasure from pacifiers. Orthodontic pacifers are better than having the infant suck on his thumb or fingers because this practice can lead to dental changes.

table 21-5 recommended immunization schedule for infants

Recommended Age	*Vaccines*
Birth, 2 mo, 6 mo	Hepatitis B (HBV)
2 mo	Diphtheria, tetanus, and pertussis (DTP #1); oral polio vaccine (OPV #1); *Haemophilus B* (Hib #1).
4 mo	DTP #2, OPV #2, Hib #2
6 mo	DTP #3, OPV #3
12 mo and older	A single dose of Varivax vaccine for chickenpox

* Coughing
* Fast, heavy breathing
* Runny nose
* Eye drainage
* Watery, frequent stools
* Pink or cloudy urine
* Less than 8 to 10 wet diapers per day
* Looks or acts sick

Fever is described as body temperature exceeding normal rectal body temperature of 37.6°C (98.6°F). A high fever (temperature exceeding 39°C or 102.2°F) does not always mean the infant has a serious infection. Acetaminophen products are recommended, such as Liquiprine, Panadol, Tempral, and Tylenol.

It is important not give an infant aspirin or products containing aspirin because aspirin is associated with Reye's syndrome, a condition affecting the brain, liver, pancreas, heart, kidneys, spleen, and lymph nodes. Reye's syndrome can be fatal (see Chap. 35). Sponge baths with water or alcohol are not recommended because they often cause the small blood vessels in the skin to constrict, causing the fever inside the body to go higher. Follow the health care agency guidelines regarding sponge baths.

✶ nursing process related to fever

Fever is described as any abnormal elevation of body temperature above normal, traditionally considered 37°C (98.6°F). Infant temperatures are typically taken rectally, making the normal reading 1 degree higher. For example, average body temperature in a 3- to 6-month-old well infant ranges from 37°C (98.6°F) to 37.5°C (99.4°F).

assessment

Subjective data include history of immaturity or neurologic dysfunction; illness or trauma, such as an ear infection or infected wound; exposure to heat; episodes of vomiting or diarrhea, increasing the risk of dehydration; and decreased fluid intake.

Objective data include sustained temperature greater than normal range. Sustained temperature readings include values of 38.8°C (101.8°F) or greater; flushed, hot, dry skin; increased respiratory rate; tachycardia; dry mucous membranes; restlessness; irritability; and loss of appetite.

nursing diagnosis

* Hyperthermia, related to illness, dehydration, or other unknown factor

planning and interventions

* Determine onset and extent of fever by monitoring temperature, pulse, and respirations (TPR) every 4 hours or more often as indicated, and document the findings.
* Administer prescribed antipyretic medications, reevaluating the TPR 30 to 45 minutes following medication administration.
* Encourage fluid intake unless contraindicated, carefully documenting ingested fluids.
* Monitor intake and output every 4 to 8 hours with attention to diminished urinary output.
* Assess infant's ability to rest, sleep, and play.
* Maintain dry clothing and bed linen to promote comfort and prevent chilling; avoid overdressing.
* Assess parents' ability to measure infant's temperature at home. Demonstrate correct technique for taking a rectal temperature using a glass mercury thermometer. For example, instruct caregiver to shake down thermometer until mercury is below 35.6°C (96.1°F), lubricate tip, and insert gently until tip of mercury bulb is inside the anus. Avoid deep insertion and trauma to infant's anus. Hold thermometer in place for approximately 3 minutes; remove, wipe clean, and read by turning it slowly until the line of mercury appears.
* Teach parents or caregivers about symptoms of elevated temperature, such as flushed, hot skin; restlessness; loss of appetite; and seizure activity.
* Teach parents or caregivers methods of decreasing hyperthermia, such as accurate administration of over-the-counter drugs that are aspirin free.
* Instruct parents to seek medical intervention if fever cannot be controlled or if infant experiences seizures, or loses consciousness.

evaluation

* Infant will maintain normal body temperature.
* Parents or caregivers will identify risk factors for hyperthermia.
* Parents or caregivers will demonstrate ability to accurately measure rectal temperature at home.

febrile seizures

Febrile seizures may occur when an infant's body temperature begins to rise suddenly. Febrile seizures occur in a small percentage of children between 5 months and 5 years. They are usually brief, lasting less than 5 minutes. This type of seizure activity does not mean a child has epilepsy.

Children experiencing febrile seizures stiffen their arms and legs; their eyes roll backward, and they may urinate or have a bowel movement during the seizure. Afterward, they may be drowsy. The caregiver must stay calm and not restrain the child in any way. The caregiver should lay the child on a flat surface, turn the head to the side, and allow the child to rest after the seizure is finished. Caregivers are instructed to seek medical intervention if the seizure does not stop within 5 to 10 minutes or if the child's lips become blue and pale.

the hospitalized infant

Hospitalization of an infant is difficult for the infant and parents. The infant may experience fear because of separation from parents or caregivers and because of pain related to illness or to diagnostic or therapeutic procedures. Infants from 1 to 6 months react primarily to changes in their routine and handling. The infant may become upset with different odors in the environment. From 7 to 12 months, infants are more responsive to a separation from parent or caregiver, reacting by crying and demonstrating behaviors of protest, despair, and detachment.

Parents of a hospitalized infant experience many concerns, including fear for the infant's life, guilt associated with illness or trauma, fear of infant rejection, guilt associated with isolation from well children, financial worries concerning long-term medical treatments and loss of work, and insecure feelings regarding child care.

Competent, compassionate nursing care can help make the hospital experience less upsetting to infants and their parents or caregivers. By teaching parents about their infant's condition and involving them in the care of the infant, the nurse helps them regain a sense of control.

key points ✳

- **Infancy, the period from 1 month to 1 year, is a time of rapid, specific, progressive, and orderly growth. Each child grows and develops at an individual pace, which is influenced by inherited genes, intrauterine environment, and extrauterine environment.**
- **Infants double their birth weight by 6 months and triple it by 12 months of age. Height increases approximately 2.6 cm (1 in) per month with a total increase of 50% over the birth length by 12 months. Most growth occurs in the trunk of the body.**
- **At birth, normal head circumference is about 35 cm (13.7 in), increasing approximately 1.3 cm (1/2 in) per month for the first 6 months and approximately 0.64 cm (1/4 in) per month between 7 and 12 months.**
- **Abdominal breathing is prevalent in infants, with a respiration rate between 20 to 40 breaths per minute.**
- **Infant motor development progresses in an orderly process, beginning with control of the head, proceeding to the trunk, and advancing to the lower extremities.**
- **An infant's sense of touch, sight, hearing, and smell are well developed by 3 months and play an important role in the infant's ability to communicate.**
- **Important developmental milestones include the ability to hold the head erect by 3 months, sit without support on a firm surface by 6 months, and bear a majority of weight on the legs by 10 months.**
- **There are 20 deciduous teeth ("baby teeth") that guide the proper positioning of permanent teeth.**
- **Teething does not cause infection but begins around the seventh month when the infant's maternal antibodies are low, making the infant less resistant to infections.**
- **The quality of the caregiver–child relationship and consistency of care are important factors in the development of infant trust.**

review questions

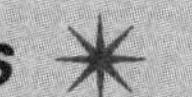

Juan Vasquez, a 6-month-old infant, is being seen in the well-baby clinic for a routine check-up. His birth weight was 8 lb according to his mother, Rosa.

1. Rosa asks the nurse how much weight Juan should have gained by now. The most appropriate nursing response would be:
   a. "All babies are different; the most important factor is that he is gaining weight."
   b. "An accepted principle of growth and development indicates that infants will double their birth weight between 5 and 6 months."
   c. "Most infants triple their birth weight around the sixth month."
   d. "Juan will gain approximately 3 lb/mo until he reaches 12 months."
2. Juan received his first immunizations of diphtheria, tetanus, and pertussis vaccine and trivalent oral poliovirus vaccine at 2 months. He is now 6 months old. what immunizations will he need?
   a. Varivax and OPT
   b. Hepatitis B and tetanus only
   c. None until he is 8 months old
   d. Diphtheria, tetanus, pertussis and oral polio vaccine.
3. Assessment of Juan's motor development at 6 months reveals an inability to sit with support. The nurse knows that this finding indicates
   a. Juan's growth is progressing in a normal pattern.
   b. Juan's motor development is abnormal, and he is most likely abused or neglected.
   c. Juan is experiencing a delay in gross motor development.
   d. Juan's ability to sit with support will be evaluated during the next visit, and if the delay is still present, he will be referred to the pediatrician for evaluation of the delay.
4. Rosa expresses concern that Juan, age 6 months, is getting spoiled. She states that she has been leaving him in his crib and ignoring his cries. The nurse knows that according to Erikson, Rosa's behaviors may cause Juan to develop
   a. mistrust of his caregiver and environment.

b. psychosexual behaviors.
c. discipline problems.
d. dislike of his mother.

5. The nurse observes Juan refusing to drink from a cup. The most appropriate nursing intervention would be to advise his mother to
   a. take him off the bottle and force him to drink from the cup.
   b. forget about cup drinking at the present time because he is not ready.
   c. withhold all liquids until he gets thirsty enough to drink from the cup.
   d. offer him diluted fruit juices from the cup, and gradually work with him until he gets used to cup drinking.

bibliography

Castiglia, P., & Harbin, R. (1992). *Child health care: Process and practice*. Philadelphia: J.B. Lippincott.

Chung, K., Olson, R., & Vinson, J. (1992). *Lippincott's review series: Pediatric nursing*. Philadelphia: J.B. Lippincott.

Eden, A. (1991). All about your baby's sleep. *American Baby, June*, 22, 86.

Gibson, J. (1992). Your loving touch. *Parents, 67*(3), 65–69.

Gulanik, M., Gradishar, D., & Puzas, M. (1994). *Ambulatory pediatric nursing*. Albany, NY: Delmar Publishers.

Jones, S. (1990) The complete guide to crying and colic. *Healthy Kids Birth, Spring/Summer*(3), 29–33.

Levine, B., & Lavi, S. (1991). Perils of childhood immunization against measles, mumps, and rubella. *Pediatric Nursing, 17*(2), 159–161.

Nettina, S. (1996). *Lippincott manual of nursing practice* (6th ed.). Philadelphia: Lippincott–Raven.

Partners Active in Learning and Sharing (PALS) (1994). *When to call the doctor*. Dayton, OH: Children's Medical Center.

Partners Active in Learning and Sharing (PALS) (1994). *Extra nutrition for extra-special babies*. Dayton, OH: Children's Medical Center.

Pillitteri, A. (1992). *Maternal and child health nursing* (2nd ed.). Philadelphia: J.B. Lippincott.

Pinyerd, B. (1992). Assessment of infant growth. *Journal of Pediatric Health Care, 6*(5), 302–307.

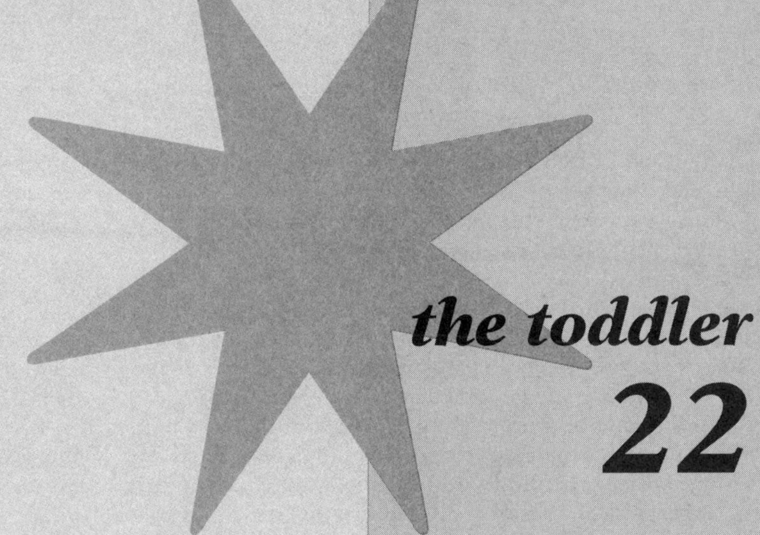

the toddler 22

outline

objectives

After studying this chapter, the reader should be able to:

* Compare the behaviors of a 1-year-old with those of a 3-year-old.
* Discuss the expected weight and height increases during the toddler years.
* Define Piaget's sensorimotor phase of cognitive development.
* Discuss the difference between egocentricism and selfishness in the toddler.
* List at least three ways a family can reinforce the toddler's sense of autonomy.
* List the three types of play typically seen during the toddler years.
* List at least four factors that influence language development in the toddler.
* Discuss the significance of bedtime rituals.
* List at least three safety factors involved with toilet training.
* Discuss factors involved in preparing the toddler for the arrival of a new baby.

key terms

autonomy
discipline
egocentrism
parallel play
punishment
separation anxiety
symbiotic play

Toddlerhood occurs between 1 and 3 years of age. The physical growth spurt seen in infancy begins to slow in the toddler years, while the individuality of the child emerges at full speed. Motor, cognitive, and psychosocial skills become more advanced. The ability to walk and talk provides the toddler with an independence that thrills and challenges the child and family. Trust established during infancy continues to develop during the toddler years as the child moves away from total dependency on caregivers.

Toddlers have a natural curiosity about life that puts them at risk for injury. Their growth and development are enhanced by providing safe learning experiences under parental guidance and control. This chapter discusses normal growth and development of the toddler, specific concerns, and health promotion.

physical growth assessment factors

Assessing the physical growth of the toddler begins with an evaluation of physical characteristics: weight and height, head and chest measurements, vision screening, dental visits, and ability to walk, run, and jump. Vital signs (see Chap. 18) and the function of various body systems (see Chapters 29–37) also are assessed.

Toddlers may be reluctant to leave the security of the caregiver during a physical examination. Allowing the toddler to sit on the caregiver's lap during the examination can reduce stress. Security objects, such as a favorite blanket or toy, also help reduce toddler stress (Fig. 22-1).

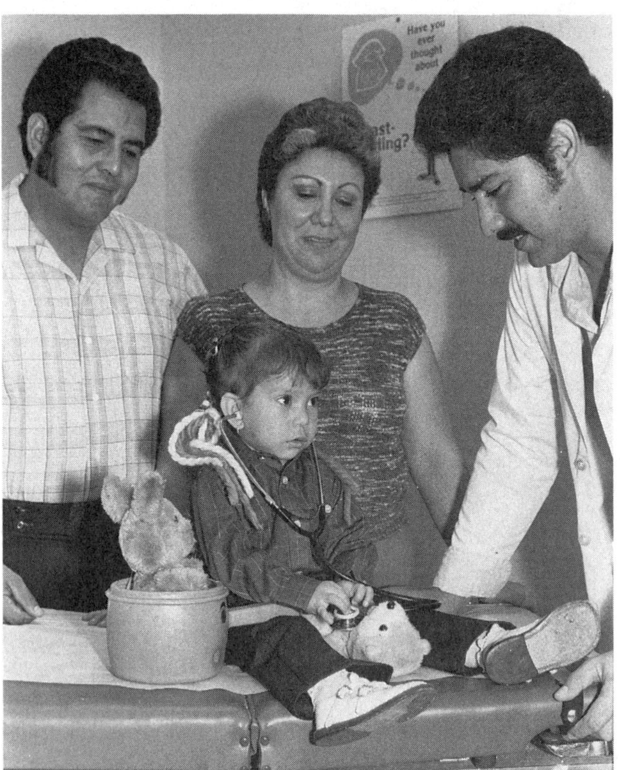

figure 22-1 *A favorite stuffed toy reduces the toddler's stress during a physical examination. (Courtesy of Texas Tech University Health Sciences Center, El Paso, Texas.)*

physical characteristics

Irregular increases are seen in the toddler's weight and height during the next 2 years, and there is no exact time when a child leaves one stage and enters another. A child can be expected to achieve certain growth and development parameters in a certain time, but these are approximations. The nurse needs to look at the physical, social, and emotional growth of the toddler as a gradual and continuous process.

weight and height

By 1 year, the toddler triples his or her birth weight. The weight begins to slow after the child's first year, with an average of 1.8 to 2.7 kg (4–6 lb) per year considered normal for the next 2 years. By 3 years, the average toddler weighs 14 to 15 kg (31–33 lb).

> **✳ nursing insight**
>
> *If the toddler is too big to weigh on an infant scale and unable to stand on adult scales, the nurse weighs herself, obtains another weight while holding the toddler, and subtracts one from the other. The difference between the two weights is the child's weight.*

The child's height increases begin to taper off after the first year with a typical gain of about 12 cm (5 in). The average height increases during the second year about 12 cm (4¾ in). Toddlers reach about half of their adult height by 24 months. A 36-month-old can be measured by standing against a growth chart or against a flat wall, marking the height, and then using a yardstick or measuring tape to obtain the correct height. Taking a height measurement on a weight scale is difficult and usually not as accurate. By 36 months, the toddler averages about 90 cm (3 ft) tall.

head and chest

Head circumference increases about 2.6 cm (1 in) between 12 and 24 months and 1.25 cm (½ in) after 36 months. This is considerably less than the 10-cm (4-in) increase seen during the first 12 months of life. The anterior fontanel (soft spot) closes between 1 and 18 months. By 2 years, the skull is about three fourths of its adult size. Chest size continues to increase during toddlerhood.

extremities

Most toddlers walk with a wide stance. Their abdomen protrudes because of weak abdominal muscles, and their legs bow due to the weight of a large trunk. The legs eventually straighten as leg muscles develop. Toddlers seem to be in constant movement and love to walk, climb, and jump. Between 2 and 3 years, long bones of the arms and legs reach approximately 34% of the body length.

display 22-1
developmental milestones of the toddler

18 MONTHS

* Walks alone
* Walks forward and backward
* Runs poorly with frequent falls
* Builds a tower of two blocks
* Scribbles spontaneously with large crayons
* Helps turn pages in a book
* Takes off clothing
* Unwraps candy or gum
* Fits one object inside another
* Turns a doorknob
* Tears paper
* Soaps hands and arms
* Uses a spoon and cup
* Recognizes familiar people and objects
* Begins to display a more difficult nature, saying "no" to most requests
* Throws temper tantrums to express anger

24 MONTHS

* Throws a ball overhand
* Kicks a ball forward
* Walks up and down stairs
* Builds a tower of four cubes
* Turns doorknobs
* Unscrews lids
* Removes shoes
* Helps with dressing and undressing
* Can be testy, stubborn, and quite verbal in stating demands
* Displays resourcefulness in getting what is wanted
* Needs praise for completing simple tasks around the house, imitating parental and sibling behaviors, and communicating specific needs

36 MONTHS

* Jumps in place
* Balances briefly on one foot
* Exercises by touching toes, knees, and shoulders
* Builds a tower of eight cubes
* Catches a large ball with arms straight
* Strings large beads
* Holds crayons with likeness of adult
* Separates more easily from caregiver
* Enjoys interactive games
* Knows gender differences
* Throws fewer tantrums
* Begins to learn cause and effect
* Bowel and bladder training is enhanced by the toddler's mature sphincter control and ability to understand simple explanations and comply with simple requests
* Bowel and bladder accidents are more common when the toddler is ill or experiences a disruption of routine

developmental assessment

developmental events

Growth and development noted during toddlerhood are separate and combined. For example, the toddler who learns to use a spoon combines motor skills, hand–eye coordination, and social imitation from watching others (Display 22-1).

✳ nursing process related to parent or caregiver risk of knowledge deficit concerning expected growth and development during toddlerhood

assessment

Subjective data to be assessed include the following:

* Parental or caregiver acknowledgement of an inadequate understanding or knowledge base of physical and psychosocial expectations during toddlerhood
* Comments about toilet training, play, and discipline reflecting an intolerance or rejection of the child
* Caregiver expectations of the child
* History of illness or trauma associated with child abuse or neglect, such as limited social or emotional stimulation or unexplained bone fractures

Objective data to be assessed include evaluation of physical, gross and fine motor development, language skills, and social and emotional growth.

nursing diagnosis

* Risk for Parent or Caregiver Knowledge Deficit, related to expected growth and development.

nursing interventions

* Observe the interaction between toddler and caregivers.
* Ask the parents or caregivers about their expectations for the toddler now and in the near future to determine age-appropriate expectations. Discuss temper tantrums, stressing that physical punishment is not the solution to control the toddler; setting consistent limits or using distraction tends to be more effective. The child can be isolated until he or she is in control, and then the

tantrum can be discussed in a calm, loving way. Distraction can be accomplished by placing a large mirror where the child can see his or her full image.

* Demonstrate proper care of the toddler related to hygiene and nutrition.
* Outline current growth and development expectations concerning toilet training. For example, stress that toilet training takes time and usually begins at 2 years, first with bowel control and then bladder control. This takes months to complete and requires consistent praise and reassurances without pressure when accidents happen.
* Provide parents or caregivers with information about child safety, including child-proofing the home by locking away dangerous chemicals and medicines, installing smoke and carbon monoxide detectors, using electrical outlet guards, removing dangling electrical cords, and guarding against falls. Car accidents are a major cause of death in children, especially when safety seats and safety belts are not used.

evaluation

* Parent or caregiver will verbalize expected developmental milestones for the toddler's age and the next level of development.
* Parent or caregiver will verbalize safety measures pertinent to the toddler.

psychosocial development

Toddlerhood is stressful for the child and caregiver as a result of the struggle between dependence and independence. This time is marked by negativism, which stems from the child's developing sense of independence. Frequently, toddlers do not comply with parental requests and respond to commands with a "no" even when they mean "yes."

Nursing assessment for lack of psychosocial development includes observing for signs of physical or neurologic disorders and absence or limitation of social and emotional stimulation provided in the home. A sense of doubt and shame can develop when toddlers are kept dependent in areas where they feel capable of using acquired skills. For example, caregivers who persist in feeding toddlers when they are capable of feeding themselves may find the toddler reluctant to eat and reluctant to try a new skill, such as self-dressing.

Because caregivers continue to be the most significant influence, toddlers often mimic parental behaviors. They are quick to realize how their behaviors affect the family. Through family interactions, toddlers learn that parents can be predictable and reliable. They begin to learn that their own behaviors have a predictable and reliable effect on others.

erikson's psychosocial development

Erikson described the psychosocial development in the toddler older than 18 months as a sense of *autonomy versus shame and doubt*. Autonomy (independent functioning) develops when parents allow toddlers to make simple choices while maintaining consistent rules for safety. According to Erikson, toddlers whose parents discourage them from trying new activities can be left with a strong sense of doubt.

Toddlers made to feel guilty for wanting independence may be left with feelings of shame and doubt. If a sense of trust is established between the toddler and parents during the first 18 months, the toddler is willing to give up dependence on the parents to assert self-control, independence, and autonomy.

A toddler's sense of autonomy is reinforced when he or she accomplishes the following tasks:

* Communicates with words
* Has control of body functions
* Separates easily from caregiver(s)
* Is mobile

sexual exploration

The toddler is a natural explorer, experimenting by trial and error, with a keen appreciation for the exploration's outcome. The toddler demonstrates increased awareness of the genital area through masturbation. Parents need to show a matter-of-fact acceptance of such body explorations and remember toddlers are involved with learning through exploring. Toddlers need to learn that all body parts are good. Parents should accept body exploration as a normal toddler process and avoid reprimanding the toddler. During toddlerhood, boys have penis erections related to physical stimulation but are usually not able to relate the erection with heterosexual or homosexual activity.

setting limits

Many behavior "mistakes" are errors in judgment because the toddler lacks knowledge or ability to grasp a more acceptable behavior pattern. Caregivers must emphasize displeasure with the behavior while still showing love for the child. Withdrawing love and affection as a punishment leads to feelings of guilt in the toddler. Although a toddler's behavior may not be appropriate or acceptable to the adult, the behavior often reflects the toddler's maturity level. Caregivers need to take behavioral cues from their toddler to help limit activities that are frustrating and require intervention, such as "friendly warnings" or an activity change. For example, a statement such as "Johnny, leave your clothing on or you will have to stay in the house" or encouraging another activity can keep the toddler from undressing.

cognitive development

Piaget refers to the age between 12 and 24 months as the *sensorimotor phase* of cognitive development. The sensorimotor phase involves the child's ability to pick up objects and explore them by looking, feeling, and tasting. The sensorimotor phase involves the tertiary circular reaction stage and the preconceptual stage.

The *tertiary circular reaction stage* involves exploring and discovering new ways to learn about the environment.

The majority of learning at this stage is achieved through trial and error, putting the toddler at risk for injury if not properly supervised.

The *preconceptual phase* depicts the toddler using images to remember the past, picture the present, and anticipate the future. During this phase, the toddler engages in pretend play and uses role playing, mimicking caregiver and sibling behaviors. An example of role playing is when the toddler watches a parent demonstrate loving gestures to a sibling and these same gestures are repeated by the toddler toward a doll. Nursing care is enhanced by using role play with the toddler.

Toddlers engage in an innocent assumption that their own view of the world is exactly the same as everyone else's. This thinking process is called *egocentrism* and should not be considered the same as being selfish (although there are some similarities). Toddlers are limited at this stage of development to viewing the world with themselves at the center. This egocentric judgment represents the inability to take anyone else's desires or rights into consideration because of limited experiences and depth of reasoning. As the toddler develops and matures, he or she naturally progresses from egocentrism to an awareness of others.

Parental understanding and guidance are essential in promoting the toddler's progress toward an awareness of others. Caregivers play a critical role in providing children with exposure to new experiences. The nurse can reassure caregivers that egocentricism is one of the many stages toddlers go through on their way to maturity (Table 22-1).

Toddlers love to be around people, and they show less fear of strangers than during infancy. During illness, toddlers may demonstrate behaviors such as clinging to the caregiver, shyness, and irritability. The nurse needs to reassure the caregiver that this behavior is normal and should direct attention away from the child and establish rapport with the caregiver before touching the child.

Toddlers are lovable and will hug and kiss familiar people and things, including pets. Adult supervision is recommended when toddlers play with pets because the child may hug the pet too firmly while showing affection, increasing the risk of injury from an animal bite. They also can display signs of jealousy and negative behavior when they perceive more attention is given to another child.

Between 18 to 24 months of age, the toddler has learned property rights and will say, "This is Mommy's," and "This is mine." Toddlers enjoy watching and imitating people. By this age, the toddler has a good memory, recalls events of the previous day, can respond to verbal directions, and can find mental solutions to problems. By 3 years of age, the toddler may count to 10 or more, compare two objects, recognize different sizes, know his or her own age, and remember fear caused by one experience and compare it with another experience. Toddlers have a limited sense of time and may dawdle and act stubborn when hurried. Their feelings are easily hurt or irritated. They eagerly seek praise, attention, and conversation with adults, asking many "why" questions and expecting answers.

moral development

According to Kohlberg, the toddler is in the *preconventional* stage of moral development, learning to conform to rules imposed by authority figures. Fear of disapproval or punishment motivates the toddler's choices of action. The child's perception of good or bad develops associated with the consequences.

Because the toddler has no internal strengths to govern behavior, caregiver supervision and guidance are important. Appropriate disciplinary actions include providing

table 22-1 emotional, intellectual, social, and physical development of the toddler

Age	Emotional Development	Intellectual Development	Social Development	Physical Development
1 y	Self-centered; unpredictable; hugs favorite toy	Loves to throw things; can say a few words; likes to imitate and pretend; can make simple drawing strokes	Enjoys talking to adults; shows affection for family; likes to be chased	Likes to stay in motion; starting to stand and walk alone; can build a crude tower of blocks
2 y	Responds to praise; sensitive to being bossed; anger is directed at responsible person	Knows where things are and where they belong; can pull a toy while walking backward; likes to feed self	Gets into everything; desires independence; enjoys playing roughly; benefits from being with other children	Walks with feet spread apart; can jump; likes to climb; can take off shoes; likes to poke fingers into holes
3 y	Is more cooperative and able to show self-control; proud of self-made items; capable of holding a grudge	Likes to repeat words; can name some colors; may compare two objects; can draw a person	Likes simple guessing games; learns to obey rules; enjoys parties	Better coordination; can hop; can string large beads

simple explanations about why certain behaviors are unacceptable, praising appropriate behavior, and using distraction. Physical punishment and restricted privileges can put the child at risk for limited or negative moral development. Fortunately, their short attention span makes distraction a useful tactic.

motor development

gross motor development

The toddler's gross motor development continues in a cephalocaudal progression, as discussed in Chapter 17. An important nursing assessment includes observing the toddler move all limbs with equal ease and range of motion. Disturbances in motor skill development may indicate neurologic or musculoskeletal disorders. Toddlers begin walking with a wide gait, progressing to walking on tiptoes, jumping, running, and balancing on one foot.

fine motor development

Fine motor skill is reflected by the toddler's ability to master fine motor skills from infancy. For example, command of the pincer movement enables the toddler to unbutton clothing, handle blocks, and hold a crayon or pencil for scribbling.

personal and social development

Toddlers can obey simple commands, such as "look at the book," and point to pictures that are familiar. They have a good memory and can remember where things belong, looking in familiar places for books, toys, snacks, and so forth. Toddlers display many advanced behaviors; however, they often stubbornly hold onto their security object (eg, blanket, toy).

Toddlers often grab desired objects and may have difficulty grasping the concept of sharing. When sharing is forced, the toddler may resort to pulling the other child's hair or biting before giving up the prized toy. Substituting a toy that is similar in size and color can be effective in distracting the toddler and solving the dilemma of ownership of the toy.

> **✳ nursing insight**
>
> *The toddler's security object becomes most important when he or she feels anxious and should be given as a comfort measure when safety and security are threatened.*

temper tantrums

Toddlers have a low tolerance for frustration when unable to complete a task and will respond with negative behavior, such as temper tantrums, which occur equally in boys and girls and throughout all ranges of intelligence. Temper tantrums are uncontrolled outbursts of anger and are a natural sequence of toddler development. Toddlers are struggling with the issues of autonomy and control while remaining dependent on their parents for care. The independent toddler may know what he or she wants but does not always have the vocabulary or the wisdom to express those wants. Consequently, angry behaviors are the result.

Developmentally handicapped and mentally retarded children are especially prone to tantrums. Children with severe limitations in expressive language may be frustrated by their inability to express their needs effectively, so they resort to temper tantrums.

A tantrum is normally preceded by an apparent aggravation that "triggers" the tantrum. The trigger may be one of the following:

* Minor trauma
* Wanting an object and not being able to get it
* Wanting to win and not succeeding
* Attempting a task beyond ability
* Being forced to do something unwanted
* Experiencing disapproval or discipline

Temper tantrums often begin with crying that accelerates. The toddler often loses control and may fall, flailing arms and legs, shouting, biting, spitting, or scratching. The angry toddler may strike out, break toys, or lie in the middle of a street, store, park, or room. The usual temper tantrum lasts from 2 to 5 minutes but may last as long as 10 minutes and may include holding the breath.

Breath holding is frightening for the parents who fear for the toddler's health. Breath holding is visible by a distended chest, air-filled cheeks, and increasing distress as the body indicates a want for oxygen. This behavior is considered harmless and should be ignored.

Although tantrums are usually harmless, their frequency and severity can increase a toddler's risk of physical injury. Tantrums also can weaken family relationships, putting the child at risk for abuse or isolation and hindering the development of friendship among peers. The management of a temper tantrum involves distraction, especially if the tantrum is pending. Distraction is used to divert the toddler's attention to another activity or toy and reduces attention on the situation that was causing the original frustration. Once the tantrum is in progress, the toddler needs to be isolated from stimuli, protected from injury, and basically ignored. Parental concern and attention during the tantrum rewards the toddler, but ignoring the tantrum tends to discourage the behavior. If the tantrum occurs in a public place, parents need to remain calm and refuse to give the toddler what is demanded. Once the tantrum has stopped, parents should interact with the toddler and compliment him or her for regaining self-control.

play

Play is an important part of the toddler's everyday experiences and is often referred to as the work of the toddler even though it is not goal directed. It is informal, spontaneous, and fun. Play is an integral part of growth and development and reflects a toddler's interests. The pleasure of play between 12 and 24 months is largely sensorimotor and includes sucking, mouthing, making sounds, listening, grasping and handling objects, crawling, walking, running, and exploring the body. Toddlers enjoy *parallel play* (play-

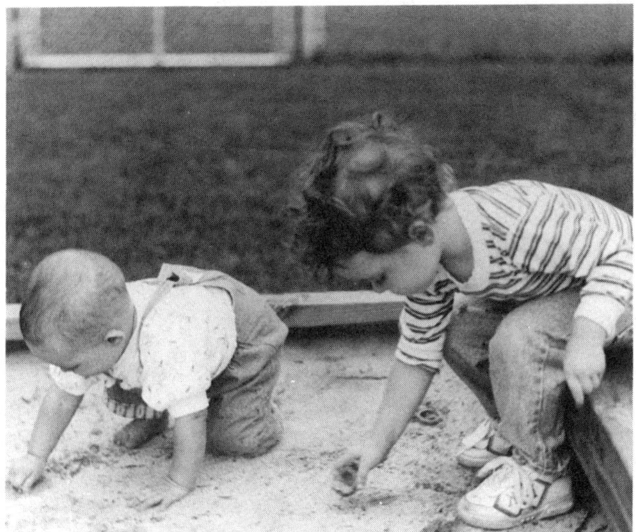

figure 22-2 *Toddlers enjoy parallel play.*

ing close to other children but individually; Fig. 22-2). See Table 22-2 for additional information on play and growth and development.

Between 2 and 3 years, the toddler tries to use objects to copy things previously experienced. For example, child-safe clay may be used to make a house. The use of objects to combine environmental experiences is known as *symbiotic play*. Toddlers love to imitate behavior and enjoy make believe or pretend play.

Pretend play can help enable the sick toddler to sort out feelings about the illness, nurses, and doctors. By using a stuffed animal, hurtful procedures can be imitated without consequence. The stuffed animal can later be cuddled by the toddler and the nurse.

Toddlers who are 3 years old are more physically and intellectually developed and able to play with other children in more cooperative type play. They can understand the significance of sharing toys and ideas to make friends. Toddlers ask a lot of questions and like simple guessing games. The 3-year-old benefits from group experiences and often enjoys going to nursery school.

language development

Language development is one of the major tasks of toddlerhood. A 2-year-old toddler normally talks in simple sentences with a vocabulary of approximately 20 to 50 words.

The development of language use goes along with the development of thinking and understanding. Language skills are learned and perfected through practice. The toddler learns frequently used adjectives, such as "good" and "bad" by 18 months. Toddlers frequently learn pronouns last because understanding pronouns is complex and confusing to the average toddler. An example of a typical toddler sentence is "Me want to play ball."

Toddlers sometimes reach a *plateau* stage in learning to talk. This occurs when the toddler is too busy growing and developing in other ways (eg, walking) to acquire new words. The toddler continues to expand understanding of new words, although he or she is too busy to say them.

Learning two languages does not confuse children or cause learning problems. When toddlers are learning two languages, they may learn fewer words in each language at first but tend to catch up by the time sentences are used.

Toddlers who have a limited vocabulary become easily frustrated and will cry more to express their feelings and wishes. Crying occurs in toddlers with a good command of language when they are too frightened, hurt, or sick to verbally express their concerns. Even when the toddler is able to speak, his or her emotions may be too great to put into words, and crying releases the anger and disappointment.

> ✱ **nursing insight**
>
> *The nurse is a stranger to the toddler, and procedures are often seen as "hurtful." It is helpful to offer simple explanations about what you plan to do and discuss the toddler's feelings concerning the procedure rather than the child's behavior.*

health promotion

The nurse plays an important role in teaching caregivers of toddlers about nutrition, daily hygiene, sleep habits and patterns, toilet training, and discipline. Providing helpful information to parents during toddlerhood can help avoid problems in later stages of life.

nutrition

Toddler growth slows at the end of the first year and is reflected in a decreased and sporadic appetite (even though the toddler is active, the need for food is less because of slower growth). Some toddlers may have a tendency to gain weight. Although this may be an inherited tendency, healthy eating habits can be learned. This is important because children can suffer physically and psychologically from the burden of carrying extra pounds.

Many toddlers are ritualistic concerning food preferences, schedules, and manners of eating. Episodes of physiologic anorexia are noted as the result of alternating periods of fast and slow growth with the toddler experiencing "food binges" (specific foods are favored exclusively or refused for no apparent reason).

Most toddlers prefer to feed themselves but need supervision because they enjoy playing in their food and may attempt to put pieces of food into their nose and ears. Self-feeding is encouraged with supervision because this increases their sense of autonomy. Giving the toddler child-sized forks, spoons, and plates aids in self-feeding. Toddlers will often assert themselves by refusing food or feeding assistance (Fig. 22-3).

Toddlers should not be given small foods that are not easily chewed (eg, popcorn, peanuts, and corn on the cob) because they can be easily aspirated. Care must be taken

table 22-2 the role of play in growth and development of the toddler

Type of Development	*Activities*	*Suggested Toys*	*Safety*
Physical	Running, jumping, and other playground activities develop muscles, wear off extra energy, and refine muscle control.	Sturdy and safe outdoor toys that allow the toddler to play "rough" but safe; small tricycle and wagon; sand box, large balls	Toddlers need adult supervision. Because a toddler's attention span is short, he or she moves freely from place to place. He or she should not be given toys that are sharp or have rough edges. Toys painted with lead paint are dangerous.
Social	Parallel play provides the toddler with social interactions and allows him or her to experience companionship and learn to cope with others. Make-believe plays a role in helping the toddler sort out feelings and understand relationships. A toddler can test the limits of right and wrong when done under the pretense of a make-believe friend.	Dolls, stuffed animals, large box or cardboard playhouse, toy cars, rocking horse, hats and dress-up clothing, hand puppet, and play dishes	Close supervision is necessary because toddlers enjoy throwing objects and picking them up. They enjoy watching other children play but have not learned group consensus. Toddlers often want what the other child has and may get verbally and physically aggressive. The play area must be free of any items onto or into which the toddler could climb. Small toys with removable parts may be swallowed or aspirated by the toddler.
Educational	The toddler begins to learn colors, shapes, sizes, and textures of play material from the selection of toys.	Cloth or plastic books, music, puppets, building blocks, large peg board, art supplies, blunt scissors, clay, and nesting toys	Supervise the toddler when or she is using scissors to make sure he or she cuts paper and not clothes, hair, self, or household articles. Toddlers love to make mud pies and may be tempted to eat them.
Therapeutic value	Allowing an angry child to vent hostilities by expressing emotions in a controlled setting is psychologically and physically helpful.	Bean bags, Nerf toys, art supplies, rubber mat, punching bag	Careful observation is needed to prevent self-injury. Once the toddler has vented frustration, he or she should be taught less aggressive ways to vent emotions. It is important to teach the child that anger is a normal emotion.
Moral value	Older toddlers begin to learn right from wrong through play. They begin to understand the importance of game rules.	Board games, card games, such as "fish"	Toddlers have a short attention span and require a variety of activities and toys to keep them involved. They can become frustrated easily with games and must be allowed to shift their attention as needed.

with hot dogs because their round and slippery shape may cause the child to choke. It is safer to cut a hot dog lengthwise and then into small pieces that the toddler can hold and feed himself or herself. Raw carrots should never be fed to young children unless shredded.

The toddler's diet includes a full range of foods that provide 100 kcal/kg per day, including milk, meat, fruits, vegetables, breads, and cereals. The toddler needs approximately 1,300 calories per day. Because body tissue, especially muscles, continues to grow rapidly, protein needs are high. Calcium recommendations are 800 mg/d. Calcium and phosphorus are important for this age group. Most toddlers do better by eating four smaller meals per day than three larger meals. The older toddler will consume approximately half the amount of food an adult consumes.

Pediatricians vary in their opinions on the use of supplemental vitamins. The toddler who is not consuming an adequate daily diet should certainly take them; however, a vitamin pill is not a substitute for good eating habits.

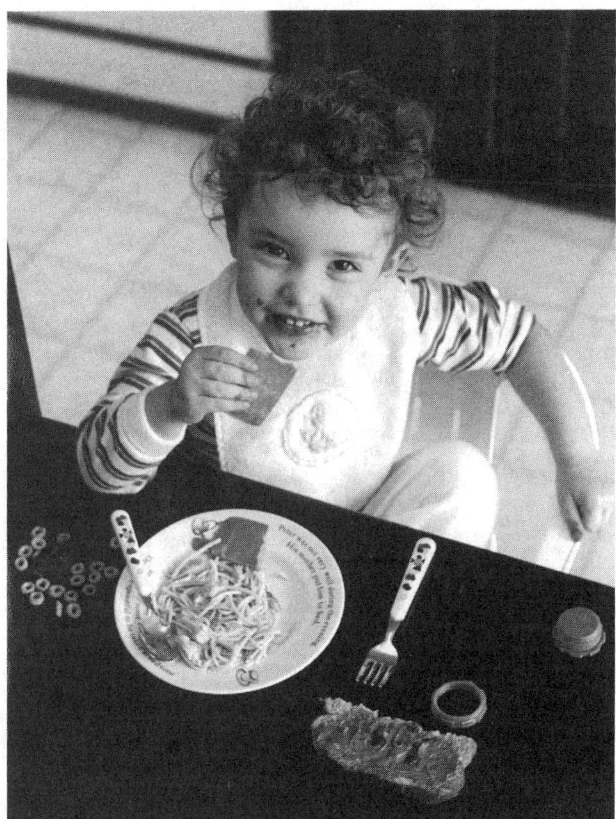

figure 22-3 *A toddler's skill in self-feeding is enhanced by using child-sized forks, spoons, and plates.*

Breakfast is frequently a toddler's favorite meal. Evaluate what the toddler has eaten in a 5- to 7-day period rather than in a 24-hour period. Survey the toddler's activity level and steady growth and development progress as indicators of normal nutritional intake. See the Teaching Guidelines on promoting positive eating experiences.

Toddlers can help with dressing and undressing themselves. They usually like water and enjoy playing in the tub but need assistance and supervision with bathing. During hospitalization, nurses must follow the toddler's bath time rituals if possible. Plastic or rubber toys suitable for the tub are recommended.

Dental care is important to prevent dental caries in the deciduous teeth. The major cause of tooth decay is lactic acid formed by bacteria that live on sugars. Candy and crackers should be avoided between meals, and if a toddler needs a bottle at night or naptime, it should be water and not milk.

Teeth require brushing with a small soft-bristled toothbrush and parental assistance after each meal and at bedtime. The toddler is taught to brush from the gum line to the edge of the teeth, including the tongue. Visits to the dentist should begin around 18 months (Fig. 22-4).

> **✶ nursing insight**
>
> *Milk is a good source of protein, phosphorus, and calcium; however, too much milk, will decrease the child's appetite for other foods and increase the risk of anemia.*

> **teaching guidelines ✶**
> **promoting positive eating experiences**
>
> * Use silverware and plates scaled to size of child.
> * Use unbreakable plastic bowls and dishes for safety.
> * Place toddler in a highchair or booster chair for meals.
> * Limit concentrated sweets and empty calories, and avoid the use of sweets as rewards.
> * Allow sufficient time for the toddler to eat, taking food away once the child starts to play with it.
> * Encourage independence by allowing the child to feed self.
> * Avoid strict table manners for toddler.
> * Avoid bribes or forced feedings reinforcing negative behavior.
> * Provide a variety of foods, especially vegetables and protein.
> * Avoid the use of food as a reward or punishment.

sleep

Sleep requirements vary with each toddler. Nightly sleeping time of 10 to 14 hours with a 1- or 2-hour daytime nap is considered average for this age. Toddlers tend not to be interested in sleep, but the normal daily cycle of sleep is a necessary physiologic process.

The toddler gains a sense of security when simple tasks are done with certain rituals (eg, reading a bedtime story). Bedtime rituals are helpful for the toddler who resists going to bed because certain habits are associated with sleep. Some children require special toys or a blanket, bedtime stories, being held or rocked, or receiving a special snack. (Bedtime bottles are often the last bottles to be given up by

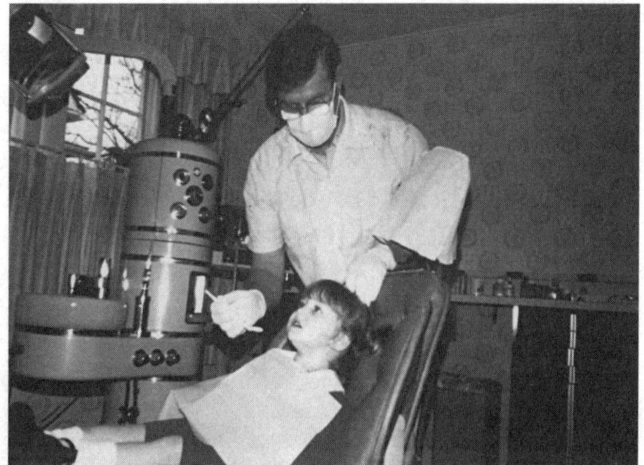

figure 22-4 *Dental visits begin around age 18 months.*

the toddler.) Lengthy, complicated bedtime rituals should be avoided. Toddlers need to know that bedtime is for sleeping, and loud talking or rowdy play is not acceptable. Toddler compliance to bedtime rules should be praised. Caregivers who work, are ill, or who have limited or no support systems may feel too tired at the end of the day to comply with the toddler's rituals. Inability to cope with the child's demands may precipitate abusive behavior.

At about 2 years, the toddler may develop a fear of the dark and may require a small night-light at bedtime. Nightmares may occur because the toddler is unable to distinguish between reality and wishes or fantasies. The toddler may have wished for "Mommy to go away" during play and now is scared that those wishes will come true.

✳ nursing insight

Discuss the toddler's bedtime routines with parents, and comply as much as possible with the child's established patterns, remembering that environmental changes, such as hospitalization, may cause nightmares.

When toddlers awaken in the middle of the night crying from fearful dreams, they need to be held until calm, encouraged to talk about their fears, given reassurances, and then returned to bed. Responding to the toddler's cries gives reassurance that his or her needs will be met. This process can be time consuming and tiring, especially if it has to be repeated several times during the night. However, it generally works better than taking the toddler out of bed. Allowing the toddler to sleep with the parents is not desirable for the following reasons:

* Toddlers tend to sleep less soundly as they get older, and their sleep will be disturbed by adult sounds, such as coughing or snoring.
* Parents and child are deprived of their privacy.
* Toddlers will not learn to conquer their fears unless they are given the chance to resolve the nightmare and return to sleep in their personal space.

The transition from crib to bed can interrupt a toddler's sleep pattern and cause night awakenings or nightmares (Table 22-3). There is no specific time to move a toddler from the crib to a bed, but safety is an important factor. The toddler who climbs over crib sides risks injury and needs to be protected by adding rails to the crib or by placing the toddler in a bed. When placed in a bed, the toddler can be protected from falling out of the bed by adding side rails to the bed. See the Teaching Guidelines promoting positive sleep patterns.

toilet training

Toilet training is a major accomplishment usually completed by 30 months; however, there is no "correct" age to begin toilet training. Most studies show that the majority of children will not develop control until after 24 months. Bowel control is usually easier to accomplish than bladder control. Toddlers who remain continent during the day may be incontinent during naptime and bedtime and have occasional "accidents." The parents and the toddler must be ready for toilet training. If this is not the case, anxiety can result, and child abuse is possible. See the Teaching Guidelines on bathroom safety and toilet training.

discipline

The toddler needs direct, well-planned discipline to achieve social and cultural acceptance. Discipline is not the same as punishment. Effective discipline enables toddlers to make some decisions about what courses of action are appropriate within the limits of their capabilities and guides the toddler's behavior in a firm but loving manner. Punishment expresses the power of personal authority used to decrease misbehavior and involves unpleasant and painful physical or mental measures in response to a

table 22-3 sleep problems

Special Sleep Problems	*Suggested Interventions*
Night fears	Avoid excitement before bedtime. Monitor television, stories, and play that depicts violence or frightening occurrences.
Sleep walking (seen more frequently in boys)	This is frequently outgrown, suggesting the behavior is maturational rather than psychological. Leave the child alone unless the child is in danger or is a danger to others. If you must awaken the child, do so by calling the child's name slowly and softly. When the child is awake, orient him or her to time and place.

teaching guidelines ✳
promoting positive sleep patterns

* Do not use the bed as punishment.
* Do not allow complicated sleep rituals.
* Do not try to force sleep if the toddler awakens early and is content to sing or play happily.
* Respond to the child's initial cry, but allow the toddler to "cry it out" after you have assessed there is no apparent discomfort. "Crying it out" allows the child to relieve frustrations and master control over emotions.
* Provide the toddler with a night light.
* Allow the toddler to sit up and look at a book quietly if not ready to sleep.
* Do not allow the child to sleep with you.

teaching guidelines
bathroom safety

Toilets can be enticing and deadly to toddlers if they fall into them. Toddlers can drown in a toilet or suffer permanent injury as a result of the fall. Avoid such dangers:

* Toddlers should not be allowed in the bathroom without supervision.
* Toilet-seat safety clamps are recommended to keep the toilet lid securely shut.

wrongdoing. Discipline teaches children how to follow the rules and expectations of society and become socialized into the broader world. In contrast, punishment teaches the toddler he or she must act a certain way to avoid pain.

Disciplinary methods for the toddler must be safety-minded and age appropriate. The toddler's need for autonomy can lead him or her to behaviors that are neither safe nor socially tolerable. Unfortunately, many caregivers use punishment measures rather than disciplinary methods for controlling negative behavior. Parents are powerful role models of what is right and expected for their children and may not realize that they are teaching their children violence when they use corporal punishment. When violence is used in the home, children tend to fear rather than learn from their behaviors.

Toddlers need encouragement to develop and use social skills. When toddlers do not learn the limits of acceptable behavior, they suffer frustration and anxiety. Setting limits during toddlerhood provides a basis for trust. Toddlers may misbehave because they do not know what is considered acceptable behavior. Effective discipline involves parental understanding of the toddler's primary personality drives associated with growth and development needs. (See Table 22-4 for additional information on discipline, punishment, and effective parenting.)

family relationships

The toddler's world is centered in the family; this is where he or she learns how to interact with others. How parents interact with their children affects how children interact with each other.

separation anxiety

The fear of separation from parents (usually the mother) peaks around the middle of the second year and ends by 3 years. A toddler's security often depends on his or her mother because she provides love, food, and security; consequently, the fear of losing this very important person is most threatening. The toddler cannot understand why he

teaching guidelines
toilet training

EVIDENCE OF TODDLER'S READINESS

* Regularity in patterns of elimination
* Ability to walk unassisted to the bathroom or potty chair
* An understanding of the importance of sitting still
* Ability to remove clothing (especially underwear)
* Ability to recognize and communicate urges to defecate and urinate by bringing attention to a soiled or wet diaper
* Display of a desire to please by cooperating, holding onto, and letting go of bowel and bladder contents

EVIDENCE OF PARENT'S READINESS

* Recognition of the toddler's readiness, displayed by specific posturing or behaviors that signal a need to urinate or defecate
* Ability and desire to invest the necessary time and energy into toilet training on a daily basis for a minimum of 3 months.

TOILET TRAINING IMPLEMENTATION

* Allow the toddler to become familiar with a potty chair by looking, touching, and sitting on it.
* Familiarize the toddler with bathroom activity by permitting observation of caregiver toileting.
* Allow the toddler to sit on the chair with clothes on because a cold potty seat can be a negative experience until he or she gets used to the feeling.
* Promote relaxation by reading books and talking while sitting on the toilet.
* Progress from diapers to training pants after successful use of the potty chair.
* Allow child to observe stool in the potty chair by taking stool from a soiled diaper and placing it in the potty.
* Allow the child to flush the potty contents unless there is fear associated with the noise of flushing (some children fear being flushed down into the toilet).
* Do not force a child to sit on the potty chair.
* Do not keep the child on the potty for more than 10–15 minutes.
* Progress to the toilet once the child has mastered the potty chair.
* Encourage the child to void each morning and before play, naptime, bedtime, and going on trips.
* Encourage boys to stand to void.
* Avoid punishment for accidents.
* Always supervise the child while in the bathroom.

table 22-4 effective parenting, discipline, punishment

Effective Parenting	*Discipline*	*Punishment*
Toddler's mutual rights are respected and acknowledged; child is aware of expected behavior.	Toddler is allowed to make choices when appropriate	No choices are permitted
Misbehavior is discussed regarding child's actions being only a part of the whole child, thus providing the child with an understanding of personal love, worth, and expectations for future behavior.	Discipline is related to the misbehavior and does not imply personal moral judgment.	Punishment is related to misbehavior and is personalized.

or she is separated from his or her mother and displays fear by crying, throwing temper tantrums, or holding the breath.

The toddler develops normal fears that go along with learning new skills and abilities. Separation anxiety is intensified by the fact that the toddler can walk and wander away from the parents. With support and reassurance of the parents, most children quickly outgrow the fear of separation.

sibling relations

When parents pay more attention to one child over another, conflicts and less friendly relationships can develop between siblings. Highly active, emotionally intense children tend to be more competitive and more negative in sibling relationships. Children who are shy or who recover quickly from emotional upsets tend to be less competitive and more positive in their sibling relationships. Researchers have observed that same-gender pairs tend to get along better than brother–sister combinations.

When confronted with strong emotions, the toddler will respond more positively to simple explanations that help him or her gain some control over the situation. Statements such as "don't cry" or "act your age" indicate a lack of understanding of the toddler's strong emotions concerning the situation.

Toddlers often have difficulty sharing parental love with siblings. The toddler may resent siblings. It is important for the toddler to be shown love by siblings. Older siblings may find it difficult to relate to the toddler and may voice strong criticism about the toddler's behavior if they do not understand this phase of growth and development.

Older siblings may act as a teacher to the toddler, who is learning new words, coloring with crayons, and playing pretend. Toddlers enjoy being included in older children's play and can experience a feeling of importance.

arrival of a new baby

A new baby requires significant adjustment on the part of the toddler. Toddlers need to be prepared for the arrival 1 to 2 months before the baby is due. This can be done by showing them their baby pictures and allowing the toddler to observe a baby receiving care. After the newborn is delivered, many hospitals permit sibling visitation. Toddlers should be encouraged to interact with the newborn under supervision (Fig. 22-5).

Regardless of careful preparation and planning, toddlers may display signs of regressive behavior when the

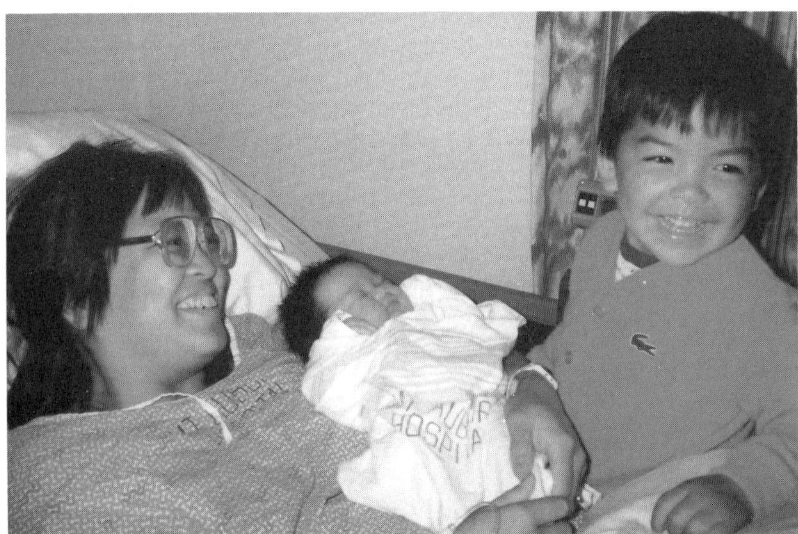

figure 22-5 *Many hospitals encourage sibling visits to facilitate bonding and to decrease rivalry.*

neonate is brought home. The regressive behavior may be demonstrated as clingy, jealous, or aggressive attempts to gain the parents' attention. The toddler may attempt to nurse or demand a bottle, suck the thumb, and even ask to wear diapers as a means of seeking attention. Parents should praise age-appropriate behavior and ignore the regressive behavior.

The new baby should not be described as a playmate for the toddler because unrealistic infant expectations may develop. With supervision, toddlers can be encouraged to help parents and older siblings care for the newborn.

health maintenance

immunizations

Immunizations during the toddler years include the following:

* Measles, mumps, and rubella at 15 months
* Diphtheria, tetanus, pertussis and oral polio vaccine at 18 months
* *Haemophilus influenzae* type b polysaccharide vaccine at 24 months
* Hepatitis B vaccine between 6 and 18 months
* Chickenpox vaccine (Varivax) one shot from 12 months to 12 years

injury

Toddlers are prone to the same injuries as infants, including falls, aspiration, poisoning, suffocation, burns, and motor vehicle accidents.

Additional information on health maintenance and health promotion is found in Chapter 18.

toddler response to hospitalization

Common fears associated with hospitalization during toddlerhood include fear of separation from parents or caregivers, loss of control, and pain. Behaviors such as protest, despair, detachment, regression, negativism, temper tantrums, and physical and verbal aggressiveness are often seen.

key points ✳

* **Children from 1 to 3 years old are considered toddlers; they exhibit slow, irregular increases in physical growth with expanding growth of motor, cognitive, and psychological skills.**
* **Physical characteristics of the toddler include birth weight tripled by 1 year, height increases reaching about half of projected adult height by 2 years, wide gait, and protruding abdomen.**
* **Cognitive development during the toddler years involves exploration and discovery of the environment with much "trial and error" learning; egocentric behavior is common during toddlerhood and involves a self-centered view of the environment.**
* **Moral development begins with the toddler conforming to rules imposed by authority figures.**
* **Psychosocial development according to Erikson involves a sense of autonomy versus shame and doubt with negative behavior common during this time as the toddler struggles for independence.**
* **A toddler's sense of autonomy is promoted with improved language skills, control of body functions, control of separation anxiety, and increased mobility.**
* **Body exploration is common during the toddler years, requiring caregivers to teach the child that all body parts are good and avoiding reprimands suggesting shame when the exploration involves genitalia.**
* **Gross motor development continues in a cephalocaudal progression with improved walking skills, crawling, climbing, and running; fine motor development involves building a tower of blocks, taking off clothing, putting one object into another, turning a door knob, and catching a large ball by age 3.**
* **Toddlers have a short attention span and can be easily distracted when displaying unacceptable behavior.**
* **Play is an important part of the toddler's everyday experiences; it promotes growth with informal and spontaneous fun progressing from sensorimotor exploration to parallel play, symbiotic play, to cooperative type play.**
* **Developmental milestones in toddlerhood include walking alone by 18 months; running by 24 months; kicking when standing by 21 months; releasing a held object by 15 months; self-feeding, drawing simple lines, and demonstrating fairly good bowel and bladder control by 36 months.**

review questions ✳

1. Ms. Gavins is a 21-year-old single mother of a 2-year-old daughter who has been awakening during the night crying and fearful. Ms. Gavins asks the nurse about this behavior. The most appropriate response would be,
   a. "This is not normal behavior, and the child should be seen by the pediatrician immediately."
   b. "She is probably having nightmares because she is going to bed hungry."
   c. "Night fears are common during this age and should be ignored."
   d. "There are several reasons why toddlers awaken at night crying. It is difficult at this age to separate fantasy from reality. Talk to your daughter about her fears."
2. Select the activity that best describes Piaget's concept of tertiary circular reaction stage.
   a. Gerry remembers his trip to the zoo over the weekend.

b. Jana refuses to share toys with her younger brother.
c. Alaina decides to see what dirt tastes like.
d. Elise refuses to play with guns because she is not a boy.

3. Mrs. Garcia's son is 2 1/2 years old and has been having temper tantrums. She asks the nurse what she can do to control his behavior. The most appropriate response would be,
   a. "Be alert for signs of impending temper tantrums and distract the child if possible. If he goes into a tantrum, ignore his behavior, and when he regains control, praise his ability to regain control."
   b. "Isolate the child, and withhold privileges."
   c. "Physically restrain the child."
   d. "Talk to him about his behavior."
4. Language development is one of the major tasks of toddlerhood, and by 2 years, the child has a vocabulary of approximately
   a. up to 10 words.
   b. less than 20 words.
   c. 20 to 50 words.
   d. 50 to 100 words.
5. A toddler's sense of autonomy can be reinforced by
   a. control of body and increased mobility.
   b. unsupervised outdoor play with playground privileges.
   c. strict rules and consistent punishment.
   d. taking care of a younger sibling or a pet.

bibliography

Castiglia, P., & Harbin, R. (1992). *Child health care.* Philadelphia: J.B. Lippincott.

Heslin, J. (1991). How to feed your picky eater. *Healthy Kids Birth, Spring/Summer*, 18–20.

Milne, N. (1991). When your baby just won't sleep. *American Baby, May*, 35–37.

Nettina, S. (1996). *The Lippincott manual of nursing practice* (6th ed.). Philadelphia: Lippincott–Raven.

Pillitteri, A. (1995). *Maternal and child health nursing* (2nd ed.). Philadelpha: J.B. Lippincott.

Taylor, C., Lillis, C., & LeMone, P. (1993). *Fundamentals of nursing.* Philadelphia: J.B. Lippincott.

Warren, H. (1991). Outdoor safety. *Healthy Kids Birth, Spring/Summer*(3), 62–69.

the preschool child

23

outline

objectives

After studying this chapter, the reader should be able to:

- Describe the differences observed in the 3-year-old, 4-year-old, and 5-year-old relative to physical, psychosocial, and intellectual development.
- State two factors that contribute to moral development in preschool children.
- Describe at least three activities of the preschooler that promote Erikson's theory of initiative versus guilt.
- Describe the underlying causes of fears, phobias, and sleep concerns.
- Discuss two factors that influence sexual identity.
- Discuss methods to manage the following preschool problems: separation anxiety, sibling rivalry, and reactions to a new baby.
- Describe the types of play observed during the preschool years.
- State normal weight gains and height changes during the preschool years.
- Discuss at least four safety concerns relevant to the preschool years.

key terms

aggression
centration
egocentricism
fluorosis
initiative
molestation
nocturnal enuresis
perception
phobia
preconceptual phase
preconventional phase
strabismus
stuttering
transductive reasoning

Neff C & Spray M. *Introduction to Maternal and Child Health Nursing,*

The preschool period is between the ages of 3 and 6 years, a time also referred to as preprimary or early childhood. The term "preschool" is somewhat misleading, however, because many children have experience in nursery school or day care by the time they reach this age.

The preschool years are fun for children as they learn, explore, experiment, and observe, discovering themselves and their expanding world. Caregivers have the task of preparing the preschooler for the transition to school. Readiness for school involves the development of language and gross and fine motor skills. These skills are important to social progress and future success of the child, not only in school but throughout life.

This chapter deals with the distinct differences in growth and development from the beginning to the end of the preschool period (Table 23-1). Physical growth tends to slow and social and cognitive development accelerates.

physical assessment

The child experiences slower growth between 3 and 6 years. Evidence of genetic influences on body measurements is often apparent by the end of the preschool period.

weight

The preschooler normally gains 1.8 to 2.3 kg (3–5 lb) per year, beginning with a typical 3-year-old weight of 14.5 kg (32 lb). By 5 years, the preschooler's 1-year-old weight doubles. For example, if the child weighed 10.88 kg (24 lb) at 1 year, the expected weight by 5 years would be 21.77 kg (48 lb).

height

The preschooler normally grows 6.5 to 7.8 cm (2½–3 in) per year, beginning with an average 3-year-old height of 96.2 cm (37 in). By 5 years, the preschooler's height is nearly double the birth length. The greater increase in height compared to weight gives preschoolers a thinner, taller appearance compared to chubby, pot-bellied toddlers.

 **nursing insight**

Day care provides new, stimulating experiences for the child, but it also increases the risk of infection. The nurse should encourage the caregiver to talk with the staff to make sure good handwashing and other safety precautions are followed.

head circumference

The average head circumference by 5 years is 50 cm (19.5") for girls and 51 cm (20") for boys. Changes in the preschooler's nose, chin, and jaw give the face a more adult-like appearance.

motor skills

age 3

gross motor skills Three-year-old children are very energetic. Their gross motor skills enable them to walk, run, kick, climb stairs, balance briefly on one foot (Fig. 23-1), catch and throw large balls, and pedal wheel toys. They are able to dress, undress, and show preference for certain types of clothing. They can follow simple directions and enjoy playing games, such as follow the leader.

fine motor skills At 3 years, the child's fine motor skills improve, making it possible to enjoy projects using paper, pencils, crayons, paste, and safety scissors. A 3-year-old can build a tower of 9 to 10 blocks, self-feed using a spoon

table 23-1 preschool growth and development

Developmental Area	*Three-Year-Old*	*Four-Year-Old*	*Five-Year-Old*
Fine motor skills	Undresses self; can cut with blunt scissors	Can lace shoes; can pour from a small pitcher into a glass	Draws a 6-part person; learns to tie shoes
Gross motor skills	Runs; climbs steps one at a time	Jumps, skips, walks slowly across a balance beam	Rides a 2-wheel bike with training wheels
Intellectual development	Short attention span; eager to learn; pretends to read books; vocabulary of 300–900 words	Matches and sorts colors and numbers; enjoys singing and simple riddles; vocabulary of 1,500 words	Can learn telephone number and street address; vocabulary of 2,000–2,500 words
Psychosocial development	Engages in symbolic play; displays jealous emotions; shows some self-control	Engages in cooperative and symbolic or "pretend" play; is bossy and talkative; needs positive, firm consistent guidance	Has strong attachment to mother; needs frequent approval; is sensitive and responds with hurt feelings to ridicule

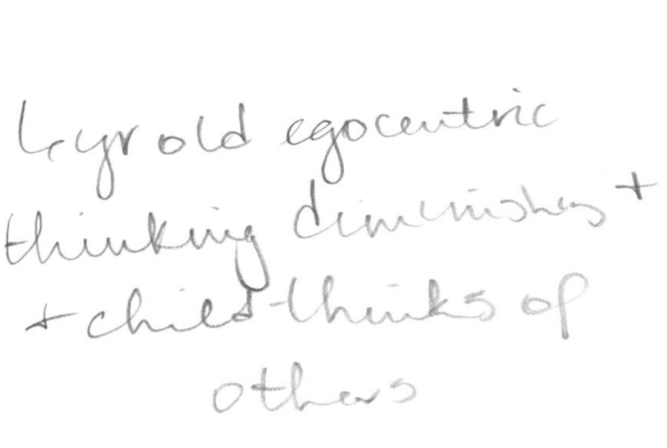

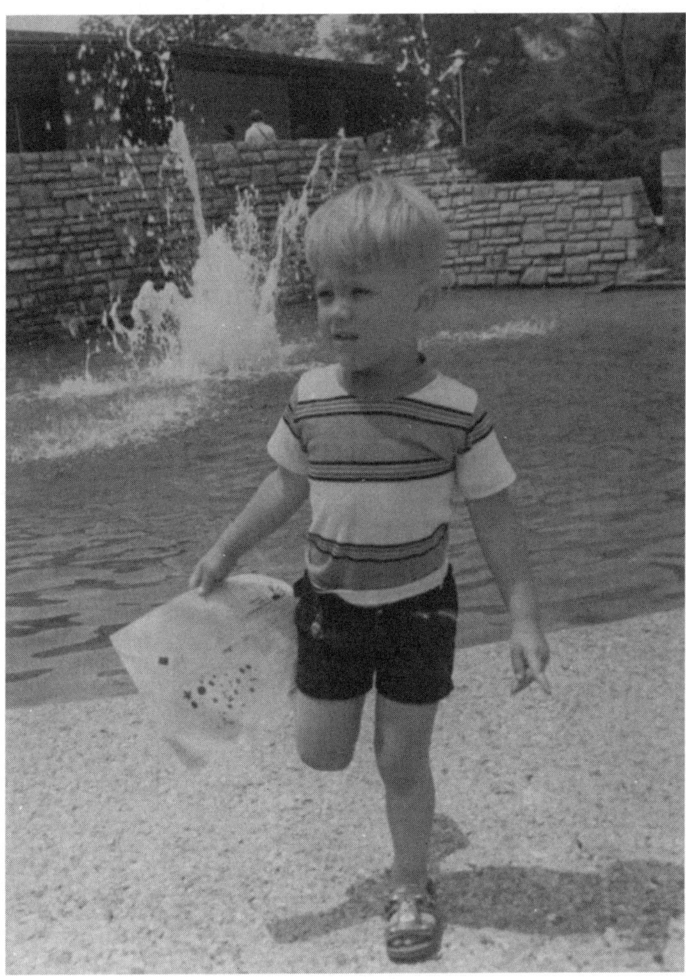

figure 23-1 *Preschoolers are able to balance briefly on one foot.*

and fork, wash his or her hands, and brush his or her teeth with supervision.

age 4

gross motor skills Four-year-old children are more boisterous. Their more developed gross motor skills enable them to refine skills learned at age 3. They can throw a tennis ball overhand, hop on one foot, climb, and walk across a balance beam.

fine motor skills Continuing development of fine motor skills enables the 4-year-old to cut out patterns on paper, using one hand for the scissors and one hand to turn the paper. The 4-year-old can make objects out of clay and button clothes.

age 5

Children at 5 years are improving gross and fine motor skills. They can ride a two-wheel bicycle with training wheels, skip, jump rope, and walk backward. Five-year-old children learn to distinguish between left and right and begin to tie their shoe laces. They can print their first name and cut their food.

✳ nursing process related to risk for altered growth and development associated with delays in gross and fine motor skills

During preschool years, the child develops important gross and fine motor control, language abilities, and social skills necessary for the school years.

assessment

The following assessment findings indicate altered growth and development in the preschooler:

* Delays or difficulties performing motor skills, such as moving all limbs with ease, pedaling a tricycle, walking up stairs by alternating feet, balancing on one foot for at least 1 second, hopping on one foot, skipping, catching a bouncing ball, jumping rope, building a tower of eight cubes, drawing a person with three to six parts, using scissors and pencils or crayons

* Delays in social or expressive skills, such as asking questions, using plurals and pronouns, story telling at age 4, sharing toys and playing with others, seating self on toilet, dressing with supervision at age 3 and without supervision by age 4, and helping with household tasks.

nursing diagnosis

* Risk for Altered Growth and Development, related to delays in gross and fine motor skills

nursing interventions

* Measure weight, height, and head circumference; plot the current data on growth charts, and compare previous measurements.
* Refer to a registered nurse or pediatrician if child falls outside the 5th and 95th percentiles for height and weight or outside the 10th and 90th for head circumference.
* Discuss possible cultural influences on growth and development specific to games, toys, and other activities.
* Observe the child's use of gross motor skills, and encourage activities promoting muscle strength, such as walking, running, and skipping.
* Promote the child's eye–hand coordination abilities by encouraging self-care activities, such as feeding, bathing, and dressing with supervision, and play activities, such as building and putting toys together with small pieces, coloring, cutting, and identifying colors.
* Assess parent's or caregiver's understanding concerning child's needs to enhance development. Encourage physical activities, such as running, jumping, climbing, and playing on child-safe outdoor toys, such as slides and swings.
* Assess toilet training progress; lack of toilet training by 5 years indicates physical disorders or problems in the home environment.

evaluation

* Weight, height, and head circumference are within normal limits on a standardized growth chart.
* Age-appropriate fine and gross motor skills are demonstrated.
* Bladder and bowel control with infrequent "accidents."

psychosocial assessment

Erikson describes the preschool period as one of *initiative versus guilt*. At this age, children begin to act on their own without prompting from others to control their own behaviors. Thus, they are learning to master the task of taking initiative and continuing to practice autonomy.

Preschool children thrive on independent activities, such as dressing and undressing. During the preschool years, the child may dress inappropriately, such as wearing mismatched clothing, a T-shirt with shorts in the winter, or nothing at all.

cognitive development

Cognitive development in the preschool years is represented by egocentrism and *animism*. Animism is defined as the belief that nonliving objects have life and perform lifelike behaviors. For example, a preschooler may explain a bicycle accident by stating "the bicycle was tired and mad at me." A preschooler may concentrate on one feature of a situation rather than on all aspects. Preschoolers think that everything has a cause. This aspect of their reasoning contributes to guilt feelings when they become ill or injured. For example, they may perceive the cause of the illness as punishment for unacceptable behavior. Their reasoning appears to be illogical and a reflection of a limited viewpoint.

ages 2 to 4

Piaget describes cognitive development of children between 2 and 4 years as the *preconceptual phase*. During this phase, the child forms concepts that are not as complete or logical as an adult's.

Preschool children are unable to attend to more than one aspect of a situation. This is a phenomenon called *centration*. They have very little understanding of past, present, or future.

The preschooler tends to see only his or her point of view rather than considering the perceptions of others, an outlook called *egocentrism*. The child assumes his or her perceptions of events are exactly the same as everyone else's. Preschoolers tend to use illogical cause and outcome reasoning. For example, a tall item is perceived as being larger (even though it is not) when compared to a similar item that is short, wide, and thick. Because the child perceives only the height rather than other dimensions, the true size of the item is not understood.

The preschooler has a short attention span and may display excitement about a new adventure. If the adventure takes a long time, such as shopping or visiting, however, the child quickly becomes bored.

The preschool child thinks in terms of specific to specific, a process called *transductive reasoning*. For example, the child reasons that if water is sucked down the toilet when it is flushed, the child also will get sucked down the toilet.

Preschoolers have difficulty understanding more than one instruction at a time. Statements like "This morning we're going to the store. Get your coat, finish your breakfast, choose what toy you want to take, wash your hands, and please don't wear those socks" may confuse the child. Thus, it is important to give only one or two instructions at a time. For example, "Please wash your hands, and brush your teeth."

ages 4 to 6

During the later part of the preschool period, the child begins what Piaget termed *intuitive thought*. Egocentric thinking diminishes as the child begins to include others in the environment. The attention span increases, and the child is able to focus on one idea at a time.

language development

An exciting development during the preschool years is the child's increased word usage and apparent understanding of words. Although the expanded ability to communicate is informative, caregivers need to be aware that conversation should remain simple and uncomplicated.

By 3 years, a preschooler's vocabulary increases to about 900 to 1,000 words. They use four- or five-word sentences, plurals, pronouns, and prepositions and articulate all vowels accurately while talking, singing, and reciting. This age is noted for talking a lot without caring whether anyone is listening (*noncommunicative language*) and asking many questions. They are fascinated with new words and enjoy imitating parents, siblings, peers, nurses, and fantasy characters.

A 3-year-old develops an interest in numbers and can count to three with ease. They take interest and pride in successfully matching colors. The preschool child is often unable to understand completely the meaning of words used to describe time and space. Terms such as "hour," "day," "month," and "mile" are only vaguely meaningful. Time and distance are best explained to a preschooler in terms of everyday activities, such as mealtime and distance to a store.

The 4-year-old child's language skills may include profanity if the child is exposed to such word usage. The child's awareness that words are an effective means of getting a response tends to generate such sayings as "I don't like you." This is a stormy age in which the child's aggression is often turned toward parents and siblings. Four-year old children tell fanciful tales outside of home with little or no restraint.

Four-year-old children can distinguish colors and enjoy combining activities, such as singing and coloring. They use a vocabulary of about 1,500 words to communicate feelings, ideas, and information. They enjoy telling stories about family members and explaining certain past and future events.

cultural influences

Language development proceeds in the same order around the world. The differences between and within countries have to do with actual sounds used by community members. Parents and siblings are models, providing experiences and interactions in language. The child mimics sounds, tones, and gestures of parents and siblings. Normal language development for preschoolers is listed in Display 23-1.

Differences in preschoolers' speech patterns may result from the following: 1) English is the language of the area, but the speakers do not follow standard English rules. 2) A large section of the community speaks another language, such as Spanish, as a first language. 3) Language differences result from differences in socioeconomic status.

delayed speech

Preschool children who do not talk or talk very little are considered having *delayed speech*. Delayed speech may be caused by physiologic, environmental, or psychological factors. Display 23-2 lists specific causes for delayed speech.

Stuttering is a common disorder in the preschool child. Stuttering can be described as a form of repetitive speech. Stuttering speech is a common behavior in young children undergoing the stress of learning to talk and usually requires no interventions. Nurses need to encourage caregivers to ignore the behavior so the child will not be overly concerned about the stutter, which is typically outgrown quickly. See the Teaching Guidelines for dealing with dysfunctional speech patterns.

display 23-1
normal language development for preschoolers

- **Mimics parental conversational styles and responses**
- **Answers appropriately to specific requests (3 years)**
- **Makes a specific request (4 years)**
- **Learns language appropriate for adults to understand, such as the use of greetings.**
- **Masters most sounds by 3–4 years but may have difficulty with a few such as "s," "l," "r," "th," and "sk."**

moral development

The child's conscience is thought to develop during the preschool years, influenced primarily by caregiver opinions about basic issues concerning right and wrong behaviors. Kohlberg describes this as the *preconventional* phase of moral development, lasting until 10 years. During the preconventional phase, children's moral standards reflect their observation of actions that earn praise or punishment.

display 23-2
factors influencing delayed or dysfunctional speech patterns

- **Cultural differences affecting the child's social contacts and use of English as first language**
- **Articulation problem or lack of comprehension**
- **Emotional and behavioral disturbances**
- **Hearing impairment, altering the child's ability to mimic words**
- **Mental retardation, ranging from mild to severe, which makes learning difficult**
- **Learning difficulties resulting from attention, memory, and perceptual problems**
- **Neurologic handicaps, such as cerebral palsy or epilepsy**

teaching guidelines
dealing with dysfunctional speech patterns

The following suggestions are provided to help caregivers and siblings of a preschooler with a dysfunctional speech pattern:

* Help the child feel accepted.
* Help the child be successful and feel important at something else.
* Try singing the words that need to be communicated, and encourage the child to do the same.
* Provide the child with verbal praise for verbal efforts.
* Do not bring attention to the child's mispronunciations.
* Do not call attention to dysfunctional speech patterns, such as "stuttering," because attention tends to make it worse.

Preschool children listen to adults and closely observe their actions. If adult words and actions contradict their teachings, children are quick to note the contradiction and may become confused or hostile.

Preschoolers are seldom spiritually neutral. Most children hear about spiritual concepts from family and friends and see churches, synagogues, or mosques and religious art. Even though preschool children may not understand spiritual or religious beliefs, they generally accept the family's religion because of family expectations.

Nurses are often confronted with questions from preschoolers dealing with holidays, especially Christmas and Easter. Common questions are "Is there really a Santa Claus?" or "Is there an Easter bunny?" The answer depends on the preschooler's age. A simple "yes" is recommended to a young child who is too young to understand abstract ideas. Older children may need to discuss their personal beliefs on the subject. Nurses can accomplish much by being good listeners.

sexual identity

Development of sexual identity or sex role is related to the biologic sex of the child and the influence of the society and culture in which the child is raised. Sexual identity in preschoolers consists of two concepts: the demonstration of particular gender-related behaviors and each child's realization that he or she is permanently a boy or girl. Gender-related behaviors often involve the use of sexually stereotyped toys (eg, dolls for girls, trucks and race cars for boys). A major difference between boys and girls is the more aggressive behavior often seen in boys.

Preschool children are aware of the difference between boys and girls. They often name their private parts using terms such as "pee pee," "tweety," or "ding dong." It is important for parents and nurses to teach the child correct terminology. Preschoolers often ask questions about genital organs in an attempt to understand the differences. By answering questions as they arise, caregivers give children a basic knowledge of physical differences and sexual roles before starting first grade.

Boys frequently ask what happened to a girl's penis. It is not uncommon for girls to try to mimic the voiding pattern of their fathers or brothers by standing to void. Myths and truths about preschoolers' need for sex information are included in Table 23-2.

Preschool boys and girls may masturbate. Masturbation is a normal activity that can help the child release tension. It is important not to shame the child for engaging in this activity. When shaming and ridicule occur, the child may have difficulties with normal sexual feelings later in life. Children need guidance concerning where and when it is appropriate to masturbate.

personal and social development

Three-year-olds are more tranquil and cooperative than toddlers. Although an occasional temper tantrum may occur, increased communication skills enable preschoolers to relieve frustrations by sharing feelings and ideas. By 3 years, children are helpful and capable of completing sim-

table 23-2 myths and truths about preschool sexual issues

Myth	*Truth*
Knowledge about sex is harmful; innocence of the young child should be preserved.	Ignorance about sex is harmful; it is better for the child to be knowledgeable about sexuality and sex roles.
Preschoolers are not old enough to understand.	Preschoolers are old enough to understand simple explanations.
Sex is too embarrassing to talk about at this age.	Sex can be an embarrassing issue at any age; honesty about embarrassment helps both child and parent. It is easier to get used to embarassment as a preschooler than at a later age.
Talking about sex at this age will give the child premature ideas about sex.	Talking about sex to a preschooler gives them the positive idea that sex is not a "taboo" subject.
Parents do not know enough about sex to inform their child.	Young children need just the simple facts about sexual issues. If needed, there are many references in the public library on the topic.

ple tasks. Increased understanding enables 3-year-olds to recognize potential dangers.

Four-year-old children are typically more aggressive and uncooperative when compared with 3-year-olds. They display rowdy, bossy, judgmental, and tattle-tale conduct.

Five-year-old children are fascinating, displaying increased patience and seriousness, especially when doing assigned tasks. The 5-year-old enjoys team play, exhibiting an understanding of game rules and social skills. Peer relations are important and typically involve friends of the same gender.

Five-year-olds often begin talking with strangers and engaging in self-disclosing conversations. This behavior poses a potential threat to the child's safety by increasing the risk of kidnapping or molestation. It needs to be discouraged by parents. It also is important to remember that molestation most commonly occurs with trusted relatives or friends rather than strangers.

play

Preschool play is a self-motivated activity through which learning occurs. Play enables the child to engage in many activities contributing to mental and physical development.

Preschoolers progress through different stages of play from 3 years to beyond 4 years. These stages include *parallel play*, involving two children playing along side each other but engaging in independent activities; *associative play*, involving children playing together with no intended purpose of the play; and *cooperative play*, involving children playing together with an intended purpose (Display 23-3).

Piaget describes two stages of play relative to the *sensorimotor period* and *preoperational period*. According to Piaget, *functional play* occurs during the sensorimotor period and is a type of practice play and exercise play. In functional play, the child repeats a behavior to master it.

display 23-3
types of play observed in the preschool years

- **Practice play: Child repeats the same activities over and over.**
- **Symbolic play: Child pretends to be a superhero or parent.**
- **Dramatic play: Child uses make-believe stories and acts out the part by dressing up.**
- **Rough and tumble play: Child runs, hops, falls over, wrestles, hits, makes faces.**
- **Play with objects: Child links self with the environment, such as feeding a baby doll.**
- **Play with language: Child plays with noises and sounds, and may include spontaneous rhyming or fantasy and nonsense.**

Symbolic play occurs in the preoperational period and provides preschoolers an opportunity to display their creativity. During symbolic play, the child "pretends" to be a character who is familiar, such as mommy or daddy (see Display 23-3). The preschooler's active imagination provides rich ideas for creative play, such as using large boxes for creating toys and adventures (Fig. 23-2).

imaginary friends

Preschoolers often develop imaginary friends. This is especially true if the child is an only child or the oldest. The imaginary friend does all of the bad things and experiences all of the good things that the preschooler dreams about. Adults need to respect the private nature of the preschooler's imaginary friend. As the preschooler becomes involved with other peers and activities, the need for imaginary friends tends to disappear.

peer relationships

Preschoolers thrive on peer relationships. They learn patterns of behavior from other children. Friendships are important, and cooperation is a critical part of friendships. Caregivers should explore the preschooler's sociability with peers. If a child is isolated by peers, there is usually a reason. Caregivers need to encourage the preschooler to have friendly relationships at this age.

fears and phobias

Children between 3 and 5 years often experience unrealistic fears due to their inability to separate fantasy from reality (*magical thinking*). As their world expands, animals, strangers, and loud noises may evoke fear. When a preschooler is frightened by a noise, hugging and giving reassurances is a good idea (Table 23-3).

Preschool children typically experience imaginative thoughts, such as believing that cats can turn into dogs and boys into girls. Television and movie shows are real to the preschooler who is unable to comprehend "make-believe" or "pretend" concepts. The preschooler relies heavily on adults to give them truthful information.

During the preschool years, children begin to develop a sense of purpose in life and a sense of comfort with their own gender. However, they are only vaguely aware of gender, racial, or religious differences. They can recognize the visual difference between black and white skin but generally do not attach cultural meaning to the differences.

family relationships

Children interpret their own behavior as either "good" or "bad," based on the reactions of other people. Caregivers and older siblings are role models for appropriate or inappropriate behavior. Family involvement helps the preschooler learn about individual strengths and weaknesses within the family relationships.

Preschoolers gain an inkling of the adult world as they try to meet adult expectations, begin to accept responsibil-

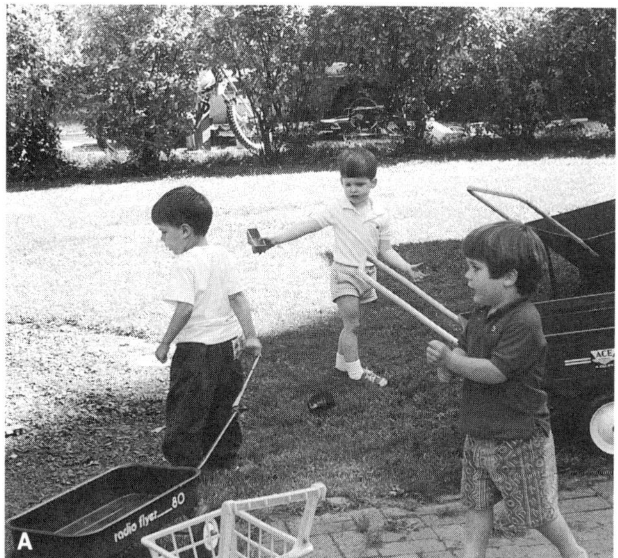

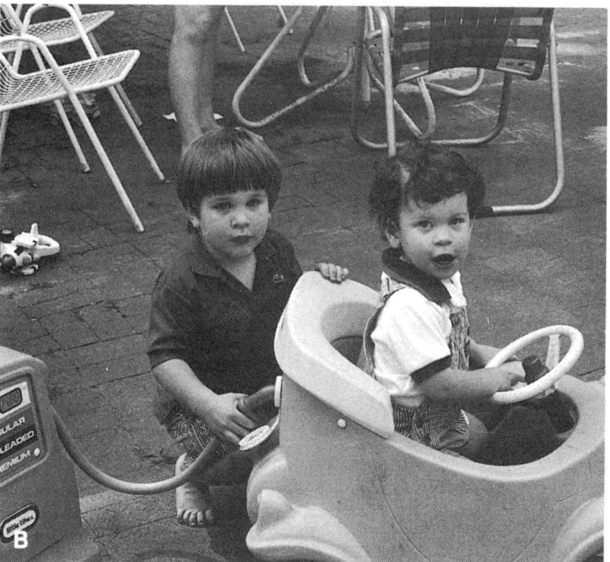

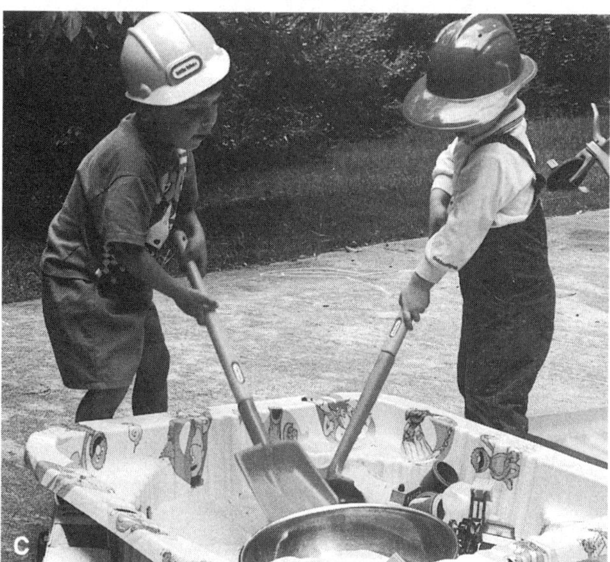

figure 23-2 *Children in the latter stages of preschool years engage in associative, cooperative, and symbolic play.*

ities, make and keep commitments, and impose some self-discipline. Preschoolers often find it difficult to live up to adult expectations, just as adults sometimes may find it difficult to live up to their own expectations.

The preschooler tends to rely less on adult caregivers for meeting basic needs and increases interactions with other family members. The child's developing sense of autonomy and initiative may result in criticism or discipline by caregivers or older siblings, leading to feelings of guilt. Preschoolers often display feelings of guilt through aggressive behaviors, seeming to ask for more rigid discipline from caregivers. Caregivers must balance their desires for perfection and obedience with the preschooler's need for independence.

When preschoolers make errors in judgment, parents need to remind them what is acceptable. Children need to know that their unacceptable behavior is disliked and how they can improve it. They also should know that they are loved, regardless of their behavior.

separation anxiety

Most preschool children are accustomed to being temporarily separated from their loved ones; however, the experience can be a source of anxiety and stress for children and parents. The pain of separation is a caregiver issue that can be handled when the safety and interests of the preschooler are guaranteed. From the child's viewpoint, separation from home is never easy at any age. However, as children grow older, peer and play opportunities balance the pain of leaving the safety of home.

> **nursing alert**
>
> *Expect powerful interactions when preschoolers are separated from parents, such as an initial rejection, followed by loss of emotional control.*

teaching guidelines
relieving separation anxiety in the preschool years

* Allow a few extra minutes to play and cuddle child.
* Permit child to express negativism, such as refusing food, delaying getting dressed, because this may give a sense of control that is not provided in day care or nursery school.
* Develop a routine of talking about leaving.
* Always tell the child you will be back.
* Do not prolong the parting.
* Expect strong emotions when reunited with the child.
* Avoid criticizing the child for crying when reunited.
* Tell the child how much you missed him or her during the day.

table 23-3 common fears and phobias and suggested interventions

Common Preschool Fears	Interventions
Darkness with monsters in the closet, goblins under the bed, and ghosts all over the house	Listen carefully to the fears, and respect whatever the child tells you.
Wind, thunder, and lightening	Tell the child that fear is natural.
Loud noises, such as fire engines, ambulances, and doors slamming	Reassure the child he or she can learn to overcome fear.
Dogs, cats, and other biting animals	Inform the child that there are no monsters, goblins, and ghosts.
Heights associated with the potential of falling	Accompany the child when looking in closets and under the bed.
Possibility of parent dying, causing the child to fear leaving home for school, parties, or a visit	Share how you overcame your fears at this age.
Stranger anxiety sometimes related to parental concern about possible child molestation	Provide opportunities for dramatic play, allowing the child to be the scary thing.
Strange places and new experiences	Help the child learn skills for coping with fear by looking at books, taking a trip to the hospital.
Failure	

sibling rivalry

Rivalry between siblings is normal and unavoidable; however, preschoolers are impressionable and easily hurt when siblings tease or ridicule. Caregivers cannot treat each child equally because each is unique. When children are valued for their individuality, they become aware of their strengths. Learning to live with others in a family provides an opportunity to respect differences.

Preschoolers can experience guilt, anxiety, and fear as a result of thoughts and actions that conflict with caregiver wishes. Caregivers need to stay out of sibling crisis if at all possible. When bodily harm is imminent, however, intervention is required. Preschoolers need to be encouraged to play independently with siblings and be rewarded for successes when learning about others (Fig. 23-3).

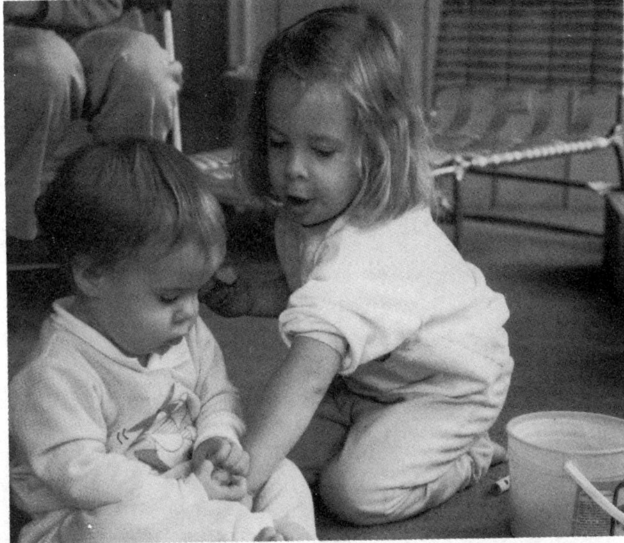

figure 23-3 *Sibling rivalry is always present to some degree as children struggle to express their identities and have their needs met.*

reactions to a new baby

It is not uncommon for the child to show anger when a new baby is introduced into the family. The older child has been the center of attention. No matter how wise and loving the parents are, they now must share their time and attention with two children rather than one. Common preschooler behaviors displayed toward the new baby include the following:

* Ignoring the baby
* Trying desperately to win back parental attention by being a model child
* Acting out behaviors or regression tendencies if good behavior does not give the desired attention
* Trying to eliminate the baby by force

Preschoolers can be helped to outgrow feelings about the new baby when parents do the following:

* Continually show love for the preschooler, regardless of what he or she does
* Enroll the child in preschool or day care before the new baby is born, thus avoiding having the older child feel deserted by the parents
* Reinforce the fact that the preschooler is growing up
* Allow the preschooler to hold the infant with supervision
* Encourage the preschooler to do small tasks that help with the infant's care and bolster his or her importance
* Spend extra time with the preschooler

preschool education

The terms *day care center*, *preschool*, and *nursery school* are often used interchangeably; however, they are different. *Day care centers* provide child care while parents work. *Nursery schools* and *preschool* programs provide social support for parents and children and include beginning education in addition to child care.

The number of children enrolled in preschool programs continues to increase. Working parents, divorce, and a belief that early schooling helps the child be educationally successful contribute to the increasing numbers attending preschool programs. Preschool or nursery schools allow the child to interact with peers and with other adult caregivers outside the home.

Many types of preschool programs are offered to socialize and educate the young child. Parents often ask nurses if preschool programs really make a difference in the child. Research studies indicate that they do make a difference:

* Preschool program children have higher academic achievement and motivation compared with children who do not attend a preschool program.
* Preschool program children are less often placed in special education classes.
* Preschool program children have fewer incidents of delinquency.

head start

Head Start programs were initiated in 1965 to provide a comprehensive developmental program for preschool children from low-income families. Head Start programs offer education, parent involvement, health services (including psychological services), nutrition, and social services.

montessori

Maria Montessori (1870–1952) developed educational programs and materials that focus on children's natural abilities and self-motivated, individualized learning. Basic beliefs of Montessori programs include early learning of reading and writing (before 5 years) and respect for all children. The Montessori method has been used in schools around the world, including some public and private schools in the United States.

programs for preschoolers with special needs

Preschoolers with special needs are those with physical and mental conditions that require special services. These include gifted children or children with physical, mental, or emotional disabilities; multicultural ancestry; or hyperactivity. Early intervention for special needs children is important to encourage growth, prevent developmental delays, reduce family stress, and decrease the need for costly services later in life.

The Education for all Handicapped Children Act (1975) provides for free and appropriate education for all children between the ages of 5 and 21 years. The Handicapped Act Amendments, passed in 1986, provide services to handicapped and at-risk children from birth to 3 years and their families.

✳ nursing considerations

Preschoolers learn and develop in a holistic manner through experiences and interactions with the physical and social environment. Nurses working with preschool children are often challenged by their many questions and complex needs. Following are suggestions for dealing with the preschooler:

* Interact with preschoolers in a friendly, nurturing way. Respect their ideas and feelings, and accept their answers as correct for their stage of thinking.
* Maximize preschool children's involvement with the physical environment by encouraging them to think about what they are seeing and experiencing ("what if" questions can be helpful).
* Respect and foster appreciation for differences among preschool children and families.
* Answer the preschooler's questions about sex education simply and honestly. Encourage the child to explain what he or she already knows, and provide only the requested information.
* Recognize the preschooler's inability to separate fantasy from reality, especially when dealing with illness. The child may feel illness results from unkind feelings and is punishment for "bad behavior."
* Recognize the preschooler's need to cover an injury or injection site with a bandage. A common fear during this age is that the child will lose all body fluids and possibly some organs if an opening in the skin is not covered.

health maintenance

Periodic health assessments are a necessity for preschool children with check-ups scheduled at least every 12 months. The preschooler's ability to ambulate and boundless curiosity and energy increase their risk of accidental injury, disinterest in eating, and sleep irregularities. The nurse can help caregivers determine a realistic sleep schedule by pointing out obvious signs of tiredness. For example, the child who is difficult to arouse in the mornings, falls asleep in school, or appears tired with dark circles under the eyes may be suffering from sleep deficit.

immunizations

Preschoolers receive diphtheria, tetanus, and pertussis; oral polio vaccine; and measles, mumps, and rubella boosters before starting to school. These are usually given between the ages of 4 and 6 years.

nutrition

The preschooler's diet should include food from all of the basic food groups. Caregivers and siblings should avoid mealtime battles. Preschoolers should not be forced to clean their plate or eat rejected food. Food servings should be kept small. Mealtime is not a good time to discuss dis-

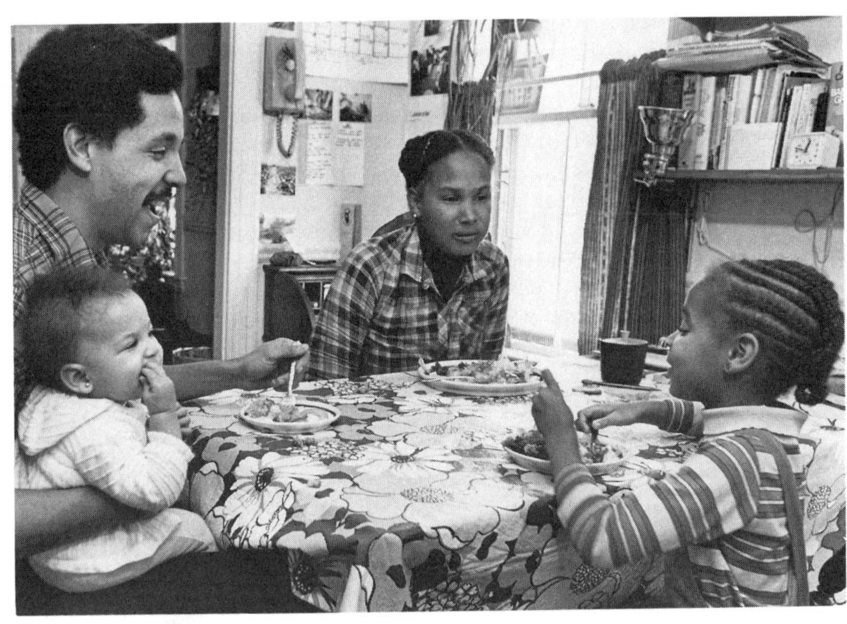

figure 23-4 *Mealtime is a good time to share daily events, with each family member taking a turn. (© Karin Rosenthal/Stock Boston)*

cipline issues. Mealtime is a good time to share daily events, with each family member taking a turn (Fig. 23-4, Display 23-4).

The recommended caloric intake for preschoolers is 85 kcal/kg or approximately 1,700 kcal/d. Many preschoolers show food "fads" and food preferences, resulting in a tendency to undereat or overeat as reflected in the child's weight and appearance. Weight gains or losses are obvious to the nurse during a routine examination when comparing previous data. The child's weight changes may not be as obvious to caregivers. Nursing intervention includes caregiver teaching about nutrition. Obesity in the preschool child contributes to obesity later in life. Weight reduction is recommended for the obese child. The amount of high-sugar foods should be limited to prevent dental caries.

display 23-4
parental do's and don'ts about preschool feeding

DO

* Expect the child to eat.
* Recognize the child's appetite will vary from day to day.
* Recognize that feelings and appetite are closely related.
* Consider the child may tire of a food and refuse to eat it.
* Prevent distractions at the table.
* Expect the preschooler to touch the food with his or her fingers.
* Serve the preschooler foods that are not too hot or too cold.
* Children like simple, unmixed food.

DON'T

* Overemphasize "manners."
* Try to introduce too many new foods too quickly.
* Force the preschooler to eat.
* Force the preschooler to clean up his or her plate.
* Make dessert a reward.
* Bring toys to the table.

daily hygiene

Dental hygiene is important in the preschool years because the permanent teeth replace the deciduous teeth. The fine motor development of preschoolers allow them to use a toothbrush properly, brushing at least twice a day. Preschoolers need supervision with brushing and flossing.

By 3 years, the preschooler will have all 20 deciduous teeth and by 5 years, will begin to lose the deciduous teeth for permanent teeth. A dental examination should be done by this age to assess the progress of dentition and reinforce good dental hygiene habits. Fluoride requirements in children 3 years and older increase to 1 mg/d and remain at that level throughout the rest of the tooth-forming years. Caries of the deciduous teeth frequently start between 3 and 6 years.

✱ nursing alert

Swallowing excess toothpaste contributes to dental fluorosis, resulting in discoloration of the teeth from too much fluoride.

Preschoolers are expected to be toilet trained and able to seat themselves on the toilet, demonstrating independent toilet activities. Boys may need encouragement to void while standing. The nurse may need to provide information to the child and caregiver about the importance of girls being taught to wipe after toileting from front to back to avoid contaminating the vaginal area with stool.

By 5 years, preschoolers can dress themselves without supervision and begin to learn to tie their shoe laces. They can bathe and shampoo with minimal supervision, but care must be taken to ensure safety in the tub. It is not uncommon for preschoolers to enjoy playing in the water so much that they forget to bathe. Hospitalized preschoolers may prefer caregiver assistance with bathing as opposed to the nurse because caregivers are accustomed to their bathing habits.

sleep

Sleeping problems that start in toddlerhood are not always solved by the time the child reaches preschool. Children this age need 8 to 12 hours of sleep each night. This means they must cycle through three periods of light sleep and rousing. When children awaken, they need to handle feelings of separation, fear of "monsters," and memories of conflicts left over from the daytime.

Stress in the preschooler's daily environment can cause nighttime fears and nightmares. When nightmares occur, the child needs parental reassurances. Reassurance is best given when caregivers provide the child with soothing words or stroking, leaving the child in his or her own bed or crib. Sleep is a major area in which the child can achieve independence, a critical goal of childhood. Children should be encouraged to learn to get themselves back to sleep.

safety

Preschoolers tend to be less accident prone than toddlers, due to better developed motor skills and greater understanding. They tend to listen to adult guidance and can understand simple safety rules. They imitate adult behavior and will readily follow the example set by the parent concerning safety.

When preschoolers are busy with play, they may forget that they are not supposed to chase a ball into the street or cross the street to play. Thus, yards and play areas should be fenced to avoid child endangerment. Refrigerators, deep holes, trash heaps, construction, and buildings can be a source of danger as the preschooler's rich imagination entices them to these sites. Falls and suffocation accidents are common in such areas.

nursing alert

Seeking adventure, the preschooler is often drawn to large containers with lids and may suffer death by suffocation.

Preschoolers are eager to use car seat belts when they see their parents using them. A child car seat can be replaced with a seat belt when the preschooler reaches 40 lb and is 40 in tall.

Preschoolers who display behavioral problems, such as hyperactivity, destructiveness, fighting, numerous temper tantrums, and aggressiveness, have a higher incidence of repeated accidental poison ingestion. Preschoolers can cover more territory than the toddler, so caregivers are advised to keep medicines and cleaning materials on a high shelf or in a locked cupboard. Candy or other edibles should not be stored near dangerous items.

Preschoolers should be instructed in water safety, especially if they have access to a swimming pool or lake. Preschoolers can be taught how to float before they learn to swim. Additional safety information is provided in Chapter 20.

abduction and sexual molestation

The incidence of abduction and sexual molestation of children has risen sharply. Although most commonly committed by a trusted relative or friend, abduction and sexual misconduct by nonfamily members have increased because more children receive care outside the home. Par-

teaching guidelines
safety measures

Preschoolers typically have more independence once they start preschool. It is important to provide the child with basic information that helps to keep them safe:

* Know your phone number and street address.
* Know how to dial 911, give your address, and stay on the line to answer qusetions when reporting an emergency.
* A stranger is someone you and your parents don't know.
* Remain a safe distance from strangers in cars; say "no" to taking rides, candy, or money.
* Run for help if you feel the person is trying to persuade you to go with them.
* Never leave school with anyone other than parents or other people who are authorized to pick you up.
* Yell loudly when in trouble.
* Say "no" to adults who want to touch your private parts.
* It is okay to disobey an adult when they tell you to do something you are uncomfortable doing (especially something related to sex).

display 23-5
appropriate interventions for disciplining the preschooler

* Acknowledge that preschoolers are keen observers and will imitate your behavior regardless of whether it is "right," "wrong," "good," or "bad."
* Provide the preschooler with options to help avoid confrontations.
* Correct the preschooler by being honest and supportive. Avoid harsh criticism that can cause the child to feel bad.
* Secure the preschooler's undivided attention (considering the child's age and experience) when discussing rules of conduct.
* Explain to the preschooler why you are saying "no" to a request, but avoid arguing.
* Encourage the preschooler to ask permission to use an item rather than taking it forcefully from another child.
* Establish rules for watching television, and reward the preschooler for following the rules.

ents or other caregivers must teach their children how to stay safe. See the Teaching Guidelines.

discipline

Discipline is different from punishment. Discipline encourages the child to learn from the misbehavior and helps the child develop self-control (Display 23-5). Punishment is hurtful and offers little learning. Instead it reflects the parent's or caregiver's loss of control in an effort to control the child. For example, when an angry child spills a glass of milk, discipline measures may include having the child clean up the spill to reinforce responsibility for one's own behavior; punishment measures include verbal or physical assault, which reinforces aggression.

preschool response to hospitalization

A preschooler's ability to comprehend the cause for hospitalization and aspects of the hospital experience is restricted by self-centered and magical thinking. The preschooler may perceive the injury or illness as punishment for misbehavior. Their fears are similar to those of toddlers and include fear of separation, loss of control, bodily injury, pain from procedures, and mutilation. Behaviors associated with these fears include protest, despair, detachment, aggression, and regression to earlier behaviors, such as bed wetting.

key points ✳

* Preschool years cover the period between 3 and 6 years.
* By 3 years, walking is an automatic process; climbing stairs and throwing objects follow predictable developmental sequences.
* Physical skills are important in the progress of intellectual, psychosocial, and language development.
* Preschool children are in the preoperational stage of intellectual development.
* Preschoolers integrate all their knowledge and skills through play.
* Play promotes problem-solving skills and social and intellectual competence, helps distinguish between fantasy and reality, promotes curiosity, and encourages communication, self-control, and language.
* Boys and girls differ based on biologic sex and how the society in which they are raised reinforces the natural differences in the sexes.
* Adults can help children overcome their fears when adults listen carefully to descriptions of fearful feelings and offer careful, thoughtful answers to the concerns.
* Language development in preschool children grows out of language experiences at home, in preschool, and in other social contacts.
* Head Start is designed to provide a comprehensive developmental program for preschool children from low-income families.
* Children participating in high-quality preschool programs tend to have higher academic achievement, greater motivation, less frequent placement in special education classes, and fewer incidents of delinquency.

review question ✳

1. Mrs. Deitrich confides in the nurse that her two children, ages 4 and 5, constantly bicker and rival with each other. An appropriate nursing response includes,
   a. "It is important to treat all your children the same; that discourages rivalry."
   b. "Rivalry between siblings is normal and unavoidable."
   c. "The rivalry is caused by the children's close birth order."
   d. "Perhaps the children need counseling."
2. An appropriate nursing assessment concerning a delay in language development in the preschool child involves
   a. noting a vocabulary of approximately 900 words in a 3-year-old.
   b. noting persistent questioning with little interest in a response.
   c. an inability to communicate ideas and feelings by 4 1/2 years.
   d. use of profanity.

3. Piaget describes the preschool child's intellectual development as the
   a. preconventional phase.
   b. initiative versus guilt phase.
   c. preconceptual phase.
   d. symbolic phase.
4. Sex role development in the preschooler includes the following concepts:
   a. Female masturbation rarely occurs.
   b. Preschoolers realize they are permanently a girl or boy.
   c. Boys are less aggressive than girls at this age.
   d. Gender-related toys are an important influence on determining sexual preference later in life.
5. An appropriate nursing intervention regarding a preschooler's imaginative friend involves
   a. respecting the private nature of the preschooler's imaginary friend fantasy.
   b. asking the child to talk about the imaginary friend.
   c. informing the parent or caregiver that the child needs psychiatric help.
   d. helping the child separate fantasy from reality.

bibliography

Betz, C., & Poster, E. (1992). *Pediatric nursing reference.* St. Louis: C.V. Mosby.

Brazelton, T. (1992). *Touchpoints: Your child's emotional and behavioral development.* Reading, MA: Addison-Wesley Publishing.

Castiglia, P., & Harbin, R. (1992). *Child health care: Process and practice.* Philadelphia: J.B. Lippincott.

Charlesworth, R. (Ed.) (1992). *Care for the developing child.* Albany, NY: Delmar.

Heiney, S. (1991). Helping children through painful procedures. *American Journal of Nursing, 11,* 20–24.

Jackson, D., & Saunders, R. (1993). *Child development.* Philadelphia: J.B. Lippincott.

Marhoefer, P., & Vadnais, L. (Eds.) (1992). *Caring for the developing child.* Albany, NY: Delmar.

Nelms, B. (1993). Discipline: What do you recommend? *Pediatric Health Care, 7*(1), 1–2.

Nelms, B., & Mullins, R. (1982). *Growth and development, a primary health care approach.* Englewood Cliffs, NJ: Prentice-Hall.

Vessey, J., Braithwaite, K., & Wiedmann, M. (1990). Teaching children about their internal bodies. *Pediatric Nursing, 16*(1), 29–33.

the school-age child

24

outline

objectives

After studying this chapter, the reader should be able to:

- ✳ *State the ages involved in the stages discussed as primary learner, middle school, and preadolescent.*
- ✳ *Discuss the differences in acceleration of physical and cognitive development.*
- ✳ *Discuss the appearance of the school-age child regarding musculoskeletal and facial growth.*
- ✳ *Describe the positive effects seen in body development, refinement, and coordination of gross and fine motor skills resulting from maturity of the nervous system.*
- ✳ *Discuss the factors involved in the school-age child's development of a sense of industry.*
- ✳ *Define the following components of Piaget's theory of cognitive development in the school-age child: conservation, classification, seriation, decentering, and reversibility.*
- ✳ *State an example of prediction, empathy, and reasoning relative to language development.*
- ✳ *Define learning disabilities.*
- ✳ *Discuss the components of moral development with reference to the importance of being the most universal task of childhood.*
- ✳ *Describe at least four family considerations specific to the school-age child.*

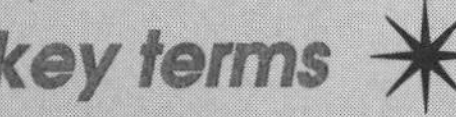

key terms

attention deficit disorder
classification
concrete learning stage
conservation
decenter
inferiority
latchkey children
preadolescent
primary learner
reversibility
seriation

Neff C & Spray M. *Introduction to Maternal and Child Health Nursing,*

School-age children are between 6 and 12 years old. Six- to 8-year-olds are often called primary learners, 9- and 10-year-olds are called middle school children, and 11- and 12-year-olds are considered preadolescents. During the school-age years, the child's physical development slows, while cognitive development becomes more pronounced (Table 24-1). As with any developmental stage, each child progresses at his or her own pace. This chapter addresses normal school-age development stages: primary learner, middle school, and preadolescent. Factors involved with the development of a sense of industry are included.

table 24-1 *growth and development chart*

Age	*Social Skills*	*Fine Motor*	*Gross Motor*	*Language*	*Cognitive*
6–7 y	Erikson's industry versus inferiority stage (continues throughout school-age years) Development of coping mechanisms	Able to use fork; begins to use knife Draws a person with body, arms, legs, mouth, eyes, nose, and hair Ties shoelaces	Runs, hops, skips, and climbs Begins to ride two-wheel bike Can walk a chalk line	Speech patterns like adults Can tell stories about monsters and other fears Vocabulary expanding	Continues preoperational thinking until 7 y Interested in birth and death Views babies as coming from females, not sure of male role Death viewed as result of outside force and seen as reversible
7–8 y	Interested in "sex"-segregated groups Follows general rules	Eye–hand coordination not fully developed May appear clumsy	Careful when trying new gross motor skills May swim, ride bicycle	Vocabulary increasing Able to say words but may not understand them	Thinking operational Begins to understand cause and effect Begins to understand concepts of past, present, and future Math and reading skills beginning to develop Collecting things as a hobby
8–10 y	Adheres rigidly to rules Still in same-sex play groups	Uses both hands independently Becoming more proficient in artistic projects	Very energetic Jumps, chases, skips, runs Engages in organized sports	Vocabulary increasing Storytelling more explicit	Able to understand others' points of view Thinking more abstract and symbolic Can reverse operations; trace the order of events backward to beginning Can tell time Reading more proficient; can add, subtract, multiply, and divide whole numbers Able to focus on more than one feature of a situation Girls become interested in menstruation
10–12 y	More in touch with peer approval Beginning of predating behaviors	Mastery of printing and cursive writing	Strength and endurance increasing, along with interest in sports	Able to define abstract terms Vocabulary influenced by intelligence, home, and school experiences	Realizes that a piece of clay, regardless of its shape, will occupy the same volume May be concerned with death issues Aware of mechanics of conception and birth

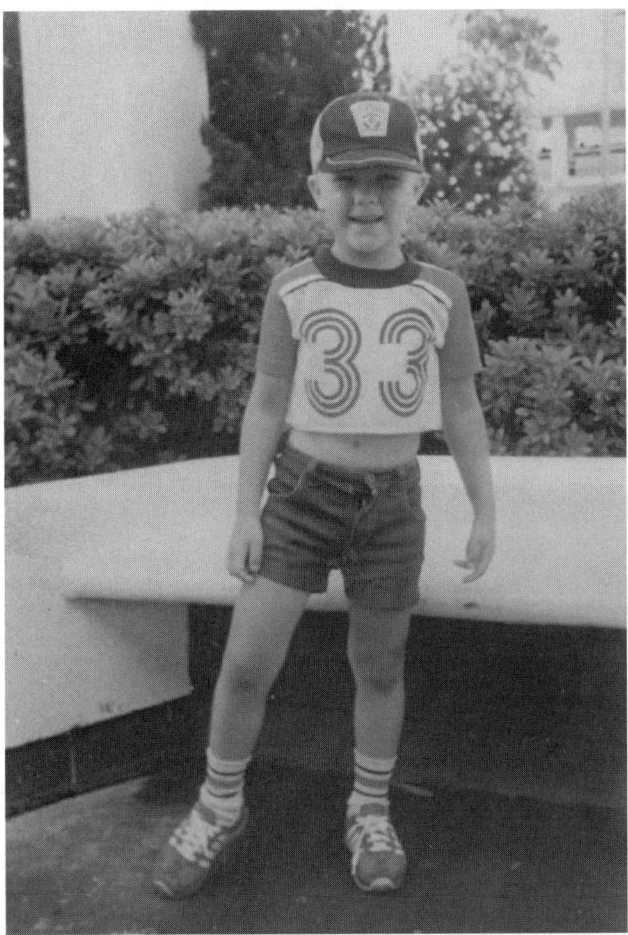

figure 24-1 *In most children between the ages of 6 and 10 years, fat diminishes, muscle and leg length increase, and they appear thin.*

physical development

growth and general appearance

Physical growth and development of the child during the school-age years is slow but steady. From 6 to 10 years, most children experience a growth plateau. Fat diminishes, muscles and leg length increase, and the child appears thin and loses the "babylike" softness of features (Fig. 24-1). Long arms and legs and large hands and feet contribute to the child's tendency to be clumsy at this age.

> ✶ **nursing insight**
> *A formula often used to predict how many pounds children from 8–12 years will weigh involves multiplying the age by 7 and then adding 5. For example, to determine the weight of a 9-year-old, you would multiply 9 × 7 + 5 = 68 lb (expected weight for a 9-year-old would be around 68 lb).*

At 9 years, girls start to pull ahead of boys in height and weight. African American children are slightly larger than white children. Asian children are smaller than white children. For more information about normal ranges for weight and height based on age and gender, refer to Appendix.

Growth patterns in school-age children are more significant than single measurements. Therefore, standardized charts are useful only as reference points. Because some parts of the body grow faster than others, school-age children may look out of proportion and uneven (asynchrony).

facial development

Between 6 and 11 years, the head appears to enlarge, and facial features show marked changes in the upper and lower jaw. The face actually grows away from the skull as the mandible moves down and away from the upper face, making the lower jaw appear elongated. About 90% of facial growth is attained by 12 years (Schuster & Ashburn, 1992).

Growth of the frontal sinuses reaches adult size by about 12 years. Sinus development strengthens the structure of the face, reduces the weight of the head, and helps provide resonance to the voice. *Sinusitis* (inflammation of the sinus cavities) is an illness seen during the school-age years.

At about 6 years, the child begins to lose deciduous teeth ("baby" teeth). These are replaced by permanent teeth, which often appear too large for the child's face. During these years, the first molars erupt, followed by the central incisors (Fig. 24-2). By the end of the school-age period, all 20 deciduous teeth have been replaced by 32 permanent teeth.

musculoskeletal development

The musculoskeletal system changes significantly during the school-age period, giving the child an adultlike posture. The spine is straight with slight lumbar and thoracic curvatures.

The rate of bone development is similar to height and weight patterns in the younger child and sexual development in the older child. The centers of the long bones continue to develop, and by 7 years, a marrow cavity has developed. Muscles of the school-age child develop at a steady rate, with a maximum growth spurt seen at puberty.

Common orthopedic problems seen during the school-age years include scoliosis, Osgood-Schlatter's disease, Legg-Perthes disease, and sports injuries, such as sprains, strains, and fractures. See Chapter 36 for additional information.

Physiologic readiness to participate in contact or competitive sports is determined by muscular strength related to biologic age and gender rather than chronologic age. Strength in muscles of the anterior and posterior surfaces of the thigh, quadriceps, and biceps helps reduce the risk of sports injuries. Knee strength is important because the knee is not protected from injury during competition.

> ✶ **nursing insight**
> *Athletic activities are best chosen according to physical abilities rather than parent, caregiver, or peer persuasion.*

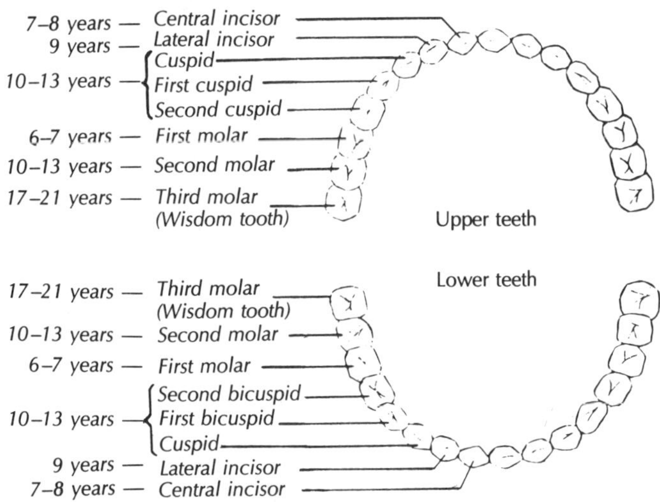

figure 24-2 *Eruption of the permanent teeth. (From Marlow, D. R. [1977].* Textbook of pediatric nursing *[5th ed.] Philadelphia: WB Saunders. With permission.)*

motor skill development

During the school-age years, the nervous system reaches maturity. The ability of this complex system to integrate all activities of the body helps develop, refine, and coordinate gross and fine motor skills. As children grow strong and tall, they show dramatic improvements in physical skills concerning timing and coordination. Development of motor control and social skills promotes positive associations with friends. Distinct differences are noted at various points in the school-age period. While the 6-year-old struggles with new responsibilities involving school, the 12-year-old struggles with physical and emotional changes involving puberty (see Table 24-1).

6 to 8 years

The active 6-year-old appears to be in constant motion. The child's improved balance allows skipping, running, hopping, jumping, throwing balls, and riding bicycles. The 6-year-old knows the right hand from the left and can recognize shapes, read, tie shoelaces, use a hammer, cut paper with safety scissors, describe objects seen in pictures, and draw a person with hands, neck, and clothing.

Seven-year-old children continue to gain control over their bodies and are able to engage in activities that require a higher degree of coordination. They can separate fact from fantasy. They are able to print and use a pencil as easily as a crayon and tend to be supercritical of their own work. Caregivers and nurses can encourage the child to be persistent with tasks by approving of and praising their efforts.

gross motor skills Six-year-old children enjoy gross motor activities using their large muscles. The child seems to have boundless energy and ignores feelings of fatigue. The 6-year-old will deny being tired and show reluctance about going to bed. Common signs of fatigue are argumentative behaviors, emotional outbursts, and decreased appetite. Six-year-old children require caregiver guidelines to protect them from excessive fatigue and possible exhaustion.

By 7 or 8 years, the child continues to have an abundance of energy. However, gross motor activities come under the control of conscious will and cognitive skills. Energies are directed toward meaningful activities. For example, bicycles are used to run errands, and running is used to get someplace quickly.

9 to 10 years

By 10 years, brain development is complete, and the child can arrange objects in order of size, engage in simple experimental science or cooking projects, build plastic or wooden models, and understand basic information about body functions. During this period, children move from printing to cursive writing, develop better hand–eye coordination, begin to understand the days of the week, and draw a person with 18 to 20 parts.

gross motor skills Middle school-age children (9–10 years) are more graceful in their movements and have increased athletic abilities. Both sexes tend to engage in sports requiring coordination skills, such as boxing, karate, track and field, or roller skating. Sufficient coordination enables the child to complete self-care activities.

11 to 12 years

Preadolescence is a time of growth spurts, and the child often appears uncoordinated. Children who have demonstrated athletic abilities between 8 to 10 years of age may experience a slight decline in athletic competence during this time. The preteen may decide to drop a sports activity because he or she feels clumsy. The caregiver may be confused about this decision because of the amount of time and effort the abandoned sports activity consumed. The nurse can reassure caregivers that this is common and will resolve itself by the time the child reaches 12 years. Channeling the child's energies in other directions is helpful. For example, playing a musical instrument and joining the school band keep the child involved with peers and school activities.

By 12 years, coordination improves, and the child is often enthusiastic about resuming a sports activity. The 12-year-old has a sense of humor and enjoys practical jokes.

gross motor skills Physical and cognitive skills enable the child to be more self-directed and controlled to engage in repetitive practice that is necessary to master a sport, musical instrument, or art project.

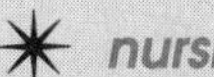 **nursing insight**

Adults are advised to slow their pace and shorten the distance when running with children younger than 14 years. Children are at risk for developing stress fractures or heat exhaustion when engaged in distance running or keeping pace with adult runners.

psychosocial development

The psychosocial development of the school-age child involves two factors: development of a sense of industry and advancement of self-concept through successful achievements. The task of becoming a productive member of society involves mastering situations through trial and error. Psychosocial development during these years means learning how to cope with failure, learning endurance, and balancing feelings of inferiority with a sense of achievement.

The developing self-concept from 6 to 12 years depends on the self-image that the child receives from significant others and on the child's own achievement ability. Positive self-concept develops when children are curious about the environment, display appropriate levels of anxiety according to the task, and experience independent behaviors. Development of the child's self-concept is influenced by parenting styles, disciplinary acts, socioeconomic settings, sex, and ordinal place in the family.

School-age children strive for increased independence from caregivers and significant adults, often rejecting adult rules and instructions. These rejection behaviors are a normal part of growth and development. Rejection of rules often stems from the child's need for independence rather than from heedless defiance of the rules. Children may feel internal conflicts over right and wrong behaviors related to adult versus peer expectations. Family support and guidance are still important, even though the school-age child tends to show contradictory conduct.

cognitive development

The school-age child is involved with two important cognitive tasks: establishment of logical or concrete thinking, enabling the child to deal with what is happening now rather than what could happen, and development of a moral code, enabling the child to deal with societal rules.

According to Piaget, children make the transition from preoperational thought to concrete operational thought between 5 and 7 years. Operational thinking is based on observation and evaluation of a situation. For example, children display an understanding of cause and effect when they throw a ball and it continues to roll away from them.

One of the hallmarks of the concrete operational stage is the appearance of *conservation*. Conservation is the ability to determine whether an item has a greater, lesser, or equal amount, regardless of how it is arranged. For example, six pennies arranged in a straight line are equal to six pennies stacked. Conservation also involves the concept that the properties of an object remain the same in spite of appearance changes. For example, 6 oz of water in a glass is the same amount as 6 oz of water in a large pitcher, although one appears larger than the other.

The development of math and science skills depends on *classification* ability. Children learn classification skills by using their senses of taste, touch, smell, sight, and hearing. Classification is the ability to identify relationships among objects, people, and events. For example, balls are round, and blocks are square.

Parents often think that children understand numbers when they are able to count; however, this is not the case. School-age children use *seriation* skills to match items and remember alphabet letters and numbers. *Seriation* is the ability to put objects into a specific order based on size, number, or shape.

A positive sign of cognitive development involves the child's ability to *decenter.* Decentering is the ability to take many aspects of a situation into consideration rather than focusing on only one particular part.

Middle school children understand the concept of *reversibility*. Reversibility is the process of going back to the beginning of an event, following the event from beginning to end, and understanding what changes could have been made to achieve a different outcome. The concept of reversibility helps children recognize that pouring water from a glass into a pitcher and vice versa does not alter the amount (Display 24-1).

School-age children younger than 10 years believe that people are responsible for all things. At about 10 years, children begin to understand the concept that people are not responsible for some events in life. Until the child accepts this idea, he or she cannot fully understand concepts such as birth, death, and the origins of life on earth.

display 24-1
cognitive development patterns of school-age children

Conservation: determining whether an item has a greater, lesser, or equal amount regardless of arrangement.
Classification: identifying relationships among objects, persons, and events
Seriation skills: putting objects into a specific order based on size, number, or shape
Decenter: experiencing from another's point of view; can see an experience from another's point of view
Reversibility: tracing the order of events to beginning

speech and language

Between 6 and 7 years, children begin to use sentences that are adultlike in grammar and length but tend to have grammatic errors. It is normal to note one or more articulation errors, particularly when deciduous teeth are missing in front, but most other speech errors disappear during this time.

Six-year-olds tend to use slang or profane words, appropriately mimicking the emotional content. They may not fully comprehend the meaning of the word being used but repeat the undesirable word for its shock value. The child must be educated about the use of acceptable and unacceptable words.

During the school-age period, language development begins to integrate the child's communication abilities and thinking processes. Children may use abstract words without fully understanding their meaning. With time, however, the use of words helps develop the understanding of abstract concepts.

Word comprehension may develop rapidly or slowly. By the time a child enters kindergarten, he or she should be able to use language for prediction, empathy, and reasoning, as shown in the following examples:

* Prediction: "Mommy will be very happy when she sees me get off the bus."
* Empathy: "My brother gets scared when he gets a shot because it hurts."
* Reasoning: "My sister gets upset when I use her make-up."

Nurses can evaluate children's language ability by inviting them to talk about themselves and events in their lives.

learning disabilities

Learning disabilities (LD) are a hidden handicap. There is no disfigurement or visible sign that initiates understanding or support. This is a disorder that affects a child's ability to interpret what is seen and heard or to combine information from different parts of the brain. *Learning disability is defined by law* as a significant gap between a child's intelligence and the skill achieved at each age. For example, a severely retarded 11-year-old who speaks like a 6-year-old would not be considered LD because the child has mastered language up to her intelligence limits. However, a fifth grader with an intelligence quotient of 100 who cannot write a simple sentence would be considered LD. Children show natural difference in their rate of development, which impacts their capacity for learning. These differences may cause learning problems but are not necessarily LDs.

Learning disabilities cause problems with schoolwork, especially in the areas of reading, writing, and mathematics. Studies indicate that children living in poverty lack motivation and experience. They also lack a general awareness to analyze past and present experiences, determine alternative actions, and engage in imaginative play. These factors interfere with academic success.

Learning disabilities encompass a combination of possible causes, symptoms, treatments, and outcomes. Because LD can appear in so many forms, it is difficult to determine the causes.

Evaluation scores from intelligence and achievement tests are used to identify learning disorders. Many learning problems result from attentional disorders, such as short attention span, distractibility, and impulsiveness, now called attention deficit disorder (ADD). Other learning difficulties are caused by reading problems, such as dyslexia. Learning problems impact nursing interventions, especially patient education (Table 24-2).

Behaviors indicating LD include delayed language or reading skills; lack of coordination in fine motor skills; frequent confusion; extreme emotional reactions; difficulty following directions and paying attention; inability to get along with others; hyperactivity; hypoactivity; lack of cultural stimulation; malnutrition; mental impairments, such as autism (child withdraws from reality); retardation; neurologic impairments, such as cerebral palsy or petit mal seizures; and physical impairments. Physical and sexual abuse also may contribute to behaviors associated with LD.

Physical impairments vary in degree, causing mild to severe learning problems, including blindness, deafness, and body deformities; diseases, such as heart disease and sickle cell anemia; and internal impairments, such as asthma and allergies. School nurses help identify learning problems by performing vision and hearing assessments. Nursing care for a child with a physical impairment focuses on independent self-care.

Children with learning difficulties require early intervention to promote potential development. Without early and appropriate intervention, these children may experience repeated failures, leading to lack of self-confidence and low self-esteem.

✳ nursing process related to attention deficit disorder

Attention deficit disorder affects the child's ability to regulate attention appropriate for the mental age. Research suggests that the sleep center of the brain is impaired. This causes the child to be on the edge of falling asleep, resulting in behaviors that are impulsive and often inappropriate in an attempt to stay awake.

assessment

Subjective and objective data to be assessed include the following:

* History of the child's inability to attend to tasks. For example, ADD children are easily distracted from activities, fail to complete projects even during play, have trouble waiting for a turn, are unable to organize tasks, and require constant adult supervision.
* Hyperactive behavior, including moving around excessively and being unable to sit still

table 24-2 learning disabilities

Types	*Characteristics*
Academic disorders include developmental * Reading (most common, referred to as dyslexia) * Writing * Arithmetic	Lag behind classmates. Dyslexic children are unable to * Distinguish or separate the sounds in spoken words * Form images or relate new ideas * Comprehend or remember new concepts * Rhyme words, such as cat and bat
Attention-deficit disorders 20% of school-age children have a type of disorder that makes them unable to focus their attention. Attention deficit often involves hyperactivity disorder (ADHD).	Attention-deficit children * Daydream often * Drift off into own world * Display inappropriate behaviors that often represent the child's attempt to stay awake ADHD children * Exhibit impulsive behaviors * Interrupt others * Display explosive energy * Are unable to follow directions, organize, or complete work * Talk excessively

nursing diagnosis

* Impaired Social Interaction, related to short attention span

nursing interventions

* Assess child's ability to interact with peers and adults, noting strengths and limitations.
* Assess parent or caregiver responses to child's behaviors, noting whether undesirable behaviors are reinforced, type of discipline techniques, and positive reinforcements used.
* Assess duration of child's attention with activities and interactions.
* Decrease environmental stimulation, and refocus child when distracted. For example, encourage child to finish one game before starting another or turn television off while talking or playing.
* Teach child age-appropriate social skills that provide positive reinforcement for appropriate interactions, for example, picking clothes up off the floor, returning toys to toy chest, and taking turns with games.
* Educate the parents or caregivers about the value of early educational intervention, such as special education classes or tutors, to increase the chance of school success. Learning disorders may or may not accompany ADD.
* Assess electroencephalogram results for abnormalities associated with ADD.
* Provide parent or caregiver with information concerning tests and medication administration, including dosage, frequency, expected results, and side effects. Stimulants may be required to increase the child's ability to stay focused on schoolwork. Methylphenidate (Ritalin) is frequently prescribed for ADD. This medication increases attention span, motor activity, and mental alertness and diminishes fatigue. Side effects include restlessness, tremors, hyperactivity, insomnia, irritability, dizziness, headache, blurred vision, tachycardia, hypertension, anorexia, and rashes. After a maintenance dose of methylphenidate is determined, the medication is often administered one to three times daily at 8-hour intervals.
* Advise parents to notify school nurse regarding medication administration.

evaluation

* The child demonstrates an age-appropriate attention span.
* The child demonstrates improved ability to interact and play with others socially.
* Parents voice understanding about medication regimen.

gifted children

According to the Education Consolidation and Improvement Act, gifted and talented children are defined as giving evidence of high performance capability in areas such as intellectual, creative, artistic, leadership capacity, or specific academic fields. In many areas of the United States, intellectually challenging programs are available for gifted children. Teachers and caregivers need to remember, however, that intellectual ability does not always equal social or psychological maturity: A gifted child is still a child.

display 24-2
primary learner's education milestones

RECEPTIVE LANGUAGE SKILLS

* **Understands opposites, such as big and little, fast and slow**

ARTICULATION AND EXPRESSIVE LANGUAGE SKILLS

* **Articulates "t," "v," "l," "th"; uses will and -ing verbs.**

READING SKILLS

* **Knows sounds of letters**
* **Recognizes common words by sight**

WRITING SKILLS

* **Prints on the line; uses letters of appropriate size**

ARITHMETIC SKILLS

* **Counts by two's**
* **Does simple addition and subtraction**

moral development

The school-age years are a critical period for moral code development in children. The development of a value system, a sense of justice or fair play, and knowledge of right and wrong are the most universal tasks of childhood; these are essential to the continuation of a civilized society. Moral values are learned and develop as an interactive process between the child and the social environment.

Moral development begins before the school-age years; however, the process of moral development is most apparent during this time. Preschool children are described as egocentric and interested mostly in their own welfare. The school-age child begins to develop decentered thinking and standards that help gain society's acceptance.

piaget's theory

Piaget's theory concerning moral development supports the thinking that morality is a system of rules for behavior set up by adults and learned by the child as a means to gain acceptance. Piaget describes the child from ages 4 to 10 years as being involved in the moral realism stage. In this stage, the child evaluates a situation based on the consequences of his or her actions.

According to Piaget, children between 7 and 8 years obey commands based on adult authority. The child lacks internal beliefs concerning justice or fair play. Children between 8 and 11 years view justice as situational; rules can be changed depending on the circumstances of the situation.

kohlberg's theory

Kohlberg describes moral development in the school-age child according to levels and stages (see Chap. 18). Level I is referred to as the premoral stage and occurs between 4 and 9 years; external control is emphasized in this level. Behavior is motivated by the wish to avoid punishment or the desire to obtain reward.

Level II occurs between 9 and 12 years and is described as the time when children conform to rules to please others. In stages 3 and 4 of this level, the child gains an internal sense of what it means to be a "nice" person.

gilligan's theory

Carol Gilligan believes that moral development in girls is different from moral development in boys. According to Gilligan, female moral reasoning is based on consideration and preservation of human relationships, whereas male moral reasoning is based on protecting the rights of others.

personal and social development

Erikson describes the major psychosocial task of the school years as industry versus inferiority. *Industry* refers to task accomplishments of the child, which may include projects of play involving creativity, completion of chores, or mastery of school projects. Children tend to measure their worth and compare their skills against peers, leading to positive feelings of accomplishment or negative feelings of inferiority.

Inferiority refers to feelings of incompetence and low self-worth. By praising the child's accomplishments and

display 24-3
caregiver guidelines for moral development

Moral development in school-age children is influenced by parental involvement:

* **Making distinctions between rules for good manners and issues of moral substance concerning justice and human relations**
* **Respecting the child's right to an apology when you have been unfair in judging the child's behavior**
* **Discussing what the child considers to be fair and unfair in family relationships and procedures**
* **Avoiding an authoritarian role when the school-age child refuses to perform even a small action, such as turning a light off, because he judges the command unfair since he didn't turn the light on**

avoiding unnecessary criticism, adults can help the child achieve a sense of industry. Helping the child achieve a sense of industry is easier than undoing feelings of inferiority once they have developed. Comparing sibling or peer performance is a common error that caregivers make. The nurse can remind caregivers that each child is unique with unique potential for achievement.

the primary learner

The primary learner interacts in a wider world that now includes school. Young children learn through experiences that provide physical, psychosocial, and intellectual developmental events (Display 24-4).

the 6-year-old

Six-year-old children are busy and excited about the transition to first grade. Preschool, nursery school, and Head Start programs help prepare the child socially and emotionally for the first grade. Most school systems require full- or part-time kindergarten attendance, reducing the likelihood of separation anxiety and conflict with school rules.

School rules encourage 6-year-olds to assume increased responsibility and self-direction. The increased accountability comes at a time when many children need practice and support in making independent judgments.

Most 6-year-olds enjoy group activities, but when tired or anxious, they prefer one-to-one contact. Caregiver–child contact is especially important at the end of the school day; however, this may not be possible for parents who work outside the home.

Six-year-old children show that they are beginning to understand abstract thinking about religious teachings. They tend to enjoy attending religious services because these experiences provide opportunities to socialize and learn.

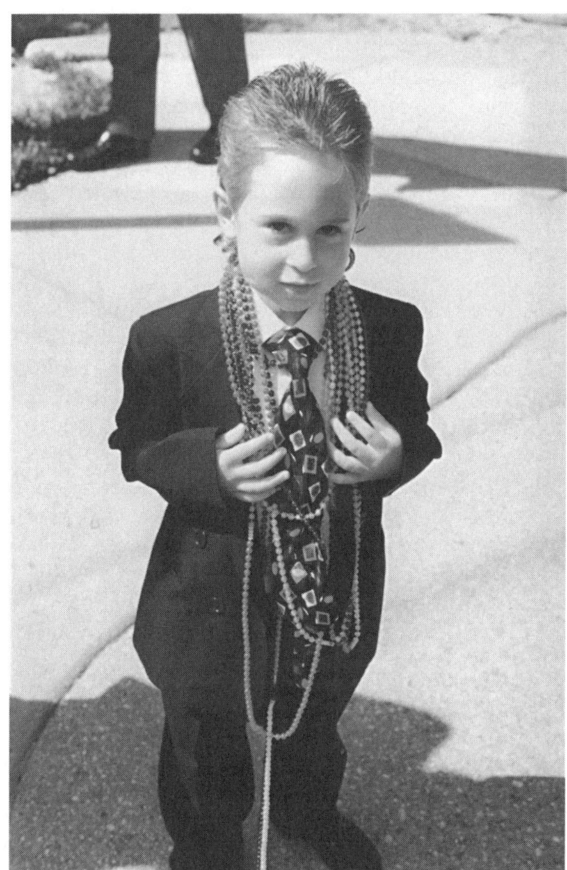

figure 24-3 *This six-year old proudly wears his collection of Mardi Gras beads.*

display 24-4
cognitive characteristics of the primary learner

Primary learner characteristics include the following:

- **Simple logical reasoning**
- **Egocentric thinking with some ability to take on the views and ideas of others**
- **Beginning skills to solve basic problems**
- **Development of strategies to complete activities or solve problems in a systematic way (searching for missing toys)**
- **Ability to plan ahead**
- **Arriving at judgments based on past**
- **Reasoning ability that is logical to the child but may not show true logic**

Six-year-olds can often be boisterous, tense, self-centered, and bossy show-offs. They also can be devastated by criticism. Adult (especially parental) love and praise are important in the child's development of positive self-image. Teasing and verbal abuse from older siblings can be especially painful to the sensitive 6-year-old.

Six-year-olds have a short attention span and tend to get involved with several projects and seldom complete any of them. They enjoy collecting things, such as leaves, butterflies, jars, bugs, and baseball cards (Fig. 24-3). They stack their collections in a haphazard manner that only they understand. They tend to voice displeasure if their belongings are disturbed by others. They enjoy using scissors to cut objects out of books, papers, and magazines but may need direction about which publications are off limits for clipping.

Six-year-old boys and girls play together in a rough house fashion. Playtime often ends in turmoil with arguments and physical battles involving both sexes. Six-year-old children enjoy pretend play and will often assume a strong gender role identity (eg, boys play policemen or cowboys, while girls play mommies or nurses).

the 7-year-old

Seven-year-old children are often quieter and less active than 6-year-olds, and they have a longer attention span. Seven-year-old children have more subdued relationships with peers, try to avoid trouble, seek parental and adult approval, and are cooperative family members. They are quick to display feelings of inferiority, become angry when experiencing failures, and take great pride in their successes.

Positive reinforcement is often more beneficial to these children than material rewards, which may be quickly discarded or consumed. Positive feelings can be recalled by the child for years to come. Seven-year-olds have a better understanding of the concept of time and demonstrate ability to read both hands on a watch or clock.

Seven-year-old children tend to spend many hours with peers of the same sex. It is common for the 7-year-old to have a "crush" on someone of the opposite sex. This feeling seldom lasts long and is usually forgotten quickly. It is important to respect the tender feelings about any relationship because a broken heart is painful at any age.

the middle school child

Children in the middle school years (8–10 years) expand their world in active, creative ways. They seek companionship and approval from their peers, joining clubs such as Boy Scouts and Girl Scouts. They want to assume responsibility, participate in group activities, and engage in hero worship (Fig. 24-4).

Most children this age are competent readers but may choose comic books as their main reading source. If comic book reading is forbidden, the child is likely to read the material without parental permission. Caregivers need to acknowledge the child's reading habits and provide guidance and encouragement with reference to desirable versus less desirable reading materials.

Middle school children are influenced strongly by what others say about them. Peer standards are more powerful than adult standards. While caregiver authority may be challenged, children have incorporated caregiver standards into their personalities and consciences by this age.

Ten-year-olds are more assertive in gaining independence, and respond more positively to suggestions rather than demands. They are courteous, well mannered with adults, self-directed, and capable of artistic accomplishments.

the preadolescent

Beginning at 10 to 11 years, physical maturation and emotional turmoil accelerate as body hormones actively prepare children for adolescence. Girls tend to display more physical maturation than boys. Children at this age are energetic, active, passionate, strong willed, opinionated, pushy, quarrelsome, and highly sensitive to peer opinions. They vacillate between dependence and independence.

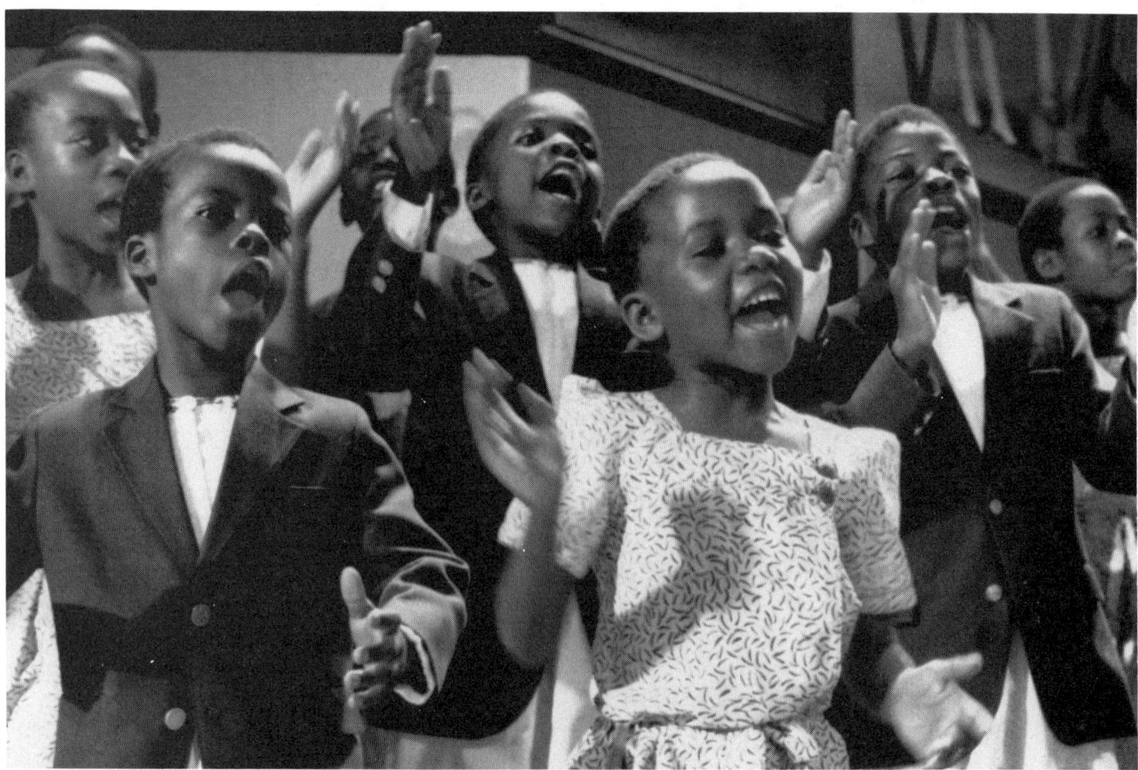

figure 24-4 *During the school years, children enjoy being part of clubs, such as church choir.*

Preadolescents tend to be less concerned with appearance in the conventional sense and more concerned with fads, peer fashion, and so forth, combining colors, styles, and articles of clothing that defy adult standards. Bathing may not be top priority for the preadolescent, even though body odors are now a concern. Preadolescent boys and girls are acutely aware of their changing bodies and body functions, which indicate signs of growing up. They are eager to learn about health and health habits.

> ✷ **nursing insight**
> *Channeling preadolescents' feelings and energies in the direction of sports and age-appropriate work can help promote positive self-esteem.*

peer relationships

Peer relationships serve many socializing functions and greatly influence the development of self-concept (Fig. 24-5). By 9 years, children expect mutual respect and affection from friends. Trusting someone outside the family helps the child learn to share feelings. Through peer group interactions, children learn that others experience many of the same feelings, fears, and frustrations about home, school, or their own abilities.

Play for the school-age child involves group interactions. Friendship groups often begin as play groups in the early school years, offering children a chance to belong and feel important. This is particularly important for children who may feel a lack of family support at home. Group membership offers the child a chance to be a leader who assigns tasks, makes up rules or rituals for the group, and dictates appropriate behavior.

This natural developmental tendency toward group interactions may lead to the formation of gangs whose main purpose is to perform illegal and destructive activities. There has been an alarming increase in these types of gangs, particularly in inner city areas. This trend has resulted in a dramatic increase in gunshot wounds and murders in children younger than 10 years. To avoid tragic, life-threatening, or even fatal consequences, caregivers are encouraged to know about their children's peer group activities.

Children who have difficulty developing peer relationships may benefit from a more structured peer group, such as Little League or Girl Scouts. Caregivers concerned about their child's choice of friends need to discuss their concerns with the child and with the child's teacher. Redirecting the child's energies into a more acceptable group can produce positive results. Some children may need professional counseling if their behavior blatantly defies parental and teacher advice.

✷ family considerations

child care

A large number of school-age children take care of themselves before and after school; they are called latch-key children. A less judgmental term is self-care. Care of children before and after school is a major issue for working parents. Various public school systems offer before- and after-school care, but families do not always have access to this resource. These families must confront the difficult dilemma of what happens to their children during this time; for many such families, child self-care is the only option.

The nurse needs to understand the context and circumstances of child care. Loneliness, fear, stress, and safety before and after school are concerns of parents and educators. Latch-key children who live in unsafe neighborhoods often are not allowed to play outside and tend to grow up in a vacuum. Children who are home alone when an accident occurs may panic or misjudge the seriousness of an injury. Fires are another concern; many children younger than 11 or 12 years cannot make sound judgments about whether to call for help or leave younger children behind. Rape, beatings, and homicides add to the list of concerns related to leaving a child home alone.

Despite these concerns, latch-key children are not always at risk. Where the child lives, the presence or absence of crime, traffic patterns, and construction activity are all factors that affect potential risk. In addition, children do not always suffer irreparable consequences from their self-care. Preparing children to meet the challenges life offers is one of the most important aspects of a family. Allowing

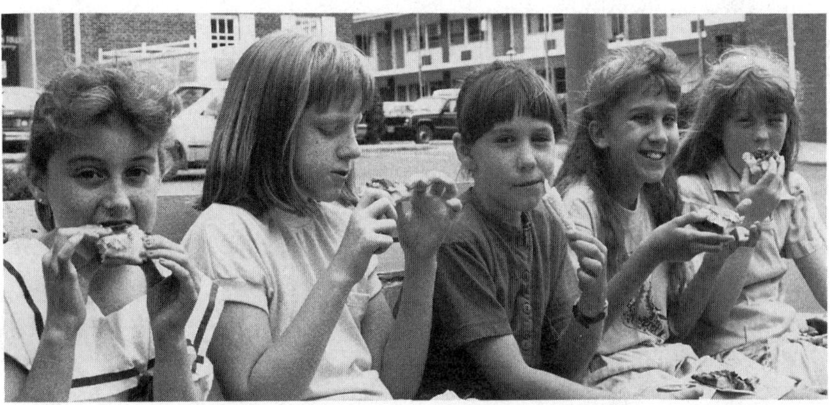

figure 24-5 *School-age children typically strive for homogeneity to support their own developing ego (eg, same gender grouping, all have bangs, long straight hair, short-sleeved tops).*

table 24-3 caregiver and child assessment for self-care responsibilities

Caregiver Factors	*Child Factors*
Confidence of child's ability to stay home alone	Ability to unlock and relock the door
Financial or work pressures that offer them no other alternative than to leave the child alone	Ability to dial a telephone and prepare a snack
Child's ability to reach the parent in an emergency	Confidence about staying alone
Workplace rules concerning emergency phone calls	Ability to read notes, field phone calls and so forth
Availability of a neighbor or relative to check on child if parent is detained at work or concerned about child's safety	Knowledge of safety factors concerning accidents, fire emergencies, choking
	Demonstration of responsible behavior and thinking patterns

children the opportunity to practice age-appropriate decision-making can become a regular part of a daily routine.

Caregiver and child readiness need to be assessed before allowing children self-care responsibilities. This assessment includes physical, emotional, and intellectual maturity. Caregiver readiness involves reasons for considering self-care, such as divorce, job responsibilities, and income. Careful assessment of the child's readiness is necessary to ensure physical and psychological safety (Table 24-3).

Family support helps the child develop a healthy self-concept, which in turn enables the child to succeed academically. Socioeconomic factors concerning differences in values held by teacher and student can cause conflicts influencing the child's self-concept and school success.

behavior problems of the school-age child

Common school-age behavior problems include trouble following directions, learning to listen, demonstrating appropriate manners, excessive television viewing, staying "on track," learning the art of confrontation, and learning to deal with others in a positive way (Table 24-4). Behavior problems and breaking rules should not be equated with failed moral development. Even though school-age children's decision-making skills have advanced, caregivers should expect mistakes to be made.

aggressive behavior

Aggression in the school-age child may be exhibited by fighting, belittling others, and displaying hostility. Aggression in the middle years may lead to problems during adolescence. The following traits are often seen in children's aggressiveness: lack of acceptable coping skills with striking out as the dominant response, especially when angry, and presence of sensitive temperament, perceiving an insult when no insult was intended. Helping children identify words that produce an emotional reaction followed by a discussion about "defusing" the word by taking the emotions away is an appropriate intervention. For example, the child who is upset about being called a "dummy" may have difficulty defining the word but is quite verbal about how the word makes him or her feel.

Aggressive behavior creates strife in the home and the health care facility. Suggestions for helping children with aggressive behavior follow:

* Treat the child with respect, establish rules for playing cooperatively, talk in an acceptable manner, and refrain from threatening other children or adults.
* Make certain the child sees the relationship between behavior and consequences, such as losing friends and privileges
* Intervene early when the child begins to argue or threaten by diverting attention to a quiet "time out" area or to another activity that helps the child release pent-up energy.

Hostile behavior in children has been linked to television, videotapes, and video games. Caregivers are encouraged to monitor subject matter and time spent in these activities.

display 24-5
child and parent exercise to reduce the "sting" of name-calling

The school-age child's ability to reason makes this simple exercise fun for dealing with sensitivities involving name-calling. After establishing rapport,

* **Call the child a name, such as "cotton ball."**
* **Ask the child if they believe they are a cotton ball and why or why not. Ask why the child believes the names other children use?**
* **Ask the child to function as a cotton ball.**
* **Use humor and playful gesturing to make the point that regardless how much the child tries, they will never be a cotton ball.**
* **Encourage child to recognize that name-calling, using words such as dummy and crybaby, is often used to get a reaction.**
* **Encourage the child to think of other ways to react to the name-calling, such as ignoring and avoiding the name-caller.**

table 24-4 common school-age behavior problems and recommended interventions

Concern	Suggested Interventions
Difficulty following directions	Establish guidelines for following directions; reward the child for following directions; allow natural consequences to occur due to the child's success or failure to follow directions.
Avoiding the truth	Establish a rule to tell the truth. Promote an open and honest line of communication. Avoid appearing shocked when child tells an untruth.
Unacceptable manners	Consider child's age; role model appropriate manners; strive for consistency.
Excess television viewing	Help the child prioritize favorite programs; establish television time after homework and chores are done; interest child in other activities (hobbies, friends); turn off the television.
Habitual tardiness	Help the child get ready for activities on time. Set an example; be sure child understands the relationship between the behavior and consequences. Establish a routine for getting ready for school, and use a timer to help the child know how much time is left.
Self-critical	Avoid being critical when correcting the child; be honest yet supportive. Help the child see good points in self and talk about them often.
Avoiding responsibility	Reward the child for accepting responsibility for problems and failures; set a good example by not engaging in blame. Avoid arguing; encourage the child to ask for help.
Avoiding homework	When possible, establish homework rules through a mutual agreement; reach agreement regarding specific study times; it may be necessary to remind the child until a pattern is established. Avoid "nagging"; write a contract with the child concerning homework rules. Discuss type of environment conducive to studying; for example, some children study better with music, while others need a quiet environment. Allow playtime between homework assignments; studying with a friend can be fun and productive.
Fearful of new situations	Avoid "forcing" a child to do fearful things; encourage the child to talk about fears. Allow time for the child to prepare for a new activity; accompany the child if possible. Encourage new activities with a peer.
Lack of sensitivity	Role model interactions by demonstrating sensitivity to family members and others; avoid teasing or saying embarrassing things when interacting with the child. Remove an insensitive child from others, and stress the importance of apologizing for "hurtful words or actions." Teach the child the difference between "friendly teasing" and "hurtful teasing." For example, "friendly teasing" does not include hurtful names or gestures but is often used to stimulate play, such as chasing each other to see who runs faster. Avoid laughing; encourage the child to role play the part of the other person.
Sibling rivalry	Treat each child with respect. Teach alternative ways to deal with anger and frustration, such as taking a walk or listening to music; reduce the emphasis on competition within the family structure; each child has strengths and weaknesses.

Nielsen reports indicate that children between 6 and 11 years watch about 26 hours of television per week. A major concern about television is the excessive amount of violence shown, even in cartoon programs designed for children.

shyness

Shy children who stand apart from others are easy to locate, but some shy children may withdraw so much that they become almost invisible. They often have difficulty interacting and making conversation with others. They play alone because the unfamiliar is a source of fear. Shy children can be influenced by inherited temperament and chronic environmental stress. When confronted with unfamiliar circumstances, such as prolonged hospitalization, death of a parent, family arguments, or mental illness in a family member, shy children show more activity in certain biologic systems, such as increased heart rate, dilated pupils, and increased muscle tension.

lying

Story telling or lying occurs during the school-age years because of the child's tendency toward egocentric thinking. This leads to a rich fantasy and make-believe world in which children have difficulty distinguishing between make-believe and reality. Lying may be the child's way of coping with failure to measure up to adult expectations. Persistent lying for no obvious reason or no apparent stress can indicate a more serious problem that requires professional counseling.

stealing

The child may take something that does not belong to him or her because of his or her inability to separate reality and make-believe. A 6-year-old may assume an object is hers because she strongly desires it. Confusion about perceived ownership can be mistaken as stealing. Sometimes stealing occurs when children give in to an impulse or to peer pressure. A more serious concern involves the child's act of stealing as a form of seeking attention because of a perceived lack of love. When stealing occurs, the child must return the items taken. Minor pirating is not a sign of delinquency. If stealing persists past 7 to 8 years or increases in frequency, counseling by a mental health professional is recommended.

Cheating is often difficult for the child to understand because it appears to be wrong in some situations but not in others. Cheating is a situational conflict, and most experts agree that children cheat under certain circumstances. Adults need to remember that children imitate the behavior of adults and often cannot understand why caregivers find their own cheating acceptable and the child's unacceptable.

school phobia

School phobia is seen in children with strong fears about separating from caregivers. School phobia can be mild, requiring parental intervention through understanding and encouragement, or more severe, requiring professional intervention. Additional information is included in Chapter 29 concerning school phobia.

divorce

Divorce is the most common major crisis in the lives of children. School-age children tend to have the most difficulty coping with divorce and often experience self-imposed guilt.

Coping with divorce can be more successful if there is continued contact with the noncustodial parent (unless that parent is abusive), frequent dependable visits, and friendly relations between divorced parents. The first year after divorce appears to be the hardest because households of divorced parents tend to be more disrupted and disorganized, with less predictable schedules for mealtimes, bedtimes, bedtime rituals, discipline, and family fun. In many cases when the mother is awarded custody of the children, the family income may drop dramatically, adding extra stress to the situation.

During the first year after divorce, boys are likely to demonstrate aggressive behaviors, and girls are likely to exhibit complaining attitudes. Children tend to nag, withhold affection, and actively ignore instructions given by the custodial parent, particularly if the mother has custody. This behavior tends to improve during the second year after divorce as households settle into a more organized routine.

✶ nursing considerations

health teaching

School-age children are generally healthy. By the sixth grade, children are actively involved in their own health care. As children mature, beliefs about health and illness become less concrete and more abstract. Studies reveal that self-esteem, gender, and parental support affect a child's health perceptions. High self-esteem contributes to healthy lifestyle practices, such as eating a balanced diet, exercising, positive peer relationships, and avoiding alcohol and tobacco products (Display 24-6 and Display 24-7)

display 24-6
developmental goals for the school-age child

* Maintenance of optimal physical growth through nutrition and exercise
* Development of a sense of industry
* Development of relationships outside the home with peers, teachers, and other adults
* Development of new cognitive and social skills
* Development of a positive self-concept
* Incorporation of safety measures in daily activities
* Development of lifestyle patterns that can promote health throughout life
* Active participation in health-promotion activities

Jackson, D.B., & Saunders, R.B. (1993). Child health nursing. Philadelphia: J.B. Lippincott.

health maintenance

immunizations

The nurse needs to inform parents that most states will refuse admittance to preschool or beginning school programs if the child has not received proper vaccination (especially for pertussis). Parents have the right to refuse immunizations for their children but need to be informed of the consequences. Diphtheria, tetanus toxoid, and pertussis vaccine or diphtheria, tetanus, acellular (reduced strength pertussis and oral polio vaccine are given at or before school entry (4–6 years). Measles, mumps, and rubella

display 24-7
goals for caregivers of school-age children

* Promote physical growth.
* Foster the development of a sense of industry.
* Encourage participation in peer group activities.
* Encourage and support school activities.
* Discuss and model moral standards of the culture.
* Foster the development of a positive self-concept.
* Foster the development of health-promotion behaviors.

Jackson, D.B., & Saunders, R.B. (1993). Child health nursing. Philadelphia: J.B. Lippincott.

vaccine is given at entry to middle school or junior high school (11–12 years) unless the second dose was given before age 11.

nutrition

Nutrition continues to be a major focus of health promotion during the school years. A 6-year-old experiencing a brief growth spurt has a good appetite but, because of the need to be in motion, often lacks the patience to sit down to eat. Obesity among school-age children is a growing concern (refer to Chap. 25).

Potential nutritional problems include small, poorly chosen, or omitted breakfasts; inadequate lunches; lack of knowledgeable adult guidance in food choices; failure to eat a well-balanced diet; and expenditure of school lunch money on junk foods, such as candy, chips, and soft drinks. School lunches are served to 60% of children in US public schools and account for 25% to 33% of total daily nutrition (Fig. 24-6).

Nursing education includes the relationship of nutrition to school performance with reference to religious, cultural, socioeconomic, and other factors impacting nutritional habits. Teaching focuses on behaviors associated with eating rather than simply providing information. Eating behaviors are learned and subject to change through various experiences.

Elimination patterns are established during the school years, and it is uncommon for the school-age child to have loss of bowel or bladder control, although bed wetting can still be a problem. About 5% of all 10-year-old children still wet their beds. The causes of enuresis and treatment are the same as those for the preschooler (See Chap. 33).

activity and rest

Sleep needs of the school-age child change with time. The 6-year-old may need 11 to 12 hours of sleep and the 12-year-old only 10. Sleep disturbances are less frequent when compared with toddler and preschool years. Night terrors or nightmares can result from seeing violent television programs or movies, discussions about death, fears about school, or personal failures and guilt. Nighttime fears experienced during the preschool years often carry over into the early school-age years, until the child is able to separate fantasy from reality (see Chap. 23). An hour or so before bedtime can be an ideal time for caregivers and children to share confidences, questions, concerns, and ideas.

Caregivers need to be alert to signs of fatigue or stress in children. Identifying emotional pressure and providing the child with guidance and support are important caregiver interventions. Younger children can become overtired easily, so it is important to maintain a bedtime hour that provides them with adequate rest.

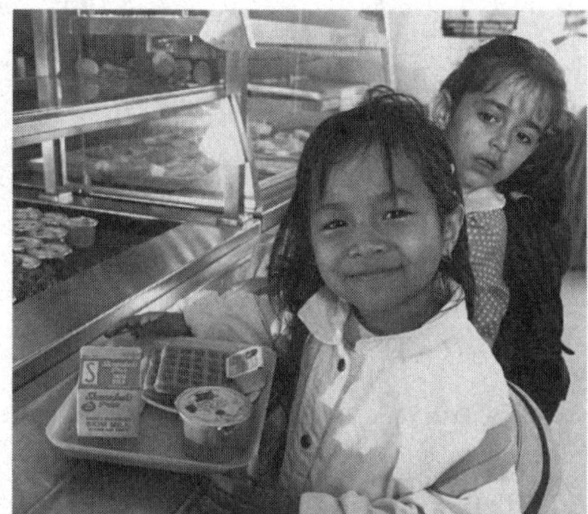

figure 24-6 *School lunch programs help children eat nutritional meals.*

dental health

Deciduous teeth are gradually lost beginning around 6 years with the eruption of permanent teeth. School-age children are proud of their "good" check-ups at the dentist. The relationship between dental caries, eating sweets, and failure to brush can be incentives for the school-age child to adhere to brushing the teeth at least twice a day.

Malocclusion is described as a notable deviation from the normal alignment of teeth, causing an overbite or underbite and requiring the attention of a dental specialist known as an *orthodontist*. Malocclusion contributes to emotional distress about the child's perception of being unattractive and may cause speech defects caused by poor tooth alignment.

Straightening of the teeth is done during the school-age years because the supportive structures are soft enough to allow gradual repositioning using braces, bands, and other orthodontic devices.

hygiene

Six- and 7-year-old children require supervision with daily care needs, such as bathing. Caregivers need to regulate the temperature of bath water, thoroughness of the bath, and the rowdiness of play in the tub or shower. Most 6- and 7-year-olds are not in tune with washing their ears, between the toes, under the fingernails, or any area considered hard to reach.

Middle school and preadolescent children do not require supervision with bathing or dressing. Modesty during preadolescence is common as the child's body begins to undergo preliminary changes associated with puberty. Middle school children and preadolescents are reluctant to accept nursing assistance with bathing while hospitalized and become embarrassed with mention of genitalia or body excretions.

Preadolescents experience body odor associated with the development of sweat glands and require the use of deodorants or antiperspirants. Manner of dress and hairstyle are closely associated with peers. Fads, such as not wear-

> **✱ nursing insight**
>
> *School-age children need to know that the risks of contracting lice is increased when they share combs, hats, headbands, safety helmets, sleeping bags, and pillows with other children.*

ing socks with sneakers, increase the risk of foot odor and athlete's foot.

safety

Death and physical disability during the school-age years is most commonly the result of motor vehicle accidents while not wearing seat belts. The use of seat belts is required by law in many states. Children are more likely to "buckle up" if their caregivers do so.

Bicycle, water, and fire safety programs are important to the school-age child (Fig. 24-7). However, parents must be aware that children may fail to practice safe behaviors even though they have been involved with safety programs. Parents must discuss emergency measures and practice specific actions necessary in an emergency situation (see Chap. 20).

Rituals for gang membership, such as being "blood sisters" or "blood brothers," puts the school-age child at risk for exposure to blood-borne pathogens, such as hepatitis and acquired immunodeficiency syndrome (AIDS). Fashion fads, such as body piercing, increase the risk of being exposed to AIDS if the needle used is contaminated.

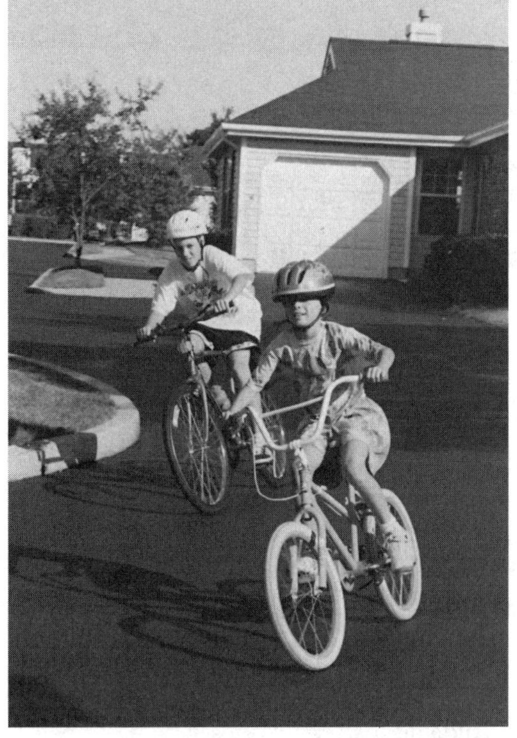

figure 24-7 *Helmets are an important part of bike safety. (Photo by Elise Dinerman.)*

substance abuse

School-age children may be tempted to experiment with substance abuse, such as alcohol or other drugs, such as airplane glue, paint thinner, and marijuana. Alcohol use may begin in early childhood and have lifelong consequences. Alcohol diminishes the ability to master developmental tasks and contributes to physical and psychological dependency. Prevention through education and example is essential. School nurses may be asked to assess a child's health status because of the teacher's concerns about behavior, such as chronic absenteeism, fatigue, and short attention span. The nurse may find the child's physical and social behaviors altered because of drugs. This requires coordinated interventions involving school, family, social services, and drug and alcohol rehabilitation agencies.

sex education

School-age children are exposed to many versions about sex (specifically sexual intercourse). *Sexuality* and *sex* can be used synonymously but do not always have the same meaning. For example, sexuality is described as the collective characteristics that indicate the differences between boys and girls. This includes such things as physical characteristics, fashion preferences involving clothing and hair style, personal feelings about self, and many more things that make a person special. Sex is used to describe male or female gender. *Sexual intercourse* is the union between a boy and girl, called *heterosexual relationships*, or between two people of the same sex, called *homosexual relationships*.

Young children are bombarded by media with sex comments and images reflecting controversy and inconsistent values. Parents, caregivers, and sex education programs help provide factual information; however, the information may be discarded if the child is not interested or views the information as irrelevant. As school-age children develop, there is a new personal investment in the business of maturing. Consequently, preadolescents try to piece ideas and facts together, often ending up with distortions. For example, a 7-year-old may appear to be listening to an open, honest discussion about sex, while thinking, "I will never do something that disgusting." However, by age 11, the information is more relevant to them, but they may be too embarrassed to ask for additional details. Material learned previously may be distorted as the preadolescent begins to sort through data relevant to them. Sex-related concerns are discussed in Table 24-5 a&b.

the hospitalized school-age child

School-age children requiring hospitalization must deal with their illness and their absence from school and peers. Prolonged absence from school may require tutoring.

table 24-5a common questions and answers about menstruation

Questions	*Answers*
Do girls start to menstruate at a specific age?	No. Each girl has her own timetable; some begin to menstruate at 10 y and others not until 14 or 15 y.
Why do girls have periods?	Girls have periods to shed the thickened lining of the uterus formed in preparation for pregnancy and discarded when there is no pregnancy. Menstruation is controlled by female hormones in the body.
What does the vaginal discharge look like?	The vaginal discharge often called "menstrual flow" or "menses" may consist of a few teaspoons to ½ cup for 3 to 7 days. The discharge can be brownish-red, dark-red, and sometimes even rusty colored. It looks like blood because there is blood in the discharge. Your body has produced extra blood that is not needed unless pregnancy occurs; menstruation allows the body to get rid of the extra blood.
Can girls wear tampons if they are virgins?	Yes. The vaginal opening has a natural opening large enough to admit a tampon.
Do tampons ever get lost inside?	Tampons will not get lost because the vaginal passage is closed at the top and if the string comes off, tampons can be removed with the fingers. Tampons must be replaced as often as sanitary pads, because the discharge is not usually visible with tampons. It is suggested you change the tampon at least every 4 hours.
Does menstruation smell?	Menstrual blood has a strong odor when exposed to air. Keeping your genitals clean, changing sanitary pads, using deodorant pads, and wearing clean underwear eliminates a great deal of the odor.
Do all girls have menstrual cramps and what causes them?	No. Not all girls have menstrual cramps, and no one knows for sure what causes them. Some experts think they are caused by an overproduction of chemicals (hormones) that cause the uterus to contract and block the menstrual flow. If you have menstrual cramps, try taking medicine, such as ibuprofen. Many girls find that exercise prevents or reduces cramp discomfort.
Why can girls get bloated and irritable during their periods?	The hormone estrogen causes the body to retain fluid. Cutting back on the intake of salt decreases bloating and irritability.
Can a girl get pregnant before she has started her period?	Yes. Ovulation takes place about 14 days before menstruation, and this is the time a girl can get pregnant.
Do you have a period every month for the rest of your life?	No. Menstruation stops during pregnancy, change of life (menopause), and after surgical removal of the uterus (hysterectomy). The menstrual cycle can be irregular or stop temporarily with severe illness, excessive exercise, stress, and while taking certain medications.

Common fears of hospitalization include disability and possible death, unknown events and procedures that may be painful, loss of control and independence, and interruption of daily routine.

perceptions about death

Dealing with death issues involves the child, family, health care providers, school nurse, teachers, and community. The increase in street violence, drive-by shootings, public and school shootings, and drug overdose exposes young children to death. Grief work of children is linked with their developmental age. Children experience grief in each stage of development. If a 4-year-old's brother dies, the child may believe that his brother will come back to life. During the next 4 to 5 years, the child will realize that his brother is not coming back, causing a renewal of sad feelings. Studies suggest children need to address "death issues" in each stage of their development until they reach mature conclusions. Nurses can help parents and caregivers better understand the child's needs and behaviors because adults may have resolved most of their personal grief after 5 to 10 years and question the child's statements or inquiries about the dead person as being unnatural.

Between 5 and 9 years, children appear to be able to accept the idea that a person has died. However, they may not understand that it is something that will happen to everyone and particularly to themselves. Around the ages of 9 and 10, the child recognizes death as an inevitable experience that will occur to them.

table 24-5b pertinent information for boys during puberty

Questions	Answers
What are some major differences between boys' and girls' sex organs?	Besides the obvious penis and vagina differences, boys have testes that continuously manufacture sperm that is stored in coiled tubes on top of of the testicles and released during ejaculation. Girls have two ovaries that produce an egg each month that is discarded during menstruation. Boys can father a child at any time, but girls only can become pregnant 2 or 3 days each month during ovulation. Boys and girls have different hormones.
What causes an erection?	An erection is nature's way to enable a boy to have intercourse. When boys are stimulated, the veins in the penis fill with blood, and the penis becomes longer and firmer.
Why do I have erections when I'm not even thinking about sexual things?	During early adolescence, unstable hormone levels contribute to spontaneous erections. Erections may be caused by a full bladder and by touching or rubbing the penis.
What is ejaculation and where does it come from?	Ejaculation is a spurt of whitish liquid called semen that comes from the opening at the end of the penis when a boy reaches sexual climax. This is the same opening that the boy urinates from, but during intercourse, the urine tubes close off so that urine and semen do not mix. Semen contains sperm and fluids that are capable of making a girl pregnant.
Does ejaculation make you weak?	No. Frequent or infrequent ejaculations do not affect stamina. Most boys experience a sense of relaxation after ejaculation and may not be able to achieve another erection for 20 to 60 minutes.
What happens when you have an erection and you don't ejaculate?	Nothing. It may be frustrating and leave you sexually anxious, but sperm does not "back up," cause the testicles to swell ("blue balls"), or anything else.
What is a wet dream?	A dream or friction that causes an erection and ejaculation during sleep. It is not the same as urinating in your sleep. The liquid that comes out of the penis is semen.

Most school-age children are acquainted with death from loss of a pet or family member. Television and movies clarify or confuse the child's concept of death. The concept of life and death is elemental to emotional development and a natural progression in life. It offers mystery to adults and children. Nurses need to understand their personal concepts about death before they can be effective with dying or grieving clients.

There is no right way to inform a child about the death of a significant person in their life; however, most experts suggest that the child be informed immediately. How the child is told about the death tends to be equal or greater in significance than what words are used. For example, Deidra, age 9, was told about her mother's death while sitting on her father's lap. They both cried and made promises to help each other. Deidra, now 22, does not remember what words her father used but remembers feeling sad and loved. Words associated with death include dead, funeral, funeral home, casket, burial, cremation, corpse, embalming, grief, mourning, viewing, grave, hearse, afterlife, and memorial services. Refer to Table 24-6 for additional information.

key points

- **School-age years are between 6 and 12; 6- to 8-year-olds are called primary learners, 9- and 10-year-olds are called middle school children, and 11- and 12-year-olds are called preadolescents.**
- **School-age years reflect a tendency for physical development to slow, while cognitive development becomes more advanced.**
- **The appearance of the school-age child results from diminished fat, increased muscle mass and leg length, and loss of "babylike" softness of features; long arms and legs and large hands and feet contribute to the child's tendency to be clumsy.**
- **During the school-age years, children show dramatic improvements in timing and coordination skills, resulting from the maturity of the nervous system, enabling body development, refinement, and coordination of gross and fine motor skills.**
- **Psychosocial development of the school-age child involves the development of a sense of industry and ad-**

table 24-6 *age-related concepts of death*

Age	*Concepts*	*Actions*	*Interventions*
Infancy	They have no concept of death. They respond to parental or caregiver emotions Older than 7 mo, infant feels separation anxiety	Irritable; crying; physical symptoms, such as vomiting, rash, anorexia	Hold infant; keep routine as normal as possible.
2–5 y	Death is reversible. Life continues regardless of death. Dead person continues to think, grow bigger, and knows what goes on in the world. Cemeteries are where dead people live. If death is explained as going to sleep, child may develop nightmares and sleep disturbances	Guilt feelings originate from "magical thinking" that the living child wished the death and it happened. May make inappropriate comments, such as "I'll die if I'm not good." May dig up dead pet for inspection. May want to touch a corpse.	Use age-appropriate language to explain death. Use correct terms, such as dead or death. Accept the child's response even though comments may not be accurate; correct without scolding. Child needs extra love and security. Be honest if you don't know the answer to a question. Discuss death as a part of life, comparing human life with nature, such as flowers or seasons of the year.
5– 9 y	Death has a personality, mostly invisible. Death is a skeleton, something ugly that takes people. Death is seen as permanent. Child fears death.	Crying anxiety, quietness	Provide security, be responsive to child's emotions without punishment or judgment. Give reassurance. Stress grief is normal. Anger may be displaced.
9 –12 y	Child recognizes death as cessation of life that operates from within the body. Death is inevitable and irreversible and ends bodily life.	Separation anxiety from parents or caregivers fearing they will die; helpful to parents in an attempt to make the situation better for the family Poor grades, self-imposed isolation from peers	Be open and honest with child. Ask if child fears death. Provide hugs and encouragement. Provide the child with the opportunity to view the body or attend the funeral.
Adolescence	Able to think in an abstract way about life and death Uses religious views in coping with a loss	May become absorbed in death issues, projecting anger and aggression May engage in risk-taking events, such as driving under the influence of drugs, Russian roulette, or other suicidal gestures	Encourage the teen to talk about the loss and concepts of death. Respond to gestures suggesting suicide in a direct and open manner. Refer for professional counseling if necessary.

vancement of self-concept through successful achievements brought about by trial and error, learning how to cope with failure, learning endurance, and balancing feelings of inferiority with a sense of achievement. Erikson defines industry as task accomplishments of the child, leading to positive feelings of accomplishment or negative feelings of inferiority, including incompetence and low self-worth.

* The school-age child is involved with cognitive development described by Piaget as conservation, classification, seriation, decentering, and reversibility; this promotes the transition from preoperational thought to concrete operational thought. It also enables the child to deal with what is happening now rather than what could happen and to develop a moral code enabling the child to deal with rules of society.
* Language development during the school years integrates the child's communication abilities and thinking processes, promoting the use of abstract words without fully understanding their meaning and using language for prediction, empathy, and reasoning.
* Learning disabilities are defined by law as a significant gap between a child's intelligence and the skill achieved at each age. They result in hidden handicaps that do not disfigure or leave visible signs but do affect a child's ability to interpret what is seen and heard or

to combine information from different parts of the brain.

- **Moral development in the school-age years includes the development of a value system, a sense of justice or fair play, and knowledge of right and wrong. These are the most universal tasks of childhood; they are essential to the continuation of a civilized society and are learned through an interactive process between the child and the social environment.**
- **Family considerations include child care before and after school and behavior problems.**

review questions

1. The 6- to 8-year-old child is called
   a. middle school age.
   b. primary learner.
   c. preadolescent.
   d. adolescent.
2. Mrs. Chinn is concerned that her 7-year-old son has stopped growing. An appropriate nursing intervention includes
   a. comparing the child's present weight and height, plotting the present values on a standardized growth chart, and noting whether the measurements fall between the 5th and 95th percentiles.
   b. reassuring Mrs. Chinn that her son is busy with motor skills rather than physical growth.
   c. reassuring Mrs. Chinn that all children experience growth "lags."
   d. reassuring Mrs. Chinn that Asian children are naturally smaller than African American children.
3. An example of positive psychosocial development in the primary learner includes
   a. trial and error learning.
   b. conservation.
   c. awareness of social injustice.
   d. ability to assume total self-care responsibilities.
4. Mrs. Mattison is concerned about her 11-year-old daughter's mood swings and development of secondary sex characteristics. Select the most accurate nursing response:
   a. "Peer relationships influence a child's moods."
   b. "Family support helps children develop healthy temperaments."
   c. "An 11-year-old is considered a preadolescent, and mood swings and development of secondary sex characteristics are normal during this time."
   d. "These concerns are normal, and the child should be seen by a specialist."
5. Select the most appropriate definition of learning disability:
   a. Dreaded fear of school reflected by complaints of physical problems and school absences
   b. Failure to develop a value system
   c. Lack of speech development
   d. Significant gap between child's intelligence and the skill achieved at each age

references

Schuster, C., & Ashburn, S. (1992). *The process of human development: A holistic life-span approach* (3rd ed.). Philadelphia: J.B. Lippincott.

bibliography

Betz, C., & Poster, E. (1992). *Pediatric nursing reference.* St. Louis: C.V. Mosby.

Castiglia, P., & Harbin, R. (1992). *Child health care.* Philadelphia: J.B. Lippincott.

Charlesworth, R. (Ed.) (1992). *Understanding child development.* Albany, NY: Delmar.

Gulanick, M., Gradishar, D., & Puzas, M. (1994). *Ambulatory pediatric nursing*. Albany, NY: Delmar.

Jackson, D., & Saunders, R. (1993). *Child development.* Philadelphia: J.B. Lippincott.

(1996). *Lippincott's review series: Pediatric nursing*. Philadelphia: Lippincott.

Marhoefer, P., & Vadnais, L. (Eds.) (1992). *Caring for the developing child.* Albany, NY: Delmar.

McIntier, S. T. (1995). Nursing the family when a child dies. *RN*, *58*(2), 50–54.

Morrison, S. (1990). *The world of child development.* Albany, NY: Delmar.

North American Nursing Diagnosis Association (1994). *Nursing diagnoses: Definitions and classification 1995-1996.* Philadelphia: Author.

Nelms, B. (1993). Discipline: What do you recommend? *Pediatric Health Care*, *7*(1), 1–2.

Steinberg, L., & Levine, A. (1990). *You and your adolescent: A parents' guide for ages 10-20*. New York: Harper and Row.

the adolescent

25

outline

objectives 

After studying this chapter, the reader should be able to:

* Define the words pubescence, puberty, and adolescence.
* Describe the physiologic changes and specific characteristics seen in boys and girls at the onset of puberty relative to body size, composition, proportions, sex organs, body hair, and menstruation in girls.
* Describe the procedures for testicular and breast self-examination.
* List four factors influencing the development of logical thinking in adolescence.
* List the three factors reflecting Erik Erikson's stage of adolescent identity.
* Discuss how adolescent morality behaviors conflict with Kohlberg's theory of moral development.
* Discuss at least four factors that influence adolescent and parental communications.
* List at least five ways parents can influence adolescent decision-making abilities.
* List at least four behaviors that depressed adolescents exhibit.

key terms 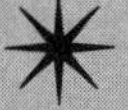

adolescence
anorexia nervosa
bulimia
identity
lactose intolerance
physiologic leukorrhea
prostaglandins
pubescence
scoliosis
thelarche

Adolescence is a difficult time because the adolescent is no longer a child but is not yet an adult. During this growth period, the body transforms in major ways. The adolescent must define who he or she is and how to relate to peers, family, and society. These years are a complex, challenging time for the adolescent, the family, and the nurse involved in their care (Display 25-1). This chapter addresses the physiologic changes and psychosocial issues associated with puberty.

Adolescence is derived from the Latin word *adolescere*, meaning "to grow up." The period of adolescence spans almost a decade, from 12 to 20 years of age. Adolescents between 13 and 19 years are called *teenagers*. Adolescence is usually described as having three separate phases: preadolescence (10–12 years, also called pubescence), early adolescence (13–15 years), and late adolescence (16–19 years). Adolescence is a period of remarkable growth and development, second only to the period between conception and birth.

During *preadolescence*, the reproductive system begins to mature, and secondary sexual characteristics appear. This is the period just before *puberty*, which is when reproductive maturity is reached. At puberty, a girl is capable of becoming pregnant, and a boy is capable of impregnating a girl.

puberty

Puberty follows an independent biologic timetable unrelated to other aspects of maturation. The adolescent may look like a child but feel like an adult or look like an adult but feel like a child. During the transition from child to adult, parents and teens may need to deal with indecision, anxiety, conflict, and rebellion. Many teenagers move through adolescence in a tranquil, responsible manner, while others experience turmoil. There are no clear-cut answers as to why one person has difficulties making the transition while another takes the changes in stride. Some experts point to the relationship between the teenager's temperament and parental expectations. Problems can occur when children fail to meet parental or societal expectations. Open, honest communication between adolescents and parents can help diminish conflict.

display 25-1
adolescent stress concerns

Friendship concerns: Peer pressure, belonging, popularity
School concerns: Grades, teacher expectations, peer competition, athletics, being trusted, being stereotyped
Family concerns: Relationship with parents, fear of disappointing parents, lack of respect from parents, divorce, step-parents, being compared with siblings
General issues: Freedom and responsibility, money, lifestyle, equating mistakes with failure, career decisions, personal decisions about drugs, sex, trust

onset of puberty

The onset of puberty varies from one adolescent to another. The anterior pituitary gland plays an important role by stimulating production and secretion of sex hormones necessary for reproductive system maturity (see Chap. 4). Genetic factors also influence the onset of puberty. Girls reach puberty between 8 and 14 years and complete the process in about 3 years. Boys begin puberty later than girls, generally between 9 and 16 years and complete the process by 18 to 20 years.

Precocious puberty or early puberty is a rare condition that results from an abnormality of one of the major glands that produce sex hormones. Delayed puberty is also an alteration of adolescent development afflicting boys more often than girls. Both conditions are discussed in Chapter 33.

Puberty triggers dramatic changes in body size, shape, composition, and proportion. Boys and girls experience muscle growth and skeletal growth accompanied by a loss of body fat. Adolescents often appear long, thin, and out of proportion because the legs, hands, and feet reach adult size before the trunk of the body. The changing appearance of sexual organs and increased levels of sex hormones also distinguish this period of transition. Teenagers have many questions about their changing bodies. They need to be reassured that puberty is a normal, natural stage of growth and development.

height changes

Boys grow between 10.2 and 30.8 cm (4–12 in) in height during adolescence. Boys' height spurt usually begins 1 year after the first testicular growth. Girls grow between 5.1 and 20.5 cm (2–8 in) in height after *menarche* (onset of menstruation). After the initial growth spurt, boys and girls average an additional ½- to 1-in height increase.

weight changes

Boys experience greater growth of muscles and bones during puberty than do girls; however, girls lose a greater proportion of body fat. Normal weight gain for girls during adolescence averages 6.8 to 25 kg (15–55 lb) during a 3-year period. Adolescent boys gain an average of 6.8 to 29.5 kg (15–65 lb) during a 4-year period.

secondary male sexual characteristics

Growth of the penis, testes, and scrotum usually occurs before pubic hair appears. With the onset of testicular growth, it is not unusual for one testicle to hang lower than the other.

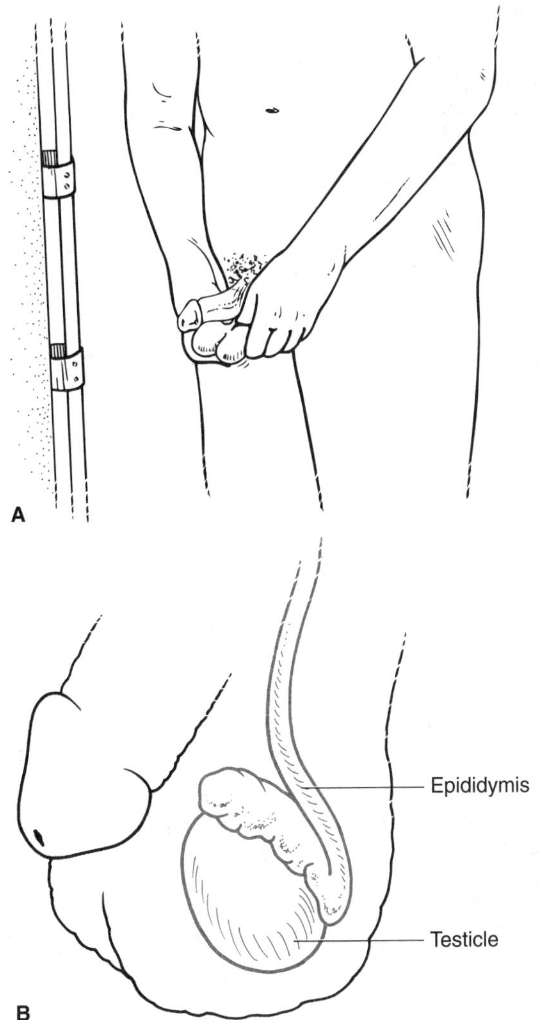

figure 25-1 *Testicular self-examination.*

Monthly testicular self-examination is recommended for early detection of cancer of the testes (see Figure 25-1 and Teaching Guidelines for Testicular Self-Examination). Testicular cancer is the most common form of cancer in males between the ages of 15 and 35 years. White males are four times more likely to develop testicular cancer than African American males. The rate among Hispanic males lies between that of African American and white males. Boys with undescended testicles and those whose testicles descended after 6 years are at increased risk of testicular cancer (National Cancer Institute, 1994).

> ✷ **nursing insight**
>
> *Adolescent boys are at risk for orchitis (inflammation of the testes) as a complication of mumps.*

> ✷ **nursing insight**
>
> *Adolescent girls are at risk for mastitis (inflammation of the breasts) and oophoritis (inflammation of the ovaries) as a complication of mumps.*

> **teaching guidelines** ✷
> *testicular self-examination*
>
> (See Figure 25-1.)
>
> * Stand naked in front of a mirror, and view the appearance of the scrotum
> * Roll each testicle gently between the thumbs and forefingers of both hands; one testicle is normally slightly larger than the other.
> * Feel along the small, firm, cordlike area on top and back of each testicle.
> * Examine the tube that comes up from the cordlike areas for normal characteristics of firmness, flexibility, and smoothness.
> * Report to parents any of the following signs:
>   Dull pain in the groin
>   Change in the appearance or firmness of the testicles
>   Any lump, particularly on the side of a testicle
>
> *Cancer can feel like a small, painless, pea-sized lump on the front or sides of a testicle.*

Male axillary and facial hair begins to appear about 2 years after pubic hair. Later in adolescence, the male voice deepens. Penile erections, occurring periodically since before birth, become more frequent and may be accompanied by involuntary release of semen during sleep, referred to as "wet dreams." During puberty, boys begin to experience unexpected, spontaneous erections. They become concerned about penis size, and boys with small penises may feel inferior to their peers. The adolescent boy needs to know that the size of a flaccid penis is no indication of how large it will be when erect and that sexual functioning does not depend on penis size.

During puberty, boys can develop a small, tender lump often described as a *kernel* beneath one or both of the nipples. This is normal and is called *male breast development*; it usually disappears within 1 year. Although breast cancer is not as common in men as in women, nurses need to emphasize breast self-examination in addition to testicular self-examination. Enlarged or tender breasts need to be reported to the parents or a physician.

secondary female sexual characteristics

Girls usually enter puberty 2 years earlier than boys. The development of breast buds *(thelarche)* and presence of pubic hair are often the first signs of puberty in the female, appearing between 8 and 13 years. As breasts enlarge, so do ovaries, uterus, vagina, labia, and clitoris. (see Fig. 4-1A)

During early puberty, it is not uncommon for one breast to be larger than the other, creating an unbalanced appearance. Extra nipples are rare, but if present, they are usually harmless except for making the breast look differ-

1. Stand before a mirror. Inspect both breasts for anything unusual, such as any discharge from the nipples, puckering, dimpling, or scaling of the skin.

The next two steps are designed to emphasize any change in the shape or contour of your breasts. As you do them you should be able to feel your chest muscles tighten.

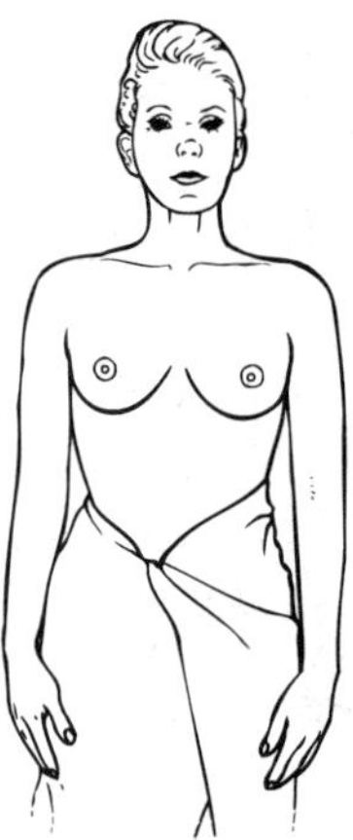

4. Raise your left arm. Use three or four fingers of your right hand to explore your left breast firmly, carefully, and thoroughly. Beginning at the outer edge, press the flat part of your fingers in small circles, moving the circles slowly around the breast. Gradually work toward the nipple. Be sure to cover the entire breast. Pay special attention to the area between the breast and the armpit, including the armpit itself. Feel for any unusual lump or mass under the skin.

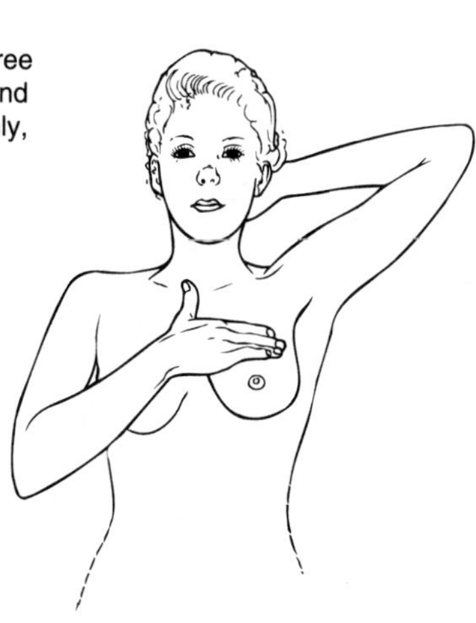

2. Watching closely in the mirror, clasp hands behind your head and press hands forward.

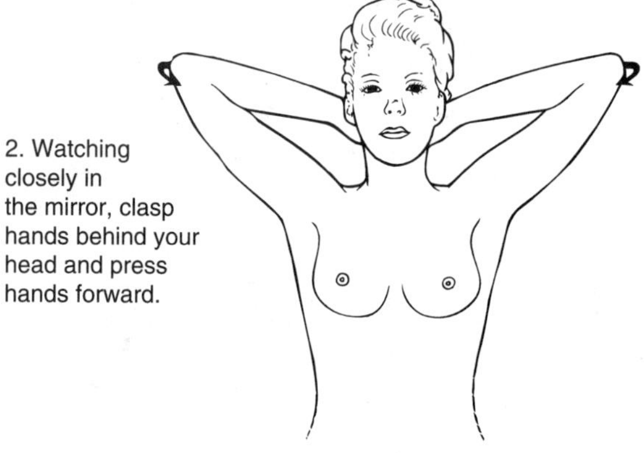

5. Gently squeeze the nipple and look for a discharge. (If there is a discharge, see your doctor.) Repeat the exam on your right breast.

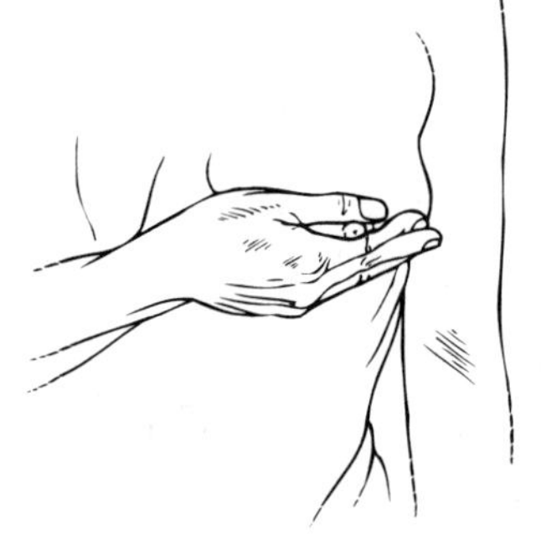

3. Next, press hands firmly on hips and bow slightly toward your mirror as you pull your shoulders and elbows forward.

Some women do the next part of the exam in the shower. Fingers glide over soapy skin, making it easy to concentrate on the texture underneath.

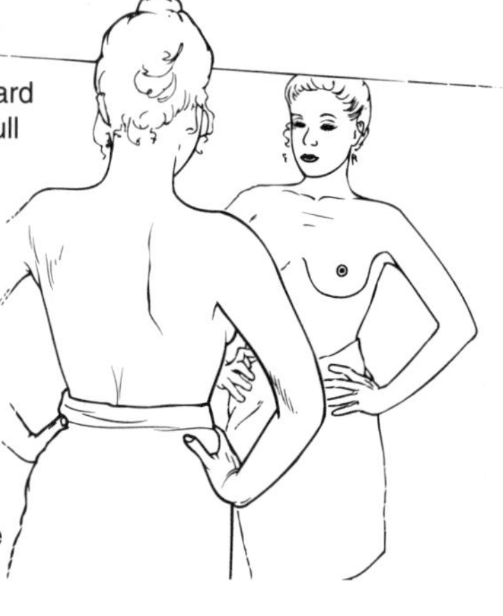

6. Steps 4 and 5 should be repeated lying down. Lie flat on your back, left arm over your head and a pillow or folded towel under your left shoulder. This position flattens the breast and makes it easier to examine. Use the same circular motion described earlier. Repeat on your right breast.

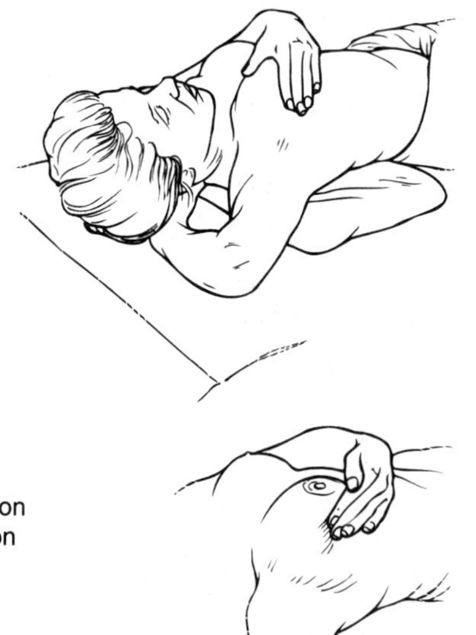

figure 25-2 *Breast self-examination should be done once a month so you become familiar with the usual appearance and feel of your breasts. Familiarity makes it easier to notice any changes in the breast from one month to another. Early discovery of a change from what is "normal" is the main idea behind BSE. If you menstruate, the best time to do BSE is 2 or 3 days after your period ends, when your breasts are least likely to be tender or swollen. If you no longer menstruate, pick a day, such as the first day of the month, to remind yourself it is time to do BSE.*

teaching guidelines
breast self-examination

* Stand in front of a mirror with breasts exposed and arms to the side. Check for dimpling or bulges in the skin, size of breasts, and any nipple changes. Move arms to back of head and then to sides of hips. Each time you reposition your arms, examine the breasts as shown.
* Check the nipple for discharge by squeezing it between your thumb and forefinger. A whitish-colored discharge is normal. Yellow or rust-colored discharge is not normal and needs to be reported to parents or a health professional.
* Lie on your back, raise one arm above your head, and examine the breast on that side, making slow circular movements with the sensitive pads of the fingers of the opposite hand. Divide the breast surface and underarm area into strips and examine each strip from top to bottom. Note any changes in the tissue or the presence of lumps. Do the same thing on the opposite side.
* Sit up, and do the same kind of examination.

ent. Surgical treatment is an option for noticeable breast size irregularities or extra nipples.

Monthly breast self-examination is an important health care measure for young women. Breast self-examination is best done 1 week after the first day of the menstrual period because breasts are less tender during this time. Many young women prefer to do breast self-examination when bathing because fingers slide over soapy, wet skin more easily (see Figure 25-2 and Teaching Guidelines for Breast Self-Examination).

The incidence of breast cancer has increased by 1% per year since the early 1970s. Because there is no known way to prevent or cure breast cancer, early detection offers the best opportunity for effective treatment. This means that monthly breast self-examination needs to become a habit for women, beginning in adolescence. It is particularly important for young women because mammography is ineffective in detecting breast tumors in women until some time after age 40. Breast cancer may occur at any age after the onset of menses and is increasing among younger women. Thirty-two percent of American women will be diagnosed as having breast cancer in 1995. There is an 18% mortality rate with breast cancer (CA, 1995).

menstruation

The first menstrual period is called *menarche* and is almost always painless, because cramping does not occur until ovulation takes place. Ovulation sometimes does not occur until months after the first menstrual period. The exact cause of menstrual cramping is unknown. Some experts think it is caused by overproduction of hormone-like substances called *prostaglandins* that cause the uterus to contract and block menstrual flow.

Vaginal discharge often occurs several months before menstruation begins and sometimes lasts 1 year or more after menarche. This discharge is called *physiologic leukorrhea* and is secreted from glands within the female genital system. Considered normal, the discharge may vary from clear to white, from watery to thick, and from small to medium amounts.

Healthy attitudes about menstruation are closely associated with a young woman's attitudes regarding sexual identity, sexual intercourse, and childbearing. Young girls are often exposed to a great deal of information concerning sexual activity without fully understanding the basics about menstruation.

cognitive development

The adolescent's developed body and brain make higher intellectual accomplishments possible. According to Piaget, the adolescent engages in logical thinking (formal operations) during puberty. Formal operational thought is a progressive process incorporating abstract reasoning, systematic problem-solving, and symbolic and logical reasoning.

Adolescents are capable of highly imaginative thinking and like to exercise their newfound intellectual abilities. They may attempt to solve long-standing problems of the world in such areas as politics, environmental issues, and religion. Adults may perceive the adolescent as being too idealistic or unrealistic in their questioning the established protocol. Adolescent idealism reflects a strong sense of hope in their efforts to make a better and safer world by correcting problems of injustice, greed, corruption, and other human foibles (Fig. 25-3).

The development of logical thinking is influenced by many factors, such as academic self-concept and interest in school, feelings of control over life, manageable stress,

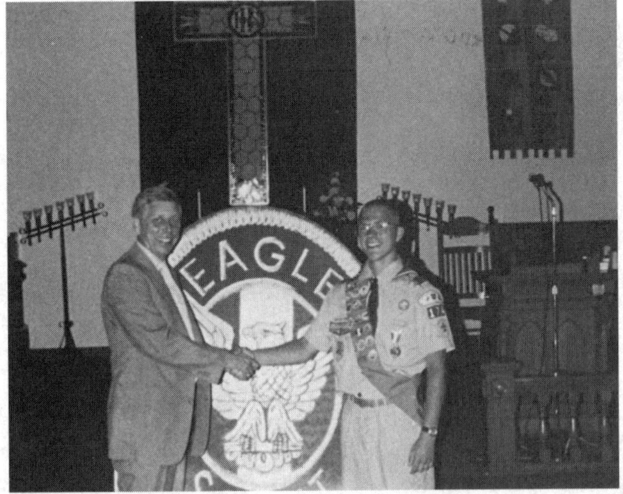

figure 25-3 *Adolescent idealism reflects a strong sense of hope to make a better, safer world by correcting problems of injustice, greed, corruption, and other human failings.*

and creativity to focus on different solutions to problems. Adolescents with personal and educational interest and training in science, logic, and mathematics demonstrate a strong ability to think logically.

school influences

School changes often occur as teenagers move from neighborhood elementary schools to large middle schools or junior high schools. Teenagers may view moving from one school to another as an exciting milestone on the road to maturity. However, such a change also can be stressful for the teen and family. Coping with changes in the school situation can be most difficult for teens who experience the following:

* Changing schools within 6 months of peak pubertal changes
* Other life changes, such as parental divorce or separation, in addition to puberty
* Low self-esteem
* Lack of popularity
* History of problem behavior in elementary grades
* Decline in grade point averages
* Decline in extracurricular activities

When stresses related to school become too powerful, students may drop out before graduation. This action can have lifelong implications. Failure to graduate from high school predisposes the teenager to low-wage jobs and impoverished lifestyles. Adolescents who drop out of school before learning to read or perform simple arithmetic skills can be hampered throughout life by these deficiencies. High school drop-outs often experience a deep sense of having nowhere to go and have little or no self-worth. Lack of interest in school is credited to many factors, including language problems, poverty, teenage pregnancy, and school versus personal and cultural differences.

Peer pressure is usually not a major deciding factor when a teenager drops out of school. Home and school influences tend to play a much more significant role in motivating students to remain in school or to drop out (Fig. 25-4; Lewitt, 1992).

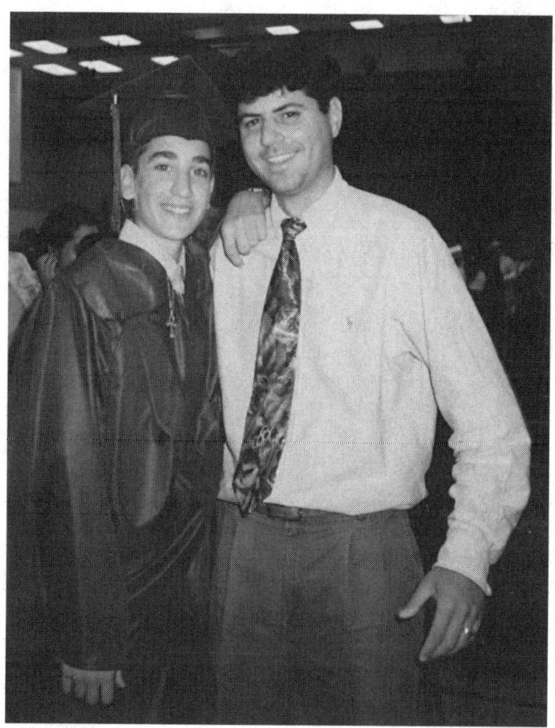

figure 25-4 *An older sibling, viewed as a role model, often encourages the adolescent to succeed in school.*

psychosocial development

According to Erikson, identity development is a lifelong process. Each previous stage contributes to a sense of being. Erikson describes events that involve crisis and result in adolescent identity development.

* Adolescents have difficulty waiting because nothing seems to come fast enough. They are tempted to take shortcuts and make premature commitments like marriage or parenthood. This delays self-discovery and identity resolution.
* Adolescents struggle for freedom from the parent, establishing rules and regulations based on self-needs. Personal doubt and insecurities are often covered up by arrogant "know it all" attitudes.
* Adolescents often have grandiose ideas and plans that do not match their skills or perseverance. They fluctuate between child-like and sophisticated adult-like behaviors.
* Adolescents begin to focus on social and career skills necessary for adult success.
* Adolescents face and resolve gender identity, gender orientation, and gender expression.
* Adolescents identify what they are against before they are able to clarify what they are for and why.

A sense of identity usually evolves gradually and involves a period of soul searching (often referred to as an identity crisis). This enables adolescents to emerge as adults with commitments that are truly their own. Adolescent decision-making involves whether to date a particular person, take a particular course, use drugs, become sexually active, become politically involved, go to college, join the Armed Forces, and so forth.

sex-role identity

Components of sexual identity include having an inner sense of being a girl or boy, behaving in accordance with one's culturally defined gender role, and determining sexual partner orientation. Children are subjected to gender typing from parents, television, teachers, and peers.

Physical and psychological growth changes noted during adolescence make gender differences more obvious compared to other stages of growth and development. Much energy is centered on learning skills that will ensure heterosexual success.

Same-sex personal relationships formed during adolescence tend to be closer and more stable than during other growth periods. Adolescent intimacies established by sharing secrets, good times, school, and sports experiences play a significant role in success with future heterosexual relationships. Ironically, the positive feelings generated by same-sex intimacies may cause stress in children (especially boys), causing homophobia. Homophobia is an intense fear and intolerance of homosexuality.

Between 12 and 16 years, it is common for adolescents to experience mixed feelings about sexual identity and relationships. For example, adolescents often spend a night out with peers of the same sex, preferring their company over that of the opposite sex.

heterosexual relationships

Relationships with the opposite sex intensify during adolescence (Fig. 25-5). Dating patterns may begin in early or late adolescence and are influenced by individual and parental attitudes, community standards, socioeconomic status, and culture. "Crowd dates" are common and provide a degree of emotional safety for young adolescents. For example, groups of boys and girls attending parties or school functions can practice social skills necessary for more serious dating without a one-to-one commitment. Peer backing and support often encourage behaviors in a crowd setting that are more forward and assertive (safety in numbers).

Double dates often originate from crowd dating. Double dating frequently involves friends pairing off into smaller group. Double dates grant teenagers an opportunity to meet and share experiences with a broad range of people.

Double dating can involve "blind dates." Blind dates occur when a girl and boy are introduced to each other through a mutual friend for the purpose of being a "couple" for an event, such as a dance, show, or party. Blind dates can be risky for the teenager, especially if car privileges are involved.

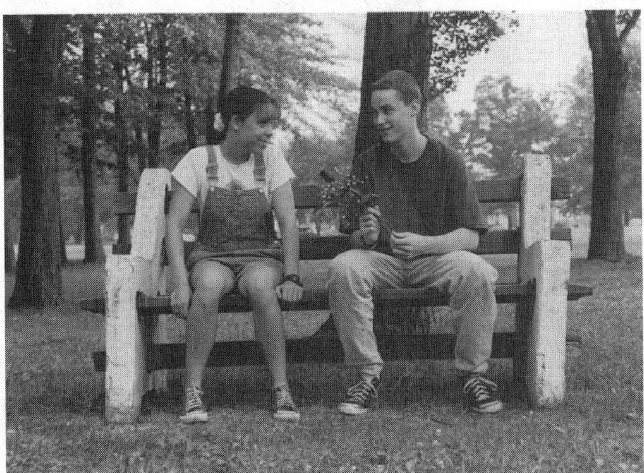

figure 25-5 *Dating is a vital part of adolescence (© Photo by Elise Dinerman).*

For example, when dates are arranged, the adolescent may not know about the blind date's background: whether the date uses drugs, drives recklessly, or is verbally, physically, or sexually abusive. The date may begin as a double date and during the evening turn into a single date, increasing the risk of intimacy. Blind dates and single dates are anxiety producing unless the two people share some common interests and are viewed as "acceptable" to each other.

Single-pair dating tends to be more frequent in adolescents with driving privileges. Single-pair dating provides the couple a degree of privacy for sharing intimacies. This aspect of single-pair dating has positive and negative qualities. A positive outcome includes the development of deeper feelings and a commitment to the relationship; negative aspects involve sexual intimacies, which increase the risk of pregnancy and sexually transmitted diseases.

homosexual relationships

Sexual preference is considered an issue during adolescence because this is a time when society recognizes sexual identity as an important part of growth and development. When adolescents continue into adulthood with a preference for their own sex, they are referred to as *homosexual.* Many young homosexuals acknowledge having distinct sexual and social orientations different from their heterosexual friends before reaching adolescence.

The pressures of dealing with sexual differences are overwhelming to many homosexual youths, increasing their risk for emotional and behavioral problems, including suicide. Young homosexuals have a difficult time sorting through issues of identity, gender role, and sexual orientation.

The desire for acceptance is important regardless of sexual preference. Judgmental nursing attitudes can be devastating to the young homosexual adolescent, who is trying to establish an acceptable identity. The nurse must inform the male homosexual adolescent of the risk of exposure to acquired immunodeficiency syndrome (AIDS) and other sexually transmitted diseases.

Adolescents are constantly making judgments about what is normal based on peer observations. Gay and lesbian youths are at risk for shame and ridicule in a society that promotes attraction to the opposite sex as normal and attraction to the same sex as abnormal.

Homosexual adolescents need reassurance that individual sexual feelings can differ and still be normal. Family counseling may be necessary to provide education and support to the adolescent and family members.

independence versus dependence

Adolescents often desire independence from parental rules yet need their continued financial support. Feelings of inadequacy or powerlessness can make it difficult for teenagers to prepare for the future. They may remain vague about future goals and try to maintain adolescent lifestyles. Individual guidance and counseling may be nec-

table 25-1 critical developmental tasks of adolescence

* ✱ Appreciate own uniqueness, accept strengths, and recognize weaknesses.
* ✱ Develop an independent identity by detaching from family and recognizing self-value.
* ✱ Define own value system; resist peer and cultural pressure to follow to their value systems.
* ✱ Acquire self-evaluation skills; develop sensitivity to personal relationships.
* ✱ Accept responsibility for own behavior reflected in management of time, money, and personal and social interactions.

essary to help with adolescent developmental tasks (Table 25-1).

peer relationships

During adolescence, teenagers continue to develop relationships with peers of both sexes. During late adolescence, interest focuses on marriage, vocation, and economic independence.

Successful development of peer relationships is important to the psychological health of the child. These relationships help the adolescent define his or her own identity, adapt to his or her changing body image, and deal with emerging sexual feelings. Alienation from peers, failure to establish a good friend relationship, or overinvolvement with peers to the point of interfering with school performance and family relationships may indicate the need for counseling.

moral development

According to Kohlberg's theory of moral development, after 9 years, children have a desire to conform to social rules of behavior by respecting authority and laws governing right and wrong acts. Kohlberg notes that the desire to conform is reflected in a majority of Americans throughout their lives. However, due to other influences in their lives, adolescent moral decision-making does not always correlate with Kohlberg's theory.

influence from peers and media

Maintaining social status through peer acceptance is equal and sometimes more important to teens than parental approval. Adolescents may disregard authority and social laws in favor of group acceptance. Positive peer interaction imposing a give-and-take response reinforces moral development in a democratic way compared with adults dictating set rules and regulations for the adolescent.

Shopping (especially in malls) provides teenagers with opportunities to socialize and be entertained. In many respects, shopping malls define social values through advertisements and product promotion. A teenager who would never have considered stealing during elementary school years may consider petty shoplifting with peers. The desire to be popular and belong to a peer group may outweigh any prior convictions of right and wrong behaviors. Teenagers reach an age when they stop wanting to be good boys and girls for parental approval and start wanting to be "cool" for peer approval.

Peer pressure can be prosocial or antisocial. Much of an adolescent's behavior reflects the kind of peer pressure being exerted. Peers tend to share similar values, attitudes, and goals. Adolescents seek reassurances from one another (Fig. 25-6). Adults may feel that peers lead adolescents astray, but teens seek out friends with similar traits.

Not all adolescents conform to peer pressure. Adolescents who have warm, affectionate relationships with family members are less likely to agree to something they do not want to do (Display 25-2).

Parental values important in the child's early years are often challenged during adolescence by outside influences, such as television, movies, videos, and advertising promoting different values. Television and other entertainment celebrities are powerful influences in shaping adolescent thoughts, behavior, language, and beliefs.

Adult respect for the adolescent's needs can help balance the influences of others and reinforce values important to the family. Teens often respond favorably to positive comments about their decision-making skills and their natural qualities of goodness. Adolescents who feel good about themselves are less likely to surrender to peer pressures. Honest evaluations and praise are appreciated by teens.

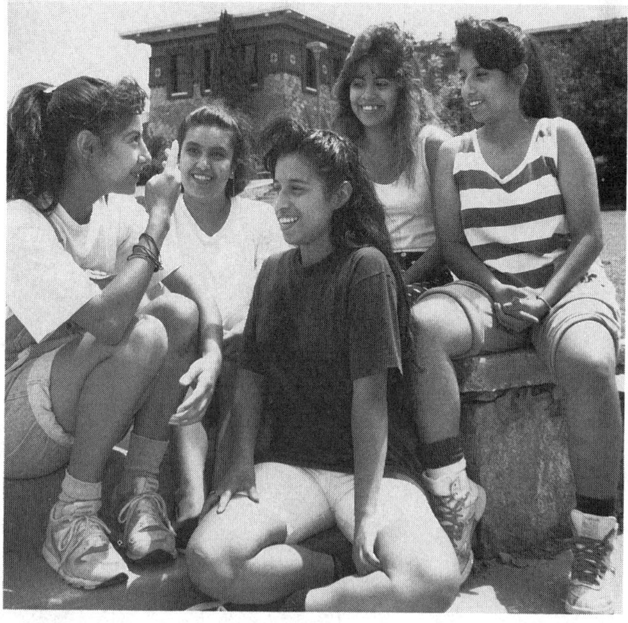

figure 25-6 *Adolescents seek reassurances from one another.*

display 25-2
tips on helping adolescents deal with peer pressure

* **Encourage teenagers to discover their own special strengths.**
* **Treat adolescents as responsible people, encouraging independence and decision-making skills.**
* **Encourage adolescents to anticipate difficult situations and plan ahead.**
* **Encourage adolescents to form associations with peers sharing similar family or cultural values**

teaching guidelines 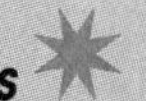
inspiring the adolescent's confidence and decision-making abilities

Adults can inspire the adolescent's confidence and decision-making abilities by the following:

* Listen and be curious about the teenager's world—it is different from an adult's.
* Keep lecturing to a minimum and boost listening to a maximum.
* Respect the teenager.
* Work on compromises rather than demands.
* Send the most important message: love.
* Share personal experiences and what you learned from them.
* Clearly inform the teen about what you expect; remember the difference between discipline and punishment.
* Decide what you need to do as a parent, and do it with dignity and respect.
* Remember to apologize when you've made a mistake; you'll be respected more for being human.
* Allow adolescents to make errors in judgment; adults make mistakes too.
* Remember mistakes are another way to learn.

The adolescent must make decisions and goals based on self-concept. A positive self-concept promotes personal development and maturation. A negative self-concept offers little hope for future accomplishments, encouraging the youth to avoid maturation.

communication

Communication is essential to any healthy relationship and is especially important during adolescence. Effective communication includes message, sender, receiver, a sign that the message was understood, and feedback.

Communicating with adolescents can sometimes be a challenge. Adults and teenagers are often acutely aware of "talking a different language." Arguments can erupt about family rules, household chores, personal habits, television, money, and so forth. There may be no easy way to avoid some disagreements, but there are ways to avoid obstacles that block effective communication.

Communication with adolescents requires sharing feelings. Using "I" messages and "you" messages can open the way to mutual understanding because these messages are nonjudgmental statements of how a person feels about a situation. Either person may think the other's reactions to a situation are ridiculous, but real feelings are involved that cannot be ignored.

Adults may use criticism in an attempt to change the adolescent's thinking. However, this often results in the adolescent becoming defensive. Adults may think that giving advice is helpful, but teenagers may see it as a sign of their inability to solve problems. The adolescent is striving toward adulthood and needs to be treated as an adult.

Active listening is an essential element in effective communication. Adolescents often complain that adults do not listen to them; adults often echo this complaint about adolescents. Active listening requires undivided attention, with the following goals: understanding another person's viewpoint, seeing the situation through his or her eyes, and sharing his or her feelings.

Adults often complain that their teenagers will not talk to them. Teenagers' unwillingness to share their thoughts may reflect a need to keep those thoughts and feelings private. An observant adult can frequently initiate conversation by commenting on the adolescent's body language. Comments such as "You look very happy" can help the teenager share feelings.

Music has traditionally been a source of communication as an expression of unity within a generation. Parents may not appreciate their adolescent's music preferences and may worry about the music's effect on the teenager's behavior. There is little concrete evidence that adolescents listen to music as a guide for behavior. Instead, music tends to be a harmless way of escaping from everyday life. Adults who are willing to listen to and discuss the music's message with adolescents can discover much about the adolescent's viewpoint concerning values, society, and life in general. See Teaching Guidelines.

physiologic growth and development

Physiologic changes during adolescence are focused primarily on changes that occur in both sexes during puberty. Accelerated growth and vast individual differences during adolescence make growth assessment a challenge. The adolescent must be reassured that growth and development vary. Physical growth concerns that require nursing interventions include growth falling outside the 5th and 95th percentiles for height and weight and notable changes in the pattern of growth.

head and face

The mandible grows rapidly during adolescence, changing the teenager's appearance. Additional facial changes result from forehead growth and changes in muscle and subcutaneous tissue.

chest and breast development

Boys have a greater increase in chest diameter than girls. Boys and girls have breast changes during adolescence, although the changes in girls are more extensive than in boys because breasts reach their adult size by late adolescence.

musculoskeletal system

Overall skeletal dimensions increase during adolescence. Leg length reaches its maximum size first, followed by hip width and chest breadth. Boys tend to grow up before growing out and generally grow taller than girls. Adolescent girls often grow up and out simultaneously, displaying wider hips than boys.

When bones grow more rapidly than muscles, fatigue, weakness, and clumsiness can result. Adolescent boys are at risk for bone development malformation in the lower extremities because of excessive weight bearing on immature bones; knee pain is a major symptom.

Postural problems are influenced by the level of development and can be corrected. Screening for *scoliosis* (curvature of the spine, more common in girls) is recommended for all adolescents (see Chap. 36).

neurologic system

The neurologic system is well developed by adolescence, and the rate of brain growth slows somewhat. The hypothalamus, part of the central nervous system, plays a key role in the onset of puberty because it triggers the increased secretion of sex hormones in the endocrine system.

health maintenance and health teaching

Health maintenance during adolescence involves health teaching and guidance because many health problems are related to changes of puberty or high-risk behaviors. Lack of, or decline in, gross or fine motor development must be investigated for significance and cause, such as muscular dystrophy.

Adolescent social and emotional development may be stormy for the teenager and caregivers. Adolescent struggles with issues of dependence and independence may contribute to threats against physical and psychological safety and well-being. For example, if the adolescent withdraws when emotionally upset and is reluctant to ask for help, adult guidance and support are inhibited.

Smoking among adolescents remains a major health concern. Studies indicate that 70.1% of American teenagers have tried using tobacco products, such as cigarettes, chewing tobacco, or snuff, increasing the risk of lung, throat, and mouth cancer (Nelms, 1993).

Adolescents often present complaints to health care workers that are unrelated to their true concerns. Common issues, such as sexually transmitted diseases, body size, anxiety about early or late maturity (penis and breast size), birth control, pregnancy, drug use, and abusive relationships, are often discussed with peers. This provides the adolescent with unclear and incorrect information because of their limited understanding. Nurses can provide valuable information to the adolescent in a private, confidential, and nonthreatening manner.

immunizations

Immunizations recommended for adolescents include tetanus toxoid booster unrelated to trauma. After the child has received five doses of diptheria, tetanus, and pertussis (DTP), tetanus and a dilute form of diptheria are recommended every 10 years. Varivax, a new vaccine currently released for the prevention of chickenpox, is recommended for children 13 years or older, given in two doses, at 4- and 8-week intervals.

screening examinations

Tuberculin skin test is recommended at 12 years of age. A complete physical examination is recommended around age 13 with VDRL screening for syphilis, complete blood count, serum cholesterol, and urinalysis. Screening for depression, suicide, substance abuse, and pregnancy are suggested for adolescents exhibiting symptoms or at risk because of dysfunctional family practices related to alcoholism or domestic violence (see Fig. 25-3).

nutrition

The recommended daily allowance (RDA) for boys during adolescence is 2,500 to 2,900 kcal. For girls, the RDA is 2,200 kcal. The adolescent's total daily energy intake should include 12% to 16% protein. Strict vegetarian diets may lead to deficiencies in vitamins and minerals (Fig. 25-7).

An increase in protein during this period is important for increased muscle mass in boys. During puberty, increased levels of the male hormone testosterone affect the extensive use of protein for the formation of lean muscle tissue and long bone growth.

Increased protein in girls is influenced by estrogen to form increased fat tissues in the abdominal area, breasts, and hips. Protein is important in the widening of the pelvic girdle (a ring of bones in the pelvic region composed of two hip bones joined to the sacrum).

The RDA for calcium and phosphorus is 50% higher during adolescence than during childhood, allowing for the increase in bone growth. Boys need 400 mg and girls need 250 mg of calcium daily during adolescence. Milk

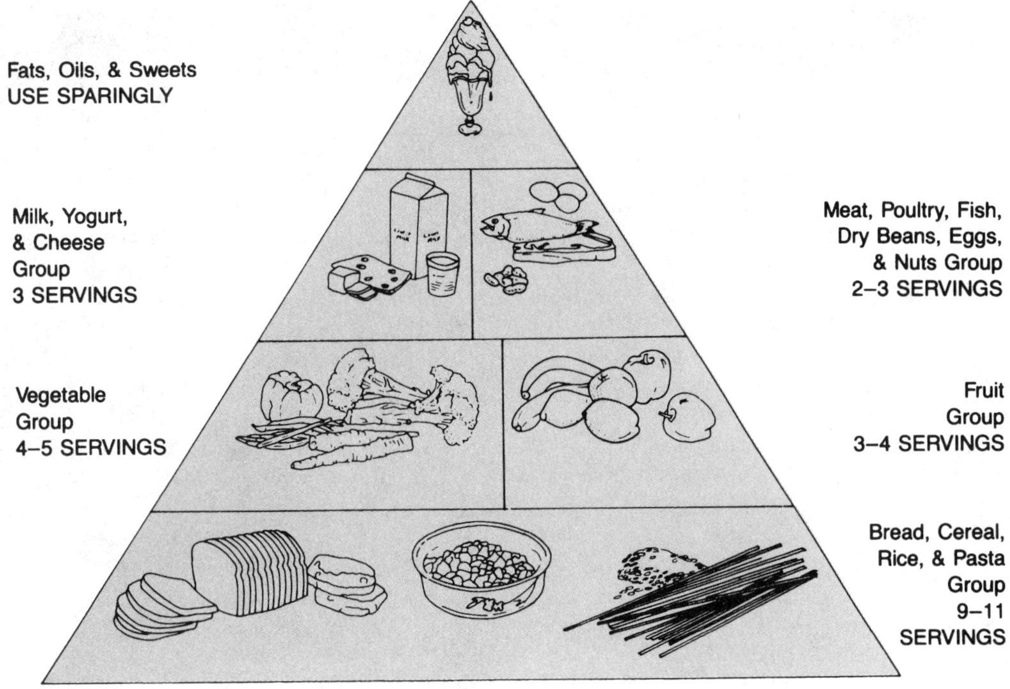

figure 25-7 *Food guide pyramid adapted for adolescents. (From United States Department of Agriculture.)*

and cheese are rich sources of calcium. Teenage girls who diet often eliminate milk and increase their risk of calcium deficit. High consumption of caffeinated soft drinks can interfere with drinking enough milk to meet calcium needs. Studies show that caffeine and sugar in a soda can cause a 30-mg calcium loss over approximately 3 hours following ingestion (Schuster & Ashburn, 1992).

Iron requirements are higher for boys and girls during adolescence. Menstruating girls need high levels of iron to replace loss during menstruation. A daily intake of 1.2 g of iron is recommended for replacement and maintenance needs. Adolescent boys need approximately 1.1 mg of daily iron. Table 25-2 provides a summary of common dietary deficiencies in adolescence. Display 25-3 shows signs of anorexia.

anorexia and bulimia

Adolescent girls may become obsessed with the idea of being thin and a fear of obesity. This may lead to fad diets and behaviors associated with anorexia nervosa and bulimia (see Chap. 34).

cholesterol

Cardiovascular disease is associated with risk factors, such as elevated blood pressure, elevated serum cholesterol level, cigarette smoking, obesity, and poor physical fitness. The average diet of children in the United States is relatively high in total fat, saturated fat, and cholesterol. Studies indicate that coronary risk factors begin during childhood, making it practical to begin preventive methods to lower blood cholesterol levels.

Adolescent and caregiver education helps evaluate eating patterns and recognize strengths and weaknesses in the diet. Fat is responsible for approximately 38% of all calories. Hamburgers are the largest single contributor of dietary fat in the United States (McCabe, 1993).

A total serum cholesterol reading of less than 170 mg/dL is considered normal; 170 to 199, borderline; and more than 200, high. Specific recommendations for cholesterol screening in children and adolescents include the following:

* Adolescents whose parents or grandparents at 55 years or younger were diagnosed as having coronary atherosclerosis, myocardial infarction, angina pectoris, peripheral vascular disease, or stroke
* Obesity

display 25-3
signs of anorexia

* Extreme fear of becoming fat, even though weight is normal or below normal
* Body image disturbance, prompting self-induced weight loss (25% or more of original body weight or 25% below normal weight ranges for age, sex)
* Denial about questionable eating patterns
* Increased susceptibility to infection
* Amenorrhea (missing three consecutive cycles)
* Use of laxatives

table 25-2 summary of common dietary deficiencies in adolescence

Nutrient	*Food Sources*	*Deficiency Symptoms*
Vitamin A	Liver, whole milk, cheese Sources of carotene, such as yellow vegetables; yellow fruits; green, leafy vegetables; and tomatoes	Diminished bone and tooth formation and visual acuity Increased risk of infections
Vitamin D	Fortified milk, fish liver oils, exposure to sunlight	Bone deformities, soft bones
Vitamin B_6 (pyridoxine)	Liver, kidney, chicken, fish, pork, eggs, whole-grain cereals, legumes, bananas	Nervous system involvement, such as irritability, tremors, and convulsions; more common in infancy
Folate (folic acid, folacin)	Green, leafy vegetables; liver; kidney; meats; fish; nuts; legumes; whole grains	Anemia identified by atypical large red blood cells, sore tongue, diarrhea
Vitamin B_{12} (cobalamin)	Animal foods, liver, other meats, dairy products, eggs	Macrocytic anemia, nervous system damage, sore mouth and tongue, anorexia, nausea, vomiting
Calcium	Milk, hard cheese, yogurt, ice cream, small fish eaten with bones, dark green vegetables, tofu, soybeans, calcium-enriched orange juice	Poor growth, fragile and deformed bones
Iron	Lean meats, liver, legumes, dried fruits, green leafy vegetables, whole-grain and fortified cereals	Anemia, fatigue, pallor, dyspnea
Zinc	Oysters, herring, meat, liver, fish, milk, whole grains, nuts, legumes	Retarded growth, declined ability to taste and smell, delayed wound healing.

- Cigarette smoking
- Elevated blood pressure
- Diabetes mellitus
- Physical inactivity

The technique for treating adolescents with elevated blood cholesterol levels is through diet therapy. The goal is to reduce blood cholesterol levels while maintaining an adequate diet. The National Cholesterol Education Program (1991) recommends drug therapy in children older than 10 years if cholesterol levels remain high after 6 months of diet therapy. Cholestyramine and colestipol are drugs that bind bile acids in the intestine. Both drugs are powders requiring water or juice to mix; they are taken immediately before, after, or during a meal when the greatest amount of bile acid is present in the intestine.

obesity

Obesity is a common nutritional problem affecting 10% to 20% of adolescents (Schuster & Ashburn, 1992). Obesity is defined as a body weight 20% or more over the recommended desirable weight for height. Usually, the cause is lack of exercise rather than excess consumption of kilocalories. Occasionally, obesity is caused by a malfunction in metabolism, such as decreased thyroid function (see Chap. 38).

The teen should try to lose excess weight before the end of adolescence. Those who do not tend to be obese throughout adult life. Dietary management consists of decreasing the consumption of kilocalories while consuming adequate amounts of essential nutrients.

Obese adolescents are at increased risk for social, emotional, and physical problems. Name-calling, teasing, and social rejection increase the teenager's risk of loneliness.

Factors that influence overeating include night eating, eating binges, eating without feeling satisfied, and excessive television viewing, which contributes to lack of exercise and consumption of snacks.

acne

More than 80% of adolescents experience some degree of acne vulgaris between 9 and 20 years. Increased androgen levels at puberty stimulate the production of sebum (oil) by the sebaceous glands of the face, neck, shoulders, and upper chest.

Most cases of acne disappear spontaneously sometime after the 20th birthday. The presence of "zits" can be an overwhelming experience for boys and girls because it alters body image.

General management of acne includes a well-balanced diet, good hygiene, avoidance of known irritants, and reduction of emotional tension. Refer to Chapter 37 for additional information.

dental health

Permanent dentition is often completed during late adolescence. The third molars tend to erupt earlier in girls. It is not uncommon for young adults to have one or more wisdom teeth removed to prevent overcrowding of teeth and malocclusion.

Malocclusion is a notable deviation of the normal alignment of teeth, causing an overbite or underbite. Malocclusion contributes to emotional distress because of the perception of being unattractive.

stress

Stress is a fact of life and is an inspiration to meet life's challenges. Too much stress can be harmful physically and mentally. Therefore, it is important to learn ways to control stress (see Display 25-4).

Teenagers are especially vulnerable to stress. They have anxieties about their body image; sexual identity; grades; athletic performance; relationships with peers, siblings, and parents; finances; and career planning. Unfortunately, the stressed adolescent may rely on drugs, alcohol, or even suicide to relieve emotional pain.

headaches

Twenty-nine percent of boys and 32% of girls have at least one headache per month during adolescence (Schuster & Ashburn, 1992). Stress-related headaches are the most common recurrent type and are called psychogenic headaches. Behaviors associated with stress headaches include the tendency to tense the muscles of the neck and scalp.

migraine or vascular headaches

Migraine headaches are referred to as vascular headaches. They often occur in adolescents who have a family history of similar headaches. Vascular headaches begin with distorted perceptual processes, such as strange sounds or lights, and difficulty thinking. The onset of headache pain is described as pounding. This pain results from dilatation of scalp vessels. Edema of the scalp vessel walls tightens the facial muscles and contributes to a steady, unmanageable, tension-type headache.

The exact cause of vascular headaches is unknown. Stress, fatigue, loss of sleep, hormonal imbalance, eye strain, use of alcohol, and ingestion of certain types of food, such as milk products, chocolate, and alcohol, may trigger vascular headaches in the adolescent. Recurrent headaches need medical evaluation.

display 25-4
stress management clues

1. Prevent stress by controlling how you respond to insignificant annoyances.
2. Recognize stress in your body, such as irritability, depression, anxiety, diminished attention, and dry mouth and throat.
3. Set goals and establish priorities; think where you would like to be in 5 years, and adapt to change.
4. Take time out for recreation, hobbies, exercise, or relaxation training to increase inner and outer strength.
5. Think positive, and have a sense of humor—laugh at yourself.
6. Communicate your feelings with family, friends, counselors, clergy, or health professionals.
7. Get support if problems or burdens are too great.

body piercing

Body piercing may include the ear, nose, tongue, nipple, umbilical region, and genitals. Health considerations include increased risk of infection and exposure to human immunodeficiency virus (HIV) transmission if piercing is done with unsterile equipment.

sleep and rest

Sleep disturbances are common during adolescence and can continue into adulthood. Most sleep difficulties originate from adolescent worries, tension, and personal, family, or school problems.

sex and intimacy

Adolescent sexual issues represent one of the most challenging areas that teenagers, nurses, and parents face. Sexual conduct originates in the complex background of the adolescent's religion, culture, social attitudes, values, and belief systems. Abstaining from sexual activity is 100% effective at preventing pregnancy, AIDS, and sexually transmitted diseases. Although abstinence is ideal, the rate of teen pregnancy and sexually transmitted diseases, including HIV and AIDS, is escalating. Nurses working with adolescents need to provide holistic care, including sex information and education (Table 25-3).

Hospitalized adolescents or those with chronic illness or disability also have sexual needs and concerns. These needs and concerns can be further complicated by such factors as pain, fatigue, motor instability, odors, and altered body image.

sex education

The amended Education Act of 1993 came into force in September 1994 and affects three aspects of sex education:

* Sex education programs are required in all state secondary schools but are optional in primary schools
* Information or reference to HIV, AIDS, sexually transmitted diseases, and aspects of sexual behavior were removed from the national curriculum science course
* Parents have the right to withdraw their children from all or part of sex education lessons that are not part of the national curriculum (Cohen, 1994).

table 25-3 *major sexually transmitted diseases*

Infection and Agent	*Transmission*	*Symptoms*	*Possible Complications*	*Prevention*
Gonorrhea—gonococcus: *Neisseria gonorrhoeae*	Sexual contact; mother to fetus during vaginal delivery	Yellow mucopurulent discharge of the genital area, painful or frequent urination, pain in the genital area; may be asymptomatic Frequent cause of pelvic inflammatory disease	Sterility, cystitis, arthritis, endocarditis	Public should be educated on safe sex practices; mother should be tested before delivery. Newborn's eyes should be treated with tetracycline ointment, erythromycin ointment, or silver nitrate. All contacts should be treated with antibiotics.
Chlamydia—bacteria: *Chlamydia trachomatis*	Sexual contact; mother to fetus during vaginal delivery	Mocupurulent genital discharge, genital pain, dysuria Frequent cause of pelvic inflammatory disease, often in combination with gonorrhea	Sterility	Public should be educated about safe sex practices. Sexual contact should be avoided when lesions are present. Infected mothers should have a cesarean delivery.
Genital herpes virus: herpes simplex type 2	Sexual contact; mother to fetus during vaginal delivery	Genital soreness, pruritus, and erythema; vesicles that usually last for about 10 days, during which time transmission of virus is likely		Public should be educated about safe sex practices. Sexual contact should be avoided when lesions are present. Infected mothers should have a cesarean delivery.
Syphilis—spirochete: *Treponema pallidum*	Sexual contact; mother to fetus through placenta; blood transfusions if donor is in early stage of disease and undiagnosed	Primary stage: genital lesion, enlarged lymph nodes Secondary stage (6 wk later): lesions of skin and mucous membrane, with generalized symptoms of headache and fever	Tertiary stage: central nervous system and cardiovascular damage, paralysis, psychosis	Public should be educated about safe sex practices. Screen blood donors; do serologic testing before and during pregnancy. Avoid contact with body secretions from infected patients.
Acquired immuno-deficiency syndrome (AIDS)—virus: human immuno-deficiency virus	Sexual contact; exposure to blood or blood products; mother to fetus	Active phase: rash, cough, malaise, night sweats, lymphadenopathy Asymptomatic phase: no symptoms, but test is positive for HIV antigens AIDS-related complex: lymphadenopathy, diarrhea, oral candidiasis, weight loss, fatigue, skin rash, recurrent infections, fever AIDS: rare infections, such as *Pneumocystis carinii* pneumonia, or rare cancers, such as Kaposi's sarcoma or B-cell lymphomas	Neurologic impairment	Public should be educated about safe sex practices, especially high-risk groups. Blood or blood products used for transfusion should be carefully screened. Intravenous drug abusers should not share needles. Universal precautions should be used consistently in all health care settings. Institute measures to avoid needlesticks among health care workers.

Adapted from Craven, R. F., & Hirnle, C. J. (1992). *Fundamentals of nursing: Human health and function.* Philadelphia, J. B. Lippincott.

display 25-5
adolescent teaching about condom use

- **Condoms decrease the risk of pregnancy, AIDS, and other sexually transmitted diseases.**
- **Safe condoms are lubricated latex with a tip or reservoir that has been pretreated with nonoxynol 9 spermicide.**
- **Unsafe condoms have been used before; are colored; are novelties, such as "glow in the dark"; have been exposed to heat; or have minute puncture holes.**
- **Using condoms is normal.**
- **Condoms can enhance sexual pleasure.**
- **Penile erections tend to last longer with a condom.**
- **Lubricant inside the condom increases sexual pleasure.**
- **Remove condom, tie a knot in the open end, discard, and wash semen or vaginal secretions from body.**

The current political and moral climate concerning sex education is complicated for school nurses concerned with the welfare of children and young people. Adult concern about sex education programs that promote condom use centers on ideas that sexual morality will decrease while sexual frequency increases. No data support these ideas. However, approximately 12 million people are infected with sexually transmitted diseases and are capable of causing serious complications and death (Kranes, 1990). The use of latex condoms during sex is the most effective preventive measure sex partners can take. Condoms are not fool-proof, but they are usually effective.

Adolescents provide various reasons for not using condoms, including inconvenience, lack of availability, lowered inhibitions, and alcohol and drug abuse. The correct way to apply a condom is discussed in Chapter 9. See also Display 25-5.

Cancer risks are increased in adolescents with sexually transmitted diseases. Studies link veneral warts (condyloma) with genital cancers. Chronic vaginitis is linked with an increase risk of cervical cancer.

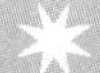

nursing alert

Adolescents need to accept their sexual feelings as normal and be aware of and responsible for the consequences of their sexual behavior.

teenage pregnancy

Pregnancy during the teenage years increases the struggle for independence versus dependence. The pregnant adolescent is faced with serious decisions relative to the future of the baby and herself. These decisions include whether to maintain or abort the pregnancy and to marry or remain single, live at home, or live with a boyfriend or other person; and to remain in school or drop out.

The pregnant teenager must cope with changes in friendships, changes in body image as the pregnancy advances, and medical costs associated with the pregnancy and childrearing (Fig. 25-8). Refer to Chapter 9 for additional information.

safety

Though most adolescents are basically healthy, they are at high risk for accidents, particularly those related to driving. Vehicular accidents are the leading cause of death between the ages of 10 and 19 years. Many of these accidents also involve alcohol and other drugs (Fig. 25-9).

The number of adolescent deaths resulting from violence, including homicide and suicide, is increasing. As more teenagers carry handguns, even to school, the spiral of violence and death increases. The death rate from violence is much higher among boys than girls and among African American than white teenagers.

substance abuse

Many adolescents experiment with alcohol and other drugs. Although drug experimentation does not necessarily mean a teenager will become a "user," regular use of drugs is cause for concern. When dealing with an adolescent drug problem, the child should be confronted directly

display 25-6
pattern of adolescent drug abuse

- ***Experimentation stage*** **involves the use of alcohol or marijuana in response to curiosity or peer influence; parents are often unaware of child's behavior.**
- ***Getting high stage*** **involves increased use of various drugs to impress others and fit into social circles where drugs are available; denial is used when confronted. Parental awareness of child's behavior often prompts actions to censure friends and eliminate the drug(s); parents may blame peers for being a bad influence.**
- ***Getting loaded stage*** **involves maintaining a steady supply of drugs; new friendships develop with peers connected to the drug scene; youth begins to violate rules at home and school and may start dealing. Parental confrontation produces a promise to cut down or quit using drugs.**
- ***Addicted stage*** **involves daily drug use with an inability to stop; youth has lost control; paranoia and suicide feelings are common. Parents feel frustration, anger, and total loss of control over the youth's lifestyle; they seek help through juvenile court or drug and alcohol counseling programs.**

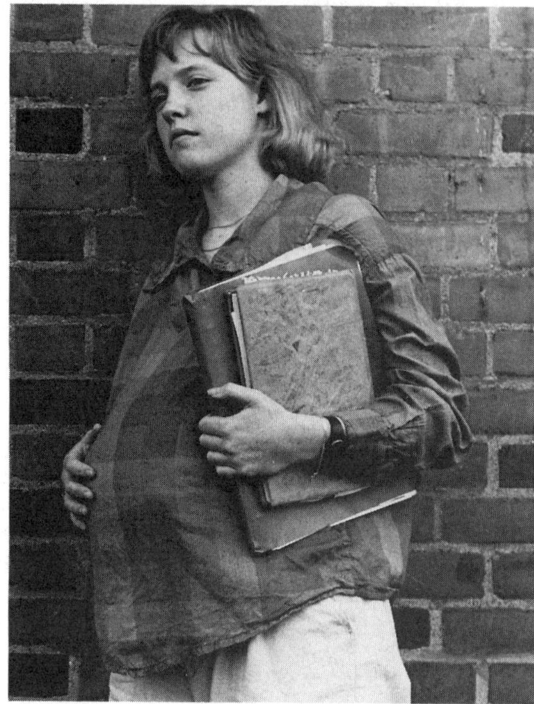

figure 25-8 *Pregnancy presents a major crisis in a young woman's life. It is important to attempt to look at all aspects of the situation when making a decision that will permanently affect the lives of all people involved (the girl, the father, the baby, and the baby's biologic grandparents). (© Gale Zucker/Stock Boston)*

with personal observations of behaviors and facts about drug use. Professional counseling may be necessary for some adolescents involved with alcohol and other drugs.

depression

Adolescence is a roller coaster of emotions, and many adolescents swing from elation to depression in a single day. Depression may be overlooked if the adolescent is perceived as simply going through a negative phase. Depressed adolescents often exhibit the following behaviors:

* Seeking constant stimulation by getting into activities with enthusiasm but quickly losing interest
* Feeling tired and complaining of headaches or stomach problems
* Disregarding appearance and hygiene needs
* Lacking the ability to concentrate
* Engaging in defiant, antisocial behaviors
* Exhibiting a dread of being alone

Depression, described as anger turned inward, is a grave concern for parents and caregivers. Health care providers must provide immediate intervention. Although extreme mood swings are considered normal, prolonged or severe depression can lead to suicide. Depression is the leading cause of suicide. Suicide rates have tripled during the last 25 years, and suicide is the third leading cause of death in 10- to 19-year-olds. (see Chap. 29)

Adolescent suicides usually follow a long history of depression or mental health problems. Adolescent suicides are usually well thought out and occur after adolescents have made repeated attempts to solve their problems. Adolescent suicides are usually accompanied by various warning signs. Any threat of suicide demands immediate professional attention. The adolescent with serious suicide plans is in a crisis situation, and professional intervention is required. See Chapter 29 for a fuller discussion of suicide.

> **nursing alert**
> *Teenage depression and suicide rates have risen dramatically because of feelings of loneliness and isolation, low self-concept, and substance abuse.*

✻ nursing process related to depression

assessment

* Subjective data to be assessed include information about familial tendencies toward depressive episodes and specific information about recent losses. These may include deaths involving friends or close family members, loss of boyfriend or girlfriend, failure in sports, or loss of status positions at school, such as class president, cheerleader, honor roll, or honor society. Withdrawal from social contacts with a loss of interest in usual activities is a sign of depression.
* Objective data to be assessed include complaints of sadness, crying episodes, impulsive behaviors, self-destruction, self-demeaning, and attention-getting. Other data include changes in sleeping patterns, including excessive sleep accompanied by complaints of tiredness, or insomnia and weight gain or loss associated with anorexia or bulimia.

nursing diagnosis

* Self Esteem Disturbance

planning and intervention

* Establish a trusting health relationship.
* Encourage the teenager to recognize and express feelings associated with shame and loss, emphasizing the stages of grieving.
* Encourage the teenager to practice forgiveness of self and others.

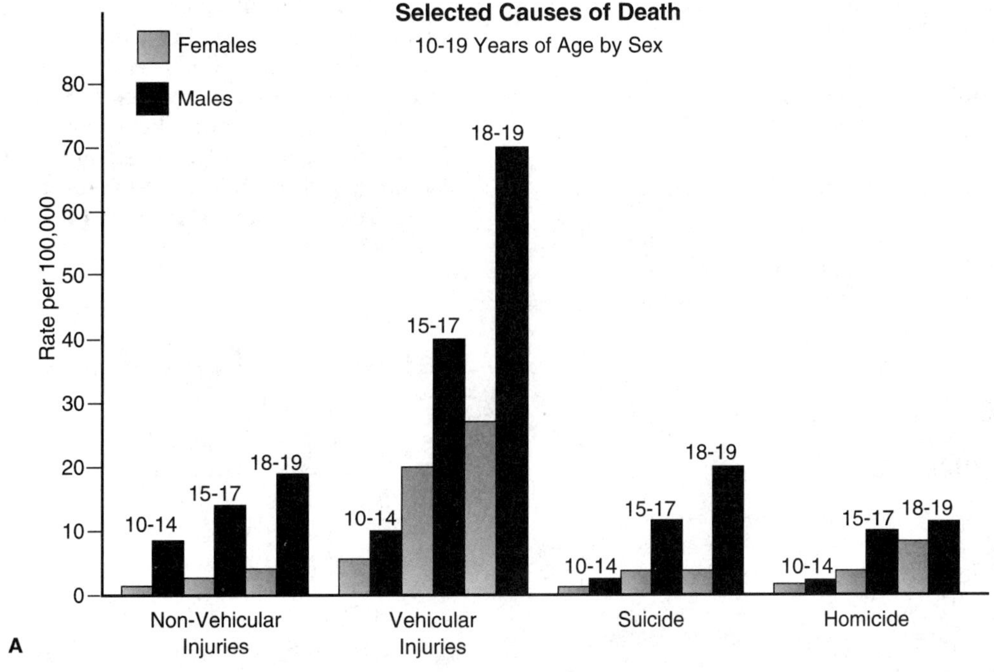

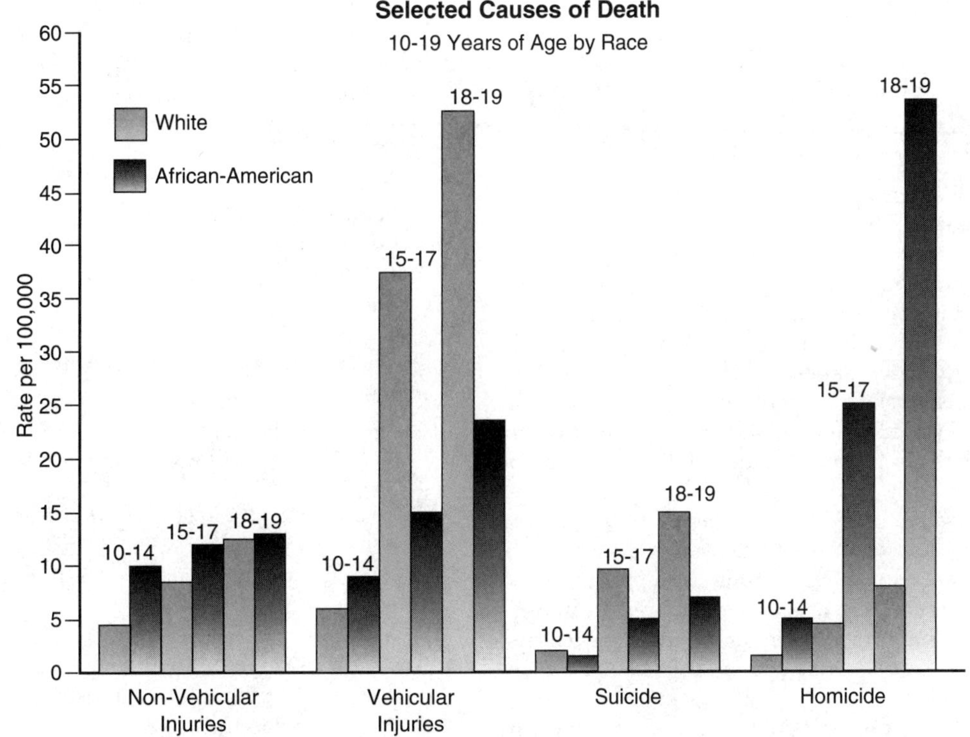

figure 25-9 *(**A**) Selected causes of death by sex. (**B**) Selected causes of death for adolescents by race.*

* Teach the teenager acceptable social skills, including communication, proper hygiene, appropriate dress, and role behaviors involving peers and family.
* Identify coping mechanisms that are appropriate or inappropriate, and help the teenager develop useful coping skills needed in times of crisis.
* Coordinate peer and family support.

evaluation

* The teenager will demonstrate an improved self-concept demonstrated by increased interest in interpersonal interactions, school, and social activities.
* The teenager will verbalize an increased ability to cope with the present and the future.

adolescent response to hospitalization

Major concerns of an adolescent facing hospitalization include the loss of control and enforced dependency on others, resulting from pain, bodily injury, and mutilation. Adolescents tend to perceive their bodies as infallible and display anger, withdrawal, or depression in response to an injury or illness. Behaviors associated with separation from peers include loneliness, boredom, manipulation, and anxiety.

key points

* **Adolescence spans the time between 12 and 20 years. Pubescence refers to the preadolescent time in which the reproductive system begins to mature and secondary sexual characteristics appear. Puberty is the period in which reproductive maturity is reached.**
* **Puberty follows an independent biologic timetable unrelated to other aspects of growth. It involves changes in sex hormones, body size, shape, body composition and proportion and occurs over 3 to 4 years.**
* **Pubertal changes in boys include the appearance of pubic hair, followed by growth of the external genitalia, appearance of axillary and facial hair, deepening voice, spontaneous erections, and wet dreams.**
* **Pubertal changes in girls include the appearance of breast buds (thelarche), followed by breast enlargement; pubic hair; enlargement of ovaries, uterus, vagina, labia, and clitoris; and onset of menstruation and ovulation.**
* **Testicular self-examination is an important measure to detect testicular cancer.**
* **Breast self-examination is important for all adolescents but particularly for females to detect breast cancer.**
* **Cognitive development during adolescence involves a progressive process incorporating abstract reasoning, systematic problem-solving, and symbolic and logical reasoning described by Piaget as formal operational thought.**
* **Development of self-identity is an important task during adolescence and is influenced by physiologic maturity, body build, body image, behaviors, peers, parental attitudes, and societal expectations.**
* **Effective communication between adults and adolescents involves sharing feelings, mutual respect, active listening, and acceptance of the teenager as an adult.**
* **Peers tend to share similar values, attitudes, and goals, seeking reassurances from one another.**

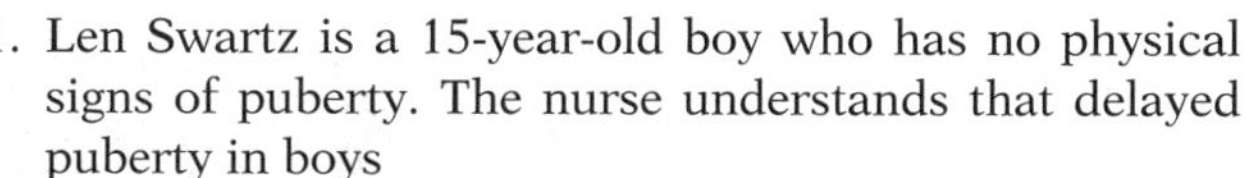

review questions

1. Len Swartz is a 15-year-old boy who has no physical signs of puberty. The nurse understands that delayed puberty in boys
   a. can cause psychological distress and interfere with self-concept development.
   b. is a natural occurrence and is nothing to worry about until after the age of 20.
   c. is reflected by increased physical growth with an absence of secondary sex characteristics.
   d. increases the boy's risk of testicular cancer.
2. Ian is a 17-year-old who has been taught to do testicular self-examinations. He asks the nurse what kind of symptoms reflect cancer. The nurse's best response includes
   a. "Cancer makes the testicles tender to touch."
   b. "Cancer makes the testicles firm."
   c. "Cancer feels like a small, painless, pea-sized lump on the front or sides of a testicle."
   d. "Cancer usually causes open sores on the testicles and penis."
3. Maria is a 13-year-old experiencing signs of puberty. The nurse understands that pubertal changes in the female include
   a. decreases in the production of estrogen hormone.
   b. slowing of weight and height gains.
   c. menarche.
   d. no change in the size of the uterus, but increased size of ovaries.
4. According to Piaget, adolescent thinking primarily involves
   a. magical, artificial thinking.
   b. logical, formal thinking.
   c. concrete, argumentative thinking.
   d. trusting, open thinking
5. Erikson describes psychological development in the adolescent as
   a. trust versus mistrust.
   b. identity versus identity confusion.
   c. autonomy versus guilt.
   d. industry versus inferiority.

references

Cancer statistics. (1995). *Journal of the American Cancer Society. 45*(1), 8–12.

Cohen, P. (1994). The role of the school nurse in providing sex education. *Nursing Times 90*(23), 36–38.

Lewitt, E. (1992). Dropout rates for high school students. *The Future of Children 2*(1), 127–130.

McCabe, E. (1993). Monitoring the fat and cholesterol intake of children and adolescents. *Journal of Pediatric Health Care* 7(2), 61–70.

Nelms, B. (1993). Teenage smoking: a major health care problem. *Journal of Pediatric Health Care* 7(2):53–54.

Schuster, C., & Ashburn, S. (1992). *The process of human development: A holistic life-span approach*. Philadelphia: J.B. Lippincott.

Taylor, C., Lillis, C. & LeMone, P. (1993). Fundamentals of nursing (2nd ed). Philadelphia: J.B. Lippincott.

bibliography

Bandman, E., & Bandman B. (1990). *Nursing ethics through the life span* (2nd ed.). Norwalk, CT: Appleton & Lange.

Berns, R. (1994). *Typical child development*. Albany: NY: Delmar.

Castiglia, P., & Harbin, R. (1992). *Child health care: A comprehensive approach to the care of children and their families*. Philadelphia: J.B. Lippincott.

Charlesworth, R. (Ed.) (1992). *Understanding child development*. Albany, NY: Delmar.

Greydanus, D. (1991). *Caring for your adolescent*. New York: Bantam.

Jackson, D., & Saunders, R. (1993). *Child development*. Philadelphia: J.B. Lippincott.

Morrison, G. (1990). *The world of child development*. Albany, NY: Delmar.

Nelson J., & Lott L. (1991). *I'm on your side: Resolving conflict with your teenage son or daughter.* Rocklin, CA: Prima Publishing.

Selekman, J., & Simpson G. (1991). Sex and sexuality for the adolescent with a chronic condition. *Pediatric Nursing, November-December*, 535–538.

Steinberg, L., & Levine A. (1990). *You and your adolescent*. New York: Harper & Row.

Weiten, W. (1992) *Psychology themes and variations* (2nd ed.). Pacific Grove, CA: Brooks/Cole Publishing.

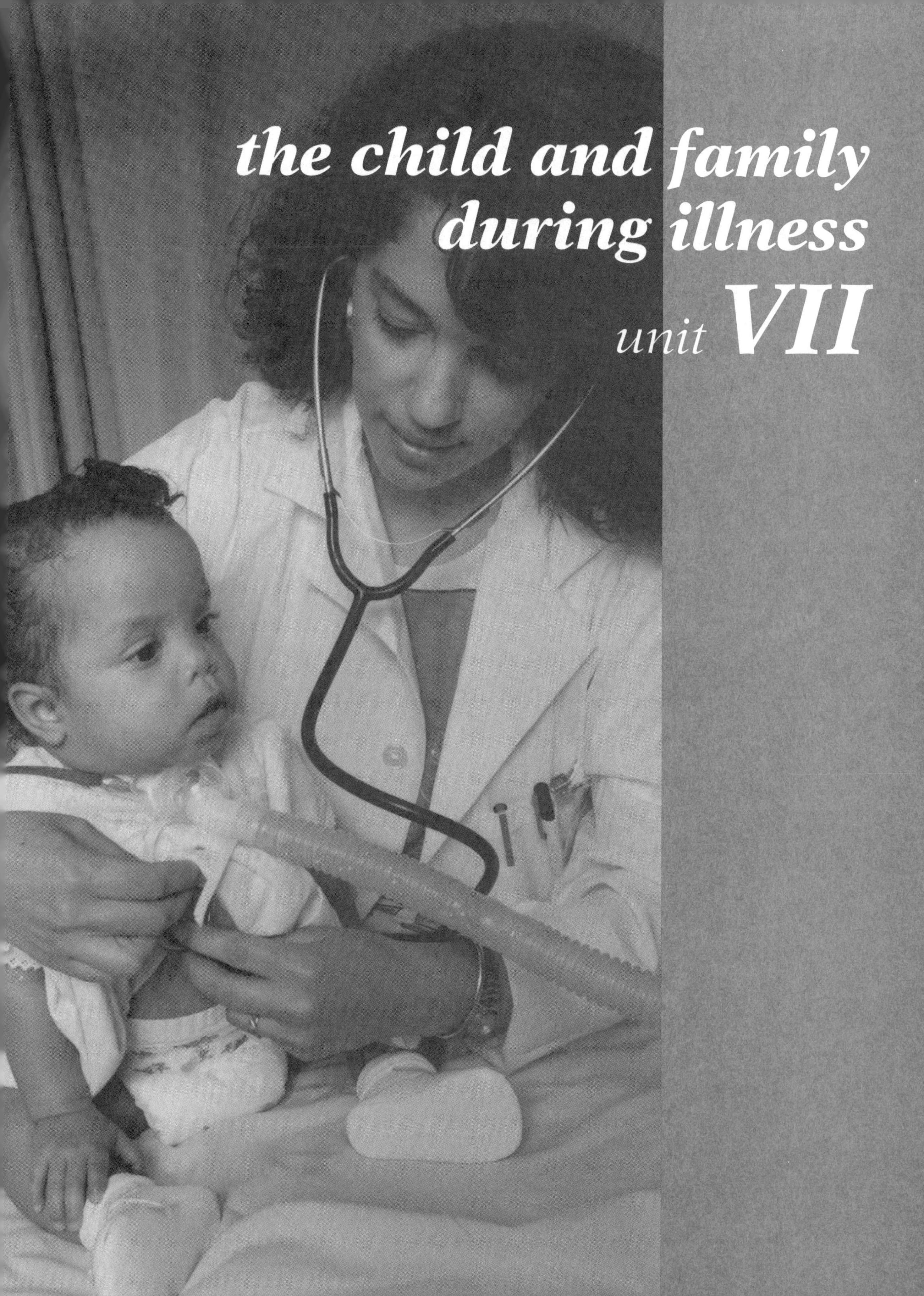

the child and family during illness

unit VII

nursing administration of medications and management of pain

26

outline

objectives

After studying this chapter, the reader should be able to:

- ✳ Administer medications safely, with attention to the child's level of development.
- ✳ Discuss poisoning prevention measures with parents and the child.
- ✳ Use the nursing process as a guide to provide safe, effective drug therapy.
- ✳ Discuss pain control measures, with and without drugs, for infants and children.

key terms

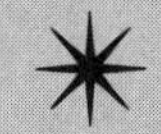

absorption
biotransformation
distribution
excretion
kilogram
medication administration record
milligram
narcotics
nonsteroidal anti-inflammatory drugs
pain management
pharmacokinetics
poisoning

Drug administration has become one of the main duties of the licensed practical or vocational nurse (LPN/LVN) and is regulated by the Nurse Practice Act in each state. Some states and institutions require that LPN/LVNs complete additional education beyond their basic program before they are permitted to administer medications; others do not require more than basic preparation. The Controlled Substance Act, a federal regulation, also affects the handling and administration of narcotics and other controlled substances.

✳ nursing considerations

The responsibilities involved with drug administration require knowledge of the drug's name, recommended dosage, routes of administration, possible side and toxic effects, primary use, and skill in the various techniques of administration and monitoring. The nurse needs to understand the client's condition and consider the age and developmental level of the child to maintain safe, effective drug therapy. Nine helpful rules for administering medications to children are included in Display 26-1.

display 26-1
nine rules in medication administration in children

1. Never give a child a choice of whether or not to receive medicine. The medication is ordered and is necessary for recovery; therefore, there is no choice to be made.
2. Do give choices that allow the child some control over the situation, such as the kind of juice, the number of bandages, or the injection site.
3. Never lie. Do not tell a child that a shot will not hurt.
4. Keep explanations simple and brief. Use words that the child will comprehend.
5. Assure the child that it is all right to be afraid and that it is OK to cry.
6. Do not talk in front of the child as if the child were not there. Include the child in the conversation when talking to family caregivers.
7. Be positive in approaching the child. Be firm and assertive when explaining to the child what will happen.
8. Keep the time between explanation and execution to a minimum. The younger the child, the shorter the time should be.
   Keep the explanation simple.
   Preparations such as setting up injection, solutions, or instrument trays should be done out of the child's sight.
9. Obtain cooperation from family caregivers. They may be able to calm a frightened child, persuade the child to take the medication, and achieve cooperation for care.

From Skale, N. (1992). *Manual of pediatric nursing procedures.* Philadelpha: J.B. Lippincott.

rights of drug administration

The nurse can reduce the risk of error in drug administration by following the six rights of drug administration: right *patient*, right *medication*, right *dose*, right *time*, right *route*, and right *documentation* (charting).

right patient

The patient must be identified either by matching name on the wristband with the name on the medication administration record (MAR) or by having the parent or caregiver identify the child.

right medication

The name of the drug on the container should match the name of the drug on the MAR. If the drug was prescribed by its trade name and the prescription was filled with a generic version, the nurse needs to look up the drug to verify that the generic and trade names match.

right dose

The right dose is always important in drug administration, but it is especially critical in children because of their smaller body weight and immature organs. Accurate liquid measure is required to ensure that the correct dose will be given. A syringe without a needle can be used to measure liquids and to administer the drug to infants and toddlers. If the dosage requires calculation, the nurse should have the math checked by another nurse to ensure accuracy.

right time

Unless military time is used, the nurse needs to make sure the time for medication is expressed as AM or PM and to check to see when the previous dose was given. Drugs usually can be given up to one-half hour before or one-half hour after the scheduled time on the MAR. Dosages given too close together can cause toxic blood levels of a drug. Generally, a drug ordered four times a day should have a minimum of 3 hours between doses. Antibiotics must be correctly timed and spaced to maintain effective blood levels of the drugs.

right route

Many drugs are recommended to be given orally, but some drugs can be given by several routes. The nurse needs to check the prescription to verify the correct route and to clarify any discrepancies with the prescriber. By reading the drug label, the nurse determines whether that form of the drug is appropriate for a particular entry route into the body. Crushing sustained-release forms of drugs or mixing several liquid medications together may alter the effectiveness of the drug. Any questions about crushing or mixing drugs should be directed to the hospital pharmacist.

right documentation

The old saying, "If is not written, it was not done" is important to keep in mind when it comes to safe drug administration. Proper recording after medication administration avoids the possibility of double dosing, which could lead to drug toxicity. Time of administration and any other pertinent information about an as-needed (PRN) medication are recorded immediately in the nurses' notes. For example, if acetaminophen is ordered PRN for fever, the nurse should include vital signs and complaints as a reason for administration, the exact time the drug was given, and follow-up documentation as to effectiveness of the drug.

✳ family considerations

Parents or other primary caregivers play a key role in a child's drug therapy. Caregiver responsibilities concerning drug administration include performing safe techniques of administration, reporting significant side effects to the doctor, and understanding how to avoid overdose. The nurse may assist in teaching or demonstrating care concerning drug administration and monitoring the child for effectiveness of the drug. Teaching needs to be at a level the parents and the child can comprehend. Having the parent or child perform a return demonstration of information or technique helps to solidify understanding. Teaching the child or caregiver also may relieve some anxiety if administration is to be an unpleasant experience, such as giving eye drops. Developmental considerations in medication administration are summarized in Table 26-1.

pharmacokinetics

To understand drug therapy, it is necessary to understand the way drugs work in the body; this is a series of processes called *pharmacokinetics*. These processes include *absorption*; *distribution*; *metabolism*, also called *biotransformation*; and *excretion* of a drug. It is important for the nurse to be aware of how the physiologic development of a child affects the pharmacokinetic processes.

absorption

Absorption of orally administered drugs can vary, depending on the child's age. At birth, gastric pH is neutral or slightly acidic but matures in 4 months. Also the diet of a newborn or an infant contains primarily alkaline foods, eaten every 2 to 4 hours. Many drugs are formulated to disentegrate for absorption in a very acid environment. A neutral or slightly acidic environment will slow medication disentegration. Gastric emptying is prolonged in newborns up to 6 to 8 hours as compared with a 2-year-old's stomach, which empties in about 2 hours. Most absorption occurs in the small intestine, so drug absorption is delayed when the stomach is slow to empty. Other factors that may slow absorption rate are irregular peristalsis and longer gastrointestinal tract in proportion to body size. Acidic drugs, such as penicillin, may be more easily absorbed in the newborn and young infant than basic drugs, such as theophylline, because of the more neutral gastric environment.

Absorption of drugs given intramuscularly (IM) or subcutaneously may be decreased due to the smaller muscle mass and erratic blood flow from the immature peripheral circulation of an infant or child. Vasoconstriction triggered by a cooler environment also can impede blood flow in body tissues. Intravenous administration bypasses absorption from the body's tissues. Therefore, oral and intravenous routes are preferred.

distribution

Drug distribution depends on the amount of water and fat in the body. The body weight of full-term newborns is about 80% water; this drops to 60% by the second year of life and remains at that level throughout childhood (Bindler & Howry, 1991). The proportion of circulating fluid compared with intracellular fluid is greater in younger children than in older children. Thus, larger doses of water-soluble drugs may be necessary to reach adequate concentrations in the blood.

Blood levels of lipid-soluble drugs depend on the proportion of fat tissue in the body. Saturation of fat tissue must occur before blood levels can increase. The varying percentage of body fat as a child grows requires different dosages to reach therapeutic levels. An infant's body weight contains about 16% fat; a 1-year-old's body contains 23% fat and a preschooler's, about 10% fat.

Drugs that bind to protein generally bind to a lesser degree in children due to a lower concentration of proteins in a child's bloodstream. This means a larger proportion of a protein-binding drug is active, enhancing the physiologic response to the drug.

metabolism (biotransformation)

Newborns and infants have lower levels of liver enzymes needed to metabolize or detoxify drugs. This decreases *metabolic* or *biotransformation* rates and means that toxic levels can be reached sooner. For example, toxic levels of chloramphenicol, a potent antimicrobial agent, can lead to "gray syndrome," a potentially fatal condition in the neonate (see Glossary). Monitoring serum drug levels in newborns and infants is extremely important to prevent serious or fatal side effects.

table 26-1 developmental considerations in medication administration

Age	Behavior	Nursing Actions
Birth–3 mo	Reaches randomly toward mouth and has a strong reflex to grasp objects	The infant's hands must be held to prevent spilling of medications.
	Poor head control	The infant's head must be supported while medications are being given.
	Tongue movement may force medication out of mouth	A syringe or dropper should be placed along the side of the mouth.
	Sucks as a reflex with stimulation	Use this natural sucking desire by placing oral medications into a nipple and administering in that manner.
	Stops sucking when full	Administer medications before feeding when infant is hungry. Be aware that some medications' absorption will be affected by food.
	Responds to tactile stimulations	The likelihood that the medication is taken will increase if the infant is held in a feeding position.
3–12 mo	Begins to develop fine muscle control and advances from sitting to crawling	Medication must be kept out of reach to avoid accidental ingestion.
	Tongue may protrude when swallowing	Administer medication with a syringe.
	Responds to tactile stimuli	Physical comfort (holding) given after a medication will be helpful.
12–30 mo	Advances from independent walking to running without falling	Allow the toddler to choose position for taking medication.
	Advances from messy self-feeding to proficient feeding with minimal spilling	Allow the toddler to take medicine from a cup or spoon.
	Has voluntary tongue control; begins to drink from a cup	Disguise medication in a small amount of food to decrease incidence of spitting out medication.
	Develops second molars	Chewable tablets may be an alternative.
	Exhibits independence and self-assertiveness	Allow as much freedom as possible. Use games to gain confidence. Use a consistent, firm approach. Give immediate praise for cooperation.
	Responds to sense of time and simple direction	Give directions to "Drink this now" and "Open your mouth."
	Responds to and participates in routines of daily living	Involve the family caregivers, and include the toddler in medicine routines.
	Expresses feelings easily	Allow for expression through play.
30 mo–6 y	Knows full name	Ask the child his or her name before giving medicine.
	Is easily influenced by others when responding to new foods or tastes	Approach the child in a calm, positive manner when giving medications.
	Has a good sense of time and a tolerance of frustration	Use correct immediate rewards for the young child and delayed gratification for the older child.
	Enjoys making decisions	Give choices when possible.
	Has many fantasies	Give simple explanations. Stress that the medication is not being given because the child is bad.
	Has fear of mutilation	
	Is more coordinated	The child can hold cup and may be able to master pill-taking.
	Begins to lose teeth	Chewable tablets may be inappropriate because of loose teeth.
6–12 y	Strives for independence	Give acceptable choices. Respect the need for regression during hospitalization.
	Has concern for bodily mutilation	Give reassurance that medication given, especially injectables, will not cause harm. Reinforce that medications should be taken only when given by nurse or family caregiver.

(continued)

table 26-1 developmental considerations in medication administration (continued)

Age	Behavior	Nursing Actions
6–12 y	Can tell time	Include the child in daily schedule of medication. Make the child a poster of medications and time due so he or she can be involved in care.
	Is concerned with body image and privacy	Provide private area for administration of medication, especially injections.
	Peer support and interaction are important	Allow child to share experiences with others.
12+ y	Strives for independence	Write a contract with the adolescent, spelling out expectations for self-medication.
	Is able to understand abstract theories	Explain why medications are given and how they work.
	Decisions are influenced by peers	Encourage teens to talk with their peers in a support group. Work with teens to plan medication schedule around their activities. Differentiate pill-taking from drug-taking.
	Questions authority figures	Be honest and provide medication information in writing.
	Is concerned with sex and sexuality	Explain relationship between illness, medications, and sexuality. For example, emphasize that "This medication will not react with your birth control pills."

From Skale, N. (1992). *Manual of pediatric nursing procedures.* (p. 118). Philadelphia, J.B. Lippincott.

excretion

Glomerular filtration rate and nephron tubular secretion of the newborn kidneys is 30% to 50% of that of the adult; however, the kidneys reach mature activity by 6 months. Longer half-life will occur for drugs excreted by glomerular filtration, such as digoxin and gentamicin. Drugs excreted by tubular secretion, such as penicillin, also will have longer half-lives. Because the newborn and infant are more prone to develop dehydration, oliguria and anuria require close monitoring, especially in relation to drug toxicity.

drug administration

dosage calculations

Pediatric dosing accuracy can be achieved by using the following computation methods. The first method can be used if the number of milligrams is ordered by the weight of the child. Dosage calculation is ordered mg/kg per day or body surface area (mg/m^2) for pediatric dosing.

The order will be written as mg/kg, for example, kanamycin 10 mg/kg IM. The frequency of each dose may be expressed either as per dose or equally divided doses given every so many hours per day. The following is an example:

1. Kanamycin 10 mg/kg IM q12h
2. Kanamycin 15 mg/kg per day IM in equally divided doses q8h

When changing pounds into kilograms, the number of pounds is divided by 2.2. The saying "You weigh 'less' if you weigh yourself in kilograms" is a reminder to divide.

When changing within the metric system, only the decimal point needs to be moved. If converting from grams to kilograms, the decimal point moves to the left three spaces, making it a smaller number. If converting from kilograms to grams, the decimal moves to the right three spaces, making it a larger number (Displays 26-2 and 26-3).

If the order is written in equally divided doses, the number of hours is divided into 24 to find the number of doses needed for a 24-hour period. For example, "in equally divided doses q8h" is calculated as 24/8 = three doses in a 24-hour period.

display 26-2
metric conversion

To convert kilograms (kg) to grams (g), move the decimal point three spaces to the right. The number should be larger in grams than kilograms. For example, 15 kg = 15,000 g; 5 kg = 5,000 g.

To convert grams to kilograms, move the decimal point three spaces to the left. The number should be smaller in kilograms than in grams. For example, 6,200 g = 6.200 kg; 25,000 g = 25 kg.

display 26-3
additional formulas for dosage calculations

Young's formula use age.

Child's approximate dose

$$= \frac{\text{age of child (years)}}{\text{age} + 12 \text{ years}} \times \text{adult dose}$$

Clark's formula uses weight.

Child's approximate dose

$$= \frac{\text{weight of child (lb)}}{150} \times \text{adult dose}$$

Fried's formula uses weight for children younger than 1 year

$$\text{infant dose} = \frac{\text{age of child (months)}}{150} \times \text{adult dose}$$

After finding the number of doses per 24-hour period, the mg/kg number is divided by the number of doses. For example, an order written for a 20-kg child written as kanamycin 15 mg/kg IM in equally divided doses q8h would be calculated as follows: 15 mg × 20 kg—3 = 300 mg—3 = 100 mg per dose.

The second method of safe dosage calculation involves body surface area expressed as m^2. The order may be written as mg/m^2. To calculate the body surface area, height and weight of the child are required; this is why the accuracy of height and weight is so important. The nomogram for calculating pediatric body surface area also is needed (Fig. 26-1).

To use the nomogram, the nurse finds the child's height on the left measure line and find the weight on the right measure line, using the same unit of measure (ie, inches and pounds or centimeters and kilograms) and connects the dots. Where the line crosses the line marked S.A., this is the body surface area (m^2) of the child. The boxed measure line is used as a quick reference or if only pounds are known. For example, the body surface area of a child weighing 24 lb with a height of 30 in is 0.5 m^2.

oral administration

Oral administration is the least traumatic route of drug administration. The infant or young child will often swallow some of the drug but then drool, spit, or choke on the rest if the taste is unpleasant. To avoid a messy wrestling match, the nurse holds the child in a bottle-feeding position, allowing the child's inner arm to go toward the nurse's back. The child's head is secured by the bend of the nurse's elbow, and the nurse holds the child's free arm with his or her supporting arm's free hand (Fig. 26-2).

If the infant or child requires restraint for drug administration, a syringe without a needle attached can be used to squirt small amounts of the drug halfway back in the mouth between the cheek and teeth. This technique may take longer, but it reduces the incidence of choking, coughing, and vomiting because it does not trigger the gag reflex. Afterward, offering a cracker or something else more pleasant tasting helps remove the medicinal taste. The experience can end on a happier note if the child is praised for his or her cooperation in swallowing all the medicine.

If the infant spits out a portion of a drug, try to determine the amount taken, and then notify the prescriber for further instructions.

Drugs should never be mixed with infant formula for several reasons. First, it will change the taste of the formula, and the infant may not finish the feeding. Second, some drugs may be altered by the formula and be rendered inactive. Third, formula may inhibit absorption of some drugs.

For the toddler and preschooler, tablets may need to be crushed if the child has difficulty swallowing them. The crushed tablets and capsule contents can be mixed in a small amount of pudding (unless the drug is incompatible with calcium, because milk is an ingredient in most pud-

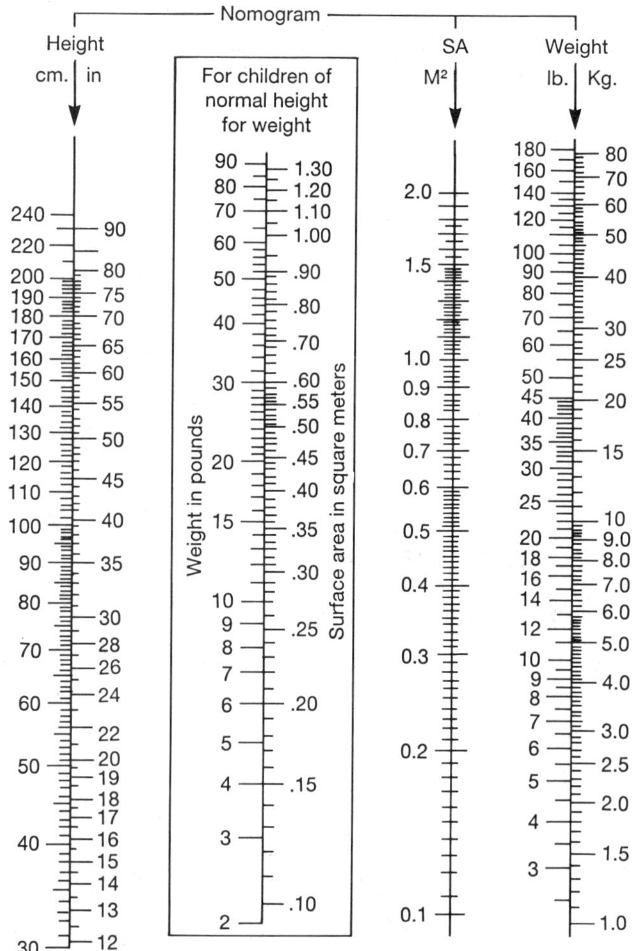

figure 26-1 *West nomogram for calculation of body surface area. (Behrman, R. E., & Vaughan, V. C. [1987].* Nelson textbook of pediatrics *[13th ed.] Philadelphia: W. B. Saunders).*

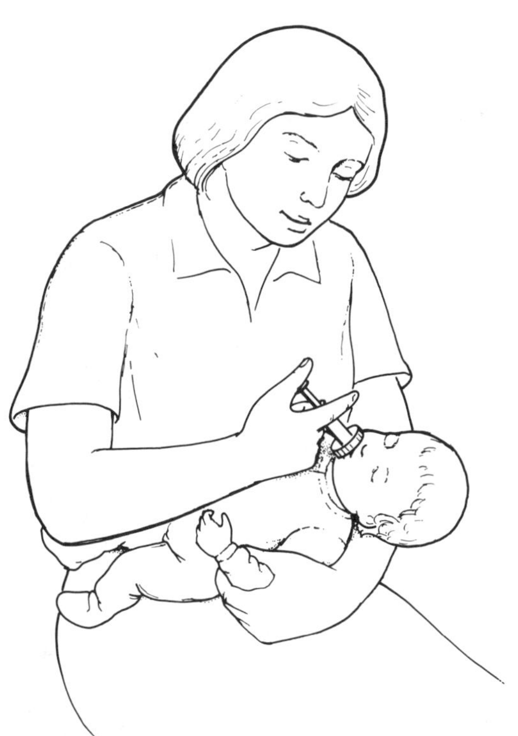

figure 26-2 *Giving medications orally to an infant.*

dings) or jelly. The nurse should avoid using an essential food, such as orange juice. Honey is not recommended for children younger than 1 year because of a possible contamination with botulism spores. An offer of pudding or jelly can be a reward for taking the medication willingly and without a fuss. The child needs to express his or her feelings about the experience and to receive praise for cooperation in taking the medication. Enteric-coated and sustained-release tablets cannot be crushed. If the child is unable to swallow these types of medications, the prescriber needs to be notified.

When caring for a school-age child or an adolescent, the nurse explains the need for the medication and its desired effect, allowing the child to make choices whenever possible. A choice of times to take the medications during the day will result in better compliance than having the child interrupt his or her schedule for the nurse's schedule. If the child is a procrastinator, setting time limits may be necessary to ensure compliance.

A child at any age may refuse to take a drug, usually due to a negative experience or to a desire for independence. The nurse needs to work with the child to overcome the negative experience. Getting the child to take the drug may require involving the parent or other caregiver.

intramuscular administration

To give an IM injection, the nurse needs to understand the anatomy and physiology of the child's level of development, carefully select an appropriate site, and use the appropriate equipment for injection. Physical and emotional trauma to the child must be minimized when giving IM injections (Fig. 26-3). Preparing the syringe out of the child's view is helpful. Otherwise, the needle can be like the fish that got away: The longer the child views it, the bigger the needle gets. Sometimes an older child may wish to see the needle before injection. Using structured play with needleless syringes may help relieve anxiety associated with injections. Rewards for cooperation, such as stickers, can make injections a more positive experience. Brightly colored, designer-print Bandaids can be applied but may represent the "war wound" from the injection, thereby reinforcing negative feelings. A regular Bandaid may be a better comfort measure for the child. Letting the child choose which Bandaid is a good distraction technique. For the neonate and the infant, cuddling and comforting after the injection help to refocus the child from the painful experience to a more pleasant feeling.

technique

The parent also may need emotional support through this procedure. Having an anxious parent assist in restraining the child may add to the child's anxiety and may not be effective; parents have been known to faint during this experience. Having another staff member restrain the child but allowing the parent to remain near can be a better alternative. Occasionally, a child may be more cooperative if the parent is not present. Secure restraint is necessary during injection to avoid injecting into the wrong site or having a needle break off or dislodge.

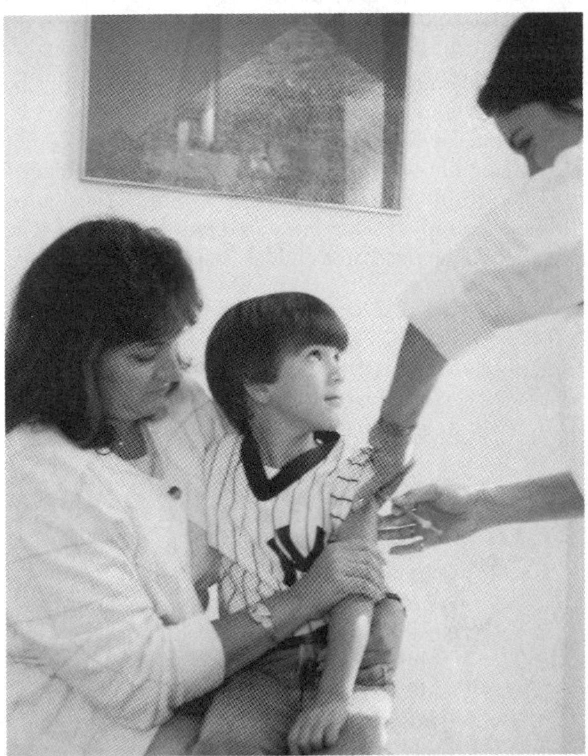

figure 26-3 *The preschool shot is made easier when accompanied by a firm, gentle hug to help the child hold still.*

The nurse can easily restrain a child younger than 6 months by positioning himself or herself above the infant, facing the legs. With the nurse's body or arms as a gentle restraint, he or she can select the exact site, pick up the muscle with one hand, and give the injection with the other (Fig. 26-4). Once the infant is able to turn over, a second person may be required during the injection. The second person should restrain the infant's arms and one leg. The nurse can then control the leg receiving the injection.

Because the child often pulls away as a natural response, the nurse firmly grasps the lower portion of the syringe when aspirating for blood and injecting the drug. A second needle should be available in case the first one becomes contaminated. The nurse can distract the child by having him or her focus on counting to 100, wiggling the big toe, or naming things in a picture on the wall.

equipment

When selecting the correct needle size, the nurse chooses the smallest gauge needle appropriate for the medication. The needle length should not exceed 1 in, except for the adult-size adolescent. Most often, 1- to 1½-in needles with gauges 20, 21, or 22 are used. The total amount of the injection should not exceed 1 mL for a child 3 years or younger and 1.5 mL for a child 3 to 6 years. By 15 years, the child could receive injections of 2 to 2.5 mL.

site

When choosing an appropriate site, the vastus lateralis muscle group can be used for all ages. The rectus femoris also is useful. The injection site is the medial to lateral aspect in the center one-third portion of the thigh. This area can be isolated by pinching up the muscle mass and inserting the needle at a right angle (Fig. 26-4).

The gluteus maximus and ventrogluteal sites may be used in a child who has been walking for at least 1 year. To avoid possible sciatic nerve damage, these sites should not be used on a child who has not been walking for at least 1 year. For a child younger than 4 to 6 years, these sites should be used only if other sites are contraindicated. The deltoid site can be used on a child 3 years or older, but the amount should not exceed 0.5 mL due to the immaturity of muscle development.

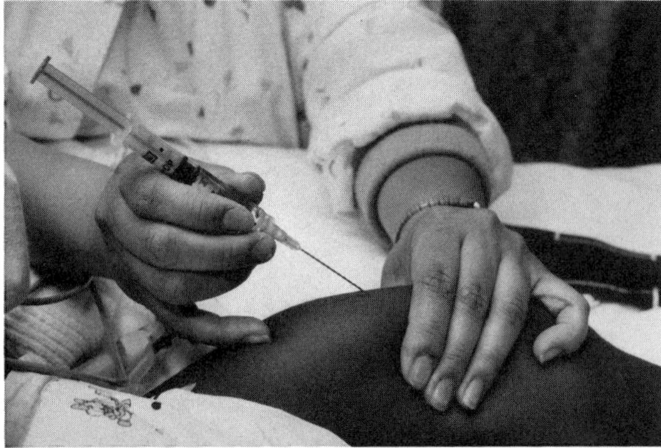

figure 26-4 *Injection site.*

intravenous administration

The LPN/LVN generally is not prepared to initiate intravenous therapy but does have the responsibility of assisting the registered nurse in maintaining the needle site and observing for complications from intravenous therapy. Intravenous therapy for children can pose some challenges for the nurse.

Parents of a neonate who requires intravenous therapy need explanations about what to expect, including possible shaving of the infant's head and the use of restraints throughout the course of therapy. The length of time necessary to perform this procedure can seem like an eternity to the waiting parent. Thus, the parent needs to know that the child can be seen as soon as the procedure is completed.

The toddler needs a brief, simple explanation just before the procedure is initiated. Instruction to the parent should include the child's limitations while receiving intravenous therapy. Restraint of the toddler will be required. The preschooler or the young school-age child and the parent can be instructed before the procedure begins. The child should know that crying is permitted. Holding the child's hand may be an effective way to help the child hold still as much as possible. The older school-age child and adolescent can hold still for the procedure; however, it is important to assess how cooperative the patient is to avoid unexpected problems.

Maintaining the needle site requires that the needle be taped securely in place. A young child's skin is sensitive and can react to the type of tape used to secure the needle. It is a good idea to ask the parent about any allergies to tape. If there are allergies or if a child shows a reaction to adhesive tape, hypoallergenic tape can be used. Plastic medicine cups may be cut, padded and placed over the site to prevent dislodging of the needle. The extremity can be restrained by pinning the armboard to the sheets or using sandbags.

The site should be checked every 15 to 30 minutes unless the intravenous pump has an alarm system. Any restlessness or complaint of pain at the site may be the first indication of infiltration or phlebitis. The site needs to be checked for signs of swelling, cool skin temperature, pain, or redness and observations reported immediately.

Another serious complication of intravenous therapy is fluid overload. Infants and children with compromised circulatory systems are extremely sensitive to the amount of circulating fluid volume. To prevent circulatory overload in these clients, intravenous tubing with a special chamber is used. This is called a volume-control chamber or measured-volume chamber and is filled with no more than twice the amount ordered to infuse in 1 hour. The parent is instructed not to adjust the rate or refill the control chamber but instead to ring the nurse.

Constant infusion pumps also are used to infuse small hourly volumes (2–3 mL/h). The battery-powered pumps allow more freedom of movement for the ambulatory patient receiving intravenous therapy. The pumps need to be observed for dry chambers, air in the tubing, and wrong infusion rates.

Careful intake and output monitoring can help prevent fluid overload. If the parent is able to be with the child, he or she can be instructed about the importance of oral intake and output; emphasizing accurate recording may prevent serious complications. Observe for signs of fluid overload. The first sign is anxiety and increased respirations; a later sign is pulmonary edema.

A cooperative older child can be instructed on how to record oral intake and output measurements. To reinforce the child's learning, the child can assist the nurse with instructing the parent on intake and output.

rectal administration

This route of drug administration is less desirable because the presence of stool in the rectum can delay or block absorption of the drug. Suppositories are the most frequent form of drug used rectally. Suppositories should not be quartered or halved because of the uncertainty of accurate dose.

equipment and technique

The nurse should wear gloves and use water-soluble lubricant and proper restraints when indicated. For the full-term infant and toddler, the pinky should be used for insertion of the suppository. For children 3 years and older, the adult index finger can be used for insertion. The preschool child can become upset during this procedure because of the age-related fear of body entry; explaining the procedure to the child can help allay fears.

The nurse puts the child in Sims' position or knee-chest position. The suppository is inserted past the anal sphincter. The child can be instructed to breathe deeply or pant like a puppy as a distraction from the procedure and the urge to defecate. The buttocks should be held together for 5 to 10 minutes or when the urge to defecate passes.

If the child defecates within 10 to 30 minutes after the suppository is given, the stool is checked for the presence of the suppository. If the suppository was not a laxative and is found in the stool, the nurse needs to notify the prescriber.

topical administration

The thin skin and larger body surface area of the neonate, infant, and small child allow increased absorption of topical medications. Thus, this age group suffers toxic effects from topical agents more often than the older client. The nurse should wash off cleansing solutions used on the infant. Any topical medication must be applied as thinly as possible to a small area.

ophthalmic administration

Eye drops and ointments can be difficult to administer to an infant and toddler, and restraint is necessary. Crying can prevent medication contact with the eye. If the child is old enough to understand, explaining the procedure can help. Otherwise, the child is asked to close the eyes. The child is then positioned so the head is lower than the body. The nurse rests the hand holding the dropper on the forehead of the child and with the other hand gently retracts the lower lid to instill the medication in the trough of the lower lid. This method allows the dropper to follow any head movement. After instillation, the child needs to be kept in that position for about 1 minute to maximize drug contact (Fig. 26-5).

If the eyelid cannot be opened, the drop can be placed near the inner canthus. When the child opens his or her eyes, blinking will distribute the drug but not as completely as with direct instillation. Light pressure over the nasolacrimal duct area (in the inner corner of the eye) for a few minutes will reduce the amount of the drug drained off the eye internally. Any excess can be blotted with a clean tissue.

Before applying ophthalmic ointment, a small amount is squeezed onto a sterile gauze and discarded. This clears any contaminated medication from the end of the tube. The child must be reminded that vision may be blurred for a while because of the ointment.

otic administration

When administering ear drops to a child, sterile technique is not necessary unless the eardrum is ruptured. Sterile technique should be used if there is drainage or a known break in the eardrum membrane.

Also, the angle of the ear canal changes with age. For the child younger than 3 years, the pinna needs to be pulled gently down and back for effective instillation. For the child older than 3 years, the pinna needs to be pulled up and back (Fig. 26-6).

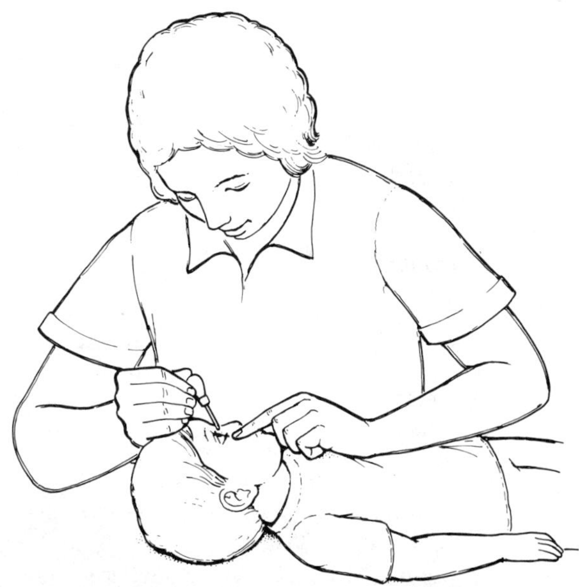

figure 26-5 *Administering eye drops.*

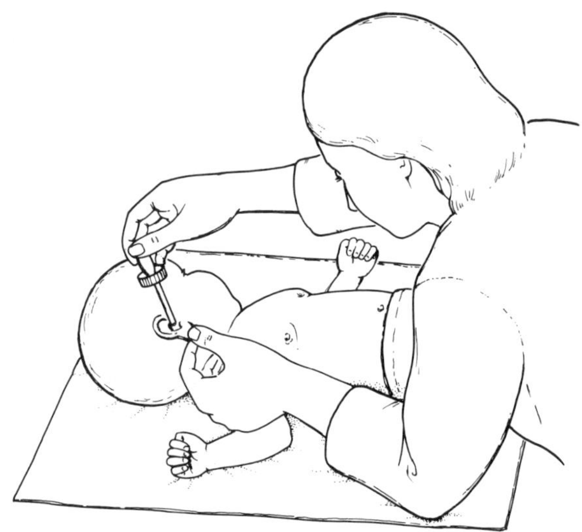

figure 26-6 *Administering ear medications.*

If the drops are cold, they can produce pain, nausea, or vertigo. Ear drops need to be warmed to body temperature before administration. A cotton ball saturated with the medication and placed in the end of the canal will prevent loss of medication from the canal.

nasal administration

The nose must be free of mucus before instillation of medication. Infants tend to breathe through the nose and will squirm in attempt to get away. The infant can be held in the football position (one arm next to the nurse's body and the infant's head in his or her hand) or in the nurse's lap with the neck hyperextended over the nurse's knees. The older child can hang the head back over a pillow or side of the bed.

The child is kept in position for several minutes after instillation. Difficulty breathing, coughing, gagging, and vomiting should be monitored because the medication may trigger one or more of these responses as it trickles down the back of the throat. Oil-based drops must be avoided because of the risk of aspiration pneumonia.

inhalation therapies

The croup or mist tent is a common type of aerosol treatment for a child with respiratory impairment. Responsibilities for the nurse include maintaining the mist level, observing the effects on the child, encouraging the child to stay in the tent, and keeping the child warm and dry.

Intermittent positive pressure breathing treatments are given by those who are specially trained to do so. One of the nurse's main responsibilities in assisting with this type of therapy is to help emotionally support the child and parent. The face mask, machines, and medications can be scary to a child who has difficulty breathing. The anxious parent tends to empathize with the feeling of being unable to breathe when child is receiving a treatment. The mask, mouth pieces, and tubing are used on one child only and cleaned according to hospital policy after each treatment to prevent cross-contamination.

Metered-dose inhalers and spinhalers are gaining popularity for treatment of the older child with respiratory disorders, such as asthma and cystic fibrosis. The medication will be drawn deeper into the respiratory tract if released midinhalation. If more than one inhalation is ordered for a dose, emphasize the importance of waiting until the recommended time between inhalations for best effect. Rebound effect can occur with overuse of some bronchodilators. This point must be stressed when instruction is given.

✱ nursing process during drug administration

assessment

Assessment of the patient receiving the drug includes collecting objective and subjective information, which encompasses a physical examination, chief complaint, and drug history, including allergies; diet habits that may influence therapy; and social history, which includes the child's favorites and dislikes, the parent-child relationship, and words used by the child to describe body parts.

nursing diagnosis

Nursing diagnoses are made from identifying problems or potential problems from the assessment data. An example of a nursing diagnosis related to drug therapy is Altered Nutrition: Less than body requirements. A common adverse effect of many medications is nausea and loss of appetite.

planning and intervention

Planning involves specific care guidelines and goals to achieve. Care guidelines in drug therapy involve using the six rights of administration, setting up the most appropriate times for the drug to be most effective, and instructing the patient or parent to improve compliance with therapy. The goals are patient oriented. If the drug is to be continued after discharge, the goal could be that the parent can demonstrate the proper technique of drug administration.

Intervention simply means carrying out the plan. In drug therapy, this includes preparing and administering the prescribed drug, documenting the procedure, checking vital signs when indicated, and reviewing data obtained on admission.

evaluation

Evaluation of drug effectiveness includes checking vital signs, inquiring if pain is relieved, measuring output, and asking for the parent's impression of effectiveness because the parent knows the child best.

managing children's pain

Nothing is more challenging for the nurse than trying to provide adequate pain management for an infant or child. Whether the pain results from an injury, an infection, or from surgery, the child experiencing pain needs comfort and relief. However, the rigid prescriptions for pain management in adults do not meet the needs of children, regardless of age.

Postoperative pain relief is a key factor in earlier mobilization of patients and reduction in postoperative complications. Thus, pain relief benefits the child, who gets to go home sooner, and the hospital, because costs are reduced.

✳ family considerations

Thorough preoperative teaching reduces anxiety in the child and the caregiver; both need to be included in the teaching plan. A clear picture of what to expect should be explained in understandable terms, not hospital language, without downplaying the amount or type of pain to expect. It is important to talk about what the equipment and rooms will look like and if possible, to show the child and parent. Neither the nurse nor anyone else should impose their feelings about the amount of pain the child will be able to tolerate.

Postoperative activities will quicken the healing process. The parent can be instructed to help with these activities with the understanding that some discomfort will be involved. Having the parent instructed on intake and output measurement may help him or her feel useful at a time when parents usually feel helpless to improve the child's situation.

✳ nursing considerations

Pain assessment needs to be geared to the child's developmental level. The nurse needs to learn what words the child uses to describe pain. For example, the child may say, "I have a bad headache in my tummy" or use such terms as "boo boo" or "ouchie." When the nurse uses these words in evaluating postoperative pain, it improves nurse–patient communication. Parents need to be included in describing how the child reacts to pain, especially if the child is in a preverbal stage of development. Children younger than 7 years depend heavily on their parents for guidance and support through painful experiences. Parental anxiety can heighten the child's pain perception. Keeping parents informed will reduce their anxiety and perhaps also reduce the child's pain.

Signs of pain can differ in children at different levels of development. Infants and toddlers often show physical reactions to pain, such as crying, rubbing an area, vomiting right after eating, fussiness, or altered sleep patterns. In older children, verbalization, facial expression, body posture, activity, and appearance can indicate pain. Television watching, playing, and sleeping a lot also may be be used as distractions to help cope with pain. Continued severe pain may be demonstrated by the child whimpering or lying still instead of crying or being restless.

The nurse can use many strategies to ease anxiety and distress and thereby relieve pain. Allowing the unrestricted presence of a parent or other family member helps provide the support and nurturing the child needs for recovery. Swaddling, rocking, and holding are helpful for the infant. Offering a pacifier, a favorite blanket, or toy can be comforting. Other comfort measures include repositioning with pillow and blankets, back rubs to relax tension caused by pain, local applications of cold or heat, and distraction (Fig. 26-7).

pharmacologic management of pain

Pharmacologic control of pain in children can be achieved when some common misconceptions concerning children and pain are abolished. First, infants and children feel pain just as adults do. Even though nerves are not fully

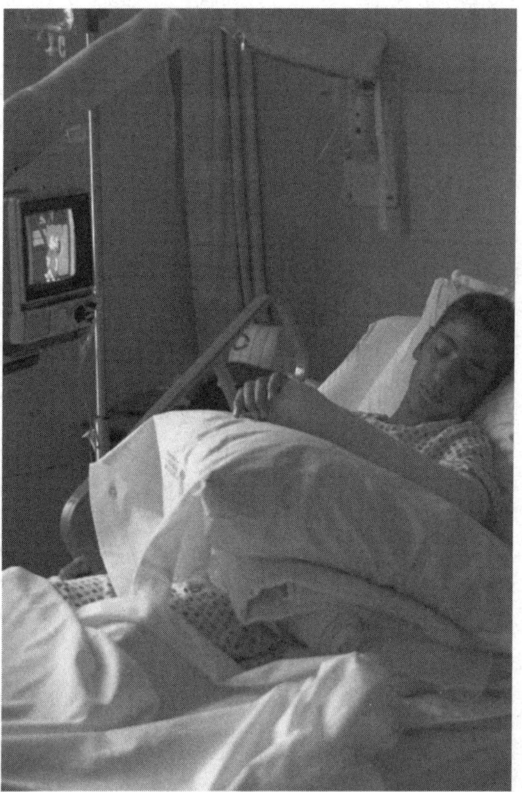

figure 26-7 *Pillows and blankets elevating the arm alleviate pain, while sleep and television distract the adolescent from concentrating on the discomfort.*

myelinated at birth, pain is still felt. Second, children are highly unlikely to become addicted to narcotics. The prevalent "just say no" programs can sometimes be misleading to the parent and child concerning narcotic use for pain. The nurse must emphasize that medication is not the same as street drugs. It has been shown that the need for intravenous narcotics for pain control tapers off on the third or fourth postoperative day. A change to oral forms of analgesics is considered when oral intake is tolerated or the amount of pain perceived has lessened. Dosage data for analgesics are included in Table 26-2.

Narcotics cause respiratory depression. A child's response to narcotics may require higher or lower doses of the drug for adequate pain control. Giving the drug around the clock with no doses omitted and documenting pain relief with vital signs on a flow sheet at timed intervals will allow the nurse to assist the physician in fine tuning the dose needed for the child's relief. Nighttime doses can be given when vital signs and assessments are scheduled to allow the child to rest in between checks.

Preferred routes of administration for pain medication are oral, rectal, and intravenous. The IM route has several

table 26-2 *dosing data for analgesics**

Drug	*Approximate Oral Dose*	*Approximate Parenteral Dose*	*Recommended Start Dose >50 kg Oral / Parenteral*	*Recommended Start Dose <50 kg Oral / Parenteral*
Codeine	130 mg q3–4 h	75 mg q3–4 h	60 mg q3–4 h 60 mg q2h (IM or SC)	1 mg/kgq3–4 h Not recommended
Hydromorphone (Dilaudid)	7.5 mg q3–4 h	1.5 mg q3–4 h	6 mg q3–4 h 1.5 mg q3–4 h	0.06 mg/kg q3–4 h 0.015 mg/kg q3–4 h
Hydrocodone (Lortab, Vicodin, others)	30 g q3–4 h	Not available	10 mg q3–4 h Unavailable	0.2 mg/kg q3–4 h Unavailable
Levorphanol (Levo-Dromoran)	4 mg q6–8 h	2 mg q6–8 h	4 mg q6–8 h 2 mg q6–8 h	0.04 mg/kg q6–8 h 0.2 mg/kg q6–8 h
Meperidine (Demerol)	300 mg q2–3 h	100 mg q3h	Not recommended 100 mg q3h	Not recommended 0.75 mg/kg q2–3 h
Methadone (Dolophine)	20 mg q6–8 h	10 mg q6–8 h	20 mg q6–8 h 10 mg q6–8 h	0.2 mg/kg q6–8 h 0.1 mg/kg q6–8 h
Oxycodone (Tylox, Percocet)	30 mg q3–4 h	Not available	10 mg q3–4 h Unavailable	0.2 mg/kg q3–4 h Unavailable
Buprenorphine (Buprenex)	Not available	0.3–0.4 mg q6–8 h	Unavailable 0.4 mg q6–8 h	Unavailable 0.004 mg/kg q6–8 h
Nalbuphine (Nubain)	Not available	10 mg q3–4 h	Unavailable 10 mg q3–4 h	Unavailable 0.1 mg/kg q3–4 h

Oral NSAIDs	*Usual Dose Adult >50 kg*	*Usual Dose Pediatric <50 kg*	*Comments*
Aspirin	650–975 mg q4h	10–15 mg/kg q4h	Interferes with platelet formation
Ibuprofen (Motrin, Nuprin)	400 mg q4–6 h	10 mg/kg q6–8 h	Suspension available
Naproxen (Naprosyn)	500 mg initial dose 250 mg q6–8 h	5 mg/kg q12h	Liquid form available
Choline magnesium trisalicylate (Trilisate)	1,000–1,500 mg b.i.d.	25 mg/kg b.i.d.	Minimal antiplatelet activity; oral liquid available
Acetaminophen (Tylenol, Panadol)	650–975 mg q4h	10–15 mg/kg q4h	No anti-inflammatory activity

*This table of recommended doses does not apply to patients with renal or hepatic dysfunction or other conditions affecting drug metabolism or excretion. Caution also should be used when combination drugs of opioid and aspirin or acetaminophen are prescribed.

Hester, N., Jacox, A., Miaskowski, C. & Ferrell, B. (1992). The management of pain in infants, children, and adolescents. *Maternal Child Nursing*, 17, May/June, 146–152.

disadvantages: Available sites are exhausted quickly, and altered tissue absorption leads to varying therapeutic levels of the drug. They also are contraindicated for children with a low platelet count. In addition, children do not like to get shots, and because of this, nurses may find it difficult to give shots. Patient-controlled analgesia can be used for older children and adolescents.

Keeping the parent and child informed about the course of treatment does several things to enhance recovery. Anxiety and fear of the unknown are dispelled. The relationship between nurse and client improves when the nurse gains the client's confidence. The nurse gains a great deal of satisfaction for a job well done when the client is kept relaxed and comfortable, and improvement is seen each day.

key points ✳

* ✳ **Administering drugs to infants and children includes the following responsibilities: observing the six rights, understanding the drug and the condition for which it has been prescribed, and understanding the developmental level of the child.**
* ✳ **Pharmacokinetics is affected by the level of physical development and by the fluid and fat percentages of total body weight.**
* ✳ **Successful administration of drugs considers the physical and cognitive development of the child and the role of the parent or other caregiver in the child's life.**
* ✳ **Drug dosage is more often prescribed as mg/kg; accuracy in dosage calculation is required to achieve therapeutic effectiveness and to prevent serious consequences of overdose.**
* ✳ **Oral and intravenous routes are used most often since the IM route is self-limiting because rotation sites are limited.**
* ✳ **Educating parents and children is the key to preventing childhood poisonings.**
* ✳ **Effective pain management means understanding that children experience pain just as adults do.**

review questions ✳

1. What is the most effective way to administer a liquid oral medication to a 6-month-old?
   a. Mix the medication into the next bottle of formula.
   b. With the child in the nurse's arms, pour the medication from the cup into the front of the mouth, and then tilt the child's head backward.
   c. Have the child restrained except for the right leg and then give the injection.
   d. Use a syringe without a needle and deposit small amounts between the cheeck and the gums, allowing the child to swallow between amounts.
2. Which site for IM injection can be used for all ages of children?
   a. Vastis lateralis
   b. Deltoid
   c. Dorsogluteal
   d. Ventral gluteal
3. How can the nurse involve the parent with the child's care when recovering from surgery?
   a. Ask the parent to check for bleeding every 2 hours and report it to the nurse.
   b. Instruct the parent on how to keep intake and output records.
   c. Reassure the parent that he or she can help in turning and repositioning the child when the nurse is unavailable.
   d. Instruct the parent to refill the IV volume controller to 30 mL when it becomes empty and call for the nurse.
4. Which of the following should be emphasized when a child is receiving a narcotic for postoperative pain?
   a. The dose of the narcotic will only be repeated if the child asks for pain medication.
   b. The pain medication will not cause addiction because the studies have shown addiction does not occur when the person is in pain.
   c. Even though the drug is like those used on the street, the dose is controlled and addiction will not occur.
   d. The narcotic should take away all the pain the child will experience.
5. Oral medications given to the newborn may have delayed absorption because
   a. Newborns often spit up after oral intake.
   b. Gastric pH of the newborn is neutral or slightly alkaline.
   c. Emptying time of the newborn's stomach is very short, causing stomach contents to pass through the bowel quickly.
   d. The newborn's diet contains primarily alkaline foods.

references ✳

Bindler, R., & Howry, L. (1991). *Pediatric drugs and nursing implications*. Norwalk, CT: Appleton & Lange.

bibliography ✳

Gay, J. (1992). A painful experience. *Nursing Times*, *88*(25), 32–35.

Hester, N. O., Jacox, A., Miaskowski, C., & Ferrell, B. (1992). Excerpts from guidelines for the management of pain in infants, children, and adolescents undergoing operative and medical procedures. *Maternal-Child Nursing*, *17*, 146–152.

Reiss, B., & Evans, M. (1993). *Pharmacological aspects of nursing care* (4th ed.). Albany NY: Delmar Publishers.

Scherer, J. C. (1995). *Introductory clinical pharmacology* (5th ed.). Philadelphia, PA: J.B. Lippincott.

Skale, N. (1992). *Manual of pediatric nursing procedures*. Philadelphia, PA: J.B. Lippincott.

Williams, B., & Baer, C. (1994). *Essentials of clinical pharmacology in nursing* (2nd ed.). Springhouse, PA: Springhouse Corporation.

nursing care of the child and family during acute illness

27

outline

objectives

After studying this chapter, the reader should be able to:

* Use principles of therapeutic communication to support children and their families who are experiencing an acute hospital admission.
* Discuss age-appropriate techniques to reduce anxiety.
* Use critical thinking to expedite the admission process while focusing on appropriate guidelines to obtain pertinent clinical information and support the child and family through their anxiety.
* Discuss legal and ethical standards related to hospital admission.
* Discuss three nursing interventions for a child undergoing surgery.
* Discuss the preparations for the child admitted to the intensive care unit.
* Name types of isolation units and psychological factors to consider.
* Discuss the principles of child development that relate to regressive behavior.
* Identify signs of mild and severe pain and ways to comfort the patient and family.
* Discuss the importance of play when implementing the nursing process.

key terms 

acute illness
discipline
emancipated minor
ICU
informed consent
isolation
play therapy
regression
separation anxiety

An *acute illness* has a rapid onset, lasts a short time, and has severe symptoms. Many health care delivery systems are available for an acutely ill child, for example, ambulatory care, public health clinics, or emergency rooms.

The nurse and family must promptly recognize the child's health care problem to expedite recovery and prevent permanent injuries. Appropriate emergency health care and medications are essential to lower the rate of morbidity and mortality of children seen in an emergency care setting. When a child is brought to the emergency room for an acute illness or injury, a systematic assessment approach is crucial to survival and the measure of health care to be delivered. Some illnesses, such as, trauma, acute respiratory and gastrointestinal disease, and infection, require hospitalization. For the acutely ill child and family, hospitalization is an abrupt unscheduled and frightening experience.

table 27-1 stages of separation anxiety

Stage	*Manifestations*
Protest	The child cries loudly and demandingly; rejects any attempts to be comforted.
Despair	The child wails rather than cries; may turn away from parent's approach; often lies on abdomen, facial expression flat; may lose weight and develop insomnia; loses developmental skills; prone to minor ailments, such as upper respiratory infections; IQ will measure lower than previous measurement.
Denial	The child is silent, face expressionless; developmental milestones deteriorate; may respond quickly but superficially to all caregivers; may have difficulty forming close relationships later in life.

✳ family considerations

fear

Fear is a normal reaction for a child who is admitted to the hospital. The nurse can be a valuable resource to help children distinguish their fears and lessen their anxiety. When children express their fears and understand that their illness is not their fault, understanding and self-confidence are demonstrated.

Parents' fears regarding the hospitalization of their children are usually related to the seriousness of the illness. Their fears are escalated by fear of the unknown and lack of information. Parents also have fears about how the current condition will affect the child in later years. The nurse must ease the fears of the parents for their well-being and for that of the child. Children are extremely astute. Although they may not fully understand the implications of their sickness, they are able to sense their parents' tension and become just as anxious.

separation anxiety

Separation from parents increases the emotional trauma felt by children who are hospitalized. Separation from rituals and attachment figures is frightening and adds to the child's confusion and frustration. Children will experience three stages of *separation anxiety* (Table 27-1). Protesting is a normal behavioral response, but it may make the parents more uncomfortable; sneaking away or lying to the child about leaving is not recommended. Comforting the child in the parents' absence will lessen their feelings of abandonment. Feelings of detachment can be avoided by placing the parents' pictures in the child's room, assisting the child with telephone calls to the parents, and encouraging the parents to provide personal audio and visual communications of their voices and activities.

scheduling

When scheduling a procedure, the nurse should consider what is best for the patient and family. The child should not be expected to remain in the hospital longer then absolutely necessary but also should not be bombarded with a day full of diagnostic tests. The nurse also needs to be aware of the strains parents face when trying to rearrange their personal schedules. They may work or have other children to care for.

visitations

Family interaction is highly recommended for the psychological wellness and physical recovery of the acutely ill child. Parents of children younger than 5 years often have unlimited visitation and remain overnight with the child. Older children appreciate having their parents around and knowing precisely when they will return. Siblings and grandparents also help comfort the child. Siblings are encouraged to visit, providing they are well supervised and the hospital room is free of hazards to young children.

✳ nursing considerations

The nurse should assess the child's and family's level of knowledge regarding the illness; anxiety will effect the child's and parents' ability to assimilate the information that the nurse shares. The nurse must communicate clearly with an unhasty approach. The nurse should follow the parents' cues as to how detailed to make the explanations; however, some parents cope better if their questions are answered methodically and with detailed explanations.

Questions should be answered honestly and in a language the child can understand. If the child is given conflicting information by another health care worker, he or she will become confused and even more apprehensive.

Scheduling nurses so that the child interacts with as few different health care workers as possible is extremely beneficial. Fear and separation anxiety are reduced when the child is able to establish a rapport with the nurse. This is most effective when one nurse follows the case from admissions through recovery and is a constant support to the child and family throughout the hospital stay.

age-specific considerations

The developmental stage of patients will determine the best way to comfort and prepare them for medical treatment.

infant

The infant in an acute care setting does not understand what is happening and becomes stressed by the caregivers' emotional reactions. Helping the infant's parents remain calm and promoting the infant–parent bond is essential to alleviate the child's anxiety.

Unable to verbalize discomfort, the infant relies on nonverbal cues to communicate. When an infant is thrashing, stiffening, and stretching the arms and limbs, he or she is nonverbally responding to disorganization. Disorganization causes the infant to be uncomfortable, stressed, or overstimulated. The nurse needs to be aware of these cues and respond accordingly. Sticking closely to the infant's typical routine and being familiar with the surroundings often calms the infant.

toddler

The toddler has three fears about entering the hospital and undergoing treatment: the unknown, abandonment, and mutilation. Nursing care of the toddler should be aimed at reducing these fears.

Toddlers need short explanations close to the time of a procedure. The toddler's imagination is vivid. The nurse must gauge the toddler's ability to communicate to elicit information and speak to the child at the appropriate level.

Toddlers' attachment to parents is heightened. Much like infants, toddlers benefit from having their parents with them as often as possible. Pictures of family members and familiar toys comfort the child while the parents are away.

school-age child

Fearful of bodily harm and extensive pain, the school-age child needs to have faith in the family and health care workers. The child should never be given intentionally inaccurate information. This can destroy their trust. School-age children should know why they are ill and need medical intervention, where they will be taken, what they will feel, and what medical equipment they will use. They need to know that the sickness is not a punishment for past misbehavior and that it does not have a magical cure. Careful, age-specific explanations of the cause and effect of an acute illness promotes a fuller understanding of medical treatment and procedures, realistic expectations, and self-worth.

School-age children can easily adapt to being separated from parents. They often spend time away from them at school, during sports practice, or while participating in other groups. School-age children still have concerns about being alone in the hospital. They can be comforted by explanations of when the parents will visit according to the daily schedule. For example, the nurse can tell the child "after you eat dinner and take your bath, your parents will be here."

adolescent

Adolescents are concerned with how an illness or treatment will affect their body image. They need information about how their body will look and function in the future. They also worry about being isolated from friends and anticipated events like school dances or football games.

The adolescent's independence and sense of control are jeopardized in the acute care setting. Relying on parents or the nurse for basic needs and expressing fears or pain may be viewed by the adolescent as immature. The nurse should not assume everything is alright merely because the adolescent is acting calm and capable. Despite their desire for independence, adolescents can still be soothed by their family's presence.

hospital admissions

preadmission teaching

Providing information regarding the disease process, treatment procedures, and expected outcome after treatment is a crucial part of preadmission teaching. Parents should know about hospital rules and regulations and what is expected of them as parents. If the child is expected to have surgery, some aspects of preoperative teaching can begin before admission (See the Nursing Care Plan: Preoperative Surgical Health Teaching). Parents should instructed about obtaining equipment and devices that may be needed postoperatively.

planned admission

A planned admission allows the child and family to be introduced to unfamiliar surroundings, procedures, and events in advance. When an admission to the hospital is planned, the child and parents are taken on a hospital tour (Fig. 27-1). The child may be anxious during the tour, but he or she will be exposed to the strange surroundings with the support of parents. Frightening areas should be avoided because the purpose of the tour is to lessen fear and anxiety.

Taking the child to a hospital room setting similar to the one where he or she will be admitted is beneficial.

emergency admission

An emergency admission is traumatic for the child and parents, especially if admission to an intensive care unit (ICU) is required. The parents and child do not have the

nursing care plan
preoperative surgical health teaching

NURSING DIAGNOSIS:
Anxiety/Fear (child and family), related to hospitalization and unfamiliar situation

GOAL: The child and family will share their concerns and feel less anxious in the hospital environment

NURSING INTERVENTIONS	RATIONALE	EVALUATION
Introduce yourself and orient the family and the child to the unit.	The child and family will feel respected and have a reference person to contact for questions.	The family and child will verbalize fears related to the surgical procedure and will feel comfortable in asking questions.
Explain to the parents the importance of their participation in care, open visiting and "rooming in" procedures.	Research supports the dangers of separation for young children and support is given for open visiting and for parents staying with the child.	The parent or caregiver will visit or stay with the child as much as possible. The child will not have signs of separation anxiety.
Encourage the parents to bring a favorite animal or toy for the child.	The familiar toy can provide comfort and security to the child.	The child will keep his favorite animal or toy with him for comfort.
Speak to the child at eye level and use age-appropriate language to orient the child to all new procedures.	Eye-level conversation is less threatening to the child, and age-appropriate terminology will increase the child's understanding and control of the situation.	The child will feel comfortable in asking questions and show signs of trust in his caregivers.
Utilize play therapy to explain all procedures and allow the child to handle equipment.	Play allows children to come to terms with new situations and helps them to deal with the "hurts" involved in hospitalziation.	The child will act out some of his fears and feel secure enough in this new environment to express negative emotions without fear of rejection.
Encourage questions from the parents and the child.	Ensuring that any question is ok lends respect to the parent and child and helps them to increase their trust in you.	The family and child will show ease in their ability to ask questions and show emotion.

opportunity to prepare or discuss the situation. Although an in-depth admission process is unlikely during an emergency admission; supporting the family's psychological needs is an integral part of nursing intervention.

When the admission process must be concise and expedient, the nurse focuses on allowing the child to participate in the process if possible and on essential components of the admission counseling. These include the following:

* the nurse should introduce himself or herself to family members.
* when referring to the child, his or her name should be used.
* the child's developmental age and ability to communicate ideas should be determined.
* information about the child's general state and chief complaint should be obtained.

admission procedures

When a child is scheduled for hospital admission, the person taking the child to the hospital should converse at the child's level of understanding. Every effort should be made to lessen the child's anxiety. Before arriving at the hospital, questions regarding what is going to happen and why should be answered.

A planned admission allows for preadmission preparation, which makes transition to hospitalization smoother and provides a less frightening experience for the child. When children are able to visit the hospital on a preadmission visit, there is an opportunity to learn about the their perception of illness and what they are expecting. Some hospitals give children masks, stethoscopes, gowns, and hair covers; they also have dolls that are used for teaching purposes and children are able to simulate medical procedures (Fig. 27-2).

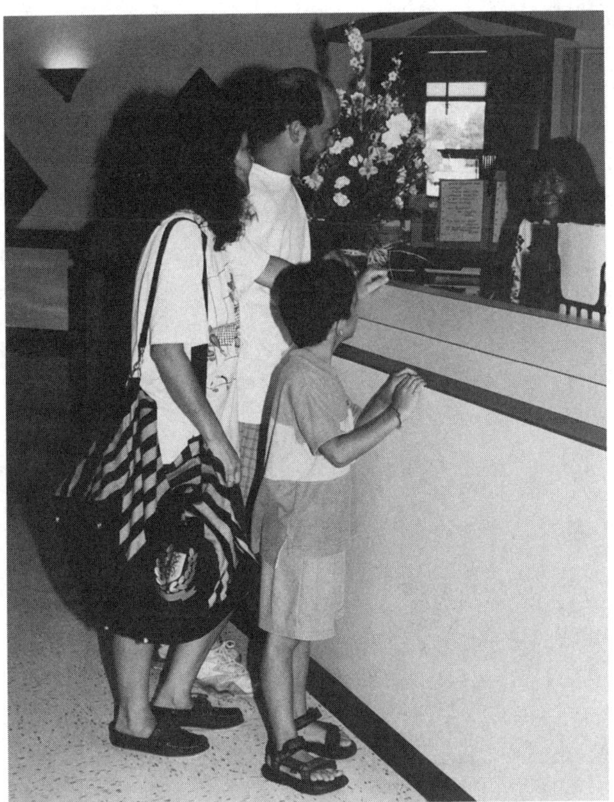

figure 27-1 *The child and family get acquainted with the hospital staff. (Photo by Elise Dinerman.)*

An interview should be conducted with the child and parents in a calm and quiet atmosphere. The child should be present at the interview.

> **nursing alert**
> *During the interview, parents should provide the nurse with a summary of all food and drug allergies.*

After the interview, the child and family should be oriented to the unit. Guidelines for orientation should include the following

* Meeting the primary nurse
* Identifying the child's room
* Introducing the child to roommates
* Touring special service rooms, such as the treatment room, playroom, and kitchen
* Explaning pediatric unit rules (Marks, 1994)

When the child returns on the day of admission, he or she will know what to expect during the admission process. Procedures such as drawing blood specimens, throat cultures, and infusion therapy will be frightening and stressful for the child regardless of preparation efforts.

The nurse should continue to support the child's emotional needs while the admission history and admission physical assessment are obtained. Afterward, the child should be placed in a room that is appropriate for age, gender, development, and type of illness.

informed consent

Consent must be given in all professional health care settings for treatment to be rendered (Erien, 1994). An *informed consent* encompasses ethical, legal, and educational aspects. It is intended to be a safeguard to protect all individuals from injury (Ruccione, 1994). Institutions require the consenting party to be informed of the intended treatment, procedures, and possible adversities to his or her health. Alternative methods of treatments also should be presented.

The nurse should consider the informed consent as a significant part of nursing process rather than a routine event; this attitude allows for information to be given thoroughly with due consideration of the individual's needs and rights (Erien, 1994).

For the consent to be valid, the consenting party must be capable of understanding the consequences of the consent and be under no overt and subtle influence. The following conditions must be met to obtain a valid consent:

* The person must be capable of giving consent: he or she must be over the age of the majority and must be considered competent (ie, possess the mental capacity to make choices and understand the consequences).
* The person must receive the information needed to make an intelligent decision. The person must act voluntarily when exercising freedom of choice without force, fraud, deceit, duress, or other forms of constraint or concern.

Traditionally, children are considered incapable of understanding the ramifications of treatment. As long as the children are minors, parents or people designated as guardians are required to give informed consent before medical treatment is rendered. Parents also may withdraw consent later.

Sensitive issues in which minors are decision makers remain controversial, such as dying with dignity and consent for abortion. Parental notification before or after an abortion remains a legal and moral issue in the United States. Presently, parental consent is not needed for treatment of a sexually transmitted disease, contraception, abortion, and drug abuse.

emancipated minors

Some minors are allowed to make decisions by law, regardless of the wishes and sometimes knowledge of their parents; these individuals are denoted as emancipated.

An *emancipated minor* is a child legally under the age of the majority but recognized as having the legal capacity of an adult under circumstances prescribed by state law. Emancipated minors are allowed to give consent for medical treatment regardless of their parent's or legal guardian's knowledge or agreement (Kelley, 1994).

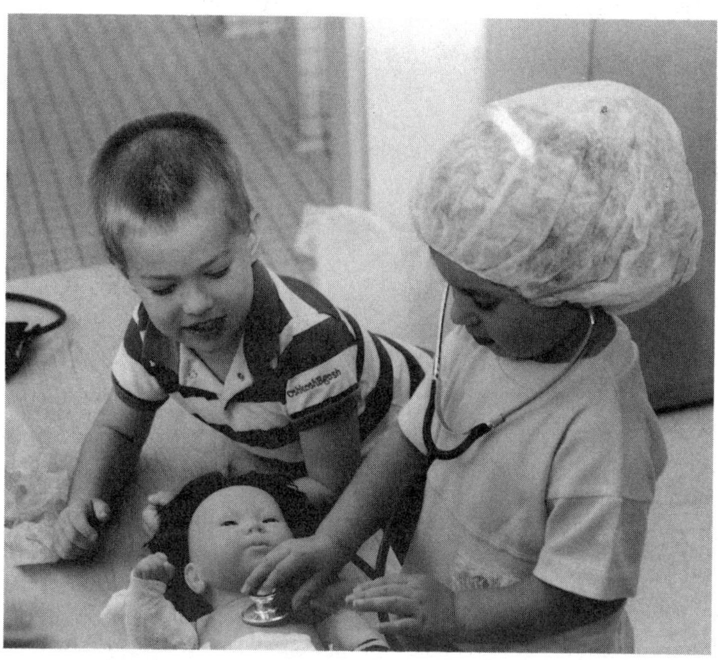

figure 27-2 *Playing with medical equipment and acting out procedures prepares children for what they will be experiencing.*

religious considerations

Cultural and religious beliefs affect how the child and his or her family respond to health care. The nurse should carefully assess the family's value system and spiritual and cultural needs; these factors will influence compliance and response to health care. Cultural and religious beliefs may be in conflict with the patient's health care practices (Kelley, 1994).

special hospital units

operating room

Safety and infection control are two relevant factors to the structure of the operating room. The temperature and humidity should be set at recommended limits to retard the growth of bacteria and prevent static electricity. Operating rooms are potential hazardous environments containing an abundance of electrical equipment and flammable materials. Surgical procedures are performed by trained professionals. Patients may receive procedures under general or local anesthesia.

recovery room

Immediately following surgery, the child is brought to the recovery room. The recovery room is an area with equipment and health care professionals for the patient who is immediately returning from the operating room. Patients remain in the recovery room until they are fully awake or are no longer drowsy from the anesthesia.

During this time, the nurse performs the following duties:

* Assesses vital signs, and the body part affected in surgery
* Checks for negative side effects of anesthesia, such as depressed respirations
* Obtains and monitors medical equipment
* Observes for bleeding, urinary output, consciousness, and airway patency

intensive care unit

The *ICU* is designed to care for children with illnesses such as acute metabolic disorders, nervous system disorders, and cardiac disorders. Children who have experienced multiple traumas or complex surgeries are candidates for the ICU. A child who is admitted for an obvious traumatic injury to one body system should be considered as having a multiple trauma until proven differently. The ICU is equipped with complex instruments designed to support metabolic process and sustain respiratory and circulatory functioning.

The child admitted to the ICU is at risk for postsurgical complications. The child's physical condition is unstable, and the health care professional must have a thorough understanding of physiology as it relates to children.

Psychological preparation should be a part of preoperative teaching when admission to the ICU is expected after a surgical procedure. The parents should be prepared for how the child will look. Ventilation support, infusion therapy, and oxygen therapy can be frightening to parents if they are not properly prepared. The child and family should be prepared for the stressors associated with ICU admission. The child will experience discomfort; he or she will not be permitted to eat or drink, and restraints may be necessary.

isolation unit

A child admitted to the *isolation* unit may experience feelings of abandonment and loss of control. The environment suddenly changes to interacting with strangers who wear a mask, gown, and gloves. They also may feel the parents have abandoned them when they leave the room.

The child's developmental age should be considered in the nursing care. Efforts to lessen regression and promote understanding of isolation should be shared by the nurse and family members. There are three common types of isolations: enteric, respiratory, and wound and skin care.

reverse isolation

Reverse isolation is used to protect patients who are immune depressed or have serious impaired resistance from pathogens. These patients may be receiving radiation treatments or steroid and antimetabolic therapy, or they may have leukemia, agranulocytosis, or extensive burns. Reverse isolation protects the patients from pathogens in the environment or pathogens carried by others. They are placed in a single room, and people entering the room should practice meticulous hand washing and use a gown, gloves, and mask.

common surgical procedures

hernia repair

A hernia is a weakening of a muscular wall, resulting in protusion of a portion of an organ or organs through an abnormal opening. Diaphragmatic, hiatal, inguinal, and umbilical hernias are common in children. Diaphragmatic hernias must be treated immediately. Inguinal hernias may also require emergency intervention if strangulation of the bowels occurs. See Chapter 34 for a fuller discussion of hernias.

appendicitis

Appendicitis is an inflammation of the veriform (or blind sac) located at the end of the cecum. It may be caused by fecalith entering the appendix and obstructing the lumen or by an anatomic defect of the cecum. Appendicitis is common in school-age children. Symptoms of appendicitis vary widely. The child may present with vomiting, periumbilical pain, anorexia, and intense pain after the abdomen is decreased and released (McBurney's point). An appendectomy (removal of the appendix) is the surgical treatment prior to rupture or other complication resulting from appendicitis.

tonsillectomy and adenoidectomy

Removal or the palatine and pharyngeal tonsils is called a tonsillectomy. Chronic tonsillitis and hypertrophied adenoids are valid reasons for a tonsillectomy and adenoidectomy. The procedure should be selectively performed after 3 years when the child's immune system is functioning adequately. Surgical correction prior to 4 years may result in regrowth or hypertrophy of lymphoid tissue.

preoperative care

Preoperative care for a child experiencing a surgical procedure is aimed at minimizing anxiety and stress. Preparing the child and family members for the surgical procedure is a psychological intervention; the psychosocial preparation can be facilitated through play, drawings, illustrations, and discussion. Anatomically correct dolls may be used to simulate surgical procedures and evaluate the child's and parents' response to the surgery.

Physical aspects of preoperative care include hygienic measures, procedural preparations (ie, preoperative antibiotic infusion, enemas, preoperative injections), and safety measures.

postoperative care

Regardless of the preoperative effort to lessen the anxiety about surgery, the child will need to adapt to an altered physical and psychological status. The child's needs should be met, and skills that were taught preoperatively will need to be reviewed. The nurse should allow the child to express feelings through play, writing, and drawing. The child's nonverbal expressions in drawings and play should be evaluated as communication.

The postoperative assessment of the child who has undergone surgery is primarily the responsibility of the nurse. Vital signs should be assessed, the child's ability to void should be evaluated, and nursing interventions and goals should be focused toward preventing postoperative complications.

special considerations in the acute care setting

pain

Children who are experiencing mild pain may have obvious signs of discomfort, such as crying, posturing, or appearing restless, quiet, listless, and uninterested in the environment.

The child experiencing severe pain may have crying episodes, insomnia, loss of appetite, and depression. More obvious signs of pain are facial grimacing, favoring body parts, or changes in pulse and respirations.

In older children, age and cultural beliefs may influence their behavioral response to pain; the nurse should consider these factors when assessing whether behaviors are pain related. (For a discussion of pain, see Chap. 26.)

comfort measures

Maintaining an open line of communication is essential to comforting the child who is in pain. Reassuring the child that the prescribed comfort measures will make him or her feel better is encouraged. Being truthful, communicating to the child the plan of care, and teaching a child what to expect are ways to reduce anxiety about anticipated pain.

Parental response directly relates to the child's response to pain. If a parent is anxious during an invasive procedure, the feelings of anxiety will be transferred to the child. Explanations about procedures will support parents and lessen their own fears about invasive procedures.

mobility

An acutely ill child's diagnosis may include immobility. Depending on the child's age, immobility could be devastating. Toddlers are exploratory; if they are suddenly restricted, they may become confused, which threatens their ability to accomplish their developmental milestones.

Activities should be directed toward self-care and independence to avoid developmental delays. Physical therapy and nursing departments should collaborate to encourage activity and prevent complications from immobility.

The immobilized child is at risk for pain and decreased muscle strength. Without frequent positioning and turning, the child will experience poor circulation and skin breakdown. Respiratory complication is a potential risk due to decreased activity and poor lung expansion.

Activities such as straw-blowing games and incentive spirometer will avoid pneumonia and increase respiratory function. Developmentally appropriate play activities should be encouraged to promote range of motion and muscle tone.

Lack of exercise and change in diet may result in constipation. Encouraging fluids and diets high in fiber will promote gastric mobility. Adequate intake of fluids also will help the patient to avoid urinary stasis and infection.

regression

When a child displays *regression* in an acute care setting, it can be upsetting for parents. Parents need help in understanding that the child's ability to return to a less mature behavior is a coping mechanism that enables the child to endure the current stressors. Some children may be potty trained before admission and regress to wearing diapers in the hospital. Supporting the child with love and compassion will help minimize the stressors that cause the regression.

✳ nursing insight

Focusing the child's attention on a regressive behavior simply enforces that behavior.

discipline

In addition to many duties, a pediatric nurse working in the acute care setting is responsible for supervising the child. *Discipline* preserves the safety of the child and provides the nurse with a measure of control. The average child does not deliberately misbehave in the hospital setting. The rambunctious child is usually bored. Focusing the child's attention on a game or event may decrease unwanted behavior. Children may act out during a procedure because they are fearful. Knowledge of the procedure ahead of time may reduce fear and encourage cooperation.

Sometimes it is necessary for a nurse to restrict the negative behavior of a hospitalized child. It is important for the nurse to understand that discipline means setting rules and guidelines and is not punishment (Marks, 1994). Punishment penalizes the child for a wrongdoing; setting limits is much more effective in helping children to control their own behavior. Though children may say that they want their own way, they feel more secure when limits are imposed on them, and they are able to assess the security of their environment.

The nurse first needs to understand the child's stage of development before attempting discipline. For example, toddlers often appear defiant and unwilling to do what is asked. In reality, they do not have an appropriate understanding of the word "no," or they may understand that the act committed is wrong, but the desire to continue is too strong to resist. Establishing rules and enforcing a "time-out" period when rules are broken is more effective than repeatedly telling a toddler "no." (See Unit VI for a better understanding of each age group's developmental stage and discipline needs.)

Although there are a many theories about discipline, the most successful methods are those suggested by the parents and caregivers. Discipline is effective when the practices are consistent. The child readily understands rules and consequences when they are similar to those imposed at home.

✳ nursing insight

Parents must be aware of the need for discipline and approve of the methods being used by the hospital staff.

provision for continuation of school work

Continuing education programs in children's hospitals are geared toward children with long-term disabilities and hospital stays. Teachers are available to help implement the teaching modality that is appropriate for each individual. They also may coordinate with public and private school teachers regarding children who are admitted for shorter periods.

When children are discharged from the acute care setting with a need for home health care, they have a definite need to remain a part of the community. Education remains a common goal in the community for people of all ages.

play

Play is the universal language of children. It enhances a child's cognitive and psychomotor skills. Through play, the child learns the social skills of cooperation and shar-

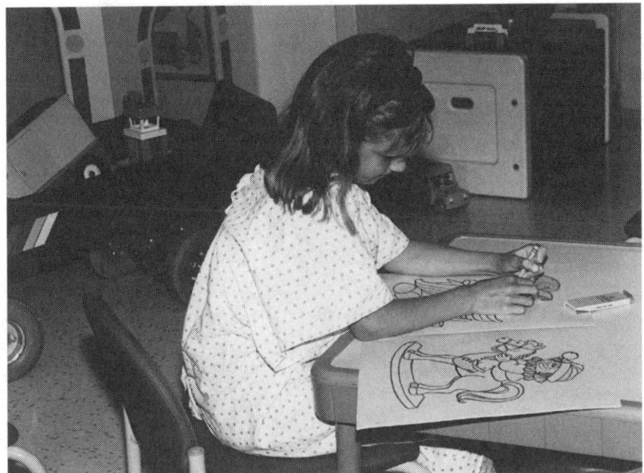

figure 27-3 *Play is an important aspect of recovery in the acute care setting. (Photo by Elise Dinerman.)*

ing. Children in hospital units should have play as a integral part of their health care.

Play for infants should allow for psychomotor exercise when possible. The toddler's desire to be active and explore the environment should be evident in the type of play that is chosen. Preschoolers are creative and enjoy manipulating toys.

School-age children enjoy coloring and puzzles (Fig. 27-3). They should be given exercises that are easily completed so that they feel a sense of accomplishment. Adolescents are more entertained with games of competition and challenge.

When the hospitalized child has a need to express anger and hostility, play can be a therapeutic vehicle to release those feelings. *Play therapy* should be reviewed by a psychiatrist to help children understand their emotions, but the nurse can use therapeutic play to understand children's feelings and thoughts. Table 27-2 list five categories of play.

table 27-2 developmental stages of play and characteristics

Types of Play	*Description*
Therapeutic (all ages)	Facilitates understanding of children's feelings and thoughts
Solitary (all ages)	Independent play with objects or toys
Parallel (2-year-old)	Plays without interaction but along side others; also observed with 4- and 5-year-olds who are able to engage in cooperative play
Associate (preschooler)	Playing together in a similar activity in a loosely structured environment
Cooperative (school age)	Tasks allocated; games structured and organized; clearly obvious whether child belongs to the activity

key points

- **Appropriate emergency health care and medications are essential to decreasing rate of morbidity and mortality of children in an emergency care setting.**
- **Supporting children to express their fears and helping them to understand that their illness is not their fault demonstrate understanding and promote self-confidence.**
- **The nurse should carefully assess the family's value system and spiritual and cultural needs because these factors will influence compliance and response to health care.**
- **Appendicitis is an inflammation of the vermiform appendix located by the cecum. An appendectomy is the surgical treatment recommended prior to rupture and other complications resulting from appendicitis.**
- **Parents and children need to know what to expect physically and emotionally in the icu.**
- **A child admitted to isolation may experience feelings of abandonment and loss of control.**
- **Parents should be supported to understand that a child's regressive behavior is a psychological defense mechanism to help him or her cope with a present stressor.**
- **Cooperation and approval from caregivers are essential for the nurse to discipline successfully.**

review questions

1. Which of the following indicates appropriate teaching–learning principles?
   a. Explaining to a toddler why he must go to sleep before anesthesia
   b. Informing the child about the frightening experiences
   c. Providing anatomically correct dolls to simulate surgical procedures
   d. Allowing the child to participate in his or her own sterile dressing change
2. When a procedure is being performed that requires a consent form, which of the following statements reflects the correct principles of obtaining the consent?
   a. A consent form can be omitted if the procedure only involves a minimal risk.
   b. The nurse must explain the procedure and obtain signed consent if the physician does not.
   c. Emancipated minors must have parental permission to sign a consent form.
   d. In single-parent families, the custodial parent must sign the consent form.
3. Which of the following measures of nursing care is appropriate for the child experiencing pain?
   a. Tell the child not to cry, because getting upset will worsen the pain.

b. Avoid answering questions that will increase the child's fear of pain.
c. Medicate the child at frequent intervals to avoid discomfort.
d. Consider how the child's culture may influence his or her reaction to the pain.

4. Safety and infection control are factors most relevant to which of the following?
a. Recovery room
b. Operating room
c. ICU
d. Isolation unit

5. Which of the following types of play should a nurse avoid when attempting to minimize the child's anxiety?
a. Associate play
b. Play therapy
c. Parallel play
d. Cooperative play

references

Erien, J. A. (1994). Informed consent: The information component. *Orthopedic Nuring, 13*(2), 75–78.

Kelley, S. J. (1994). *Pediatric emergency nursing* (2nd ed.). Norwalk: Appleton & Lange.

Marks, M. G. (1994). *Broadribb's introductory pediatric nursing* (4th ed.). Philadelphia: J.B. Lippincott.

Ruccione, K. S. (1994). Informed consent in pediatric oncology: A nursing perspective. *Pediatric Oncology Nursing, 11*(3), 128–133.

bibliography

Long, B. C., Phipps, W. J., & Woods, N. F. (1979). Medical surgical nursing. St. Louis: C.V. Mosby.

McCaleb A., & Edquil, A. (1994). *Journal of Pediatric Nursing, 9*(4), 233–238.

Mott, S R., James, S. R., & Sperhac, A. M. (1990). *Nursing care of children and families.* Redwood City, CA: Addison-Wesley.

Pillitteri, A. (1995). *Maternal and child nursing* (2nd ed.). Philadelphia: J.B. Lippincott.

Southard, P. A. (1994). *Pediatric emergency nursing: Legal issues* (2nd ed.). Norwalk, CT: Appleton & Lange

Steele, S. (1981). *Child health and the family.* New York: Masson Publishing.

Wong, D. L. (1995). *Whaley & Wong's Nursing care of infants and children*. St. Louis: Mosby–Year Book.

Wong, D. L. (1995). *Essentials of pediatric nursing* (5th ed.). St. Louis: Mosby-–Year Book.

outline

care of the child and family during chronic, life-threatening, or terminal illnesses

28

objectives

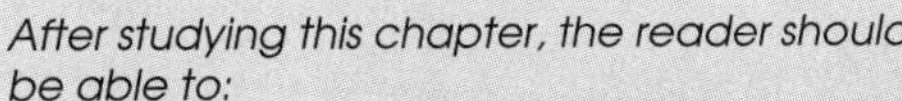

After studying this chapter, the reader should be able to:

* Verbalize the scope of chronic, life-threatening, and terminal illness.
* Define the terms chronic, life-threatening, and terminal illness.
* List the three causes of chronic, life-threatening, and terminal illnesses.
* Verbalize social and financial concerns for the family of a child with a chronic, life-threatening, or terminal illness.
* Describe grief and the grieving process.
* Discuss nursing goals and interventions that may help the family during crises.
* Discuss cultural and religious implications of chronic, life-threatening, or terminal illness.
* Discuss five coping strategies that can be observed in the dying child.

key terms

chronic illness
life-threatening illness
terminal illness
home care
grief
loss
death and dying
organ donation

Neff C & Spray M. *Introduction to Maternal and Child Health Nursing,*

The number of children living with a chronic, life-threatening, or terminal illness is increasing. This is due in part to advances in medicine and technology that have dramatically increased survival rates in children. It also is a result of the increasing incidence of infectious diseases, such as tuberculosis and acquired immunodeficiency syndrome (AIDS), in the pediatric population. Specialized care is required for the child and family in these situations. These children and their families must cope with and accept this crisis of illness and the possibility of death. The nurse is in a position to assist them in this process if he or she has an understanding of the impact that a chronic, life-threatening, or terminal illness has on the child and family.

By focusing on the child's strengths and abilities rather than on the disability or the illness, the nurse can help meet the child's individual physical and emotional needs. This chapter does not discuss specific illnesses, diseases, or treatments because they are covered in detail in other chapters in this text. The purpose of this chapter is to help the nurse develop the skills necessary to ensure comprehensive care throughout a chronic, life-threatening, or terminal illness.

display 28-1
examples of chronic illnesses

GENETIC

Muscular dystrophy
Asthma
Sickle cell anemia (usually considered a chronic illness but many children die before they reach adulthood)
Cystic fibrosis (usually considered a chronic illness but many children die before they reach adulthood)

CONGENITAL

Malabsorption syndromes
Bronchopulmonary dysplasia
Spina bifida

ACQUIRED

Spinal cord trauma
Progressive central nervous system disease (tumors, encephalitis)

incidence of chronic, life-threatening, and terminal illness in children

Approximately 30% of all children younger than 18 years will experience some form of chronic, life-threatening, or terminal illness (Newacheck & Taylor, 1992). Two thirds of these chronic illnesses involve asthma and congenital heart defects. Accidents, such as poisoning and near-drowning, are common childhood life-threatening conditions. The leading terminal illness is cancer. It is the number one cause of death in children 1 through 14 years (American Cancer Society, 1992).

chronic illness

A chronic illness is one that is long lasting or recurrent. It interferes with daily functioning for at least 3 months of the year or causes hospitalization for at least 1 month of the year. Causes can be genetic, congenital, or acquired. Display 28-1 gives examples of illnesses according to their cause.

special considerations for the child with a chronic illness

When a child has been diagnosed with a chronic illness, many important things must be considered. The child will have to adapt his or her lifestyle to include daily or weekly therapies, special procedures will have to be followed exactly, special equipment may be needed, and the child and family will need to learn about the nature of the illness and what can be expected as a result of the illness. In addition, developmental considerations explain how the illness may affect the normal development of children. These developmental considerations are discussed later in this chapter.

life-threatening and terminal illness

A life-threatening or terminal illness has the potential to cause death in the individual. Depending on the illness, death is likely or certain. Causes can be genetic, congenital, or acquired. Display 28-2 gives examples of illnesses according to their cause.

special considerations for the child with a life-threatening or terminal illness

When a child has been diagnosed with an illness like cancer or AIDS or has had a serious accident involving head trauma, the child's and the family's whole world is affected. There are often feelings of despair and fear. The child is forced to undergo extensive treatments and procedures similar to those experienced by the child with a chronic illness. In addition, the child with a life-threatening or terminal illness faces the same developmental hurdles to overcome as the child with a chronic illness. However, in these cases, there is always the possibility that despite daily medications and therapy and being aware of and confronting developmental problems, death will occur.

✳ family considerations

Chronic, life-threatening, and terminal illness affects each family member. It has the potential to disrupt the function and integrity of the family unit. It isolates, increases stress and financial burdens, and has the potential to alter family developmental tasks.

display 28-2
examples of life-threatening and terminal illnesses

GENETIC

Osteogenesis imperfecta (type II or III)
Cancer (Wilms' tumor, chronic myelogenous leukemia)
Renal failure

CONGENITAL

Heart defects
Neuroblastoma
Retinoblastoma

ACQUIRED

Acquired immunodeficiency syndrome
Tuberculosis
Head trauma
Cancer (thyroid, types of leukemia)
Near-drowning
Poisoning
Near-miss sudden infant death syndrome

communication

Communication among family members is encouraged to discuss feelings and the impact of the child's chronic illness or ultimate death. This is especially important for the parents because the illness can place stress on a marriage. In addition, other children may feel neglected or unloved because of the attention placed on the sick child.

financial

Most families of children with a chronic, life-threatening, or terminal illness face financial hardships. Insurance programs usually do not cover the multitude of medical bills involved with these illnesses. If both parents have been working to support the family, it is often necessary for one to quit to provide primary care to the ill child. While this is vital to provide emotional support and coping skills to the ill child and the family, it increases the financial strain.

social

The family will have to spend large amounts of time in health care facilities, caring for the child at home, and supporting each other (Fig. 28-1). Unfortunately, the family becomes isolated from friends, coworkers, and the rest of society. It is sometimes necessary for the family to relocate to be near a specialized health care facility. This means being away from family and established social support systems. Sometimes fear of contracting the disease, while unfounded, may keep family and social contacts away. In addition, the child may need to be isolated from others to prevent him or her from contracting an additional illness that may add stress to the existing one.

family functioning

Balancing normal family functioning and the needs of the child can be difficult. Factors that impact on this balance include the family's and child's developmental needs, coping abilities, past experiences, adaptive abilities, and amount of time the family has been a unit.

Discipline is another important family function for the child with a chronic or terminal illness. For example, when the ill child is treated differently from the rest of the family, resentment and jealousy can occur. The ill child may learn early in the disease how to manipulate siblings

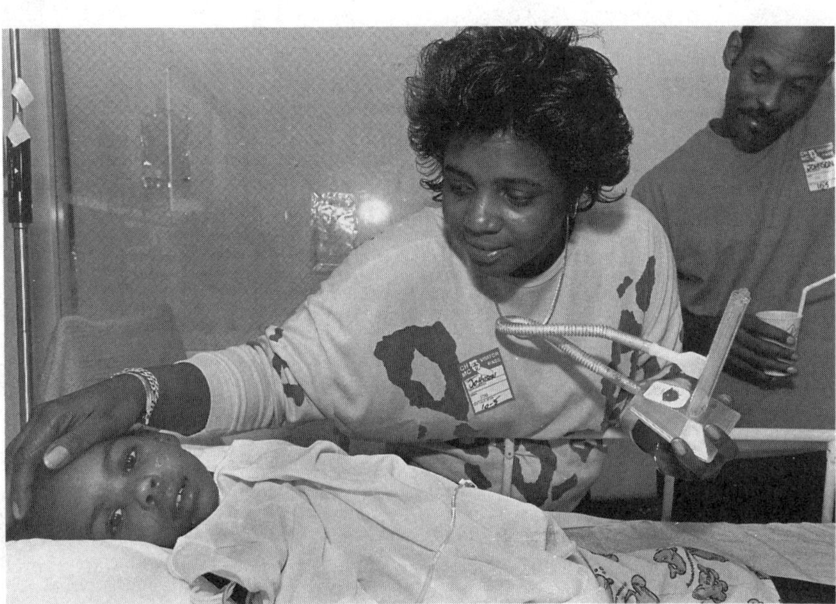

figure 28-1 *The amount of time parents spend in the hospital caring for the chronically ill child may isolate them from their social support systems.*

and parents to gain extra attention or privileges. Later, when the child attends school, he or she may become stressed and frustrated when peers and teachers do not respond favorably to the manipulative behaviors.

grief

The family and the child progress through various stages of grief, which depends on the nature of the illness and its long-term prognosis. Understanding that stages of grief and reactions to illness are normal and expected may help the child and family handle the situation. The nurse can support the child and family by evaluating their grieving process (see "Grieving and Loss in Chronic, Life-Threatening, and Terminal Illness" on page 452).

✳ nursing considerations

The nurse is often with the child and family when the initial diagnosis is made and is thus in a position to offer support and direction at a critical time. The nurse's attitude of acceptance, rejection, hope, or despair is an important factor in the family's adaptation. It may be the nurse's role to ease the adaptation of the child and family. This may be accomplished by helping the child and family understand the diagnosis (see the Nursing Care Plan).

In addition, because chronic and terminal illnesses are usually long term, nurses play an important role throughout the illness. They can help make the various procedures and necessary tests easier and less painful for the child. Nurses should encourage the child to engage in therapeutic play using dolls and equipment, such as syringes, to help vent frustrations about the illness (Fig. 28-2). Decorative bandages can be distractors when used to cover the stick site.

Children who are given permission to cry during painful or frightening experiences tend to feel a sense of strength that promotes control. Receiving praise following a painful experience promotes self-confidence, especially in preschool and older children. Stickers and special treats promote positive feelings in toddlers and older children.

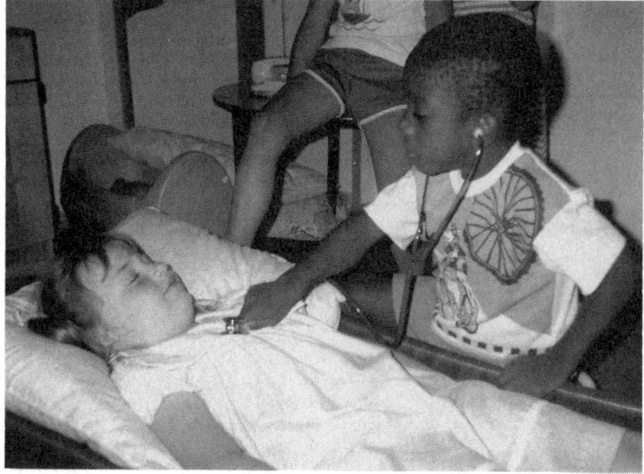

figure 28-2 *Sociodramatic play may help the child cope with a growing awareness of death.*

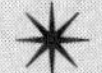 **nursing insight**

A family focus is an essential element for an effective plan of care.

nursing interventions

promote psychosocial well-being

The nurse can accomplish this by developing realistic goals, encouraging appropriate independence, promoting self-worth, and developing open, honest communication.

promote growth and development

The nurse can promote growth and development by performing an assessment based on the child's developmental level.

promote use of appropriate resources

The nurse should provide information concerning the resources available from the hospital, community, and government and should encourage the family to use these resources.

cultural and religious considerations

The attitudes, values, behaviors, and beliefs of various cultures and ethnic groups have an impact on the manner in which chronic, life-threatening, and terminal illnesses are viewed. The child's response to the illness and the response of the family and community depend on these factors. However, the nurse should be careful not to generalize certain characteristics across a population because many times individuals have adapted their beliefs and behaviors to the area in which they live.

Diagnosis of a chronic or terminal disease or the occurrence of a life-threatening accident often enhances the spiritual needs of the child and family. A representative of the clergy should be available to the family and child. Children with a serious illness need reassurance about love, forgiveness, and life meaning. Assistance in identifying all that they have accomplished in life rather than on what they could have done may meet these needs of the child.

developmental considerations

The age at which the child is diagnosed with an illness greatly influences how the child will develop mentally, socially, emotionally, and physically. The child, family, and nurse must be aware of these concerns so that they are prepared for special challenges and able to overcome developmental hurdles to live a full life despite the illness.

infancy

Prolonged separation from family due to hospitalization may damage the infant's sense of trust. In addition, if

nursing care plan
for the family and child with leukemia

NURSING DIAGNOSIS

Ineffective Management of Therapeutic Regimen: Families, related to insufficient knowledge of the disease process, treatment, and side effects

GOAL: Family and child will understand the disease and all aspects of the treatment

NURSING INTERVENTIONS	RATIONALE	EVALUATION
Educate the family and the child regarding the new diagnosis of leukemia and recommended treatment. Include information on pathophysiology of disease, options in treatment, side effects, and reduction of risk factors.	Providing specific information about the leukemia and its treatment can assist the family's understanding of the disease and increase their understanding of the importance of compliance with treatment.	The family will state an understanding of the disease, ask appropriate questions regarding treatment, and exhibit risk-factor reduction behavior, such as infection-prevention strategies
Explain to the family that the child will be fatigued and review energy-conservation plans.	The anemia associated with inadequate RBC production related to decreased WBC can quickly cause fatigue; therefore, energy conservation is important.	The child will incorporate rest periods into his or her day and energy-expending acitvities will be limited/replaced with more sedentary activities (such as checkers).
Teach parents and child information regarding signs of infection, anemia, and bleeding.	These life-threatening side effects indicate additional treatment may be necessary.	The family and child will state the importance of and recognize these signs of complicaitons.

NURSING DIAGNOSIS

Altered Growth and Development, secondary to long-term treatment of leukemia

GOAL: Normal growth and development will be maintained

NURSING INTERVENTION	RATIONALE	EVALUATION
Promote normal growth and development within the individual child's physical capabilities.	Activities may be limited, secondary to fatigue or limitations imposed by the leukemia or treatment.	The child will gain confidence from appropriate developmental tasks that remain safe for the child.
Encourage reading or increasing computer skills.	Giving the child an obtainable goal can assist in increasing his or her self-confidence.	The child will improve reading skills and learn a new computer program.
Inform the parents to promote normalcy of activities as much as possible during the maintenance phase of treatment.	This will lead to the child's maintaining a level of independence.	The child will maintain ADL indepencence and continue at an age-appropriate level.

physical contact with the parents is decreased as a result of the disability, the infant's sensorimotor response may decrease. Finally, if the infant's parents or caregivers are overly protective, the infant will become dependent and less willing and able to separate to accomplish tasks on his or her own.

toddler

A chronic, life-threatening, or terminal illness may decrease the toddler's ability to master tasks and prevent mobility. As a result, the toddler may fear doing things alone and may have low self-confidence.

preschool

Preschool children with a chronic, life-threatening, or terminal illness may have a decreased ability to achieve in task-oriented activities. They also will be slower to develop a positive body image because they are focusing on their illness, there is disfigurement due to the illness, or they are dependent on mechanical devices because of the illness.

They also may have anxiety and pain. In addition, children at this age may have feelings of guilt because they think they caused their condition.

school-age

The school-age child may be unable to participate in work or play activities at home and at school. This decreases the chance of achievement in certain areas. Children with illnesses may be labeled "different." This limits their relationships with peers and their sense of belonging. To compensate for this, the school-age child may demonstrate independence with refusal to do certain things, resentment, or risk-taking behaviors.

adolescence

As the child approaches adulthood, the realization of the impact of the condition can be detrimental to continued growth and development. The adolescent may have difficulty establishing a personal identity. This also is a difficult time for the adolescent with a chronic, life-threatening, or terminal illness because many times these teenagers are rejected by their peers and cannot "fit in." Teenagers with these illnesses may be less future oriented and less independent.

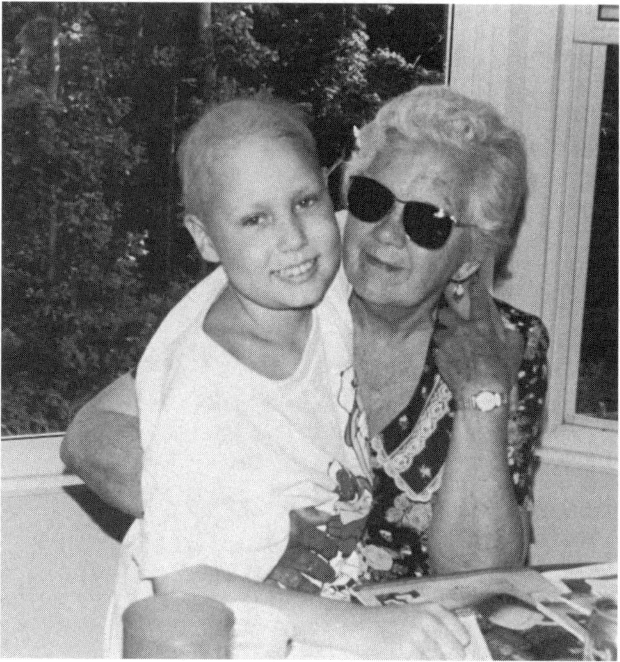

figure 28-3 *Being at home with loved ones is a comfort to the terminally ill child.*

home care for the child with a chronic, life-threatening, or terminal illness

The decision to care for a child with a chronic, life-threatening, or terminal illness at home is difficult. It should be discussed with the entire caregiving team—physician, nurse, parents, child, respiratory support services, home health agencies, hospice coordinator, and so forth. Caring for a child at home requires a physical and emotional commitment. The task can be monumental.

It is often more comfortable for a dying child to be in familiar surroundings with family and friends (Fig. 28-3). When the family cares for a child who is terminally ill, it helps them and the child. Many parents feel helpless watching their child die. Knowing that they are caring for their child and keeping their child comfortable and pain free will help them feel that they are doing something when there is little hope of recovery.

The advantage of home care is that the child can feel more a part of the family and will be encouraged to develop physically and emotionally. Home caregivers must be given explicit instructions on their role. They must fully understand how to use any necessary equipment. The nurse should give exact instructions and require caregivers to demonstrate procedures of routine care. Often children with multiple handicaps or ventilator-dependent children who receive care in the home require support from home health nurses, aids, and other support people. Caregivers must know how to contact these support people. In addition, caregivers must know the signs and symptoms that indicate that the child requires hospitalization.

tracheostomy care

A typical situation for home care is a child with a tracheostomy that requires suctioning. Caregivers need to know the functioning of the tracheostomy and how to trouble shoot problems. A tracheostomy is a small opening in the child's windpipe (trachea) to help the child breathe better. The material needed for care at home includes suctioning equipment, emergency equipment, a humidifier, and oxygen.

The air that enters the trachea directly has bypassed the nose and mouth. Therefore, it is not warmed, humidified, or filtered before entering the lungs. Daily care of the child with a tracheostomy requires additional fluids by mouth and humidification and filtering of the air being breathed. In addition, the area around the tracheostomy should be kept clean and dry, and the ties that hold the tube in place must be changed to ease irritation, prevent excess moisture, and prevent skin breakdown. These procedures take time and skill. Suctioning is often done in conjunction with these procedures, but it may be necessary several times a day. See Display 28-3 for tracheostomy care and suctioning.

grieving and loss in chronic, life-threatening, and terminal illnesses

Grief is a normal psychological reaction to loss. It may be a reaction to a perceived loss or an actual loss. In the case of chronic, life-threatening, or terminal illnesses, the child often has to give up certain activities that were a large part of his or her life before becoming sick. The child may be

display 28-3
tracheostomy care and suctioning

EQUIPMENT

Sterile saline
Suction equipment
2×2 gauze pads
Sterile cotton-tipped swabs
Half-strength hydrogen peroxide
Water
Ointment or stoma adhesive (if prescribed)
Tracheostomy ties (twill tape)

PROCEDURE

Wash hands thoroughly.
Assess lung sounds before beginning and between each suctioning.
Bag with oxygen before and during procedure if required.
Instill sterile saline (1–2 mL) into tracheostomy tube.
Attach sterile suction catheter to suction device set at 80–100 mm Hg pressure.
Insert sterile suction catheter the length of the tracheostomy tube.
With a rotating motion, remove catheter using intermittent suction.
Allow child to rest.
Repeat as needed after reassessment of lung sounds.
Assess color, quantity, odor, and consistency of secretions.
Inspect the area around the tube.
Dip cotton-tipped swabs in peroxide and clean gently around base of tube at insertion site.
Rinse with cotton-tipped swabs tipped in clear water.
Dry with gauze.
Place a dry piece of gauze around the tube at the insertion site only if necessary (usually required only if irritation from tube or copious secretions).
Apply ointment or stoma adhesive sparingly, if needed.
Prepare clean tracheostomy ties (at least 2½ times the neck circumference is a good guide).
Fold the clean tie in half, inserting the loop end through the wing hole next to the old tie. (If necessary, loosen old tie slightly before beginning.)
Pull the loose ends of the tie through the lop and pull snug (see Fig. 28-1).
Take the two loose ends, and wrap around the neck in opposite directions and tie securely at the *side* of the neck with a square knot (avoids confusion with back ties of clothing).
Remove old tie.
Repeat on other side.

unable to perform a task that was easily done before the illness. A child with a terminal illness may experience additional grief because of the knowledge that sometimes children with these sicknesses die. Another example of loss is a significant change in physical appearance as a result of illness. For example, the child undergoing chemotherapy to treat leukemia may lose all of his or her hair, or the child with juvenile rheumatoid arthritis may be confined to a wheelchair. The nurse must be empathetic to the personal meaning behind each child's loss.

the grief process

Children with chronic, life-threatening, and terminal illnesses experience grief and loss when their illness is diagnosed or after an accident has occurred. However, because these illnesses are typically long term, the various stages of grief may be repeated throughout the course of the illness or throughout the life of the individual. For example, an 8-year-old child diagnosed with muscular dystrophy will have an intense experience with grief and loss during initial diagnosis. Throughout the next few years, the child may appear to be adjusting to the illness and coping well. However, the child may experience a new phase of grief during the adolescent years when he or she realizes that this illness prevents participation in contact sports or dancing at the prom.

The typical first reaction to diagnosis of a chronic, life-threatening, or terminal illness is shock and disbelief. The child may experience periods of numbness and immobility or anguish and acute pain. The child often asks, "why me?" or "what did I do to deserve this?" Parents are often in disbelief that something like this could happen to their perfect child.

The child then begins to become aware of the diagnosis and will progress through a period of intense mourning. They may mourn the loss of bodily function or because they are scared of dying. The child should be allowed and encouraged to cry and grieve. A child's inability to cry interferes with the grieving process.

The intense mourning eventually subsides to feelings of sadness about the loss. The child begins to be able to talk about the illness and is able to receive comfort and support from family and friends. Finally the child and the child's family are able to accept the reality of the illness and the loss (potential or actual) and continue living as best as possible. There are no time limits put on the various phases of grief—each child is different. However, the nurse must be aware of signs of severe depression. A child with a chronic, life-threatening, or terminal illness who is experiencing extreme depression for extended periods needs professional counseling.

experiencing death

Death is a distinct possibility in children with life-threatening and terminal illnesses and even in children with chronic illnesses. Working with children who are facing death is demanding. It is emotionally, physically, intellectually, and spiritually draining to work with dying chil-

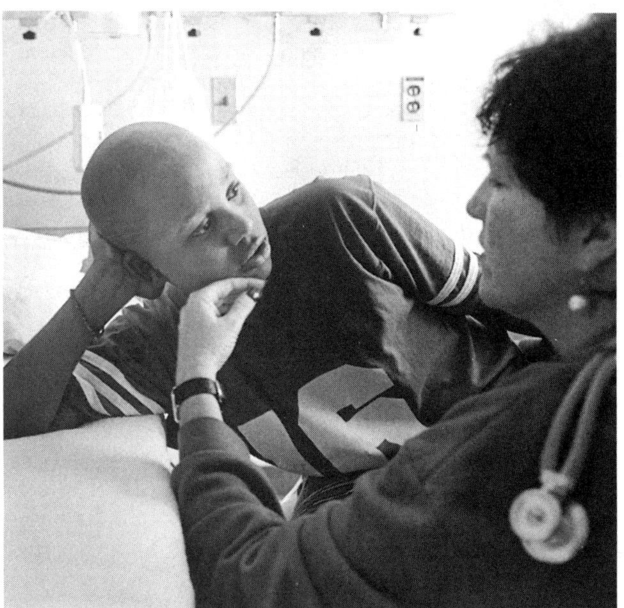

figure 28-4 *The consistent support, encouragement, and friendship the nurse provides for the patient and the life lessons the nurse learns from this individual make the difficult task of working with a dying child worthwhile. (Kathy Sloane© Courtesy of Children's Hospital, Oakland, CA.)*

dren who have critical physical needs and intense fears of what is going to happen to them. The nurse is put into the position of meeting the emotional and physical needs of distraught family members and friends. However, there are rewarding experiences in working with these children. There is a great deal to be learned about the joy of life, the process of death, and how to help people deal with moments of intense loss (Fig. 28-4). The nurse should be aware of a child's understanding of death to provide the best possible care and the best answers to the child's many questions about what is happening to him or her. Table 28-1 describes children's concepts of death according to their age and stage of development.

coping strategies for death and dying

Elizabeth Kübler-Ross was a pioneer in the study of responses to death and dying (Kübler-Ross, 1969). She identified five coping strategies that can be observed in the child facing his or her own death or the death of those they love.

denial and isolation

This phase begins with the child being told that he or she is going to die or that someone close to them is going to

table 28-1 a child's concept of death

Developmental Stage	*Concept of Death*	*Typical Reactions*
Infancy	A child younger than 2 years has no concept of death or its permanence. The infant is only aware that death means separation.	Clingy behavior, excessive crying, withdrawal, upset stomach
Toddler	Separation is a major fear. The child can sense anxiety and fear but lacks the understanding of the finality of death.	Nightmares; is easily frightened; fear of the dark; acts out or internalizes aggression
Preschool	Death is believed to be temporary. There is a magical view of death. The cause of death may be related to themselves or may be viewed as punishment.	Wants to hear the story of death repeatedly; makes silly or inappropriate comments; acts out death through play activities
School-age	Begin to understand that death is permanent and that they are capable of dying. Death is feared and associated with pain, sadness, and separation. There is realization that everyone has to die at some point, but death is viewed as a horrible fact of life. They may think death is punishment for bad behavior.	Anger, guilt, worry about abandonment, death, and pain; uses play acting or art to express feelings; tries to understand the meaning of life; heaven, and life after death; fear of being buried alive
Adolescent	Has an adult understanding of death. May try to break away from parent's view of death (religious or secular) to form their own ideas about death. Death threatens adolescent tasks of identity and independence.	Anger at need for dependence in coping with death; may withdraw; deny the loss, or feel hopeless; may feel that no one cares; may reject funeral customs

die or has died. Typical coping strategies are shock, disbelief, denial, a "no, not me" or "it is not true" response. This is a normal reaction, and caregivers should not be concerned unless denial becomes a chronic behavior. During this time, the nurse must be supportive.

anger

Denial quickly turns to questioning like "why me?" or "why my sister?" There is often serious depression and feelings of guilt followed or accompanied by outbursts of anger. These displays of anger may be shown to strangers, health care workers, spouses, siblings, parents, and so forth.

bargaining

The next stage is bargaining. Many times the child will use this manipulative coping mechanism when denial and anger are not working. They may make agreements in an attempt to postpone their own death or to bring someone back to life. For example, A child may say "If I make the honor role in school, I won't get sick and die."

depression

When children realize they have no control over when they or their loved one will die, they begin to mourn. They may turn their feelings inward and blame themselves, or they may act on their feelings of depression and helplessness by lying, cheating, or fighting. Nurses must realize these actions are a natural part of grieving, and they should provide minimal intervention.

acceptance

This phase occurs when the child admits that he or she is going to die or that a loved one has died. The child accepts it as reality. The child will continue to experience sadness and may want only to be with family members or close friends. The child's self-concept will improve with the realization that he or she is not to blame for what is happening. The nurse should allow privacy but should not abandon the child or family.

special considerations in death

organ donation

Approaching a grieving family about organ donation is a difficult but important task because viable organs must be harvested soon after brain death. Technologic advances have increased the success of organ transplantation, but the need for organs far outnumbers available organs. Some families will view organ donation as an ultimate good arising out of the tragedy of their child's death. Other families may view organ donation as a violation of their child's body and will not permit it. Whatever decision the family makes must be respected.

States may have laws requiring that the family be asked about donation whenever a person is considered "brain dead." (See Chapter 35.) Many localities have organ procurement agencies. However, it may be the nurse's responsibility to approach the family. The laws for organ donation differ in each state, and updated government information on organ donation may be obtained form the Office of Organ Transplantation in Washington, D.C.

summary

Care of the child with a chronic or terminal illness is complex. The social and financial impact on the family can be devastating. In addition, the child and the family have to cope with treatments, hospitalization, anxiety, uncertainty about the outcome of the illness, and possible death. Grief and loss are real, important, personal, and painful concepts for the child and family. The nurse is in a position to assist the family in focusing on coping strategies to ease the impact of a chronic or terminal illness. Death is a distinct possibility for many terminally and chronically ill children. Caring for children who are dying is emotionally and physically demanding. To work effectively with these children, the nurse must understand the child's developmental concepts of death and coping strategies used to deal with death.

key points ✳

- **The number of children afflicted with chronic or terminal illnesses is growing. There are estimates that 30% of children younger than 18 years will experience a chronic or terminal illness.**
- **Chronic illness interferes with daily functioning and involves loss.**
- **Terminal illness also interferes with daily function and involves loss, but death is an added dimension and a real possibility.**
- **Chronic and terminal illnesses can be genetic, congenital, or acquired.**
- **Family communication is vital to help direct the family focus during crises.**
- **Chronic and terminal illnesses have a significant social and financial impact on the family.**
- **Grief is normal and has predictable patterns.**
- **Specific interventions can direct the family focus during crises and provide information about the resources available from the hospital, community, and government.**
- **Attitudes, values, behaviors, and religious beliefs have a significant impact on how one views the chronic or terminal illness.**
- **Five coping strategies that can be observed in the dying child include denial and isolation, anger, bargaining, depression, and acceptance.**

review questions

1. The majority of families caring for a child with a chronic illness experience:
   a. Financial hardships.
   b. An alteration in bonding with the ill child.
   c. An increase in positive family interactions.
   d. Adaptation to the child's illness within 1 month following the diagnosis.
2. Augustin is a 9-year-old suffering from a serious congenital heart defect. The mother is concerned about his depressed mood. An initial nursing assessment would include:
   a. The degree of Augustin's depression and the time period involved.
   b. Augustin's reaction to his diagnosis.
   c. The amount of time and energy spent on physical play.
   d. The family's acceptance of the child's diagnosis.
3. The number of children living with a chronic, life-threatening, or terminal illness is increasing because:
   a. Prenatal care is accessible to a large population of pregnant women.
   b. Diseases typically fatal to newborns have declined.
   c. Advances in medicine and technology have increased survival rates in children.
   d. National infant mortality rate has increased.
4. A primary nursing consideration in caring for children with a terminal illness is:
   a. Discuss aspects of grief with the child and family.
   b. Focus on the child's strengths and abilities rather than on the disability.
   c. Educate the family about community support groups.
   d. Encourage children with chronic illness to attend school.
5. The nurse can expect an 8-year-old diagnosed with muscular dystrophy to experience intense grief during the initial diagnosis and a new phase of grief when he or she is:
   a. An adult and desiring to have children.
   b. An adolescent and wanting to participate in sports and social events, such as dancing.
   c. A year older and realizing how much life has changed.
   d. Dismissed from the hospital and receiving care at home.

references

American Cancer Society (1992). Cancer facts and figures. New York: Author.

American Cancer Society (1992). Cancer facts and figures. Atlanta: Author.

Kübler-Ross, E. (1969). *On death and dying*. New York: Macmillan

Newacheck, P. W., & Taylor, W. R. (1992). Childhood chronic illness: Prevalence, severity, and impact. *American Journal of Public Health, 82*(3), 364–371.

bibliography

Betz, C. L., Hunsberger, M., & Wright, S. (1994). Family-centered nursing care of children. Philadelphia: W.B. Saunders.

Engel, G. (1964). Grief and grieving. *American Journal of Nursing, 64*, 93.

Erikson, E. (1964). *Childhood and society* (2nd ed.). New York: W.W. Norton.

Freud, S. (1957). Mourning and melancholia. In J. Strachey (Ed. and Trans.), *The standard edition of the complete psychological works of Sigmound Freud* (Vol. 14). London: Hogarth Press.

Giger, J. N., & Davidhizar, R. E. (1991). *Transcultural nursing: Assessment and intervention*. St. Louis:; C.V. Mosby.

Grollman, E. (1990). *Talking about death: A dialogue between parent and child* (3rd ed.). Boston: Beacon Press.

Jackson, D. B., & Saunders, R. S. (1993). *Child health nursing*. Philadelphia: J.B. Lippincott.

Johnson, B. S. (1995). *Child, adolescent, and family psychiatric nursing*. Philadelphia: J.B. Lippincott.

Oltjenbruns, K. (1991). Positive outcomes of adolescents' experience with grief. *Journal of Adolescent Research, 6*, 43–53.

Piaget, J. (1969). *The early growth of logic in the child.* New York: W.W. Norton.

(1992). *Webster's 21st Century Dictionary*. Nashville: Thomas Nelson.

Wong, D. L. (1993). *Whaley & Wong's essentials of pediatric nursing* (4th ed.). St. Louis: Mosby–Year Book.

nursing care of the child and family with a mental health problem

29

outline

objectives 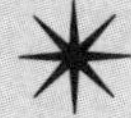

After studying this chapter, the reader should be able to:

* Discuss the impact of family on a child's mental health status.
* Discuss developmental considerations in relation to mental health.
* Discuss nursing considerations for the child with mental retardation.
* Define learning disorders.
* Discuss nursing care for children with attention deficity hyperactivity disorder.
* List three types of anxiety disorders.
* Discuss treament for childhood depression.
* List risk factors for suicide.
* Discuss the characteristics of the child at high risk for substance abuse.
* Define schizophrenia.

key terms 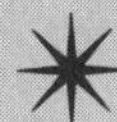

counselor
delusions
deviant behavior
emotional abuse
empathy
family preservation programs
maladaptive behavior
pediatric psychiatrist
personal distress
psychologist
system
temperament

Mental health disorders in children include mental retardation, autism, separation anxiety, and substance abuse. These disorders can be genetic, behavioral, or a result of environmental influences like poverty, teenage pregnancy, drug abuse, violence, and homelessness. In addition, a lack of financial and emotional support takes a heavy toll on the child's ability to develop useful mental health concepts.

Many different professionals work with children who have mental health disorders. A *pediatric psychiatrist* specializes in the study, prevention, and medical treatment of mental disorders in children. A *psychologist* is trained in methods of psychological analysis, therapy, and research. A *counselor* is trained in specific areas of expertise to help guide the client through stressful events. Table 29-1 describes three different types of mental health therapies that are used in the child with mental health disorders. For example, a guidance counselor in the school system works with children experiencing age-related problems, such as relationships with peers, teachers, career choices, situational crises involving child abuse and suicide, and referrals to appropriate agencies.

✳ family considerations

Environmental systems help to shape the child's development. These systems include the family, school, and neighborhood. A *system* is described as an organized grouping of related parts. The family system (an organized group of individuals, roles, and interactions) furnishes the child with a safe harbor to learn what is expected as a member of society.

Maladaptive behaviors learned by the child within one functioning system frequently extends to another system. For example, parental respect fosters respect for teachers. Disrespect for parental authority is imitated by blatant disrespect for authority figures at school and in the community.

Childhood behavioral, emotional, and mental health problems have often been linked to struggles, turmoil, and emotional and physical abuse within the family.

In the past, children were removed from their families in an attempt to address their mental health needs in a more stable environment. The trend today is to focus on building therapeutic communication skills and effective parenting skills within the child's natural environment. Collaboration with families has proven to be more effective. Holistic care focuses on the child, family, health care provider, and professional counselor as "partners" in a mental health treatment plan. *Family preservation* programs have been designed to offer therapeutic services for the entire family in the home. The therapy is goal oriented and time limited, typically lasting from 4 to 12 weeks.

Support is fundamental for family success because it increases coping stamina. Families of children with emotional and behavioral problems are not always "dysfunctional." Many times they simply lack appropriate, affordable, and accessible community-based support services.

The American family today often has less of a support system than in the past. There are more single parents, parents who both work, and families who have relocated and cannot rely on nearby relatives for advice and support. In addition, there are more teenage parents and more parents who have immigrated to the United States and do not speak English. Recognizing children and families at risk prompts early intervention with positive results. School nurses and guidance counselors provide an important link between comunity services offered by schools, social services, and mental health care facilities.

table 29-1 types of mental health therapies

Therapy	*Description*
Psychotherapy	Client talks with a therapist to gain assistance in altering emotions, thinking, or behaviors that are distressing.
Behavioral therapy	Child's behavior is modified or changed based on the idea that all behavior is learned, and emotional disorders are conditioned responses that can be modified by "unlearning." Unacceptable behaviors result in negative consequences; acceptable behaviors result in positive reinforcement.
Pharmacologic therapy	Specific drugs are used to control or modify behaviors, correct imbalances, and promote participation in group or individual counseling sessions.

✳ nursing considerations

The nurse must use empathy when working with children with mental health disorders. *Empathy* is an objective awareness and understanding of the feelings and behaviors of another person.

Children with mental health problems have feelings, many of which are hidden. The nurse can help children discover and understand hidden feelings by encouraging expression in a nonjudgmental atmosphere. Building trust is based on the nurse's ability to listen and understand what the child is saying verbally and emotionally, acknowledge willfully the child's feelings, and realize that useful communication helps the child apply information toward a decision-making process. The goal in a helping relationship is to enable the client to achieve personal decision-making skills by using his or her own values and attitudes to problem solve. The nurse's role involves empowering the client to work through a dilemma.

developmental considerations

personality development

Personality development parallels physical growth and development. Theorists such as Maslow, Erikson, and Piaget organize personality development in a sequential way, emphasizing the importance of mastering a primary level before moving on to a more complex level (see Chap. 18). For example, newborns do not have a concept of morality because their reflex actions are based on the wants of satisfying basic needs, such as food, rest, and elimination. Trust is developed when adults meet the infant's needs.

Throughout the first years of life, children learn right and wrong behaviors from their parents. When relationships and bonding between the mother, father, and the children are impaired, there can be serious psychological consequencess.

Young children typically blame themselves for their parents' failures. Unfortunately, this practice is likely to result in the development of inadequacies that may affect them for life.

emotional abuse

Parents are not always aware of how critically they behave toward their children and how intolerant they are of allowing their children to make mistakes. Emotional abuse is as painful as physical assault and may have longer lasting consequences. Although scars are not visible, they exist psychologically.

Emotional abuse is not a single event. It is a long-term pattern of behavior that reduces a child's self-concept to feelings of unworthiness. The child feels unworthy of respect, friendship, natural birthright, love, and protection.

Emotional abuse can be deliberate with no apparent causative factors. A typical abusive statement might be "you are no good." It also can occur during prolonged stressful periods, such as divorce battles involving child custody. For example, a woman full of anger and bitterness toward her husband may project her feelings onto her child with statements like "you are ugly like your father." Emotional abuse can be active ("I can't stand you; get away from me!") or passive (withholding emotional support). In other cases, parents attempting to modify or channel a child's unacceptable behaviors may describe the child as "bad" rather than addressing the behavior as a single event. The child develops a sense of guilt and loss of self-esteem or decides to give up trying to please the parent(s).

Children react to abuse by trying to "explain" the conduct of the abusers. The child typically ends up struggling for survival in a sea of self-blame. Emotionally abused children grow up with altered perceptions about their own and others' behaviors. They often become involved in relationships that are abusive because they are eager for love but are convinced they do not deserve it.

displacement of feelings

Children experiencing anxieties often have difficulty taking ownership of their feelings. This is reflected by denying feelings, avoiding discussion of feelings, blaming others, detachment, and minimizing feelings by talking about them in an abstract or superficial way.

The nurse can help children take ownership of their feelings by encouraging them to identify their immediate feelings clearly and genuinely, express the intensity of their feelings, and specify the potential source of their feelings. For example, when a statement is made, such as "I hate my parents," the nurse can be effective by addressing the expressed emotion with a statement, such as, "You sound very angry at your parents."

Children can be afraid to solve their problems because of secondary gains they receive from indulging in self-pity, getting sympathy from others, not having to accept responsibility for oneself, or experiencing the thrill of living in constant turmoil.

Nurses must recognize road blocks. *Road blocks* are behaviors (positive and negative) and secondary gains that inhibit a change in behavior. The child may need help in evaluating why they do or do not feel a need for change in behaviors. By listening to ideas about positive and negative benefits of change, the nurse can help the child focus on a small workable part of a problem rather than the entire dilemma. For example, a teenage girl being physically and emotionally abused by her boyfriend may indicate a desire to dissolve the relationship but comments that "my boyfriend is the most popular guy in school, and if we break up, I will lose all my friends." Helping the teenager recognize the controlling forces of the relationship and safety issues involved with an abusive relationship is an important nursing intervention.

temperament

Temperament can be described as how a child's behavior is expressed or how easily the child "fits" into the family. Temperament and character are often used synonymously.

Parental understanding of a child's temperament helps individualize expectations and parenting methods appropriate for the child. Understanding the child's character encourages recognition of the connection between difficult temperamental tendencies and behavior problems in childhood.

abnormal behavior

All children exhibit behavior at certain stages in their development that may be considered abnormal when compared with adult behavior. A knowledge deficit concerning age-expected behaviors of the child may be the problem rather than an actual mental health alteration. Asking the parents to describe their expectations allows the nurse to evaluate how realistic the parents' expectations are. The following are types of abnormal behavior:

* Deviance—behavior that varies from what society considers tolerable. Cultural standards vary from one group to another, but all cultures have what is considered normal or expected patterns of behavior.
* Maladaptive behavior—behavior that limits everyday living. An example of this is drug abuse that prevents

the child from functioning effectively with peers and family and in school.

* Personal distress—children troubled by depression or anxiety disorders that are circumstantial or internally induced from an imbalance of body chemicals. For example, circumstantial depression or anxiety can result from poor preparation for a major examination, resulting in failure of a course.

mental illness

Mental illness is an alteration of mental thought processes affecting the behaviors and emotions, making it difficult for the client to function independently in society. The diagnosis of a psychological disorder is often based on *value judgments*, in contrast to physical disorders, which are diagnosed using value-free criteria. For example, children with pneumonia are diagnosed by symptoms and laboratory and x-ray findings regardless of their personal values. Decisions about mental illness reflect cultural values and social trends. They often are not diseases in a strict sense and tend to support inaccurate stereotypes (Table 29-2).

Children and adults will experience times when their behaviors can be described as deviant, maladaptive, or distressing. An important consideration in determining mental illness is the *degree* and *frequency* of expressing deviant, maladaptive, and distressing behaviors.

psychological disorder classification

The *Diagnostic and Statistical Manual of Mental Disorders, IV (DSM-IV)*, a manual of the American Psychiatric Association, classifies psychological disorders. The manual is frequently updated with data based on research and psychiatric expertise. It describes more than 200 types of psychological disorders.

This chapter discusses the following disorders that according to the DSM-IV are commonly diagnosed in infancy, childhood, or adolescence: mental retardation, learning disorders, motor skill disorders, communication disorders, pervasive developmental disorders, attention deficit and disruptive behavior disorders, and separation anxiety disorder.

The following additional DSM-IV mental disorders are discussed as they pertain to the pediatric population: overanxious disorders, avoidant disorders, depression, suicide, substance abuse, and schizophrenia.

✳ nursing process for a child with a mental disorder

Children experiencing alterations of mental health undergo an initial evaluation to determine if the problems are of a psychiatric nature or related to a medical condition. Admission into a mental health care facility or intervention program parallels a crisis situation. Providing client and parental support is vital at the admission stage and helps promote compliance to treatment programs.

assessment

Subjective data to be assessed include the following:

* Description of self (if age appropriate) or parental description of child's moods; anxiety level; stress factors; relationship status; cultural factors; lifestyle; suicidal thoughts or behaviors; past and present losses, such as

table 29-2 facts about psychological disorders

Psychological Disorders Are Not	*Psychological Disorders Are*	*Nursing Considerations*
A sign of personal weakness	Influenced by genetic factors, family background, and exposure to stress	Evaluate self-biases concerning mental disorders; recognize family history of mental illness as significant.
Incurable	Resolved with therapy and at times spontaneously	Encourage client and parents to seek early intervention and maintain a positive attitude toward the prognosis.
Always violent and dangerous	Occasionally linked with violence	Threats of violence can be a way to manipulate parents and others. Recognize age-appropriate behaviors; adolescence symbolizes a time of acting out.
Different in their actions and easily recognized	Similar behaviors as "normal" children; infrequent display of bizarre behaviors	Recognize age-appropriate behaviors. For example, toddler temper tantrums are normal, whereas passive, compliant behavior in toddlers may reflect a loss of hope.

death of family member or peer; degree of insecurity; current or past experience with delusions or hallucinations; type of medication (if any) being taken; onset of puberty in adolescents; abnormal behaviors; and past and present medical or surgical diagnoses

Objective data to be assessed include the following:

* Level of consciousness, emotional status, consistency of behavior, use of defense mechanisms, psychomotor activity, appearance, affect, mood, intellect, thought processes, concentration, reasoning, motor ability, nutrition and hydration status, level of fatigue, skin condition (presence of "track" lines, which indicate intravenous drug use)
* Neurologic examination of age-appropriate reflexes, limb strength, meningeal signs, such as stiff neck, headache, and irritability; gait; and past and present vital sign measurements

nursing diagnoses

* Self Esteem Disturbance, related to low self-esteem
* Risk for Violence: Self-directed or directed at others, related to the inability to cope with negative feelings
* Altered Growth and Development, related to Down syndrome or autism
* Risk for Altered Parenting, related to inability to communicate with child
* Risk for Sensory/Perceptual Alterations, related to inaccurate interpretation of environmental stimuli resulting from psychotic disorder
* Risk for Impaired Social Interaction, related to severe anxiety, dependent behavior, social isolation
* Risk for Altered Thought Processes, related to anxiety and depression

nursing interventions

The following interventions are appropriate for promoting self-concept:

* Establish a trusting relationship with the child, and encourage open verbalization about fears, anxieties, and stressors.
* Encourage the client to recognize feelings by listening in a nonjudmental way.
* Encourage the child to use acceptable social skills through communication, hygiene and dress, and relationships with family members.
* Accept and support client's feelings; use clarification, and stress reality. Avoid arguing or agreeing with inaccurate communication.
* Praise socially acceptable behavior.
* Encourage client to identify self-related positive characteristics.
* Encourage client to persue a hobby.

The following interventions are appropriate for promoting self-control:

* Provide the client with explanations about procedures and restrictions.
* Assess the child's coping mechanisms, and encourage alternative methods of dealing with stress.
* Assess the child's potential for violence, and take precautionary safety measures, such as hourly or more frequent observation, removing potentially harmful objects from room, bathroom privileges with assistance only, and administering prescribed medication.
* Encourage the client to follow treatment plan, and assess behavioral responses to therapy. Behavior modification methods increase the client's awareness of "cause and effect" behavior. For example, the client decides to fight with another teenager and is denied television privileges for 1 week as a result of lack of control. Set limits on behavior.
* Discuss your observations with a client who is hallucinating. For example, make a statement, such as "You appear to be listening to something." Make frequent but brief remarks to interrupt the hallucinations.
* Administer prescribed medications, and monitor for effectiveness and side effects.

The following interventions are appropriate for promoting interpersonal relationships:

* Use clear, simple, concrete terms when defining acceptable behavior.
* Assist client to evaluate personal behavior realistically.
* Encourage noncompetitive activities.
* Promote healthy lifestyle practices, such as adequate nutrition, exercise, safe sex (if applicable), and positive family relationships.

The following interventions are appropriate for promoting education:

* Assist client and family to evaluate past and present family interactions that are positive and negative.
* Provide client and family with information about the mental health disorder, procedures, treatments, medications and side effects, and prognosis.
* Discourage blaming, but assist with appraisal of the situation, such as what is wrong, what the causes are, and what the options are.
* Encourage client compliance and family support of treatment plan and follow-up care.

evaluation

* The child will exhibit a positive self-concept by demonstrating an increased interest in interactions and activities.
* The child will demonstrate increased self-control demonstrated by a decrease in aggressive behavior to self and others; he or she will verbalize a realistic perception of self with strengths and limitations and identify consequences of personal behavior.
* Child will demonstrate an improved ability to express self and feelings. He or she will share concerns regarding responses of others and engage in noncompetitive activities with peers.
* Child and parents will identify factors that contribute to anxiety, identify alternatives to present coping pat-

terns, and describe rationale and procedure for treatments, medication schedule, and positive and negative effects of medication.

diagnostic tests

basic laboratory examination

* Blood chemistries, such as electrolytes, glucose, calcium, albumin, blood urea nitrogen, and liver function
* Blood count, including hematocrit, white count and differential, and sedimentation rate
* Drug levels for toxic screen and medication blood levels
* Arterial blood gases, urinalysis, electrocardiogram, and chest x-ray

laboratory examination based on clinical symptoms

* Electroencephalogram determines seizures; computed tomography detects normal pressure hydrocephalus, stroke, and space-occupying lesions.
* Additional blood chemistries, such as heavy metals (especially lead), thiamine (essential for normal metabolism of carbohydrates and fats; moderate deficiency causes impaired functioning of the nervous, circulatory, digestive, and endocrine systems), thyroid battery levels, and lumbar puncture, detect infection or intracranial bleed.

mental retardation

Mental retardation is characterized by subaverage intellectual functioning in children younger than 18 years reflected by an intelligence quotient (IQ) of 70 or below. Mental retardation is described in degrees, such as mild, moderate, severe, and profound (Table 29-3). The incidence of mental retardation is estimated at approximately 1% and is more common in boys (American Psychiatric Association, 1994).

The major predisposing factors of mental retardation include the following:

* Heredity factors, such as inborn errors of metabolism
* Early alterations of embryonic development, such as chromosomal irregularities (Down syndrome), infections, maternal alcohol consumption, and trauma
* Gestational problems, such as malnutrition, prematurity, hypoxia, and trauma
* Infant- and childhood-acquired illnesses, such as infections, trauma, and poisoning (especially lead)
* Environmental influences, such as withholding physical and emotional care and stimulation

characteristics

Mental retardation is diagnosed when a person demonstrates subaverage intelligence in at least two skill areas, including communication, self-care, home living, social and interpersonal skills, community resource application, self-guidance, functional academic skills, work, leisure, health, and safety. Onset of symptoms must develop before 18 years for a child to be diagnosed with mental retardation.

Mentally retarded children often display passive, placid, and dependent behaviors. However, disruptive or aggressive behavior may be seen in the child with deficient communication skills. Some children with mental retardation display self-injurious behaviors, such as head banging. Mentally retarded children may be at risk for physical abuse because caregivers may become angry and frustrated while caring for these children. In addition, sexual abuse may occur because the child is not able to understand what is happening to him or her and has difficulty communicating the abuse to an authority figure.

table 29-3 classification of mental retardation

Degree	*IQ Level*	*Description*
Mild	50–55 to 70	Considered educable; acquire academic skills up to sixth grade level; social and vocational skills for minimum support; need supervision and guidance
Moderate	35–40 to 50–55	Considered trainable; adapt well to life in a supervised community setting
Severe	20–25 to 35–40	Can be trained in elementary self-care skills; learn sight reading; perform simple tasks in closely supervised settings
Profound	below 20–25	Impairments in sensorimotor reflexes; some motor development, self-care, and communication skills possible with training in closely supervised and sheltered environment

From American Psychiatric Association (1994). *Diagnostic and Statistical Manual of Mental Disorders* (4th ed.). Washington, D.C.: Author.

✳ nursing considerations

The nurse is in a position to counsel, educate, and provide resource information to the family who has a child diagnosed with mental retardation. Initially, the family is in shock or grieving, and they are concerned about their child's immediate and long-term future. The nurse can provide information on education, special health needs, home care versus institutional care, and sexual considerations.

education

Children with mental retardation are able to learn and require stimulation just as much as other children. Depending on their degree of impairment, children with mental retardation should be mainstreamed into preschool programs and regular public schools as much as possible. The nurse should encourage caregivers to be patient when they teach children self-care tasks and safety information. Mentally retarded children should be given simple short-term memory instructions one step at a time.

special health needs

Children with mental retardation may have difficulty explaining what hurts. The nurse should teach caregivers to look for signs of pain, for example, the child holding his or her head or rubbing his or her ear. When children with mental retardation are hospitalized, it is important for nurses to try to stick to the child's normal everyday routine as much as possible to prevent stress and anxiety in the child. The nurse also should explain every procedure or nursing activity to the child in simple terms.

home care versus institutional care

Although in the past many children with mental retardation were placed in institutional care, this is not encouraged today. Children with mental retardation have much more opportunity for stimulation and interaction in a home setting surrounded by parents and siblings. However, these children have special needs and often require constant surveillance. Caring for these children can be demanding and exhausting. The nurse should provide information on resources and support groups available for families with children who have mental retardation.

If the child has severe mental retardation or if the parents are physically or emotionally unable to care adequately for the child, group and foster homes are an option. The nurse should evaluate the family's coping skills, needs, and feelings before making recommendations for care.

sexual considerations

As children with mental retardation become adolescents, the child's physical body is that of a teenager, yet the mental thinking is much younger. Menstruation can be a trying experience because mentally retarded girls are often not knowledgeable about the process and are frightened by the blood and cramping. Mentally retarded teenagers often fail to understand that masturbation should be performed in private and may act out their sexual feelings whenever they feel an urge. In addition, they often do not have the same opportunities as other teenagers to masturbate in private due to close parental restrictions, supervision, and group home living arrangements. Therefore, this normal activity becomes an issue.

If the teenager is sexually active or plans to be sexually active, principles of safe sex must be addressed, which include specific information about condoms and birth control. See Display 29-1 for points to consider when planning a sex education program for mentally retarded youths.

down syndrome

Down syndrome is the most common chromosomal abnormality in children resulting from a trisomy of 21 chromosomes. The condition is associated with maternal age, especially mothers older than 35 years.

pathophysiology

Physical characteristics of Down syndrome include a flat, broad, nasal bridge; inner epicanthal eye folds with upward and outward slanting of the eyes, giving the child an oriental look; a protruding tongue; short neck; transverse palmar crease; and hyperextensible and lax joints. Problems associated with Down syndrome include cardiac defects, respiratory infections, feeding difficulties, delayed developmental skills, and mental retardation.

medical management

Medical management is aimed at promoting optimum growth and development abilities. Treatment of cardiac and respiratory involvement is directed at prevention.

nursing care

Initially nursing care centers on the emotional needs of the family. Feeding difficulties are compounded by the child's large tongue and poor sucking reflex, requiring

display 29-1
points to consider when planning a sex education program for mentally retarded youths

- **Maintain the teenager's complete attention through eye contact, physical contact, and short education sessions.**
- **Use pictures, models, and child's terminology to teach about body parts and sexual activity.**
- **Evaluate the teenager's understanding by asking simple questions about the material.**

time and parental teaching to ensure the infant receives proper nutrition. Feeding to the back and side of the mouth enables better swallowing. Parents should be informed about the signs of respiratory infections because Down syndrome children can quickly become seriously ill with pneumonia. The child's cardiac status is monitored for signs of congestive heart failure with the presence of tachycardia, dysrythmias, and edema. Families may need referral to infant-stimulation programs, nutritionist, speech therapist, physical therapist, and occupational therapist (Fig. 29-1).

Growth hormone has been used on a limited number of children to treat Down syndrome and has had positive results. Growth hormone administration requires instruction to prepare the parent or caregiver to administer it at home. Synthetic growth hormone is given subcutaneously 3 days a week. Parents require information about sterile technique, selection and rotation of injection sites, and proper positioning of the child. Follow-up nursing care involves assessment of growth and development and comparing growth grid results. (See the Nursing Care Plan.)

 **nursing insight**

The main objective in caring for a Down syndrome child is to help him or her achieve the highest level of functioning.

learning disorders

Children are diagnosed as having a learning disorder when they score below normal on standardized tests in reading, math, or writing. Age, schooling, intelligence, and cultural considerations must be taken into account when administering the tests. Learning disorders can continue into adulthood.

Learning disabilities may be caused by genetic factors, perinatal injury, neurologic disorders, or other medical conditions, such as lead poisoning or fetal alcohol syndrome. Impaired vision or hearing also can affect learning ability and must be investigated through audiometric or visual screening tests. Approximately 5% of students in public schools in the United States are identified as having a learning disability (American Psychiatric Association, 1994).

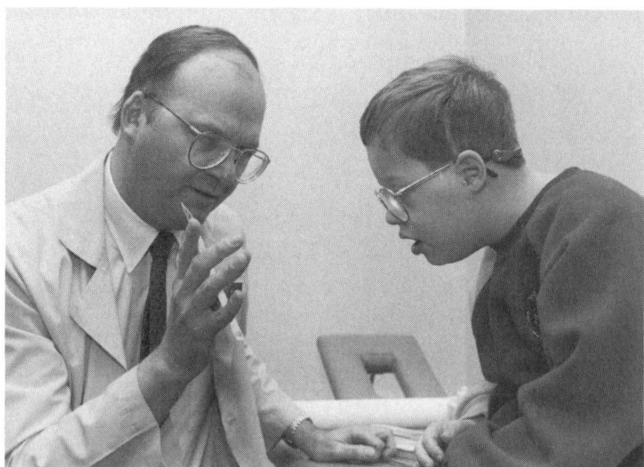

figure 29-1 *Therapy enables the adolescent with Down syndrome to work toward autonomy.*

nursing care

Children with learning disabilities tend to have low self-esteem and deficits in social skills; they are easily discouraged. The school drop-out rate for children or adolescents with learning disabilities is reported at nearly 40% (1.5 times greater than the average student).

motor skills disorder

Developmental coordination disorder is an impairment in the development of motor coordination that interferes with academic success or activities of daily living. Younger children often display clumsiness and delays in walking, crawling, sitting, and tying shoelaces. Older children have problems with assembling puzzles, building models, playing ball, or printing.

Developmental coordination disorder occurs in children from 5 to 11 years. This disorder is diagnosed independent of a general medical condition, such as cerebral palsy or muscular dystrophy.

communication disorders

Expressive language disorder is an example of a communication disorder and is characterized as an impairment involving verbal and sign language. Language difficulties limit academic and occupational success. Speech is limited, new words are difficult to acquire, and the child uses short sentences with grammatic errors. The disorder is typically recognized by 3 years. Approximately 50% of children with this disorder outgrow it.

pervasive developmental disorders

Pervasive developmental disorders are exhibited by severe and extensive impairment in several areas of development, including reciprocal social interaction skills, communication skills, or stereotyped behavior and activities. Infantile autism is an example of a pervasive developmental disorders.

infantile autism

Infantile autism is manifested by the presence of markedly impaired development in social interaction, communication, activity, and interests. Autistic children are inclined

nursing care plan
for the family with a child diagnosed with Down syndrome

NURSING DIAGNOSIS

Health Seeking Behaviors, aimed at learning more about the care of the child with Down syndrome

GOAL: Parents will describe the care and options necessary for the child with Down syndrome

NURSING INTERVENTIONS	*RATIONALE*	*EVALUATION*
Describe diagnosis, prognosis, home care needs, and potential treatment needs to the parents.	The parents will need to understand the wide range of possibilities and alternatives to make an informed decision regarding the child's care.	The parents will verbalize feelings regarding the diagnosis and their ability to use resources and provide care.
Discuss options in care such as institutional vs home care.	Nonjudgemental discussion around individual family's circumstances regarding the ability to keep the child at home vs. in a suitable foster home can help the parents to evaluate options.	The parents will openly discuss their feelings regarding options for care.
Discuss the child's physical well-being and mental retardation in regards to lifetime effect on health care and educational needs.	This will teach awareness of the associated physical anomalies, such as cardiac defects, respiratory infections, and feeding difficulties. The family will need to understand the varying educational abilities and the new programs being developed for the child with Down syndrome.	The family will state need for continued follow-up treatment concerning physical anomalies. Parents will discuss educational options and show an understanding of the advancement of newer programs.

to have an intense interest in nonfunctional habits and rituals and often become upset if there is any deviation from routine.

Behavior common to most children with autism includes body movements, such as hand clapping, body rocking, or walking on tiptoe. They may be hyperactive, impulsive, and aggressive. Children with autism usually have a short attention span, often exhibit a peculiar response to sensory stimuli, and are often self-injurious with a high threshold for pain. In addition, they may be fascinated with the movement of a spinning wheel or electric fan for hours and feel intense attachment to an inanimate object, such as a rubber band.

diagnosis

Diagnosis of autism is marked by delays or abnormal functioning in at least one of the following areas before 3 years: social interaction, language used in social communication, or symbolic or imaginative play. Autistic children usually experience mental retardation in the moderate range (IQ of 35–50).

Autism is more common in boys than girls. Treatment recommendations combine multiple disciplines and therapies.

attention deficit hyperactivity disorder

Attention deficit hyperactivity disorder (ADHD) is the newest term applied to a persistent pattern of inattention, hyperactivity, or impulsivity that is frequent and severe. Etiology is uncertain and may be related to any illness or trauma affecting the brain at any stage of development. Multiple causes are probably involved. A biologic theory has been suggested because many people with ADHD respond to central nervous system-stimulant drugs.

characteristics

Behavior exhibited by these children is not unusual childhood behavior. The difference is the quality of motor activity and developmentally inappropriate inattention, impulsivity, and hyperactivity that the child displays. Behavior manifestations may vary in number and severity. Most behaviors are noted at an early age, but learning disabilities may not be noticed until the child is in school.

diagnosis

A child is diagnosed with ADHD when he or she has six or more behavioral symptoms of either inattention, hyperactivity, or both. See Display 29-2 for a list of behavioral symtoms of inattention and hyperactivity.

Additional diagnostic criteria include the presence of some symptoms before 7 years; some symptoms present in two or more settings (eg, home, school); clear evidence of social, academic, or occupational dysfunction; occurrence of symptoms outside of an episode of pervasive developmental disorder; schizophrenia or other psychotic disorder; and inability to find any other mental order to which the symptoms can be accounted. The disorder can be classified as predominately inattentive, predominately hyperactive, or combined (most common).

management

Management usually involves a multiple approach, including medication (methylphenidate [Ritalin], dextroamphetamine [Dexedrine], magnesium pemoline [Cylert], and tricyclic antidepressants), family counseling and education, behavioral and psychotherapy, proper classroom placement, and environmental manipulation.

nursing care

Nurses are active participants in all aspects of management of the child with ADHD. They are a liaison between other health care professionals and education professionals. Nurses should encourage parents to vent their feelings and assist them in understanding the importance and longevity of treatment. The nurse should teach the parents and the child about the nature of the disorder, provide reading material, and refer the family to support groups.

Parents must be taught about the nature of the medications. Some medications (Pemoline) require 2 to 3 weeks to achieve the desired effects; others must be given in low doses at first and then increased until the effect is achieved. Parents should be informed of possible side effects, such as anorexia, blurred vision, and sleeplessness. Small, frequent meals and finger food snacks are helpful for anorexia induced by methylphenidate. Sleeplessness may be reduced by administering medications earlier in the day. Methylphenidate may cause depressed growth. To limit this effect, growth must be carefully monitored, and the child may be placed on medication "holidays" or "vacations" on weekends and during the summer. Tricyclics cause increased dental caries and warrant meticuluous dental care. Parents should keep all medications out of children's reach. Nurses must evaluate the effectiveness of the child's medication by directly observing and questioning parents, child, and teachers.

Assist families in learning environmental manipulation, using organizational charts, decreasing distractions, and modeling positive behaviors. The nurse can encourage consistency at home and school, appropriate placement in classrooms equipped for special training, and counseling for children and families who demonstrate anxiety or depression.

display 29-2
behavioral symptoms of inattention or hyperactivity in the child with attention-deficit hyperactivity disorder

* **Fails to pay close attention to details or makes careless mistakes**
* **Difficulty sustaining attention to tasks or play**
* **Does not seem to listen when spoken to**
* **Does not follow through on instructions**
* **Has difficulty organizing**
* **Avoids or dislikes tasks that require sustained mental effort**
* **Loses things necessary for tasks**
* **Is easily distracted**
* **Forgets daily activities**

HYPERACTIVITY OR IMPULSIVITY

* **Fidgets or squirms**
* **Leaves seat in classroom**
* **Runs or climbs excessively or during inappropriate times**
* **Has difficulty playing quietly**
* **Is often "on the go"**
* **Talks excessively**
* **Impulsively blurts out answers before questions are complete**
* **Has difficulty waiting turn**
* **Interrupts or intrudes on others**

anxiety disorders

Anxiety disorders are indexed in three groupings: separation anxiety, avoidant disorder, and overanxious disorder. Many of these are family related.

separation anxiety

Developmental crisis related to Erikson's stage of development described as "trust versus mistrust" occurs as early as 6 to 12 months, resulting from separation from parent(s). Severe and persistent anxiety is noted when the child is separated from a parent (usually the mother), home, or other intimate environment. As the child develops, anxiety increases when subjected to traveling independently from home or spending time at a friend's house (especially overnight), attending camp, or going to school (school phobia).

Common symptoms include complaints of headache, nausea, vomiting, and stomach ache coinciding with the child's apprehension of separation or actual separation. The child may refuse to leave the house, becoming house bound or disabled from severe separation anxiety reflected by morbid fears of illness, injury, danger, or death. Before a diagnosis of separation anxiety is made, the disturbance must last at least 2 weeks.

avoidant disorder

Avoidant disorder may be evident as early as 2 1/2 years. Stranger anxiety occurring between 6 to 12 months is usually resolved before 2 years when the child learns to trust people and begin to develop autonomy.

When fear of strangers is unresolved, the child may begin to avoid contact with strangers, displaying an unreasonable obsession for affection and acceptance with family members. Behaviors such as clinging, crying, withdrawing, or mute behavior are common and increase the risk of positive social interactions. Diagnosis is made when symptoms persist for 6 months or more.

overanxious disorder

Overanxious disorder is described as unreasonable anxiety about future events, minor procedures, personal competency, and social acceptance. The child has an excessive need for reassurance.

Somatic ailments, such as headache, dizziness, shortness of breath, and a "lump-in-the-throat" feeling, and feelings of tension are common. This condition must be evaluated based on degree and severity of symptoms.

Preschool children typically have a worrisome nature that is considered normal but not restricting. At the school-age level, it is important to assist children in recognizing individuals who can give them the social supports needed to deal with stressors.

childhood depression

Depression in general is "anger turned inward." Primary depression is due to a problem unrelated to a real life event, situation, or illness. Secondary depression is a result of a life event. A typical characteristic of depression is grief. *Grief* is described as an inability to perceive joy.

Certain types of depression tend to run in families, which indicates a biologic vulnerability that can be inherited.

treatment

Depression is treated with a variety of antidepressants and psychotherapies. Medication offers quick symptom relief, and psychotherapy helps the client learn more effective ways to cope with life's problems.

Antidepressant medications include tricyclics, monoamine oxidase inhibitors, and lithium (used for bipolar (manic depressive) disorder. Antidepressant drugs are not habit forming but must be carefully monitored for correct dose and possible side effects.

nursing care

The nurse should warn the child not to mix medications with any over-the-counter medications or with any medications prescribed by the dentist or another doctor. In addition, the child and family should be informed about the side effects of antidepressants, which include dry mouth, constipation, blurred vision or dizziness, and bladder problems, such as difficulty emptying the bladder. See the Teaching Guidelines for care tips when taking antidepressant medications.

suicide

Suicide is the act of taking one's own life voluntarily. Alcohol, drug abuse, depression, and behavioral problems contribute to the high rate of suicide in school-age children and adolescents. Serious terminal illnesses, such as acquired immunodeficiency syndrome and cancer, also contribute to the suicide rate in children and adolescents.

risk factors

Risk factors for suicide include the following:

* Previous psychiatric problems, such as depression, alcoholism and schizophrenia, that required professional intervention (may or may not involve hospitalization)
* History of drug abuse, behavioral problems, or depression
* Gender. Boys are three times more successful with suicide; girls make more attempts.
* Age. Adolescents are the most likely to commit suicide.
* Race. White people have a higher risk factor than African Americans.
* Prior suicide attempts
* History of a recent interpersonal loss, such as death of a friend, family member, or parent; family stress seen with divorce
* Uncontrolled anger toward someone close with a desire to make them feel sorry and guilty
* Low self-esteem and feelings of hopelessness, powerlessness, shame, guilt, and self-hatred

warning signs

The child or adolescent who exhibits marked personality changes, such as sadness, withdrawal, apathy, or anxiety, should be closely watched for a suicide attempt (Fig.

teaching guidelines
care for antidepressant medication administration

Care for common side effects from antidepressant medications include:

* Drink plenty of water, chew sugarless gum, and brush teeth often for dry mouth.
* Eat bran cereals, fruit, and vegetables (especially salads); drink extra water and fruit juice; take walks; and engage in exercise for constipation.
* Rise from bed or chair slowly when experiencing dizziness; tell someone you feel dizzy; do not drive your car.

29-2). In addition, angry outbursts, hyperactivity, aggressiveness, or obnoxious behaviors in a child who is not normally like this are warning signs. Other warning signs include a decline in school work performance and a decreased participation or performance in sports or other activities. Finally, the child who talks, thinks, writes, or dreams about harming or killing himself or herself must be closely monitored. See Display 29-3 for a list of suicide precautions for children who exhibit these warning signs.

> **nursing alert**
> *Children who suddenly appear less depressed and more energetic after a period of serious depression are more at risk for suicide because they have more energy to commit the act than children who are still in a depressed and despondent mood.*

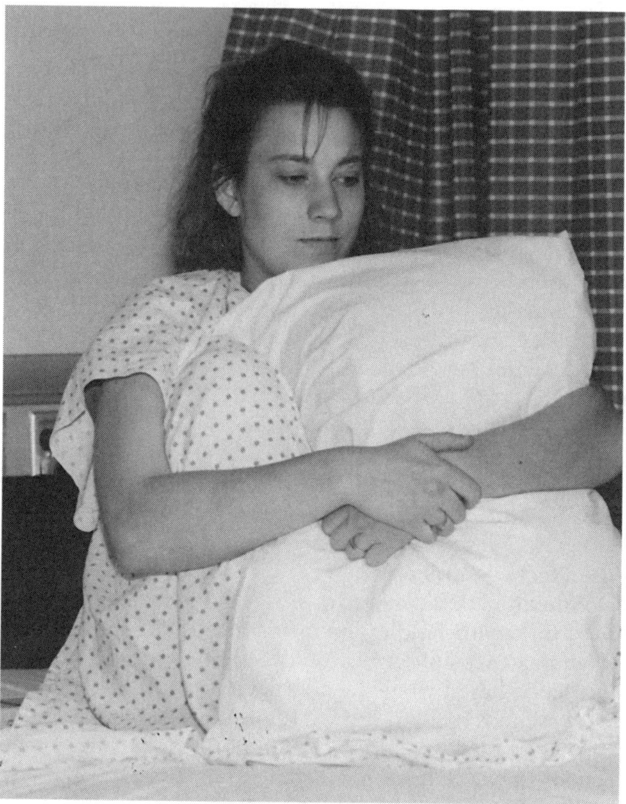

figure 29-2 *Withdrawn behavior may be a suicide warning. (Photo by Elise Dinerman)*

substance abuse

Surveys indicate that 9 out of 10 adolescents have tried drugs or alcohol at least once. Abuse occurs when the child's functioning is impaired by the substance for more than 1 month and repeated attempts to cut back or stop using the substance have failed.

Studies indicate that many adolescent substance abusers experienced clinical depression before drug use was started. Children who submerge their emotional pain in alcohol or drugs are often unable to identify their emotional state on a daily basis and need help recognizing anger, fear, and frustration.

Substance abuse withdrawal produces physical and emotional symptoms. Although these may vary according to the drug used, common signs include sleeplessness, exhaustion, irritability, and depression. The child going through withdrawal faces the emotional trauma of dealing with everyday problems without a chemical crutch.

developmental characteristics of children at risk for drug abuse

In general the "high risk" individual shows significant inadequacies in one, several, or all of the following areas:

* Identification with viable role models. The child vulnerable to drug abuse does not see himself or herself as like (or the same as) people whose attitudes, values, and behaviors allow them to "survive" in their environment.
* Identification with and responsibility for "family" processes. A child with poorly developed identification does not identify with things greater than himself or herself (eg, relationships with another person, mankind, God). He or she does not see that what he or she does affects others.
* Problem-solving skills. Children lacking problem-solving skills are not able to work through problems or do not believe that problems can be solved through application of personal resources. They turn to drugs (usually alcohol) to take away their problems.
* Intrapersonal skills. Children weak in this area have an inability to cope with personal stresses and tensions. They are often dishonest with themselves, deny themselves, are unable to defer gratification, and have low self-esteem.
* Interpersonal skills. Children lacking these skills tend to have difficulty expressing themselves, are dishonest with others, lack empathic awareness, are resistant to feedback (highly sensitive to criticism), and are unable to share feelings or give or receive love and help.
* Systemic skills. Children lacking in this area refuse to accept the consequences of their behavior. Instead, they tend to see themselves as victims of circumstances.
* Judgmental skills. Children lacking these skills demonstrate repetitious self-destructive behaviors, such as unprotected sex and shared drug equipment use.

nursing care

A major goal of nursing care is to make the child feel comfortable and secure enough to be able to talk about the addiction. The nurse must listen and not make judgmental comments. Scare tactics, such as "using drugs will destroy your brain," should not be used when caring for a child

display 29-3
suicide precautions

* *Never* leave the suicidal child alone.
* Take the suicide threat seriously. Children who talk about it do it.
* Suicidal behavior is a cry for help.
* Be willing to give and get help sooner rather than later.
* Listen to what the child is saying without passing judgment.
* Encourage a child who is talking about harming self to talk with a trusted friend, health care professional, crisis hotline, or emergency response for help.
* Ask the child if he or she has a plan to commit suicide. Encourage the child with a suicide plan to talk about the plan.
* If the child is found semiconscious or unconscious, maintain an open airway, and call for emergency care. Note if any medication or drugs are near the child.

with an abuse problem. Instead, the nurse should focus on counseling the child and helping him or her gain self-confindence. The nurse should encourage and help the child set realistic goals of discontinuing drug use.

childhood schizophrenia

Schizophrenia is described as a group of mental disorders identified by disruption of thinking, mood, behavior, and a varied concept of reality. Ideas and feelings tend to be isolated from one another. For example, the child may relate a sad experience in a happy manner. The disorder is incorrectly called a "split personality."

Schizophrenia affects boys and girls equally. Onset is usually adolescence or early adulthood, but it occurs occasionally in children as young as 5 years. The exact cause is unknown. Genetic factors are a possibility because this disorder tends in run in families. Studies indicate a possible link between nutritional and immunologic deficiencies and a potential viral infection influence.

Symptoms include delusions (false beliefs that are usually bizarre and absurd), hallucinations (false sensory perceptions), severe anxiety, inappropriate affect, incoherent speech or invention of new words, morbid thoughts, absence of friends, and concrete thinking.

Brain studies performed on schizophrenics have revealed a loss of brain tissue, abnormalities in brain density, brain asymmetry, and atrophy of the cerebellum. Studies also have indicated an excessive number of receptors for *dopamine*, a brain chemical involved in controlling body movements.

medical treatment

Treatment includes antipsychotic medications that block the action of dopamine in the brain, such as phenothiazine, butyrophenones, and thioxanthenes. Treatment with medication and psychotherapy enables many children with schizophrenia to live independent to moderately independent lives.

key points ✳

* The origins of childhood behavior and mental health problems are linked with hereditary influences, family struggles, and turmoil. In the past, children were removed from their families; the trend today is to focus on the strengths of families, building therapeutic communication and effective parenting skills within the child's natural environment.
* Developmental considerations include the child's developing personality and temperament and factors such as emotional abuse, displacement of feelings, and if and at what developmental stage the child exhibits abnormal behavior.
* Nursing considerations for the child with mental retardation include education, special health needs, home care versus institutional care, and sexual considerations.
* Learning disorders are diagnosed when a child scores below normal on standardized tests in reading, math, or writing. Age, schooling, intelligence, and cultural considerations must be taken into account when administering the tests.
* Nursing care for children with ADHD includes teaching the parent and child about the disorder, providing reading material, referring the family to support groups, teaching about necessary medications, and assisting families in learning environmental manipulation, such as using organizational charts, decreasing distractions, and modeling positive behaviors.
* Separation anxiety, avoidant disorder, and overanxious disorder are three types of anxiety disorders seen in children.
* Treament for childhood depression includes antidepressant medications and psychotherapy.
* Risk factors for suicide include previous psychiatric problems, history of drug abuse, behavioral problems, depression, gender (male), age (adolescents), race (white people), prior suicide attempt, history of recent interpersonal loss, uncontrolled anger toward a loved one, and low self-esteem, guilt, or self-hatred.
* A child at high risk for substance abuse is weak in the following areas: identification with role modes, identification with family processes, problem-solving skills, intrapersonal skills, interpersonal skills, systemic skills, and judgmental skills.
* Schizophrenia is described as a group of mental disorders identified by disruption of thinking, mood, and behavior with a varied concept of reality; ideas and feelings tend to be isolated from one another.

review questions

1. An adolescent considered at risk for drug abuse can be described as having a/an:
   a. Below 50 IQ.
   b. Above 120 IQ.
   c. Belief in miracle solutions to problems.
   d. Autistic temperament.
2. The ultimate goal in caring for a mentally retarded child is to encourage:
   a. Socialization skills.
   b. Self-care skills.
   c. Dependency.
   d. Education.
3. Select the environment that is best for providing care to children with mental disorders.
   a. Family home.
   b. Children social service facilities.
   c. Mental health facilities.
   d. Isolation.
4. Select the most appropriate statement concerning emotional abuse.
   a. Emotional abuse prevents the child from peer interactions.
   b. Emotional abuse often involves threats to harm, followed with physical harm.
   c. Emotional abuse destroys the child's self concept and self worth.
   d. Emotional abuse involves denying the child basic care.
5. Select the most important nursing measure when caring for a child with mental illness.
   a. Recognition of the family's importance to the child's welfare.
   b. Assessment of the child's eating patterns.
   c. Promotion of the child's weaknesses.
   d. Restricted acceptance of the child's beliefs.

references

American Psychiatric Association (1994). *Diagnostic and statistical manual of mental disorders* (4th ed.). Washington, D.C: Author.

bibliography

Anglin-Levieux, L., & Sawyer, E. (1993). Incorporating play interventions into nursing care. *Pediatric Nursing, 19*(5), 459–462.

Barron, C., & Yoest, P. (1994). Emotional distress and coping with a stressful relationship inadolescent boys. *Journal of Pediatric Nursing, 9*(1), 13–19.

Clark, L. (1989). *The time-out solution.* Chicago, IL: Contemporary Books.

Clunn, P. (1991). *Child psychiatric nursing.* St. Louis: Mosby–Year Book.

Hathaway, W., Hay, W., Groothuis, J., & Paisley, J. (1993). *Current pediatirc diagnosis and treatment* (11th ed.). Norwalk, CT: Appleton & Lange.

Karp, N. (1993). Collaboration with families: From myth to reality. *Federation of Families for Children's Mental Health, Winter*, 21–23.

Keller, M., Lavorie, P., Beardslee, W., Wunder, J., Schwartz, C., Roth, J., & Biederman, J. (1992). The disruptive behavioral disorder in children and adolescents: Comorbidity and clinical course. *Journal of the American Academy of Child and Adolescent Psychiatry, 31*(2), 204–218.

Knitzer, J. (1992). Children's mental health policy: Challenging the future. *Journal of Emotional and Behavioral Disorders, 1*(1), 8–16.

Looney, J. (1988). *Chronic mental illness in children and adolescents.* Washington, D.C.: American Psychiatric Press.

Newcorn, J., & Strain J. (1992). Adjustment disorder in children and adolescents. *Journal of the American Academy of Child and Adolescent Psychiatry, 31*(2), 318–325.

Rogers, C. (1964). Approach to values: The valuing process in the mature person. *Journal of Abnormal and Social Psychology, 8*, 135–151.

Sharrer, V., & Wenger-Ryan, N. (1995). A longitudinal study of age and gender differences of stressors and coping strategies in school-aged children. *Journal of Pediatric Health Care, 9*(3), 123–130.

Shives, L. (1990). *Basic concepts of pyschiatric-mental health nursing* (2nd ed.). Philadelphia: J.B. Lippincott.

Teeter, R. (1993). *Young people.* Danbury, CT: Grolier Electronic Publishing.

Weiten, W., & Lloyd, M. (1994). *Psychology applied to modern life adjustment in the 90s.* Pacific Grove, CA: Brooks/Cole Publishing.

Wylie, M. (1992). The evolution of a revolution. *Networker, Janurary/February*, 17–29.

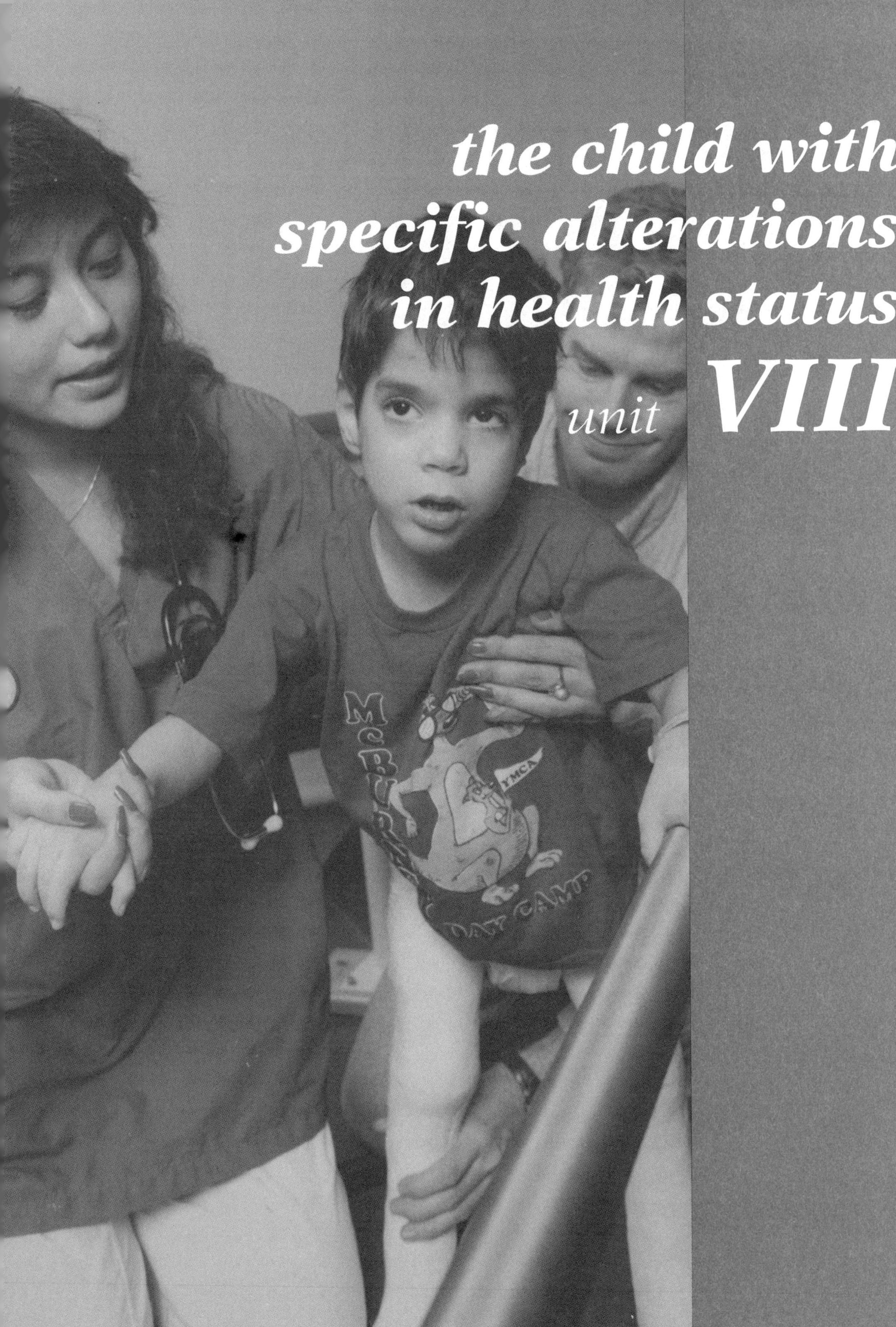

the child with specific alterations in health status

unit VIII

the child with an alteration in respiration 30

outline

objectives

After studying this chapter, the reader should be able to:

- ✳ Discuss the anatomy and physiology of the respiratory system, acknowledging age-specific differences.
- ✳ Identify no fewer than three family considerations concerning respiratory diseases.
- ✳ Discuss the nursing process related to promoting normal breathing patterns, maintaining an open airway, maintaining normal body temperature, promoting hydration, and promoting activity and home care.
- ✳ List diagnostic tests pertinent to viral and bacterial respiratory infections.
- ✳ Explain why young children are more prone to upper airway obstruction than older children.
- ✳ List at least three infections caused by the respiratory syncytial virus.
- ✳ Discuss similarities and differences in nursing care for acute lower respiratory conditions, including bronchiolitis, pneumonia, and tuberculosis, and nursing measures appropriate to chronic respiratory conditions, including cystic fibrosis and asthma.
- ✳ Discuss the condition of sudden infant death syndrome, and list at least four predisposing factors.
- ✳ Discuss medical and surgical management of children experiencing tonsillitis and adenoiditis, noting at least two common complications seen in recurrent infections and two common postoperative complications.
- ✳ Describe safety factors involved in chest physiotherapy.

key terms

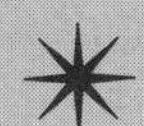

apnea
atelectasis
cor pulmonale
cyanosis
dyspnea
diuretic
hypoxemia
percussion
postural drainage
rales
retractions
stridor
tachypnea

Respiratory diseases are common in children and can range from mild disorders to life-threatening events. Early diagnosis and intervention are essential in preventing minor illnesses from becoming serious. Understanding the prevalence and transmission of respiratory infections helps the nurse administer competent care to the child and pertinent information to the family caregiver.

Nursing care of children with respiratory conditions is based on understanding age-related anatomy and physiology of respiration. This chapter discusses respiratory anatomy and physiology, age-related differences, common diagnostic tests, parental and nursing considerations, specific respiratory disease information, and procedures pertinent to pediatric respiratory care.

anatomy and physiology of the respiratory system

The respiratory system is responsible for the continuous supply of oxygen needed to sustain life in the body's millions of cells and for the removal of carbon dioxide from the body. The respiratory system works with the cardiovascular system to provide for gas exchange, that is delivery of oxygen (O_2) to the cells and removal of carbon dioxide (CO_2) by way of the bloodstream. Dysfunction of the respiratory system interferes with this exchange of gases, depriving cells of oxygen and causing cell death.

Respiration occurs at two levels: external and internal. *External respiration* occurs at the alveolar level in the lungs. Gas moves from an area of higher pressure to an area of lower pressure by a process called *diffusion.* For example, O_2 in the lungs moves out of alveoli into capillaries and into body tissues, while CO_2 moves from pulmonary capillaries into alveoli to be exhaled through the mouth and nose. *Internal respiration* occurs at the cellular level and involves the chemical combustion of food and O_2 to form CO_2 and water, producing energy.

Ventilation (breathing) is the process that moves air into and out of the lungs. The act of breathing brings oxygen into the body from the environment and releases carbon dioxide from the body into environment. This exchange of gases helps control the levels of oxygen and carbon dioxide in the blood, which helps maintain normal acid-base (pH) balance in the body. An increase in oxygen can result in respiratory alkalosis, while an increase in carbon dioxide predisposes to respiratory acidosis.

Respiratory alkalosis is an abnormal condition of the body characterized by a pH level greater than 7.44. Normal pH is rarely 7.4 in the clinical setting. The normal range is 7.35 to 7.45 with allowance for ± 0.02 error in either direction. Respiratory alkalosis may be caused by an excessive intake of oxygen through hyperventilation or related to oxygen administration. Signs and symptoms tend to be vague and include dizziness, prickling, tingling and numbness of the extremities, muscle cramps, cardiac arrhythmias and loss of alertness. Treatment involves correcting the cause of hyperventilation or excessive O_2.

Respiratory acidosis results from respiratory retention of CO_2 and is characterized by a pH level falling below 7.25. Any severe physiologic disorder, such as upper and lower airway obstruction, respiratory depression, ineffective coughing, and deep breathing due to poor effort or pain, can result in respiratory acidosis. The symptoms depend on the severity of the problem. For example, a slight increase of retained CO_2 causes mild dyspnea, increased heart rate, and drowsiness. As CO_2 levels increase because of ventilatory failure, symptoms become more severe and include increasing dyspnea, restlessness, loss of alertness, and coma. Treatment involves administration of supplemental oxygen to correct decreased blood oxygen levels and correct the underlying cause.

Respirations are promoted by movement of the diaphragm and external intercostal muscles. Small children experiencing difficulty in breathing often retract the sternal and intercostal muscles during respirations in an attempt to take in as much air as possible.

age-specific considerations

The rate of respiration decreases as an individual matures. Normal newborn respiration ranges from 40 to 60 breaths per minute (at rest). Respiration in toddlers ranges from 20 to 30 breaths per minute. For the school-age child, the rate is 18 to 26 breaths per minute; for a teenager, the rate is 12 to 20 breaths per minute, the same as in an adult (Table 30-1). The rate and depth of respirations are controlled by the respiratory center in the brain, located in the medulla oblongata and lower portion of the pons. Respirations also are stimulated by the levels of oxygen and carbon dioxide in the blood, acid–base balance (pH) within the body, activity, and emotions.

Compared with adults, children (especially infants and toddlers) have smaller anatomic structures and lower resistance to infection. For example, an adult's throat, referred to as the *pharynx*, is approximately 5 in long, while that of an infant is approximately 2 in. The *pharynx* has three subdivisions: 1) *nasopharynx* (the superior part of the throat), 2) *oropharynx* (found behind the mouth), and 3) *laryngopharynx* (area around the voice box). Air enters the nasopharynx, then moves down into the oropharynx. The oropharynx receives food from the mouth. Air passes through the laryngopharynx, enters the pharynx, and is moved downward into the bronchiole tree (Fig. 30-1). The infant's tongue is larger in proportion to the mouth than that of an adult, increasing the risk for airway obstruction. Obstruction of any one of these areas is a serious concern and could result in respiratory arrest (see Fig. 30-1).

Children have a tendency to develop edema of the air passages, making them easily obstructed. The potential for edema of the respiratory soft tissue in newborns and infants is greater because they have small airways with large amounts of soft tissue. Irritation from environmental pollution and infections contributes to the development of edema. Viruses and bacteria are the most common causes of acute respiratory infections in children.

table 30-1 *respiration rates and assessment factors*

Respiration Rate According to Age	*Technique*	*Consideration*
Infant—30–50 per minute	Count for 1 full minute.	Abdominal muscles are used for breathing.
Toddler—20–30 per minute	Count for 1 full minute. Small child may prefer to be held by caregiver. Easier to auscultate respirations with a stethoscope placed on chest front or back.	Abdominal muscles are used for breathing. Irregular breathing patterns are normal with short (less than 10-sec) periods of apnea.
School-age child—18–26 per minute	Count for 30 seconds and multiply by 2.	Thoracic breathing patterns are used after age 7 y.
Adolescent—12–20 per minute	Count for 15 seconds and multiply by 4.	Note rate, rhythm, and depth of breathing. Rate is 14–20 per minute.

Chronic respiratory disorders in children, such as cystic fibrosis (CF) and asthma, can be linked to prenatal development, hereditary factors, or allergies. For example, CF is genetically linked with a protein deficiency that contributes to the production of thick mucus in the respiratory, gastrointestinal, and reproductive systems. Asthma is often triggered by allergens in the child's environment.

Sinus infections commonly seen in adults are usually not a problem until the child is 6 to 8 years old, because the frontal sinuses, the structures most affected by sinus infections, do not develop until this age. However, it is not uncommon for infants to experience nasal discharge and stuffiness for several weeks due to their small nasal passages and their susceptibility to become reinfected with the cold virus.

School-age children have a natural tendency to experience enlarged *tonsils*. Enlarged tonsils require no intervention unless respiration is compromised or infection is

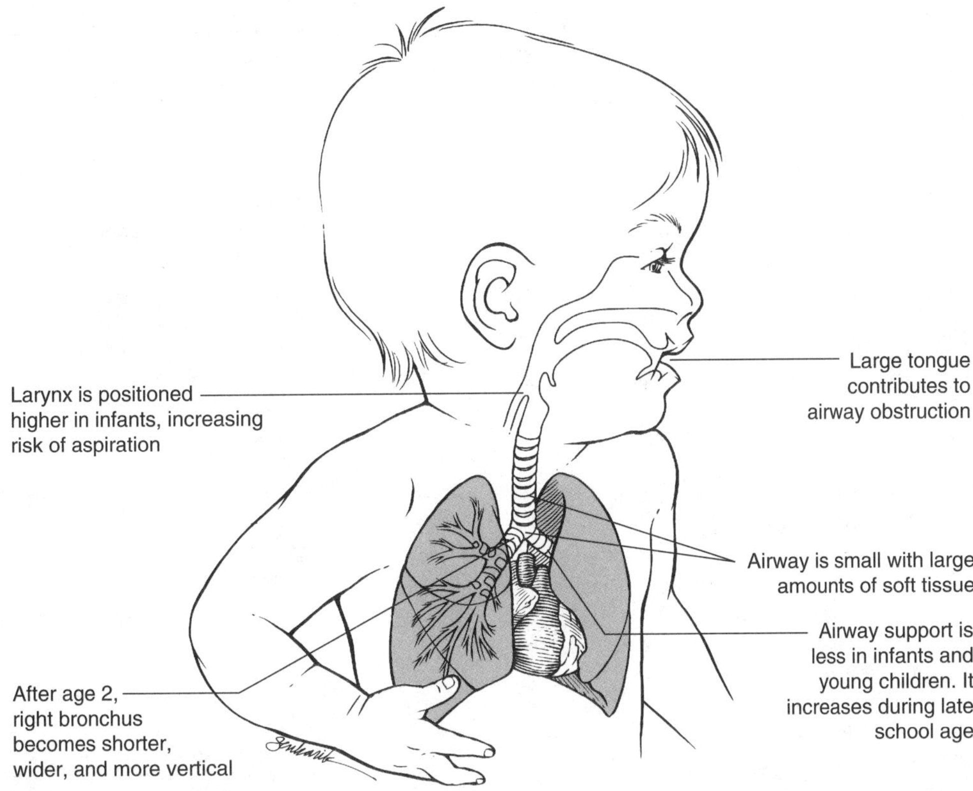

figure 30-1 *Child's respiratory system.*

present. Snoring noises made while sleeping indicate a potential airway clearance problem related to large tonsils.

Newborns lack the ability to clear mucus from the respiratory tract effectively, making them more susceptible than older children to respiratory infection or respiratory obstruction. During toddlerhood, the maturity of the bronchi is similar to that of the adult. The right bronchus is larger in diameter and more vertical in descent compared with the smaller and slightly horizontal left bronchus. The size and position of the right bronchus contribute to a higher incidence of pneumonia and foreign body aspiration into the right lung.

Infants use their abdominal muscles for breathing. Thoracic breathing patterns begin at 2 to 3 years and become complete by 7 years. Lung alveoli increase in size and number until 3 years. After 3 years of age, growth of the respiratory tissue corresponds to the child's age and size, with adult proportions noted in late adolescence.

The structures of the respiratory system increase in size during adolescence. In boys, the larynx and trachea are typically larger than girls and are comparable to adult sizes. Breath sounds are softer in adolescents when compared with younger children due to an increase in chest wall size. The chest circumference is more cone-shaped during the preschool years, reaching adult proportion by 6 years.

✶ family considerations

Viral and bacterial respiratory diseases are common in young children and are easily transmitted from one sibling to another. Caregivers often share stories about how one child infected all of the other family members. Many respiratory diseases are associated with elevated temperature, increased mucus production, and irritability. While not necessarily life-threatening, these symptoms can cause the child to be restless and cross. Infants become frustrated when they are unable to suck because of thick mucus blocking their nose. Older children with colds can be discontented and irritable because they do not feel like playing, but they are not sick enough to be in bed. It is easy to understand why caregivers sometimes feel anxious and frustrated.

The life-threatening potential of respiratory disorders produces high anxiety within the family, especially when small children are concerned. Seeing a small infant struggle to get his or her breath while being placed in an oxygen tent can be an overwhelming experience for a parent. Parents often express feelings of helplessness and guilt concerning the child's crisis and hospitalization.

Parents' lack of knowledge about the disease, procedures, medicines, and the hospital environment can cause them great concern. They may feel responsible for the child's illness and question their parenting skills. They may blame each other for the illness and provide little or no support to each other.

Personal lifestyle patterns, such as the use of tobacco, can contribute to a child's respiratory problems. Children subjected to second-hand smoke tend to have a higher incidence of respiratory illnesses than children living in smoke-free environments. Children attending day care centers and nursery schools are more likely to be exposed to a variety of respiratory diseases.

Caregivers and older siblings of children with chronic respiratory problems may need to learn cardiopulmonary resuscitation (CPR) if the respiratory condition poses life-threatening risks. School-age children with chronic respiratory problems leading to repeated or lengthy absences may need special assistance to keep up with their school work. Tutoring may be necessary if the child is required to be away from school for an extended time.

✶ nursing considerations

Infants and small children have an intolerance to nasal congestion, a susceptibility to ear infections, and increased severity of respiratory symptoms due to smaller airway diameters. A serious complication of respiratory disorders is respiratory arrest, making emergency measures, such as CPR, necessary.

The nurse must be alert to family concerns regarding the child's illness, providing accurate information and explanations to help reduce caregiver anxiety. Financial concerns regarding hospital cost, home health care, and medication expenses can be referred to social service departments.

Safety is a major responsibility in providing child care. Oxygen equipment must be monitored for safety. A small hole in an oxygen tent can decrease its effectiveness. All toys left in the crib must be inspected to guarantee safety from aspiration of small removable parts.

Toys with long strings are dangerous to infants because they can get wrapped around the neck or swallowed, causing strangulation. Friction toys are not allowed under oxygen or oxygen mist tents because a spark can cause a fire in the high-oxygen environment. Noisy alarm systems from monitoring equipment, such as apnea monitors and pulse oximeters, can cause sensory overload, making children irritable and fussy.

Infant respiratory problems are often linked to three factors: 1) a microorganism's ability to cause disease; 2) environmental factors, such as nutrition, hygiene, psychosocial stimulation, and exposure to environmental toxins, such as cigarette smoke; and 3) the infant's body responses to biologic, chemical, or physical injury and stress.

✶ nursing process in respiratory disorders

assessment

Assessment of children with respiratory diseases includes an interview and physical examination. Respiratory illnesses can begin at birth. Low Apgar scores can indicate infant risk for developing respiratory illnesses. Knowledge of familial tendencies to respiratory diseases helps the nurse identify other risk factors, such as CF, asthma, and sudden infant death syndrome (SIDS).

subjective data

Subjective data are often obtained from parents or caregivers unless the child is old enough to provide the information accurately.

objective data

assessment of respirations

Count the number of respirations for 1 minute. Because infants have a shallow and irregular respiratory pattern, using a stethoscope gives a more accurate rate. *Tachypnea* is an increased respiratory rate and can be the first evidence of respiratory distress in children.

Note rate; pattern; presence of expiratory grunting; widening of the nostrils; hypothermia; bluish discoloration of the skin (*cyanosis*), which may be present even after oxygen administration; decreased breath sounds or abnormal lung sounds (wheezes, crackles, or rhonchi); nasal congestion; coughing; and hoarseness. A decrease in respiratory rate following an episode of tachypnea may indicate exhaustion and potential shock.

Note the presence of sternal retractions in infants and small children. Retractions are seen more frequently in newborns and infants because the intercostal tissues are weak and underdeveloped. When respiratory obstruction is present, children will inspire more forcefully than normal to inflate their lungs, using their subcostal, substernal, intercostal, supraclavicular, and suprasternal muscles. Retractions are seen when the intercostal spaces constrict (Fig. 30-2). Retractions in children can easily cause fatigue and exhaustion followed by respiratory arrest.

Note the strength of the child's cry.

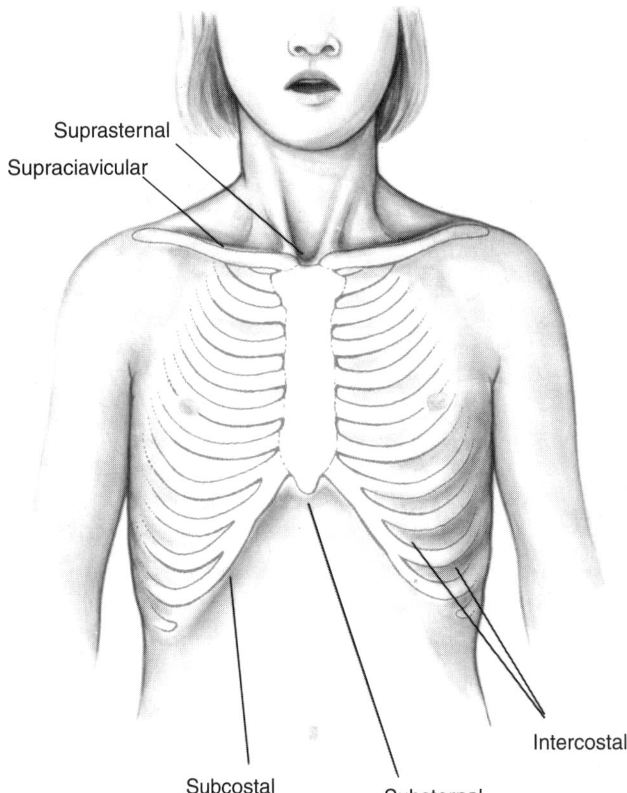

figure 30-2 *Sites of respiratory retraction.*

assessment of vital signs

Establish a baseline for respirations, pulse, and temperature.

An elevated temperature, pulse, and respiration rate indicates infection.

An elevated pulse and respiration rate with normal temperature readings might indicate congestive heart failure.

Blood pressure does not usually drop until the child is in critical condition: therefore, care is not based totally on the blood pressure reading.

assessment of skin

Note coloring of the skin and mucous membranes. Pinkish skin and mucous membranes in white children and reddish skin and mucous membranes in children with darker skin indicate normal exchange of oxygen and carbon dioxide.

Observe for alteration of oxygen and carbon dioxide exchange, causing a build-up of carbon dioxide, which is reflected by a bluish discoloration of the skin and mucous membranes known as *cyanosis*. In darker skinned children, cyanosis is indicated by a dusky gray skin tone.

Check the mouth, lips, cheekbones, nail beds, and ear lobes for signs of cyanosis.

Check the results of the red blood cell count because children with low red blood cell counts (hemoglobin below 5 mg) may not look cyanotic even though they have a serious breathing problem. Cyanosis is not always a true indicator of airway difficulty.

Observe for clubbing of the fingers reflected by a change in the angle of the nail to the fingertip (Fig. 30-3), commonly seen in children with chronic respiratory disease.

Observe the chest appearance for visible deformities.

assessment of cough

Note when coughing occurs because it is a reflex that is produced by stimulation of the respiratory tract nerves by irritants and mucus. Coughing helps to mobilize secretions, promote lung expansion, prevent mucus retention, and expel foreign bodies from the respiratory tract.

Note the child's actions during and after a coughing episode because coughing increases chest pressure and decreases blood return, increasing the risk of fainting.

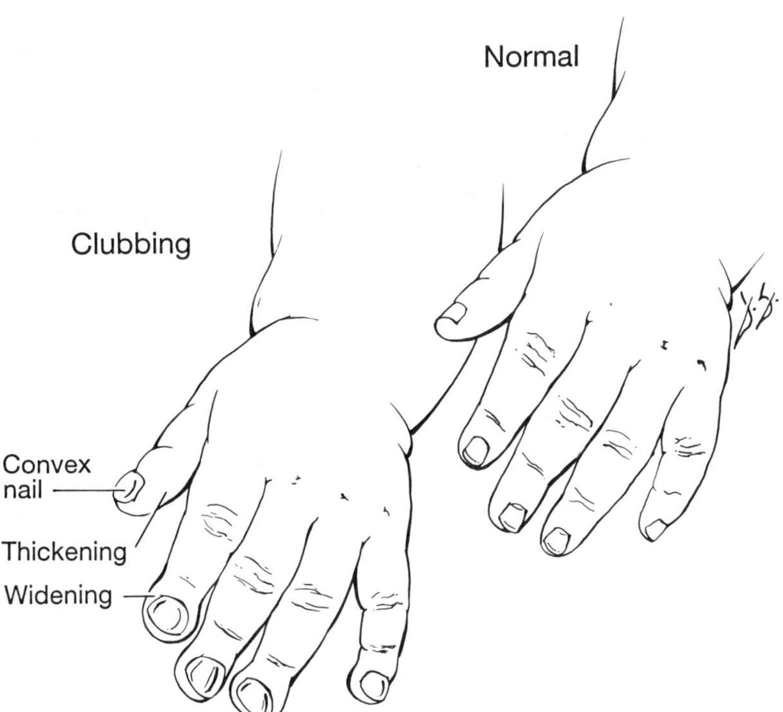

figure 30-3 *Clubbing of the fingers.*

Young children often vomit following a coughing episode and may be suspected of having gastrointestinal problems rather than respiratory problems.

Clarify statements made by caregivers concerning the child "spitting up." Make certain the spit up is from the lungs and not the stomach.

assessment of activity

Observe for signs of restlessness and anxiety; they are often the first signs of airway obstruction.

Note child's level of orientation because a decrease of oxygenated blood (*hypoxemia*) may cause impaired judgment, disorientation, combativeness, fatigue, motor incoordination, apathy, listlessness, irritability, and coma.

assessment of mucous discharge

Note the amount, color, consistency, and source of mucous drainage. An increase in thin, watery, clear, mucous discharge is expected when the mucous membrane is inflamed. Thick white, yellow, or green mucus is typical when children have respiratory infections. Scant, stringy, and sticky mucus is noted in children who are dehydrated.

history of illness

Question the caregiver as to when the child's symptoms first appeared.

Determine if previous medical attention was obtained and the compliance with prior treatment.

Question the child's general health status and health status of siblings.

Question caregiver as to the child's breathing patterns, especially periods of apnea. Discuss child's eating patterns and strength of child's crying.

nursing diagnoses

Ineffective Breathing Patterns, related to cellular oxygen deficit

Ineffective Airway Clearance, related to airway inflammation and increased mucus production

Risk for Altered Body Temperature, related to viral and bacterial infections

Risk for Fluid Volume Deficit, related to insensible fluid loss from increased respiration, diaphoresis, and reduced fluid intake

Activity Intolerance, related to disease process altering oxygen transport

Altered Growth and Development, related to repeated or prolonged hospitalization and isolation due to disease processes

Altered Family Processes, related to illness of child, expense of medications, and treatments

Knowledge Deficit, parents, related to disease, life-saving techniques, management of convalescence, and prevention of disease recurrence

Altered Health Maintenance, related to apnea in high-risk infants

Anxiety, related to respiratory distress

Anxiety of parents, related to child's illness

planning and intervention

The exchange of oxygen and carbon dioxide are essential to life; consequently, it is important to plan the nursing care around increasing respiratory effectiveness.

promoting normal breathing patterns

Enhance the child's respiratory effectiveness by administering prescribed medications and oxygen therapy.
Monitor respiration rate and breath sounds.
Place in a semi-Fowler's position.
Elevate the head of the crib or bed, and place infants older than 6 months in infant seats to facilitate breathing. It is more appropriate to elevate a small infant at approximately a 90-degree angle with adequate support to back and head so that the infant is not able to slump and put pressure on the diaphragm.
Avoid overstretching the neck in a backward direction (hyperextension).
Observe for periods when the child is not breathing, known as apnea. If apnea occurs, stimulate the infant by stroking soles of feet, back, and chest.
Provide a cool environment, because cool, moist air promotes easier breathing than warm, dry air. A fan used to circulate room air may benefit older children.

promoting oxygen therapy

Administer and monitor oxygen as prescribed by the doctor.
Comply with agency's safety protocol for use of incubator and oxygen equipment.
Carefully assess ordered liter flow, blood gas reports, pulse oximetry, and equipment safety.
Monitor pulse oximeter sensor placement on the hand, finger, feet, or toe. Oxygen values should not drop lower than 95%.
Observe the pulse oximeter sight for circulation impairment. Be alert for burns and blisters from the electrode and skin reactions to the adhesive ring. The pulse oximeter sensor must be wrapped tightly enough to reduce sensitivity to movement yet not too tightly to constrict blood flow.
Provide humidified air as ordered to help relieve dyspnea and laryngospasm and thin mucous secretions.
Check for a build-up of mist inside a mist tent or croupette.
Comply with agency safety protocol for use of oxygen equipment.
Follow agency protocol for care of a child who has been intubated. Intubation is insertion of an endotracheal tube through the nose or mouth to maintain an open airway and is most always done by a doctor or a specially trained registered nurse.
Inspect the child's facial area for signs of irritation when an endotracheal tube or oxygen equipment is secured with tape.

promoting effective airway clearance

Suction child if the gag and coughing reflexes are weak. Nose or mouth suctioning is typically done on an as needed basis to remove excessive or thick mucus and in the presence of noisy breath sounds. Bulb syringe suctioning is recommended for nose and mouth suctioning of infants. Normal saline nose drops are effective for thinning mucus before suctioning. When suctioning an infant, first suction the mouth, then the nose. Suction mucus from the nose before bottle or breastfeedings.
Change position frequently; this helps promote coughing.
Provide postural drainage and chest physiotherapy (Fig. 30-4).
Encourage fluids to keep secretions from becoming thick and sticky.

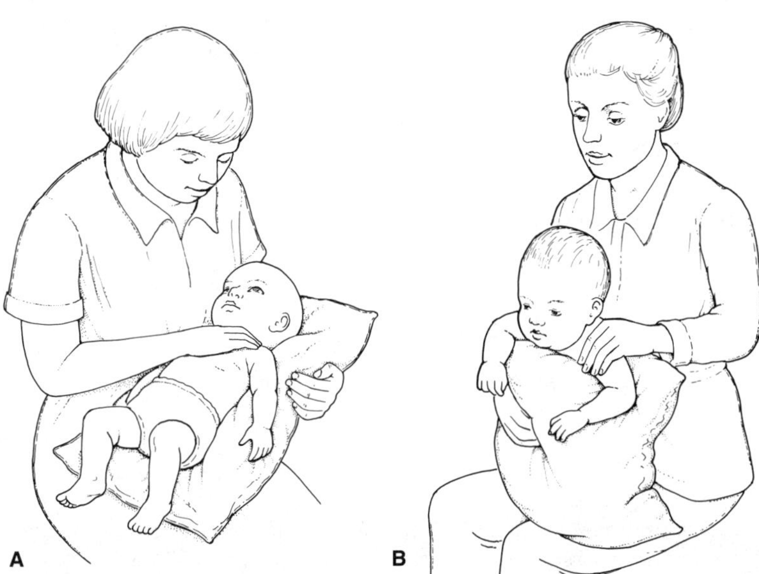

figure 30-4 *Postural drainage/chest physiotherapy relies on positioning of the body to enhance mucous drainage.*

The following actions can cause bronchospasm or blockage and must be avoided:
Making a child lie flat
Forcing a child to drink
Looking down a child's throat using a tongue depressor

promoting normal body temperature

Monitor and document temperature every 2 to 4 hours. Encourage the use of cool cotton clothing, and remove extra clothing or blankets that may hold in body heat if temperature is elevated.
Change wet clothing and bed linen to keep the child dry.
Maintain room temperature between 20° and 21°C (68° and 70°F).
Administer antipyretics and tepid water sponge baths as ordered. Tepid sponge baths may be ordered for temperature readings more than 39.4°C (103°F) unless contraindicated by physician. Sponge baths have not always proven to be an effective way to lower the temperature; in some cases, a tepid bath can actually increase the child's temperature from the chilling effect it has on the body. Increases in pulse and respiration rates are noted with temperature elevation.
Observe for seizure activity with temperature elevations above 38.8°C (102°F). Seizure precautions include padding crib sides or side rails and having oxygen and suction equipment available.
Administer antibiotics as prescribed.
Monitor white blood count and blood, throat, or sputum cultures.
Monitor the temperature of incubators and warmers because they are often used during respiratory distress in newborns and small infants. A neutral thermal environment helps the neonate maintain a normal core temperature of 36.0° to 36.5°C. (96.8°–97.7°F) with minimal oxygen consumption and caloric expenditure. Heat loss in small children contributes to shock. The temperature of incubators varies with the amount of time portholes are open.
Warming an infant too quickly can cause periods of apnea. Proper warming can be done by setting the incubator temperature 1.2°C (2°F) above the infant's body temperature.

promoting hydration

Monitor and record accurate intake and output as ordered. Routine intake and output are documented every 8 hours.
Monitor and document signs of dehydration by checking skin turgor, fontanel (sunken fontanel reflects dehydration in newborns and infants), dark circles under the eyes, and mucous membrane integrity.
Note specific drugs that have a diuretic action, such as theophylline.
Assess the parenteral fluid infusion site, and report and record any redness or edema and complaints of pain. When a scalp vein is used as an infusion site, shaved hair is saved for the family caregiver.
Weigh infant every 8 hours, and record (using the same scale if possible to reduce possibility of errors).
Be aware of electrolyte imbalances associated with fluid loss (especially sodium and potassium; see Appendix for normal values).
Report vital sign changes, such as low blood pressure and increased heart or respiratory rate seen in hypovolemic shock, to the charge nurse.

promoting activity

Monitor child's activity and agitation level; report any changes to the charge nurse.
Handle the infant gently with support to the head and neck.
Turn and reposition the child every 1 to 2 hours to promote bronchial drainage and expansion of all lung fields.
Place crib mobiles in different parts of the crib to stimulate interest and encourage movement.

promoting normal growth and development

Teach parents about normal growth and development patterns, and emphasize importance of continued family attachment. Provide age-appropriate toys and activities.

promoting home care

Recognize parent anxieties.
Encourage parents to express feelings and concerns about home care.
Observe for parental fatigue, and intervene by offering to stay with the child while parents take a break.
Assist family to identify support people and establish a support system.
Encourage parents to discuss the child's disease and possible emergency situations.
Observe parents' involvement with the child and type of coping skills used.
Demonstrate infant care techniques, such as holding, feeding, diapering, soothing, and stimulating respirations.
Provide parents, older siblings, and other caregivers with information about CPR.
Answer questions concerning discharge planning, including how to reach the pediatrician or nurse practitioner 24 hours a day; reach available emergency services in the area; measure the infant's temperature and weight; detect signs of respiratory distress, such as dyspnea and cyanosis; administer prescribed medications; and maintain a safe environment when home oxygen administration is ordered, especially the importance of not smoking when oxygen is on and avoiding friction toys and nylon clothing.
Emphasize the importance of keeping follow-up appointments with the physician.

evaluation

Respiratory status is improved. The child has no signs of respiratory distress.

The child is afebrile and well hydrated with moist mucous membranes; intake and output are balanced, and weight gain is evident.

Parents verbalize an understanding of diagnosis, treatment, home care, and follow-up care of the child.

Parents demonstrate minimal anxiety by their relaxed behavior toward treatments and medication administration.

diagnostic tests

Diagnosis of respiratory infections is usually based on a complete history, physical examination, and pertinent laboratory tests. Nasal secretion cultures are often used to confirm a diagnosis of *respiratory syncytial virus* (RSV; see p. 484). Throat cultures and rapid identification tests determine the presence of beta-hemolytic streptococcal infections when the child complains of a sore throat.

> **nursing alert**
> *Nose and throat cultures only reveal organisms present in the upper respiratory tract. Pneumonia cannot be diagnosed by this means.*

Sputum cultures can be used to determine bacterial infections in older children. However, expectorated sputum is rarely available from children younger than 5 to 6 years. Young children tend to have difficulty understanding the concept of expectorating mucus and are more likely to swallow it.

A *complete blood count* (CBC) is ordered to determine the body's response to infection. An elevated white count is expected in the presence of an infectious process. The normal number of white blood cells is higher in infancy and early childhood (5,000-19,000) than later in life (see Appendix).

Pulmonary function tests are usually not done on small children because most children are not able to perform the maneuvers before the age of 5 to 7 years. These tests are often ordered for older children diagnosed with CF or asthma.

Bronchoscopy examination is visualization of the bronchi through a bronchoscope, enabling the doctor to visualize the bronchial tree. A bronchoscopy is often necessary when a child aspirates a foreign object into the upper respiratory tract. The foreign object can be removed with forceps that fit down into the bronchoscope. The bronchoscopic examination requires that the child's throat be anesthetized. After the bronchoscopic examination, the child's gag reflex needs to be checked before giving liquids, food, or medication by mouth.

> **nursing alert**
> *The absence of a gag reflex can be noted 30 to 60 minutes after a bronchoscopy, putting the child at risk for aspiration.*

Chest x-ray examinations are ordered for children suspected of having pneumonia because the x-ray will reveal areas of infiltration or consolidation of the lung. Chest x-rays also are used to locate foreign objects in the lower respiratory tract. Infants and small children are often unable to take a breath and hold it when instructed, making it difficult to obtain a clear image on a chest x-ray.

Blood gas studies are used to determine the effectiveness of the child's breathing. Arterial blood gases (ABGs) indicate PO_2, partial pressure of oxygen in arterial blood; PCO_2, partial pressure of carbon dioxide in arterial blood; O_2 saturation, the percentage of hemoglobin-carrying oxygen; pH, the acid–base balance of the blood; HCO_3, the bicarbonate concentration in blood; and base excess, bicarbonate available for buffering (Table 30-2).

table 30-2 arterial blood gas information

Measurement	*Definition*	*Normal Range*	*Special Considerations*
PaO_2	Partial pressure of oxygen in arterial blood	80–100	Readings <80 indicate hypoxemia or hypoxia; O_2 therapy needed.
Sao_2	Percent saturation of hemoglobin with oxygen in arterial blood	Greater than 95%	Determined by blood gasses and pulse oximetry; less than 95% stimulate respirations or give O_2 as ordered.
$PaCO_2$	Partial pressure of carbon dioxide in arterial blood	35–45 mm Hg	Changes in $PaCO_2$ cause an equal and opposite change in PaO_2 (eg, $>PaCO_2$, $<PaO_2$).
pH	Hydrogen ion concentration in the blood	7.35–7.45	Lower pH reflects respiratory acidosis; higher pH reflects respiratory alkalosis.

Specimens for blood gas studies are obtained from the umbilical cord in newborns. The temporal artery may be used as a site in young infants, and the radial artery is often used for older children. In small children, when it is impossible to obtain arterial blood directly, heel or finger sticks may be used.

Oxygen therapy is based on ABG readings. The percentage of oxygen in normal room is approximately 21%. When adequate oxygen cannot reach the bloodstream because of obstructive lung disease, the amount of oxygen in hemoglobin is decreased. When children cannot rid the body of carbon dioxide, they show an increase in the partial pressure of carbon dioxide, often reflected by cyanosis of the skin and mucous membranes.

acute upper airway obstruction

Upper airway obstruction is always critical in young children because they have proportionately smaller airways than adults. Typical upper airway disorders of children are the common cold and acute laryngotracheobronchitis, more commonly known as croup.

Young children tend to be more susceptible to inflammation of the upper respiratory tract than older children, increasing their risk for airway narrowing and obstruction. Male infants tend to have a more difficult time with respiratory infections and airway obstruction than female infants. The exact reason is unknown, although young girls are thought to have larger airways than boys.

Obstruction of the upper airway in children may be caused by swelling due to viral infections, bacterial infections, or the presence of a foreign body in the nose or mouth. Young children have a tendency to place small toys, beans, marbles, and so forth in their noses and mouths as a means of exploring the world.

nursing alert

Tiny fingers can remove glued eyes on stuffed toys and place them in the mouth, increasing the risk of aspiration.

acute nasopharyngitis (common cold)

The common cold is one of the most frequent viral infectious conditions of childhood. Infants and preschool children have the highest incidence of colds, occurring more frequently in the early spring and fall. Ear and lung infections result from secondary bacterial invasion of the tissues. Congested nasal passages interfere with breathing and nutritional intake.

pathophysiology

Rhinoviruses account for approximately one third of all colds. There are more than 200 other viruses that can cause a cold. Group A hemolytic *Streptococcus* is the chief cause of bacterial colds.

Viral infections are spread by droplets and direct contacts by the infected child's sneezing, coughing, or spitting mucus. Cold viruses can live up to 72 hours. Infections can be spread by young children sharing toys that have been contaminated by a cold virus or by bacteria.

medical management

Medical intervention for a cold is aimed at relief of symptoms, which include elevated temperature, anorexia, vomiting, diarrhea, sneezing, runny nose and eyes, sore throat, and coughing. Antipyretics, such as acetaminophen (Tylenol), are given for temperature elevation; aspirin and aspirin products are contraindicated. Nose drops and gentle suctioning are used to thin and remove mucus in the nose. Most children experiencing a cold are managed at home.

nursing insight

When preschool children have a runny nose and have not learned how to blow, have them hold a tissue to their nose, and ask them to blow out a pretend candle through the nose instead of the mouth.

nursing alert

The use of aspirin is not acceptable for children because of the link between the ingestion of salicylates and Reye's syndrome, an acute and frequently fatal illness in children.

acute laryngotracheobronchitis (croup)

Most cases of *croup* are caused by viral infections; a few cases are caused by allergens and bacteria. Croup is a common syndrome involving inflammation or edema of the subglottic tissue (Fig. 30-5).

Croup is frequently seen in children 3 months to 3 years of age. There is a slightly higher tendency for boys to be affected than girls. Croup occurs all year, but the number of cases tends to increase in cold weather and in areas with cold climates, such as the northeastern United States, because children are exposed to dry room air caused by forced air heating. Croup can be classified as *viral* or *spasmodic*. A lateral neck x-ray will confirm the diagnosis by showing a narrowed airway in the subglottic area, which looks like a church steeple or sharpened pencil point. This is often referred to as the "steeple sign" or "pencil sign."

pathophysiology

Viral croup has a gradual onset following a 2- to 3-day history of upper respiratory infection. The respiratory distress caused by viral croup is due to swelling in the sub-

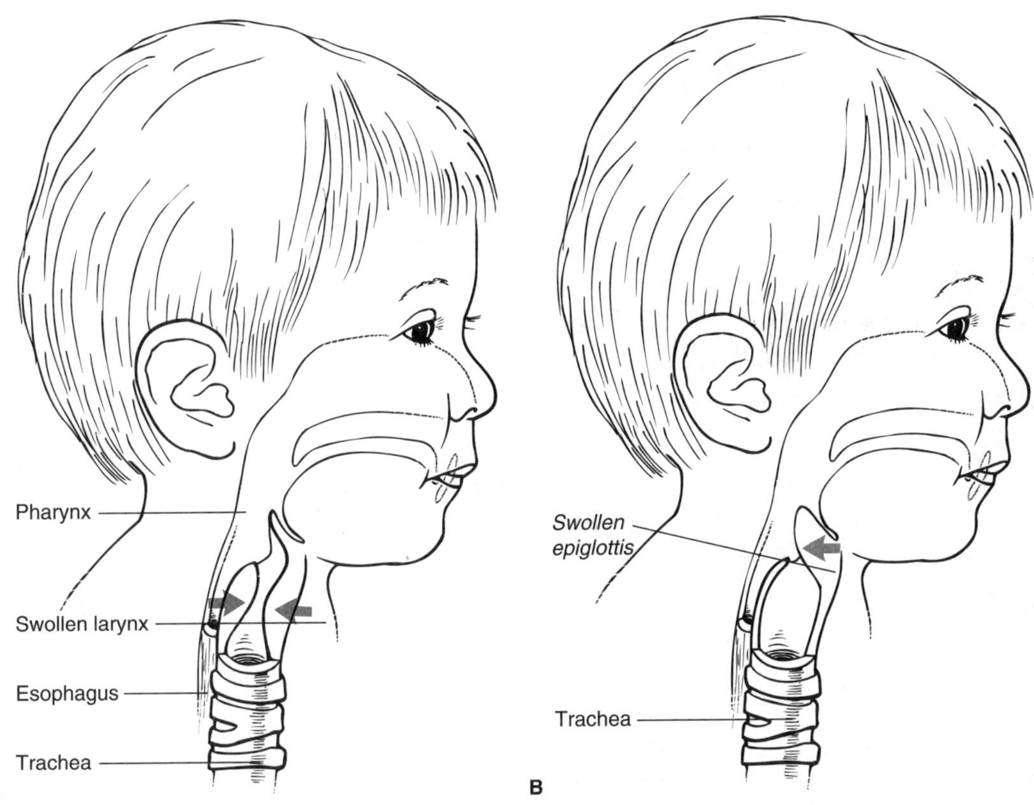

figure 30-5 *Airways in croup and epiglottitis.* ***(A)*** *Croup is a virus that causes swelling of the larnyx lining and results in airway obstruction.* ***(B)*** *Epiglottitis is a bacterial infection that causes severe swelling of the epiglottis.*

glottic area, which is normally the narrowest part of the respiratory tree in infants.

Spasmodic croup has a sudden onset without an upper respiratory tract infection preceding the illness. The etiology is believed to be allergic; however, viruses may be a cause.

Croup is characterized by drooling, indicating difficulty swallowing (*dysphagia*); nasal congestion; and mucus drainage, interfering with the infant's ability to suck. Other symptoms include a harsh, barky cough; hoarseness; and *stridor* (a harsh, shrill sound caused by obstructed airflow in the larynx or trachea, audible during inspiration).

medical management

Most children with croup are managed at home with a cool mist vaporizer and careful observation of fluid intake to prevent dehydration. Antipyretic medication (nonaspirin, such as acetaminophen) is given if fever is present. Epinephrine may be ordered by the physician and is usually given by nebulization. Nebulized epinephrine provides temporary relief of airway obstruction by constricting the blood vessels and reducing edema (see Table 30-4 on page 491). Antibiotics are not indicated unless a bacterial infection is present. Hospital admission with oxygen therapy is necessary when the child experiences severe respiratory distress.

 **nursing alert**

Water left in vaporizers is an excellent reservoir for bacteria growth and can lead to reinfections. Vaporizers need to be emptied and cleaned thoroughly after use.

influenza (flu)

Type A influenza is the most fatal form of this viral infection. It occurs every 2 to 3 years with a new strain appearing every 10 to 15 years. *Haemophilus influenzae* type B (HIB) is the most common cause of infection in children between the ages of 3 months and 3 years.

pathophysiology

The incubation period for influenza is from 1 to 3 days. A child with influenza is contagious up to 24 hours before symptoms appear and until 7 days after the onset of symptoms. Influenza is transmitted either directly, through inhalation of respiratory droplets from an infected person, or indirectly, through contact with a contaminated object, such as a toy. The symptoms include fever, sudden onset of chills, malaise, headache, muscle ache, a nonproductive cough, conjunctivitis, laryngitis, and runny nose. Frequently, the major symptoms subside in about 5 days, but a cough and weakness may continue.

medical management

Diagnosis of HIB is based on history and physical examination, nose and throat cultures, and increased serum antibody titers. Hospitalization is seldom required unless there are complications. Complications include meningitis and epiglottitis.

Treatment is supportive and includes bed rest, increased fluid intake, and administration of analgesic-antipyretics and expectorants. Acetaminophen is given for fever. Prophylactic antibiotics are sometimes used to prevent secondary infections. Amantadine (an antiviral agent) is helpful in reducing the severity of type A influenza.

Immunization with HIB conjugate vaccine is given at 2, 4, and 6 months of age. The number of HIB cases has declined since 1985 when the vaccine was introduced.

nursing care

Nursing measures include palliative care, such as rest, increased fluid intake, proper nutrition, and administration of prescribed medications for complaints of discomfort, presence of elevated temperature, and cough. Patient, parents, and siblings are instructed about the importance of handwashing after contact with body secretions, not eating or drinking after each other, and covering the mouth and nose when coughing or sneezing.

epiglottitis

Epiglottitis is a bacterial infection of the epiglottis commonly caused by HIB. Epiglottitis causes airway obstruction. It is an acute and potentially fatal infection causing edema of the epiglottis and obstruction of the airway (see Fig. 30-5*B*).

This disease is seen mostly in toddlers and school-age children. It accounts for about 10% of laryngeal infections in young children. It can be seen more commonly in boys than in girls at any time and in any geographic location.

pathophysiology

Epiglottitis occurs in children who have been well or mildly ill with an upper respiratory infection. The disease has a sudden onset and rapid progression of respiratory difficulty, often within 2 to 4 hours after onset. The appearance of the epiglottis is cherry red and swollen. Dysphagia causes drooling. Temperature elevation may be noted with readings of 39° to 40°C (102.2°–104°F). Septicemia can develop as a secondary problem.

medical management

Epiglottis is a serious and deadly condition unless diagnosed quickly. The diagnosis is based on history, physical examination, and direct visualization of the epiglottis under anesthesia. A throat culture is not done because it may stimulate laryngospasm, resulting in respiratory obstruction. A lateral neck x-ray will show an enlarged round epiglottis that looks like an adult thumb print, called "thumb sign."

A patent airway must be established quickly, either by endotracheal tube or tracheostomy. Intravenous antibiotics are instituted for 7 to 10 days. Oxygen administration is based on ABG reports and pulse oximetry data.

lower respiratory conditions

respiratory syncytial virus infections

Respiratory syncytial virus is a myxovirus that accounts for the majority of lower respiratory infections, including bronchiolitis and pneumonia, in children younger than 2 years. RSV infections almost always require the child to be hospitalized. Unfortunately, RSV is highly contagious and can be easily spread by contact with infected secretions. The virus can live up to 30 minutes on inanimate objects. RSV infections can occur in epidemics during winter and early spring. The infection can be seen at any age but most often is seen in infants and children younger than 2 years. Transplacental passage of maternal antibodies against RSV does not appear to provide complete protection for the newborn.

pathophysiology

RSV begins as an upper respiratory infection with symptoms of fever, otitis media, and conjunctivitis. The disease can progress quickly to include the lower respiratory tract. Symptoms of croup, bronchiolitis, bronchitis, and pneumonia are common. Often, there is a related *otitis media* (infection of the middle ear).

Exposure to the RSV can occur during coughing or sneezing. It is not an airborne disease but is communicable by direct contact, such as playing with contaminated toys.

medical management

Diagnosis of RSV can be made on clinical symptoms, although it is sometimes difficult to differentiate between other viruses during peak seasons for virus infections (especially winter). A specific test called *enzyme immune assay* can be done on nasal secretions for a confirmed diagnosis of RSV. Results of this test can be obtained within 6 hours in most hospitals.

The treatment of RSV depends on the severity of the disease. The treatment for mild, uncomplicated RSV is palliative. Assisting the child to breathe is a major goal. Hospitalization of the child is indicated if the respiration rate exceeds 50 to 60 per minute, hypoxemia is present, and nutrition is altered.

Hypoxemia is treated by the administration of moisturized oxygen through oxygen mist tents (croupettes) or humidifiers. Analgesics and antipyretics are ordered for discomfort and temperature elevation. Medications, such as antihistamines, expectorants, and sedatives, are usually not given because they are ineffective. Antibiotics may be given to prevent or treat the presence of secondary bacterial infections. Fluids are given either by mouth or intravenous infusion to prevent dehydration and loosen respiratory secretions. Severe cases of RSV may require intubation, mechanical ventilation, invasive monitoring, and intensive care nursing.

The medication ribavirin (Virazole) is given to high-risk children with serious RSV infections and children at high risk for getting the virus. Ribavirin is a broad-spectrum antiviral agent that inhibits viral reaction. This drug is administered in aerosol form through oxygen equipment, such as oxyhoods, mist tents, masks, or mechanical ventilators.

nursing care

When administering ribavirin, it is important to inspect the oxygen delivery system because the small particles of medication tend to clog tubing, obstructing the flow of oxygen. The child's reaction to ribavirin and any adverse reactions need to be noted and reported. Signs need to be posted to alert caregivers or visitors who are pregnant that aerosol ribavirin is considered harmful to the unborn child.

bronchiolitis

Acute bronchiolitis is often referred to as *acute interstitial pneumonia*. There tends to be a high incidence of bronchiolitis in young children who have been exposed to upper respiratory viral infections. RSV is a causative agent in more than 50% of bronchiolitis infections.

pathophysiology

Bronchiolitis causes the bronchi and bronchioles to become plugged with thick mucus, making it difficult for the child to inhale or exhale. Breath sounds are diminished and an expiratory wheeze can be heard. The onset of bronchiolitis is marked by sudden dyspnea with cyanosis and a dry, persistent cough. There is often a low-grade temperature of 38.3° to 38.9°C (101°–102°F).

medical management

Diagnosis and medical management for bronchiolitis are similar to that for RSV infections. Treatment includes administration of oxygen using a hood or tent. Nasal oxygen and mist tents are not indicated because they may cause reflex bronchoconstriction. Bronchodilators are prescribed to relieve bronchospasms, and ribavirin is used to inhibit the viral reaction. Postural drainage may be ordered to promote drainage of pulmonary secretions (see Fig. 30-4).

pneumonia

Pneumonia is a lower respiratory tract infection that can be caused by bacterial, viral, fungal, or mycoplasmal organisms. Early recognition of pneumonia can make the difference between simple home treatment or more intensive care requiring hospitalization. Older children with pneumococcal pneumonia tend to receive care at home; infants or young children are typically admitted to the hospital for treatment. Pneumonia requires prompt treatment to avoid serious complications.

There is a higher incidence of pneumonia in infancy and early childhood and a lower incidence noted in school-age children and teenagers. Pneumococcal pneumonia is the most common form of bacterial pneumonia found among infants and children. Infants with pneumococcal pneumonia have bronchial involvement rather than the lobar type seen with older children.

pathophysiology

Pneumonia is an inflammation or infection of the pulmonary tissue. Significant clinical symptoms of pneumonia include cough, dyspnea, tachypnea, cyanosis, diminished breath sounds, and crackling breath sounds (*rales*). The course of the illness depends on the causative agent, age, and reaction of the child and the degree of bronchial obstruction. Chest x-ray findings may not support the clinical findings of pneumonia until later in the disease process. During the initial onset of pneumonia, abnormal breath sounds are audible, indicating the presence of respiratory disease, although visible changes in lung tissue are minimal. During the latter stages of pneumonia, abnormal breath sounds are minimal or not present, although the x-ray findings clearly demonstrate pulmonary changes resulting from pneumonia. The white blood cell count usually is not elevated in viral and mycoplasmal pneumonia but is elevated in bacterial pneumonia (see Appendix).

Bacterial pneumonia is caused by *Streptococcus pneumoniae*, *Staphylococcus*, and *Chlamydia*. Pneumococcal and staphylococcal pneumonias are the most common. The alveoli become inflamed in bacterial pneumonia, and fluid containing fibrin, bacteria, leukocytes, and erythrocytes leaks into the interstitial space, filling the alveolar sacs. The sputum expectorated is rust colored and considered a cardinal symptom of pneumonia.

Pneumocystis carinii pneumonia occurs as an opportunistic infection in children with altered immunity resulting from congenital immunodeficiency, cancer treatment, or infection with human immunodeficiency virus (HIV) or acquired immunodeficiency syndrome (AIDS). This type of pneumonia is transmitted from person to person. Symptoms include a diffuse pneumonitis with dyspnea at rest, tachypnea, cough, fever, and decreased ability to exchange oxygen and carbon dioxide. Chest radiographs show infiltration of both lungs.

medical management

Treatment of pneumonia is symptomatic. The child is given antipyretics for fever and discomfort. Intravenous therapy may be ordered if symptoms of dehydration are present. Intravenous infusion of antibiotics also may be indicated in the treatment of bacterial pneumonia. Antibiotics are usually not ordered for viral pneumonia unless as a prophylaxis to prevent secondary infection.

The sudden onset of high fever seen in pneumonia can cause "fever convulsions." Medical management is aimed at reducing the child's fever and controlling seizure activity. Oxygen therapy is based on clinical findings of cyanosis, oxygen blood levels, and pulse oximetry data. Postural drainage is ordered to facilitate drainage of purulent secretions.

chronic respiratory conditions

cystic fibrosis

CF is a complex, inherited disorder. It is genetically transmitted as an autosomal recessive trait and is considered the most common severe autosomal recessive disease in the white population. One in 20 Americans is a silent carrier of the defect, and if two carriers conceive a child, that child has a one-in-four chance of having CF. As carriers, the parents are not directly affected by the disease.

CF occurs in approximately 1 in 2,000 white children in the United States. The incidence in African Americans is 1 in 17,000 (Marks, 1994). The male to female ratio is 3 : 1. CF is a generalized disorder causing major dysfunction of all *exocrine glands* (glands that secrete externally through one or more ducts, such as sweat glands). Although the disease affects multiple organs, approximately 50% of CF children have lung involvement, resulting in *bronchiectasis* (dilatation and destruction of the bronchial walls) and eventually death.

Cardiovascular system involvement in CF includes right-sided heart enlargement and congestive heart failure resulting from obstruction of pulmonary blood flow, known as *cor pulmonale.* As infants mature, their problems related to CF increase to include gallbladder dysfunction with gallbladder stone formation; reproductive system dysfunction, such as infertility in males due to decreased sperm production and infertility in females due to the presence of thick, tenacious cervical mucus; and visual field defects, such as optic atrophy.

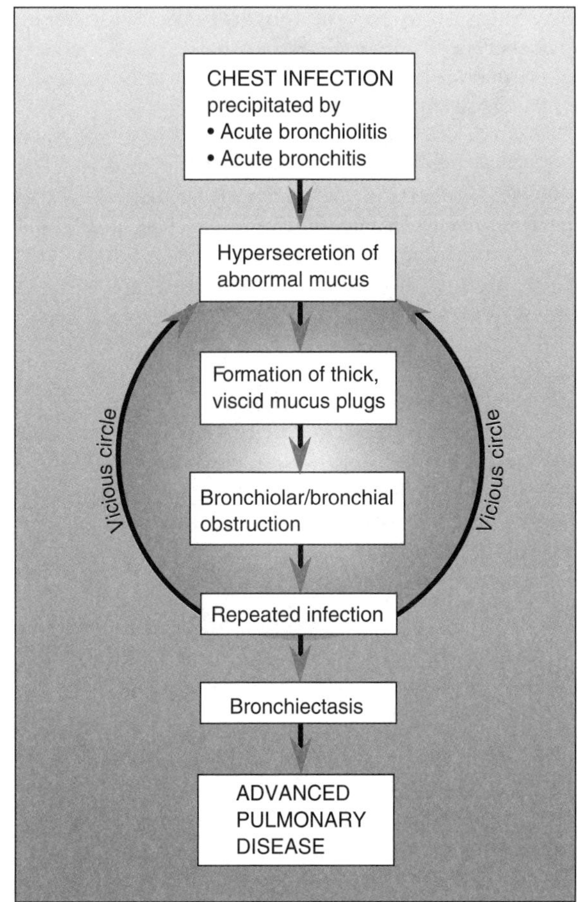

figure 30-6 *Basic pathophysiology of cystic fibrosis.*

pathophysiology

CF occurs when the child lacks CF protein. CF protein normally directs the flow of chloride molecules across the cell membrane. Lack of CF protein causes the following changes: The movement of chloride and sodium molecules in the body is disrupted, the body's water balance is disrupted, potassium and calcium levels are elevated, and mucus builds up to dangerous levels in the lungs and in the organs of the gastrointestinal system (Fig. 30-6).

In children with CF, large volumes of thick, dry secretions are produced by the bronchial mucous glands. These thick secretions obstruct the airways, contributing to the development of *bronchiectasis.* Meconium ileus is the presenting symptom of CF in newborns who later develop additional symptoms. The presence of thick, sticky meconium resulting from depletion or absence of pancreatic enzymes causes a bowel obstruction.

Sodium and chloride become trapped in the lung cell lining in CF children. The trapped salt draws water from airways and dehydrates the mucus to a thick sticky consistency. Infectious bacteria thrive in the mucus and destroy fragile tissue, eventually leading to pulmonary failure and death. CF is described in stages, beginning with an acute phase and progressing to a chronic phase.

In 1992, researchers conducted studies on a gene linked with CF. Researchers claim evidence that CF genes can be efficiently transferred into the CF patient's airway to correct the physiologic effects of CF disease. This information gives hope to all people affected by the disease. More research is needed with human subjects, but the future for CF patients is much more promising than in the past. At present, the average life span for an infant with CF is approximately 28 years.

diagnostic tests

Diagnosis is primarily based on clinical findings that include a family history of CF. A positive *sweat chloride test* result confirms the diagnosis. *Pilocarpine iontophoresis sweat test* results indicating high sodium and chloride levels in perspiration indicate CF (>60 mEq/L). Chest x-ray findings may be normal initially but later show increased areas of infection and generalized obstructive emphysema. Stool analysis is positive for steatorrhea (bulky and greasy stools with a distinctively foul odor). Newborns suspected of having CF are tested with a meconium strip test for increases of lactose and protein content. Blood gas studies often show a decreased oxygen saturation in children with CF.

Frequent respiratory infections, chronic cough, and poor growth can indicate a CF condition. Parents may report that the infant's kisses taste salty. Infants with CF are always hungry, tend to swallow air during feeding, and are often diagnosed as having colic. An important differentiation from colic and CF is the characteristic bulky, foul-smelling stools.

medical management

Currently, children with CF are treated with palliative measures directed to four major goals:

1. Maintaining a patent airway through postural drainage, chest percussion, and bronchodilator therapy
2. Controlling pulmonary infections with antibiotic therapy
3. Maintaining electrolyte balance, especially sodium and chloride, by adding extra salt to the diet or using salt tablets
4. Maintaining adequate nutritional status by giving predigested protein formulas high in carbohydrates and protein with no restriction of fats, commercially prepared pancreatic enzymes during meals or snacks to aid digestion and absorption of fat and protein, and supplemental vitamins (especially fat-soluble vitamins) to promote growth

Future treatment of children with CF will include CF replacement.

nursing care

assessment Assessment of the child with CF includes the assessments discussed on page 476 for respiratory diseases plus close observation of any side effects of drug therapy.

Objective assessment data include the child's reaction to prescribed medication; amount, color, frequency, consistency, and presence of fat (steatorrhea) in the stools; and dietary management.

nursing diagnoses

* Risk for Ineffective Airway Clearance, related to inability to clear mucus from tract
* Altered Nutrition: Less than body requirements, related to inability to digest fat
* Impaired Gas Exchange, related to thick respiratory system secretions
* Risk for Respiratory Infection, related to thick mucus blocking air passages

planning and intervention

* Perform chest physiotherapy (postural drainage and chest percussion) every 4 hours per order between meals (avoid treatment before and after meals).
* Provide high-protein, high-calorie, carbohydrate and sodium diet, and keep calorie diary. Administer prescribed medications, such as salt tablets and antibiotics, and pancreatic enzymes (given with food).

> **✳ nursing insight**
>
> *Postural drainage for young children can be a game if the child is physically strong enough. The game involves playing "wheelbarrow." The child gets into a crawling position, and the nurse grasps the child's legs and moves him or her around the floor like a wheelbarrow.*

evaluation

* Child's airway will remain patent during the course of the illness.
* Child's height and weight follow percentile growth curves.
* There is no fat in the stool.

sudden infant death syndrome

SIDS is the sudden, unexpected death of an apparently healthy infant in which autopsy fails to identify the cause. SIDS is the leading cause of death in babies older than 1 week and has affected infants for thousands of years. The infant with SIDS apparently stops breathing during sleep and dies. There are no cries or other sounds of distress before death occurs.

The cause of SIDS remains a mystery, despite 20 years of research. Although SIDS can strike without warning, some infants at risk can be identified. Risk factors include prematurity, a history of apnea (possibly related to seizures, gastroesophageal reflux, anemia, sepsis, or maternal substance abuse, especially cocaine or methadone addiction), and a family history of SIDS. Infants at risk can be placed on apnea monitors so that parents will be alerted if the infant stops breathing and can begin resuscitation.

Until recently, many pediatricians advised parents to put their infant to sleep on its stomach. In 1994, however, the National Institute of Child Health and Human Development recommended that infants be placed on their backs or on their sides to sleep, rather than on their stomachs. This recommendation was based on studies in New Zealand, Britain, Australia, and Norway indicating that SIDS deaths could be reduced by 50% by placing infants on their backs. Parents and other family caregivers need to be cautioned about the importance of the infant's sleeping position.

Soft, fluffy pillows, blankets, mattresses, and comforters also are believed to increase the risk of SIDS. As babies breath into the soft bedding, they saturate it with carbon dioxide and then inhale the trapped gas. Parents need to understand the importance of this simple precaution about bedding.

Apneic episodes are nonbreathing periods of more than 20 seconds accompanied by a heart rate below 100 with cyanosis of the skin and mucous membranes; the episodes require stimulation or resuscitation to restart breathing and maintain life.

SIDS occurs most frequently in infants between 2 and 3 months of age and is often preceded by a history of recent cold or upper respiratory infection. It seldom occurs before 2 weeks or after 6 months of age. SIDS is more common in boys than girls and occurs more often among twins and triplets, African Americans, Native Americans, and infants born into households of lower socioeconomic status.

pathophysiology

Most researchers agree that no single factor is responsible for a SIDS death. A 1994 study suggests that a genetically weak diaphragm may be responsible. Another study suggests that SIDS is linked to an immune system reaction. Research continues to seek more answers about the cause or causes of this tragic phenomenon (Fig. 30-7).

The SIDS infant is found by parents or other caregivers to be limp, cyanotic, without respirations, cold, and flaccid. Death from SIDS occurs most frequently between midnight and 9 AM. An autopsy is performed to verify the diagnosis.

medical management

Medical intervention is aimed at preventing SIDS, which includes identifying infants at risk and placing them on cardiopulmonary monitoring, assessing ABG values to determine abnormal oxygen and carbon dioxide exchange, chest x-ray study to assess presence of upper respiratory infections, and upper gastrointestinal study to detect reflux apnea. When stomach contents reflux into the esophagus, respirations are altered as the infant attempts to swallow the contents.

nursing care

assessment Objective data include general appearance, behavior, developmental milestones, chest examination, respiratory status, and chest auscultation.

Subjective data include caregiver's knowledge of appropriate sleeping positions and bedding for infant and ability to manage home apnea monitoring, perform CPR, and use coping mechanisms.

nursing diagnosis

- Altered Family Processes
- Knowledge Deficit, related to SIDS
- Anticipatory Grief

planning and implementation

- Provide instructions regarding home apnea monitoring.
- Inform caregivers that monitoring does not prevent SIDS.
- Refer caregivers and older siblings to appropriate community-based support groups.
- Instruct caregivers and older siblings how to initiate CPR.

• History of apnea
• Maternal substance abuse
• Placing child on stomach
• Soft fluffy pillows capable of becoming saturated with carbon dioxide
• Weak diaphragm
• Immune system reaction
Improper position
Weak diaphragm

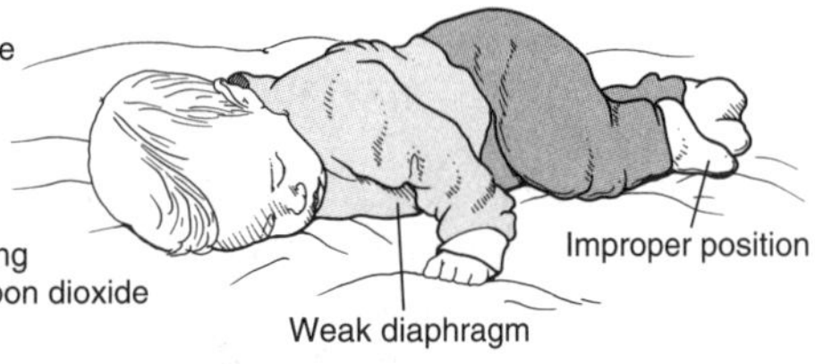

figure 30-7 *High-risk factors for sudden infant death syndrome.*

evaluation

- Family members will participate in care of the infant, demonstrating knowledge of correct sleeping position and appropriate bedding; ability to use apnea equipment, attach electrodes, and set the alarm system; and perform CPR.
- Family will maintain functional system of mutual support for each other.
- Family will seek appropriate community support as needed.

bronchopulmonary dysplasia/idiopathic respiratory distress syndrome

Bronchopulmonary dysplasia (BPD) is a chronic pulmonary disease of infancy and is a common complication of idiopathic respiratory distress syndrome. Respiratory distress syndrome of the newborn also is known as hyaline membrane disease and is caused by immaturity of the lungs at birth commonly seen in premature infants.

Infants at risk are usually premature (<32 weeks' gestation); weigh less than 1,500 g; have characteristics of tachypnea, dyspnea, hypoxemia, and hypercapnia (excess carbon dioxide in the blood); and require oxygen of more than room air (21%) at 28 days of life. Symptoms of BPD may last 1 to 2 years and sometimes longer. The mortality rate is high. Most deaths of infants with BPD result from cor pulmonale, respiratory infection, and SIDS.

The exact cause of BPD is unknown. Risk factors include the premature infant who has been mechanically ventilated, given prolonged use of high oxygen exposure and positive airway pressures, suffered meconium aspiration, or experienced persistent pulmonary hypertension. The incidence of this disorder is slightly higher in white male infants.

pathophysiology

Oxygen toxicity and trauma caused by positive-pressure ventilators are two factors considered in the development of BPD. The alveolar sacs and small airway lining become scarred, portions of lung tissue collapse, and enlargement of smooth muscle in the airway causes bronchospasms. Endothelial cell damage leads to edema. BPD usually progresses from an acute to a chronic condition.

medical management

Medical intervention is primarily aimed at preventing pulmonary hypertension, respiratory infections, and enlargement of the right ventricle of the heart as a result of hy-

nursing alert

Monitor the oxygen concentration in incubators and warmers to avoid complications from high oxygen concentrations. Oxygen concentration levels over 80 mm Hg can cause retinal vessels to constrict, resulting in hemorrhage, retinal detachment, and eventually a type of blindness known as retrolental fibroplasia. *Retrolental fibroplasia is a formation of fibrous tissue behind the lens of the eye.*

pertension of the pulmonary circulation known as *cor pulmonale.* Because pulmonary hypertension and right-sided heart failure occur in the chronic stage of BPD, fluid restriction and diuretics, such as furosemide (Lasix), are usually ordered. Research studies on infants receiving furosemide, a potent loop diuretic, have found an increase in dynamic lung compliance, decrease in total pulmonary resistance, and possible improvement of gas exchange. Long-term use of furosemide can cause adverse effects, such as urinary loss of electrolytes, diminished levels of chloride in the blood (hypochloremia), and metabolic alkalosis (pH >7.45) with secondary hypoventilation. Children taking furosemide need extra potassium, either through foods high in potassium, such as bananas or orange juice, or through potassium replacement medications.

In the acute phase, inspired oxygen concentrations, ventilator settings, and blood gas values must be carefully monitored. The infant may require additional calories to sustain weight gain of at least 10 g/kg per day and prevent growth retardation. Intravenous fluid therapy is monitored carefully to avoid overhydration. Respiratory infections must be prevented if possible.

nursing care

Subjective data include history of premature birth and repeated respiratory problems.

assessment Objective data include symptoms of right-sided heart failure, including edema of the extremities, full or edematous fontanel, periorbital edema, tachycardia (increased heart rate), feeding difficulties, weakness, weak cry, abdominal distention, rales, and wheezing.

intervention Nursing interventions specific to BPD include the following:

Gentle handling and frequent rests during postural drainage, percussion, vibration, and suctioning to help reduce trauma to the upper airway and minimize periods of hypoxia

Use of strict aseptic technique when caring for the infant with BPD to protect from infection

Careful monitoring of intake and output and daily weighing while infant is on diuretic therapy

Careful monitoring of electrolytes (especially potassium and chloride) and child's reaction to electrolyte replacement therapy.

asthma

Asthma is an obstruction or blockage of the airways that is reversible either spontaneously or with proper medication. Asthmatic children experience narrowing of the airways with difficult breathing and an audible wheezing sound on expiration from air being forced through blocked air passages. Asthma affects only the air passages, not the air sacs, as seen in emphysema.

Part of the nurse's role is to educate the child with asthma and the family in management of this chronic illness. This means helping them to separate the facts from the myths about asthma (Table 30-3).

pathophysiology

Asthma is the most common chronic medical problem in children younger than 17 years. It affects approximately 5% to 10% of the children in the United States. *Extrinsic asthma* is the allergic form of the disease; *intrinsic asthma* is the nonallergic form. In children younger than 10 years, boys have a higher incidence of asthma than girls.

table 30-3 asthma myths and facts

Myths	*Facts*
Asthma is "all in your head."	Asthma is not a psychosomatic illness. Emotional upset can trigger asthma symptoms.
Asthma is curable with proper medication.	Asthma is not curable but can be well managed with medications, such as bronchodilators.
Asthma is always due to an allergy.	The exact cause of asthma is unknown. Precipitating factors include allergies, infections, aspirin and tartrazine, exercise, irritants, foods, emotional upsets, weather conditions, and pregnancy.
Asthma is always cured by moving to another geographic location.	Factors that precipitate an asthma episode are found everywhere.
Everyone who "wheezes" is suffering from asthma.	Not everyone who wheezes has asthma. Wheezing can occur as a result of other medical conditions, such as heart problems.
Asthma is never a cause of death.	Status asthmaticus can cause death.
Asthma symptoms occur when the child is active.	Asthma symptoms tend to "flare" at night and in the early morning hours.
All children with asthma should take allergy shots.	Allergy shots are indicated when a known allergen exists.

Approximately half of all children with asthma outgrow it by 15 years as the size of the airways increases with maturity. Heredity determines whether a person has the potential for developing asthma; however, environment and allergens are predisposing factors, not causes. Allergies, infections, aspirin products, tartrazine (yellow food dye), exercise, irritants, foods (food additives such as sulfites), emotional upsets, weather conditions, and even pregnancy are among the more common factors that can precipitate asthma symptoms. The main symptom during an acute episode is shortness of breath accompanied by coughing and wheezing. The following processes are noted with an asthma attack:

* Airways become narrowed and blocked
* Bronchospasms occur as a result of muscle constriction surrounding the airways
* Airway lining becomes inflamed and edematous
* Production of mucus increases, clogging the airways
* Gas exchange is altered

medical management

Diagnosis is based on family history of allergies and history of recent infections. Information about the child's environment and exposure to irritants (especially cigarette smoke) is important. About 40% of children with severe asthma have one asthmatic parent (Jackson & Saunders, 1993). Children may show evidence of hyperinflation of the lungs, use of accessory muscles, and appearance of hunched shoulders and "pigeon chest." Eosinophil and immunoglobulin E levels used to determine allergic response are elevated in asthmatic children subject to allergies.

There are three approaches to treating asthma:

1. Administration of proper medications, such as bronchodilators (Fig. 30-8), corticosteroids, and antibiotics (Table 30-4)
2. Avoidance of substances that trigger an asthma attack
3. Desensitization to allergens using allergy injections

Treatment plans for children are based on the occurrence and severity of asthma symptoms. According to the

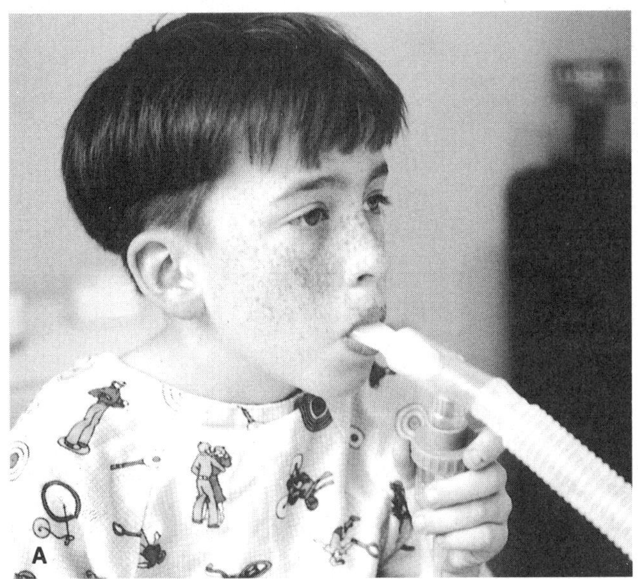

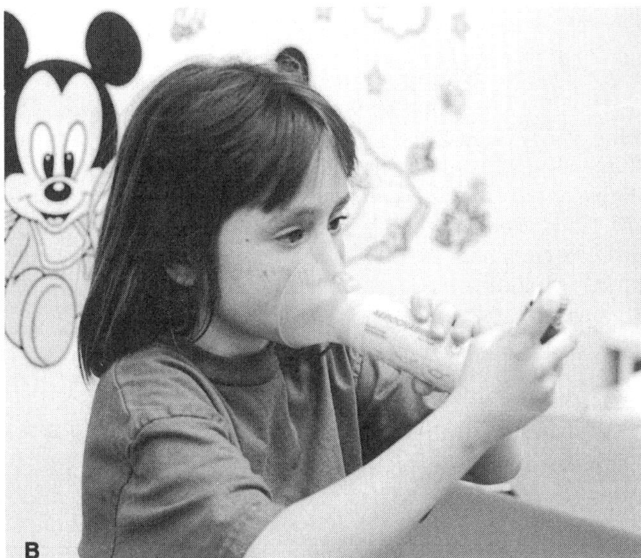

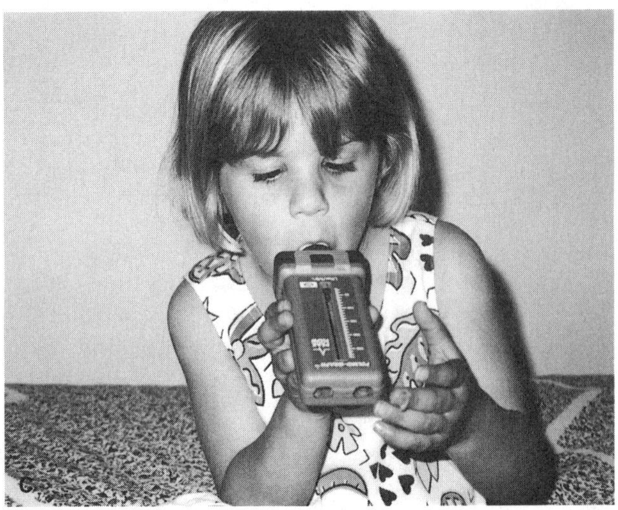

figure 30-8 *(**A**) Hand nebulizer. (**B**) Metered-dose inhaler bronchodilator with a spacer device. (**C**) Peak flow meter.*

table 30-4 asthma medications

Classification Drug/Dose/Route	*Drug Effect*	*Nursing Implications*
BRONCHODILATORS		
Epinephrine—0.01 mg/kg given subcutaneously. Epinephrine inhaler—1–2 inhalations of 1:100 or 2.25% racepinephrine (0.2 mg/dose); repeat q3h	Bronchodilation, vasoconstrictions, cardiac stimulation. Give promptly at onset of bronchospasm. Provides instant relief with short duration.	Monitor blood pressure for hypertension, pulse for tachycardia, and respiration rate. Note relief from symptoms. Note amount, color, and character or sputum.
Isuprel—1:400, 1:200, and 1:100 given per nebulizer	Bronchodilation and cardiac stimulant	Medication may tinge sputum pink or red.
Albuterol oral (liquid or tablets), age 2–6 y—0.1 mg/kg three times daily (not to exceed 4 mg 3 times daily) Inhalation—1–2 puffs q4–6 h or 2 puffs 15 min prior to exercise	Relaxes smooth muscle of bronchiole. Prevents exercise-induced bronchospasm. Does not stimulate the heart as much as adrenalin.	Assess lung sounds, pulse, and blood pressure before administration. If dose is missed, do not double dose. If child is taking more than one inhalation, albuterol must be given first, wait 5 min, and administer other medications. Have child rinse mouth with water following inhalation to reduce dry mouth.
Theophylline oral (liquid, tablet, capsule), I.V. Oral route does not give prompt bronchodilation and is used as a continuous rather than an acute mode of therapy.	Bronchodilation; relaxes muscles around the air tubes; prevents mast cells from releasing histamine, which can lead to asthma symptoms in the allergic child. Stimulates nervous system, and acts as a mild diuretic.	Monitor vital signs, blood theophylline levels. Observe for side effects, such as nausea, vomiting, diarrhea, headache. Monitor intake and output. Theophylline capsules can be broken and medication "sprinkled" on food to be tolerated better by children. Do not crush enteric-coated or time-released tablets or capsules. Force fluids to at least 2,000 mL/d.
ADRENERGIC		
Metaproterenol sulfate (Alupent) betaagonist aerosol inhalers—per order, usually 1–2 puffs q4h or prn	Relaxes bronchospasms; reduces in-flammation, edema; and mobilizes secretions. Action starts within 10 min and lasts up to 4–6 h.	Check vital signs, lung sounds. Ad-minister with food to decrease gastrointestinal upset. Force fluids. If cortisone inhaler also has been ordered, use metaproterenol first.
Terbutaline sulfate (Brethine) pill form or liquid given q6–8 h	Dilates bronchioles.	Tablet can be crushed and given with food. Can cause tremors in skeletal muscles, and child may experience an increased awareness of the heartbeat.
CORTICOSTEROID		
Prednisone, (Solu-Medrol oral), inhaled, IV—Onset of action for oral corticosteroids is approximately 3 h	Anti-inflammatory; Interrupts the development of bronchial inflammation.	Record intake and output. Assess child for edema (moon face); monitor vital signs (especially blood pressure for elevation), gastrointestinal symptoms (peptic ulcers are common), and elevated blood sugar levels. Cortisone therapy requires tapering over 5–7 d and not abruptly discontinued.
ANTIBIOTICS		
	Used for respiratory infections.	Administer antibiotic at scheduled times to maintain proper blood levels. Observe side effects specific to drug administered, such as skin rashes, especially hives.
Cromolyn sodium (Intal)—inhalation, capsules	A prophylactic agent used for bronchial asthma. Not recommended during an asthma attack—can worsen symptoms and increase risk of status asthmaticus. Decreases daily wheeze and exercise-induced asthma attacks.	Assess for signs of diarrhea, flushing, headaches, vomiting, abdominal pain, and itching. Check eyes for redness, tearing, and irritation and nose for stuffiness. Child may dislike taste of medicine; can be dissolved in water but do not mix with fruit juice, milk, or foods. Give 30 min prior to meals. Side effects are minimal unless sensitive to cromolyn sodium.

teaching guidelines
how to use a metered-dose inhaler

* Shake the inhaler vigorously with cap in place.
* Remove the cap.
* Have the child stand and remove gum or food from the mouth.
* Hold the inhaler so the mouthpiece is facing the child in a downward position, 1–2 in from the lips.
* Instruct the child to blow breath out normally, then open mouth and begin to breathe in as you press the top of the medication container.
* Instruct the child to hold his or her breath as long as possible, at least for 10 seconds. School-age children can make a fist and use their fingers to count to 10 mentally and physically; when all their fingers are pointing out, they blow their breath out. When children are having difficulty holding their breath, they can be encouraged by saying, "You did five fingers yesterday. Can you try for more today?"
* Let breath out slowly through the nose or puckered lips without straining.
* Instruct the child to relax, then repeat as many times as the physician orders.
* Remember that morning and evening treatments are especially important to help open the airways and clear the lungs for daytime activities and a good night's sleep.

symptoms, asthma is classified as *chronic mild, chronic moderate,* and *chronic severe*. *Status asthmaticus*, a severe episode of asthma that does not respond to ordinary therapeutic measures, such as ordinary bronchodilator medications, occurs in a small percentage of patients with severe asthma. This condition is a medical emergency requiring prompt intervention to prevent death.

nursing care

The onset of an asthmatic attack can be gradual or sudden. Gradual onset is noted by nasal congestion, sneezing, and watery nasal discharge present before the attack. Sudden onset often occurs at night with the child awakening with wheezing (especially noticeable on expiration), diaphoresis, coughing, and dyspnea that is increased during expiration. The nurse's main concern is to relieve the child's respiratory distress during an attack. Maintaining an open airway is essential and may require suctioning if the child is too weak to cough and expectorate thick mucus.

Because asthma is a chronic disorder controlled predominately with medication, it is important to educate children and their caregivers about prescribed medication, expected results, and potential side effects. The use of some inhalators, nebulizers, and peak flow meters requires specific instructions, and compliance is improved when the nurse provides verbal and written instructions. Caregivers must be given clear and concise information in their dominant language (see Teaching Guidelines: How to Use a Metered-Dose Inhaler).

A reliable early sign of an asthma episode is a drop in the child's peak expiratory flow rate. Children older than 4 years can learn to use a peak flow meter. A peak flow meter reading of 80% to 100% reflects no symptoms and full breathing reserve; 50% to 80% reflects mild-to-moderate symptoms with diminished reserve; below 50% reflects serious distress with significantly impaired pulmonary function.

The use of oxygen equipment can be frightening to the child and parents. The child may respond more positively to the equipment if allowed to examine it within the limits of safety. The prescribed oxygen therapy should be administered before cyanosis appears. Providing caregivers with appropriate information about oxygen therapy can help relieve some of their anxieties.

Breathing exercises are most often done in the morning before breakfast and at night before going to bed. During abnormal breathing patterns, muscle groups seem to work together, alternating their levels of activity to prevent total exhaustion by any one muscle group. Asthmatic children

teaching guidelines
promoting the child's asthmatic condition and emotional growth

The child's asthmatic condition and emotional growth can be promoted when caregivers do the following:

* Use a positive approach regarding restrictions by stressing what the child is able to do rather than what he or she is not able to do.
* Encourage the child to lead an active, healthy life, emphasizing the importance of taking prescribed medications.
* Check with the American Lung Association, The Asthma and Allergy Foundation of America, and the National Asthma Education program for current information and locally sponsored services, such as Asthma Camp.
* Educate the child about the cause of the asthmatic condition.
* Inform the child's schoolteacher, physical education teacher, school nurse, babysitter, and others who are responsible for the care of the child about asthma, medications, and treatments appropriate during an asthma attack.
* Encourage the child to consider a water sport, such as swimming, because the moisture from the water helps the breathing process.
* Explore the idea of a "hairless" pet, such as a goldfish, snake, or turtle. Animals with hair usually are contraindicated.

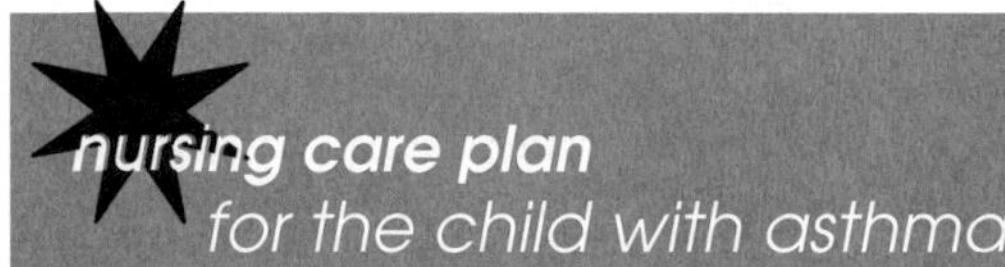

nursing care plan for the child with asthma

NURSING DIAGNOSIS

Ineffective Airway Clearance, related to retained pulmonary secretions and bronchospasm

GOAL: promotion of adequate airway clearance

NURSING INTERVENTIONS	RATIONALE	EVALUATION
Educate the child and parent on administration of bronchodilators, corticosteriods, and antibiotics, if prescribed.	Bronchodilatos will be used in treatment of bronchospasm; corticosteriods are directed at airway inflammation that can obstruct airflow, and antibiotics may be prescribed to treat retained secretions that are infected.	The child and family will demonstrate appropriate use of metered-dose inhalers, and state purpose and side effects of the prescribed medications.
Have the child drink fluids that he or she enjoys, and teach the family about the importance of hydration.	Adequate hydration will help to keep pulmonary secretions thin and prevent mucous plugging.	The child will have an adequate oral intake, maintain good skin turgor, and have a stable daily weight.
Inform the child and the parents on the importance of avoiding substances that trigger an allergic reaction.	Environmental control and use of desensitization to allergens with allergy injections can help prevent an allergic bronchospastic reaction.	The child's environment will be assessed for potential allergens. The child will be tested for allergic responses, and appropriate desensitization will be done.

NURSING DIAGNOSIS

Fear, related to sudden onset of breathlessness

GOAL: The child will have less apprehension

NURSING INTERVENTIONS	RATIONALE	EVALUATION
Provide information to the child and family on the cause and effect of the disease and the best ways to decrease asthma attacks.	Giving the family and the child information will promote greater involvement in their care and lessen their anxiety by increasing their knowledge and control of the disease.	The family and the child will state an understanding of the disease process and list preventive risk factors.
Encourage family to express their fears regarding care of the child.	Using a focused assessment of the cause of the fear by having the family verbalize their feelings will direct the nurse in devising suitable instructions.	The family and the child will discuss exact fears comfortably with the nurse.
Discuss emergency procedures with the family and the child.	Having a plan for emergencies is not only necessary for the health of the child but also will increase the family's control and help them to feel less anxious.	The family and the child will state the plan of action for emergencies.
Give the family references for local support groups for families of asthma patients.	Sharing common concerns with others experiencing similar feelings and problems can alleviate anxiety.	The family will join a support group or state comfort in a strong network of families of children with asthma.

are taught abdominal breathing, which is accomplished by using abdominal muscles to compress the abdomen when the chest cage and pelvis are fixed (see Teaching Guidelines: Promoting the Child's Asthmatic Condition and Emotional Growth). This process aids exhalation and coughing by forcing the diaphragm upward, emptying the air out of the lungs. See the Nursing Care Plan For the Child With Asthma.

tuberculosis

Tuberculosis (TB) is an infectious disease caused by the tubercle bacillus *Mycobacterium tuberculosis.* It is a public health problem throughout the world and is considered an important chronic infectious disease in terms of illness, death, and cost.

The incidence of TB had been declining until 1986,

when it began to rise sharply. Although this increase was initially attributed to the HIV/AIDS epidemic, a 1994 study linked TB more directly with the increase in poverty and homelessness. TB has long been acknowledged as a disease of poverty, most often affecting minorities and the homeless. It also is common in refugees from Asia and Central America, and in alcoholics and intravenous drug users. It is estimated that between 10 and 15 million people in the United States are infected with *M. tuberculosis,* and more than 20,000 new cases are reported annually.

More than 80% of childhood cases occur in minority populations. Reports indicate that transmission occurs in children younger than 15 years, with a higher incidence in children younger than 5 years.

Deaths from TB occur in about 5% of all cases, usually due to noncompliance with treatment. Nearly all properly treated patients with TB are cured, although certain strains of TB have become drug resistant.

pathophysiology

TB is spread by airborne droplets from the cough or sneeze of a person with untreated TB of the lungs or larynx. Children repeatedly exposed to contaminated air may become infected. The tubercle bacilli travel into the air sacs of the lungs and multiply. Within 2 to 10 weeks after the initial infection, tubercle bacilli spread through the lymphatic channels to regional lymph nodes and then through the bloodstream to other tissues and organs. The TB lesion may heal, leaving scar tissue, or continue as a mass of soft, pink, fleshy tissue that forms during the healing process, referred to as a *granuloma*; it eventually causes necrosis, sloughing, and cavity formation.

TB can live in the body without making the individual sick. Most individuals who become infected do not develop clinical illness because the body's immune system brings the infection under control. Individuals who are infected but do not have clinically active pulmonary or laryngeal disease are not normally infectious. People with compromised immune systems, such as those infected with HIV, are at increased risk of developing clinically active TB.

medical management

Preventive therapy reduces the risk of developing clinically active TB in infected people. There are two types of tuberculin testing: purified protein derivative (PPD), using an intracutaneous stick, and old tuberculin (tine and Mono-Vac tests), injecting dried or liquid tuberculin on multiple puncture prongs. TB is diagnosed primarily through the PPD (Mantoux) method of screening. The Mantoux test should be used for a high-risk population and if the tine or Mono-Vac test is positive.

A positive reaction to the Mantoux test is characterized by redness and swelling with the size of reaction measured against a scale (Table 30-5). A reaction of less than 5 mm is considered negative; 5 to 9 mm results requires retesting, and 10 mm or greater indicates positive results. A suggestive reaction on a TB test indicates that a child has been exposed to *M. tuberculosis* and does not necessarily mean that active disease is present in the body.

TB screening includes a sputum smear and culture for the presence of acid-fast bacilli. Chest x-ray is used to determine presence and extent of the disease. The child with TB may be asymptomatic or have insidious symptoms that can be easily overlooked.

The current preventive therapy regimen is recommended for high-risk groups within the population, regardless of age, and consists of 6 to 12 months of daily isoniazid (10 mg/kg up to 300 mg/d). Children who are in close contact with infectious cases are given the preventive therapy regardless of their skin test reaction. After 3 months of preventive therapy, the initial skin test is repeated. Therapy may be discontinued if the skin test is again negative, and there is no longer contact with the infectious person.

Breast-feeding is not discouraged when the mother is on anti-TB drugs. Because there is such a small concentration of the drugs found in breast milk, no toxicity is produced in the nursing newborn.

The duration of therapy depends on the drugs used. TB is treated with at least two drugs. The most common drugs used for the initial treatment of TB in children are isoniazid, rifampin, pyrazinamide, and streptomycin. It is often difficult to obtain culture confirmation of disease in children; therefore, the choice of drugs may depend on drug susceptibility. TB in an infant is much more likely to spread; thus, prompt, vigorous treatment must be started as soon as the diagnosis is suspected.

Bacillus Calmette-Guérin (BCG) vaccine is used to introduce artificial immunity against TB and may be recommended for infants and children with negative tuberculin skin tests in a high-risk population. The practice of protecting high-risk children with BCG has decreased because equal or greater protection is provided though daily isoniazid administration.

 **nursing insight**

Using a nontoxic pen, draw a happy face over the tuberculin skin test site to ease the child's discomfort and make it easier for the caregiver to locate the site and detect any reaction.

nursing care

Objective data include the child's cough and expectoration of mucopurulent sputum. Symptoms of acute febrile illness with chills and night sweats are commonly seen in children with TB.

Subjective data include fatigue, anorexia, indigestion, chest pain, aching, knowledge about disease (if age appropriate). Caregivers need knowledge concerning prescribed medications, how TB is spread, and the proper discarding of secretions from the mouth and nose.

It is important that the home be well ventilated. Family members must be screened for TB. The child usually ceases to be infectious 2 to 4 weeks after the start of drug therapy.

table 30-5 oxygen administration methods, effectiveness, and nursing considerations

Oxygen Device	Percent of Oxygen	Effectiveness	Nursing Considerations
Oxygen hood/oxyhood	22%–100%	Preferred method for newborns. Gives a mix of O_2 and CO_2. Maintains O_2 concentration around infant's head. Allows access to body care. Hood must fit firmly around head.	Check hood temperature; avoid overheating—can cause minimal apnea and dehydration. Keep noise level down to prevent hearing loss. Check neck for pressure from hood.
Venturi mask	24%–50%	Highly accurate; mixes air and O_2. Does not dry mucous membranes. Set O_2 flow rate per order Set venturi valve for desired amount of inspired O_2.	Check mask for proper fit, tubing for kinks and blocked intake ports. Provide information and reassurances. Common complaints include feeling confined and skin irritation around mask.
Nasal cannula	Up to 40%	Used for low O_2 concentrations. Nasal prongs fit most any face. Allows moving, eating, and talking. Cannot be used if nose is blocked. Dries mucous membranes. Can dislodge easily.	Avoid applying too tightly. Check patency of nostrils with flash-light. Check for irritation below nose, above ears, and around chin.
Mist tent/croupette	Up to 60%	Provides cool, high humidity. Maintain O_2 flow rate at 10 L/min or greater depending on doctor's orders. Check tent for holes or tears. Keep tent tightly tucked under the mattress.	Monitor for hypothermia. Check for wetness of linens and stuffed toys that collect moisture, creating a reservoir for germs. Avoid friction toys.
Isolette/incubator	40%–100%	Difficult to maintain high levels of O_2. Temperature must be managed. Increased risk of bacteria growth inside incubator.	Monitor temperature—hypothermia uses energy; hyperthermia causes increased O_2 use and apnea.
Continuous positive airway pressure mask		Allows spontaneous breathing. Provides continuous positive airway pressure; noninvasive. Child can talk and cough.	Check for skin irritation around mask because it requires a tight fit. Assess respiratory, circulatory, and gastrointestinal function qh for increased risk of aspirating vomitus, pneumothorax, decreased cardiac output, gastric distention.

tonsillitis and adenoiditis

Tonsillitis is inflammation of the tonsils. Each tonsil is a ring of lymphoid tissue that forms a protective barrier against upper respiratory infections. The tonsils are located on either side of the mouth cavity, behind the tongue, and are easily seen when enlarged.

Adenoiditis is inflammation of the adenoid glands. The adenoids are located in the back of the nasal passage and upper throat near the opening of the eustachian tube. They cannot be seen because they extend from the roof of the nasal pharynx to the edge of the soft palate.

pathophysiology

Lymphoid tissue normally enlarges in childhood between 2 and 10 years and decreases in size during puberty. The lymph tissue acts as a part of the body's defense against infection; however, sometimes this tissue itself can be a site of acute or chronic infection. Occasionally the tissue becomes so hypertrophied that it interferes with breathing. Partial deafness has been attributed to chronic tonsillitis and adenoiditis. These infections can occur at any age but are seen most frequently in the preschool child.

Enlarged tonsils without symptoms usually do not indicate tonsillectomy. The adenoids, when enlarged, may cause mouth breathing, snoring, and recurrent ear infections.

medical-surgical management

Medical management is aimed at controlling the infection by means of drug therapy. Palliative measures are used to relieve the pain and may include throat irrigations, gargling, ice packs or heat, and administration of analgesics and antibiotics.

If tonsillitis and adenoiditis become chronic, surgery may be necessary. Surgery is aimed at reducing the incidence of severe, recurrent sore throats; mouth breathing; snoring; and frequent earaches. Tonsillectomy does not prevent sore throat or "strep throat."

Prior to tonsillectomy, blood studies are ordered, including CBC. The hemoglobin, hematocrit, prothrombin time, and partial thromboplastin time values are especially significant because any bleeding tendencies make the child a serious surgical risk.

Surgical removal of tonsils (tonsillectomy) and adenoids (adenoidectomy) is a short procedure (about ½ to 1 hour). The most frequent complication following a tonsillectomy and adenoidectomy is bleeding at the time of surgery or immediately afterward. The bleeding may require the insertion of packing and depending on the amount of blood loss, administration of blood transfusions. A small amount of bleeding can occur approximately 1 week postoperatively and results from the crust (scab) coming off at the operative site. Such bleeding is scant and stops within a few minutes.

nursing care

Most children scheduled for surgery are invited to tour the pediatric unit, surgical suite, and recovery room. The tour provides children and nurses an opportunity to interact in a relaxed, somewhat nonthreatening environment. Unless there are additional health problems, children are admitted to the hospital on the day of the scheduled surgery and stay for approximately 12 to 24 hours postoperatively. The time of discharge is based on ability and willingness to drink liquids and void, stability of vital signs, and absence of bleeding, nausea, vomiting, and temperature elevation.

assessment

Preoperative data include reaction of parents and child to hospital environment, parental knowledge base and coping style, and vital signs and temperature data, NPO status and laboratory test results.

Postoperative data include signs of hypovolemic shock: hypotension, tachycardia, tachypnea, frequent swallowing, restlessness, and anxiety; and malignant hyperthermia: muscle rigidity, immovable joints, tachycardia, fever, hyperkalemia and acidosis. Malignant hyperthermia is a hypermetabolic condition and a potentially fatal complication of anesthesia.

nursing diagnoses

- Pain, related to surgical procedure
- Risk for Infection, related to surgery
- Risk for Fluid Volume Deficit, related to blood loss during surgery, fluid restriction preoperatively and reluctance to swallow because of painful throat
- Knowledge Deficit, related to home care

planning and intervention

- Monitor vital signs (pulse, respirations, and blood pressure), and document. When bleeding occurs, a pulse increase is usually noted before the blood pressure drops.
- Monitor intake and output q 8 hrs.
- Monitor temperature, report progressive temperature elevation to charge nurse and initiate prescribed "cooling" methods.
- Inspect the back of the throat with a flashlight for signs of bleeding. Frequent swallowing can indicate the child is swallowing blood. Restlessness can be a sign of increased bleeding.
- Do *not* use a tongue blade when inspecting the child's throat because this may stimulate the gag reflex, initiate vomiting, and increase bleeding.
- Instruct parents to save all tissues used by the child, any mucus expectorated, and any emesis so that blood loss can be assessed. Inform parents that if the child vomits old blood, the emesis will have the appearance of coffee grounds.
- Elevate head of bed to semi- or high-Fowler's position. Position child on side or abdomen (Fig. 30-9); avoid flat prone position until the child is alert to reduce the risk of aspiration if vomiting occurs. Allow the child to assume a position of comfort when alert.
- Have suction equipment readily available.
- Administer analgesics and antipyretics as ordered 30 minutes before meals.
- Apply an ice collar to the child's neck for 10 to 15 minutes at a time if prescribed by the doctor.

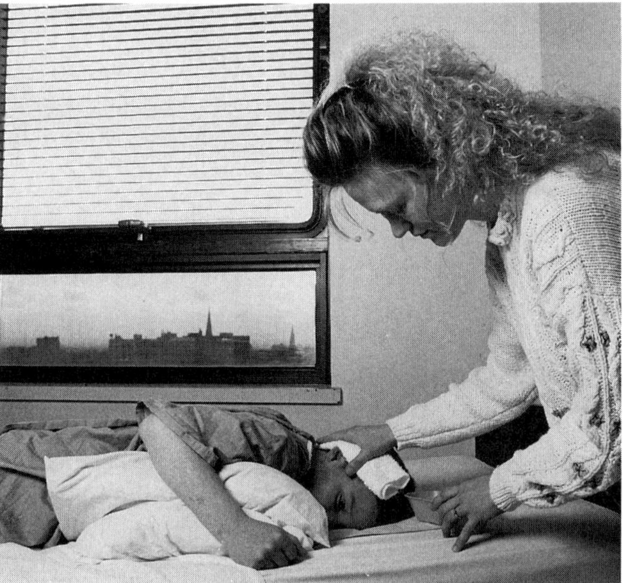

figure 30-9 *Positioning a child following tonsillectomy. The pillow under the chest makes secretions flow out of mouth. (Courtesy of the Department of Medical Photography, Children's Hospital, Buffalo NY.)*

* Ice chips, popsicles, or other cool liquids are given when child is awake enough to request liquids. If no vomiting occurs, a soft diet is given.
* Remind the child not to cough or clear the throat.
* Encourage family caregivers to stay with the child. Surgery is a frightening experience, and additional love and support from a caregiver can help alleviate the child's fear and anxiety.
* Keep crying and coughing to a minimum.
* Provide home care instructions. The nurse needs to receive feedback from the caregivers indicating that they understand the information provided. The information located in the Teaching Guidelines display can help the caregiver to understand the difference between normal recuperation and complications that may require medical intervention.

teaching guidelines

distinguishing between recuperation and complications requiring medical intervention

* The child may run a fever (between 99°–100°F; 37.2°–37.8°C) 1–2 days following surgery. If temperature exceeds 102°F, notify the surgeon.
* A white membrane forms where the tonsils were removed. This is usually not a sign of infection, although the breath may have a bad odor until the white membrane comes off. The child should not gargle.
* The child may complain of pain in the throat, cheeks, neck, and ears that worsens when swallowing. If pain is severe, application of a warm wet washcloth to the neck for about 15–30 minutes every 4 hours may help, along with administration of acetaminophen (Tylenol) liquid (appropriate dose for age). Ear ache may result from removal of tonsils and adenoids; however, this is temporary and resolves with healing. The child should be encouraged to eat because swallowing helps keep the throat moist and promotes healing. Avoid foods that have a high acid content, such as orange juice, and foods that are extremely hot, cold, or spicy.
* If bleeding from the nose occurs, apply an ice pack to the neck and nose. If bleeding from the throat occurs, apply an ice pack around the neck. Swallowing ice chips helps control minor bleeding. Have patient sit up and spit blood into tissues or basin; save all specimens. If bleeding does not stop in 10 minutes, contact physician and take to emergency department.
* Do not restrict the child's activities. Playing outside is permitted if the weather is warm. Children should not be permitted to swim for 2 weeks following surgery because of the risk of infection.

evaluation

* Child will have no signs of bleeding, as evidenced by stable vital signs and pertinent observations.
* Child will display adequate pain control reflected by decreased irritability.
* Child will have normal temperature readings.
* Parents will verbalize an understanding of home care instructions.

procedures related to respiratory diseases

oxygen therapy

Oxygen therapy involves the administration of supplemental oxygen at concentrations greater than room air (21%). Oxygen administration is ordered for *hypoxemia*, insufficient oxygenation of the blood. The degree of hypoxemia is monitored with ABG levels, pulse oximetry, or transcutaneous monitoring.

Oxygen is administered by nasal cannula, Venturi masks, simple face masks, oxygen hoods, isolettes, mist tents or croupettes, endotracheal tube during mechanical ventilation, or through an inflatable anesthesia bag with a mask (Fig. 30-10).

A *mist tent* is a plastic canopy over the child's bed or crib. Oxygen enters the tent through a hose carrying nebulized water. The air is cooled by an ice chamber or electrical cooling unit and circulates in the tent providing the child with moist cool air. Bed linen and gowns need to be changed frequently to avoid chilling from wet clothing. Monitor the child for low body temperature because the mist tent temperatures are approximately 6° to 15°F below room temperature. Encourage parents to put their heads into the tent to provide comfort to the child.

nursing alert

To ensure proper oxygenation of a mist tent and prevent suffocation, set oxygen gauge according to doctor's order (usually 10 L/min or greater). Allow unit to run for 5–10 minutes before placing the child inside.

The *oxygen hood* is an efficient device for maintaining oxygen levels in young infants; the *nasal cannula* allows the infant greater freedom of activity, but is difficult to maintain. Oxygen concentrations are given in Table 30-5.

humidifiers and vaporizers

Humidifiers and vaporizers are units that disperse water into the air to increase the moisture content. Humidifiers and vaporizers can provide a cool mist or heated mist of air and are used primarily to relieve a humidity level deficit.

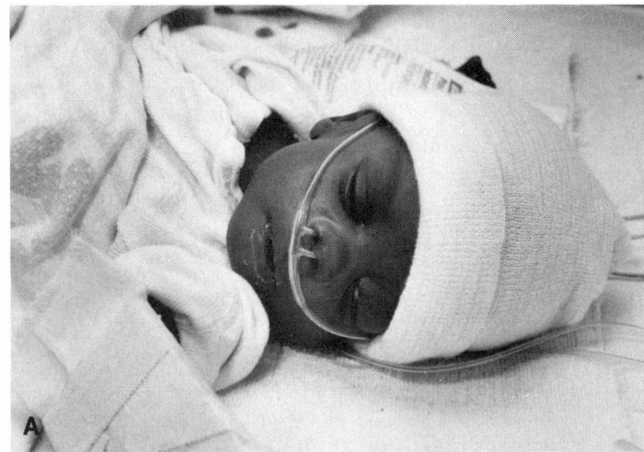
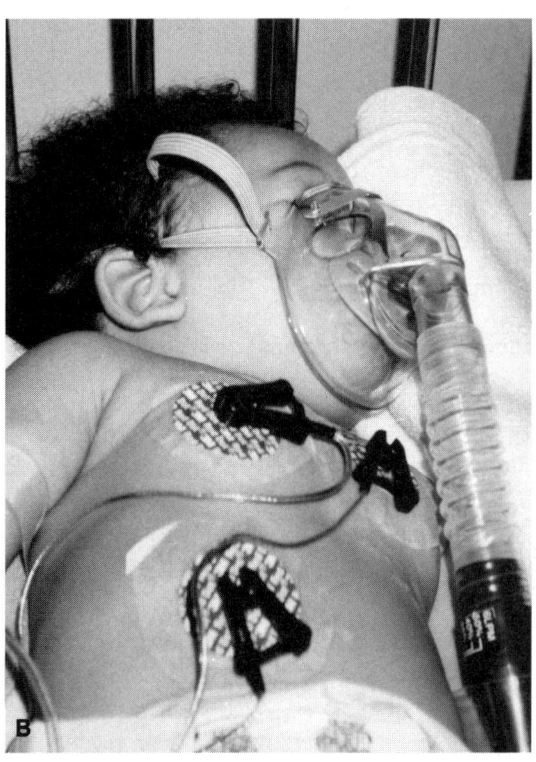
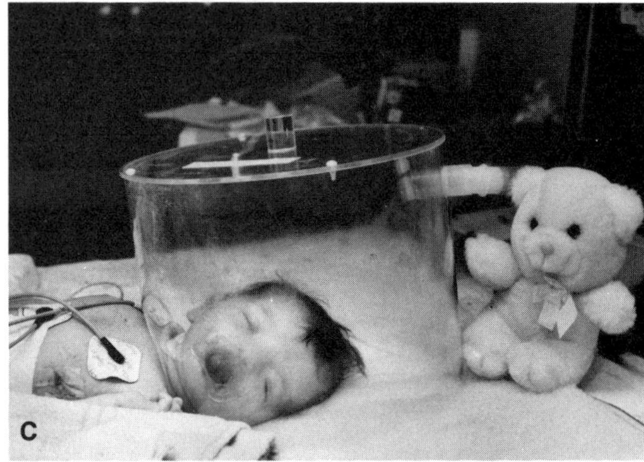
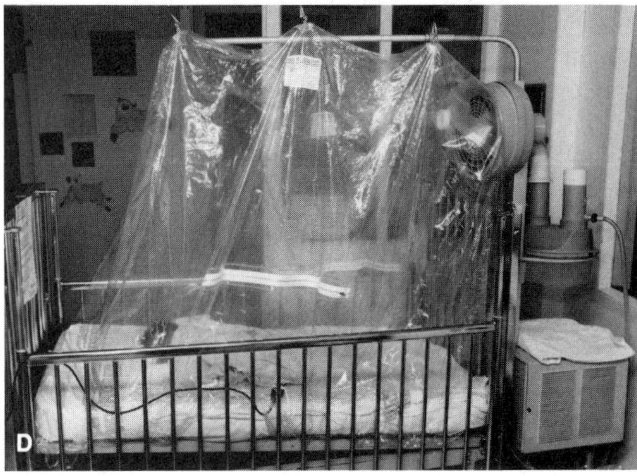
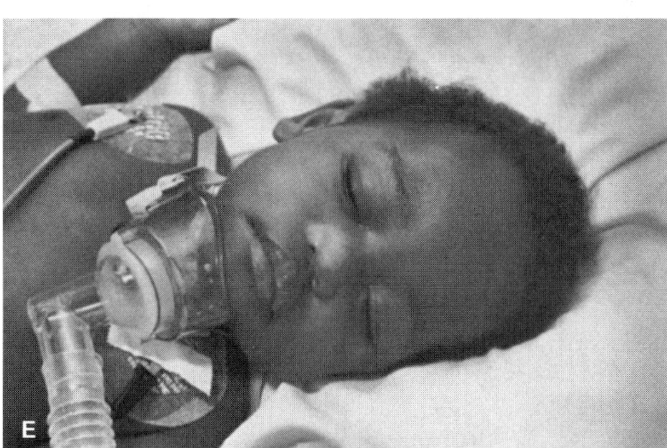

figure 30-10 *Several types of oxygen therapy for children.* ***(A)*** *Nasal cannula.* ***(B)*** *Face mask.* ***(C)*** *Oxygen hood.* ***(D)*** *Mist tent.* ***(E)*** *Pediatric tracheostomy tube. (Source: Skale, N.* Manual of pediatric nursing procedures. *Philadelphia: J. B. Lippincott.)*

> **nursing alert**
>
> *Humid heat may be uncomfortable to a patient who is breathing through the nose or mouth. Adjust equipment for patient's comfort. Take care that equipment is out of the reach of younger children to avoid injury.*

atomizers (metered dose)

Atomizers are hand-held aerosol generators that produce a flow of gas through a pressurized canister. The medication is forced through a small jet, and a mouthpiece directs the medication flow locally into the patient's upper airway. This procedure is most often used to relieve bronchospasms. The child is instructed to hold the mouthpiece about 2 in from the mouth and inhale deeply. After initiation of inspiration, have the child compress the mouthpiece and canister. Have the child hold his or her breath for l0 to 15 seconds and exhale slowly.

✶ nursing insight

Help a child relax during an aerosol nebulizer treatment by pretending to be an astronaut on an outer space adventure, with the mask as a space mask.

chest physiotherapy and postural drainage

Chest physiotherapy involves *percussion* and *vibration* to dislodge and mobilize secretions into larger airways and enable the child to cough and expectorate the mucus. Chest percussion uses the hands in the cupping, clapping, or tapping position to set up vibrations over various segments of the chest wall. This procedure helps loosen secretions and promotes expectoration. The time spent over each lung segment is approximately 3 to 5 minutes.

nursing alert

Do not percuss on bare skin, sternum, spine, stomach, or kidneys. Do not percuss if child has tuberculosis or empyema.

Postural drainage involves positioning the patient so that gravity helps drain various lung segments. Postural drainage is contraindicated if hypoxemia is present (Display 30-1).

intermittent positive pressure breathing treatment

Intermittent positive pressure breathing (IPPB) refers to the inhalation of a gas by an intermittent pressure. The gas is delivered in 15- to 20-minute treatments, with humidity, medication aerosol, or both, depending on the physician's order. IPPB improves alveolar ventilation and lung expansion, decreasing the risk of atelectasis and pneumonia. IPPB improves the delivery of aerosol medications, coughing, and expectoration, minimizing the risk of airway obstruction or chronic airflow limitation. Coughing is expected after an IPPB treatment. Careful assessment and documentation of type of cough and presence of expectorated mucus is important.

The use of home IPPB respirators has increased, as has the number of children with serious respiratory conditions receiving care in the home. The Bennett respirator is the most popular because it is durable, easy to operate, flow sensitive, and uses a nondisposable breathing circuit. Nurse and family caregivers must be familiar with the knobs and tubes of the respirator for safe use.

display 30-1
clinical signs of hypoxemia

- **Cyanosis (bluish discoloration) of the lips, mucous membranes of mouth and tongue, nailbeds, soles of feet in dark-skinned children**
- **Clubbing of the fingers**

pulse oximetry

Pulse oximetry measures the arterial oxygen saturation of blood in a noninvasive way. Saturation is obtained by measuring the amount of light that is reflected from two wavelengths in the vascular bed in the child's ear, nose, foot, toe, or finger (Fig. 30-11). This noninvasive procedure is being used more frequently and has been proven reliable. Probe placement on fingers, toes, and feet can easily dislodge and must be checked frequently. It is equally important to change the monitor site to prevent skin breakdown at the sensor site. Pulse oximetry will

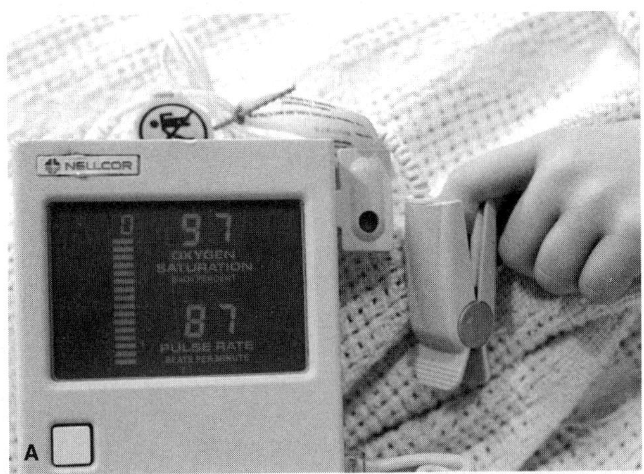

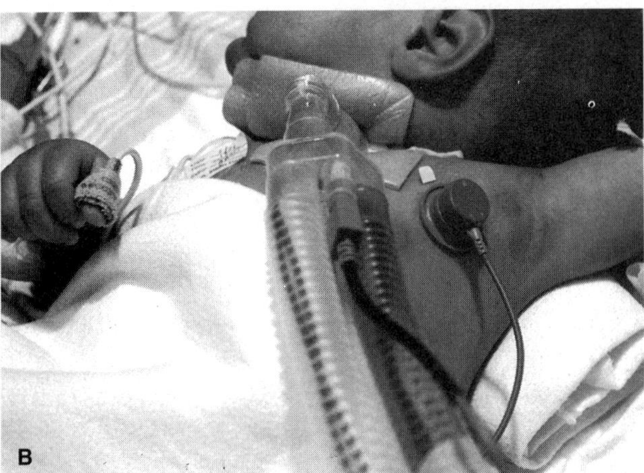

figure 30-11 *(**A**) An example of a pulse oximeter (SpO_2). (**B**) An infant on mechanical ventilation, on a noninvasive thumb), and transcutaneuos CO_2 monitor (upper chest).*

measure only oxygen saturation. If a child has a low hemoglobin, the pulse oximetry may give a false high-percentage reading because the oxygen concentration of available hemoglobin is high (see Fig. 30-11).

transcutaneous monitoring

Transcutaneous monitoring uses specially designed electrodes that attach to the chest and measure oxygen and carbon dioxide as they diffuse through the skin. Transcutaneous monitoring differs from oximetry because it measures oxygen pressure, while oximetry measures oxygen saturation (see Table 30-5).

apnea monitors

The apnea monitor uses an electrode that is placed on the infant's chest to obtain an electrical current with respiratory motion. A major disadvantage is that the monitor cannot distinguish between patient motion and true respiratory motion. Most systems have an alarm system that is usually set for 15 to 20 seconds to detect apnea.

what would you do?

Tai is a 5-year-old Vietnamese boy recently diagnosed as having tuberculosis and assigned to you as a home health nurse. He lives with his parents, grandmother, and a younger brother. The entire family sleeps in one bedroom. Meals are served in several large serving dishes in the middle of the table. The grandmother has responsibility for rearing Tai. She seldom leaves the house and has limited understanding of English. Tai missed his last appointment at the Health Department. After checking his medicines, you suspect that he may not be taking the medications as prescribed because too much medicine remains in the bottles. No one in Tai's family has received a tuberculin skin test, even though Tai was diagnosed 2 weeks ago.

key points

* Diseases of the respiratory system are common in children, ranging from mild disorders to life-threatening events, and are caused by viral and bacterial infections, genetic factors, and allergies.
* The respiratory system provides the continuous supply of oxygen needed to sustain life, excretes carbon dioxide (a waste product of tissue metabolism), and helps maintain the body's acid–base balance.
* The anatomy of the respiratory system in children differs from that of adults; children's immature respiratory structures increase respiration rates and the risk of airway obstruction.
* Family caregivers of children with respiratory diseases experience anxiety and concern about many factors, including possible hospitalization; the disease process; care of well siblings; cost involved in treatment, medications, and equipment; possible lifestyle changes; transmission of disease to other family members; separation of child from family members; home care; and potential threat to child's life.
* Nurses caring for children with respiratory diseases need to be aware of normal growth and development behaviors because respiratory infections are common during infancy and early childhood.
* Safety is a major responsibility in providing respiratory care and consists of checking equipment (especially oxygen) for maximum efficiency, discouraging toys with long strings and friction toys in oxygen tents, keeping crib sides and side rails up to prevent falls, and changing wet clothing and linen to prevent chilling, especially when a mist tent is being used.
* Pink skin and mucous membranes indicate normal exchange of oxygen and carbon dioxide in white children; a reddish skin undertone and pink mucous membranes are normal in well-oxygenated dark-skinned children.
* Children with altered breathing patterns typically respond to oxygen therapy; medication administration, such as bronchodilators and antibiotics, if infection is present; positioning with head elevated; and circulation of cool moist air.
* Complications resulting from respiratory disease or its treatment include risk for "fever seizures" when temperature elevations are above 38.8°C (102°F), periods of apnea progressing to respiratory arrest, retrolental fibroplasia from excessive exposure to high concentrations of oxygen, fluid and electrolyte imbalances, altered physical and psychosocial growth and development, status asthmaticus seen in asthma, and death.
* Diagnostic tests related to respiratory function include viral cultures and antigen detection assays of mucous secretions, sputum and throat cultures, rapid identification tests determining the presence and type of bacterial infection and sensitivity of organism to medication, CBC, pulmonary function tests, bronchoscopy examination, chest x-rays, and blood gas studies.
* Most children with respiratory problems are managed at home, with caregivers being responsible for part or all of the care.
* Researchers have identified the gene responsible for causing CF, offering hope for a cure in the immediate future.
* *H. influenzae type B* conjugate vaccine is recommended for infants older than 2 months to prevent *H. influenzae* pneumonia.
* The increased incidence of TB is associated with the increase in poverty and homelessness.
* Hemorrhage is the most common complication following surgical removal of the tonsils and adenoids.

review questions

1. Children's anatomy and physiology of the respiratory system differ from the adult's. Select the most accurate statement about these differences from the following:
   a. Compared with adults, children have a greater tolerance to nasal congestion.
   b. Children tend to experience more severe respiratory symptoms due to smaller airways, ineffective clearing of mucus, increased risk of edema of soft tissue, and weaker muscles controlling the diaphragm.
   c. Viral and bacterial infections of the respiratory system are more common in adults.
   d. A child's hyaline membrane gives some protection against severe respiratory infections.
2. Mikey is an 8-month-old admitted to the hospital for possible RSV infection. Select the most appropriate nursing interventions for this disease.
   a. Monitor oxygen equipment for possible clogging from medication administration.
   b. Give nothing by mouth except medications.
   c. Assess the skin for signs of jaundice and small bleeding areas.
   d. Maintain isolation precautions.
3. Ian is a 7-year-old with CF who is receiving replacement enzymes. What body system will be unaffected by the enzymes?
   a. Respiratory
   b. Neurologic system
   c. Reproductive
   d. Gastrointestinal system
4. Jerri is an active 8-year-old with asthma. Jerri's mother asks the nurse what sports activity would be appropriate for her daughter during the winter months. A pertinent response includes the following:
   a. Swimming
   b. Track
   c. Basketball
   d. Skiing
5. Children suffering from asthma are often treated with the following medications:
   a. Antibiotics, antihistamines, and analgesics
   b. Bronchodilators, cortisone, and antipyretics
   c. Allergy injections, antibiotics, and diuretics
   d. Bronchodilators, antihistamines, and cortisone

references

Marks, M. (1994) *Broadribb's Introductory pediatric nursing* (3rd ed.). Philadelphia: J.B. Lippincott.

bibliography

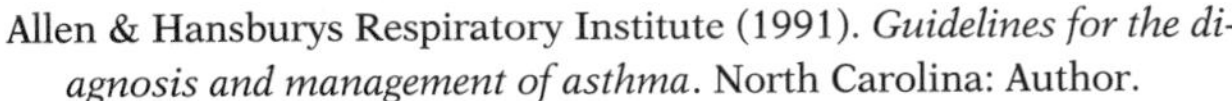

Allen & Hansburys Respiratory Institute (1991). *Guidelines for the diagnosis and management of asthma*. North Carolina: Author.

Bucher, H., Fanconi, S., Baeckert, P., & Duc, G. (1989). Hyperoxemia in newborn infants; Detection by pulse oximetry. *Pediatrics, 84*(2), 226–230.

Carpenito, L. (1995). *Nursing diagnosis application to clinical practice.* Philadelphia: J.B. Lippincott.

Castiglia, P., & Harbin, R. (1992). *Child health care.* Philadelphia: J.B. Lippincott.

Chung, K., Olson, R. & Venson, J. (1992). *Lippincott's pediatric nursing review*. Philadelphia: J.B. Lippincott.

Cystic Fibrosis Foundation (1991). Cystic fibrosis cells corrected in laboratory dishes. *Commitment, July*.

Deglin, J., & Vallerand, A. (1993). *Davis's drug guide for nurses* (4th ed.). Philadelphia: F.A. Davis.

Erbstoesser, M. (1995). Care of the patient with malignant hyperthermia. Journal of Post Anesthesia Nursing, 4(2):71–73.

Gomberg, S. (1990). Mistaken identity... is it epiglottitis or croup? *Pediatric Nursing, 16*(6) 567–570.

Hathaway, E., Hay, W., Groothuis, J., & Paisley, J. (1993). *Current pediatric diagnosis and treatment* (11th ed.). Connecticut: Appleton & Lange.

Jackson, D. & Saunders, R. (1993). *Child development*. Philadelphia, PA: J.B. Lippincott.

Jess, L. (1992). Your patient has asthma. *Nursing 92, 4,* 48–51.

Mayers, M. (1991). *Clinical care plans: Pediatric nursing.* Philadelphia: Markham-McKenzie Publishers.

Quillen, T. (1994) Tips and timesavers, "moon gas" medication. *Nursing 94, 7,* 14.

Ray, J., Booth, J., & Rojeski, T. (1990). *Medical and surgical interventions, parental instructions, tonsillectomy and adenoidectomy.* Zanesville, OH: Southeastern Ohio Otolaryngology.

Speer, K. (1990) *Pediatric care plans.* Springhouse, PA: Springhouse.

Suddarth, D. (1991). *The Lippincott manual of nursing practice* (5th ed.). Philadelphia: J.B. Lippincott.

Taber's Encyclopedia, 17th ed. (1992). Philadelphia, PA: FA Davis.

Thompson, E., & Ashwill, J. (1992). *Pediatric nursing: An introductory text* (6th ed.). Philadelphia: W.B. Saunders.

U.S. Department of Health and Human Services (1991). *Core curriculum on tuberculosis*. : Author.

the child with an alteration in cardiovascular function
31

outline

objectives

After studying this chapter, the reader should be able to:

* Discuss several concerns of the family when a child has a cardiovascular system disorder.
* Discuss nursing considerations for children with cardiovascular system disorders.
* State the components of the cardiovascular system.
* Describe the changes that take place when a newborn's circulation changes from placental to pulmonary.
* Describe heart catheterization and the adaptations necessary according to the child's age.
* Discuss at least five nursing interventions for care of the child with a cardiovascular system disorder.
* List the contributing factors for congenital heart defects.
* Describe the typical symptoms of congestive heart failure.
* Discuss nursing care for the child with rheumatic fever.
* Discuss prevention of hypertension in the child.

key terms

cardiomegaly
chorea
collagen
commissurotomy
compensated heart failure
cyanosis
decompensated heart failure
diaphoresis
dyspnea
dysrhythmia
endocarditis
polycythemia
primary hypertension
secondary hypertension
valvuloplasty

The child with a cardiovascular system disorder is at high risk for psychosocial and additional physiologic problems. Disorders of these systems tend to be chronic and, in children, usually occur in utero or at birth if the fetal (placental) circulation does not undergo changes necessary for pulmonary circulation. Many of the diseases and disorders are serious and potentially fatal unless treated promptly. Alterations of cardiovascular function include congenital heart defects and acquired heart disease.

✶ family considerations

Parents of children born with cardiovascular system disorders, such as congenital heart defects, must deal with the serious nature of the problem immediately after birth. The threat of losing the baby can overshadow concerns of overwhelming long-term care, future surgery, and developmental delays. However, once the infant is stabilized, these long-term concerns become more apparent, and long-range planning should begin.

Developmental delays are common in children with cardiovascular system disorders. Poor sucking ability increases the risk of altered growth. Heart disease is a major cause of organic failure to thrive, and the child's small stature can be a worry for parents. *Dyspnea* (difficulty breathing), especially on exertion, is common in children with cardiovascular disease. This limits their ability to develop gross motor skills.

✶ nursing considerations

Early indications of heart disorders include difficulty with lying flat, intolerance to activity, or assuming a squatting position not related to play.

Nursing considerations for children with cardiovascular disorders include addressing the age and developmental level fears of the child (Table 31-1). Client and caregiver teaching is a major nursing function. The sick infant may require tube feedings to conserve energy normally used for sucking. Holding and cuddling the infant during feeding strengthens bonding and infant trust. The chronic nature of many of these disorders increases the child's risk of delays in growth and development.

Frequent finger, heel, and venipuncture sticks for blood component determination can cause discomfort and anxiety in the child. Allowing the child to vent anger is important.

anatomy and physiology

The cardiovascular system also is called the circulatory system and consists of the heart, blood, and blood vessels. The major role of the heart is to pump oxygenated blood to tissues and remove metabolic waste products from tissue cells. Blood and blood vessels exchange materials, such as oxygen and carbon dioxide, between the blood and tissues.

the heart

The heart is a hollow organ made up of three layers of tissue. The inner layer that lines the valves of the heart is called the endocardium. The middle layer or muscle layer is called the myocardium, and the thin outermost layer of the heart wall is called the epicardium. The pericardium is a combination of the epicardium and a serous lining of the fibrous sac that encloses the heart.

The heart is divided in half. The right and left sides are separated by a partition called the septum. Each side has two chambers, an atrium and a ventricle, that are separated by valves. The valves keep blood from backing up into the heart chambers (Fig. 31-1).

conduction system of the heart

The heart rate is regulated by the sinoatrial node, also known as the pacemaker of the heart; atrioventricular node (AV); AV bundle, right and left bundle branches; and Purkinje fibers. The sinoatrial node generates an electrical impulse that begins the heartbeat and stimulates atrial contraction. The AV node stimulation carries the current through the bundle of His and through the ventricular walls by way of the bundle branches and Purkinje fibers.

table 31-1 developmental stages and age-related fears in children with cardiovascular system disorders

Age	*Developmental Stage*	*Major Fear*
Infants	Trust versus mistrust	Separation
Toddler	Autonomy versus shame and doubt	Separation, loss of control, physical limitations, loss of routine
Preschoolers	Initiative versus guilt	Separation, loss of control, body injury and pain, fear of procedures and body mutilation
School-age	Industry versus inferiority	Separation from parents and peers, loss of control, body injury and pain

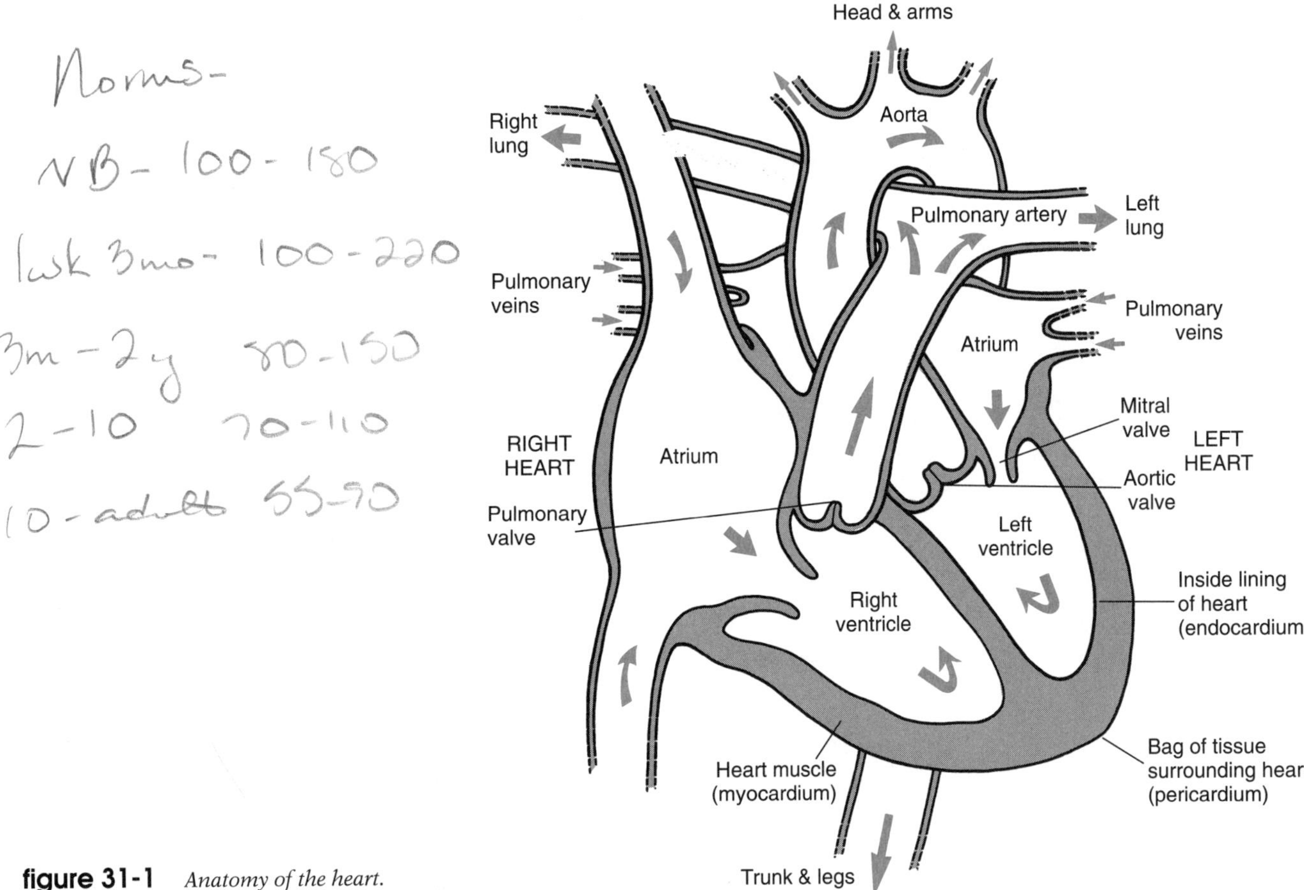

figure 31-1 *Anatomy of the heart.*

An electrocardiogram (ECG) is a recording of the heart's electrical impulses. Each heartbeat displays three major deflections on an ECG reading (see Fig. 31-2):

1. P wave represents atrial contraction.
2. QRS complex represents the electrical impulse going through the ventricles.
3. T wave represents a resting period between beats.

great vessels of the heart

The two great vessels of the heart are the pulmonary artery and the aorta. The pulmonary artery divides into left and right branches and delivers deoxygenated blood from the heart to the lungs. The aorta delivers blood that has been oxygenated by the lungs to the body through the systemic circulation.

blood vessels

Arteries, veins, and capillaries are the three types of blood vessels. Arteries carry oxygenated blood away from the heart. They are large vessels made up of three layers of elastic tissue. Arteries branch into arterioles, which determine blood flow distribution and resistance. The capillaries are tiny vessels that branch off from arterioles. Their function is to supply oxygenated blood and nutrients to all tissues and to remove waste products from the blood. Venules carry blood from the capillaries to the veins. Veins are large vessels that carry the deoxygenated blood back to the heart.

age-specific differences in the cardiovascular system

The newborn's first breath symbolizes an important milestone in the cardiovascular system. At this point, placental circulation changes to pulmonary circulation.

Anatomic changes noted at birth or shortly after involve closure of fetal structures, including the following:

* The *umbilical cord* connects the fetus to the placenta where oxygen, carbon dioxide, nutrients, and other wastes are exchanged by diffusion from the fetus to the mother; it is severed immediately after birth when the cord is cut.
* The *ductus venosus* allows fetal blood to circulate through the liver, with the majority of blood going to the inferior vena cava, and right atrium; it constricts after the cord is cut and becomes nonfunctional.
* The *foramen ovale* is an opening in the interatrial septum that allows blood to flow from the right atrium to the left atrium; functional closure occurs after birth, with anatomic closure resulting in several weeks.

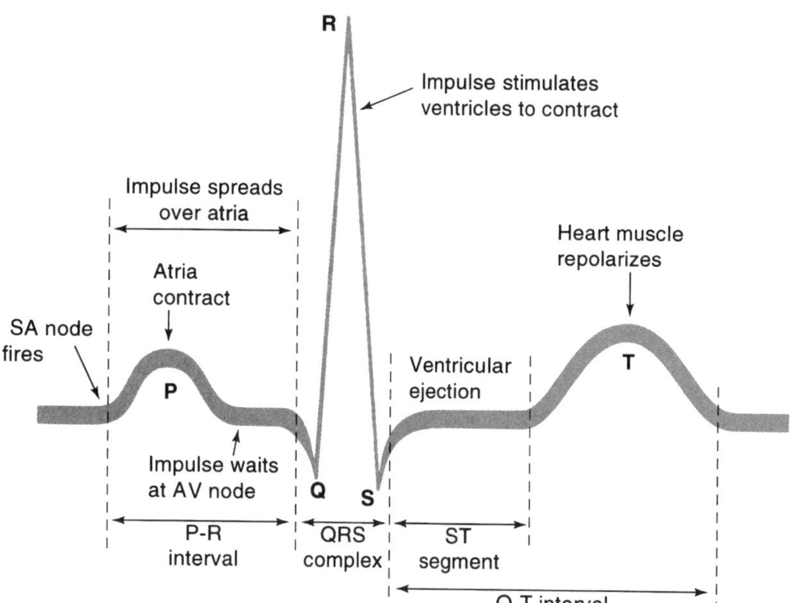

figure 31-2 *ECG waves, electrical and mechanical events. Electrical impulse is initiated by the SA node and spreads throughout the conduction system of the heart, causing the P, Q, R, S, and T waves. If the heart responds normally, the atria and then the ventricles contract.*

✱ The *ductus arteriosus* is a short vessel that shifts most of the blood in the pulmonary artery to the aorta, bypassing the fetal lungs; it constricts 15 to 20 hours after birth, marking the beginning of pulmonary circulation.

Failure of fetal circulatory structures to close at birth constitutes the majority of congenital heart defects.

diagnostic tests

Diagnostic testing for cardiovascular system disorders involves specialized tests and general testing performed for various other body system diseases.

Only the more common tests involved in cardiovascular system evaluation are included in this chapter. Normal values for tests are included in the Appendix.

blood tests

Complete blood count with differential and platelet count provides information about the blood through a series of tests. These tests determine the number, variety and percentage, concentrations, and quality of blood cells.

Hematocrit measures the percentage of total blood volume, which consists of packed red blood cells. Hematocrit values are elevated in cyanotic heart disease and lowered in congestive heart disease.

Hemoglobin measures the iron-containing pigment of the red blood cells that carry oxygen from the lungs to the tissues. Hemoglobin values parallel the red blood cell count. Hemoglobin values are elevated in cyanotic heart disease and lowered in congestive heart disease.

Erythrocyte sedimentation rate measures the sedimentation rate or settling of erythrocytes. This test is helpful in diagnosing inflammatory conditions. The values are increased in congestive heart failure (CHF).

Blood cultures identify specific microorganisms causing a clinical infection.

Arterial blood gas studies analyze the adequacy of oxygenation, ventilation, and acid–base status by measuring blood pH and partial pressures of oxygen and carbon dioxide.

heart function tests

An ECG records the electrical forces of the heart. Ambulatory ECGs record the heart's electrical activity for 24 hours or more during the child's activities of daily living. See the teaching guidelines display about ECGs.

ultrasound imaging

Heart sonogram, heart echogram, echocardiogram, and Doppler echocardiogram are noninvasive procedures that visualize and record on a video screen or videotapes information concerning cardiac structures; these include the heart's position, size, movement of heart valves and chamber walls, and blood flow. A typical examination takes 30 to 45 minutes. Prepare the child for the test by telling him or her that it is important to remain still, the test is painless, and occasionally he or she may feel a vibrating sensation.

x-ray imaging

Routine chest x-ray provides images of the thorax, mediastinum, heart (especially size, shape, and position), and lungs, providing information about the heart size. Nurses

teaching guidelines
electrocardiograms (ECGs)

Tell the child who will be undergoing an ECG the following:

* A special test has been ordered to watch your heartbeat.
* Your heart beat gives off an electrical current.
* You do not feel the electricity, but a special machine can record it, similar to a radio picking up signals and playing your favorite music. The difference is that the machine recording your heartbeat does not make a sound but makes a special drawing.
* A sticky jelly and small round patches called electrodes are put on your skin to help the machine pick up the beat.
* The test does not hurt and takes only 5 to 10 minutes after the electrodes are applied.
* After the test is done, the sticky jelly is washed off and you can rest, watch television, or play.

must wear protective lead aprons to decrease exposure to radiation. X-rays are contraindicated in teenagers during the first trimester of pregnancy.

x-ray imaging with contrast

Cardiac catheterization, also called heart catheterization or angiography, is an invasive test that detects abnormalities in the heart chambers, valves, and blood vessels; it does this by threading arterial and venous catheters into the right and left sides of the heart, injecting contrast media, and viewing the heart structures. The site of heart catheterization differs with the child's age as follows: umbilical vessels are used in the neonate, the right or left femoral artery and vein is used in the infant, and the antecubital vessels of the arm or femoral artery are used in the older child.

nursing care before a heart catheterization

Explain the purpose and procedure to children (as age appropriate) and parents. Describe sensations the child will feel, such as pressure with the catheter insertion, momentary "hot flashes," or nausea, headache, or cough when the contrast medium is injected. Sedatives enable the child to rest but are not intended to make them unconscious.

nursing alert

Complications following a heart catheterization include heart irregularities, bleeding, perforation, phlebitis, and obstructions at catheterization entry site.

Nothing is given by mouth for at least 4 hours prior to the test.

A consent form must be signed by the child's legal guardian.

nursing care following a heart catheterization

* Assess level of consciousness and complaints of discomfort.
* Monitor vital signs, including temperature, every 15 minutes for 1 hour, then every hour. Do not take blood pressure on heart catheterization extremity.
* Assess bleeding at catheterization site. Keep extremity straight; maintain placement of pressure dressings or sandbags.
* Assess neurovascular status of catheterized extremity.
* Record intake and output.
* Evaluate child's and parents' understanding of discharge instructions.

nursing insight

Neurovascular assessment of an extremity following a heart catheterization involves the five P's: pulselessness, puffiness, pain, paresthesia, and pallor.

magnetic resonance imaging

Magnetic resonance imaging (MRI) is a noninvasive, computer-based procedure providing images of detailed views of fluid-filled soft tissue on a magnetic field. It provides information about many aspects of heart function, such as cardiovascular anatomy, congenital heart defects, blood clots, and infections.

nursing care

The following nursing care applies before the test:

* Explain the procedure to the child and parents. The machine used for MRIs can be explained by comparing the gantry to a tunnel. The test is painless; sedation is used for infants and small children to keep them still during the test. Most facilities allow parents to accompany the child to the MRI area. The equipment has a two-way communication system that allows the child and operator to talk during the test.
* Offer clear liquids only for 4 hours before the examination, depending on the health care facility's protocol.
* Remove all metal from the child, such as jewelry, dental retainers, and brassieres, because metal can interfere with, alter, or distort the magnetic field and decrease the quality of the images.

Following the test, the child should resume pretest diet, medications, and activity unless the doctor orders a change.

✳ nursing process for children with alterations of the cardiovascular system

assessment

Subjective data to be assessed include the following:

* Family history of cardiovascular system disorders, especially congenital heart defects
* Information concerning unusual events during the pregnancy and birth, for example, maternal infections during pregnancy, difficult labor or complicated delivery, low newborn Apgar scores.
* Information about activity patterns, position assumed at rest that facilitates breathing, for example, an infant seat or "squatting" position assumed by infants and young children

Objective data to be assessed include the following:

* Thin appearance, indicating poor nutrition, such as poor feeding with frequent regurgitation and poor weight gain; large appearance associated with fluid retention noted in the face and extremities
* Delayed physical, emotional, and developmental growth
* Heartbeat irregularities, including heart murmur
* Tachycardia even during sleep (pulse ranges are given in Table 31-2)
* Alterations in blood pressure, such as hypotension or hypertension, and unequal blood pressures in arms and legs
* Respiratory difficulties, such as dyspnea, chest retractions, and nasal flaring. An infant or young child normally breathes with the diaphragm, making it necessary to look at the abdomen while assessing the respiration status.
* Pallor, cyanosis, and clubbing of digits (seen more often after 2 years of age)
* Activity intolerance, fatigue

table 31-2 pulse rate differences depending on age and activity

Age	Awake, Quiet Inactive State	Sleeping	Actively Playing, Emotionally Upset, or Has a Fever
Newborn	100–180	80–160	Up to 200
1 wk–3 mo	100–220	80–200	Up to 220
3 mo–2 yr	80–150	70–120	Up to 200
2–10 yr	70–110	60–90	Up to 200
10 y–adult	55–90	50–90	Up to 200

Adapted from Castiglia, P. & Harbin, R. (1992). *Child health care* Philadelphia: J.B. Lippincott, (p. 572).

> **✳ nursing insight**
>
> *Benign abnormal heart rates, called sinus dysrhythmia, are common during infancy and in young children. They are detected by increases in the heart rate during inspiration and slowing during expiration. Have the child hold his or her breath while you auscultate the heart, and sinus dysrhythmia should temporarily disappear..*

nursing diagnosis

* Anxiety, related to serious nature of illness and potentially poor prognosis
* Anticipatory Grief, related to possible death of the child and limitations on normal lifestyle
* Altered Growth and Development, related to chronic nature of cardiovascular disorders
* Activity Intolerance, related to decreased oxygenation of tissue
* Knowledge Deficit
* Altered Nutrition: Less than body requirements, related to poor sucking in infants, general decreased energy reserves, and special diets
* Self Esteem Disturbance, related to chronic fatigue and discomfort, restricted activities, surgical scars, lack of privacy, and parental overprotection

nursing interventions

promotion of understanding aimed at relieving anxiety

* Orient the child and parents to hospital and hospital routines, such as visitor restrictions, visiting hours, and special procedure areas.
* Explain necessary procedures and diagnostic tests, and encourage the child and parents to ask questions.
* Encourage parents to participate in the child's care.
* Provide emotional support.

promotion of hope

* Encourage sharing of concerns.
* Promote the integrity of the child and parents by recognizing strengths.
* Promote family cohesiveness by encouraging effective family communications.
* Supply accurate information about the child's present condition, future interventions, and statistics on prognosis. Resist the temptation to give false hope.
* Recognize the various stages of grief, including denial, isolation, depression, anger, guilt, fear, and rejection.
* Encourage the child and family to focus on and support their social network of relationships. Respect religious and spiritual beliefs.

promotion of growth and development and nutrition

* Encourage the family to provide as normal a life (within the limits of the disorder) as possible for the child by age-appropriate activities for stimulation. Stress the importance of understanding normal developmental tasks; explore ways of avoiding overprotecting the child through overstrict activity limitations, and encourage sibling involvement.
* Provide small, frequent meals to decrease the workload on the heart. Provide the child with favorite foods, and schedule feedings or meals after rest periods, providing a calm, nonstressful environment during mealtime.
* Position child in semi-Fowler's position during feedings to facilitate swallowing. Administer prescribed oxygen during feedings.
* Assess intake and output.
* Follow health care agency's protocol for tube feedings if that method of feeding is required.
* Monitor laboratory values for red blood cells, hematocrit and hemoglobin for decreases indicating anemia, and electrolyte values for hypokalemia (Display 31-1) or hyponatremia (Display 31-2). Administer iron preparations and potassium as ordered; fluid and sodium restriction may be necessary.

promotion of activity

* Organize nursing care to provide for periods of uninterrupted rest; intervene promptly when infants are crying; provide diversional activities that do not overtire older children. Play is alternated with rest periods.
* Administer oxygen as ordered, and place child in a semi-Fowler's position to facilitate breathing. Chalasia seats or infant carriers can be used for infants and small children.
* Assess the shape of fingernails; a thick, wide appearance is typical of chronic hypoxia and is referred to as "clubbing."

promotion of child and parental knowledge

* Provide child and parents with information about the anatomy and physiology of the cardiovascular system; complicated surgical interventions; home care management, including administration of medications and recognition of adverse side effects; special diets; special procedures; and emergency interventions, such as cardiopulmonary resuscitation.
* Encourage the parents to participate in the child's care by helping with medication administration, treatments, and activities of daily living.
* Teach parents how to monitor the child's pulse rate, administer prescribed medications, and recognize effectiveness.

promotion of self-esteem

* Establish a trusting nurse–client relationship, and encourage child to ask questions about health, treatments, progress, and prognosis.
* Promote social interactions by encouraging socialization with other children on the unit.
* Provide age-appropriate toys, games, and books.
* Encourage child to express feelings about the defect or disorder and treatments required; support positive coping mechanisms. Discuss realistic expectations.
* Question child's feelings about being a girl or a boy. Assess gender-based role expectations currently and in the future.
* Refer to community resources for counseling as indicated.

evaluation

* Child (if age appropriate) and parents verbalize knowledge about defect, disorder, treatments, and potential complications; they express realistic expectations and feelings of hope.
* The child maintains or gains adequate weight and demonstrates age-appropriate growth and developmental skills.
* Activity tolerance is improved, reflected by decreased or absence of fatigue, dyspnea, pallor, and cyanosis during activities of daily living and nonstrenuous play.
* The child voices positive feelings about self and realistic plans to compensate for limitations.

display 31-1
symptoms of hypokalemia

* **Serum potassium level below 3.5 mEq/L**
* **Muscle weakness and cramps**
* **Diminished bowel sounds**
* **Hypotension**
* **Heart irregularities with electrocardiogram changes**
* **Drowsiness, lethargy, and coma**

display 31-2
symptoms of hyponatremia

* **Serum sodium level below 136 mEq/L**
* **Water intoxication**
* **Weakness, irritability, fatigue**
* **Tremors and convulsions**
* **Headache**
* **Hypotension**
* **Decreased skin turgor**

congenital heart defects

Congenital heart defects include conditions resulting from abnormal heart development. In more than 90% of congenital heart defects, the cause is unknown (Pediatric Nursing, 1992). Contributing factors include maternal infections during the first trimester, maternal alcoholism or use of other drugs considered toxic to the fetus, maternal dietary deficiencies, insulin-dependent diabetic mothers, and maternal age greater than 40 years.

Children with congenital heart defects will often exhibit *dysrhythmias*, cyanosis, pallor, heart murmurs, decreased blood pressure, frequent respiratory infections, and fatigue.

classification of congenital heart defects

Congenital heart defects are usually classified as an anatomic abnormality, hemodynamic abnormality, or tissue oxygenation abnormality.

Anatomic abnormalities can develop as valvular, septal, or great vessel defects. Hemodynamic alterations are caused by one or a combination of anatomic abnormalities. The result is *increased* or *decreased* blood flow through the pulmonary or systemic circulatory systems or the *mixing* of pulmonary and systemic blood. Tissue oxygenation classification is determined by the presence or absence of *cyanosis*, a bluish discoloration of the skin that indicates that tissues are not getting enough oxygen (Fig. 31-3).

This discussion classifies congenital heart defects according to whether they are acyanotic or cyanotic. However, the discussion of the defect will include a description of the specific abnormality and the hemodynamic status. Refer to Figure 17-5 for anatomic views of congenital heart defects.

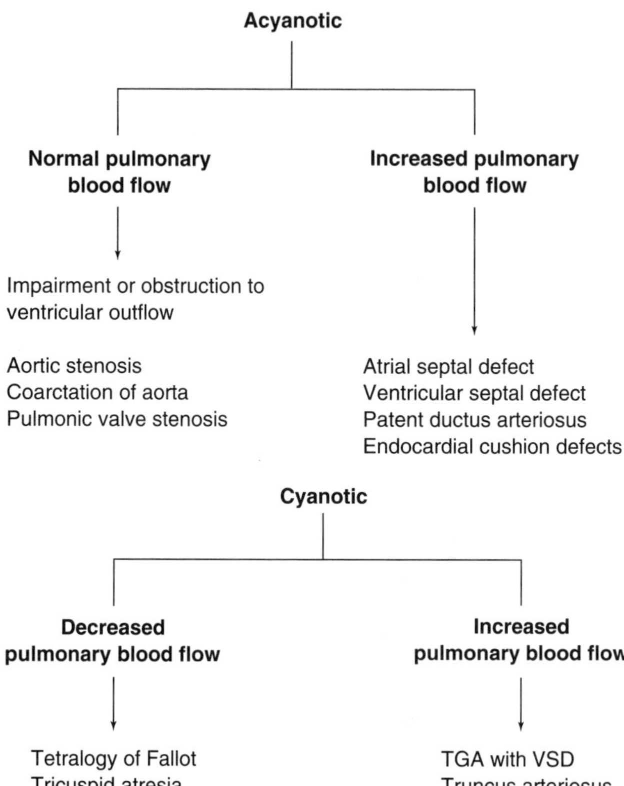

figure 31-3 *Classification of congenital heart disease based on the direction of pulmonary blood flow.* (ASD, *atrial septal defect;* TGA, *transposition of great arteries;* VSD, *ventricular septal defect.)*

acyanotic heart defects

patent ductus arteriosus This defect occurs when the ductus arteriosus fails to close after birth. Oxygenated blood is shunted into the pulmonary circulation, resulting in increased pulmonary blood flow. Symptoms include a continuous loud murmur, pallor, widened pulse pressure (greater difference between the systolic and diastolic blood pressure), feeding problems, repeated respiratory infections, and *cardiomegaly* (enlarged heart). In addition, children with patent ductus arteriosus commonly experience pulmonary edema and CHF. Treatment includes medication therapy for CHF and surgical repair of the ductus by 1 year.

atrial septal defect This defect consists of an abnormal opening in the atrial septum, which allows oxygenated blood to be shunted from the left atria to the right atria through the ASD, resulting in increased pulmonary blood flow. Symptoms include slow weight gain, intolerance to activity, dyspnea on exertion, and ECG changes. These symptoms may not be noticed until the child is a toddler. The opening can be closed when the child is between 4 to 6 years old. The open heart surgical procedure involves suturing or patching the opening.

ventricular septal defect Ventricular septal defect consists of an abnormal opening in the ventricular septum, which shunts oxygenated blood from the left ventricle to the right ventricle, resulting in increased pulmonary blood flow. Symptoms are seldom seen at birth if the opening is small. It is usually detected during the preschool years by the presence of a murmur. Small openings may close spontaneously. If the defect is large, feeding problems, frequent respiratory infections, dyspnea, and CHF may result. Surgery is usually delayed until the child is a few years old to allow for growth of the heart and lower surgical risks. Until that time, CHF is controlled medically. A synthetic Dacron™ patch is usually used to close the hole during an open heart procedure.

endocardial cushion defects These defects can occur anywhere along the septum of the heart where the atria meet the ventricles. The mitral and tricuspid valves also may be involved. These defects usually result in blood being shunted left to right between the atria and ventricles, thereby increasing pulmonary blood flow. Newborns with this disorder are usually asymptomatic until a few months after birth. Symptoms include pulmonary congestion and CHF. It is the most common congenital heart defect in children with Down syndrome. Surgical repair of the defect is required.

aortic valvular stenosis Because of narrowing or blockage of the aortic valve, blood flow from the left ventricle is obstructed, and left ventricular hypertrophy results. Pulmonary blood flow is normal. Symptoms are generally not seen during infancy. Older children may develop chest pain, dyspnea, a loud systolic murmur, and ECG changes. Treatment consists of surgical prosthetic valve replacement.

pulmonary stenosis Pulmonary stenosis occurs when the pulmonary valve is narrowed, causing obstruction of blood flow out of the right ventricle. Pulmonary blood flow is normal. The condition can range from mild to severe. Symptoms include dyspnea, edema of the extremities, and CHF. Immediate surgery to correct the obstruction is necessary in symptomatic newborns.

coarctation of the aorta A narrowed aorta obstructs the outflow of blood from the left ventricle, causing increased left ventricular pressure. Pulmonary blood flow is normal. A child with coarctation of the aorta will experience growth retardation, fatigue, headache, epistaxis (nosebleed), leg cramps, cardiomegaly, and possibly CHF. Emergency care involves giving prostaglandin E to dilate the narrowed vessel. Surgical repair is usually performed when the child is 2 to 4 years old.

cyanotic heart defects

tetralogy of fallot This defect actually consists of four defects: ventricular septal defect, overriding of the aorta, pulmonary stenosis, and right ventricular hypertrophy. With severe blockage, blood is shunted from right to left. The results are decreased pulmonary blood flow and decreased oxygen in the systemic circulation (cyanosis). A child with this disorder will appear cyanotic, and the cyanosis will worsen with age. Other signs and symptoms include clubbing of fingers and toes, squatting posture to help with breathing, dyspnea on exertion, failure to thrive, heart murmur, and increased red blood cells and hematocrit values. Surgery is performed when the child is 18 to 36 months old.

tricuspid atresia The primary defect of tricuspid atresia is an abnormally closed tricuspid valve, accompanied by an atrial septal defect, right ventricular hypoplasia, and varying degrees of pulmonary stenosis. As a result of the combination of these defects, pulmonary blood flow and oxygen in the systemic circulation (cyanosis) are decreased. The infant with this defect will exhibit severe cyanosis, respiratory distress, CHF, and ECG changes. A surgical procedure is performed to create an aorticopulomonary or atrioventricular connection. Survival rates of 10 to 15 years have been documented (Woods, 1995).

transposition of the great vessels This defect occurs when the pulmonary artery and the aorta switch sites of origin during development. As a result, the pulmonary artery originates form the left ventricle, and the aorta originates from the right ventricle. This results in two closed systems. Oxygenated blood flows continually through the pulmonary circulation and deoxygenated blood flows continually through the systemic circulation. An infant will not survive until surgery can be performed unless there is some mixing of blood through the foramen ovale, a ventricular septal defect, or the ductus arteriosus.

At birth, the neonate will experience cyanosis and activity intolerance. An emergency cardiac balloon catheterization procedure is performed to increase mixing of blood through the foramen ovale. Surgery is performed as soon as possible to reroute blood flow.

truncus arteriosus This defect consists of the formation of one large artery instead of a separate aorta and pulmonary artery. This causes a combination of oxygenated and deoxygenated blood to eject from the left and right ventricles into the pulmonary circulation and the systemic circulation. Pulmonary blood flow is increased. Symptoms include pronounced cyanosis with exertion and CHF. The CHF is treated medically, and surgery is performed to correct the defect before the child is 2 years old.

nursing care of the child with congenital heart disease The child and parents must be provided with information about the defect and treatment plan. Parents may feel extremely anxious about the heart specialist's plan to wait for surgical intervention until the child is older, fearing that the child may die before the surgery. Reassure parents that delaying the surgery until the child is older allows heart structures and other body systems to stabilize and reduces some surgical risks.

Allow parents to provide care for, hold, cuddle, and touch the child as often as possible. Children with heart defects are candidates for surgical intervention at larger regional hospitals, making it necessary for some parents to travel long distances. Information about low-cost room and board facilities is usually available through the hospital. For example, lodging at the Ronald McDonald House is available for families with chronically ill children and provides an opportunity to socialize with other parents facing similar experiences.

When children with chronic heart problems are admitted to local hospitals for conditions such as recurring respiratory infections or from complications following corrective surgery, it is important to obtain as much information as possible about the treatment plan recommended by the cardiologist. Assessing the client's and parents' compliance with previous treatment plans provides an insight as to possible knowledge deficit or possible denial of the serious nature of the problem. The Nursing Care Plan provides further information on the care of the child and family with congenital heart disease.

congestive heart failure

Increased blood flow to the lungs seen in many congential heart defects contributes to CHF. Congenital heart defects are the major cause of CHF in children up to 3 years of

nursing care plan
for the child with a congenital heart defect

NURSING DIAGNOSIS

Decreased Cardiac Output, related to structural anomaly of the heart

GOAL: *The child will have adequate tissue perfusion*

NURSING INTERVENTIONS	RATIONALE	EVALUATION
Provide rest periods for the child.	This will decrease the workload of the heart and decrease the metabolic needs of the child.	The child will conserve energy as evidenced by comfortable, uninterrupted rest periods throughout the day.
Respond quickly to the infant crying.	Excessive crying will stress the already compromised heart by increasing myocardial oxygen consumption.	The child will not tire from excessive crying and will be soothed quickly by caregivers.
Administer medications such as digoxin as prescribed to increase cardiac output.	Depending on the type of anomaly, a positive inotropic agent may be used to improve cardiac output.	The child will receive appropriate medications safely (such as monitoring apical pulse and digoxin levels) and will have improved cardiac output.

NURSING DIAGNOSIS

Altered Family Process, related to life-threatening heart defect in the child

GOAL: *The family will understand the stress of the illness and identify appropriate resources*

NURSING INTERVENTION	RATIONALE	EVALUATION
Communicate to the family an understanding of the impact the diagnosis has had on the entire family system.	Sharing an understanding of the stress will assist in facilitating a trusting relationship that further promotes communication and verbalization of feelings.	The family will verbalize their feelings regarding the diagnosis and prognosis of the congenital heart defect.
Explore normal family dynamics and establish the effectiveness of present coping mechanisms.	The family under stress will undergo various changes in dynamics. It will be important for the nurse and family to realize if the changes and coping mechanisms are adaptive or maladaptive.	The family will identify their strengths and weaknesses and incorporate healthy coping mechanisms that will positively affect the family structure and dynamics.
Advocate the use of outside resources to assist the family in emotional support.	Relatives, friends, and clergy can aid the family at this time and assist in reducing the stress of the situation by helping with the emotional upheaval, financial concerns, and the logistic planning of eventual home care for the child.	The family will identify appropriate resources that they are able to use when the time is necessary.

age; CHF also can be caused by chronic lung disease, severe anemia, blood transfusion reactions, fever, drugs, excessive intravenous fluid administration, and other heart disorders that weaken the heart's pumping ability.

pathophysiology

Congestive heart failure occurs when the heart cannot pump enough blood to meet the body's demands, and blood backs up into the chambers of the heart, causing many organs to become congested with blood and fluid. It can affect the right side, left side, or both sides of the heart.

In right sided heart failure, blood backs up from the chambers of the right atria and ventricle into the *superior and inferior vena cava* (major vessels that return deoxygenated blood from body cells to the right atrium). The backflow of blood causes gross edema of the extremities and contributes to enlargement of the liver.

Left sided heart failure occurs when the left ventricle fails to pump blood out of the aorta, causing the oxygenated blood to back up into the left atrium and lungs. Lung congestion is called pulmonary edema. Edema in the extremities is not a major symptom with left sided heart failure unless the condition progresses to include the right side.

Complete heart failure involving right and left sides is common in infants and young children. It is characterized by gross edema of the extremities, liver congestion, pulmonary edema, and decreased cardiac output. The body produces an increased amount of red blood cells (*polycythemia*) to compensate for the lack of oxygenated blood circulation caused by cyanotic heart disease. Unfortunately, polycythemia contributes to clot formation, increasing the child's risk of cerebral vascular accident (CVA).

medical management

The major goal in treating CHF involves improving the heart's ability to pump effectively. *Compensated* heart failure occurs when treatment stabilizes the heart and improves cardiac output. *Decompensated* heart failure is the failure of the heart as an effective pump.

Medication, such as digoxin, is used to slow and strengthen the heart beat and increase cardiac output. Accumulation of excessive body fluid is reduced by administration of diuretics, fluid restriction, and decreased dietary sodium. Oxygen and pain medications are administered to treat pulmonary edema. Morphine sulfate, a frequently used pain medication, requires close monitoring because it may cause decreased respiratory rates.

✱ nursing process for congestive heart failure

assessment

Subjective data to be assessed include the following:

✱ History of congenital heart defect, anemia, blood loss, infections, occurance and type of heart surgery (*open heart surgery* requires cardiopulmonary bypass; *closed heart surgery* can be done without cardiopulmonary bypass), child's general health status, medications being used and for what purpose, feeding difficulties, and failure to thrive
✱ Information about maternal difficulties during pregnancy or delivery, newborn's Apgar score (if known), and family history of heart disease

Objective data to be assessed include the following:

✱ Tachycardia, decreased peripheral pulses, generalized edema (right sided failure), dyspnea, substernal and intercostal retractions, nasal flaring, crackles, and dry cough (left sided failure)
✱ Decreased urinary output (less than 1 mL/h), fatigue (especially with feedings), and *diaphoresis* on forehead noted mainly when crying or eating
✱ Presence of edema. This is often considered a late sign of CHF and is seen around the eyes, in the genital area, and as generalized body puffiness. Edema can be assessed by applying gentle pressure on an area for up to 5 seconds. If edema is present, a depression of the skin is noted (often called pitting edema).

nursing diagnosis

✱ Decreased Cardiac Output, related to heart structure defects
✱ Fluid Volume Excess, related to alteration of blood circulation
✱ Impaired Gas Exchange, related to pulmonary edema
✱ Risk for Injury, related to medication dosage or adverse reaction to medication
✱ Knowledge Deficit, related to disease process and home care

nursing interventions

promotion of cardiac output

✱ Assess and record apical heart rate and rhythm, presence and strength of peripheral pulses, blood pressure, capillary refill time (less than 3–5 seconds), skin color, presence of edema, increased or decreased temperature readings (hypothermia often indicates a decrease in cardiac output), and diaphoresis.
✱ Assess cardiac monitor for electrode placement. Report and document any significant changes noted on cardiac monitor. Assess electrode placement sites for signs of irritation.
✱ Decrease cardiac demands by keeping the child warm, organizing care to provide child with periods of uninterrupted rest, avoiding infant feedings that last more than 45 minutes, and providing small, frequent feedings. Adhere to health care agency's safety measures when administering tube feedings, such as checking for tube placement, measuring residual, and holding feedings based on residual amounts.

promotion of hydration

✱ Monitor intake and output, daily weights, and intravenous fluid administration.
✱ Maintain fluid restrictions if ordered. Assess skin turgor, fontanels, mucus production, and urine characteristics for signs of dehydration.

promotion of respiratory status

✱ Assess and record rate, character, and regularity of respirations.
✱ Auscultate breath sounds; note presence of cough and mucus production.
✱ Place child in semi-Fowler's position.
✱ Administer prescribed oxygen. The use of cool mist or

humidified oxygen delivered in a noninvasive way, such as a tent or oxygen hood, is more effective with small children.

* Morphine sulfate may be ordered for children with severe CHF for its sedative effect and effectiveness in pulmonary edema. Respiration status must be evaluated before administering morphine because it decreases respiration rate. An overdose can cause respiratory arrest.
* Administer diuretics, and monitor for signs of hypokalemia (see Display 31-1).
* Monitor pulse oximeter readings; report findings if oxygen saturation falls below 95%.

promotion of safe drug administration

* Check apical pulse before administering digoxin (refer to Display 31-3 for age-appropriate ranges).
* Monitor for side effects of digoxin, including bradycardia, irregular heart beat, anorexia, nausea, vomiting, and diarrhea. When digitalis toxicity is suspected, a serum digoxin level will be ordered. Nontoxic serum digoxin levels vary according to the health care facility but typically are in the range of 1.1 to 2.2 ng/dL (see Appendix).
* Double check all dosage calculations for accuracy.
* Monitor heart rate and rhythm and electrolyte levels for signs of hypokalemia from diuretic use.

promotion of home care

Teach parents the signs and symptoms of CHF, including shortness of breath, wheezing, blue discoloration of the skin, fast pulse, fatigue, poor feeding, restlessness, perspiration noted on face during feeding or crying, and rapid weight gain.

* Encourage the parents to weigh child daily and record. Notify the doctor if weight gain is more than 2 pounds in a 24-hour period.
* Teach parents how to take the child's pulse using the carotid or radial pulse sites.
* Provide emotional support. Suggest the use of home health care services.

display 31-3
nursing safety measures for digoxin administration

* **Count apical pulse for 1 minute.**
* **Hold digoxin when pulse is below**
  110 in infants.
  90 in small children
  70 in older children
* **Do not**
  Skip or make up doses.
  Mix with formula or food.

* Provide information about medication administration. Diuretics must be given in the morning to avoid interruption of an older child's sleep from frequent voiding at night. Caution parents never to increase or decrease the digoxin dose unless the doctor orders a change. The need to increase the dose of digoxin is often necessary as the child continues to grow.
* Encourage the family to plan ahead by refilling the digoxin prescription before the bottle is empty.
* Stress the importance of giving the medication as ordered. If a dose of digoxin is missed, the next dose is to be given at the regular time. The medication should not be doubled. If the child vomits the medication more than one time, the doctor needs to be notified.

nursing alert
Parents should be informed that digoxin must be kept out of reach of young children—digoxin overdose can be fatal.

* Inform parents about the signs of digoxin toxicity, including loss of appetite, diarrhea, and vomiting.
* Evaluate the parents' understanding of dietary guidelines, which may include restricted sodium (sodium is not the same as salt) and increased potassium intake if child is taking medication such as furosemide (Lasix) as a diuretic.
* Stress the importance of follow-up care with a health care provider. Typical childhood immunizations may be delayed until the child is older. Remind parents to keep the pediatrician informed.

evaluation

* The child demonstrates improved cardiac status by maintaining stable heart and respiratory rates and normal laboratory values.
* The child maintains adequate respiratory function, reflected by normal skin and mucous membrane color, normal capillary refill, and less dyspnea with natural respiration pattern.
* The child has normal fluid and electrolyte values and decreased edema.
* The child suffers no injuries or adverse effects from medication dosages.
* The parents verbalize an understanding of the disease process; complications; home care instructions, especially concerning drug administration; and follow-up care.

acquired heart disease

rheumatic fever

Rheumatic fever is an inflammatory disease of the *collagen* (connective tissues), which can cause inflammation of, and often permament damage to, the heart. It is a common cause of acquired heart disease in children between 5 and 15 years old.

pathophysiology

Studies have indicated that there is a connection between rheumatic fever and infection with group A hemolytic *Streptococcus*, which causes common childhood illnesses like "strep" throat and ear infections. The hemolytic *Streptococcus* is thought to trigger antibody formation and an autoimmune reaction. These antibodies attack the heart valves, causing rheumatic *endocarditis* (inflammation of the endocardium). The mitral valve becomes inflamed, thickened, and hardened (mitral valve stenosis). This prevents it from opening and closing properly and hinders blood flow from the left atrium into the left ventricle (Fig. 31-4). This often causes symptoms of CHF.

symptoms

Rheumatic fever usually develops about 1 to 4 weeks after infection with hemolytic streptococci. In addition to heart damage and symptoms of CHF, common symptoms include the following:

* Fatigue
* Fever ranging from mild to severe
* Migratory large joint pain
* Subcutaneous nodules over bony prominences
* Erythema marginatum (skin rash on the abdomen)
* *Chorea* (St. Vitus' dance; irregular, involuntary movement seen more often in girls)

medical–surgical management

Diagnosis of rheumatic fever includes an elevated white blood cell count and erythrocyte sedimentation rate. Echocardiography, ECG, and heart catheterization confirm the diagnosis. Medical treatment is aimed at preventing or treating symptoms of CHF using medications such as digoxin and diuretics. Penicillin (or erythromycin) is initially given to rid the body of the *Streptococcus* infection and is continued on a long-term basis to prevent recurrence of rheumatic fever. Children who have had rheumatic heart disease are at increased risk of developing subacute bacterial endocarditis. Therefore, antibiotic therapy is especially important before any type of dental or medical procedure that has the potential to cause bleeding or infection. Surgical intervention involves enlarging the mitral valve (mitral *commissurotomy*), plastic repair of the mitral valve (*valvuloplasty*), and valve replacement.

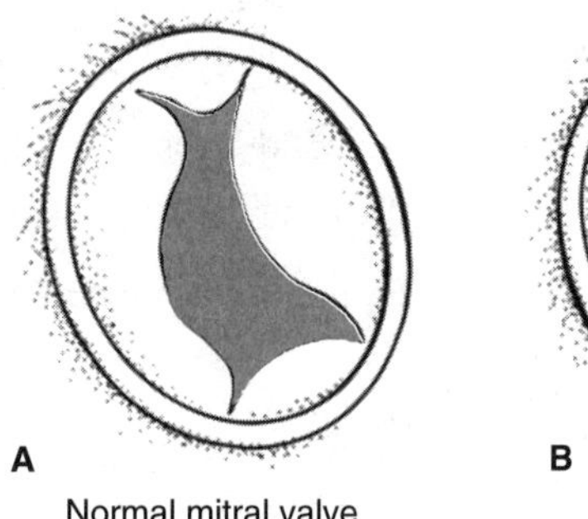

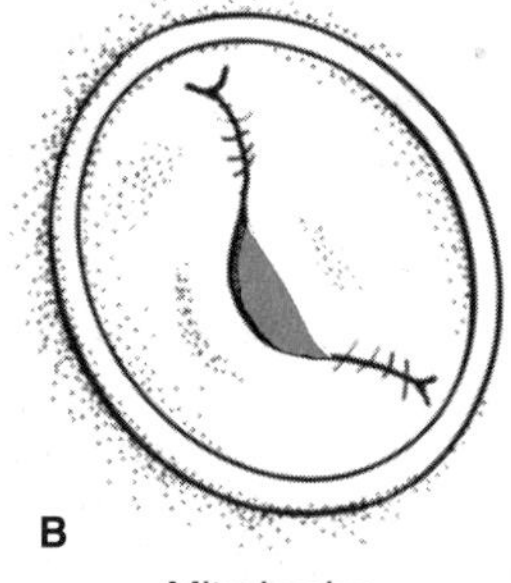

figure 31-4 *(**A**) The normal mitral valve opens widely to allow blood to pass from the left atria to the left ventricle. (**B**) Following what is generally an infectious process, the mitral valve leaflets become thickened, causing a partially obstructed pathway for the passage of blood.*

nursing care

During the acute period of the disease, the child must have complete bed rest to ease the workload of the heart. The nurse should record fluid intake and output, temperature, pulse and respiration rate, and blood pressure as ordered. The child should be handled gently because of swollen, painful joints.

Another goal of nursing care is to provide the child and parents with education about the disease. This includes stressing the importance of following the prescribed medication schedule to prevent recurrence. The nurse also must provide emotional support for the child and family, especially if the child is scheduled for heart surgery.

> **nursing alert**
>
> *Prophylactic antibiotics must be given to children with a history of rheumatic fever before any dental or invasive procedures to reduce the risk of endocarditis.*

hypertension

Hypertension (high blood pressure) is a result of either increased cardiac output or increased peripheral resistance. If the hypertension is caused by an existing renal, vascular, endocrine, or congenital disorder, it is termed *secondary*. *Primary hypertension* has no known cause but is believed to be influenced by a combination of factors, including obesity, age, race (hypertension is more prevalent in African Americans), smoking, diet, activity level, heredity, and anxiety. Although hypertension is normally considered an adult disease, children and especially adolescents are becoming increasingly susceptible to it. In addition, behaviors and habits practiced in childhood greatly influence adult health.

symptoms

A child with hypertension usually does not exhibit symptoms. Sometimes headaches, dizziness, and vision problems will occur. Uncontrolled hypertension in the child may eventually lead to heart disease, stroke, or renal disease as an adult. Hypertension is diagnosed when the child's blood pressure measurement is consistently between the 95th and 99th percentile for sex and age (Jackson, 1993). If the measurment is consistently above the 99th percentile for sex and age, the child has severe hypertension (Fig. 31-5).

treatment and prevention

Nonpharmacologic treatment for hypertension in the child consists primarily of diet and lifestyle modification and stress reduction. The overweight child is encouraged to be more active and eat foods that are low in fat and salt. Smoking is discouraged. Pharmacologic methods of treating hypertension include diuretics or beta-adrenergic

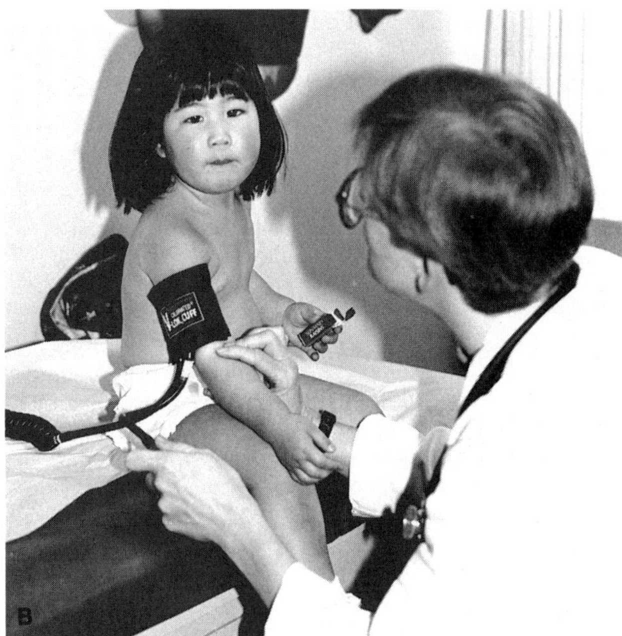

figure 31-5 *Assessing blood pressure is vital in detecting hypertension.*

blockers. However, these medications should be used cautiously because long-term effects of these drugs on children are not known.

Prevention consists of routine screening, especially for children with a family history of the disease. In addition, because birth control pills have been linked to high blood pressure, adolescents taking this medication should be carefully screened. The nurse should encourage children to start practicing good health and eating habits when they are young.

key points

* **Parents of children born with cardiovascular system disorders must deal with many serious concerns. These include the threat of losing the baby because congenital heart defects are often serious and require open heart surgery; day-to-day uncertainties about the child's failure to thrive because poor sucking ability increases the risk of altered growth; fear of the child contracting an infection; social isolation; and overwhelming drains on the family's emotions, energies, and finances.**
* **The infant with cardiovascular system disorders may require alternate feeding methods, such as tube feedings, to ensure proper nutrition.**
* **The newborn's first breath symbolizes an important milestone in the cardiovascular system as the newborn changes from placental circulation to pulmonary circulation.**
* **Cardiac catheterization detects abnormalities in the heart chambers, valves, and blood vessels. Arterial and venous catheters are threaded into the right and left sides of the heart, and contrast media is injected to view the heart structures.**
* **General nursing intervention for care of the child with a cardiovascular disorder includes promotion of understanding aimed at relieving anxiety, child and parental hope, growth and development, activity, absence of infection, child and parental knowledge, and self-esteem.**
* **The exact cause of congenital heart defects is unknown. However, contributing factors include maternal infections during the first trimester of pregnancy, maternal alcoholism, drug use considered toxic to the fetus, maternal dietary deficiencies, insulin-dependent diabetic mothers, and those older than 40 years.**
* **Typical symptoms of CHF include gross edema of the extremities and liver enlargement (right sided failure); pulmonary edema (left sided failure); and gross edema of the extremities, liver congestion, pulmonary edema, decreased cardiac output, and polycythemia (complete heart failure).**
* **Nursing care for the child with rheumatic fever includes monitoring and recording vital signs; carefully handling the child with swollen, painful joints; providing education about the disease; stressing the importance of taking the prescribed medications; and providing emotional support.**
* **Prevention of hypertension in the child consists primarily of routine blood pressure screening and encouragement of healthy living and eating habits.**

review questions

1. Fatima Torres' son, Pat, was born with an AV septal heart defect. He is being seen in the clinic for a routine examination. Pat is busy playing while the nurse takes subjective data from Fatima. She confides that she feels trapped caring for Pat and perceives him to be a difficult child compared with her other children. Select the most appropriate nursing intervention.
   a. The nurse should acknowledge Fatima's statement and encourage her to explore negative feelings toward Pat.
   b. The nurse should refer Fatima and her son to Children's Social Service because the family is at risk for child abuse.
   c. The nurse should provide Fatima with information about Home Health Care Agencies or respite care available in the community.
   d. The nurse should suggest Fatima seek professional counseling.
2. Mrs. Calland's 1-week-old son has a congenital heart defect. She asks why her son requires a tube feeding. Select the most appropriate nursing response.
   a. "Your son may have other problems in addition to the heart defect, and the doctor wants to provide nourishment in the safest manner."

b. "Most seriously ill infants get more nourishment from a tube feeding."
c. "Why do you ask? Did you want to breast-feed?"
d. "Your son needs to conserve his energy and by getting nourishment through a tube, he does not have to use energy sucking."

3. Terry is a 5-year-old with a heart murmur. He is scheduled for an electrocardiogram (ECG) and asks the nurse for information. Select the most appropriate nursing actions.
   a. Tell Terry the test measures and records the electrical current going through his heart.
   b. Show Terry an ECG machine and encourage him to ask questions.
   c. Explain that when the heart beats, energy from the heartbeat will be recorded by a machine. Small round patches are placed on the chest during the test but are removed afterward. Provide reassurance that the procedure is not painful and that his parents can stay during the test.
   d. Provide Terry's parents with instructions about the test and encourage them to talk to him and calm his fears.
4. Assessment data for a child with left-sided heart failure include
   a. squatting position, dyspnea, and abnormal blood gasses.
   b. orthopneic position, peripheral edema, and elevated blood pressure.
   c. tachypnea, hyperthermia, and increased appetite.
   d. Decreased urinary output, enlarged liver, and ascites.
5. Children with chronic heart problems are at increased risk for:
   a. Respiratory infections.
   b. Obesity.
   c. Mental retardation.
   d. Diarrhea.

references

(1992). *Lippincott's review series: Pediatric nursing.* Philadelphia: J.B. Lippincott.

McCance, K. (1994). *Pathophysiology: The biological basis for disease in adults and children* (2nd ed.). St. Louis: C.V. Mosby.

Woods, S. (1995). *Cardiac nursing* (3rd ed.). Philadelphia: J.B. Lippincott.

bibliography

Allen, H., Teske, D., & Davis, J. (1993). The primary physician and patients with congenital heart disease. *Pediatric Directions Children's Hospital, Spring/Summer*, 24–27.

Carpenito, L. (1995). *Handbook of nursing diagnosis* (6th ed.). Philadelphia: J.B. Lippincott.

Castiglia, P., & Harbin, R. (1992). *Child health care.* Philadelphia: J.B. Lippincott.

Club, R. (1991). Chronic sorrow: Adaptation patterns of parents with chronically ill children. *Pediatric Nursing, 17*(5), 461–465.

Fischbach, F. (1995). *Quick reference to common laboratory and diagnostic tests.* Philadelphia: J.B. Lippincott.

Gulanick, M., Gradishar, D., & Puzas, M. (1994). *Ambulatory pediatric nursing*. Albany, NY: Delmar Publishers.

Jackson, D.B. & Saunder, R.B. (1993). *Child health nursing*. Philadelphia: J.B. Lippincott.

Jensen, C. (1992). Nursing care of a child following an arterial switch procedure for transposition of the great arteries. *Critical Care Nurse, December*, 51–57.

Marino, B., & Lipshitz, M. (1991). Temperament in infants and toddlers with cardiac disease. *Pediatric Nursing, 17*(5), 445–448.

Memmler, R., Cohen, B., & Wood, D. (1996). *The human body in health and disease* (8th ed.). Philadelphia: Lippincott–Raven.

Pillitteri, A. (1995). *Maternal and child health nursing* (2nd ed.). Philadelphia: J.B. Lippincott.

Scherer, J., & Timby, B. (1995). *Introductory medical-surgical nursing* (6th ed.). Philadelphia: J.B. Lippincott.

Smeltzer, S., & Bare, B. (1992). *Brunner and Suddarth's textbook of medical-surgical nursing*. Philadelphia: J.B. Lippincott.

(1992). *Taber's encyclopedia* (17th ed.). Philadelphia: F.A. Davis.

the child with an alteration in hematologic or immune system function

32

outline

objectives

After studying this chapter, the reader should be able to:

* Discuss several family considerations relating to the child with an alteration in hematologic or immune system function.
* Describe the composition of the blood.
* List the ways in which the body protects itself against foreign substances.
* Discuss how jaundice may develop in the newborn.
* Discuss the pathophysiology of sickle cell anemia.
* Describe aspects of nursing care for the child with hemophilia.
* Discuss the medical and surgical management of leukemia.
* List ways in which the child with allergies and the family can environmentally control allergies.
* Define autoimmunity.
* Discuss the ways in which infants and children aquire human immunodeficiency virus.

key terms

albumins
antibodies
antigens
basophil
dyscrasia
eosinophils
fibrinogen
globulins
hemarthrosis
icterus
leukocytes
macrophage
neutrophils
prothrombin
thrombocytes

Neff C & Spray M. *Introduction to Maternal and Child Health Nursing,*

Alterations of hematologic or immune function in the child are usually chronic disorders requiring lifelong treatment. Many of these disorders are life-threatening. They affect blood components and immune function, causing problems throughout the entire body. Alterations of hematologic function include anemia, sickle cell anemia, hemophilia, and leukemia. Alterations of immune function include allergies, autoimmunity disorders, immunodeficiency disorders, and acquired immunodeficiency syndrome (AIDS).

✷ family considerations

In children with hematologic or immune system disorders, parents may fear interaction with other children due to the child's lowered resistance to infection and tendency to bruise. The limited exposure to social experiences contributes to limitations on age-appropriate play.

If a child is diagnosed with anemia, parents may feel responsible for having caused the problem or for failing to recognize it. In addition, important food sources for the child with iron-defiency anemia can be expensive for low-income families and may increase the parents' frustration about the child's condition.

Certain blood disorders, such as hemophilia, are inherited. If the parents blame each other or themselves, guilt and anger can cause friction within the family. If the family does not seek counseling to resolve these issues, the family may break up.

Parents must create an appropriate allergen-free environment for children with allergies. This may involve not having pets or keeping the house free of dust, rugs, and feather beds or pillows. In addition, the child may require special laundry detergent and bath soap.

Guilt and despair are common feelings in parents of children with an immune disorder like AIDS because many children contract the disease directly from the mother. In addition, many times the mother or both parents are sick with the disease and have to deal with their own sickness and eventual death as well as the sickness and death of their child.

Parents and siblings often accommodate the sick child's needs over their own. Fear that the child is too fragile to enjoy a long life encourages family members to indulge the affected child.

✷ nursing considerations

Children with disorders of the hematologic or immune system are usually scared about their diagnosis and do not know what to expect. The nurse must provide factual information about the disease, explain necessary treatments for the disease, and teach the child preventive measures to stay as healthy and active as possible.

Frequent finger, heel, and venipuncture sticks for blood component determination can cause discomfort and anxiety in the child. Allowing children to vent anger without chastising them is important.

Children with chronic disorders of the hematologic and immune system are at increased risk of developmental and growth delays. The nurse should be aware of this and promote growth and development by encouraging interaction with peers and family, encouraging school attendance whenever possible, and providing the child with age-appropriate activities.

Children with AIDS are sometimes shunned because of their illness. The nurse must be completely accepting of these children by treating them like every other child. These children need to be touched, hugged, and reassured that they are normal.

anatomy and physiology

blood components

Blood is composed of plasma and formed substances called blood cells. Plasma is approximately 90% water and 10% dissolved elements. The disolved elements are predominately proteins classified as *albumins*, *globulins*, or *clotting factors*. Albumin regulates the flow of water and solutes through the capillaries. Globulins are plasma proteins associated with antibodies and created in the lymphoid organs and lymph nodes. *Fibrinogen* and *prothrombin* are clotting factors found in plasma.

The three kinds of blood cells include erythrocytes (red blood cells); leukocytes (white blood cells), which help the body fight infection; and thrombocytes (platelets) that aid in blood clotting.

Erythrocytes are formed in the red bone marrow of flat and irregular bones. These cells make up the greatest percentage of the total blood volume. Their primary function is to transport oxygen and carbon dioxide to and from all tissues of the body. Erythrocytes are continually created and destroyed. Their average lifespan is 120 days.

There are five kinds of leukocytes. Granular leukocytes are produced in the red bone marrow and include neutrophils, eosinophils, and basophils. Agranular leukocytes are produced in the lymphatic tissue of the spleen, lymph nodes, thymus, and red bone marrow. Two types of agranular leukocytes are lymphocytes and monocytes.

Platelets are not whole cells but are pieces of cells originating in the red bone marrow. Platelets prevent blood loss by causing vasoconstriction of blood vessels and initiating the formation of a clot (Display 32-1).

lymphatic system

The lymphatic system plays a major role in immune function. It is responsible for returning tissue fluid to the blood and protecting the body against foreign material. Most organs of the body are drained by the lymphatic system with the exception of the brain, eyes, and ears. Lymph, lymph vessels, lymph nodes, spleen, and thymus gland are included in the lymphatic system. Movement of lymph involves smooth muscle contraction of the lymph vessels because the lymphatic system does not have a pump.

display 32-1
steps in the blood clotting process

A blood clot forms in response to the following events:

* Tissue damage occurs, causing bleeding.
* Platelets rupture, producing coagulation factors known as thromboplastin and thrombokinase.
* Prothrombin accompanied by calcium and thrombokinase generate thrombin. Vitamin K must be present for the manufacture of prothrombin.
* Fibrinogen (a protein essential for blood clotting) converts thrombin into fibrin. Fibrin makes up the strands that entangle red blood cells to form a clot.
* A clot forms after all the above factors are completed.

Lymph formation takes place in tissue spaces throughout the body called lymph nodes. Lymphocytes and monocytes are made by lymph nodes for the primary purpose of filtering foreign content, such as bacteria, out of the bloodstream.

the immune response

Immunity refers to the body's ability to create protective antibodies to resist foreign substances. Cell-mediated immunity, humoral immunity, B-cell immunity, complement fixation, and immunoglobins are ways in which this occurs.

cell-mediated immunity

Cell-mediated immunity occurs when T cells respond directly to antigens. Activated, antigen-specific *helper T cells* multiply rapidly and produce several different types of T cells, such as *memory T cells*, *killer T cells*, and *suppressor T cells*. Memory T cells "remember" the specific foreign antigen and quickly activate when the antigen enters the body again. Killer T cells chemically destroy antigens by disrupting their cell membrane. Suppressor T cells stop the immune response once foreign antigens are destroyed (Display 32-2). These responses occur without the formation of antibodies and are effective against viruses, fungi, and malignant cells.

humoral immunity

Humoral immunity occurs when B cells produce antibodies in direct response to stimulation by an antigen. Antigens entering the body are presented to B cells by sensitized helper T cells. Activated B cells divide rapidly into memory B cells and plasma B cells. Memory B cells "remember" the foreign antigen and keep the information on "file" for future reference. Plasma B cells multiply rapidly and produce antibodies specific to the foreign antigen. This detoxifies invading antigens, making them harmless.

complement fixation

Complement fixation is a group of 14 proteins present in the blood that are activated by exposure to antigen-antibody reaction. These special proteins attach to an invading antigen and make holes in the antigen's membranes by exerting enzyme action.

immunoglobins

Antibody formation by lymphocytes and plasma cells includes serum proteins called immunoglobulins (Ig). Classes of immunoglobulins are shown in Table 32-1. Two major categories of immunity are genetic and acquired. Antibodies join with antigens in a lock-and-key manner (Fig. 32-1).

age-specific considerations

The long bones of the infant's body contain red marrow that produces red blood cells. During early childhood, yellow marrow replaces the red marrow, and blood cells are produced primarily in the ribs, scapulae, vertebrae, and skull bones.

Large numbers of red blood cells are needed during fetal circulation to provide sufficient oxygen to fetal cells. These extra red blood cells are not needed in pulmonary circulation. As a response, the infant's body begins destroying the extra erythrocytes. The waste product that results is bilirubin.

Increased bilirubin is responsible for the condition known as physiologic jaundice. A yellowish discoloration of the skin (*jaundice*) results from an excessive amount of bile pigment in the blood. Bile pigmentation of the tissues, membranes, and secretions is called *icterus*. *Icterus neonatorum* is the medical term for physiologic jaundice and is described as hemolytic jaundice occurring in the newborn. It is considered mild, self-limiting, and usually requires no treatment.

The immune system parallels the growth of the lymphatic system. Infants and toddlers have an increased risk of infections compared with preschoolers. This is due to a lack of IgG and IgA growth until the child is 2 or 3 years

display 32-2
mechanisms of immunity

* Foreign substance enters the body as an antigen.
* Body recognizes the presence of a foreign antigen.
* Macrophage cells eat the foreign antigen.
* Parts of the antigen are presented on the macrophage's cell membrane.
* Helper T cells encounter the macrophage, becoming sensitized to the foreign antigen.
* Helper T cells become specific in their response to the foreign antigen, initiating either or both cell-mediated immunity or humoral immunity.

table 32-1 classes of immunoglobulin/antibodies

Name	Site	Role
IgM	Intravascular fluid	Initial defense
IgG	Blood	Long-term immunity following specific disease recovery or immunization
IgA	Saliva, tears, breast milk	Primary defense; passive immunity to breast-fed infants
IgD	Circulating B lymphocytes	Unknown
IgE	Serum, surface membrane of basophil and mast cells	Releases histamine, immediate response in allergic reactions

old. This growth continues to increase through adolescence. Breast-fed infants receive some immunity from their mothers, equipping them with a stronger immune system than formula-fed infants.

diagnostic tests

Many general and specialized tests are used to diagnose hematologic and immune disorders. General blood tests, skin testing for allergies, and testing for human immunodeficiency virus (HIV) are discussed below.

blood tests

* Red cell count: Decreased values indicate anemia or leukemia. Increased values indicate polycythemia (increased red cell mass), dehydration, and hemorrhage or immediately after hemorrhage.
* White cell count: Increased values (leukocytosis) indicate infection, hemorrhage, or leukemia. Decreased values (leukopenia) indicate hypersplenism; bone marrow depression due to cancer chemotherapy; primary bone marrow disorder, such as leukemia; aplastic anemia; and myeloma.
* Hematocrit values: Decreased levels indicate anemia, leukemia, significant blood loss, and hemolytic reactions to incompatible blood transfusions. Increased levels are found in polycythemia, erythrocytosis, severe dehydration, and shock.
* Hemoglobin values: Decreased levels are found in anemia, severe hemorrhage, and hemolytic reactions to transfusions of incompatible blood, infections, or systemic diseases. Increased levels are found in hemoconcentration of the blood.
* ESR levels: Erythocyte sedimentation rate levels are increased in diseases such as autoimmune disorders, infections, cancer, and severe anemia. They are decreased in sickle cell anemia.
* Bone marrow test: Examination of the bone marrow is used to diagnose leukemia, blood deficiencies, decreased production of white blood cells (agranulocytosis), and platelet disorders.

skin testing for allergies

Skin testing involves three methods: intradermal injection test, which are injections of allergens given in the intradermal skin layer; scratch test, in which a scratch is made on the skin, and a small amount of liquid antigen is applied to the scratch; and patch test, in which a concentrated form of the suspected allergen is applied to the skin for 48 hours and covered with an inclusive dressing. A positive reaction is noted by a hive or localized redness or swelling in the site.

Children are often apprehensive about skin testing and fear the pain of multiple scratches or injections. The nurse should provide explanations and reassure them that the testing is more annoying than painful. Intradermal injections are similar to tuberculosis screening.

testing for human immunodeficiency virus

In adults, anti-HIV IgG antibodies in serum are detected by using enzyme-linked immunosorbent assay and Western blot tests. These standard, commercially available serologic tests are not reliable in diagnosing HIV in newborns and young children because they will detect maternal transplacental acquired anti-HIV IgG up to 15 months of age.

Polymerase chain reaction, HIV culture, and detection of antigen HIV-specific antibodies of a class that does not cross the placenta provide a more accurate diagnosis of HIV infection in newborns and young children. New tests detect the virus rather than the antibody. The new testing method detects the presence of IgA, which is produced by the infant in response to the HIV infection and cannot be transmitted from mother to fetus because IgA does not cross the placental barrier. A positive IgA test confirms that the infant is infected. Diagnosis of HIV infection can be made in infants as young as 3 months.

✳ nursing process for the child with alterations of hematologic and immune function

assessment

Subjective data to be assessed include the following:

* History of infections (especially respiratory and fungal infections)
* Family history of genetically acquired hematologic diseases or immunologic disorders

Objective data to be assessed include the following:

* Presence of skin rashes, petechiae, or bruising
* Severe, persistent fungal infection
* Fatigue, lethargy, pallor
* Presence of opportunistic infection

nursing diagnosis

* Risk for Infection, related to alterations of hematologic or immune system, decreased activity, intravenous access sites, surgical interventions, and invasive diagnostic procedures
* Anxiety, related to serious nature of illness and potentially poor prognosis
* Client and Parental Knowledge Deficit
* Self Esteem Disturbance, related to chronic fatigue and discomfort, skin rashes, bruises, infections, restricted activities, lack of privacy, and parental overprotection

nursing interventions

reducing risk of infections

* Reduce the risk of infection through careful handwashing, avoiding contact with infected people, maintaining current immunizations, and providing adequate nutrition and rest.
* Monitor temperature and white blood cell laboratory values for elevations above normal limits based on age.
* Assess wound and intravenous sites for evidence of redness, odor, edema, and purulent drainage. Change dressings as ordered using sterile technique.
* Provide child and parents with information about symptoms of infection; teach technique for taking temperature, and stress the importance of notifying the doctor for temperature elevations above 38.4°C (101°F).

relieving anxiety

* Encourage parents to be involved in the child's care.
* Provide emotional support to the child and family.
* Refer the child and family to support groups or counseling if needed.
* Explain all necessary procedures, tests, and treatments, and answer all questions that the child or family may have.

promoting knowledge

* Provide the child and parents with information on the components of the hematologic or immune systems and facts about the specific disease.

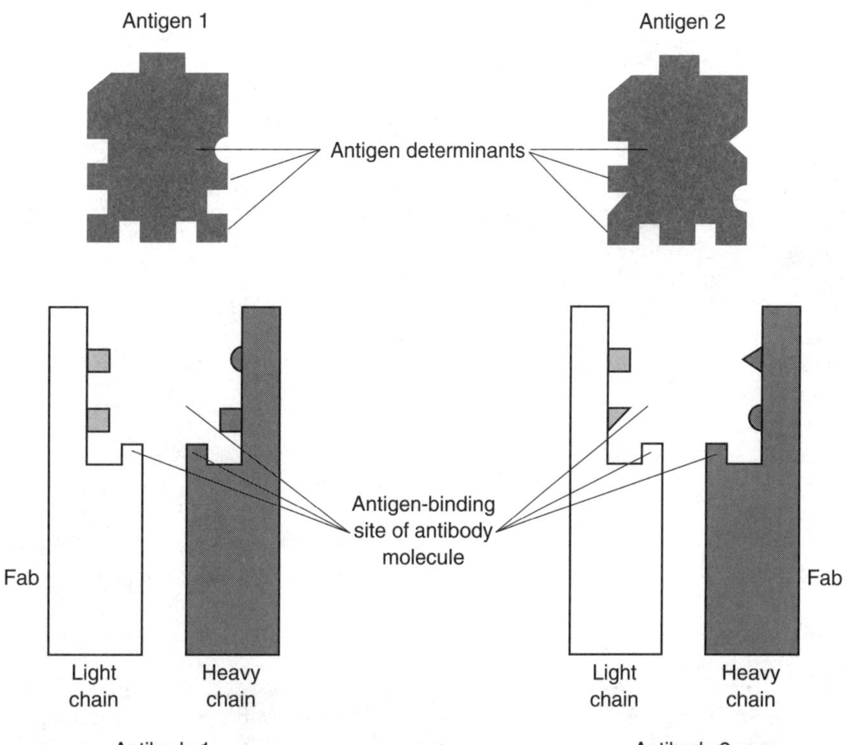

figure 32-1 *Antigen-antibody binding. The specificity required for antibody binding with an antigen is determined by the shape of the combining site on the antibody.*

* Explain all treatment plans, necessary medications and side effects, special diets, and limits on activity.
* Teach parents and child (if able) how to administer required medications and how to monitor their effectiveness.

promoting self-esteem

* Establish a trusting nurse–client relationship; listen to the child's fears and concerns, and provide emotional support.
* Encourage interaction with family, friends, and peers within the hospital setting.
* Allow the child to talk about the disease or disorder and how it has affected their life and relationships with their parents, family, and friends.
* Provide time for the child to be private; allow the child to play a role in decision-making, and encourage the parents to allow the child some independence.

evaluation

* The child remains free from infection.
* The child and the family voice reduced anxiety related to the child's illness, hospitalization, treatments, and medications.
* The child and family demonstrate knowledge about necessary medication administration.
* The child expresses feelings about the disease or disorder, voices positive feelings about self, socializes with others, and participates in making decisions about his or her care.

hematologic disorders

Hematologic disorders involve a large group of illnesses affecting blood components, sometimes called *dyscrasias*. Blood dyscrasia is an old term that implies "bad mixture" of the blood cells. Blood cell excesses or shortages can be life-threatening because normal blood cell counts are necessary to sustain life.

Blood disorder symptoms are not easily recognized. The child appears pale, complains of tiredness, and often experiences a lowered resistance to infections; this is often attributed to being tired from vigorous play, school activities, or being "run down" from irregular eating and lack of sleep.

Children with hematologic disorders undergo a host of invasive diagnostic tests, procedures, and treatments. These can lead to anxiety and stress for the child and parents. The child should be encouraged to express or act out anger and frustration through puppets, role playing, and drawing pictures.

anemia

Anemia is a condition in which the number of red blood cells (erythrocytes) is decreased, or hemoglobin levels fall below normal. Normal hemoglobin levels range from 10 to 14 g/d in infants to 12 to 14 g/d in older children. *Hemoglobin* is the iron-containing pigment of the red blood cells responsible for carrying oxygen from the lungs to the tissues. Anemia is the most common hematologic problem of infancy and childhood.

pathophysiology

Anemia in children is usually associated with the following:

* Blood loss associated with trauma, invasive procedures, or surgery
* Decreased or impaired red blood cell production, suppression of bone marrow, or dietary deficiencies of protein and green, leafy vegetables (eg, iron-defiency anemia)
* Abnormality of the red blood cells with increased cell destruction inside and outside of the cell (eg, sickle cell disease)

medical management

Medical management of anemia is directed at reestablishing normal red blood cell and hemoglobin values. This involves diagnosing the cause of the anemia, correcting it, preventing complications, and taking measures to restabilize the blood components. Nutritional support, vitamin and mineral supplements, and rest are usual methods of treatment. Blood transfusions may be performed for some types of anemia.

✳ nursing process for the child with anemia

assessment

Subjective data to be assessed include the following:

* History of deficient dietary intake or *pica* (an appetite for nonfood substances), contact with lead through lead-based paints or plumbing, surgery resulting in excessive blood loss
* Family history of genetically transmitted diseases (eg, sickle cell anemia)

Objective data to be assessed include the following:

* Pallor, tachycardia, muscle weakness, fatigue, hypotension, and increased respirations

nursing diagnosis

* Altered Tissue Perfusion, related to decreased hemoglobin
* Activity Intolerance, related to increased potential of hypoxia

nursing interventions

* Support child's need to limit activities by avoiding strenuous play.
* Provide rest periods by organizing care around scheduled treatments.

teaching guidelines
oral iron administration

* Give iron supplement on an empty stomach for better absorption.
* Give with citrus juices because vitamin C helps iron absorption.
* Use a dropper straw when giving liquid iron to avoid discoloring the child's teeth.
* Black stools are common.
* Keep medication away from children; an overdose can cause brain damage and death.

* Avoid high altitudes.
* Avoid infections.
* Administer vitamin and oral supplements as ordered (see the Teaching Guidelines above).
* Provide the older child and parents with nutritional guidelines for iron-deficiency anemia. Caregivers must limit infant milk intake to less than 32 oz/d, providing iron-fortified formula (not cow's milk) and cereal for children younger than 1 year, and encouraging a diet rich in proteins, such as meat, liver, whole grains, legumes, and green, leafy vegetables.
* Refer parents to a nutritionist or to Women, Infants and Children (WIC; a nutrition program) if available in the community. If anemia is genetic, refer the child and parents to a genetic counselor.

evaluation

* Child has adequate tissue perfusion, as evidenced by warm extremities, stable vital signs, normal skin tone, and increased energy level.
* Dietary patterns reflect adequate intake of iron-rich nutrients.

sickle cell anemia

Sickle cell anemia is an inherited disorder of the hemoglobin that primarily affects African Americans and people of eastern Mediterranean origin. One in 12 African Americans carries the gene. Carriers of the gene have *sickle cell trait*, an asymptomatic condition that causes the blood to have normal and sickled hemoglobin (hemoglobin S). *Sickle cell disease* occurs when a child receives the sickle cell trait from both parents. It results in the replacement of normal hemoglobin with hemoglobin S. Sickle cell disease is a serious condition requiring treatment and frequent hospitalization.

pathophysiology

Hemoglobin S replaces all or part of the normal hemoglobin, altering the appearance of red blood cells when oxygen is released to the tissues. The red blood cells have a sickled look rather than the characteristic round appearance of a normal cell (Fig. 32-2). This irregular shape prevents them from flowing through capillary beds.

Symptoms can be mild to severe. Major symptoms include chronic anemia related to decreased lifespan of the sickled red blood cell (less than 40 days), painful and swollen joints, ulcers, and abdominal pain.

diagnosis

The *sickle solubility test* is used to diagnose sickle cell disease by confirming the presence of hemoglobin S in peripheral blood; *hemoglobin eletrophoresis* determines the amount of hemoglobin S in red blood cells in a person diagnosed with sickle cell disease.

sickle cell crisis

Sickle cell crisis is a sudden, severe onset of sickling. Several types of crises have been identified. A *vaso-occlusive crisis* occurs when sickled cells merge in vessels and cause tissue hypoxia. A type of crisis seen only in the young child is called *sequestration crisis.* This occurs when large amounts of blood pool in the liver and spleen. The spleen may be removed (splenectomy) if the child experiences repeated crises.

The child in sickle cell crisis will have severe worsening of symptoms. In addition, the crisis may cause infarctions in the spleen, bone, liver, kidney, and central nervous system. These infarctions may result in vomiting, fever, severe abdominal pain, paralysis, infection, blindness, severe headaches, stroke, and coma.

Dehydration, fever, exercise, and respiratory infections that lower blood oxygen levels have been indicated as precipitators of a sickle cell crisis.

medical management

Medical management for sickle cell anemia is palliative when the symptoms exacerbate. A major goal in managing the child with sickle cell anemia is to avoid a sickling crisis. Intravenous fluid administration increases the fluid

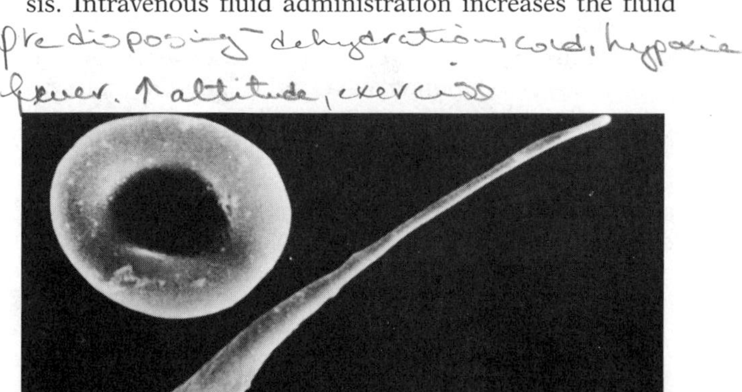

figure 32-2 *A normal and a sickled red blood cell.*

volume and decreases the cell's potential for sickling and development of thrombosis. Analgesics are often necessary to control the pain. Strong emphasis is placed on keeping immunizations current to reduce the risk of infections. Blood transfusions are given for severe anemia. Administering packed red cells may be required to maintain the hemoglobin above 12 g/d.

nursing care

The primary goal of nursing care is to provide the family with ways to prevent a sickle cell crisis. This includes advising the child to avoid strenuous exercise, high altitudes, and contact with people with infections. Vaccines are an important part of health maintenance in children with sickle cell anemia. The vaccines that are administered include the pneumococcal vaccine, meningococcal vaccine, *Haemophilus* B vaccine, and hepatitis B vaccine.

In addition, the nurse should provide the child with plenty of fluids and should not withhold liquids at night for bed wetting—enuresis is a complication of the disease. When fluids are restricted, the risk of sickle cell crisis is increased. Maintaining hydration can be accomplished by giving the child a drink every hour. Inform school-age children to take fluids to school, on hikes, and on special outings. Care must be taken to avoid dehydration in the summer.

Inform the child to avoid contact sports that increase the risk of dehydration and increase the risk of injury to an enlarged spleen. Encourage the child to balance activity with rest. The nurse should administer prophylactic penicillin as ordered and encourage the child to eat a well-balanced diet containing necessary vitamins and iron.

When children are hospitalized with a vaso-occlusive crisis, the nurse must monitor intravenous fluids, electrolytes, and intake and output. Bed rest is encouraged during the acute phase of the illness. Vital signs, especially temperature, must be monitored for signs of infection. Children receiving blood transfusions are at risk for blood-borne pathogen diseases, such as hepatitis B and AIDS.

Administer prescribed analgesics for pain. Acetaminophen is used for mild pain, and meperidine and morphine are used for extreme pain. Safety measures should be instituted when administering meperidine or morphine. This includes assessing respiration rate, raising side rails, and keeping the call light within child's or parent's reach. Applying warmth to the affected site also can be comforting.

hemophilia

Hemophilia is an inherited bleeding disorder transmitted by an X-linked recessive chromosome. Therefore, it is a male disease transmitted by carrier females (Fig. 32-3). The incidence is approximately 1 in 8,000 live male births (Pediatric Nursing, 1992).

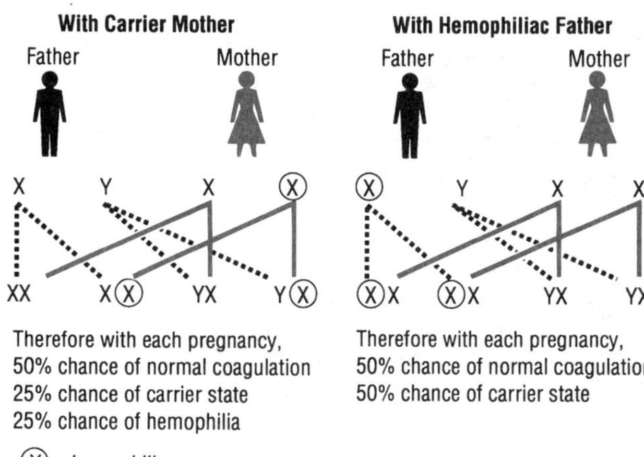

figure 32-3 *Genetic transmission of hemophilia.*

pathophysiology

Hemophilia involves abnormalities of clotting factors and causes impaired ability to form a fibrin clot. Hemophilia A, the most common form of the disease, involves a defect or deficiency of factor VIII. Hemophilia B (also called Christmas disease) involves a defect or deficiency of factor IX. A deficiency of these factors results in extensive bleeding that can be spontaneous or caused by injury. The most frequent site of bleeding is in the joints (*hemarthrosis*), causing pain and loss of joint motion.

diagnosis

Diagnosis of hemophilia is based on family history, child's health history, and presenting symptoms. Prothrombin time is used to screen for factors II, V, VII, and X deficiencies. Normal value range is 12 to 14 seconds. Partial thromboplastin time is used to screen for factors II, V, VIII, IX, X, XI, and XII; normal value is less than 30 seconds.

medical management

Medical management of hemophilia is palliative. The only treatment for hemophiliacs is to replace the missing factors in their blood to prevent bleeding. This is accomplished by transfusion of plasma concentrates or fresh frozen plasma containing the missing factors. A concern with this treatment is the potential for contracting AIDS and hepatitis. However, this risk has been significantly lowered during the last few years because of vigilant screening of blood donors and due to testing and heat treatments of all blood products. Corticosteriods are administered to reduce inflammation caused by bleeding.

nursing care

Hemophiliacs are usually not strangers to health care. They often have multiple hospital admissions starting at a young age. The nurse should be aware that age-related growth and development activities make children more vulnerable to bleeding episodes. For example, the toddler with an unsteady gait is more likely to fall, causing minor injury that can result in prolonged bleeding.

The nurse also should be aware of terminology used by children with hemophilia. This includes describing bleeding episodes as "regular bleeds" versus "bad bleeds." Bad bleeds are often described according to the amount of blood; the color of the blood; the amount of swelling; bleeds into the bones, head, or stomach; bleeds that occur in the same place in the body; or the amount of pain (Spitzer, 1992).

The nurse should measure and mark the circumference of the bleeding site. This will help evaluate whether the bleeding has stopped when future measurements are made. The nurse must be aware that the risk of hypovolemic shock is increased with blood loss and is reflected by low blood pressure, increased pulse rate, and increased respiration rate.

Child and parental teaching is a major part of nursing care for the hemophiliac. See the teaching guidelines for home care of the child with hemophilia.

leukemia

Leukemia is a malignant disorder of the blood-forming tissues. It is often categorized according to the primary cell type and level of maturity. The ranking includes lympho, involving the lymphatic system; myelo, involving the bone marrow; blastic and acute, involving immature cells; cytic and chronic, involving mature cells.

Acute lymphoblastic leukemia accounts for 80% of leukemia seen in children (Pediatric Nursing, 1992). Acute lymphocytic leukemia is classified by whether it is T lymphocytic, B lymphocytic, or null cell (neither T cell nor B cell). More than 75% of children with acute lymphocytic leukemia have null cells. This has the best prognosis.

Children between 3 and 4 years have the highest incidence. The exact cause of leukemia is unknown; however, certain factors increase a child's risks. These factors include Down syndrome, siblings of a child with leukemia, and exposure to radiation during fetal development. Children are considered long-term survivors when they have been disease free for at least 5 years and have been off therapy for 2 or more years (Hobbie & Hollen, 1993).

pathophysiology

Immature white blood cells (lymphocytes) replace normal cells in the bone marrow. These immature white blood cells ineffectively fight infection, decreasing the child's resistance to disease.

Leukemic cells suppress bone marrow, resulting in decreased red blood cell and platelet formation and leading to anemia and a tendency to bleed. Diagnosis is made by an extremely high white blood cell count, decreased red blood cells and platelets, and bone marrow aspiration revealing 80% to 90% immature white blood cells.

medical–surgical management

Treatment of leukemia has three medical phases, described as induction, sanctuary, and maintenance. Surgical management consists of bone marrow transplantation.

induction This phase involves reducing the number of leukemic cells by a combination of chemotherapy drugs and radiation administration. Drugs commonly used include steroids, such as prednisone, intravenous vincristine, and intravenous L-asparaginase.

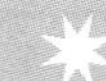

nursing alert

Risk of anaphylactic shock is increased when administering L-asparaginase. Epinephrine and oxygen must be available.

sanctuary therapy This therapy includes attacking leukemic cells shielded by the blood–brain barrier in the central nervous system and leukemic cells in the testes that are protected by their peripheral site from systemic chemotherapy treatment. To seek out cancer cells that have sanctuary, chemotherapy drugs are administered into the spinal canal, which is known as *intrathecal* therapy. Radiation is often used for about 6 to 8 weeks after diagnosis of leukemia in conjunction with chemotherapy treatments.

maintenance therapy Maintenance therapy includes keeping the child in remission while continuing to reduce the number of leukemic cells. Therapy continues for 1 to 3 years and is based on normal laboratory values.

Negative effects of cancer therapy result from a lack of nourishment to healthy cells, chronic cell injury, and scar tissue formation. Lung damage, heart dysfunction, liver damage, cognitive impairment, additional malignancies, and cosmetic changes are a few of the possible effects of chemotherapy and radiation. Most consequences are

teaching guidelines
home care of the child with hemophilia

* Early signs of bleeding into the joints include swelling, loss of function, and pain.
* Other signs of bleeding include tarry, black stools or emesis with coffee-grounds appearance; airway obstruction due to bleeding into the neck; and hematomas in the spinal cord, resulting in paralysis.
* Basic first aid information for minor bleeds includes applying pressure and ice and elevating and splinting extremities.
* Factor replacement must be administered correctly and as prescribed.
* Acetaminophen—***never*** aspirin products—is used for pain.
* Preventive care includes using a soft toothbrush for dental hygiene, playing with soft toys, using padded bed rails, and wearing a medical alert identification.
* Dietary information concerns intake of protein and vegetables and avoiding weight gain, which can be stressful to the joints.

noted several months to several years following completion of therapy.

bone marrow transplantation Children who are critically ill and facing imminent death from poor response to chemotherapy or radiation treatment may be candidates for a bone marrow transplant. This procedure can be performed by using one of three types of bone marrow transplants ranked according to donor. The types of bone marrow transplants include *autologous*, reinfusion of the child's own bone marrow; *syngeneic*, using bone marrow from an identical twin; and *allogenic*, donation of bone marrow from a sibling, relative, or another person who is considered an antigen-matched donor.

Prior to bone marrow transplantation, aggressive chemotherapy and possible total body irradiation are required to destroy leukemic cells and enable the new bone marrow to provide healthy cells. The necessity for strong chemotherapy before the procedure can be fatal before the transplant is given. The child is kept in a sterile environment before and immediately following bone marrow transplantation to reduce the potential risk of death from infection. Long-term survival after a bone marrow transplant is 25% to 50%.

✶ nursing process for the child with leukemia

assessment

Subjective data to be assessed include the following:

- History of recurrent infections, easy bruising, bone and joint pain, headache, anorexia, vomiting, tiredness, weakness, and lethargy
- History of opportunistic infections, such as thrush (*Candida*) and herpes simplex
- Family history of cancer conditions

> **✶ nursing insight**
> *Acute leukemia may be mistaken for an acute infection, such as rheumatic fever.*

Objective data to be assessed include the following:

- Pallor, petechia, epistaxis, bruising and bleeding from minor trauma, enlarged lymph nodes, vomiting, fever, weight loss, poor wound healing, and enlarged lymph nodes

nursing diagnosis

- Risk for Infection, related to anemia and ineffective white blood cells
- Activity Intolerance
- Pain
- Fear, related to unknown and pain from procedures
- Knowledge Deficit (parental), related to disease process and treatment plan, such as chemotherapy and radiation.

nursing interventions

prevention of infection

- Provide a private room, visitor restrictions, and in some cases, reverse isolation to reduce the risk of infection because bone marrow suppression is common during chemotherapy drug administration. Monitor for increased temperature, indicating infection. Keep infant's diaper area clean and dry, avoiding rubber or plastic pants. Powder with talc must not be used, and cornstarch is not recommended because it "clumps" and provides a growth medium for bacteria.
- Instruct parents to postpone live virus vaccines, such as polio, measles, and varicella because they can precipitate the disease in an immune-suppressed child. Immunization may be continued 6 to 12 months after chemotherapy is stopped and the child's blood count values are within normal range.
- Assess the mouth for signs of thrush, which include white patches on the mucous membrane of the mouth that are painful, cannot be rubbed off, and may bleed. Herpes simplex blisters also may be noted.
- Monitor complete blood count and hemoglobin values for deviations from normal.

> **✶ nursing insight**
> *Careful handwashing by nurses, parents, visitors, and others associated with the child's care decreases the child's risk of contracting infections.*

promotion of activity

- Turn the child on bed rest at least every 2 hours, and use pillows to support extremities. Promote adequate rest by providing a calm, quiet environment. Schedule care time to allow child uninterrupted rest.
- Provide for age-appropriate play according to child's energy level.
- Monitor platelet count because decreases in platelets increase the child's potential to bleed or bruise easily. Instruct children to avoid contact sports, bicycling, skate boarding, and playground equipment until platelet counts return to normal.

promotion of adequate hydration and nutrition

- Assess for nausea and vomiting often occurring 2 to 6 hours after administration of chemotherapy drugs and lasting up to 48 hours. Nondrug therapy can be effective and involves relaxation techniques, distraction with quiet play, videos, or music.
- Offer clear liquids, such as diluted apple juice, Jello water, Kool Aid, popsicles, and uncarbonated beverages.
- Encourage rest prior to meals.
- Administer drugs, such as phenothiazine, an effective antiemetic, when nondrug therapy is unsuccessful. Antiemetics are scheduled during waking hours while the child desires activity. Monitor blood values for electrolyte disturbances that can result from untreated nausea and vomiting.

* Monitor intake and output at least every 8 hours. Provide oral hygiene using a soft brush or lemon and glycerine swabs because the child's mouth may be painful because of stomatitis or herpes simplex lesions. The oral mucous membrane is often affected by chemotherapy. Oral lesions develop 5 to 14 days after the administration of chemotherapy agents and last up to 10 days. Encourage children to suck on ice chips, popsicles, snow cones, milk shakes, or frozen liquids to ease lesion pain. Provide small, high-protein and carbohydrate meals using the child's favorite foods.

> **✱ nursing insight**
> *Discourage gum chewing in children complaining of nausea because it increases gastric juices and feelings of nausea.*

promotion of power

* Provide age-appropriate explanations about disease, procedures, and treatments. Preschool children have a short attention span, so long, complicated explanations should be avoided. Provide information about the disease and treatments by showing pictures and other types of visual aides, such as dolls. Encourage the child and parents to ask questions and express emotions.
* Adolescents must be helped to accept the physical changes associated with cancer therapy and puberty. It is important to promote the adolescent's own creative power so that he or she can cope with hardships. Encourage the adolescent to break away when cancer treatment routines become overwhelming. Attending a camp or taking a family vacation allows teenagers to put some distance between themselves and drug administration, blood testing, and clinic appointments, providing a better perspective when they return.
* Encourage family's and child's involvement in routine care, treatments and test results. Include young children in discussions about care. Preschoolers are frequently ready to learn about their disease and its management.
* Provide information about side effects of chemotherapy, stressing that they are temporary (Table 32-2).
* Promote self-esteem by stressing the child's strengths. Loss of hair (alopecia) and severe weight loss contribute to alterations in body image.
* Provide emotional support for the child and family. Encourage interaction with other children with leukemia and their parents. Identify support systems available to the family. Consult spiritual leaders as indicated by family need and preference. Provide palliative care, and assist child toward a comfortable, peaceful death if the condition proves fatal.
* Assist the ill child and family as they deal with the consequences of cancer therapy. Provide available information for concerns about return of the cancer; risk of second type of cancer; vital organ function; physical, intellectual, and psychosocial growth and development; and sexual maturation and fertility.

evaluation

* Child shows no signs of infection; temperature is within normal range, and blood count is normal.
* Child engages in activities appropriate for age.
* The child's discomfort is decreased, enabling more activity and play with appropriate rest periods.
* Child and parents voice understanding of care and engage in self-promoting activities.

immune function disorders

Disorders of immunity include allergies, autoimmune disorders, and immune deficiency disorders. Allergies and autoimmunity disorders can be serious and chronic. They include mild but annoying allergies to cat hair or pollen, serious alleries to bee venom, and the chronic, autoimmune disease of lupus erythematosus. On the other hand, immune deficiency disorders are often fatal and include AIDS.

allergies

An allergy is described as an acquired hypersensitivity to a substance that normally does not cause a reaction in the body. Allergens are protein antigens, such as animal dander, pollen, drugs, or food. Repeated exposure to the allergen causes tissues to become sensitized.

pathophysiology

Antibodies are produced in the tissues as a response to the allergen. The antibody-antigen reaction occurs in the tissue, not the blood. Histamine released from injured tissue sets up a local or systemic reaction. For example, pollen allergies typically cause rhinitis, itchy eyes, and sneezing in response to histamine release. Severe drug allergies result in respiratory difficulties that can be fatal (eg, anaphylactic shock). Common allergic reactions in children include allergic rhinitis and lactose (milk) intolerance.

Diagnosis of an allergic reaction is based on history of sensitivities, symptoms, and types of exposure to suspected allergens and an increased eosinophil count. The cause of allergies is determined by skin testing.

medical management

Children with allergies often require desensitization of the allergy when avoidance of the allergen is not possible or not effective. Desensitization is accomplished by administering subcutaneous injections of dilute allergen extract at frequent intervals, which sensitize the child's immune response. The allergen's extract strength is increased until the child develops a tolerance to it; this is a maintenance dose. The child is given the maintenance dose on a regular basis. Desensitization is based on exposure to the offending allergen and may require injections during a particular season (such as during late summer and fall for ragweed allergies) or throughout the year in the case of allergies to mold or animal dander.

table 32-2 side effects of chemotherapy and nursing considerations

Side Effect	*Nursing Intervention*
Photophobia	Stress the importance of avoiding prolonged exposure to the sun up to 2 days following chemotherapy by using sunscreen with an SPF of 15 or greater and a protective hat.
Nausea and vomiting; food and odor dislikes, food cravings, altered taste perceptions	Encourage relaxation techniques, distraction through play, and clear liquids to ensure hydration; administer prescribed antiemetics. Monitor intake and output.
Hemorrhagic cystitis	Force fluids, encourage voiding, check urine-specific gravity, and monitor red blood cells in urine. Monitor urine for color, odor, amount, sediment, or mucus.
Fever	Monitor temperature above 38.3°C (100.4°F) for longer than 24 hours unrelated to chemotherapy—indicates infection.
Bone marrow suppression	Monitor blood counts (decreased blood cell count seen 14 days after therapy). Inform child and parents about risk factors, such as anemia, bruising, bleeding, and increased risk of infection. Avoid aspirin products, constipation, crowds, shopping centers, and sometimes school until count is normal. Sexually active teenagers must refrain from sexual intercourse.
Stomatitis	Assess mouth for ulcerated areas or presence of herpes simplex blisters. Provide mouth care with soft brush or swabs. Irrigate mouth or swish with water mixed in a small amount of table salt and baking soda. Apply a mixture of equal parts (5 mL each) of aluminum hydroxide (Amphojel), diphenhydramine (Benadryl), and lidocaine (viscous Xylocaine) directly to sores or have patient swish and spit out. Provide ice chips, popsicles, and milk shakes. Monitor daily weight; assess for signs of malnutrition and dehydration.
Alopecia and skin changes	Explain that hair loss occurs frequently with chemotherapy and is not permanent; it may grow back a different color and texture. Hair loss may occur weeks to months after drug therapy. Suggest hair cut prior to chemotherapy. Wig fitting (if used) is best down prior to hair loss. Encourage use of caps, hats, or scarves. Acne and rashes are common with prednisone administration and clears when medication is stopped.
Neurologic complications	Evaluate for paresthesia, peripheral nerve inflammation or degeneration, and motor weakness.
Liver complications	Monitor liver function tests. Assess skin and mucous membrane color for jaundice.
Psychosocial concerns	Assess child's anxiety, fears, depression, and helplessness. Assess family's reaction to the diagnosis and child; refer for counseling. If child and parents are in the denial stage of grief, do not intervene—support the denial.
Pain	Assess origin of pain (eg, invading tumor pressing on nerves, muscle, or pain); chemotherapy induces pain, such as headache, abdominal, or limb discomfort. Administer analgesics, encourage self-hypnosis, progressive relaxation, guided imagery.

nursing care

Following an injection of allergen extract, the child is at risk for an anaphylactic reaction. The nurse must monitor the child carefully during the injection and for 20 minutes following the injection for signs of respiratory difficulties escalating to respiratory arrest. Epinephrine 1:1,000 is given subcutaneously as an emergency measure for signs of anaphylactic reaction.

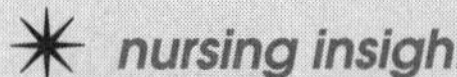

Milk-sensitive infants are often sensitive to soy.

Less serious local reactions include redness or edema at the injection site. The nurse should apply cool compresses and administer oral antihistamine as prescribed.

Another nursing goal includes educating the child and family about allergies and teaching them ways to control symptoms. If the allergy is environmentally influenced, the nurse can provide the child and family with methods of limiting exposure to allergens by keeping the child's living space free from dust, mold, and dander (see the teaching guidelines).

autoimmunity

Autoimmunity is an abnormal reaction to one's own tissues. T cells fail to recognize "self" and set up an attack as if "self" were a foreign antigen. Autoimmune hypersensitivities tend to run in families.

pathophysiology

Autoimmunity may be triggered by a variety of factors. Certain self-antigens may have never been exposed to the developing immune system. If these antigens are detected by the immune system later in life, an immunologic reaction is initiated because the self antigens are recognized as foreign. Other factors that have been implicated as potential triggers include certain drugs and drug reactions, viruses, complications of an infectious diseases, supressor T-cell dysfunction, or genetics.

Disorders associated with autoimmune factors include juvenile rheumatoid arthritis, juvenile diabetes (insulin-dependent diabetes mellitus), systemic lupus erythematosus, and glomerulonephritis.

immune deficiency diseases

Immune deficiency disorders involve faulty immune mechanisms resulting from genetic or acquired factors. Immune deficiency disorders are often fatal.

Genetic immune deficiency disease is a rare condition in which the child is born without a properly functioning immune system. Children are prone to overwhelming infections and require a near-sterile environment to survive. Attempts to provide a safe environment for the child have created a life within a "bubble."

nursing care

Nursing care for the immune-deficient child involves minimizing the risk of infections. The nurse must protect the child in many different ways. For example, bananas must be peeled before giving them to the child because bacteria can grow on the peelings.

Growth and developmental delays are common because children use so much energy fighting infections. In addition, parental bonding may be strained if the parents are unable to hold the infant, and psychosocial growth may be impaired if the child is unable to socialize with siblings or peers. The nurse should be aware of these potential developmental problems and assist the family and child in developing as normally as possible. The nurse should provide emotional support for parents who grieve the loss of rearing a normal child. Financial concerns are common, and the nurse should refer the family to any available community services.

teaching guidelines
environmental control of allergies

* Use washable rugs.
* Avoid banners, shelves with books, trophies, and pictures that tend to collect dust.
* Provide the child with washable dolls and stuffed animals.
* Provide foam pillows rather than feather pillows.
* Avoid stuffed furniture in the child's bedroom.
* Restrict family pets to animals that do not cause an allergic reaction in the affected child, or keep pets outside.
* Schedule frequent changes of filter in hot-air heating systems.
* Protect the child from exposure to cigarette smoke, aerosol sprays, strong cleaning agents, such as Clorox, and paint.

acquired immunodeficiency syndrome and human immunodeficiency virus

The fifth leading cause of death among children 1 to 4 years old is AIDS. It is caused by HIV. Perinatal transmission of the disease from an HIV-positive mother accounts for 30% to 50% of children afflicted with the disease. Babies born to infected mothers are tested for anti-HIV antibodies after 3 months. Children also can be infected through blood products (especially hemophiliacs), breast milk, sexual abuse, or unsafe sexual activity and intravenous drug use during adolescence.

Extended family members often assume the role of caregiver for the child with AIDS because the parent(s) may be debilitated by the disease or disease-related activities, such as drug abuse, or they may be dead. Uninfected siblings of children with AIDS are forced to witness the deterioration and destruction of their families.

Pediatric AIDS is increasing in poor, African American, and hispanic children of the inner city. Parental lifestyles, such as intravenous drug use by the mother or her partner, are the major risk factors for perinatal infections.

Adolescents have recently emerged as a risk group for HIV infection. Risk behaviors related to HIV include early age of sexual activity, lack of condom use during vaginal and anal intercourse, increased number of sex partners, increased frequency of sexual intercourse, homosexuality, intravenous drug use, sharing drug needles, and history of pregnancy (for girls).

pathophysiology

The disease is caused by a retrovirus that is attracted to T_4 lymphocytes, macrophages, and cells of the central nervous system. The virus is capable of entering body cells and replicating their genetic make up (DNA). Symptoms of HIV usually occur within 3 weeks of initial exposure to HIV. Destruction of the T_4 cells reduces the body's ability to fight infection.

In children younger than 1 year, HIV progresses rapidly to AIDS; HIV attacks the child's immature immune system, which has not formed antibodies against common infectious organisms. Children younger than 1 year with fewer than 1,500 CD_4 cells (known as T helper cells) and older children with less than 400 CD4 cells are at risk for opportunistic infections. Children infected with HIV can transmit the virus to others anytime after infection has occurred whether or not they are symptomatic.

When a child tests seropositive on antibody tests and develops certain illnesses, such as *Pneumocystis carinii*, lymphocytic interstitial pneumonia, or other opportunistic infections, AIDS is diagnosed. In comparison with AIDS in adults, children seldom develop Kaposi's sarcoma, toxoplasmosis, tuberculosis, cryptococcoses, or histoplasmosis.

medical management

The antiviral drug zidovudine (AZT) attacks HIV and slows the progress of HIV in children. Zidovudine syrup needs no special handling or refrigeration, does not have a bitter aftertaste, and can be mixed with juice, ice cream, or strained fruit. Side effects of the drug include anemia and neutropenia, decreased activity, pallor, increased respiration rate, and cyanosis.

Dideoxyinosine (Videx), is given to children with an intolerance to zidovudine. The action of this drug is to inhibit strains of HIV that resist zidovudine. Side effects include peripheral neuropathy and pancreatitis.

Another treatment is administering intravenous immune globulin. Studies conducted by the National Institutes of Health indicate that children with AIDS who receive monthly doses of intravenous immune globulin have fewer bacterial infections and longer infection-free periods than children not receiving the immune globulin.

Children with AIDS who have low white blood cell counts are often given antibacterial drugs on a regular basis to help prevent infections, such as *P. carinii* pneumonia.

respiratory involvement

P. carinii pneumonia is the most frequent opportunistic infection. It affects up to 50% of HIV-infected children younger than 1 year (Boland, 1991). Symptoms include a sudden fever, dyspnea, dry cough, hypoxia, and abnormal breath sounds. Diagnosis is based on symptoms, endotracheal suction, or lung biopsy. Reduced T_4 cell count indicates the extent of damage to the immune system.

Treatment includes oral trimethoprim-sulfamethoxazole (Bactrim and Septra). Intravenous infusion of pentamidine is infused for at least 1 hour. It is important to watch for side effects of hypoglycemia and hypotension. Blood glucose monitoring is done before and after administration of pentamidine.

nursing care Assess the child's baseline respiratory status to determine normal ranges. Encourage ambulation, position changes, coughing, deep breathing, avoiding overexertion, and maintaining adequate hydration.

central nervous system and sensory involvement

Children with AIDS often experience seizure activity, neck stiffness, muscle rigidity, irritability or lethargy, meningitis, encephalopathy, cytomegalovirus, and central nervous system lymphomas; HIV damages the nerves and increases tumor formation. Infections with HIV affect the brain. The extent of brain involvement is based on computed tomography scan or magnetic resonance imaging results. Treatment includes surgical intervention, chemotherapy, or radiation for tumors.

Neurologic involvement includes developmental delays, loss of developmental milestones, and loss of reflexes, coordination, and memory. The child is often irritable and may experience hearing loss and visual disturbances.

nursing care Assess the child's need for physical, occupational, and speech therapy. Instruct the child and caregivers about sign language and lip reading. Encourage age-appropriate self-care, especially in school-age children. Establish a daily routine for care to foster a sense of trust in infants and young children. Provide developmentally appropriate activities and toys geared at increasing stimulation. Encourage regular school attendance.

gastrointestinal involvement

Children with HIV tend to lag behind other children their age in physical growth. Slow growth may be attributed to using extra energy to fight the virus and other infections. When an infant eats well but does not gain weight, gastrointestinal infection is often suspected. Symptoms such as diarrhea may not respond to ordinary treatment. The treatment for most opportunistic gastrointestinal infections is lengthy and complicated.

Children with HIV are considered at risk for failure to thrive. Contributing factors include loss of appetite, chronic diarrhea, painful oral and esophageal lesions (candidiasis), dental caries, nausea and vomiting, painful sucking and swallowing, malabsorption problems, and damage to the intestinal flora.

nursing care Monitor daily weights and track progress on a graphic record or growth charts. Encourage children to select foods they like. Engaging the child in meal planning provides an opportunity to build self-confidence and independence. Avoid giving the child citrus fruits (acid stings the mouth). Lactose-free formulas tend to be better tolerated than milk-based formulas.

Prior to eating, provide anesthetic agents for oral cavity lesions. Provide consistent, gentle oral hygiene. Thrush and herpes simplex blisters are common in children with AIDS and are very painful. Administer antiemetics and pain relievers to facilitate the child's comfort and promote intake of food. Dietary supplementation with multivitamins is best given in a liquid or chewable form.

Recovery from an acute illness in normal children involves catch-up growth. This process involves an acceleration of weight gain followed by sluggish growth until the normal growth curve is reestablished. Children with HIV tend not to follow this pattern.

cardiac involvement

The child with HIV or AIDS experiences activity intolerance related to decreased cardiac output. Heart muscle changes are related to repeated infections. Symptoms of congestive heart failure are common and include tachycardia with fluid retention.

nursing care It is important to assess for a baseline of cardiac status, including vital signs, temperature, appearance of skin, skin color, presence of edema, and pulmonary congestion. Plan care and activities to avoid overexertion. Monitor intake and output, maintain fluid restriction when ordered, and assess for signs of dehydration resulting from restricted fluids. Administer glycoside and diuretics per order, noting any signs of hypokalemia.

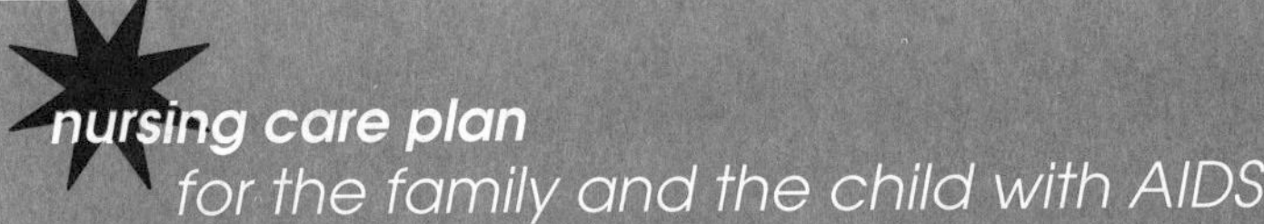

nursing care plan for the family and the child with AIDS

NURSING DIAGNOSIS

Ineffective Family Coping, related to the diagnosis of a terminal condition in a child

GOAL: The family will exhibit increasing ability to care for the child and maintain family functioning

NURSING INTERVENTIONS	RATIONALE	EVALUATION
Support family and the child in verbalization of their feelings and perception of the situation.	Honest discussion may help decrease feelings of guilt and mobilize family members to support each other and the child.	Family verbalizes their feelings and states their ability to continue to care for the child.
Evaluate available family, community, and hospital resources.	The shame associated with AIDS and the altered family coping may prevent the family from investigating necessary resources.	The family can identify resources to seek when needed.

NURSING DIAGNOSIS

Self Esteem Disturbance, related to social isolation

GOAL: The child will be able to identify positive attributes about himself and identify a positive support system

NURSING INTERVENTIONS	RATIONALE	EVALUATION
Encourage the child's expression of feelings about social isolation.	Providing a listening ear can assist the child in coping with feelings.	The child will share negative experiences and feeling about his diagnosis of AIDS.
Assist the child in finding positive attributes about himself.	Reminding the child about his positive qualities can help him to better perceive the whole picture.	The child will view himself in a positive light.
Educate the child on the public's lack of knowledge and fear of the disease.	This will help the child to see that it is the public's ignorance of the facts and fear of the disease that are the cause of their treatment toward him, not his personal qualities, which are causing the social isolation.	The child will state an understanding of the public's fear and will promote education toward understanding more about the disease process.
Assist child in identifying age-appropriate support systems and encourage the child and the family in their use.	Support groups can help to teach and support the child in dealing with the crises of his illness.	The child and family maintain close ties with a support group throughout the course of the child's illness.

Monitor laboratory tests, such as blood gas values, electrolytes, and blood urea nitrogen.

common childhood diseases

Typical childhood diseases, such as diaper rash, bacterial otitis media, or sinusitis, progress to perianal abscesses, pneumonia, and septicemia quickly in HIV-infected children. *Haemophilus influenzae* type b, pneumococcal pneumonia, and influenza virus vaccines offer some protection. The usual childhood immunizations are given, along with subcutaneous inactivated polio vaccine instead of the live oral vaccine.

nursing care Prompt treatment of any infection is important. Skin protection includes keeping the skin moisturized every day and administering consistent and thorough hygiene. Encourage caregivers to report fever, pain, altered activity levels, difficulty breathing, poor appetite, weight loss, vomiting or diarrhea, skin rashes, or developmental regression immediately so that intervention can be initiated.

psychosocial concerns

Parents of HIV-infected infants may not be able to care for the child because of their own poor health resulting from

display 32-3
basic aspects of physical and psychosocial care for the child with human immunodeficiency virus

* Nutritional support
* Aggressive measures to prevent pneumonia, such as coughing or suctioning, deep breathing, postural drainage and thumping, and immediate intervention for signs of respiratory infections.
* Consistent, thorough oral and personal hygiene
* Pharmacologic interventions for immune system support and antibiotic therapy
* Developmentally appropriate child life and educational activities
* Individual or family psychosocial counseling as needed
* Client advocacy with client or family education
* Support for reintegration into the community.

AIDS. If the mother's or father's lifestyle involves drug abuse and casual sex, the sick infant will probably not receive adequate care. In addition, the child may be abandoned if treatment for drug abuse is being sought.

Many infants receive care by extended family, foster parents, or in hospitals. If the caregiver has not obtained legal guardian rights, issues concerning consent for treatment, code status, and financial responsibilities become legally unclear.

Parents caring for an HIV-infected infant may have to overcome feelings of guilt and denial. In addition, children with AIDS and their families may face extreme predjudice and social stigmatization by neighbors, school peers, and even extended family members. The Nursing Care Plan addresses issues of family coping and self-esteem for the family and child with AIDS.

Nurses often must calm fears and teach about the disease when a child with AIDS returns to school. Children with HIV can safely attend school and day care if care is taken not to expose other children and personnel to the child's body fluids, such as blood and stool. School personnel must be taught to wear latex gloves when tending to an open wound, nose bleed, bloody vomit, or diarrhea. Teachers are encouraged to take the hepatitis B vaccine as a precautionary measure (Display 32-3).

Depression, withdrawal, emotional lability, and aggressive behaviors are noted in children with AIDS. Social isolation, chaotic family situations, abandonment, and medication side effects influence the child's emotional turmoil. See Display 32-4 for basic aspects of physical and psychosocial care for the child with HIV.

display 32-4
safety measures for care of the child with acquired immunodeficiency syndrome

* Treat all blood or other bodily fluids as if they were infectious.
* People performing needle sticks or skin testing associated with bloodshed must wear disposable rubber gloves; those with open wounds or skin lesions must be extremely cautious even while wearing rubber gloves, in case the glove tears.
* Spilled blood, semen, or body fluids containing blood are considered risky and must be wiped up with paper towels and gloved hands. The area of contamination must be flooded with 1:10 bleach, such as diluted Clorox, for 15 minutes and then wiped dry.

key points ✳

* Parents may fear their child's interaction with other children or feel responsible or guilty for causing a disease or genetically passing a disease to their child. In addition, parents may need to create an appropriate environment for their child with allergies. Parents with children who have HIV may have to deal with their own sickness and eventual death as well as the sickness and death of their child. Parents often have the tendency to indulge their chronically sick child.
* Blood contains plasma and blood cells. Plasma is 90% water and 10% disolved proteins. The three types of blood cells are red blood cells (erythrocytes), white blood cells (leukocytes), and platelets (thrombocytes).
* The body has a strong defense system that protects against foreign invaders. It accomplishes its defense through cell-mediated immunity, humoral immunity, B-cell immunity, complement fixation, and immunoglobins.
* Extra red blood cells required during fetal circulation are unnecessary after birth, and the body usually destroys the extra red blood cells. The waste product is called bilirubin. If there is an excessive amount of bile pigment in the blood, jaundice results.
* Sickle cell anemia results when oxygen is released to tissues and abnormal hemoglobin (hemoglobin S) replaces all or part of normal hemoglobin. These sickled cells get stuck as they attempt to flow through capillary beds.
* When caring for a child with hemophilia, the nurse should be aware of age-related growth and development activites and terminology used by children with the disease. In addition, the nurse should always measure and mark the area of bleeding, monitor the child for shock, and teach the child and parent about the disease.
* Medical management of leukemia consists of induction, sanctuary, and maintenance. These steps in-

clude chemotherapy, radiation, intrathecal therapy, and long-term follow up care. Bone marrow transplants are surgically performed if the child is facing imminent death.

* Environmental control of allergies includes using washable rugs, avoiding furniture decorations and toys that collect dust, using foam pillows rather than feather pillows, restricting certain pets, cleaning air conditioning vents and heating system filters, and keeping the child away from cigarette smoke, aerosol sprays, and cleaning agents.
* Autoimmunity is an attack against one's own tissues. There are many factors that may trigger an attack.
* Thirty to fifty percent of infants and children with HIV perinatally acquired the disease from their mother. Blood products tainted with HIV, breast milk, sexual abuse, and unsafe sexual practices or intravenous drug use during adolescence are other ways children can acquire the infection.

review questions

1. An expected outcome for children following treatment for lymphocytic leukemia includes
   a. blood values, especially white blood cell values, within normal range.
   b. positive response to the drug AZT.
   c. compliance to fluid restrictions.
   d. erythrocyte sedimentation rates within normal limits.
2. Veronda is 4½ years old and suffers from sickle cell anemia. She asks the nurse why the disease is called sickle cell. Select the most appropriate nursing response.
   a. "You will need to ask the doctor."
   b. "The blood cell is sickle shaped, clumps easily, and causes clot formation, making your legs hurt."
   c. "Because of the way a special cell is shaped."
   d. "Because the disease can cause strokes from the blood cells clumping together."
3. Janelle, 6 months old, is HIV positive. Select the most pertinent subjective data necessary to provide her with effective nursing care.
   a. History of blood dyscrasia
   b. Maternal lifestyle practices relative to unprotected sex and drug abuse
   c. History of physical and developmental delays
   d. Apgar scores at birth
4. Cassandra is surprised to learn her 9-month-old has anemia and states "There must be a mistake, my baby drinks milk all the time—just look how fat she is!" Select the most appropriate nursing assessment.
   a. Assess the infant's skin coloring, mucus membrane, and cry response.
   b. Obtain nutritional data, including the amount of milk intake and baby food or pureed table food.
   c. Question how often the mother weighs her infant and the type of scale used.
   d. Inquire about the infant's birth weight and mother's prenatal care.
5. Select the complaint requiring immediate nursing action following the administration of an allergy injection.
   a. Redness, itching, and swelling at injection site
   b. Voice hoarseness, difficulty swallowing, and slight dyspnea
   c. Rash on the trunk of the body
   d. Fever

references

Boland, M., & Czarniecki, L. (1991). Starting life with HIV. *RN, January*, 54–58.

Hobbie, W., & Hollen, P. (1993). Pediatric nurse practitioners specializing with survivors of childhood cancer. *Journal of Pediatric Health Care*, 7(1), 24–30.

(1992). *Lippincott's review series: Pediatric Nursing.* Philadelphia: J.B. Lippincott.

Spitzer, A. (1992). Children's knowledge of illness and treatment experiences in hemophilia. *Journal of Pediatric Nursing*, 7(1), 43–51.

bibliography

Clark, J. (1991). Cholesterol: Is it important in childhood? *Modern Medicine*, *59*, 10–13.

Club, R. (1991). Chronic sorrow: Adaptation patterns of parents with chronically ill children. *Pediatric Nursing*, *17*(5), 461–465.

DiClemente, F., & Ponton, L. (1993). HIV-related risk behaviors among psychiatrically hospitalized adolescents and school-based adolescents. *American Journal Psychiatry*, *150*(2), 324–325.

Ellis, J. (1991). How adolescents cope with cancer and its treatment. *Maternal Child Nursing*, *16*, 157–160.

Fischbach, F. (1995). *Quick reference to common laboratory and diagnostic tests*. Philadelphia: J.B. Lippincott.

Heins, H. (1992). AIDS in babies: Prevention and treatment update. *American Baby*, *January*, 14–15.

Jemmott, L. (1993). AIDS risk among black male adolescnets: Implications for nursing interventions. *Journal of Pediatric Health Care*, 7(1), 3–11.

McCance, K. (1994). *Pathophysiology: The biological basis for disease in adults and children* (2nd ed.). St. Louis: C.V. Mosby.

Nicholas, S., & Leung, J. (1991). Guidelines for nutritional support of HIV-infected children. *The Journal of Pediatrics*, *July*, 59–62.

Pillitteri, A. (1995). *Maternal and child health nursing* (2nd ed.). Philadelphia: J.B. Lippincott.

Shannon, K. (1990). Recombinant erythropoietin in pediatrics: A clinical perspective. *Pediatric Annals*, *19*(3), 197–206.

Smeltzer, S., & Bare, B. (1992). *Brunner and Suddarth's textbook of medical-surgical nursing*. Philadelphia: J.B. Lippincott.

White, J., & Cunningham, A. (1991). Ryan White: My own story. New York: Dial Books.

the child with an alteration in urinary or reproductive system function

33

outline ✷

objectives ✷

After studying this chapter, the reader should be able to:

- ✷ Discuss the relationship between the urinary system and reproductive system.
- ✷ List four functions of the urinary system.
- ✷ Describe how the kidneys regulate fluid, electrolytes, and blood pressure.
- ✷ Discuss at least four ways a family affects the care of a child with a genitourinary condition.
- ✷ Discuss age-related considerations for nursing care of an infant, toddler, school-age child, and adolescent with a genitourinary condition.
- ✷ Define precocious puberty.
- ✷ Compare the differences between congenital anomalies, such as hypospadias, epispadias, and testicular torsion.
- ✷ Describe Wilms' tumor, staging, and interventions required.
- ✷ Discuss the relationship between vesicoureteral reflux and urinary infections.
- ✷ Discuss the impact of renal failure on the body and the benefits of hemodialysis, peritoneal dialysis, and kidney transplantation.

key terms ✷

androgen
anuria
ascites
anticholinergic
azotemia
bruit
creatinine
dialysate
dialysis
dysuria
enuresis
exstrophy of the bladder
hematuria
hydronephrosis
hypoplastic kidneys
nephron
oliguria
orchiopexy
phimosis
pseudohermaphrodite
reflux
rejection
shunt
urea
uremia
uremic frost
urethral "stents"
vesicoureteral reflux

Neff C & Spray M. *Introduction to Maternal and Child Health Nursing,*

The genitourinary system consists of organs involving reproduction and urination. Even though the functions of these two systems differ, the closeness of specific anatomic structures makes it logical to study them simultaneously. For example, a man's urethra is a passageway for urine and for sperm to exit the body. Consequently, an abnormality in the male urethra affects the ability to excrete urine and reproduce.

Genitourinary disorders often require care administered by a *urologist*. Specific kidney diseases are treated by a *nephrologist*. Alterations of the reproductive system may require care by a *gynecologist*.

The reproductive system is discussed in detail in Chapter 4, and sexually transmitted disease (STDs) are detailed in Chapter 13. Genitourinary system and anatomy and physiology with age-specific considerations, specific disorders and diseases, and nursing care are included in this chapter.

nursing alert

Universal precautions must be observed when handling body fluids.

✳ family considerations

Parents or caregivers who are comfortable discussing genitourinary concerns with an older child are more likely to become aware of problems at the onset of an infection or disease, enhancing early health care intervention. Symptoms of many urinary tract disorders are misleading. For example, mild abdominal pain is a common symptom and could apply to a variety of childhood disorders, especially constipation. Parents may not bring the child into a health care facility as early in the disease as they might if symptoms were more pronounced. Parents' inability to recognize symptoms can lead to feelings of guilt and confusion.

Congenital or chronic kidney disease can affect the family's ability to cope with the ill child and other siblings. Siblings can feel left out and express their wish to be sick. Sick children are sometimes not required to follow the family rules, and parents often become overly permissive. Alternative child care may be necessary while the ill child and parents keep frequent clinic appointments.

Stress and anxiety about the disease, recommended medical and surgical interventions, and financial costs can undermine the family's stability. Kidney disorders that are chronic with repeated hospitalizations can be financially overwhelming. Blood transfusions may be necessary but may not be allowed by a family's religion.

Time-consuming procedures, such as continuous ambulatory peritoneal dialysis, contribute to isolation for the child and caregivers. Caregivers are often concerned about the child's ability to live a normal life and experience normal social interactions with peers. Parental anxieties involve distress about the child's discomfort from frequent blood tests required with hemodialysis. Family counseling may be necessary.

✳ nursing considerations

Physical examination of the genitourinary system includes inspection and palpation of the external genitalia. This may be uncomfortable for the child and parents. Preschoolers and school-age children may be hesitant for the nurse to examine their genitals and may act aggressively, fearing the nurse's intentions. Children are taught not to discuss or show their "privates" to strangers. The nurse may often be a stranger to the child and therefore must try to develop a trusting relationship. Respecting the child's privacy helps establish rapport and decrease anxieties. The child should be provided with age-appropriate explanations before beginning the examination. The use of slang words followed by the proper medical term is most effective when describing an examination to a child. Parents can help by explaining the difference between a medical examination and unwelcomed talk or touch.

Teenagers may seek intervention alone or accompanied by a teenage support person. They may be fearful that they have contracted an STD and want to avoid parental knowledge of their sexual activity. Nurses must follow agency policy regarding notification of parents. However, many agencies regard adolescent sexual information as private and confidential to the teenager.

Special consideration for age-appropriate concerns, fears, and anxieties about modesty are necessary when examining a child's genitalia (Table 33-1).

Encouraging caregivers of the same sex to be with the child during genitourinary examinations and other procedures can be reassuring to the child. Preschool and young school-age children tend to fantasize about body mutilation and may have difficulty understanding procedures such as catheterization or vaginal examinations unless they are explained using visual aids.

Holding the child's hand and offering reassurances help decrease anxieties. Feelings of anxiety are common in older school-age children and adolescents because they tend to perceive the nurse's examination as a violation of their most private parts.

Older school-age children and adolescents may not want caregivers present during genitourinary examination because of embarrassment about having the genitals exposed. During this age, teenagers can become easily embarrassed with even a discussion about genitals. Nurses who feel uncomfortable examining the child's genitals will need to resolve these feelings to avoid increasing the child's anxieties.

Most children and young adolescents think in concrete terms, making it difficult for them to think beyond the present or understand what they have not experienced. For example, the nurse may find the child inattentive when discussing long-term consequences of repeated urinary infections that can lead to the need for dialysis. However, the child may show much interest if the nurse talks about missing school, sports, and social functions.

anatomy and physiology of the genitourinary system

urinary system

The urinary or renal system consists of two kidneys, two ureters, one bladder, and one urethra. The functions of the urinary system include urine production from waste products of cell metabolism, excess salts, toxins, and extra fluid; maintenance of fluid and electrolyte balance; regulation of acid–base balance; and production of hormones that help control blood pressure, manufacture blood cells, and sustain bone formation.

table 33-1 age-related considerations for genitourinary examination

Age	*Child's Reactions and Nursing Considerations*
Infant (1 mo–1 yr)	Small genitalia makes assessment difficult. Infants cry in response to being bothered. Provide parental explanations.
Toddler (1–2 y)	The toddler has a fear of pain. Stranger awareness and shyness are common. The toddler has increased anxiety related to being held for the examination. Lack of understanding makes the toddler a challenge to examine, requiring at least two nurses to complete the examination. Evaluate parents' presence as to positive or negative effects on child's behavior.
Preschool age (3–5 y)	Stranger awareness and fear of the unknown are common . Provide simple, factual explanations to child. Preschool and young school-age children fantasize about body mutilation and may have difficulty understanding procedures, such as catheterization or vaginal examinations, without the use of visual aids.
School age (6–12 y)	Embarrassment and modesty are common. Simple factual explanations with visual aides and teaching videos are beneficial. Encourage child to ask questions. Avoid using complicated medical terminology.
Adolescence	Fears are similar to school-age child; they may fear parental discovery if sexually active.

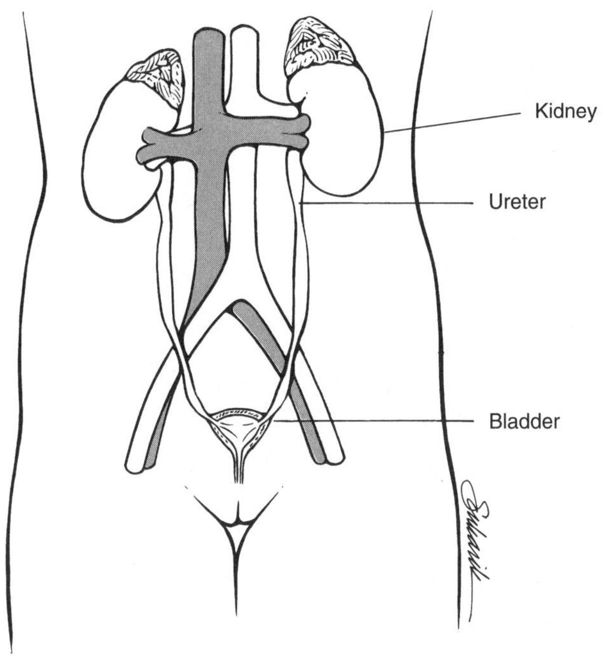

figure 33-1 *The urinary tract.*

urinary production and excretion

The kidneys are the major organs of the urinary or renal system. The kidney pelvis is responsible for collecting and transporting urine from the kidney (Fig. 33-1). Nephrons are microscopic units of the kidney, responsible for producing urine. Each nephron consists of a glomerulus and a tubule. Glomeruli are clusters of capillaries.

Substances not needed by the body, such as excess fluid, hormones, bacteria, end-products of food digestion (urea), and drugs are passed out of the body as urine. *Urea* is the chief nitrogen constituent of urine and the final product of protein metabolism in the body. Urinary output according to age is discussed in Table 33-2. Excretion of urea is increased in fever and diabetes.

table 33-2 24-hour urinary output expectations according to age

Age	*24-Hour Output*
Infant	400–500 mL
Toddler	500–600 mL with 8–10 voidings
Preschool	600–750 mL with 90–10 voidings
School-age child	700–1,500 mL
Adolescent	1,500 and greater, depending on fluid intake

The ureters, urinary bladder, and urethra are responsible for the routine elimination of urine. *Ureters* are tubes that originate in the kidney pelvis, terminate in the bladder, and carry urine from the kidney to the bladder. Ureters move urine toward the urinary bladder by peristaltic waves.

The *urinary bladder* is a muscular sac that is a reservoir for collected urine. As urine is collected, the bladder muscles stretch to store urine. Nerves located in bladder muscle tissue relay a message up the spinal cord to the brain that the bladder needs to empty. In response to this message, the brain sends a message to the bladder sphincters to relax; at the same time, the urinary bladder contracts, allowing urine to flow from the body. Children with spinal cord damage or brain dysfunction typically have an altered ability to empty the bladder. When the bladder fills, it enlarges and squeezes the lower ends of the ureters, preventing a backflow (reflux) of urine into the ureters. Urine reflux increases the child's risk of urinary tract infections.

The *urethra* is a tube leading from the bladder to the outside of the body. The urethra in the male extends through the entire length of the penis; the female urethra is found between the clitoris and vaginal opening. The opening of the urethra to the outside is known as the *urinary meatus*.

maintenance of fluid and electrolyte balance

The kidneys form urine from blood plasma. The blood flow through the kidneys is a major factor in regulating urinary output. The expected urinary volume varies with each child and is influenced by the amount of fluid intake; water needs of the lungs, skin, and gastrointestinal tract; amount of waste products to be excreted by the kidneys; ability of the kidneys to concentrate urine; and blood volume, hormonal influences, and age.

Fluid and electrolyte balance in the body is altered when kidney function is altered. For example, when the kidneys fail, there is no mechanism for maintaining fluid, electrolyte, and acid–base balance. Damage to the cluster of blood vessels within the kidney limits the organ's ability to filter, allowing excess fluids and electrolytes to build up in the blood. Sodium, chloride, potassium, calcium, and phosphorus that are normally reabsorbed by the tubules according to body requirements are excreted instead.

Fluid and electrolyte imbalances are caused by conditions associated with decreased fluid intake, excessive fluid elimination, and kidney failure. Renal diseases that cause fluid and electrolyte imbalances include acute or chronic renal failure, pyelonephritis, glomerulonephritis and obstructive disorders.

regulation of acid–base balance

The kidneys play a major role in maintaining acid–base balance in the body. They accomplish this by excreting electrolytes that are not required and by retaining those that are needed by the body. When an acid factor is in excess, the kidneys excrete hydrogen ions and conserve basic ions; when an alkaline factor is in excess, the kidneys excrete basic ions and retain hydrogen ions.

The kidneys are important in maintaining the pH of blood and tissue fluid within normal ranges. The kidneys help keep the body's pH balance by controlling plasma bicarbonate (a buffer). A deficiency of base bicarbonate is associated with diabetes mellitus and excessive infusion of isotonic saline. An excess of bicarbonate occurs when the child is vomiting (loss of stomach acids); has ingested alkaline substances, such as sodium citrate; or has gastric suctioning.

Chloride moves in and out of red blood cells in exchange for bicarbonate to support the body's acid–base balance. Chloride is controlled by the kidneys, level of secreted aldosterone (a hormone secreted by the kidneys), and diet or intravenous infusions.

Potassium is one of the most important body electrolytes. A reduced serum potassium level affects the heart muscle, causing heart beat irregularities and possible heart block. Potassium is found within the cells and is present in cellular and extracellular fluid. Extracellular fluid loss contributes to potassium loss.

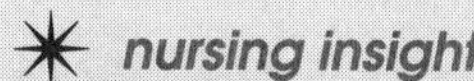

nursing insight

Fluid moving from inside of the cell to the outside is influenced by sodium intake. Water goes where salt is.

production of hormones

The kidneys produce three hormones: renin, antidiuretic hormone, and prostaglandins. Renin is secreted in response to a decrease in blood pressure, production of erythropoietin, and activation of vitamin D. Altered kidney function predisposes the child to hypertension, anemia, and disruption of bone growth.

Renin initiates the renin–angiotensin mechanism to raise blood pressure. Angiotensin causes vasoconstriction and stimulates the adrenal cortex to secrete aldosterone, both of which help maintain normal blood volume and blood pressure. Aldosterone enhances sodium reabsorption and causes an increase in plasma sodium. The kidneys help ensure that the heart has enough blood to pump to maintain cardiac output and blood pressure.

Antidiuretic hormone determines whether urine will be concentrated or dilute.

Prostaglandin hormones are produced by the kidney and act as vasodilators. Kidney disease interfering with the production of the prostaglandin hormones results in hypertension.

Vitamin D is activated in the cortex of the kidney, converted to *calciferol* by the kidneys, and considered the most active form of vitamin D. Calciferol stimulates calcium and phosphate absorption in the intestine. Vitamin D deficiency increases a child's risk of the bone disease known as *rickets*. Rickets causes abnormalities in the shape and structure of bones. Children with kidney disease usually require oral vitamin and mineral supplements to improve their calcium levels.

Erythropoietin is a hormone secreted by the kidneys whenever the blood oxygen level decreases. Erythropoietin stimulates bone marrow to produce erythrocytes. The increase in red blood cell production can be compared with a safety net for the kidneys because kidneys require a sufficient supply of oxygen-rich red blood cells to maintain function. Children with chronic or end-stage renal disease have a decreased ability to produce this hormone and are at high risk for anemia.

✶ nursing considerations

The patient's state of hydration can be assessed by monitoring urine production, skin turgor, presence of tears, amount of mucus production, the fontanel in infants, and urine-specific gravity.

A highly concentrated urine indicates water deficit; a dilute urine indicates adequate hydration or overhydration. Urine-specific gravity measurement can help differentiate the scanty urinary output of acute renal failure from that of water deficit. In acute renal failure, the specific gravity is fixed at a low level, while in water deficit, the specific gravity is high.

There is a close association between metabolic alkalosis and potassium deficit. Potassium deficit makes it difficult for the kidneys to excrete alkali for reasons unknown. The correction of potassium deficit allows the kidney to retain needed acids and excrete alkali. Early symptoms of potassium deficit are generalized weakness, diminished or absent reflexes, weak pulse, decreased blood pressure, shallow respirations, and vomiting.

reproductive system

The female reproductive system consists of mammary glands (breasts), labia majora, labia minora, clitoris, vaginal opening, cervix, uterus, ovaries, fallopian tubes, and perineum. The male reproductive system consists of penis, scrotum, testicles, epididymis, vas deferens, ejaculatory ducts, urethra, seminal vesicles, urethral gland, and prostate gland. The function of the reproductive system is to create life. The reproductive system is discussed and illustrated in Chapter 4.

✶ nursing process in genitourinary disorders

nursing assessment

Subjective data to be assessed include the following:

* A detailed history of genitourinary function, including family history of kidney disease, diabetes, hypospadias (urethral opening on the underside of the penis), and *enuresis* (involuntary urination in toilet-trained children); prenatal history of maternal injury, number of abortions, medications, exposure to toxins, drug or tobacco use, presence of increased or decreased amounts of amniotic fluid, number of umbilical cord vessels, and neonatal voiding problems; developmental history concerning toilet training, age of puberty, girl's age of menarche, and terms used by child and family for genitourinary parts and functions; history of genitourinary disease, urinary tract infections, STD, vaginitis or epididymitis; present illness, including precipitating factors, duration, location, severity of symptoms, changes in feeding or fluid intake, change in appetite, alteration of sleeping patterns, vaginal or penile discharge, genital pruritus, gastrointestinal complaints, and sexual contacts if STD is suspected

assessment of self-image

* Question older children and caregivers of younger children about their feelings concerning sexuality and reproductive function. Adolescents may be concerned that peers and family will view them as "abnormal" or "dirty" because of their disorder. Determine the adolescent's knowledge about sexual functioning, self-care, hygiene practices, and if sexually active, their knowledge about contraception, STDs, and pregnancy.

Objective data to be assessed include the following:

* Assessment of urine: Normal urine is clear to slightly hazy and pale yellow to amber (refer to Table 33-2). Foods, vaginal discharge contamination (especially menstrual flow), and degree of hydration or dehydration may affect urine appearance. Alteration in urine color is discussed in Table 33-3. Abnormal odor may be due to foods (asparagus, garlic), medications, bacteria, and ketones. *Oliguria,* a diminished amount of urine formation seen after profuse perspiration, diarrhea, or renal failure, may be noted. *Anuria* is an absence of urine formation associated with total renal failure. The presence of red blood cells (*hematuria*) often indicates lower urinary tract infections, glomerulonephritis, or hemophilia. Alterations in normal voiding patterns include straining, frequency, and *dysuria* (painful urination) or a burning sensation with start of urine flow.
* Assessment of genitalia: Inspect the external genitalia, including the presence of odorous vaginal or penile discharge. The nurse must remember to use good handwashing technique and wear examination gloves when examining the genitals and handling body fluids. Prepubertal girls normally do not have vaginal discharge or odor. Penis discharge or odor is not normal in boys. Adolescent girls may have a clear mucus-type, odorless vaginal discharge, known as physiologic leukorrhea. Menstrual flow may be noted at menarche and during menstruation. Purulent, foul smelling vaginal or penile discharge suggests infection. Normal genitalia in children before puberty appear smooth and flesh colored. Appearance of genital hair signals puberty changes. Bruises or skin eruptions, such as blisters and skin tags, are viewed as abnormal and may indicate trauma, precocious sexual activity, sexual abuse, or STD. Masses in the inguinal region indicate possible lymph node enlargement or inguinal hernia. Penis size and appearance are noted for abnormalities. A penis shorter than

table 33-3 alteration in urine color

Urine Color	Contributing Factors	Nursing Implications
Straw (dilute)	Anxiety, diabetes insipidus, diabetes mellitus, overhydration	Assess specific gravity for range of 1.000–1.010. Monitor intake and output; assess child for hypokalemia.
Dark yellow or amber (concentrate)	Fever, dehydration	Assess hydration status. Monitor intake and output and vital signs.
Cloudy	Blood, pus, fat, phosphate, sperm, bacteria, or vegetarian diet	Collect clean-catch or catheterized specimen in morning for urine culture. Send specimen to laboratory quickly or keep cold. Note odor. Monitor child for increased temperature, C/O burning, or pain with urination.
Red or brown	Hemoglobin, erythrocytes, drugs such as phenytoin (Dilantin)	Test urine for presence of blood. Rule out factors such as strenuous exercise, menstruation, drugs. Assess vital signs.
Orange	Drugs such as phenazopyridine (Pyridium)	Note medications, and reassure child and caregiver urine color is caused by drug.
Yellow, green-brown	Bilirubin	Test urine for presence of bile pigments. Urine bilirubin is abnormal. Collect fresh midstream urine specimen. Assess skin and sclera for jaundice.

Fishbach, F. (1995). *Common laboratory and diagnostic tests.* Philadelphia: J. B. Lippincott.

2 cm in a newborn indicates an increased risk of ambiguous sex anomalies. The foreskin of an uncircumcised penis is usually fully retractable by 2 years. A deviation from this would indicate phimosis, a defect of the geniturinary system discussed later in this chapter. The nurse checks the skin for irritation and excoriation around the genitals. Children receiving antibiotics and sulfonamides are at increased risk for fungal infections around the genitalia.

* Assessment of hydration: Note weight gains and losses associated with body fluids. Signs of fluid retention include weight gain, moon-faced appearance, bulging fontanel in infants, and generalized edema. Signs of electrolyte imbalance include muscle cramping, paresthesia, cardiac rhythm disturbances, and disorientation.
* Assessment of skin: Note skin color, turgor, and integrity. Pallor indicates a low hemoglobin and hematocrit value. A decrease in skin turgor (the elasticity of the skin) in the presence of dry, flaky skin represents dehydration. Skin tears, lesions, or burns contribute to fluid loss and increased risk of infection. Skin lesions in the perineal area are often associated with STDs. Adhesions of the labia are seen with chronic irritation of the genital area in girls. Vaginal tags are noted occasionally in newborn girls but are considered harmless unless infected. *Uremic frost* (a fine powder of uric acid crystals) is a serious symptom of kidney failure. The collection of uric acid crystals causes pruritus, increasing the child's risk of secondary skin infection related to scratching.

✳ nursing insight

In some African and Moslem cultures, female circumcision is practiced to promote adhesions and virginity.

nursing diagnosis

* Risk for Impaired Skin Integrity, related to irritation from concentrated urine, discharge from genitals, and tissue edema
* Altered Urinary Elimination, related to urinary infection and renal failure
* Pain, related to genitourinary infections, painful procedures, diagnostic tests, and surgical interventions
* Risk for Fluid Volume Excess, related to kidney failure
* Body Image Disturbance, related to catheters, fistula, scars, altered onset of puberty
* Self Esteem Disturbance, related to chronic kidney disorders, sexually transmitted diseases, and isolation
* Risk for Knowledge Deficit, related to normal anatomy and physiology, and procedures and treatments required at home

planning and implementation

promotion of urine elimination

* Provide toilet-trained children with the opportunity to use a potty chair or commode unless contraindicated. Provide privacy for the older child. Encourage fluid intake, and monitor intravenous therapy to dilute urine.

If a urinary catheter is in place, keep the catheter tubing patent and secure. Instruct the child to avoid pulling on catheter (see the teaching guidelines). Administer prescribed antimicrobial therapy, such as nitrofurantoin (Furadantin) given to children older than 1 month and urinary analgesics, such as phenazopyridine hydrochloride (Pyridium).

promotion of skin care

* Check infant's diapers, and change when wet; cleanse urine from skin to reduce the amount of bacteria that is likely to grow in the warm, damp environment of a soiled diaper, and apply topical creams and lotions to diaper rash areas. For example, Desenex can be used if the child has a fungal rash around genitalia.
* Vitamins A and D ointment is effective for uncomplicated redness in diaper area. Cloth diapers must be washed and rinsed thoroughly to reduce the risk of skin irritation and possible genitourinary infection.
* Educate girls using age-appropriate language to cleanse the genitalia from front to back to avoid contaminating the urethra and vaginal openings with stool.
* Educate adolescent girls about the importance of feminine hygiene, including changing sanitary napkins every 3 to 4 hours during menstruation and proper insertion and frequent changing of tampons.
* Uncircumcised boys (older than 2 years) are taught to retract the foreskin of the penis for thorough cleansing.
* The genitalia are carefully inspected every shift for signs of irritation or discoloration, discharges, and odor. Sitz baths are soothing to the child with painful urination or excoriation of the genitalia.

teaching guidelines
care of the child with a urinary drainage tube

* Make a bed cradle with disposable bed pads, rope, and a large cardboard box open on one side.
* Place open side of box facing down with an opening large enough to fit over the child's waist on one side.
* Cut a small hole in the top of the box to inspect the dressing and catheter.
* Punch one hole on either side of the box; thread the rope through the holes, and tie the ropes to the bed frame to keep the box securely in place.
* Make a small hole near the bottom of one side of the box to allow the catheter to hang free.
* Pad the outside of the box with disposable bed pads.
* Encourage the child or caregivers to draw pictures on the box to provide sensory stimulation.

promotion of hydration

* Monitor intake and output at least every 8 hours and more frequently if ordered. Weigh the child at the same time each day using the same scale and with the child wearing the same amount of clothing.
* Monitor compliance with sodium-restricted diet. Administer prescribed diuretics. Assess the color, consistency, and specific gravity of the child's urine. Assess the child's skin turgor and mucous membranes every 8 hours.
* Monitor serum electrolyte and creatinine levels. Normal levels indicate the return of normal kidney function. Assess the child for edema, and measure abdominal girth every 8 hours.
* Monitor intravenous therapy to avoid fluid volume deficits or excesses. Microdrip chambers are often attached to the primary intravenous bag or bottle to ensure accurate measurement of infusion. The nurse is responsible for checking the intravenous site for signs of infiltration, such as redness or swelling. When extremities are used for intravenous placement, it is important to check circulation because tape and restraints could alter circulation.
* Fluid restriction must be explained to the child (as appropriate) and parents to ensure compliance. The child must be reassured that he or she is not being punished. Children older than 3 years are more likely to show compliance with fluid restriction if allowed to make selections from a list of fluids allowed. Older children can be taught to calculate their own intake and output, with nursing assistance to ensure accuracy, to promote compliance and encourage feelings of independence.

promotion of positive self-image

* Encourage the child and parents to discuss feelings and fears associated with the diagnosis. Help the child focus on assets and positive features. Professional counseling may be necessary. School-age children are encouraged to have peers visit. During peer visits, catheter tubing and drainage bag may need to be camouflaged to prevent embarrassment to the patient. This can be done by attaching a leg bag or by emptying the bag so that the flat bag and curled tubing are hidden under the child's robe or bed linen.

promotion of home care

* Teach child (if age appropriate) and caregiver the importance of proper hygiene, regular voiding, signs of fluid retention, and proper medication routine.
* Teach the parents how to take the child's blood pressure and how and when to administer antihypertensive medications. Assess the parents' understanding of the disease and prescribed treatment. Teach the parents and child the signs and symptoms of infection, including fever, color of urine, increased pain, and increased white blood cell count. Nurses can promote the child's sense of control by talking about how the child can assist with procedures.

* Teach home catheterization early in the hospitalization (if possible) or include it in the plan of care for home health nursing. Older children and adolescents can be taught self-catheterization. Caregivers are responsible for younger children or older children with physical or mental limitations. Most public school systems have special programs using nursing personnel to help children with specific needs attend classes and interact with other children.

evaluation

* The child achieves a normal elimination pattern.
* The child's skin lesions and wounds heal in a timely manner and without complications.
* Pain is relieved illustrated by child resting, playing, and eating.
* Fluid volume is stabilized; intake and output are balanced, vital signs are within normal limits, weight is stable, and edema is absent.
* The child recognizes and incorporates changes into self-concept without revoking self-esteem; he or she seeks information about disease process.
* The child participates in age-appropriate learning process, verbalizes understanding of condition or disease process and treatment, performs necessary procedures correctly, and explains reasons for the actions.

diagnostic tests for kidney function

Urine and blood are important media for determining normal versus abnormal kidney function. When kidney function is altered, components that are normally retained in the body enter the urine. For example, albumin, glucose, blood, bile pigments, and casts are not usually seen in normal urine.

Careful examination of the blood provides valuable information about the urinary system and reproductive system. Because all blood is filtered through the kidneys to remove waste products from the body, an elevated blood urea nitrogen level indicates a degree of kidney failure. A list of tests specific to kidney function is provided in Table 33-4.

Urine studies include the following:

* *Routine urinalysis* determines normal and abnormal components of urine from a voided specimen, specific gravity, and pH. Normal urine is clear; cloudy urine indicates increased white cells and possible urinary infection. Normal urine has a characteristic musty odor; strong or foul urine odors are associated with infection or dehydration. Healthy urine is sterile but will quickly decompose at room temperature, developing an ammonia odor from the breakdown of urea.
* *Twenty-four hour urine collection* determines a more accurate evaluation of creatinine clearance than a spot urine test.
* Urine culture determines the specific cause of infections of kidneys, ureter, bladder, and urethra obtained from a clean catch midstream or catheterized specimen collected in early morning when bacteria count is highest.
* *Urea clearance* measures urine levels of urea.
* *Phenolsulfonphthalein* (PSP) excretion determines renal blood flow by determining the amount of time for the kidneys to excrete PSP. It is important to push fluids after the PSP test.

> **nursing alert**
>
> *The nurse needs to ask if children or parents are allergic to iodine or sea food because contrast media (dyes) may contain iodine, which can trigger severe allergic reactions in some children. The reaction starts with itching, sneezing, wheezing, and flushed skin within minutes after the injection, progressing to anaphylactic shock and death.*

Blood chemistry studies include tests to determine the following:

* *Blood urea nitrogen and creatinine tests* determine the kidney's ability to remove nitrogen body from the blood.
* *Creatine clearance test* determines glomerular filtration rate of the kidney. The test involves a blood specimen and 24-hour urine sample. Young children must wear a urine collection device so that all urine is collected during the 24 hours.
* Complete blood count. Elevated white blood cells indicate infection. Decreased hemoglobin and red blood cells indicate anemia often seen with kidney diseases.
* Serum electrolyte levels (especially sodium, potassium, calcium, and chloride), aldosterone level, and creatinine determine kidney function; arterial blood gases determine acid–base balance.
* Serology testing screens for syphilis, hepatitis B infections, and acquired immunodeficiency syndrome (AIDS).
* *Candida* antibody test detects the presence of antibody to *Candida albicans* and is helpful in diagnosis of systemic *Candida* infection. The blood test is indicated when positive cultures are obtained from specimens with high potential for urine contamination.

Cultures of the genitalia include the following:.

* Vaginal and penal discharge in sexually active teens or sexually abused children is associated with STDs. Any body discharge must be handled using universal precautions, especially when dealing with children. Vaginal discharge is obtained during a pelvic examination by inserting a vaginal speculum and swabbing the vaginal and cervical areas. Penis drainage is obtained by inserting a small wire swab into the urethra.

Imaging studies include the following:

table 33-4 kidney function tests

Test	Explanation
Blood urea nitrogen (BUN) <100 mg%	The BUN is a waste product of protein breakdown. The level reflects dietary intake of protein, glomerular filtration rates, and infection.
Creatinine (CR) (0.6–1.2 mg/ 100 mL)	A waste product of muscle breakdown, CR is normally removed from the blood by healthy kidneys. High levels of CR can cause nerve damage, pruritus, and numbness and tingling of toes.
Serum potassium (3.5–5.4 mEq/L)	This is an intracellular electrolyte that regulates muscle action. Too much or too little potassium can cause the heart to stop. Blood levels reflect compliance to diet, drug therapy, or losses from vomiting and diarrhea.
Serum sodium (135–145 mEq/L)	Found in extracellular fluids, serum sodium helps kidneys regulate body fluid. The higher the levels in the blood, the more water is retained by the body, causing thirst, edema, and dyspnea. Extra sodium and water cause increases in blood pressure.
Chloride (98–106 mEq/L)	Found in extracellular fluid, chloride is necessary for nerves and muscle to work together
Serum calcium (8.5–10.5 mEq/L)	Calcium helps to keep bones strong and growing. Adequate amounts of calcium are provided by foods, such as dairy products.
Phosphorus	Made by protein breakdown. It is a chemical that works with calcium to keep bones strong. High phosphorus levels will cause a low calcium level and vice versa. Prolonged increased phosphorus levels lead to bone disease.
Hematocrit (HCT)	The amount of red blood cells compared to water (plasma) in the blood is HCT. Chronic renal failure causes a decrease in the HCT because the kidneys can no longer make the hormone that helps to build red blood cells.

* *Kidney-ureter-bladder radiography* determines the kidney size, position, structure, and presence of stones.
* Excretory urography, also known as intravenous pyelography, allows visualization of the kidney structures, ureters, bladder, and urethra with the use of a contrast media. The child must be told that there will be a general feeling of warmth while the contrast material is put through the intravenous tubing.
* *Computed tomography scan* constructs an image of the kidneys from a series of cross-sectional slices without exposing children to radiation. Computed tomography scans identify obstructions, polycystic kidney disease, congenital anomalies, and hydronephrosis.
* *Voiding cystourethrography* determines urinary *reflux* (backward flow of urine), chronic urinary tract infections associated with strictures, and incontinence. A urinary catheter allows instillation of a contrast medium into the bladder; x-ray pictures are taken as the child voids. Some children may have difficulty voiding in the presence of others and need reassurances to do so.

Endoscopic procedures include the following:

* *Cystoscopy examination* involves direct visualization of the bladder, ureters, and urethra using a lighted tubular lens. *Cystourethroscopy* involves the insertion of two scopes (cystoscope and urethroscope) into the urethra and bladder to visualize the structures and determine abnormalities, such as urethral stricture, diverticula, or polyps. General anesthesia is used. Following the procedure, assessment includes vital signs, level of consciousness, ability to void, color of urine, and complaints of discomfort. Some burning with urination is expected. Nursing care includes forcing fluids (unless contraindicated) to dilute the urine and reduce the burning sensation during voiding and maintaining fluid balance.

Percutaneous renal biopsy involves the following:

* *Renal needle biopsy* involves inserting a needle into the kidney to excise tissue, distinguishing glomerular from tubular renal disease, and detecting the presence of Wilms' tumor. Children are sedated before the procedure, and the biopsy site is numbed with 1% lidocaine. Children are usually awake during the procedure and need to be reassured that they will feel pressure. When a child's anxiety is high, pain and pressure can be interpreted as being the same. Preparing the child in advance by asking them to describe the difference between pain and pressure helps the nurse understand the child's perspective. For example, pain can be reported in terms of a "pinch" on the skin, while pressure can be described as "pushing" on the skin. Following the biopsy procedure, the biopsy site must be carefully assessed for bleeding, hematoma formation, redness, edema, and heat, indicating infection.

congenital anomalies

hypospadias

Hypospadias is a relatively common birth defect affecting 1 in 300 male infants. It is identified by the abnormal position of the urethral meatus on the underside of the penis. It rarely is seen in girls and is more difficult to diagnose. Hypospadias in girls often creates a rectal fistula, resulting in urine flow into the rectum.

pathophysiology

The penis may display a downward curvature, narrowing of the meatus, and an incomplete ventral foreskin. Hypospadias is classified by the position of the urethral meatus and is stated as glandular, penoscrotal, scrotal, or perineal (Fig. 33-2).

surgical management

Surgical management for hypospadias is aimed at straightening the penis, bringing the meatus to the tip of the penis, and creating a cosmetically acceptable appearance of the genitals. Surgical intervention is typically done between 6 and 12 months of age, depending on the severity of the problem and preference of the urologist.

Performing the surgical repair at an early age helps spare the child and family undue psychological trauma related to separation anxieties, toilet training problems, and altered gender identity.

Surgical technique depends on the severity of disease and the surgeon's selected procedure. Skin and bladder tissues are often used for free grafts. The tissue is rolled into a tube and used to extend the urethral meatus to the tip.

Complex variations of hypospadias may require a two-stage repair. The first stage consists of release of the downward curvature of the penis and creation of a perineal urethrostomy. The second stage, performed about 6 months later, is aimed at bringing the urinary meatus to the tip of the penis and using foreskin to cover the exposed shaft of the penis.

Three types of urinary drainage catheters are used in hypospadias repair, depending on the surgeon's preference and child's age. They include urethral and suprapubic catheters, suprapubic tubes, and urethral stents.

For older children who are toilet trained, catheters or suprapubic tubes are used. These catheters and tubes keep the child dry without the use of a diaper. Suprapubic cystostomy, perineal urethrostomy, and urethral catheters are used to divert the urine for 7 to 14 days. Urethral stents are placed into the urethra or bladder and left in place for 7 to 10 days, depending on the surgeon. Urethral stents are often allowed to drain into a diaper (Fig. 33-3).

Postoperative complications are seen in approximately 5% to 10% of cases. Complications include stenosis, fistula formation, infection, and graft loss.

✱ nursing process for hypospadias

assessment

Preoperative objective data to be assessed include the following:

- Absence of ventral foreskin
- Dimple or groove at tip of penis
- Urethral opening on the ventral side of penis

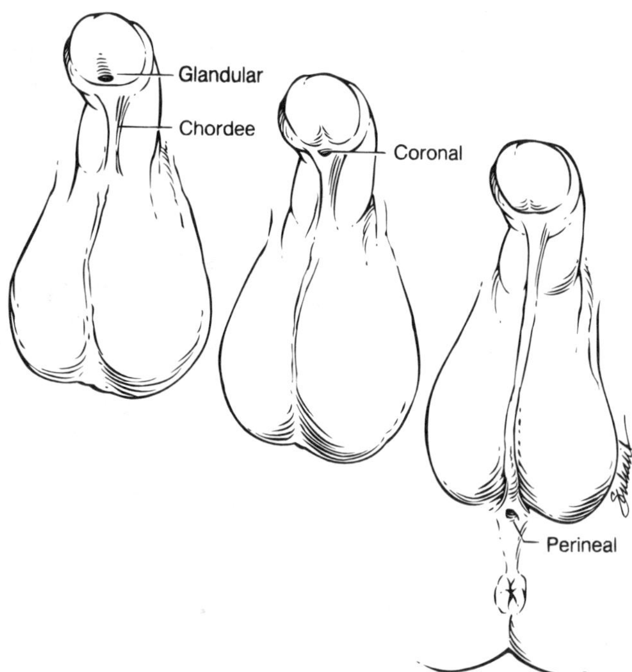

figure 33-2 *Typical hypospadias. The defect is described by anatomic location of the aberrant urethral meatus and its association with the chordee.*

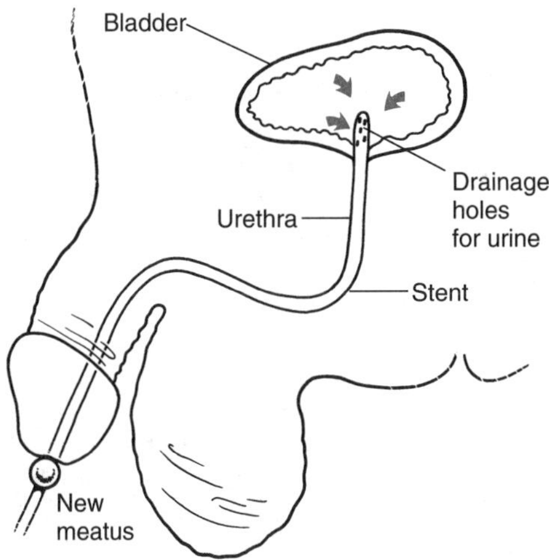

figure 33-3 *Urethral stent for urinary drainage.*

Postoperative objective data to be assessed include the following:

* Penile swelling
* Bleeding at surgical site
* Dysuria (painful urination)
* Irritability
* Restlessness

nursing diagnosis

* Anxiety, related to surgical procedure
* Risk for Infection, related to placement of indwelling catheter
* Altered Comfort, related to pain due to surgery
* Parental Anxiety, related to the physical imperfection of the child's penis after surgery
* Knowledge Deficit, related to home care

planning and implementation

* Promotion of child and parental understanding of surgical procedure: Provide explanations in appropriate terms about the surgical procedure and expected postoperative care. Use pictures and dolls when explaining to the child. Allow child to act out fears and fantasies with puppets or dolls.
* Promotion of catheter care: Secure catheter patency by keeping the catheter drainage bag below the child's bladder level and tubing free of kinks and loops. Use aseptic technique and universal precautions when emptying the catheter bag. Monitor the child's urine for cloudiness. Monitor intake and output at least every 4 to 8 hours. Monitor surgical dressings for foul odor or purulent drainage every 4 hours. Encourage the child to drink 2 to 3 oz or more per hour. Administer prescribed antibiotics, such as gentamicin or ampicillin, and monitor for adverse effects, such as oral and diaper area candidiasis, diarrhea, or a blotchy skin rash.
* Promotion of comfort: Administer prescribed medications, such as analgesics for pain (Tylenol or Tylenol with Codeine for children older than 2 years). Limit activity for the first 48 to 72 hours postoperatively. Moderate restrictions are maintained for 7 to 10 days until the suprapubic tube and larger dressings are removed.

> **nursing insight**
> *Forewarn parents that frequent administration of codeine can increase the risk of constipation, which results in increased bladder spasms.*

* Promotion of parental acceptance of child's defect: Encourage the parents to express their feelings and concerns about the child's condition. Assist the parents through the normal grieving process. Refer the parents to an appropriate support group.
* Promotion of home care: Instruct the parents about the following: 1) catheter care, proper positioning and taping to avoid disturbing the incision, and avoidance of catheter kinks or twisting; 2) how to place the penis so it is pointed in the caudal (tail) direction and taped securely along the catheter; 3) regular emptying of the urinary leg bag; 4) catheter irrigation in case the catheter becomes obstructed using sterile technique; 5) bed cradle to keep linens from rubbing against the catheter and penis; 6) administration of prophylactic urinary antibiotics, such as cefaclor (Ceclor) or sulfamethoxazole (Bactrim), to prevent urinary infections; 7) importance of keeping follow-up appointments for the removal of penis dressings approximately 4 days postoperatively; 8) how to bathe the penis twice daily for 5 to 10 minutes and then apply an antimicrobial ointment, such as bacitracin or mupirocin (Bactroban), after the penis dressing is removed by the surgeon. Telfa pads are used to cover the penis and avoid irritation of the incision from the diaper. Restrict child's activities to avoid straddle toys, such as baby bouncers or bicycles, and gym or contact sports for older children. Instruct parents to report the following situations to the doctor immediately: temperature elevation, incision site drainage (yellow or green indicates infection; bright red indicates bleeding) and redness, decreased urinary output compared with the previous day, and trauma to the genital region.

evaluation

* Child and parent will be less anxious and will verbalize an understanding of the surgical procedure.
* Child will remain free of infection.
* Child will have decreased amounts of pain reflected by ability to rest, socialize, and play.
* Parents will verbalize acceptance of child's defect.
* Parents will verbalize an understanding of home care instructions.

epispadias

Epispadias is a condition in which the urethral meatus is located on the dorsal side of the penis. The condition is rare and often associated with exstrophy of the bladder (discussed below).

Surgical intervention for epispadias is required if the penis is curved dorsally and smaller than usual. Surgical repair occurs between 2 and 3 years and consists of reconstructive surgery of the penis and urethra. Nursing care is similar to the child undergoing repair of hypospadias.

exstrophy of the bladder

Exstrophy of the bladder occurs when the anterior wall of the bladder is positioned on the abdominal wall instead of being enclosed within the abdomen (Fig. 33-4). This is the result of an in utero defect. The exposed bladder allows for urine leakage. This may lead to skin ulceration and infection. Exstrophy of the bladder requires surgical intervention within the first 48 hours of life. As time passes, reconstructive surgery may be required. If the bladder cannot function, it must be surgically removed and replaced with an artificial bladder, or segments of the bowel may be connected to the ureters; a stoma is then created and covered by an ostomy bag for drainage.

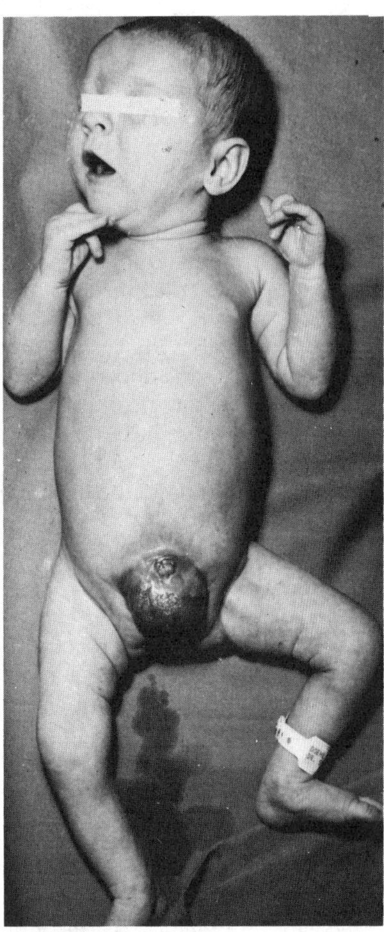

figure 33-4 *Exstrophy of the bladder. The anterior surface of the urinary bladder lies open on the lower abdomen.*

phimosis

Phimosis is an abnormal narrowing of the foreskin that prevents foreskin retraction. As a result, urinary output is obstructed. The child is at an increased risk for infection and urine leakage. *Circumcision* is the surgical intervention for phimosis (refer to Chapter 16: Nursing Care of the Normal Newborn).

testicular torsion

Testicular torsion is a twisting of the spermatic cord, occurring more frequently in adolescent boys with inadequate testicular support. Occasionally newborns are born with testicular torsion. Symptoms include scrotal edema with a unilateral red or bluish discoloration, reflecting a loss of blood supply. Older children complain of scrotal pain and tenderness, lower abdominal pain, nausea, vomiting, and fever. Neonates may fail to display symptoms.

Diagnosis of testicular torsion is based on symptoms and physical examination. The condition often requires emergency surgery in an older child because the diminished blood supply to the testes can cause irreversible tissue damage. If the testis must be removed, a prosthesis is often inserted for psychological reasons.

vesicoureteral reflux

Vesicoureteral reflux is a backward flow of urine up the ureters during voiding (Fig. 33-5). The condition is often associated with urinary tract infections (UTIs). Vesicoureteral reflux occurs 10 times more often in girls than boys and is more common in white people than in African Americans (Pediatric Nursing, 1992).

pathophysiology

A backflow of urine occurs when the pressure of a full bladder forces urine up into the ureters. Normally, urine flows from the ureters into the bladder and from the body during voiding; however, because the valve that guards the entrance from the bladder to the ureter is defective, urine is able to push back into the ureters and be retained, creating a good reservoir for bacteria growth.

Vesicoureteral reflux is classified according to the degree of reflux of urine from the bladder into upper genitourinary tract structures (Table 33-5). Vesicoureteral reflux increases the child's risk of renal damage because the refluxed urine exposes the collecting tubules of the nephrons to microscopic organisms, and stasis of the urine results in inflammation and scarring.

medical–surgical management

Vesicoureteral reflux is often diagnosed when investigating a urinary tract infection, including during urinalysis, voiding cystourethrogram, and cystoscopy. Once the diagnosis is made, a major goal is to maintain renal function and prevent renal scarring and urinary tract infections. Long-term administration of prophylactic antibiotics,

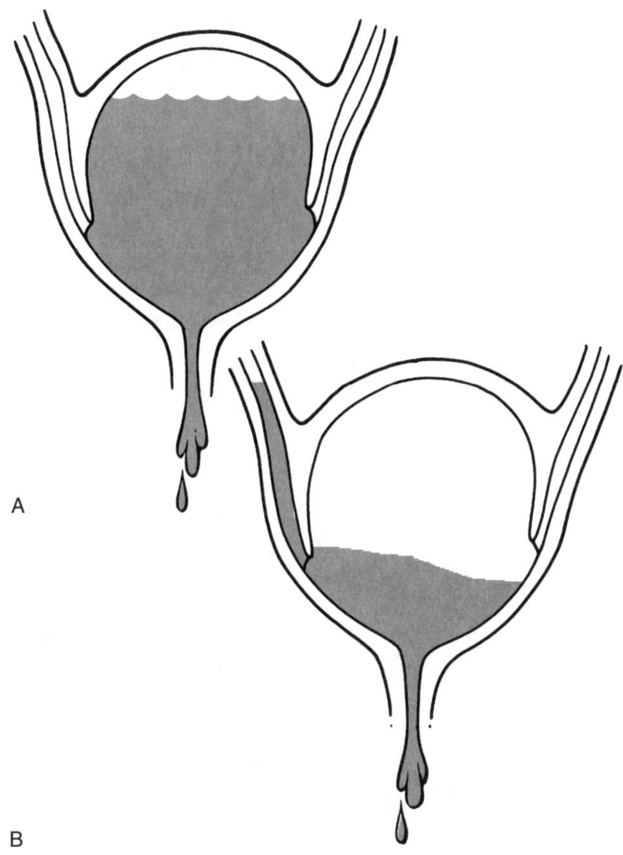

figure 33-5 *Bladder reflux **(A)** Normal voiding pattern. **(B)** Reflux into ureters with voiding.*

such as ampicillin, reduces the occurrence of bladder infections.

Invasive treatment for vesicoureteral reflux includes endoscopic examination with a cystoscope and Teflon paste to stabilize the ureter valves. This procedure is used for minor vesicoureteral refluxes. When ureters need more extensive repair, surgical intervention includes reinsertion of the ureters into the bladder at an oblique angle, creating a normal valve effect. Surgical success is high.

A suprapubic catheter is used following surgery to drain urine from the bladder, reducing the potential for pressure at the surgical site. Stent catheters are threaded through the ureters into the kidney pelvis, draining urine directly from the kidneys.

preoperative nursing care

* Assess child's voiding pattern for small, frequent voidings of foul-smelling, cloudy urine with reports of a sense of urgency or pain.
* Monitor intake and output.
* Administer prescribed antimicrobial medication, such sulfamethoxazole or amoxicillin; note positive response to the drug, such as becoming asymptomatic and having negative urine cultures. Stress the importance of giving the medication around the clock until completely finished, even if the child is feeling better. Parents need to be advised to notify the doctor if the child develops diarrhea stools, vaginal discharge, or skin rash. Sexually active female adolescents must be advised to use a nonhormonal method of contraception while taking ampicillin.
* Monitor laboratory tests, such as elevated white blood count indicative of infection. Urine cultures are done every 4 to 8 weeks to assist with the assessment of infection. Complete blood counts are ordered every 3 to 8 months to monitor bone marrow depression, a rare side effect from the use of sulfamethoxazole.
* Teach the child and parents about proper hygiene; regular voiding; increased fluid intake, especially water and fruit juices; avoiding soda; medication administration; and signs of urinary tract infection.

postoperative nursing care

* Assess operative site for signs of bleeding and infection, such as redness, edema or purulent drainage, and pain.

table 33-5 vesiculoureteral reflux (VUR): grade, action, and nursing implications

Grade	*Reflux Action*	*Nursing Implications*
I	VUR into the lower ureter	Teach child and caregiver importance of taking prophylactic antibiotics; administer medications at bedtime; monitor for bone marrow suppression.
II	Ureteral and pelvic filling, no caliceal dilation	Same as grade I.
III	Ureteral and pelvic filling with mild caliceal blunting	Preoperatively assess child's and parents' reactions to surgery. Postoperatively, assess urine, incision site.
IV	Marked distension of pelvis, calices, and ureter	Same as grade III.
V	Hydronephrosis	Same as grade III. Monitor blood urea nitrogen, complete blood count, and arterial blood gases.

- Change sterile dressings over suprapubic catheters per physician's orders. Care must be taken to keep ureter stents in place if they are used as part of the operative procedure.
- Assess urinary output, including urine from all tubes and dressings. Urine draining from the stents should be equal on both sides, indicating bilateral kidney function. *Hematuria* is expected for 1 to 2 days.
- Administer prescribed analgesics for operative pain. Antispasmodics are often prescribed to reduce bladder spasms. Phenazopyridine hydrochloride (Pyridium) produces a local anesthetic effect on the mucosa of the ureters and bladder approximately 30 minutes after oral administration, relieving burning, pain, urgency, and frequency associated with urinary tract infections and irritation. Phenazopyridine tends to cause a yellowish tinge in the sclera of the eye and turn urine reddish orange.
- The child must be instructed not to touch or move the suprapubic tube because this will trigger bladder spasms.

home care

- Home care instructions include avoiding tub baths until the suprapubic tube site is completely healed. Instructions concerning dressing changes to drain site must include proper cleaning and dressing application. Girls must use good perineal hygiene, such as cleansing from the urethra back toward the anus after toileting to reduce the risk of exposing the urethra to stool and infection. Stress the importance of reporting signs of infection, such as temperature elevation, cloudy urine, malaise, and anorexia. Fluids are encouraged with knowledge about the importance of drinking cranberry juice or apple juice to maintain acidic urine. Children and parents are encouraged to comply with follow-up appointments.

tumors and other acute conditions of the kidney

wilms' tumor

Wilms' tumor is a malignant tumor of the kidney (*nephroblastoma*) frequently diagnosed in young children between 2 and 3 years, although some children are diagnosed as early as 6 months and others during adolescence.

pathophysiology

Wilms' tumor is often associated with other congenital anomalies of the genitourinary tract. The tumor may be genetic. At first, the tumor is asymptomatic. As it grows or hemorrhages, a firm mass may be felt in the child's abdomen. Parents are usually the first to notice the mass, often thinking it is the result of severe constipation. Wilms' tumor is classified by the National Wilms' Tumor Study in a staging system ranging from I to V according to tissue involvement. Stage I involves one kidney, while stage V involves both kidneys (Table 33-6).

medical–surgical management

Diagnosis of Wilms' tumor is based on a complete physical examination. The tumor is palpated as a firm, nontender mass. The child's urine contains blood. The child often has a fever, hypertension, abdominal pain, anorexia, and vomiting.

Treatment is based on the stage of the tumor. Stage I through III are almost always surgically removed with favorable prognosis. Stage IV involves metastasis to the lungs and is treated with radiation or chemotherapy. Surgical intervention for stage V is more serious because both kidneys are involved. If the bilateral tumors are small, they can be removed, leaving functioning kidney cells intact. Often bilateral tumors are treated initially with radiation to shrink them, making surgery less extensive. Prognosis after treatment is good.

Complications following radiation therapy often involve scarring, resulting in small bowel obstruction, nephritis, sterility in girls from damage to the ovaries, development of a second tumor, and increased risk of leukemia.

preoperative nursing care

- Provide the child and caregivers with explanations about preoperative and postoperative care, stressing that the child will receive pain medication as needed.
- Provide information about chemotherapy, preparing child and caregiver for the start of treatments immediately following surgery. Information about the side effects of chemotherapy and radiation is important, especially when hair loss is a concern. Hair loss can be traumatic to young children, and the effect is less severe when the child understands that the hair will grow back once treatments are finished.
- Avoid abdominal palpations prior to surgery to decrease the risk of metastasis. Abdominal girth measurements are taken and recorded daily, tracking tumor growth.
- Monitor the blood pressure to determine the degree of hypertension common to the tumor. Children often complain of headache associated with hypertension.

postoperative nursing care

- Monitor vital signs, especially blood pressure, because hypotension occurs when the pressure is released from the mass pushing against the renal artery.
- Assess bilateral breath sounds at least once every shift to check for normal respiratory function.
- Encourage the child to cough and deep breathe, decreasing the risk of atelectasis or hypostatic pneumonia.

> **nursing alert**
>
> *Hypotension is frequently noted following removal of a Wilms' tumor because pressure is relieved from the renal artery; vital signs indicating shock include increased pulse and respirations with decreased blood pressure.*

table 33-6 Wilms' tumor staging

Stage	Description	Surgical Intervention
1	Involves one kidney	Complete removal
2	Extends beyond the kidney into adjacent tissue	Complete removal, possible radiation
3	Confined to the kidney and abdomen with no signs of metastasis	Complete removal, possible radiation as a prophylactic measure
4	Metastatic involvement, often to the lung	Surgery, radiation, and chemotherapy
5	Both kidneys involved	Surgical removal, dialysis, candidate for kidney transplant

✳ Assess surgical site, noting the presence of bleeding, approximation of skin edges, presence of sutures or staples, redness, edema, and purulent drainage.

nephrotic syndrome

Nephrotic syndrome is associated with glomerular disease and is characterized by severe proteinuria, hypoalbuminemia, and edema. The cause is unknown. Nephrotic syndrome affects children between 2 and 7 years and is twice as common in boys.

pathophysiology

Children with nephrotic syndrome have a physiologic change in the glomerular membrane, increasing its permeability to protein. Blood protein passes into the urine, causing a loss of serum protein.

Fluid collects in body cavities, especially the abdomen, because of decreased osmotic pressure in the capillaries. *Ascites* is a common symptom of nephrotic syndrome and is described as fluid in the abdominal cavity.

Hypovolemia occurs when fluid shifts from intracellular spaces to interstitial spaces; however, the body's perception of the fluid loss prompts the release of antidiuretic hormone and aldosterone. This leads to sodium and water reabsorption and increased edema. Potential complications include renal disease, renal failure, and congestive heart failure.

medical management

The focus of care includes fluid and electrolyte balance, decreasing edema and hypertension, providing a high-protein and low-sodium diet, and administering steroids, such as prednisone. Prednisone is often prescribed for children with nephrotic syndrome to reduce the loss of protein in the urine. Taking prednisone involves maintaining a schedule and recognizing common side effects, such as a full, round face often referred to as a "moon face"; fluid retention; headache; intracranial pressure, bruising; peptic ulcer formation; muscle wasting; and muscle pain. Children must avoid exposure to people with infectious diseases because the drug can cause immunosuppression, increasing their risk of contracting infections. Vaccinations may be held during administration of steroids, and the pediatrician must be informed so that the child's vaccination schedule is monitored. Morning administration coincides with normal body secretion of cortisol. Steroid administration must never be discontinued abruptly, so a "weaning" method is used. For example, the frequency is gradually decreased until all the medication is taken.

Cholinergic drugs, such as bethanechol (Urecholine), are often used to treat urinary retention and neurogenic bladder. The drug is typically administered on an empty stomach and can cause gastrointestinal distress. Vital signs must be monitored because orthostatic hypotension is a common adverse reaction.

nursing care

✳ Administer prescribed medications, and note side effects. Typical drugs used are steroids (prednisone), immunosuppressant therapy (usually cyclophosphamide or methotrexate) for children who are unresponsive to steroids, and broad-spectrum antimicrobial agents (such as cephalosporins) to reduce the risk of infection.
✳ Monitor fluid retention by keeping an accurate intake and output record, weighing daily measuring abdominal girth (increased values can indicate ascites), and assessing the presence of edema in the face, extremities, and lumbar-sacral region. Monitor child for decreased urine-specific gravity, indicating diuresis.
✳ Assess skin integrity. Provide proper skin care, including daily baths with moisturized soap and position changes. Support edematous areas with pillows. Use powder to prevent skin surfaces from rubbing.
✳ Maintain nutritional status by providing small, frequent meals consisting of high-protein foods. Instruct patient and family about the importance of following a sodium-restricted diet.
✳ Monitor for signs of infection because children are at an increased risk of secondary infections due to the loss of immunoglobulin (a protein) in the urine. Educate child and parents about the signs and symptoms of infection, including temperature, urinary discomfort, and nausea and vomiting. Do not allow visits from anyone with an acute infection.
✳ Conserve the child's energy by encouraging bed rest and quiet play. Perform passive range-of-motion exercises during the acute phase of the disease.
✳ Support the child and parents or caregivers by keeping them informed about the condition, providing explana-

tions about ordered tests and procedures, and encouraging open communication.

acute poststreptococcal glomerulonephritis

Acute poststreptococcal glomerulonephritis (APSGN) is a type of nephritis described as a self-limiting autoimmune disease occurring after a streptococcal (beta-hemolytic) infection, such as pharyngitis, otitis media, or impetigo. It is one of the most common types of acute glomerulonephritis in children and affects boys between 5 and 10 years twice as often as girls. The exact cause is unknown.

pathophysiology

Acute glomerulonephritis affects the glomeruli and filtration rate of the kidneys, resulting in water and sodium retention and hypertension. Long-term effects on the renal system seldom occur with APSGN.

Protein and blood are not normally found in urine but will show up in the urine of children with APSGN. Serum tests on children with APSGN show elevated blood urea nitrogen and creatinine levels. Positive serum antistreptolysin-O titers indicate a recent steptococcal infection.

The onset of APSGN is sudden and usually occurs within 7 to 14 days after a streptococcal infection of the respiratory tract or skin. Urine output appears reddish brown with an increased specific gravity from blood cell sediment.

The child often complains of abdominal pain, a low-grade fever, anorexia, and headache. Generalized edema from sodium and water retention contributes to dyspnea, heart enlargement, and pulmonary edema. Hypertension results from the increase in circulating fluid volume.

Most children with ASPSGN recover completely. Serious complications include hypertensive encephalopathy, pulmonary edema, and acute renal failure.

medical management

Acute glomerulonephritis typically runs its course in 1 to 2 weeks. Medical treatment is focused on palliative care. Urinalysis screening for protein and blood is recommended for children 2 weeks after a streptococcal infection. Oxygen and medications specific for congestive heart failure (digitalis) and hypertension (diazoxide) are given.

nursing care

* Monitor and document blood pressure readings every 2 to 4 hours during the acute phase.
* Institute seizure precautions, including suction and oxygen equipment at the bedside and padded side rails. Seizure activity can result from hypertensive encephalopathy.
* Administer diuretics (such as Lasix) as ordered. Diuretic agents are administered in the early morning to avoid the frequency of nighttime voiding. Assess serum potassium levels for signs of hypokalemia resulting from loss of potassium during diuresis.
* Monitor and record intake and output. Assess color, consistency, and specific gravity of urine.

✳ nursing insight
Renal failure is most commonly reflected by a decrease in urinary output.

* Provide small, frequent meals that are high carbohydrate (needed for caloric demands associated with fever), low sodium with no added salt (to reduce edema), and potassium enriched or decreased depending on serum potassium levels and diuretics used. Children with diminished urinary output often require a low-potassium diet.
* Schedule rest periods to follow play activities.

renal failure

When both kidneys fail to function, waste products and water build up in the body, causing uremia. *Uremia* is a toxic condition associated with the retention of urinary waste products in the blood. Renal failure (often referred to as kidney failure) can occur suddenly or over many years and can be acute or chronic. Maintaining blood chemical balance and waste product removal is accomplished by *dialysis* (treatment of removing waste products from a patient's blood by using an artificial kidney through a blood vessel shunt) during kidney failure.

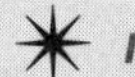
nursing insight
*Three cardinal signs of uremia are the three A's: **a**nemia, **a**cidosis, and **a**zotemia (collection of urea, creatinine, and other nitrogenous wastes in the blood).*

acute renal failure

Acute renal failure is a sudden and complete loss of kidney function in children with potential life-threatening consequences. A decrease in circulating blood is directly linked with acute renal failure. The condition is reversible, and prognosis is favorable with early diagnosis and treatment.

pathophysiology

Acute renal failure in children is due to a number of causes, such as decreased blood flow to the kidneys, resulting from massive fluid loss seen in diarrhea and vomiting, burns, or nephrotic syndrome; diseases that damage the kidney, such as glomerulonephritis; and obstruction of the urinary tract below the kidneys, involving a calculus, clot, tumor, or kinking of the ureters.

medical management

Children with acute renal failure typically have anemia, altered platelets, and fluid and electrolyte abnormalities. The chief symptom is oliguria. Medical management focuses on correcting the anemia, maintaining a normal platelet count and pH balance, restoring fluid and electrolyte balance, managing hypertension, and treating the underlying cause.

nursing care

* Nursing care involves critical care skills in an intensive care unit.
* Support parents or caregivers because they can easily feel intimidated with the highly technical equipment used to monitor cardiac and respiratory status.
* Encourage active family participation in the care of the child.
* Instruct child and caregivers about home health care, which typically includes a diet low in protein, sodium, potassium, phosphorus, and fluids; administration of medications, such as multivitamins, calcium supplements, and iron; and hemodialysis or peritoneal dialysis administration.

chronic renal failure

Chronic renal failure (also called end-stage renal disease, ESRD) is a decrease of kidney function in both kidneys that occurs over time. When the kidneys stop functioning in chronic renal failure, they will usually not function again.

pathophysiology

The most common reasons for ESRD between birth and 5 years include poorly formed urinary tract systems that fail to remove urine correctly, causing kidney failure; small kidneys, called hypoplastic or dysplastic; and hydronephrosis associated with congenital blockage of the ureters.

From 6 to 12 years, the most common cause of kidney failure is a defect in the urinary tract. After 13 years, glomerulonephritis (inflammation of the small blood vessels in the glomeruli of the kidney), repeated pyelonephritis, and hypertension are the major causes of renal failure.

medical–surgical management

The goals of treating children with ESRD are to provide a normal lifestyle while living with the problem and promoting growth and development. Short stature or stunted growth is a common problem among children with chronic renal failure, and early treatment is important to enable the child to reach normal limits.

Transplantation is the best treatment for children with chronic renal failure. When a transplant is not readily available, medical management includes dialysis treatment. Hemodialysis and peritoneal dialysis are the two kinds of dialysis. Hemodialysis uses a dialysis machine and an artificial kidney; peritoneal dialysis uses the abdomen's peritoneal membrane as a filter.

nursing care

Children with kidney failure have special medical, social, and emotional needs.

* Inform the child and caregivers about the condition and treatment in age-appropriate language.
* Encourage child to maintain as normal a lifestyle as possible by going to school, playing, and traveling. School provides the child with necessary education and social interaction opportunities.
* Assess children for feelings about sexuality compared with same-sex peers. For example, determine whether catheters, fistulas, and multiple scars affect the child's self-image and to what degree.
* Discuss dietary restrictions with child and caregiver, and refer to dietitian. Dietary restrictions include restricted amounts of protein (care must be taken to provide enough protein for growth and development needs while not giving so much that urea builds up in the blood), sodium, potassium, phosphorus, and fluids.
* Encourage caregivers to discuss financial concerns. Medicare is available for children with chronic renal disease who require dialysis or kidney transplantation.
* Encourage family to give the child continued love and support.

hemodialysis

Hemodialysis removes wastes and fluids from the blood through an artificial kidney or dialyzer specially made for children. The process takes 4 to 6 hours and is done two to three times per week at a hospital or dialysis center until normal kidney function returns or a renal transplant is possible.

Hemodialysis is administered through a blood access, such as a shunt, subclavian catheter, fistula, or synthetic graft or conduit (Table 33-7). The needle insertion is uncomfortable at the start of hemodialysis, but the treatment is not painful. Children are able to read, do homework, watch television, or sleep while being hemodialyzed (Fig. 33-6).

The artificial kidney in hemodialysis has two compartments. One compartment lets blood flow through it, while the other permits a solution called dialysate or bath flow through. A thin membrane separates the compartments, allowing the blood and dialysate to flow in opposite directions.

Waste products from the blood go into the dialysate and are drained from the machine while clean blood returns to the body. Blood goes through the artificial kidney at a rate of approximately ½ pint per minute, allowing the blood in the body to go through the artificial kidney twice every hour.

nursing care

* Assess shunt, fistula, and graft sites with a stethoscope for a rushing sound called a *bruit* (pronounced "brew-ee"). The rushing sound is made as venous and arterial blood connect. Assess for presence and strength of the pulse. If the bruit or pulse is absent, notify the doctor immediately.
* Assess vital signs. Blood pressure always drops during hemodialysis, but a sudden drop needs to be reported. Do not take blood pressure in the arm with the shunt.
* Sterile technique must be used when cleansing and applying shunt site dressings. An antibiotic ointment, such as mupirocin, is often applied to the shunt site to reduce the risk of infection.

table 33-7 types of blood accesses used in hemodialysis

Type	Description	Nursing Implications
Shunt	A temporary external device consisting of a plastic-like tube with one end attached to an artery and the other end attached to a vein	Avoid taking blood pressures or drawing blood from the arm with the shunt. Monitor shunt placement, and keep child from touching shunt.
Subclavian catheter. The subclavian catheter is a temporary blood access.	Special plastic-like tube inserted through the skin at the collar bone	A sterile dressing covers the insertion site and must be kept dry and free from pulls or tugs.
Fistula. The fistula is a permanent blood access.	Requires a surgical procedure that connects an artery and a vein, usually in the forearm	This procedure allows the vein to increase in size and the wall to thicken because of the increased blood flow. Avoid taking blood pressures or drawing blood from arm with the fistula.
Synthetic grafts	Require surgery; connected in a horsehoe shape and attached to an artery and a vein	Graft placement is under the skin and considered a permanent blood access. Avoid taking blood pressures or drawing blood from arm with the graft.

home dialysis

Home dialysis allows flexible treatment schedules and is often more acceptable to the child and caregivers. Home dialysis requires training; programs last several hours, two or three times weekly for approximately 6 to 8 weeks or until the caregiver is comfortable with the procedure.

peritoneal dialysis

Peritoneal dialysis is the oldest method of removing waste from the body. The peritoneal membrane surrounding the intestines and other abdominal organs is used as a filter or artificial kidney. The different types of peritoneal dialysis are discussed in Table 33-8.

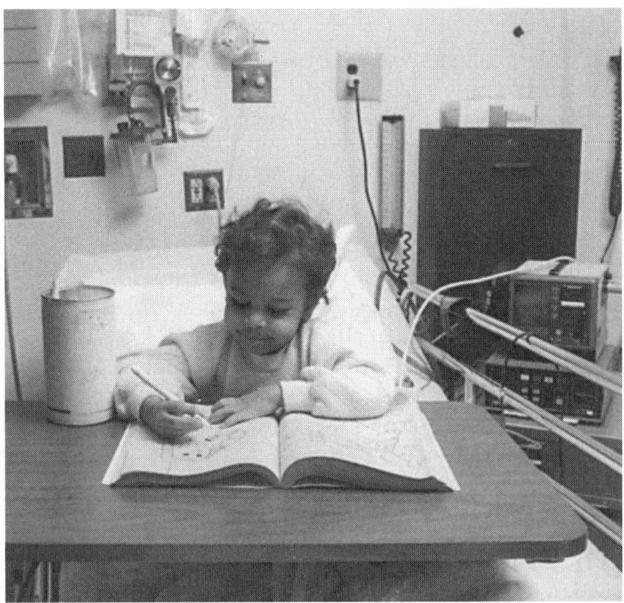

figure 33-6 *A young boy plays while he is having hemodialysis.*

The peritoneal dialysis procedure involves draining a specially prepared sterile solution (dialysate) into the peritoneal cavity through a catheter. The dialysate bathes the peritoneal membrane; waste products and excess water flow out of the blood, through the peritoneal membrane, and into the dialysate. The dialysate and waste products from the abdomen are drained into an empty solution bag and discarded.

Continuous ambulatory peritoneal dialysis is an endless, daily treatment that can take place while the child goes to school, plays, travels, or is busy with activities of daily living. Most children can master this by 12 years.

The major drawbacks to peritoneal dialysis involve an increased risk of infection of the peritoneal cavity (peritonitis) and infection at the catheter site. Cardinal signs of infection include elevated body temperature, malaise, redness, purulent drainage, and tenderness at the catheter site.

nursing care

- Warm the dialysate bag to body temperature, but no higher than 37.8°C (100°F) to prevent lowering the child's core temperature. Avoid using a microwave oven to heat the bag because the temperature of the solution is prone to be uneven. UL-approved heating pads can be used.
- Monitor vital signs. Blood pressure during peritoneal dialysis tends to remain constant, unlike hemodialysis. If the blood pressure drops too low, the child can be placed in a sitting position and given salty broth to eat (this helps stabilize fluid volume by increasing fluid retention).
- Assess the drained fluid for color and clarity. Normal

table 33-8 types of peritoneal dialysis

Type	Description
Continuous ambulatory peritoneal dialysis	Bags of dialysate remain attached to the tubing at all times and can be folded and secured at the waist. Dialysate is drained into the peritoneal cavity where it remains for 4–6 h and then is drained. This exchange process is completed three to five times per day, every day. At night, the dialysate remains in the peritoneal cavity for up to 8 hours.
Continuous cycling peritoneal dialysis	Exchanges are made while the child sleeps. A machine warms, fills, drains, and weighs the solution at intervals throughout the night.
Intermittent peritoneal dialysis (IPD)	A machine regulates the infusion and drainage of dialysate. A typical IPD schedule is a treatment often taking 12 hours at least three times per week.

fluid is crystal clear and very pale yellow. Report cloudy fluid immediately because this indicates infection.
* Wear a mask while in the room with a patient receiving treatment.

kidney transplantation

Transplantation is the treatment of choice for nearly all children with ESRD. Dialysis is used until the transplant surgery is possible. Kidney transplantation increases the child's chances of attaining normal growth.

Adult kidneys can be transplanted to small children, but it is better to use a smaller kidney when possible. Transplants are possible from donors as young as 1 year.

Potential donor kidneys can come from related or nonrelated people or from a cadaver. Parents and siblings older than 18 years can be donors. The child receiving a living relative's kidney has a lower chance of rejection, requires fewer drugs, and has better kidney survival.

The operation takes about 3 hours, with discharge from the hospital within 1 to 3 weeks following the operation. After the operation, the child remains in a sterile area. Sometimes he or she is restricted to a plastic-enclosed bubble. Parents must wear gowns, gloves, and masks while visiting the child. Such procedures may make the caregivers and child feel isolated. The nurse can help by explaining that there is an increased risk of infection due to surgery.

Rejection of a donor kidney occurs when the child's cellular or humoral immunity attacks the kidney as a foreign invader with the intent to destroy it. Rejection symptoms include signs and symptoms of inflammation reflected by increased white blood cells, temperature elevation, increased pulse and respirations, and absence of kidney function with elevated blood urea nitrogen, decreased urinary output, and generalized edema.

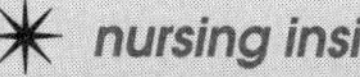
nursing insight

Following a kidney transplant, children may fantasize about the donor, imagining their body has been invaded by another person's spirit.

contraindications for a kidney transplant Occasionally children are not transplant candidates because they have severe heart disease, serious infections, cancer, or lack the ability to comply with the doctor's orders in taking the immunosuppressive drugs needed after a transplant.

Immunosuppressive drugs must be taken daily for the rest of the child's life to prevent the new kidney from rejection. Immunosuppressant drugs, such as azathioprine and cylosporine, are used with glucocorticoids to inhibit cell-mediated immune responses. Children must be carefully observed for signs of infection, and care must be taken to avoid contact with contagious people and those who have been vaccinated with live polio vaccine. Vaccination schedules must be monitored closely, avoiding the use of live virus vaccines.

genitourinary infections

Genitourinary infections can involve the urinary or reproductive system and frequently affect both. Genitourinary infections include inflammation, usually caused by bacteria of the urethra (urethritis), bladder (cystitis), ureters (ureteritis), kidneys (pyelonephritis), epididymis (epididymitis), and vagina (vaginitis).

urinary tract infections

Girls between the ages of 2 and 6 years develop UTIs more often than boys. Sexually active adolescents are at risk for UTIs. In boys, UTIs may be linked with STDs.

pathophysiology

The major cause of UTI is *Escherichia coli*, the bacterium commonly found in stool. Viral infections are not as common in the urinary tract as organisms such as enteric streptococci, *Klebsiella* and *Enterobacter*, and *Staphylococcus epidermis*. Obstruction of urinary flow from the body, such as vesicoureteral reflux, renal calculi (stones), urinary stasis, and obstruction, contributes to UTIs. Bacteria grow rapidly in the warm, moist, dark environment of urine.

Inflammation is typically restricted to the lower urinary tract involving the urethra and bladder. Chronic bladder infections (cystitis) produce change in the ureters, contributing to vesicoureteral valve weakness, increasing the risk of backward flow (also called reflux) of urine. Kidney infections often occur from an infection starting in the lower urinary tract moving up to the kidney pelvis.

Chronic infection leads to scarring and loss of normal renal tissue.

medical management

Diagnosis is based on a complete physical examination. Urine often contains blood (hematuria), appears cloudy with strands of mucus or pus, has a foul odor, and causes pain and burning during urination. Back (flank) pain is common. Urine cultures and sensitivity evaluations identify specific organisms responsible for the infection and the most effective drug against the organism.

Urinary antiseptic agents, such as nitrofurantoin, are effective for local urinary tract infections but are not effective in systemic bacterial infections. Nitrofurantoin causes the urine to be rusty brown and is best administered with food to decrease the risk of gastrointestinal upset. It is never crushed if ordered in pill form because crushing may increase the drug absorption time, altering urine concentration. It can be added to juice, water, or formula if given in liquid form. Care must be taken to rinse the child's mouth following administration of liquid nitrofurantoin to avoid staining the teeth.

Systemic bacterial infections respond to antibiotic agents, such as sulfisoxazole, ampicillin, and cephalexcin. Cefaclor is used to treat resistant UTIs. Oral fluids and intravenous therapy are recommended to dilute the urine and maintain fluid balance.

nursing care

Children with lower urinary tract infections are seldom hospitalized but are cared for at home. The teaching guidelines list ways caregivers can reduce the risks of the child developing a UTI. Home care includes the following:

* Providing parents or caregivers information about medication dosage and administration techniques, follow-up visits for urine cultures, and preventive measures, including good perineal hygiene.
* Educating sexually active adolescents about the importance of safer sex practices and voiding before and immediately after intercourse.
* Stress the importance of follow-up with repeat urine cultures. Urine collected at home must be refrigerated until brought to the office or laboratory for evaluation.

See the Nursing Care Plan.

teaching guidelines
urinary tract infections

Reduce the risk of urinary tract infections by doing the following:

* Avoid bubble baths
* Avoid tight-fitting clothes, tight-fitting diapers for infants
* Go to the bathroom when you have the urge
* Avoid being constipated
* Wipe from front to back after urinating or having a bowel movement (applies to girls)
* Drink fluids, such as water, orange juice, or cranberry juice
* Avoid drinking soda pop or tea
* Wear cotton underpanties rather than nylon
* Rinse pubic hair at the end of a shower or bath to rinse away residual soap.

epididymitis

Epididymitis is an inflammation of the epididymis. It is often associated with urine reflux through the vas deferens in boys. Less common causes include trauma, gonorrhea, syphilis, or spread of a distant infection, such as tuberculosis. Without prompt treatment, it may result in chronic, irreversible epididymitis or sterility.

Inflammation causes swelling and thickening of the spermatic cord and testicular swelling. Pain, tenderness, high fever, and sometimes urethral discharge resemble symptoms of cystitis. The patient's scrotum is enlarged, hot, and reddened. Antibiotics, such as nafcillin and chloramphenicol, are used to treat the infection. Scrotal support is worn continuously until the edema is reduced and sitz baths every 4 to 8 hours and as needed help relieve the discomfort.

vaginitis

Vaginitis is described as an inflammation of the vagina and the vulva, marked by pain, itching, and discharge. There are several types of vaginitis, and effective treatment involves accurate diagnosis of the causative organism. The three major infecting organisms include bacteria, *trichomonas,* and *Candida albicans* (Table 33-9). Vaginal infections are often caused by more than one organism at the same time. Additional types of vaginitis are discussed in Chapter 4.

pathophysiology

Normal vaginal discharge includes mucous secretions from the cervix and vagina plus discarded vaginal cells. Vaginal discharge is present in adolescent girls but not normally in girls before puberty. The vagina of a healthy girl contains organisms that are necessary to keep the many bacteria in the vagina in normal balance. When the normal balance is upset, one or more organisms that reside in the vagina can multiply, changing the normal bacterial flora and causing vaginitis.

The excess bacteria produce excess waste products discarded as vaginal discharge. The abnormal discharge tends to irritate tissues, causing itching, edema and burning of the vulva, increased frequency of urination, and an unpleasant odor.

The resistance of the vagina, like the resistance of the rest of the body to infections, is affected by a poor diet, lack of sleep, or the presence of another disease or infection. There is an increased risk of vaginitis when girls take

nursing care plan for the child with urinary tract infection

NURSING DIAGNOSIS

Altered Urinary Elimination, related to pain of pyelonephritis

GOAL: *Discomfort will decrease and urinary elimination will remain adequate*

NURSING INTERVENTIONS	RATIONALE	EVALUATION
Document severity of pain on a pain scale understandable by the child (such as the face scale)	A developmentally appropriate pain scale can assist the child in subjective measurement of pain.	The child will use the pain scale and improvement will be evaluated on the same pain scale after treatment.
Encourage intake of fluids to decrease dysuria if not contraindicated.	Intake of adequate fluids will help to flush the urinary tract of infection.	The child will have an adequate intake of fluids.
Administer a mild analgesic.	This may help reduce pain.	The child will state an improvement in his pain.
Administer antibiotics as prescribed.	An antibiotic is often employed to combat the infection.	The child will take the oral antibiotic for the prescribed number of days.
Monitor intake and output and daily weights.	These are reliable indicators of fluid status.	The child will have a balanced intake and output and remain with a stable weight.

antibiotics, hormones, or engage in excessive douching. Tight-fitting clothing and intercourse without enough lubrication contribute to cuts or abrasions of the vagina, increasing the risk of vaginitis. Diabetic girls have a higher risk fo *C. albicans* vaginits when the urine contains sugar. Vaginitis in girls is linked with cystitis.

medical management

Diagnosis is based on appearance and culture of the discharge. Treatment is specific for the organism responsible for the infection (see Table 33-8). A pelvic examination may be necessary if any of the following symptoms occur: a heavy vaginal discharge that itches, burns, or smells; no signs of puberty, such as breast growth, underarm hair, or pubic hair by 14 years; no periods by 16 years; no periods for more than 4 months; menstrual cramps that cause absence from school; vaginal bleeding that lasts more than 10 days; heavy vaginal bleeding; or any signs of pregnancy. The teaching guidelines can help prepare the young woman for her pelvic examination.

table 33-9 specific organisms causing vaginitis, symptoms, and treatment

Organism	*Symptoms*	*Treatment*
Bacterial (most common is *Haemophilus vaginitis, Gardnerella)*	Gray, yellow, sometimes blood-streaked, watery discharge with a foul odor; edema and redness of vulva	Administration of oral or vaginal instillation of metronidazole (Flagyl). Administer oral medication with food or milk. Tablets can be crushed. Avoid intake of alcohol; avoid intercourse during treatment with vaginal gel.
Trichomonas	Yellow-green or gray, thin, foamy discharge with foul odor	Administration of oral or vaginal metronidazole. Douching with weak vinegar helps relieve pruritus. Sexual partner requires treatment to avoid reinfection.
Candida albicans fungus considered opportunistic	Thick, white cottage chesse consistency discharge; vulvular itching	Administration of antifungal medications, such as Nystatin or Monistat. Bathing genitals with dilute sodium bicarbonate helps relieve itching. Common in diabetic teenagers with glycosuria. Monitor for relief of symptoms.

teaching guidelines
pelvic examinations

A young woman's first pelvic examination is an event that marks another step toward maturity. Feeling some anxiety is normal if the woman does not know what to expect. Tell the woman the following:

* The health care provider will ask questions about your menstrual cycle.
* You will be asked to undress and put on a gown for the examination.
* Your breasts will be examined for lumps by pressing gently in a circular motion around the breast and underarm area.
* You will be asked to lie on a table with stirrups, which will expose your genital area.
* Relax by taking deep breaths (close your eyes if you want). You will feel an instrument called a speculum being inserted into the vagina. It is normal to feel pressure.
* The physician may insert one or two fingers into your vagina while putting pressure on your stomach. This is done to check your uterus, ovaries, and fallopian tubes.
* Keep your arms down to your side and breathe through your mouth to relax your stomach muscles.

nursing care

* Instruct the patient to use the prescribed medication as directed and not to stop during menstruation or when the symptoms disappear. Vaginal medication tends to leak, requiring the use of a sanitary pad to keep dry and avoid staining clothing. Not using the medication long enough is a common cause of vaginitis recurrence. Sexual partners must be told about the vaginitis because treatment may include them. Sexual abstinence or use of condoms is suggested during the time of infection.
* Stress the importance of follow-up examinations to confirm that the infection is gone.
* Instruct the adolescent to avoid scratching the perineal area because scratching can further irritate the area and spread the infection.
* Stress the importance of keeping the vulva dry because infection spreads in moisture and heat. Measures promoting dryness include drying the body thoroughly after bathing, wearing cotton underpants, avoiding tight jeans or slacks, and changing out of bathing suits soon after swimming.

toxic shock syndrome

Toxic shock syndrome (TSS) is a life-threatening *Staphylococcus aureas* infection associated with tampon insertion at the time of menstruation. It is thought that during the tampon insertion, bacteria on the girl's fingers and irritation from the insertion method contribute to the infection.

Symptoms of TSS include fever with diarrhea, vomiting, severe hypotension, increased pulse and respirations, impaired renal function, confusion, severe muscle pain, decreased platelet count, and severe headache during the menstrual period. Treatment includes administration of penicillinase-resistant antibiotics and intravenous fluids to maintain fluid and electrolyte balance.

sexually transmitted disease

Sexually transmitted diseases are disorders of the reproductive system commonly seen during the adolescent years. The effects are numerous and varied. These diseases have serious implications on quality of life, mortality, sociologic issues, maternal–newborn health, reproductive health, and psychological factors. Chapter 9 defines and describes each of the common STDs. Sexual education regarding STDs is discussed in Chapter 25. In this chapter, the consequences on reproductive health and the psychological well-being of pediatric clients are discussed.

One of the biggest threats to reproductive health is the lack of treatment for an STD. There are many reasons adolescents would not seek medical intervention. Many STDs are asymptomatic or have mild indications. Gonorrhea, chlamydia, genital herpes hidden within the cervix or vagina, nongonococcal urethritis, first-stage syphilis, and human immunodeficiency virus (HIV) are often asymptomatic or go unnoticed in women. Untreated, these diseases may spread to the fallopian tube, cause scarring, and possibly result in sterility. Gonorrhea (in 20% of men), trichomoniasis, first-stage syphilis, and HIV are usually asymptomatic or go unnoticed in men. In time, they may lead to infections in the testes and possibly cause sterility. Even STDs that have obvious signs may go untreated, particularly in adolescents. Teenagers are often afraid to confide in their parents, embarrassed or unable to seek intervention independently, or uneducated about their bodies and the signs of STDs.

Sexually transmitted diseases may compromise the mental status of adolescents. Young women dealing with sterility may become depressed or grieve for the loss of future children. Genital warts and herpes may cause adolescents to be insecure about their bodies. This is especially true for young men who have visible warts or blisters on the penis. Discussing a chronic STD with a new partner is an uncomfortable situation for most people, regardless of age. Teenagers may be more reluctant to share this information, fearing peer rejection or ridicule. They also may become anxious about intimacy, which may have a long-lasting effect on their impressionable self-image. Adolescents or children who are HIV positive or have AIDS may be isolated by their peers. Often they are cut off from the social network, which is vital to their development.

nursing care

Nurses need to be particularly sensitive to adolescents seeking medical care for an STD. An understanding and nonjudgmental attitude is imperative. The nurse will gain more information by asking teenagers specific questions, rather than relying on them to offer details. During an examination, the nurse can continue to provide support. Many young women may never have had a gynecologic examination. The nurse can help relieve apprehensions by remaining with them and talking them through the examination. Sexually transmitted diseases diagnosed in prepubescent children may indicate sexual abuse. By law, medical practitioners are required to investigate and report any suspicions of sexual abuse.

Nurses can be most effective in educating adolescents about STDs. Adolescents will benefit by knowing how to practice safe sex. They need to learn the symptoms that signify an STD. They also need to know the importance of overcoming their fears and discussing STDs with partners to reduce the risk of contracting and spreading diseases. Nurses can hand out pamphlets regarding STDs and sexual health and provide resources to contact when an STD is feared.

disorders associated with menstruation

The most frequent reproductive disorders in adolescent girls involve menstrual irregularities. Menstrual disorders are classified as painful or irregular.

mittelschmerz

Mittelschmerz is pain associated with ovulation. The pain is benign and of limited duration and intensity. Pain experienced from ovulation in the right ovary may be suspect for appendicitis but lacks the associated symptoms of nausea, vomiting, fever, abdominal guarding, and rebound tenderness seen with appendicitis.

dysmenorrhea

Dysmenorrhea is painful menstruation associated with feelings of abdominal "bloating," or severe cramping 24 hours before onset of menstrual flow. Mild breast tenderness, diarrhea, nausea and vomiting, and headache may be present. Dysmenorrhea may also exist with another disorder or infection of the reproductive system. Symptoms are generally controlled by an over-the-counter analgesic.

menorrhagia

Menorrhagia is an abnormally heavy menstrual flow. Menorrhagia increases the adolescent's risk of anemia from excessive iron loss. Treatment may include the administration of a low-dose oral contraceptive, which decreases menstrual flow.

metrorrhagia

Metrorrhagia is bleeding between menstrual periods and includes the normal spotting experienced by some girls during ovulation, breakthrough bleeding associated with oral contraceptives, or vaginal irritation. Adolescents with metrorrhagia for more than 1 month are referred to a gynecologist because vaginal bleeding is an early sign of ovarian or uterine cancer.

endometriosis

Endometriosis is abnormal growth of extrauterine endometrial cells found in the cul-de-sac of the peritoneal cavity, the uterine ligaments, and the ovaries. The abnormal tissue responds to estrogen and progesterone stimulation by swelling and then sloughing its layers similar to the response of the uterine lining during menstruation.

Adolescent girls with endometriosis fail to ovulate or ovulate irregularly and may experience blockage in the fallopian tubes, increasing their risk of infertility. Medical treatment involves administration of estrogen- and progesterone-based oral contraceptives that help diminish the amount of tissue sloughing and a synthetic androgen called danazol that helps shrink the abnormal tissue. Danazol has marked side effects, including weight gain, hirsutism, and acne. Surgical intervention involves laparotomy and excision of the tissue by laser surgery.

amenorrhea

Amenorrhea is an absence of menstrual flow normally noted with pregnancy. Additional factors associated with amenorrhea are tension, fatigue, chronic illness, extreme dieting, or strenuous exercise. Amenorrhea may or may not require treatment and is considered *primary* if the girl has never menstruated; it is *secondary* if it occurs after established menstrual cycles.

premenstrual syndrome

Premenstrual syndrome (PMS) occurs during the luteal phase of the menstrual cycle and affects women physically and emotionally. The cause is generally unknown, but PMS has been linked to hormonal imbalance and dietary influences. Although symptoms vary in degree and number, the common ones are identifiable. Physical manifestations of PMS include bloating, breast tenderness, headaches, and fatigue. Psychological indications include anxiety, irritability, depression, and cravings, particularly for salty or sugary foods.

Because PMS occurs in many women, it is often trivialized by health care workers and loved ones. However, PMS is real to the woman and can interrupt her life significantly. Teenagers who are just beginning to experience PMS and do not easily recognize their symptoms may be especially distressed. The sympathetic nurse will appreciate the client's complaints and teach methods to alleviate the pain and discomfort. Eliminating or decreasing the intake of caffeine, salt, alcohol, and tobacco can significantly decrease the effects of PMS. Increasing exercise and taking oral contraceptives can be helpful as well. The nurse can help the adolescent learn her cycle by having her record physical and emotional changes on a calendar. This will allow her to know when and what to expect, thereby decreasing anxiety about her symptoms. In more severe cases of PMS, hormone therapy might be prescribed.

onset of puberty

During toddlerhood, preschool, and school-age years, genital growth corresponds with overall body growth. The reproductive function of the organs remains inactive until the onset of puberty. The onset of puberty marks the beginning of the ability to procreate.

The onset of puberty marks dramatic changes in the characteristics of genitalia (see Chap. 25). Early or delayed pubertal changes often cause anxieties for children and caregivers. Pubertal changes alter self-image and hormone production, contributing to emotional and psychological confusion. A child's anxieties range from worry about what is normal and how peers will view the body changes to grief about the loss of how they perceived themselves. Caregivers' anxieties focus on the child's emerging sexual maturity, emotional immaturity, amd potential for premature sexual activity and unwanted pregnancy.

precocious puberty

Precocious sexual development refers to the onset of puberty before 8 years in girls and before 10 years in boys. Early production of gandotrophins stimulates the growth and development of secondary sex glands and menses (Fig. 33-7). Precocious sexual development happens twice as often in girls as in boys. Although the cause is unknown in approximately 80% to 90% of the cases, precocious puberty has been linked to pituitary tumors, trauma near the pituitary glands, or ingestion of oral contraceptives (in girls).

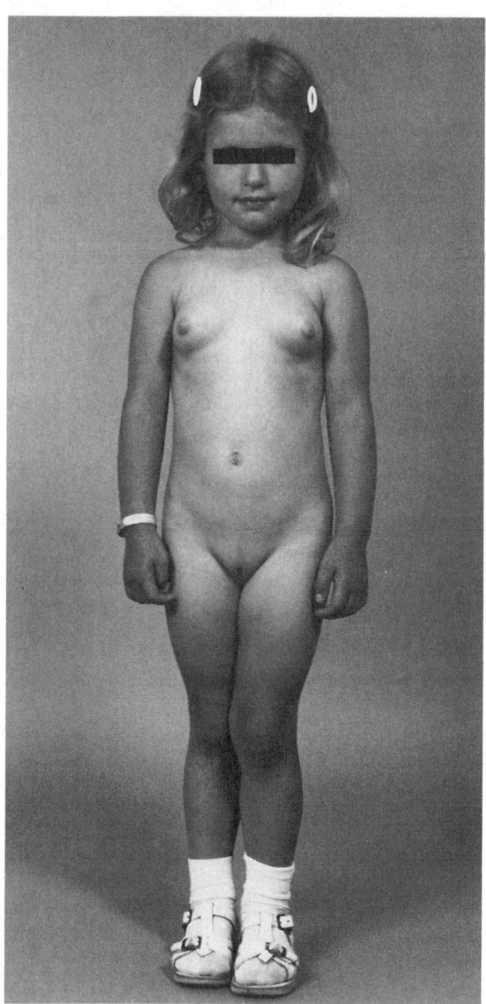

figure 33-7 *An 8-year-old with precocious puberty. (Courtesy of Brian Smistek.)*

When children begin puberty early, they are much younger than expected but seldom have any abnormalities requiring medical intervention. Treatment depends on whether there is an abnormality of one of the major glands producing sex hormones and specifically what the abnormality is. When appropriate, luteinizing hormone-releasing hormone may be administered to decrease the effects of precocious puberty.

Early puberty can create problems for children, such as self-consciousness and vulnerability to sexual abuse. Children exhibiting adjustment problems to early puberty changes need a lot of parental love, support, and guidance. Professional counseling is advised for serious and prolonged anxieties. Preschool children may feel guilty about body changes, perceiving the changes as their fault. A school-age child at the concrete level of cognitive development may experience anxiety when the body does not comply with what they have been told would happen. Educating parents about responses typical of the child's growth and development level helps them be more supportive and educational.

The child experiencing precocious puberty needs information about sexuality, reproduction, and STDs. It is important to keep in mind the child's chronologic, emotional, and cognitive age when providing this information.

delayed puberty

Boys and girls can experience delayed puberty, but it occurs more often in boys; it causes stress, anxiety, and adjustment difficulties. Pediatricians do not always agree as to what age marks delayed puberty. Girls are considered delayed if they fail to develop breast buds by 13 years; boys are considered delayed if testicular enlargement has not occurred by 13 years.

A complete physical examination is necessary to eliminate possible organic causes. Boys are given male hormone injections once a month for 3 months if there are no signs of disease and bone age is less than chronologic age. Male hormone injections speed up growth of the pubic hair and genitals. A major benefit of the treatment is restoration of the boy's self-image and reduction of anxiety.

Girls with delayed puberty are seldom treated with medication. Pediatricians tend to reassure girls that delayed onset of menstruation is not a problem or concern unless they want to become pregnant.

other genitourinary conditions

imperforate hymen

Imperforate hymen is a condition in which the membranous ring normally found at the vaginal opening totally blocks the vagina, preventing the escape of vaginal secretions and menstrual flow. Before menarch, girls often do not have symptoms. In girls who have begun to menstruate, the blocked flow may build up in the vagina and cause abdominal pain. The treatment is surgical removal of the hymen tissue.

fibrocystic breast changes

Fibrocystic breast changes are common in adolescents, appearing at puberty when estrogen levels increase. Sometimes called fibrocystic breast disease, these changes are normal. Round, fluid-filled cysts form in the connective breast tissue. The cysts frequently are palpable in the upper outer quadrants of the breast. The density of the lesions varies with the menstrual cycle and ingestion of foods high in caffeine. The lesions can be painful. Diagnosis of the cysts is made by sonogram.

Danazol (a synthetic androgen) sometimes is used to reduce the pain of fibrocystic breast changes. The adolescent needs reassurances that fibrocystic breast changes do not lead to cancer. Health teaching includes teaching the teenager how to do breast self-examinations (see Chap. 25).

enuresis

During infancy, voiding is a spontaneous and automatic function when the bladder volume reaches approximately 30 to 60 mL of urine. By 3 years, kidney function is considered mature. Complete bladder control can be expected of a 5-year-old; however, most children begin to stay dry at night by their fourth year. Girls achieve complete bladder control slightly before boys.

Enuresis is the medical term for bed wetting and is described as an involuntary passage of urine after the age when a child would be expected to be toilet trained. Enuresis is associated with 5- to 7-year-old children. *Nocturnal enuresis* is an involuntary discharge of urine occurring during night sleep. Functional nocturnal enuresis occurs more often in boys than girls and is thought to be familial.

Careful assessment must be made to rule out urinary infection or undue stress as a cause of the enuresis. Regression in bladder training is associated with the following:

* Separation from parent(s)
* Onset of illness
* Birth of a sibling
* Ingestion of fluids immediately before bedtime

When caregivers limit fluid intake after the evening meal as a way to control nocturnal enuresis, there is an increased risk of exposing the child to dehydration. Several medications are prescribed for enuresis, including the following:

* Desmopressin—a hormone taken through the nose to control frequent urination and bed-wetting
* Imipramine hydrochloride (Tofranil)—an anticholinergic drug that retains urine; may cause seizure activity in children prone to seizures

cryptorchidism (undescended testes)

Cryptorchidism, a common congenital anomaly in boys, is the failure of the testes to descend to the scrotum. It occurs more frequently in premature infants because the descent of the testes from the inguinal canal of the lower abdominal cavity typically occurs in the last trimster of gestation. The cause is multifactorial but is believed to be due to the understimulation of hormones. Common problems associated with cryptorchidism may include an increased probability of developing testicular cancer, a decrease in fertility, and an increased likelihood of developing an inguinal hernia or undergoing testicular torsion.

Theraputic management is aimed at correcting the undescended testes and other associated problems. Surgical intervention is usually delayed until 1 year of age with the hope that the testes will spontaneously descend by the ninth month of life. It is also thought that the surgical procedure, orchiopexy, is safest for the child at around 1 year. Postoperative care concentrates on keeping the incision area clean and infection free. If the child is not toilet trained, an indwelling catheter may be needed to avoid urine infecting the incision.

Undescended testes can be stressful for the patient and family. The nurse must provide support to the parents during the child's first year and additional support if surgery is required. The caregivers must be reassured that this is common, especially in premature infants. At the same time, the nurse needs to educate the family about early detection of a testicular neoplasm and inform them about other possible complications.

ambiguous genitalia

Pseudohermaphrodite is the medical term to describe ambiguous genitalia (Fig. 33-8). The cause of this rare condition is complex. Many chromosomal abnormalities have been associated with the defect. Gender may differ from sex based on the level of male versus female hormones.

Parents begin gender identification in the delivery room with the birth of their baby boy or girl. Anything that threatens gender identification can have serious psychological developmental consequences. Parental support is important, especially when an infant's genitalia do not appear normal.

When an infant is born with ambiguous genitalia, it may take a few days to determine whether the baby is an incompletely developed boy or a masculinized girl. The birth certificate is not completed until information about the newborn's genetic, gonadal, and internal body sex is determined.

After identifying the true sex of the infant, reconstructive surgery is considered. Intervention includes correction of a hpospadias or undescended testes, removal of labia adhesions or an enlarged clitorus, or construction of an artificial vagina. (Pillitteri, 1995). Parents need to contemplate the consequences of treatment on the child's future sexual enjoyment. Decisions to remove a female's clitoris or to raise a chromosomal male as a female are serious. Parents need the benefit of knowing all their options.

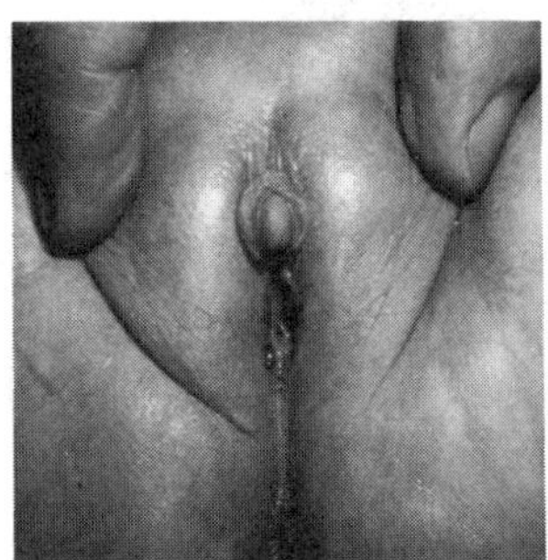

figure 33-8 *Ambiguous genitalia. It is difficult to tell if the child has an underdeveloped penis or an enlarged clitoris.*

penile trauma

Traumatic rupture of the corpora cavernosa, commonly known as fracture of the penis, occurs exclusively during erection as a result of direct blunt trauma that bends the erect organ in an unphysiologic manner. Usually, the fracture occurs when the penis slips out of the vagina and is thrust against the perineum or symphysis pubis. The patient may report hearing a popping noise during intercourse followed by severe pain, swelling, and possible difficulty with urination. It is a rare but significant injury.

Penile fracture may rupture one or both corpora cavernosa, and the tear may involve partial laceration or complete transection of the urethra. Conservative treatment consists of splinting the penis, applying a pressure dressing over a Foley catheter, using ice packs, and administering sedatives. However, with this approach, complications, such as persistent hematoma, abscess, or penile angulation are possible. The surgical approach, aimed at immediate repair of the tear, is often the treatment of choice because it offers fewer follow-up complications.

✷ specific procedure for urinary system

urinary catheterization procedure

Careful observation of the child's urinary output gives the nurse valuable information about urinary function. Catheterization is often ordered to provide the child with an outlet for urine, promote comfort, and provide accurate output recordings.

The nurse follows the institution's catheterization procedure guidelines and maintains sterile technique. The equipment for catheterization in children is basically the same as for an adult. Patient preparation includes age-appropriate teaching. Infant catheterization requires a small size 8 or 10 French catheter. An infant's bladder is higher and more anterior than an adult's, and the urethra lies under and around the symphysis pubis, making the meatus difficult to see in girls. When the catheter is inserted into the female infant, it is directed downward. Male infants are easier to catheterize. The penis is held in an erect position while the catheter is gently inserted.

Maintaining proper infant positioning and avoiding contamination of supplies typically require restraining the infant, either with the help of a parent or an additional health care worker. Caregivers need to be informed that infant crying can be expected, not necessarily from discomfort but from temporary restraints on activity.

Teenagers, especially boys, may fear discomfort but are reluctant to voice their concerns. The visual knowledge concerning the size of the urinary meatus limits a boy's comprehension of how the smallest rubber catheter would not cause excruciating pain during insertion. Providing a thorough explanation with the use of visual aids helps the teenager understand and cooperate.

Explaining about the importance of assessing the urine contributes to increased teenager compliance with saving urine specimens. Feelings of control are reinforced when an older child or teenager empties the urinary drainage bag and keeps urinary output records.

key points ✷

- ✷ The genitourinary system consists of organs involving reproduction and urination. The closeness of specific anatomic parts makes it logical to study them simultaneously; for example, a boy's urethra is a passageway for urine and sperm to leave the body.
- ✷ The function of the urinary system includes urine production from waste products from cell metabolism, excess salts, toxins, and extra fluid; maintenance of water balance; regulation of acid–base balance; and production of hormones that help control blood pressure, manufacture blood cells, and sustain bone formation.
- ✷ The kidneys form urine from blood plasma. Blood flow through the kidneys is a major factor in deciding urinary output; hormones such as aldosterone and antidiuretic hormone influence the reabsorption of water and help maintain normal blood volume and blood pressure. Water balance in the body is altered when kidney function is altered.

* Family considerations include a willingness to discuss genitourinary concerns with older children, promotion of an early awareness of problems and early intervention, knowledge of symptoms of urinary tract disorders, and financial support for the care of children with congenital or chronic kidney disease, an ability to cope with the ill child and other siblings, and complicated home health treatments.
* Nursing considerations include the importance of establishing rapport with children and families by using familiar slang words associated with genitourinary function and anatomy followed by the correct medical terms, respecting the child's privacy, and maintaining confidentiality.
* Congenital anomalies include hypospadias, a relatively common birth defect in which the urethral meatus is on the underside of the penis. It is rarely seen in girls and is more difficult to diagnose. Epispadias is a condition in which the urethral meatus is located on the dorsal side of the penis. Testicular torsion is a twisting of the spermatic cord, occurring more frequently in adolescent boys with inadequate testicular support and occasionally in newborns.
* Wilms' tumor is a malignant tumor of the kidney (nephroblastoma) associated with other congenital genitourinary anomalies and classified by the National Wilms' Tumor Staging System from I to V according to tissue involvement. It is frequently diagnosed in children around 2 to 3 years old with surgical removal based on the stage of the tumor. Prognosis after surgical intervention, chemotherapy, or radiation treatment is good for stage I, II, and III.
* Vesicoureteral reflux, a backward flow of urine up into the ureters during voiding; vaginitis; and epididymitis contribute to urinary tract infections.
* Renal failure occurs when both kidneys fail to function, and waste products and water build up in the body, causing uremia. The condition can be acute or chronic and requires hemodialysis or peritoneal dialysis to remove the wastes from the blood. Most children experiencing chronic renal failure are candidates for kidney transplantation.
* Precocious puberty refers to the growth of the child's genitals with the onset of puberty before 8 years in girls and before 10 years in boys; it occurrs twice as often in girls. The cause is unknown in approximately 80% to 90% of the cases. It is rare and develops when there is an abnormality of one or more of the major glands producing sex hormones.

review questions

1. Raphael is a 2-year-old boy with recurring urinary tract infections. His mother's dominant language is French; she understands limited English. Raphael has been treated during the last 2 months with antibiotics. The most appropriate nursing assessment to determine the cause of the recurrences includes
   a. determining if Raphael drinks from a bottle or cup.
   b. determining the mother's understanding and compliance to the prescribed antibiotic administration.
   c. determining if Raphael is toilet trained.
   d. determining if Raphael has any congenital anomalies.
2. Adam is 17 years old and sexually active with complaints of foul-smelling penile discharge. An appropriate nursing intervention includes
   a. washing the penis daily with a weak sodium bicarbonate solution.
   b. testing for an STD.
   c. using universal precautions when administering care.
   d. Forcing fluids.
3. Bradley, 12 months old, is recovering from surgical intervention for hypospadias. An expected outcome immediately following surgery includes
   a. establishment of normal voiding.
   b. improved sexual image.
   c. stabilization of catheter and ureteral stents.
   d. resuming normal activities.
4. Rita is a 10-year-old with acute renal failure requiring hemodialysis treatments. She has a temporary shunt in her left arm. When planning her care, it is important to
   a. take all blood pressures in the right arm.
   b. monitor bowel movements.
   c. push fluids to dilute urine.
   d. report any signs of edema immediately.
5. Characteristics of uremia include symptoms of
   a. anemia, acidosis, and azotemia.
   b. hypertension, excessive urine production, and thirst.
   c. hypotension, alkalosis, and hypokalemia.
   d. dehydration, confusion, and elevated blood urea nitrogen.

references

Chung, K., Olson, R., & Vinson, J. (1996). *Lippincott's review series: Pediatric nursing.* Philadelphia: Lippincott–Raven.

Pillitteri, A. (1995). *Maternal and child health nursing* (2nd ed.). Philadelphia: J.B. Lippincott.

bibliography

Carpenito, L. (1995). *Handbook of nursing diagnosis* (6th ed.). Philadelphia: J.B. Lippincott.

Centers for Disease Control and Prevention (1993). Sexually transmitted diseases treatment guidelines. *Morbidity, Mortality Weekly Report, 42*(RR-14), 99–102.

Cohen, B. (1991). Children's compliance to dialysis. *Pediatric Nursing, 17*(4), 359–365.

Dunn, S. (1993). How to care for the dialysis patient. *American Journal of Nursing, 93*(6), 26–33.

Fishbach, F. (1995). *Common laboratory and diagnostic tests.* Philadelphia: J.B. Lippincott.

Gulanick, M., Gradishar, D., & Puzas, M. (1994). *Ambulatory pediatric nursing.* Albany, NY: Delmar Publishers.

Lehman, E., & Kremer, S. (1990). Fracture of the penis. *Surgery, Gynecology & Obstetrics, 171*, 148–150.

(1994). *Living with kidney disease. A patient manual.* Indianapolis: Tri-State Renal Network.

Memmler, R., & Wood, D. (1996). *The human body in health and disease* (8th ed.). Philadelphia: Lippincott–Raven.

Stark, J. (1994). Interpreting B.U.N./creatinine levels. *Nursing 94, 24*(9), 58–61.

Sugar, E., Firlit, C., & Reisman, M. (1993). Pediatric hypospadias surgery. *Pediatric Nursing, 19*(6), 585–588.

Thomas, C. (1992). *Taber's encyclopedia* (17th ed.). Philadelphia: F.A. Davis.

the child with an alteration in gastrointestinal function

34

outline ✱

outline (continued)

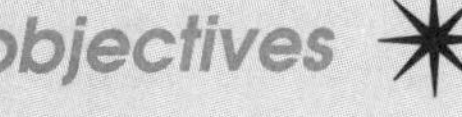

objectives

After studying this chapter, the reader should be able to:

✱ *Discuss at least four caregiver considerations when dealing with a child experiencing an alteration in GI function.*
✱ *Discuss the warning signs associated with anorexia nervosa or bulimia.*
✱ *Identify four nursing considerations for the child with an alteration in GI function.*
✱ *List diagnostic tests commonly ordered for altered GI function.*
✱ *Describe the anatomy and physiology of the GI system from infancy to adolescence.*
✱ *Discuss how weak gagging and swallowing reflexes put the infant at risk for aspiration pneumonia.*

objectives (continued)

✱ *List six nursing assessments for the child with an alteration in GI function.*
✱ *List three reasons infants and small children are at a higher risk for dehydration.*
✱ *Describe two types of failure to thrive.*

key terms

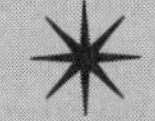

abdominal girth
absorption
anorexia nervosa
appendicitis
barium enema
bulimia
chalasia
chyme
colonoscopy
digestion
esophagogastroduodenoscopy
ingestion
malnutrition
pyloromyotomy
steatorrhea

Alteration in gastrointestinal (GI) function can affect any or all of the following processes: ingestion, digestion, absorption, and elimination. Such alteration can interfere with the child's ability to process food effectively, delaying or inhibiting growth and development.

Gastrointestinal function may be altered by congenital, hereditary, and psychological factors and by bacterial and viral infections and parasitic infestations. This chapter deals with family considerations, anatomy, and physiology of the GI system; disorders of the GI system; nursing care of the child with an alteration in GI function; and procedures relating to the disorders. Child and caregiver information is provided to promote physical and psychosocial growth.

✶ family considerations

Caregivers have a major responsibility for meeting the child's nutritional needs. These needs change as metabolism, age, sex, growth periods, stress, and physical conditions change. Proper nutrition is emphasized with each health maintenance check-up because physical growth and development are closely associated with diet. It is easy to understand why parents become anxious when the child's nutritional needs are not being met due to refusal to eat or inability to retain food.

Caregivers of infants who are "colicky" may have difficulty recognizing changes in the infant's behavior that signal a GI disorder. The infant's established behaviors of irritability, unexplained crying, poor eating, excess flatus, and posturing with legs drawn to the abdomen, may be so routine that caregivers do not suspect a serious problem.

culture

Feeding rituals begin in infancy, based on caregivers' culture and personal preferences. Infants who are fed when hungry and cuddled during feedings learn to trust, a basic developmental task. Learned eating habits in childhood often continue into the adult years. Eating disorders, such as obesity, have been linked with early feeding practices.

Although white Americans place a high value on being thin, other cultures have a different viewpoint. For example, African Americans do not stigmatize overweight women to the same degree as American society in general. African American girls are called "big" or "healthy," rather than "fat."

Cultural customs and beliefs about food must be considered when discussing a child's nutritional needs. Child and caregiver compliance with proposed changes in the diet is much more likely when the nurse respects existing food customs and ideas when communicating with clients.

food safety

Food safety issues include proper food labeling, the freshness of food ingredients, and nutritional content. Foods containing high fat and sugar are not recommended.

Food safety includes other health risk factors. The use of pesticides in food production is linked with increased cancer risk for children and adults (see Chap. 19).

Microbiologic contamination of food sources, such as meat, eggs, and milk, can occur before consumer purchase and can be a major, even life-threatening health risk in children. Nausea, vomiting, and diarrhea are common symptoms of food poisoning, increasing a child's risk for dehydration. Food contamination can occur when food is handled by people with unclean hands, prepared in soiled cooking utensils, or not cooked properly.

Children need to be taught to wash fresh fruits and vegetables before eating them. Washing helps remove chemicals used in agriculture. Chemical residues persist even after washing, however, making organically grown produce a better choice.

poverty

One out of every five American children lives in poverty; nearly half of all African American children live in poverty. Families living in poverty are more concerned with obtaining enough food to relieve hunger than with the nutritional content of that food. They may not understand the significance of recommended daily food allowances or the importance of checking food ingredients.

Families living in poverty often lack adequate refrigeration or cooking facilities, increasing their risk of eating poorly cooked or spoiled foods. They may not have access to clean water to wash food, dishes, and hands, thus increasing their risk for bacterial and viral infections.

Drainage from outside toilets increases the risk of stool contamination in well water, reservoirs, and garden foods. Poverty puts the entire family at increased risk for contracting infections from each other because of crowded living space.

✶ nursing considerations

Proper nutrition affects the health of all body systems. Knowledge about nutrition and diet therapy is necessary for all nurses but especially for those working with pediatric clients. When nutritional needs are not adequately met, GI function is impaired, interfering with the child's normal growth and development.

communication with caregiver and child

The nurse establishes rapport with children and caregivers by listening to their views on proper nutrition and health. Based on these views, the nurse can then provide factual nutritional information in a stimulating but nonthreatening way. For example, some families consider a chubby, milk-fed baby to be a healthy baby. Information about milk-fed infants being at increased risk for obesity, heart disease, and anemia may not seem important to caregivers if they perceive their child as healthy. However, facts about nutrition may interest the caregiver who wishes to keep the baby healthy.

The nurse should provide children and caregivers with information about age-appropriate diet expectations. For example, toddlers enjoy finger foods and resist sitting for long periods. They may eat a few bites and run off to play. Keeping nutritious snacks available so the child has access to food throughout the day may prove more beneficial than expecting the child to eat three large meals.

nutrition and the hospitalized infant

Hospitalization of a breast-fed infant need not interfere with the mother's continuing to breast-feed. Mothers who continue to breast-feed strengthen maternal–infant attachment and established routines. When a nursing mother is unable to stay with the infant, electric or manual breast pumps can be used to keep breast milk available during her absence. Nurses need to reassure the nursing mother that the child will not go hungry. Pediatrician-prescribed formula is sometimes given to breast-fed infants to supplement or replace breast milk.

anatomy and physiology of the gastrointestinal system

The adult digestive tract is a tube about 8 meters (23 ft) long. It includes the mouth, pharynx, esophagus, stomach, and small and large intestines. Other organs involved in GI function are the liver and gallbladder.

The four major functions of the GI system include ingestion, digestion, absorption, and elimination. *Ingestion* involves taking food into the mouth, chewing, and then swallowing. Teeth help break down food so it can be swallowed and moved down the pharynx (throat) and esophagus into the stomach for *digestion*. Peristalsis moves food through the GI tract, where *absorption* takes place and then to the rectum for *elimination* of undigested and unabsorbed foods from the body (Fig. 34-1).

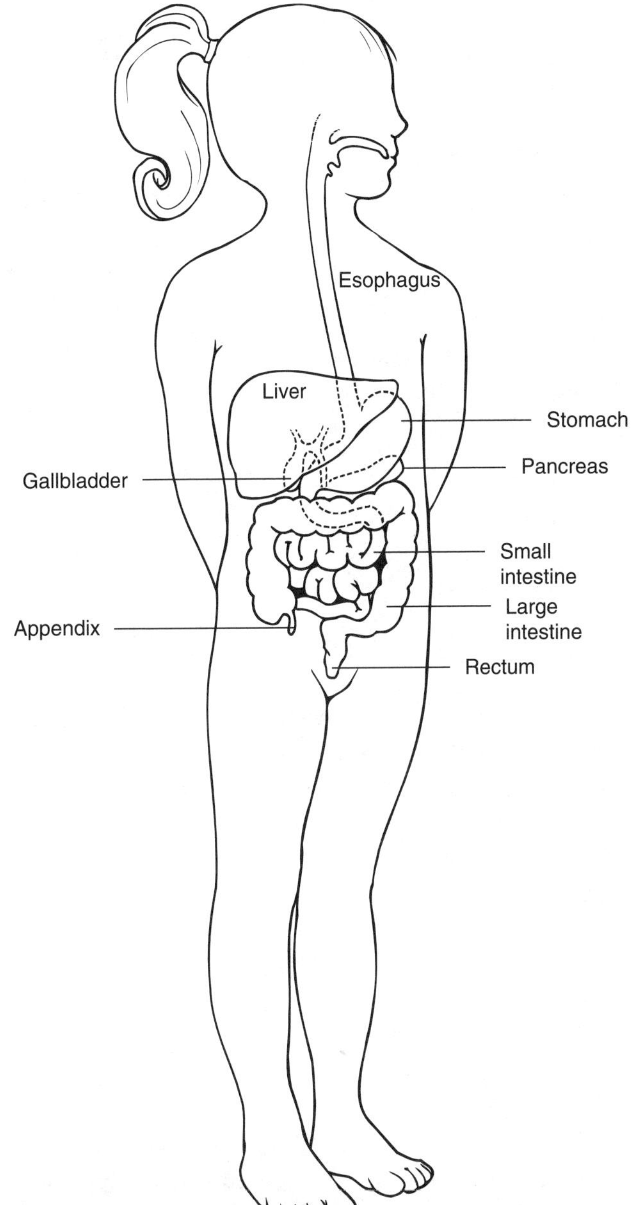

figure 34-1 *Anatomy of pediatric GI system.*

esophagus

The esophagus is a tubular passageway to the stomach. The *cardiac sphincter* at the lower end of the esophagus prevents stomach contents from flowing back into the stomach. In some newborns and infants, the cardiac sphincter does not close properly and allows regurgitation of fluid into the esophagus. This condition is called *chalasia* or reflux and can be serious if stomach contents are aspirated into the lungs.

stomach

The stomach is a muscular organ with a sphincter at the lower end called the *pyloric sphincter*. The stomach is a reservoir for food and the site of digestion. Glands found in stomach tissue secrete mucus, enzymes, hydrochloric acid, and the intrinsic factor responsible for vitamin B_{12} absorption. The stomach churns food particles with gastric juices into a mixture known as *chyme*. Chyme passes into the small intestine through the pyloric sphincter. Some infants are born with a narrowing of the pyloric sphincter (*pyloric stenosis*), which delays stomach emptying and is characterized by projectile vomiting (refer to page 580).

small intestine

The small intestine has three divisions including the duodenum, jejunum, and ileum. Most of the digestion and absorption of food takes place in the small intestine. Absorption involves the transfer of digested food through the wall of the intestine and into the circulatory system. The small intestine lengthens by 50% during the child's first year.

large intestine

The large intestine includes the *cecum* with its pouchlike projection called the *appendix*, *ascending colon*, *transverse colon*, *descending colon*, *sigmoid colon*, and *rectum*, where elimination occurs. The functions of the large intestine include the completion of absorption, formation and removal of feces, and manufacture of vitamins. Bacteria that normally live in the colon act on the food residue stored there to manufacture vitamin K and some of the B-complex vitamins. Water from the digested food is absorbed in the large intestine and excreted through the kidneys. Solid waste is excreted as feces through the rectum.

liver and gallbladder

The liver and gallbladder are considered accessory organs of the GI system. The liver manufactures and secretes bile necessary for the digestion and absorption of fat, and the gallbladder stores the excess bile. The liver also has the following responsibilities:

* Removing waste products from the bloodstream and secreting them into bile
* Receiving nutrient-rich blood directly from the GI tract and storing or transforming the nutrients into chemicals to meet the body's metabolic needs
* Regulating glucose and protein metabolism
* Storing vitamins A, B_{12}, other B-complex vitamins, and D
* Synthesizing blood proteins, such as albumin, fibrinogen, globulin, and clotting factors

enzymes

Carbohydrate digestion is influenced by enzymes known as *amylases* found in saliva and pancreatic juices. Fat digestion is achieved primarily by *pancreatic lipase*. Protein digestion is influenced by *protease* found in gastric juices, such as pepsin.

development of gastrointestinal function

the GI tract is functional at birth, although the elastic and muscle tissues are not fully developed, and neurologic control is incompetent, increasing the infant's risk of aspirating food. For example, as food moves through a mature digestive tract, gagging and swallowing reflexes prevent aspiration of food into the lungs. These reflexes are present at birth, but swallowing coordination is not strong until the infant is about 6 months old.

infant

Most digestive enzymes are present at birth, with the exception of pancreatic amylase and lipase. Thus, the newborn is able to digest protein and carbohydrates found in breast milk or formula. *Pancreatic amylase*, responsible for starch digestion, and *lipase*, responsible for fat digestion, are secreted at adult levels by 3 months. By 1 year, the child's liver is able to secrete bile and store it in the gallbladder. Bile combines with lipase by 1 year, enabling the child to digest fat much as an adult does.

Regurgitation (spitting up small quantities of milk) is common in young infants and results from air bubbles in the stomach, feeding too quickly, or overfeeding. Regurgitation often stops spontaneously around 2 to 3 months with maturity of the cardiac sphincter. Inconsistencies with peristalsis tend to slow stomach emptying. Hiccups are common and usually occur when the infant is fed too quickly without adequate burping. Increased peristalsis in the lower ileum increases stool frequency to one to six stools per day.

Stomach capacity varies with each child. Typically, a newborn's stomach capacity is 10 to 20 mL (less than 1 oz), increasing to 90 to 150 mL (3–5 oz) by 1 month and to 210 to 360 mL (7–12 oz) by the first birthday.

toddler

By 2 years, the toddler's GI system is mature enough to handle any foods that are included in an adult diet. The salivary glands are mature and functional. Stomach capacity increases to about 500 mL (more than 16 oz), enabling the toddler to eat three meals a day. Stomach secretions become more acidic, tending to reduce the risk of GI infections. The gastric emptying time remains less than the average adult's emptying time of 4 hours. Bowel movements become more regular and less frequent, anal sphincter control matures, increasing the likelihood of successful toilet training.

school-age child

The GI system of the school-age child performs similar to that of an adult with a stomach capacity of between 750 and 900 mL (25–30 oz). The position of the intestines is lower in the abdomen, similar to the adult. Gastric, pancreatic, and hepatic juices are produced in proportions comparable to adult proportions.

adolescent

During adolescence, gastric acid increases, especially free hydrochloric acid. The liver is fully functional and continues to grow. The increase in liver size enables the body to store greater amounts of vitamins. Lactase deficiency may appear during adolescence, leading to lactose intolerance, which is more prevalent among African Americans and Native Americans. Children with lactose intolerance experience diarrhea, abdominal pain, abdominal distention, or increased flatus associated with the ingestion of milk and milk products.

development of teeth

Deciduous teeth continue to erupt during toddlerhood with lower incisors, first molars, and canine teeth emerging between 1 and 2 years. By 1 year, the toddler has six teeth. By 18 months, eight teeth have emerged, and by 2 years, 12 to 16 teeth are present. Most 3-year-olds have all 20 deciduous teeth, including the second molars. Around 6 years, permanent teeth erupt, and deciduous teeth fall out.

dental caries

Dental caries are described as tooth decay resulting from plaque formation on the teeth, interaction of bacteria (usually *Streptococcus*), diet, and tooth susceptibility. Tooth decay increases the child's risk of *gingivitis* (inflammation of the gums).

The most common causes for dental caries are infant or child feeding habits, lack of adequate oral hygiene, and lack of adequate fluoridation in drinking water (< 0.7 ppm). The presence of tooth decay in young children, better known as *bottle caries*, is associated with infants' sleeping with a bottle in the mouth or the consumption of large amounts of sugary liquids.

Measures to prevent dental caries include brushing the teeth using fluoridated toothpaste, regular dental checkups, and avoiding cariogenic foods (eg, candy, soda pop). Dental fluoridation treatments and fluoridation of drinking water promote healthy teeth (Display 34-1). Children can begin brushing with a small soft-bristled toothbrush, under the supervision of the caregiver at approximately 2 years. Gums in a newborn and teeth in an infant and young toddler should be wiped clean with a cloth or gauze or brushed by the caregiver before 2 years.

By 6 years, the child should brush at least twice each day. Brushing after meals and before bedtime is ideal but not always practical when children are in school. The child's growth in fine and gross motor coordination makes brushing possible without caregiver supervision.

display 34-1
fluoride information

Fluoride has been found to prevent dental caries when taken into the system or by using fluoride toothpaste. The exact way fluoride helps is unknown but it is thought to make enamel less soluble, reduce cariogenic (cavity producing) bacteria, and restrict bacteria from clinging to tooth enamel.

Dental caries can affect the normal eruption of permanent teeth seen around 5 years. Children are at the greatest risk of developing cavities between 4 and 8 years and 12 and 18 years.

During adolescence, regular preventive dental checkups are advised. Many adolescents wear orthodontic appliances that require special brushing and flossing methods to clean the teeth effectively.

✳ nursing process in altered gastrointestinal function

nursing assessment

subjective data

* Determine the chief complaint, onset of the problem, symptoms, health of other family members, and if any home remedy measures have been used.
* Note past GI illnesses, treatments, and consequences.
* Record any surgeries, genetic or congenital disorders, low Apgar scores, current medications, allergies, and eating habits.

objective data

assessment of growth

* Use standard measures of weight, height, and frontal-occipital circumference for infants younger than 36 months. Plot findings on a growth chart and screen out measurements above the 97th percentile or below the third percentile in height and weight for referral.

assessment of the abdomen

* Examine the abdomen of small children while they are being held by the caregiver. Older children can lie down on an examination table. Note the symmetric shape of the abdomen. Children experiencing urinary retention will display fullness above the symphysis pubis, making the abdomen appear asymmetric. Note the presence of of abdominal bruising (may indicate child abuse), scars, rashes, lesions, abdominal distention or depression, visible peristaltic waves, and tenderness.
* Assess the appearance of the umbilicus, and note if flat, inverted, or protruded outward slightly. Umbilical stumps dry in about 5 days after birth and drop off by 2 weeks.

assessment of bowel sounds

* Auscultate bowel sounds in the four quadrants of the abdomen for frequency and character. Bowel sounds reflect the noise of air and fluid moving through the GI tract. Normal bowel sounds are high pitched and gurgling and occur about 5 to 34 times each minute. Listen to each quadrant for at least 5 minutes before assuming bowel sounds are absent. Prepare children for bowel sound auscultation by allowing them to touch the stethoscope. During the auscultation, a game can be

played with comments such as "Is that cereal or toast I hear in there?"

nursing insight

Warm the stethoscope before listening to the abdomen to prevent the child from tightening the abdominal muscles.

assessment of vomiting

* Assess the characteristics of emesis for the presence of undigested food or uncurdled milk, which indicates an obstruction, or a congenital absence or closing of the esophagus. Presence of milk curds in the emesis can indicate a formula intolerance. Presence of blood in emesis (*hematemesis*) will resemble coffee grounds and indicates GI bleeding. In small children, vomitus may come from the mouth and nose.
* Note complaints of nausea. Young children are often unable to describe a feeling of nausea before vomiting.
* Assess the child's pattern of vomiting relative to food intake and desire to eat immediately following a vomiting episode.

assessment of stool

* Assess what the child or caregiver perceives as "normal" stool elimination.
* Assess stool color, consistency, and odor. Constipated stools are described as hard and difficult to pass. Diarrhea stools are typically frequent, watery, or loose and often accompanied by urgency and abdominal cramping.
* Explore what foods or activities trigger the child's bowel movements.
* Note caregiver toilet training methods. If these methods are harsh, toileting can cause tension and anxiety during elimination.

assessment of skin

* Assess skin pallor, jaundice, or carotenemia. Pallor is associated with anemia, while jaundice is associated with liver disease.
* Note the presence of bruising, indicating injury or abuse.
* Note the presence of *striae* described as fine, pinkish-white or gray lines seen in parts of the body where skin has been stretched. Striae is common on thighs, abdomen, and breasts of girls who are or have been pregnant and children who have been obese.
* Assess the genitals and anal area for outward signs of inflammation, lesions, scars, skin tags, fissures, lumps, swelling, or excoriation.

assessment of hydration

* Assess mucous membranes for moisture and presence of mucus in the mouth.
* Assses the fontanels in an infant (sunken anterior fontanel indicates dehydration).
* Assess for other signs of dehydration, such as the presence of dark circles under the eyes, loss of skin elasticity, pallor, decreased tear production, and decreased urinary output.

assessment of the mouth

* Assess an infant's mouth during crying episodes. Pearly white cysts are commonly seen along an infant's gumline, disappearing by 2 to 3 months. Infants who are teething tend to have a white line in addition to gum swelling before the tooth erupts. Healthy oral mucous membranes appear moist and without lesions, inflammation, patches, or swelling. Healthy mucous membranes are pinkish in white-skinned and patchy brown in dark-skinned children. The tongue is found in the midline and should be able to extend as far as the alveolar ridge to allow for normal speech. Look for dental caries. Toddlers and preschoolers like to show off their teeth and will enjoy different games, providing the nurse a chance to inspect the mouth. For example, games that involve seeing who has the widest open mouth, the longest tongue, or can growl the loudest provide good visualization of the oral cavity. School-age children tend to be cooperative when they understand the purpose of the examination. Lesions or burns around the mouth are seen when young children ingest corrosive substances.
* Assess for herpes stomatitis caused by Type 1 herpes simplex virus. Note the presence of a thick white coating in the mouth, indicating thrush.

assessment of pain

Pain assessment involves subjective and objective data.

* Note abdominal pain described as progressive, severe, or colicky that persists without improvement for more than 6 hours; this may signal an emergency situation.
* Assess the presence of abdominal tenderness, rigidity, and rebound tenderness (typical symptoms of peritoneal irritation associated with appendicitis and peritonitis). *Rebound tenderness* is described as pain felt when abdominal structures rebound following finger pressure to the abdomen. To check for rebound tenderness, push fingers gently but deeply into a region, then rapidly remove them (start on the side or area where tenderness is not expected). Rebound pain may occur as a sharp, stabbing pain at the inflammation site.

nursing insight

Palpate rebound tenderness at the end of the abdominal assessment to avoid producing pain and spasms that may interfere with the rest of the abdominal examination.

* Note the location of pain (pain in the lower right quadrant is typical of appendicitis).
* Abdominal pain will most likely be described by young children as a "tummy ache." Young children tend to have difficulty describing the exact location of abdom-

inal pain. When asked where their pain is located, they often point to the entire abdomen.

* Note the child's body positioning (children experiencing abdominal discomfort tend to assume a fetal position with legs drawn up toward the chest).
* Assess patterns of restlessness and crying in relation to the ingestion of food. For example, infants may appear eager to nurse, take the nipple in their mouth, and continue to cry. They may or may not suck or swallow the feeding.
* Note the expulsion of flatus orally or rectally. Colon pain is often described as a "cramp" associated with passage of gas.
* Assess the menstrual cycle of girls past puberty because pain may be related to the menstrual cycle rather than the GI system. Pain associated with ovulation is usually experienced about 2 weeks prior to the menstrual flow and can mimic appendicitis. Ovulation pain is often described as sharp with moderate to severe intensity. Pain that worsens during menstruation may indicate endometriosis.
* Note a pattern of chronic pain. Chronic abdominal pain is often vague and nonspecific. Usually the pain is episodic, unrelated to meals, and centrally located in the abdomen. Recurrent abdominal pain is more common in school-age children. The precise cause of chronic abdominal pain is unknown and thought to be more functional than organic. The "rule of three" is often used to describe chronic abdominal pain in children: 3 years or older; three or more episodes of abdominal pain; 3-month span in which the child experiences abdominal pain episodes.

nursing diagnoses

* Altered Growth and Development, related to impaired GI function
* Altered Nutrition: Less than body requirements, related to vomiting, diarrhea, food intolerance, sore mouth, and disease process
* Altered Nutrition: More than body requirements, related to undesirable eating patterns, intake in excess of metabolic requirements, and sedentary activity patterns
* Pain, related to abdominal cramping and GI dysfunction
* Risk for Fluid Volume Deficit, related to vomiting and diarrhea
* Impaired Tissue Integrity, related to diarrhea and dehydration
* Risk for Aspiration, related to vomiting, weakness, and disease process
* Diarrhea, related to disease process or food intolerance
* Ineffective Breathing Patterns, related to abdominal distention
* Risk for Infection, related to weakness, anatomic defects, and disease process
* Family Coping: Potential for Growth, related to hospitalization of child with an acute or chronic illness, home care of the child with special needs, and interruptions of family life due to treatment regimen
* Altered Family Processes, related to knowledge deficit, illness, economic problems, and separation from the child
* Diversional Activity Deficit, related to activity restrictions, isolation, and lack of parent–child attachment

planning and implementation

promotion of nutrition

* Feed infants every 4 hours unless contraindicated. Use feeding techniques such as cereal-thickened formula, large nipple openings, and small, frequent feedings. Burp the infant after each 1 to 2 oz. Feed the infant slowly in small amounts, and place the infant in a right-sided Fowler's position or in an infant seat for at least 1 hour after feeding. Place older infants and toddlers in a highchair for feedings, and encourage finger foods. Explain to the older child the importance of eating nutritious foods. Encourage the child to eat with others (if possible). Try a surprise, such as a jello-tasting party (unless contraindicated). Plan care to decrease or eliminate nauseating odors or procedures near mealtime. Offer frequent, small feedings (six per day plus snacks) with highest protein and calorie nutrients when the child feels most like eating. Provide the child on a restricted diet (especially a reduction diet) encouragement and praise for following the diet. Administer tube feedings and monitor intravenous (IV) hyperalimentation.

promotion of comfort

* Assess infant for signs of pain, such as continuous crying regardless of the intervention and body positioning.
* Administer prescribed analgesics, and assess the effectiveness 30 minutes later.
* Explain and discuss painful procedures to children and caregivers. Suggest the use of a pacifier for infants who are allowed nothing by mouth or who cannot suck their fingers because of restraints. Though infants may not understand explanations, they respond to a soothing voice. The child may be soothed by a nursery rhyme or story.
* Encourage caregivers to stay with the child during procedures (unless contraindicated). Discuss caregiver understanding of the child's pain origin and relief measures.
* Explain if child is taken to another room for a procedure. Painful procedures are usually performed in a treatment room rather than the child's room. Reassure the child that he or she will be returned to his or her room after the procedure.
* Praise the child for enduring the discomfort. Rock and cuddle children following painful experiences.

promotion of hydration

* Maintain strict input and output (weigh diapers if ordered). Measure emesis and liquid stools, monitor IV fluids, monitor vital signs (especially body tempera-

ture) every 2 to 4 hours, and check urine specific gravity and serum electrolyte values.

* Encourage fluids, such as Pedialyte for infants and water and ice chips for older children. Preschoolers and young school-age children may find it fun to have a tea party (an effective way to increase fluids) using doll cups and tea pot.

promotion of skin integrity

* Inspect skin for redness, blanching, warmth, and open areas. Turn and reposition child every 2 hours. Care of excoriation in the perineal area includes the use of cotton diapers as liners in disposable diapers if disposable diapers irritate the area, the use of disposable diapers if cloth diapers cause irritation, and cleansing and applying prescribed ointments or creams to genitalia after each urine and stool. Older children may find relief in taking sitz baths, wearing cotton underwear, and using special wipes to soothe rectal irritation from frequent stools.

prevention of complications

* Assess abdominal distention and associated respiratory distress. Monitor signs of respiratory distress, especially after feeding. Burp or bubble infants during bottle feeding to decrease the risk of "gas bubbles." Clear excess secretions from an infant's mouth using gentle suction with a bulb syringe.
* Assess breath sounds. Observe and record the color and character of sputum for signs of respiratory infection associated with aspiration of food.
* Monitor the level of consciousness. Food and fluids must be withheld if the child is unconscious.
* Provide explanations to parents about the child's condition, treatments, and diagnostic tests. Teach children and caregivers about proper nutrition, and help them recognize the importance of diet to maintain weight and prevent obesity.
* Describe and demonstrate required home care skills to parents, and evaluate their return demonstrations. Involve the parents in the child's care and play.
* Include family members in patient care conferences when appropriate. Expand caregiver knowledge by providing a list of information, such as signs and symptoms of disease, community agencies available to help with the family's and child's special needs, step-by-step instructions for procedures and medication administration, and dates and times for follow-up appointments.
* Encourage family members to verbalize feelings of guilt, anger, blame, and hostility, and appraise family stress created by child's illness. Assist family members to develop realistic expectations for the ill child.
* Explore with parents probable causes of diarrhea and vomiting, such as dietary indiscretions, contaminated foods, and food allergies.
* Discuss stress and ways of coping related to age and circumstances.

evaluation

* Child retains feedings, gains weight, appears comfortable and satisfied after feedings, and responds to being held and cuddled.
* Child shows no signs of complications from GI disorder, such as aspiration pneumonia, anemia, skin breakdown, or hypovolemia.
* Vital signs (especially temperature) are within normal range limits, and no signs of infection are present.
* Child is well hydrated with moist mucous membranes and tear production. Fluid and electrolyte balance is maintained.
* Bowel habits return to normal pattern.
* Parents verbalize knowledge of signs and symptoms of disease process, complications, home care, and follow-up care. Parent–child attachment is established or maintained.
* Child engages in diversional activity appropriate for age.

diagnostic tests

Many tests are used to help diagnose GI diseases and disorders in children. The most common specimens collected are blood, urine, and stool. Universal precautions must be observed when handling body fluids. Collected specimens must be labeled carefully.

stool analysis

Collection of stool for examination is usually a one-time collection (Display 34-2). Because the collection is done at random, signs reminding the patient, family, and nurses to save all stool are important reminders. Most stool specimens are sent to the laboratory immediately because a fresh specimen produces the most accurate results. When stool cannot be sent to the laboratory in a timely manner, it must be refrigerated. If necessary, stool can be frozen.

> **nursing alert**
> *Universal precautions must be practiced when handling the stool and emesis. The amount, color, consistency, and odor are included in a stool assessment.*

Routine stool examination helps detect GI bleeding and disease. Stool consistency, content, odor, and color are important nursing assessments. Normal stool appears brown and soft; formed, hard stool indicates constipation, and nonformed stool reflects diarrhea (Table 34-1).

Stool cultures detect certain disease-producing bacteria, such as pathogenic *Escherichia coli, Salmonella, Shigella, Campylobacter jejuni*, and *Clostridium difficile.* Ova and parasite tests detect parasites or their eggs, such as hookworm, whipworm, tapeworm, and pinworm.

Stool pH and presence of blood can be tested by using commercial tapes, dip sticks, and solutions according to the manufacturer's instructions. Blood in stool and emesis

display 34-2
stool specimen collection information

* Include stool containing blood, mucus, or pus in the stool specimen sent to the laboratory.
* Avoid sending stool containing barium or other enema solution.
* Do not contaminate the outside of the specimen container with stool.
* Remember to label the specimen with child's name, room number, age, physician's name, date, time of collection, and specific test ordered.

can be occult (hidden) and not readily seen by the nurse. Hematest and guaiac tests are used to determine occult blood.

Timed stool specimens can be started with the first stool passed by the child. Every stool is saved within the collection period, and the specimen is sent to the laboratory according to agency instructions.

When stool specimens are ordered for children who are not toilet trained, the stool is obtained directly from the diaper. Older children with bathroom privileges are instructed to use a potty chair, bedpan, or commode with a collection hat placed so that stool does not come in contact with toilet water.

nursing insight

In the absence of a bowel movement, stool cultures can be obtained by swabbing the inside of the anal sphincter.

pinworm screening

Pinworms are tiny parasites that live in the lower intestines. They are usually harmless and produce few symptoms except for severe anal itch. This disease is common and affects people of all social and economic levels.

Worm eggs are swallowed or inhaled and develop into adult worms in the intestinal tract. Female pinworms travel at night down the intestine and lay eggs on the perineum, causing anal itch. When the child scratches, eggs get on the fingers and under fingernails and are easily transferred to other people or objects. Shaking bedlinen can project the eggs into the air and increase the risk of inhaling them.

The use of clear cellophane tape helps determine the presence of pinworms. Pieces of cellophane tape are pressed over the anal and perineal area for about 1 minute during the night or early morning hours, then taped onto a glass slide and sent to the laboratory.

other laboratory tests

Additional laboratory tests to determine GI system disease include complete blood count with differential, hemoglobin, hematocrit, cholesterol, transaminase, am-

table 34-1 stool assessment

Stool Profile	*Implications*
Brown, soft formed	Normal
Narrow ribbonlike	Spastic or irritable bowel and possible partial bowel obstruction
Hard, formed	Constipation due to diet or medications
Soft, nonformed, or liquid	Diarrhea due to a spastic bowel or viral infection
Nonformed stool with blood and mucus	Bacterial infections or colitis
Yellow or green nonformed stool	Seen in prolonged diarrhea
Black stool	Suggests GI bleeding, intake of iron supplements, or ingestion of raw to rare meat
Tan or white stool	Liver or gallbladder duct blockage, hepatitis, or cancer
Red stool	Indicates colon or rectal bleeding; medications and foods can cause red stool.

teaching guidelines
obtaining a specimen for pinworm screening

The pinworm is one of the most common intestinal parasites affecting humans. The child with pinworms is often restless at night and has itching around the rectum from the worms laying their eggs.

* The specimen is best collected at home after the child has gone to sleep or first thing in the morning before the child awakens.

Specimen collection involves the following:

* Obtain a cellophane tape preparation from the doctor's office or clinic.
* Separate the child's buttocks during sleep.
* Place a strip of tape on the rectum and the area around the rectum.
* Remove the tape and place it on the glass slide. Wash your hands.
* Place the slide in a sealed envelope and wash your hands again.
* Return the specimen to the office or clinic as directed.

monia, lipase, and urine-specific gravity (refer to Appendix for normal values). The hydrogen breath test is used to determine lactose intolerance and malabsorption disorders. Liver function tests are discussed on page 575. Endocrine function tests are discussed in Chapter 38.

endoscopy

Endoscopy is the direct visualization of the lining of a hollow body organ using a long, flexible tube equipped with a camera that photographs the organ lining. Endoscopic examinations are invasive procedures and require that the caregiver sign an informed consent form, indicating that they understand the potential risks and benefits of the procedure. An endoscopic procedure allows the physician to examine the mucosa, blood vessels, and specific organ parts and take a biopsy of tissue for closer examination if necessary. Common endoscopy examinations include esophagogastroduodenoscopy, colonoscopy, and proctosigmoidoscopy (Table 34-2). Child must not be given food until the gag reflex returns.

imaging studies

Imaging studies of the GI system include x-ray and fluoroscopy of the upper GI system and small bowel, nuclear scans, and x-ray of the large intestine. Nuclear imaging analyzes concentrations of injected or ingested radiopaque substances.

table 34-2 endoscopy procedures

Test	*Purpose*
Esophagogastro-duodensocopy	Assists in diagnosing inflammatory, ulcerative, and infectious diseases; tumors; structural deformities; and removal of foreign objects from the esophagus, stomach, or duodenum
Colonoscopy	Permits visual examination of the large intestine to determine cause of constipation, diarrhea, rectal bleeding, inflammatory and ulcerative bowel disease, colonic stricture, and tumors
Proctosigmoid-oscopy	Allows visual examination of the lining of the distal sigmoid colon, rectum, and anal canal to determine the cause of changes in bowel habits, lower abdominal pain, presence of blood, mucus or pus in stool; assists in determining inflammatory, infectious, and ulcerative bowel disease; tumors; hemorrhoids; polyps; fissures; fistulas; and abscesses inside the rectum

nursing alert

* *Children's cells are vulnerable to ionizing radiation used in x-ray and fluoroscopy procedures.*
* *Shield genital area and breasts during all x-ray and fluoroscopy procedures to avoid exposing children to unnecessary radiation.*
* *Radiation has a cumulative effect on the cells of the body, increasing the risk of cancer in later life. For example, girls who were treated for scoliosis as adolescents have an increased risk for developing breast cancer.*

radiologic examination of the upper gastrointestinal tract

Gastric x-ray radiography, upper GI study, esophagus and stomach x-ray, and small bowel study use fluoroscopic and x-ray techniques to visualize the upper GI tract, allowing the physician to view the size, contour, motility, and peristaltic patterns.

The x-ray procedure requires giving the child nothing by mouth (NPO) for approximately 8 hours prior to the examination and giving an oral contrast agent, usually barium, to outline the GI contents. Follow-up x-rays are performed after the fluoroscopic examination to detect the cause of swallowing difficulties and signs of GI bleeding or small-bowel disease. Radiologic studies are useful in diagnosing strictures, ulcers, tumors, malabsorption syndrome, hiatal hernia, and motility disorders.

radiologic examination of the lower gastrointestinal tract

Barium enema (also called large bowel study and colon x-ray) uses x-ray and fluoroscopic techniques to show the normal position, contour, filling, and patency of the large bowel. The child is given a contrast agent (usually barium) using an enema per rectum or ostomy.

A barium enema x-ray is used to detect congenital deformities; bowel obstruction; stenosis; lesions, such as diverticula, polyps, tumors, fistulas, and hernia; and inflammatory changes, such as colitis. The barium enema procedure is used to treat intussusception (telescoping of the bowel) discussed on page 597.

gastric emptying nuclear scan

A milk or gastric scintiscan is used to determine gastric reflux or gastric emptying associated with stomach anomalies that are often congenital. Sedation may be given to an infant or small child. The isotope is mixed with food or formula and given to the child. The scan can take up to 1½ hours.

nursing precautions related to contrast media

The nurse follows agency protocols involving the use of contrast media. Radiopaque contrast agents, such as iodine and barium, have the potential for causing mild (skin rash) to severe (respiratory arrest) reactions. Assessment for iodine allergies includes determining a child's allergy to seafood. Conditions that contraindicate the use of io-

teaching guidelines
x-ray of the upper gastrointestinal tract

* An upper GI x-ray involves drinking a chalky mixture called barium.
* Barium appears white on x-ray, outlining the throat, stomach, and bowel, allowing the doctor to watch the barium on a special x-ray television.
* The test takes between 30 and 40 minutes.
* Sometimes the doctor will order a "small bowel follow-through" so that he or she is able to see the barium go all the way through the small bowel. This requires more x-rays and may take an additional 1 to 2 hours.

dine includes syphilis, pheochromocytoma, multiple myeloma, pregnancy, asthma, renal failure, and long-term steroid use.

Prior to contrast administration, children are NPO for several hours (time can vary depending on the agency) to prevent nausea, vomiting, and increased risk of aspiration of gastric contents. The most common complication following contrast media administration is constipation, which can be prevented by giving adequate fluids and mild laxatives as prescribed. Medications such as narcotics that slow elimination are avoided.

Immediately following a contrast media x-ray, stool will be light but should return to normal color within 2 days. Infants must have bowel aspiration following the procedure because the infant's digestive system is not developed enough to excrete this foreign substance.

biopsy of the small bowel

A small bowel biopsy is indicated when an abnormality of the small bowel mucosa is suspected. Small bowel biopsy is often done during an endoscopy examination.

Another type of small bowel biopsy involves the use of a Watson-Crosby capsule visualized through fluoroscopy. The capsule is attached to a rubber tube and swallowed by the child.

A tissue sample is taken by using suction on the end of the tubing as capsule and tube are guided into the small bowel. A similar procedure is used for rectal biopsies. Precautions are important to prevent children from unnecessary exposure to radiation during fluoroscopy procedures (see Nursing Alert, page 574).

liver function tests

Liver function is evaluated through blood, urine, and tissue examination. Children with liver disorders may have various signs and symptoms requiring a number of diagnostic tests. A common symptom of liver dysfunction is *jaundice,* described as a yellowish skin discoloration resulting from bilirubin deposits in body tissues. Evaluation of serum and urine bilirubin is important because a major function of the liver is to produce and excrete bile. Liver function tests are described in Table 34-3.

liver biopsy

Liver tissue is often obtained by a percutaneous needle liver biopsy. This test is used to determine diffuse and local liver disease. Prior to the test, coagulation studies are done, blood is typed and cross-matched in case it is needed, and the child is NPO for about 6 hours before the procedure (depending on agency's policy). During the procedure, the child is asked to hold his or her breath during needle insertion to prevent pleural cavity puncture. Following the test, the child is positioned on the right side for the first 2 hours and maintains bed rest for up to 24 hours. Vital signs are monitored every 1 to 2 hours for signs of hemorrhage.

nursing procedures

intravenous therapy

Children are likely to lose a greater proportion of body fluid with vomiting and diarrhea than adults, thereby increasing their risks for dehydration, pH imbalances, and death.

Intravenous therapy is a common intervention when children are at risk for dehydration. Referring to the IV equipment as the child's "friend," with the explanation that the liquid going into the body helps make him or her better, is a positive way to deal with the therapy. Children often respond to the nurse's humorous suggestion that they are getting strong from the "supercharged" IV solution.

gavage feedings

Gavage feedings provide nourishment directly through a nasal or oral tube passed into the stomach. Infants and small children are not good candidates for this type of tube feeding because they tend to pull on the tube unless their hands are restrained.

After the original insertion, before each feeding or drug instillation and at least once a shift, the nurse must confirm that the nasogastric tube is in the right place. The most reliable method is to take an x-ray. However, this exposes the child to radiation, requires pediatrician translation, and is difficult to do in outpatient settings.

Conformation of tube placement is often done by measuring the pH of fluid aspirated from the tube. Gastric juice pH ranges between 1.0 and 5.0. Comparison of the latest pH reading to the initial one helps verify position. Another method to check for tube placement is listening with a stethoscope over the stomach area while 1 to 5 mL of air is instilled. Drawbacks of this procedure include loud breath sounds and the fact that vigorous peristalsis may be mistaken for moving air. It also is difficult to instill enough air in small-bore tubes.

Aspiration of stomach contents determines the child's ability to handle the prescribed amount of feeding. When

table 34-3 liver function tests

Test	Test Purpose	Special Considerations
Serum bilirubin (direct—0.1–0.4 mg; indirect—0.2–0.8 mg/dL; total—0.3–1/3 mg/dL)	Checks liver's ability to secrete and excrete bile	NPO before specimen collection (agency policy); keep specimen from light.
Urine bilirubin (negative)	Measures excreted bilirubin	Protect specimen from light.
Urine bilinogen (0.3–3/5 mg/dL)	Detects biliary tract obstruction and red blood cell destruction	Collect specimen at peak production time (12–4 PM). Protect specimen from light.
Bromsulphalein (BSP) dye excretion test (Normal liver removes (0% or more BSP from blood within 45 minutes).	Determines liver function by its ability to store and excrete dye	NPO for up to 12 hours (agency policy) prior to the test; make sure child has not undergone any other dye procedures in last 48 hours. Weigh child; note any allergies.
Indocyanine green dye excretion test (Normally dye clears within 20–30 min.)	Determines liver function based on absorption and excretion of dye; defines blood flow to liver	Dye is injected by IV based on child's weight. Child is NPO for 8–12 (agency policy) hours prior to test. Note any allergies.
Aminopyrine breath test (Normally disappears in 2 h after IV injection of isotope-labeled aminopyrine.)	Measures liver's ability to metabolize compounds	Child is NPO prior to the test (agency policy); weigh. Encourage resting during test.
Serum enzymes (SGOT—3–36 U; SGPT—12–32 U; LDH—70–195 U)	Detects liver damage and disease	Explain blood will be drawn for the test.
Serum proteins (total proteins—6.8 g/dL; albumin—3.5–5.5 g/dL; globulin—1.5–3 g/dL)	Detects liver disease	Child is NPO prior to the test.
Prothrombin time (11–16 sec or 100%)	Determines vitamin K formation	Observe needle puncture site for bleeding.
Alkaline phosphatase (Normal values vary depending on method used.)	Detects inability to excrete bile due to obstruction; indicates bone disease	Explain procedure. No other preparation necessary.

stomach contents are aspirated, the amount is subtracted from the amount to be given for that particular feeding, avoiding the risk of overdistending the child's stomach. Aspirated stomach contents are always reinstilled into the stomach because the aspirate contains important stomach enzymes.

Nasogastric tube feedings may be performed by gravity or feeding pumps. Gravity tube feedings take approximately 15 to 20 minutes. Following the feeding, the infant will need to be burped and placed on the right side for up to 1 hour to prevent regurgitation and aspiration of the feeding. Feeding pumps must be programmed to deliver the correct amount of formula as ordered by the physician.

gastrostomy tube feedings

Gastrostomy (G) tube feedings involve the surgical insertion of a feeding tube through the abdominal wall into the stomach. The procedure is not without risk because anesthesia is required, and potential for infection exists. The G tube insertion site requires a sterile dressing until it heals. The insertion site needs to be assessed for signs of infection and irritation. Gastric juices may leak out around the G tube, especially if the child pulls on the tube. The skin exposed to gastric juices will become irritated, requiring skin preparations, such as zinc oxide or Stomadesive. New types of G tubes include the button or MIC-KEY tubes, which are skin level (reducing the child's ability to pull on the tube) and can be left in place for longer periods (Fig. 34-2).

percutaneous endoscopic gastrostomy tube feedings

The percutaneous endoscopic gastrostomy (PEG) tube is used as an effective nutrition delivery system for children who are at high risk for chronic nutritional deficiency. High-risk children are those with multiple disabilities, brain damage, cystic fibrosis with chronic food intolerance, failure to thrive, short bowel syndrome, congenital heart defects, and complex congenital oropharyngeal and laryngotracheal malformations. The PEG procedure uses endoscopy to place the G tube properly, reducing the risk of complications due to anesthesia. Internal and external crossbars stabilize the PEG tube perpendicularly between the gastric mucosa and abdominal wall. The feeding procedures for G tube feedings and PEG feedings are similar to the nasogastric tube feedings. See Table 34-4 for a comparison of nasogastric, G, and PEG tube feedings.

✶ nursing insight

Pediatric considerations specific to gastrostomy tube feedings include the following:

- *Surgical placement of a gastrostomy tube with an antireflux procedure decreases the child's stomach capacity.*
- *Small stomachs tend to benefit from small but continuous feedings.*
- *5–10 mL of water or 3–5 cc of air is used to flush tubing for infants; 15–30 mL of water is needed for children.*
- *Maintain open tube for the infant or child who is unable to burp or bubble.*
- *Viokase or carbonated beverages may help dissolve clogs that form in gastrostomy tubing.*

total parenteral nutrition

Parenteral nutrition, also called total parenteral nutrition, hyperalimentation, or hyperal, is a method of feeding a child through the veins. Nourishment is given through an IV tube or catheter that is threaded into the superior vena cava. The formula contains sugar, protein, vitamins, minerals, and lipids and usually provides 1 kcal/mL (Table 34-5).

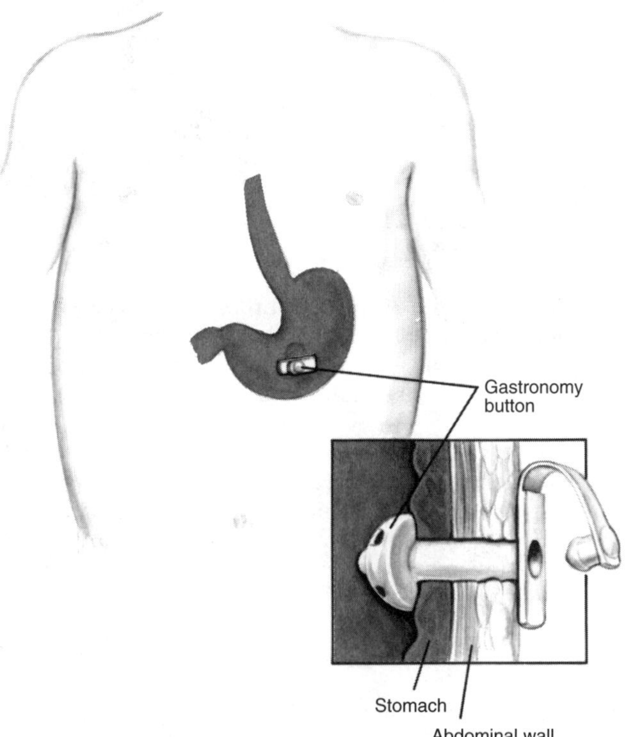

figure 34-2 *Gastrostomy button. Surface appearance is slightly raised, flat, and rectangular. It requires daily skin care with mild soap and water. Antireflux valve can fail, causing leakage of stomach contents.*

eating patterns and related disorders

Children's eating patterns are affected by many factors, including family size, caregiver schedules, family income, and cultural factors. Some children are picky or fussy eaters or usually have a good appetite but suddenly start to eat less or not at all. Instead of eating at mealtime, they may just play with their food. On certain days, they may eat regularly, and on other days refuse food for no apparent reason. If the child is growing in spite of lags in eating, the picky eater stage will likely be short lived and unimportant. Providing children with food choices, child-sized servings, and opportunities to try one new food at a time and offering healthful desserts helps children get through this stage.

fast food and junk food

Teenagers often prefer "fast food" and "junk food." These foods contain empty calories, mostly from sugar and fat, but little protein, vitamins, or minerals. Such foods contribute to teenage weight gain without adequate nourishment, increasing the risk of developing iron deficiency anemia and heart disease. When teenagers are also parents, "junk food diets" affect the entire family.

obesity

Obesity describes excess adipose tissue relative to lean body mass, reflecting a long-standing imbalance between food intake and energy used for activity. An estimated 10% to 30% of adolescents in the United States are obese (Lippincott's Pediatric Nursing Review, 1992). Obesity that is unrelated to overeating and underactivity is associated with endocrine disorders, such as hypothyroidism (see Chap. 33). Social, psychological, hereditary, and family factors contribute to obesity. Homeostatic mechanisms maintain obesity once it is established.

Obesity contributes to increased risk of heart disease, musculoskeletal disorders, and psychosocial problems. Obesity in adolescence can affect developmental tasks related to identity and self-esteem. It is not uncommon for obese adolescents to experience chronic low self-esteem.

Researchers believe there is a genetic disorder, nicknamed syndrome X, that increases the risk of obesity and other health problems, especially in African Americans (Sackor, 1994). Obesity carries the same health risks for African Americans as for people of other racial groups.

Treatment for obesity includes a diet plan that provides for weight loss with no metabolic complications or excessive hunger, preservation of lean body mass, promotion of normal growth and development and regular exercise, and behavior modification concerning social and behavioral aspects of eating. Support groups involving teenagers experiencing the same weight problems are helpful. Diet pills and fasting are discouraged. Surgical bypass procedures to treat obesity are controversial in adolescents.

table 34-4 comparison of nasogastric, gastrostomy, and percutaneous endoscopic gastrostomy

Tube	*Advantages*	*Disadvantages*	*Complications*	*Nursing Care*
Nasogastric	Insertion of tube is less traumatic and ideal for short-term needs (<6 wk).	Tube can be easily dislodged if child is active and pulls on it. Feedings can be instilled into the lungs if tube placement is not verified. Proof of tube placement may be unreliable except for x-ray.	Aspiration pneumonia, tissue trauma	Confirm tube position by instilling air into tube and listening over the stomach for gurgling sounds. Measure pH of fluid aspirated from the stomach. Check for residual before each feeding, and reinstall aspirated contents. Remove tube after feeding and discard.
Gastrostomy	No risk of tube dislodging into the lungs. Decreased risk of aspiration pneumonia. Good for long-term use. Skin-level tubes can be used, such as the Button or MIC-Key. The skin-level tubes are not easily removed by the child.	Requires an anesthetic for placement. Tube may pivot and enlarge the stoma; leakage around the tube can cause skin breakdown and increased risk of infection. Button tubes are good for 6 mo, and insertion and removal are painful. The MIC-Key can be inserted and removed with less pain.	Infections, tube dislodgment, leakage, cellulitis, pain at site, clogging of the tube, septicemia, and anesthesia risks	Carefully assess skin around tube site; and change dressing. Measure the length of tube protruding from the abdomen following placement, and check the tube's external length at each feeding.
Percutaneous endoscopic gastrostomy	Insertion per endoscopy requires no anesthesia. Can be altered to provide jejunal feedings. Activity is unrestricted.	Not recommended for children with peritonitis, ascites, or severe gastroesophageal reflux. Risk of skin breakdown around tube.	Infections, tube dislodgement, leakage, clogging of the tube	Sterile dressing for first day postinsertion, then no dressing is needed. Rotate PEG tube crossbar 90 degrees q4h and tape. Cleanse insertion site with ½ st. H_2O_2 or soap and water q8h and prn.

dieting

Fad dieting is common among adolescents and some adults. While such eating patterns may be harmless if used temporarily, they can impair health if extended for a long period.

In recent years, the fashion industry has promoted the idea that being thin is more attractive. In an attempt to become thin or maintain a thin appearance, some children, especially girls, develop serious eating disorders. The two most common are *anorexia nervosa* (compulsive dieting to the point of starvation) and *bulimia* (a destructive cycle of binge eating followed by self-induced vomiting to prevent weight gain). The psychodynamics of both conditions are complicated.

anorexia nervosa

Anorexia nervosa is a complex psychological disorder characterized by a pathologic fear of weight gain and distortion of body image, leading to faulty eating patterns, malnutrition, and extreme weight loss. The disorder has developmental and psychological consequences. The typical child with anorexia is female, a high achiever in school, a perfectionist, and a model child with a low self-esteem.

Treatment of anorexia involves family and individual therapy. Behavior modification has proven helpful in changing anorectic eating patterns. Goals of therapy include resolution of psychological issues, restoration of normal eating patterns, increase in self-esteem, and promotion of self-control.

bulimia

Bulimia is an eating disorder characterized by episodes of binge eating followed by self-induced vomiting. Bulimia tends to begin late in adolescence and affects girls more than boys.

Treatment for bulimia is similar to that for anorexia nervosa. Vomiting gastric acids increases the teenager's risk for metabolic alkalosis; thus, appropriate interven-

table 34-5 total parenteral nutrition (hyperalimentation)

Indications	Maintain nutritional status in children with malnutrition or altered GI function
Formula composition	Protein, carbohydrates, electrolytes, vitamins, and fats
Administration	Indwelling, Broviac, or Hickman subclavian vein catheter
Nursing measures	Keep solution refrigerated, warm to room temperature before infusing.
	Keep administration rate steady. Use sterile technique for dressing changes. Measure growth, and follow blood and urine tests
Complications	Thoracic puncture during insertion
	Air embolism during line change
	Infection, electrolyte imbalance, dehydration, essential fatty acid deficiency from inadequate fat intake, and hypoglycemia after total parenteral nutrition is stopped

tions to treat this complication include close monitoring for at least 1 hour after eating.

alterations in gastrointestinal function

diarrhea

Diarrhea is described as *acute* or *chronic*, inflammatory or *noninflammatory*. *Acute* diarrhea is a common disorder of children with serious complications, including dehydration, acid–base imbalance, and hypovolemic shock. Diarrhea related to an inflammatory process is frequently associated with *gastroenteritis*, an inflammation of the stomach and intestinal lining. Infants are predisposed to diarrhea when they are malnourished, immune suppressed, or exposed to poor hygiene methods. Chronic diarrhea may result from laxative abuse in older children.

pathophysiology

Diarrhea is not a single disease but can result from a variety of diseases or disorders, causing copious, watery stools. Diarrhea occurs in the following conditions:

* Bacterial infections that invade the intestinal mucosa and cause dysenteric diarrhea. *Clostridium Difficile* causes watery, mucous, foul-smelling, and sometimes bloody diarrhea. It can occur at any age and is seen more often in children who have extended illnesses or recovery from abdominal surgery. Vancomycin is a medication often used to treat *C. difficile*.
* Viral infections, such as rotaviruses, enteric adenoviruses, astroviruses, and calicivirus. The most common viral pathogen is *rotavirus*, which accounts for up to 50% of diarrhea cases requiring hospital admission, especially during winter and spring. There is a high incidence of rotavirus in children 6 to 24 months. Children experience green, liquid, and mucous stools and low-grade fever (up to 100°F).
* Parasitic infections such as *Giardia lamblia* and cryptosporidium, common in day care centers
* Infections outside the GI tract, such as those affecting the middle ear, urinary tract, and respiratory system
* Food or milk allergies
* Side effects from medications, especially antibiotics

medical management

Management of diarrhea focuses on the child's hydration status. Infants who are more than 10% dehydrated and experiencing hypernatremia will be admitted to the hospital for IV rehydration. *Oral rehydration therapy* includes the physiologic replacement of fluids, feeding, and close observation of the child's hydration status (Display 34-3). Oral hydration is recommended unless the child is in hypovolemic shock requiring immediate fluid replacement

teaching guidelines
anorexia nervosa or bulimia

When caregivers suspect an eating disorder, early intervention is important in preventing serious complications related to malnutrition.

* Question the child about noticeable weight loss or weight gains, skipped meals, or excessive eating.
* Express concern if a sudden weight gain or loss of 20% occurs (based on growth charts reflecting sex, age, and height).
* Listen closely to comments about child's perceptions of body image and concerns about being fat or thin.

Observe for the following:

* Erosion of tooth enamel and increase in dental caries from frequent vomiting
* Preoccupation with exercise and prolonged vigorous exercise
* Diarrhea associated with the (often-hidden) self-administration of enemas or laxatives
* Bizarre preoccupation with eating
* Preoccupation with cooking or preparing food, often fixing elaborate meals for others without actually eating
* Abdominal pain following consumption of large amounts of food
* Absence of menstruation not related to pregnancy
* Appearance of fine body hair
* Susceptibility to infections

display 34-3
oral rehydration therapy solution

CEREAL SOLUTION RECIPE

½–1 cup infant rice cereal
2 cups water
¼ teaspoon table salt

1. Accurately measure salt with a measuring spoon; level with a knife.
2. Gradually add cereal to the water until the mixture is as thick as is drinkable. Mix well.
3. Give the child the solution after each diarrheal stool. Infants need about ½ cup; older children need a full cup.
4. Discard the mixture after 6–8 hours or if it becomes too thick to drink.
5. If the child vomits, offer the mixture in small amounts, ½ to 1 teaspoon every few minutes.
6. Continue breast-feeding or bottle feeding during diarrhea.
7. Allow older children to eat solid foods in small, frequent meals, but avoid fruit juices and food high in sugar.

by IV fluid administration. Feeding and drinking are encouraged during the beginning stage of diarrhea because the rapid fluid loss during diarrhea does not interfere with intestinal tract functions. Pain and a significant amount of cost can be avoided if feedings are maintained.

nursing care

Appropriate early feeding during diarrhea can prevent dehydration. However, it is advisable not to give a child anything to eat or drink for 1 hour after vomiting.

The American Academy of Pediatrics suggests the following foods and liquids be given if the child is not experiencing dehydration:

- Breast milk or half-strength formula or milk in children younger than 1 year
- Commercial oral electrolyte solutions, such as Pedialyte or Ricelyte
- Precooked infant rice cereal and rice-based formulas, which tend to decrease stool duration and output
- A BRATTY diet, which is well tolerated once the child is able to retain liquids. (BRATTY is an acronym for *b*ananas, *r*ice, *a*pplesauce, *t*ea, *t*oast, and *y*ogurt.)
- Drinks made with unsweetened yogurt, vegetable juices, and half-strength unsweetened orange juice
- Mashed bananas or banana flakes to supply potassium
- Starchy foods, such as mashed potatoes with plain water

The following foods and liquids are to be *avoided* or given in small amounts.

- Sugar-sweetened solutions, such as soft drinks and juicelike drinks, which promote diarrhea
- Chicken broth containing high amounts of sodium and little or no carbohydrate

Children with diarrhea need to conserve their energy. Bed rest is indicated until their status improves. Nursing activities need to be organized to allow intermittent rest periods. Universal precautions are necessary when handling stool or emesis to reduce the risk of spreading infection. Diarrhea stools contain a large amount of acid, which contributes to skin breakdown. Air fresheners and proper room ventilation reduces the odor common with most diarrhea.

vomiting

Vomiting is the ejection of stomach contents (*emesis*) through the mouth. Children who are vomiting are at an increased risk for dehydration, shock, and disturbance of acid–base balance.

Projectile vomiting is an explosive type of vomiting that propels emesis approximately 3 to 5 ft and is a classic symptom of pyloric stenosis. When projectile vomiting follows a head injury, it usually indicates a concussion. *Nonprojectile vomiting* is a milder type that propels emesis 12 to 15 in and is seen with gastroenteritis.

Regurgitation is a nonforceful expelling of food from the stomach without abdominal muscle contractions, often referred to as "spitting up" and associated with feedings. *Rumination* is a deliberately induced regurgitation and reswallowing of some of the regurgitated food. Rumination is seen in infants between 3 to 6 months, usually disappearing by 2 years.

Bile is normally found in all emesis. If bile is present, emesis left in the open air will turn green. Bile is absent in vomitus of infants with pyloric stenosis. Emesis that has a fecal odor indicates bowel obstruction.

nursing care

The care of a child who experiences vomiting is similar to that of a child with diarrhea. A major concern is to prevent respiratory distress and aspiration of vomitus into the lungs.

Stomach contents contain hydrochloric acid and other enzymes caustic to the mucous membranes, resulting in inflammation, scar tissue formation, decreased respiratory function, and increased risk of chronic lung disorders. Vomiting increases the child's risk of metabolic alkalosis resulting from loss of stomach acids. An inability to retain ingested food increases the risk of malnutrition.

dehydration

Dehydration is defined as a condition resulting from an excessive loss of body water and is called fluid volume deficit. Water is an essential component of all body reactions. The majority of water is found within the cells and is called *intracellular fluid*. Fluid found outside of cells is referred to as *extracellular fluid*. Signs and symptoms of dehydration vary with severity of the fluid loss. Children who are mildly dehydrated do not show outward signs of dehydration; their skin usually remains warm and pink, and their chief complaint is thirst.

Clinical dehydration appears in children who are 5% to 10% dehydrated. Signs of dehydration include cool, pale skin; decreased urine output; irritability; and decreased tear production. Severe and life-threatening dehydration occurs in children who have lost 15% to 20% of their body fluids.

Infants and small children experiencing diarrhea and vomiting are at increased risk for water and electrolyte imbalance. Large liquid stools can deplete the infant's extracellular fluid volume. Additional factors that place infants at high risk for dehydration include the following:

* Increased metabolic rate about three times that of an adult
* Larger body surface in relation to weight
* Inability to conserve water because of immature kidney function
* Rapid loss of fluids and electrolytes in the presence of diaphoresis, increased respirations, and burns
* Fluid restriction related to GI tests and GI surgery

During treatment of fluid loss, it is essential to observe for fluid volume excess (overhydration). *Overhydration* describes an excess in the amount of extracellular fluid with symptoms of edema and increased risk of heart failure. A common cause of overhydration is excessive quantities of IV fluid administration.

types of dehydration

Dehydration can be described as *mild, moderate*, or *severe*; nursing assessment and management are based on the degree of dehydration (Table 34-6). There are three types of dehydration, described in terms of water loss and electrolyte levels (primarily sodium): isotonic, hypertonic, and hypotonic.

Isotonic dehydration involves a proportionate loss of water and electrolytes. *Hypertonic* dehydration involves greater loss of water than electrolytes. *Hypotonic* dehydration involves a greater loss of electrolytes than water.

electrolytes

Sodium is the major electrolyte found in extracellular fluid and an excess *(hypernatremia)* or deficit *(hyponatremia)* produces noticeable symptoms. Symptoms of sodium deficit include apprehension, convulsions, abdominal cramps, and diarrhea. Symptoms of sodium excess include excitement; convulsions; dry, sticky mucous membranes; decreased urine; and firm tissue turgor.

Potassium is the major electrolyte found in intracellular fluid. Potassium deficit *(hypokalemia)* can occur with severe diarrhea. Symptoms include loss of appetite, intestinal distention, and soft muscles.

medical management

Medical management of the child with dehydration is primarily fluid replacement to prevent hypovolemic shock. Care is focused on correcting the primary cause of fluid loss, such as diarrhea, vomiting, excessive respirations, burns, or kidney dysfunction. Establishing normal electrolyte balance requires close monitoring of serum electrolyte values with appropriate electrolyte replacement. Refer to medical management of diarrhea and vomiting (page 579) for additional information.

nursing care

Nursing care for dehydration is similar to the care described for children with diarrhea and vomiting (page 580). Fluid and electrolyte imbalances require prompt interventions to prevent life-threatening complications, such as shock. Nursing care of children with dehydration includes the following:

* Assess urine output, and monitor intake and output at least every 8 hours. A sign of dehydration is failure to urinate for more than 6 hours or scant urinary output.
* Assess for obvious signs of dehydration, such as absence of tear production, sunken anterior fontanel in infants, dark circles under the eyes, dry mucous membranes, sticky saliva, irritability, hyperactive reflexes, dry skin, and loss of skin turgor (Fig. 34-3).
* Assess results of electrolyte reports, especially potassium and sodium (an elevated serum sodium reflects dehydration).

table 34-6 assessment of patients with dehydration

Degree of Dehydration	*Symptoms*	*Percent of Weight Loss*	*Nursing Interventions*
Mild to moderate	Restless, irritable, sunken eyes, no tears, dry tongue and mouth, thirsty and drinks eagerly	3–9	Monitor weight, I&O, offer oral fluids 1–2 oz qh; measure specific gravity.
Severe	Lethargic or unconscious, rapid, thready pulse, cyanosis, cold extremities, rapid breathing, sunken and dry eyes, no tears, dry mouth and tongue, drinks poorly or not able to drink	Greater than 10	In addition to nursing care for mild to moderate dehydration, monitor IV replacement therapy, checking the IV site, rate, and solution.

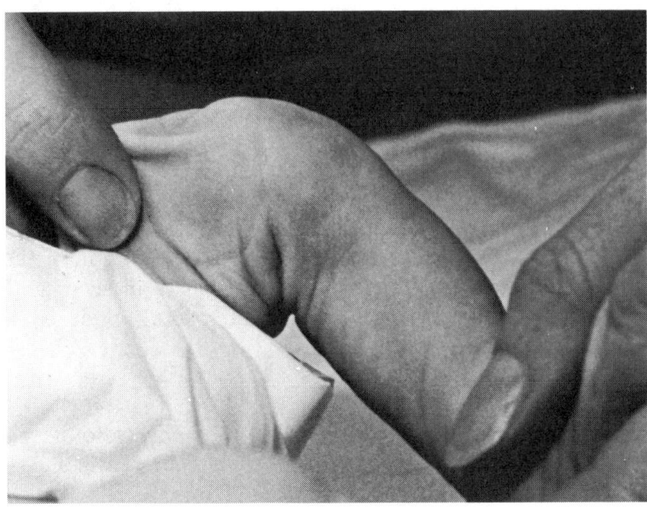

figure 34-3 *In a child with fluid volume deficit, pinched skin may remain raised for a short time.*

- Monitor daily weights; loss of weight is often noted.
- Assess fluid replacement therapy for needle placement, correct flow rate, and signs of fluid volume overload, such as sudden weight gain, edema, and signs of congestive heart failure (see page 581).
- Avoid rectal temperatures or rectal medications if diarrhea is a factor.
- Provide comfort measures for children who are NPO, such as pacifiers for infants and oral hygiene every 2 hours for older children. Caregivers can provide comfort by rocking infants. If the IV needle placement prohibits holding or rocking, gentle stroking can be soothing. Diversion in the form of board or card games can be positive distractors for older children with IVs.
- Soothe dry lips with an application of lip balm in older children.

constipation

Constipation is defined as the passage of infrequent, hard stools. Constipation can originate from organic or functional causes. The condition affects 10% of children and is found in all age groups.

pathophysiology

Ninety-eight percent of all constipation problems in infants are considered functional. In late infancy, an excessive amount of cow's milk contributes to constipation. Voluntary stool withholding (sometimes learned in toilet training) causes the rectosigmoid colon to distend and fill with excessive amounts of stool before the impulse to defecate is triggered. The distended rectum becomes less sensitive, decreasing the sensation to defecate. Passage of these stools is painful and difficult. Awkward body positioning can make defecation difficult. Physical examination frequently reveals a distended abdomen and large rectal vault.

medical management

Medical intervention includes an enema to evacuate the stool found in the colon. After the stool is expelled, nonstimulating laxatives are used to establish bowel movement regularity. Dietary management includes increased fluid and bulk intake.

nursing care

Enemas may be ordered as a nursing measure for constipation. An enema is a rectal injection of a liquid for cleansing the bowel. Cleansing enemas are used to empty the lower intestine. Isotonic saline or commercially prepared solutions also may be used. The amount of fluid instilled varies according to the age and size of the child (Table 34-7). The enema tubing or tip should never be forced into the child's rectum.

Constipation can produce stools that are rock hard from lack of water. Children often experience pain, hemorrhoids, and occasional small amounts of rectal bleeding when passing the stool. Positions for enema administration are shown in Figure 34-4.

table 34-7 instillation fluid for enema procedure

Age	*Amount of Fluid*
Infant (5–10 kg)	100–200 mL
Small child (11–30 kg)	200–300 mL
Large child (31–50 kg)	300–500 mL
Adolescent (over 50 kg)	500–700 mL
CATHETER ADVANCEMENT	
Infant (5–10 kg)	1 in
Small child (11–30 kg)	2 in
Large child (31–50 kg)	3 in
Adolescent (over 50 kg)	3–4 in

Note: Never force the catheter into the anal canal. If a well-lubricated catheter does not advance easily, stop the enema.

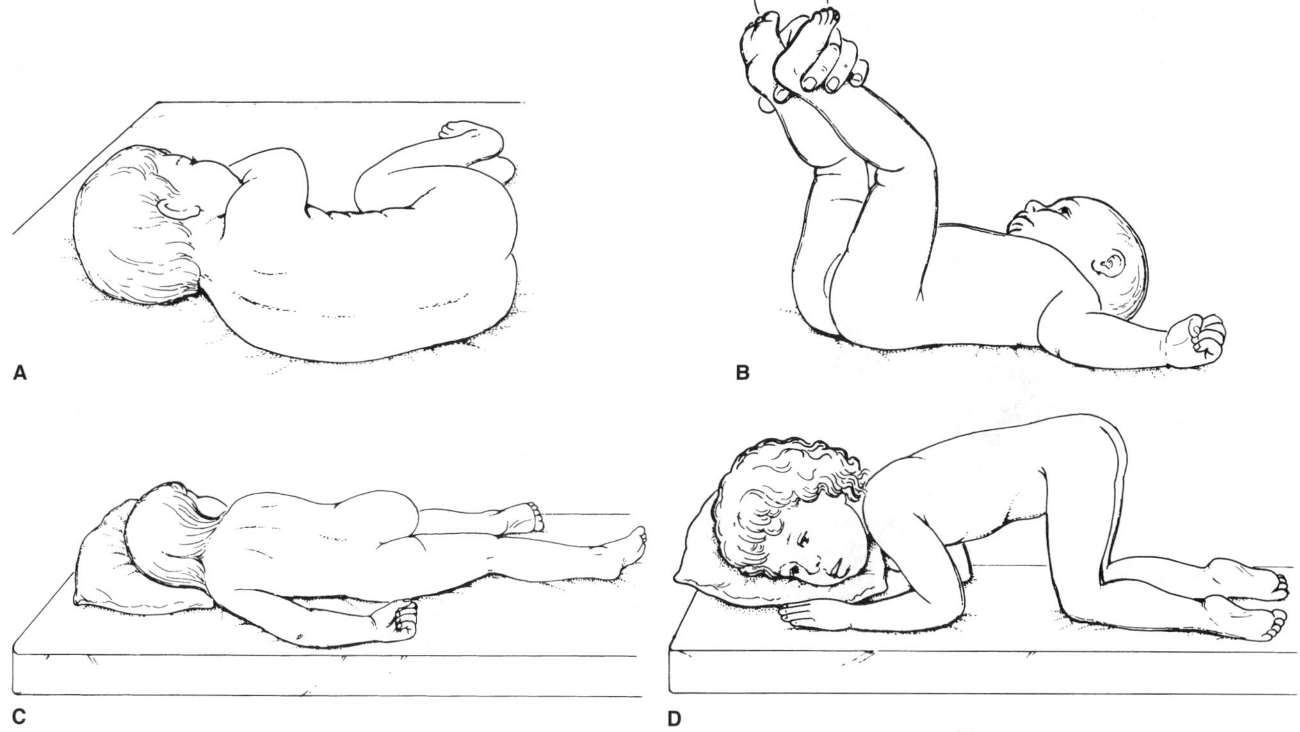

figure 34-4 *Position for enema administration.* ***(A)*** *The child lies on the left side in the lateral recumbent position with knees drawn up to the chest.* ***(B)*** *The infant is placed on the back, and the legs are lifted to expose the anal orifice.* ***(C)*** *The Sims' position is used for the older child who lies on the left side, with the right thigh flexed about 45 degrees to the body axis.* ***(D)*** *The knee–chest position may be used for the older child. The child balances on the knees and chest, resting the head on the forearms.*

Caregivers may require instructions to give the child an enema at home. Caregiver education includes the importance of proper nutrition, fluid intake, exercise, and privacy for promoting bowel elimination.

malnutrition disorders

Malnutrition is a condition caused by inadequate nutrition with deficiency of one or more nutrients essential for health. These nutrients include proteins, vitamins, and minerals.

protein malnutrition (kwashiorkor, marasmus)

Kwashiorkor (local name in Gold Coast Africa meaning "displaced child") is a protein malnutrition resulting from severe protein deficiency. Marasmus is a condition in which there is deficiency of both calories and protein. Kwashiorkor and marasmus can be seen as problems secondary to other chronic conditions or as the primary result of lack of food substances (especially protein) in the child's diet. Kwashiorkor has a high incidence among children 4 months to 5 years.

pathophysiology

Infants experiencing protein malnutrition develop swollen abdomens, generalized edema, delays in growth and development, muscle wasting, apathy, and mental changes. Marasmus is characterized by gradual wasting and atrophy of body tissues, causing the infant to have a wrinkled appearance. In untreated cases of either disorder, mortality rates are as high as 30% or more.

medical management

Medical intervention consists of dietary management with administration of protein-rich formula and supplemental vitamins and minerals. For children who are unable to tolerate food by mouth, IV nutritional therapy (hyperalimentation) and tube feedings are ordered (see page 575). Diarrhea, tuberculosis, and dysentery are common complications of protein malnutrition.

vitamin deficiency (rickets)

Rickets is a vitamin deficiency disorder caused by a lack of vitamin D. Children living in climates where sunshine is rare are more prone to this disorder.

pathophysiology

The deficiency of vitamin D interferes with the absorption of calcium and phosphorus, resulting in bone softening (especially occipital bones). Tooth eruption is delayed with defects of tooth enamel noted and an increased incidence of dental caries. Bones in the thoracic region are deformed, and shafts of long bones become soft and porous. Delays in standing and walking result from muscle weakness.

medical management

Medical intervention is aimed at proper dietary intake, especially of vitamin D. Infants and children require approximately 400 U of vitamin D daily to prevent rickets. Supplemental vitamin D is provided in synthetic vitamins, fish liver oil, and whole and evaporated milk fortified with vitamin D.

nursing care of the child having gastrointestinal surgery

Gastrointestianl surgery is indicated when the child experiences appendicitis and hereditary and congenital anomalies unresponsive to medical interventions. When newborns and small infants undergo surgical intervention, the risks are increased because of the immaturity of body systems.

School-age children typically fear surgery related to their fear of mutilation, pain, and loss of control. Elective surgery allows the child to visit the hospital and surgical suite. It is important to use correct medical terminology when describing expected procedures and treatments. Explain pain management and the child's role. Explain hospital policies concerning peer visits, telephone access, television viewing, and so forth.

Caregivers are often unable to think clearly when children face emergency surgery. Fear for the child may be compounded by their experiences or lack of experience with surgery. The nurse's calm, reassuring attitude helps support the child and caregiver. The nurse needs to remember to give factual and age-appropriate information to help alleviate the child's anxieties. Caregivers will need concise, factual information along with a great deal of compassion and understanding.

> **✳ nursing insight**
> *Magical thinking in young children may lead them to believe surgery is punishment for "bad" thoughts or wishes, causing depression as a response to the guilt.*

preoperative care

Preoperative nursing care focuses on the physical and psychosocial preparation of the child and the psychosocial needs of the caregivers. Infants' level of cognitive development prevents them from understanding explanations about surgery. Parents are encouraged to bring security objects, such the child's special blanket or toy. Caregiver anxieties are often focused on surgical risks, discomforts of the child, and outcome of surgical intervention.

Preoperative preparation for children includes accurate weight and height measurements; vital signs; skin assessment for signs of infection and dehydration; complaints of discomfort, either voiced or indicated by body positioning; NPO status for 4 to 6 hours before surgery to decrease the risk of aspirating stomach contents during intubation (a pacifier can help meet infants' sucking needs); removal of nail polish, hairpins, nylon underwear, and contact lenses; and obtaining information about any allergies to food or medication.

nursing diagnoses

- Anxiety (of child or caregiver), related to the surgical procedure and unknown outcome
- Hypothermia, related to ineffective thermoregulation associated with surgery

planning and implementation

- Explain procedures and routine care in age-appropriate terms. Infants benefit from the nurse discussing care, even though they are too young to understand the words. They are soothed by the tone of voice.
- Listen to the family's concerns about the disease, anesthesia, and surgical interventions. Help parents identify misconceptions about the infant's condition. Instruct family about the location of lounges, dining areas, chapel, phones, and so forth.
- Provide warm blankets to prevent chilling.

evaluation

- Child and caregivers verbalize understanding of preoperative events with decreased anxiety noted in relaxed facial expressions and verbal communication.

postoperative care

Postoperative care of the child is aimed at pain management associated with the surgical procedure, proper hydration, tolerance of diet advancement, signs of bleeding or infection, tolerance of activity, caregiver understanding of surgical procedure and postoperative management, and child's knowledge about procedures and recovery.

nursing diagnosis

- Pain, related to surgery
- Ineffective Breathing Pattern, related to anesthetic administration
- Risk for Infection, related to surgical incision
- Risk for Dehydration, related to preoperative and postoperative fluid restrictions

planning and implementation

- Note pain indicators, such as crying that is undiminished by soothing techniques; grimacing; increase in blood pressure and apical pulse rate; agitation; body position, such as drawing up legs; and abdominal tenderness. Administer analgesics as ordered. Assess the effectiveness of the analgesic 30 minutes after administering, and note side effects. Hold and cuddle infants.
- Monitor respiration rate every 15 minutes and oxygen saturation (normal levels are considered above 95%).

Child's respiratory control center is easily fatigued after surgery. Place the child in a semiprone or lateral position unless contraindicated. Observe for postintubation croup related to edema of the small airway, such as crouplike cough, hoarseness, inspiratory stridor, and cyanosis.

* Inspect dressings and incisional area for signs of bleeding and infection (redness, drainage, and edema). Monitor temperature, pulse, respirations, and blood pressure. Note complete blood count results for signs of bleeding and infection. Collect cultures if infection is suspected, and note the results. Maintain strict handwashing techniques and universal precautions. Use sterile technique when changing dressings. Keep tape measure in place if frequent measurement of abdominal girth is needed. A small dressing often covers the surgical incision. Changing the child's dressing takes time and patience. If the child has a stuffed animal or doll, putting a small dressing on the toy can help establish rapport. Following some surgical procedures, drains are placed beside the incision to help drain infectious material from the abdomen. The child is kept in a semi-Fowler's position to facilitate downward drainage into the pelvis rather than upward to the lungs. Provide safety measures to keep children from removing dressings or tubes.
* Monitor IV fluids. Keep an accurate record of intake, output, and weight. Advance diet as prescribed by the physician and tolerated by the child. Nutritional management of the surgical patient is complicated by the child's metabolic response to the stress and trauma of the operation, affecting nutritional requirements and management. Follow hospital protocol for nasogastric or G tube feedings.

evaluation

* Child rests easily with diminished crying and irritability.
* Child maintains effective breathing patterns and an adequate level of oxygenation.
* Nutrition and hydration of child improve. Bowel elimination is established postoperatively.

hereditary and congenital disorders

celiac sprue disease (gluten-induced enteropathy)

Celiac sprue disease is a disease of the small intestine characterized by chronic inability to tolerate foods containing gluten or protein portions of wheat, barley, oats, or rye flour. Probable causes of celiac sprue are an inborn error of metabolism or an abnormal immunologic response. The disease affects approximately 21 per 100,000 births. The first onset of celiac sprue takes place in early infancy when the child's diet advances from mainly milk to the addition of cereals.

pathophysiology

Malnutrition and secondary deficiency diseases occur from atrophy of the intestinal villi, resulting in a reduction of absorption in the intestine. Symptoms of celiac disease appear as early as 6 months and include fatty, foul, frothy, bulky stools (steatorrhea); general malnutrition with muscle wasting; abdominal distention; peripheral edema of the lower extremities; and secondary vitamin deficiencies (Fig. 34-5).

Endoscopic examination reveals a flat mucosal surface of the intestines with an absence or atrophy of intestinal villi confirmed by a small bowel biopsy. Low levels of vitamin D can interfere with calcium absorption, resulting in the reduction of bone mass *(osteoporosis)* and a softening of the bone *(osteomalacia)*. Impaired calcium absorption related to low levels of vitamin D can cause rickets or tetany. Epistaxis, ecchymosis, or intestinal hemorrhage can occur due to disturbed blood coagulation caused by vitamin K deficiency. Inflammation of the tongue and mouth result from failure to absorb water-soluble B vitamins.

celiac crisis

A serious complication of the disorder is *celiac crisis*. The major symptom of celiac crisis is diarrhea, which may be accompanied by anorexia, vomiting, weight loss, dehydra-

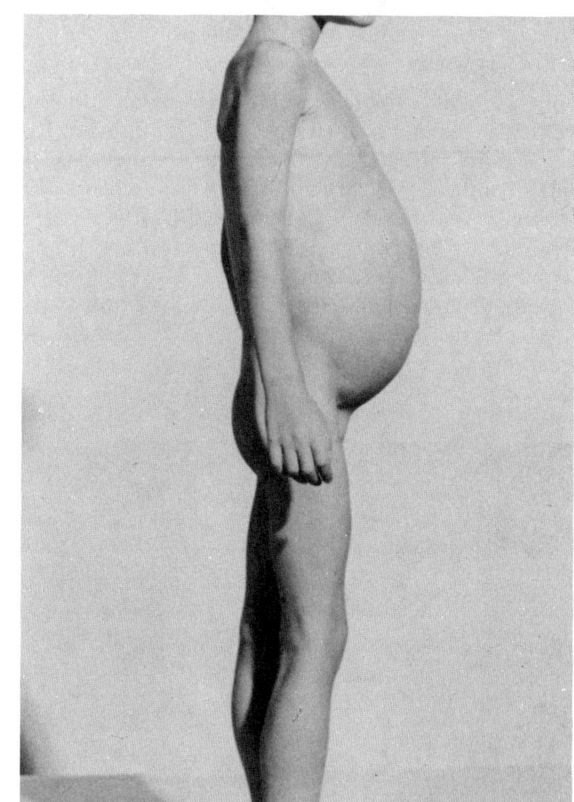

figure 34-5 *A child with celiac disease. Notice the extremely enlarged abdomen and the wasted extremities. (From Pillitteri, A. [1995].* Maternal and child health nursing. *Philadelphia: J.B. Lippincott.)*

tion, and distended abdomen. Celiac crisis is triggered by infections (often respiratory), prolonged fasting, ingestion of gluten, or exposure to anticholinergic drugs. Celiac crisis can lead to electrolyte imbalance, rapid dehydration, and severe acidosis.

medical management

The main treatment is dietary management with a relatively "gluten-free" diet. The word relatively is important to keep in mind because it is impossible to remove every source of gluten protein. The prescribed gluten-free diet will be as low in gluten as possible (Table 34-8). Studies reveal that most infants can tolerate a small amount of gluten.

The gluten-free diet consists of simple sugars (monosaccharide and disaccharides). Complex sugars (polysaccharide) are prohibited. Corn and rice are used as substitute grain foods. Dietary management must provide the child with adequate caloric intake for normal growth and development. Reintroduction of gluten in the diet is recommended after 2 years of dietary management.

Calcium replacement is indicated if tetany occurs or if loss of bone density is noted. Temporary hyperalimentation may be necessary if the child is seriously malnourished. Supplemental vitamins are given to prevent or correct deficiencies, especially vitamins A and D. Cortisone therapy is used conservatively. Cortisone produces remission of symptoms but can cause exacerbation after the medicine is discontinued.

nursing care

Monitor the child's tolerance to prescribed diet and weight increases. Promote optimal nutrition through reinforcement of parental education concerning gluten-free diet, supplemental vitamins, calcium, iron, and folate.

Observe child for muscle tremors indicative of tetany. Use noninvasive procedures, such as Chvostek's sign, to determine calcium deficiencies. *Chvostek's sign* is assessed by tapping the muscles on the side of the face over the area of the facial nerve. When calcium levels are significantly decreased, facial spasms occur.

table 34-8 nutritional considerations for gluten-free diet

Foods Allowed	*Foods to Avoid*
Meat: beef, pork, poultry, fish Eggs Milk, cream, cheese All fruits and vegetables Grains, such as rice, corn, gluten-free wheat, puffed rice, corn flakes, corn meal	Commercially prepared ice cream, malted milk, prepared puddings. Anything made from wheat, rye, oats, or barley, such as bread, rolls, cookies, crackers, cereal, spaghetti, macaroni, noodles, beer, and ale.

Determine parental knowledge about disease condition and ability to manage care, including medications, and to reduce the risk of celiac crisis. Discuss dietary restrictions of gluten. Impress caregivers with the need to read food labels because gluten is frequently added to processed foods as thickeners or fillers. Refer parents to American Celiac Society for information and support.

hirschsprung's disease (congenital aganglionic megacolon)

Hirschsprung's disease is a congenital absence of parasympathetic ganglion nerve cells in the intestine. Symptoms may be present at birth or appear in infancy. This disease occurs in 1 in 5,000 live births and is at least four times more common in white boys than in girls or African Americans. Hirschsprung's disease can be acute in some children and considered a chronic, progressive condition in others. The exact cause is unknown.

pathophysiology

Hirschsprung's disease is characterized by a lack of autonomic parasympathetic ganglia in the smooth muscle wall of the colon, causing intestinal function to be sluggish with inadequate peristalsis, leading to intestinal obstruction. The distal end of the descending colon is most often affected. The involved portion of the intestine has a narrow lumen and lacks peristalsis. The portion of colon above the affected area appears dilated and hypertrophied with an accumulation of feces and gas. Symptoms include an inability to pass stool; severe, watery diarrhea; abdominal distention; vomiting; and anorexia. The muscular coat of the dilated colon may become thin and ulcerated (Fig. 34-6).

medical–surgical management

The management of Hirschsprung's disease is directed at relieving intestinal obstruction, restoring peristalsis, and preserving the external anal sphincter function. A low-residue diet, laxatives, and enemas control the symptoms when the disorder is mild.

Failure to respond to medical management indicates the need for surgical intervention. Surgical intervention usually involves a colostomy and resection of the affected bowel.

Preoperative care of the child prior to a colostomy procedure involves a diet of clear fluids for 24 to 48 hours, bowel emptying with enemas or laxatives, and reduction of the normal bowel flora by antibiotic administration.

Colostomy is described as bringing part of the large intestine outside of the body through an opening in the abdomen, creating a stoma. *Stoma* is described as the part of the intestine visible on the outside. The stoma is shiny, red, and wet. The stoma does not have nerves to feel pain. However, it can bleed if irritated or rubbed too vigorously.

The colostomy procedure is often performed as a temporary measure to decompress the intestine; divert fecal material, allowing the bowel time to rest and resume normal function; and enable the infant to gain the physical stamina necessary to undergo extensive surgery.

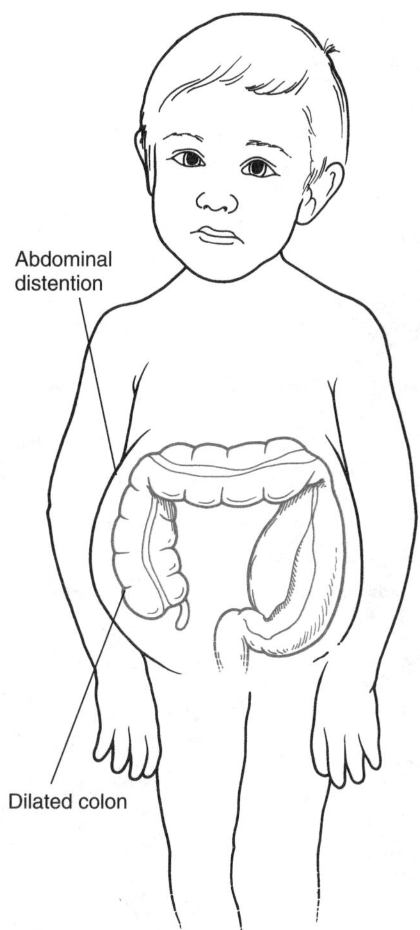

figure 34-6 *Hirschsprung's disease.*

A colostomy is made on the distal portion of the colon where a collection of normal sensory neurons is found. A major goal of surgery is to establish future fecal continence. Surgical prognosis is good. Consultation with an ostomy nurse can be helpful in teaching caregivers.

preoperative nursing care

nursing assessment

* Assess the child's response to hospitalization, knowledge of surgical procedure, recent exposure to illness, vital signs, level of consciousness, level of hydration, weight, respiratory status, and blood counts.
* Assess child's developmental level and coping mechanisms and caregiver's ability to cope with surgical procedure

nursing diagnosis

* Anxiety, related to surgical procedure for colostomy, postoperative pain, altered self-image

planning and implementation

* Orient the child and caregivers to nursing unit.
* Discuss surgical procedure with child in an age-appropriate manner and with caregivers; evaluate understanding.
* Complete preoperative checklist, addressing issues such as removal of fingernail polish, dental appliances, jewelry, and contact lenses; noting the presence of loose teeth; assessing vital signs; having the child void; ensuring the surgical procedure consent form has been signed; including laboratory results with the chart; and giving preoperative medication.

evaluation

* The child and caregivers will demonstrate an understanding of the disease process, purpose of hospitalization, goals and possible complications of surgery, and the planned postoperative colostomy management.

postoperative nursing care

Postoperative care of the child is aimed at managing pain associated with the surgical procedure, monitoring hydration, assessing the stoma, and facilitating the return of bowel elimination.

nursing assessment

* Assess colostomy stoma for color, moisture, and drainage in the pouch. Prepare caregivers for the appearance of the colostomy. A bluish colostomy indicates compromised blood supply and must be reported immediately.
* Assess vital signs. Temperature elevation indicates infection. Increase in pulse and respirations with a decrease in blood pressure indicates shock.
* Assess bowel sounds in all four quadrants; advance diet as prescribed by surgeon.

nursing diagnosis

* Risk for Infection, related to surgery on the bowel
* Risk for Dehydration, related to preoperative and postoperative fluid restrictions
* Knowledge Deficit, Child and Parental, related to colostomy care

planning and implementation

* Control pain with medication administration. Monitor pain relief approximately 30 minutes after medication is administered. Patient-controlled analgesia pumps may be used and require caregiver understanding (see Chap. 26).
* Monitor IV therapy for correct infusion rate, presence of redness, or edema at needle site, indicating infiltration. Check skin turgor, fontanels, saliva, and urine output for signs of effective hydration.
* Teach caregivers proper care of ostomy, such as cleansing and applying pouch.

evaluation

* Child rests easily with diminished crying and irritability.
* Nutrition and hydration improve.

* Temperature, pulse, respirations, and blood pressure are within normal ranges.
* Bowel elimination is established.
* Caregivers demonstrate understanding of ostomy care.

teaching guidelines 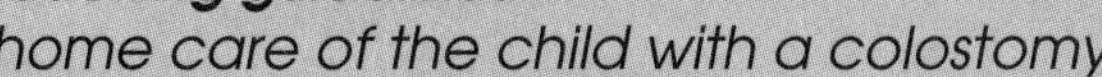
home care of the child with a colostomy

Care of the child with a colostomy:

* Allow the child to bathe or shower with or without the colostomy pouch. Water does not harm the ostomy.
* Avoid soaps that contain perfume, cold cream, oils, or lanolin. (Dial soap can be safely used.)
* Encourage the child to eat a balanced diet. Observe what foods affect the child's ostomy function, and avoid them.
* Encourage a school-age child to stay involved with peers. It is the child's choice whether to tell friends. The colostomy pouch will be hidden under clothing.
* An ostomy presents no barriers to any types of exercise and sports. Weight lifting may be limited (consult the surgeon).

Prevent infants from pulling at the colostomy pouch:

* Tuck the ostomy pouch into the diaper, and pin the undershirt to the diaper.
* Sleepers or overalls that snap at the neck and between the legs keep the pouch away from the infant.
* Make sure elastic bands on clothing do not rub across the stoma.
* There is no need to restrict the infant's activity by keeping him or her off the abdomen; however, check the position of the pouch afterward.

Caring for a child with special needs is a lot of work. Ask several family members and friends to learn the care so that you can take a break.

ostomy care for children

Ostomy care in children is basically the same as for an adult with the following exceptions:

1. Normally the colostomy of a small child is not irrigated. Irrigation should be done only in preparation for diagnostic tests or surgery and sometimes for constipation. The nurse never irrigates a child's colostomy without a physician's order.
2. The amount and consistency of drainage are monitored closely. Dehydration can occur quickly in infants and small children.
3. Because infants or young children eliminate more frequently, skin breakdown can occur.
4. Children are active, and collection bags may not stay in place.

cleft lip and palate

Cleft lip is a congenital anomaly of one or more clefts in the upper lip and results from an incomplete fusion of the oral cavity (Fig. 34-7). Cleft lip occurs in approximately 1 in every 1,000 births and is more common in boys.

Cleft palate is a congenital anomaly that can occur with cleft lip or as a single irregularity and involves an incomplete fusion of the partition separating the nasal and oral cavities (see Fig. 34-7). Cleft palate occurs in 1 in 2,500 births and is more common in girls.

pathophysiology

The clefts in the lip can be seen as small dimples or larger gaps involving nasal structures. Large clefts alter the infant's facial appearance and dental development. Cleft palate varies in severity from a cleft involving the soft palate to extensive openings in the hard palate and portions of the upper jaw (maxilla). Diagnosis is based on visible evidence of the clefts. These infants cannot create suction for effective sucking. Food often returns through the nose. They are subject to nasal crying and frequent bouts of otitis media.

medical–surgical management

Surgical correction of cleft lip occurs between 1 and 2 months, depending on the defect's severity and the infant's general health status. Bilateral cleft lip defects require a two-stage procedure because of the difficulty in correcting both clefts at once (see Fig. 34-7).

Surgical correction of cleft palate is performed between 6 and 18 months and may require several operations performed in stages. Early repair of cleft palate facilitates normal development of the infant's speech pattern.

preoperative nursing care

Nursing care goals for a child with cleft lip and cleft palate include taking steps to ensure adequate nutrition and hydration and prevent aspiration of secretions. Caregiver support may be needed to promote maternal–infant attachment. Caregivers need reassurance that reconstructive surgery is possible to correct the congenital defect.

nursing diagnosis

* Ineffective Airway Clearance, related to pooling of secretions in the mouth
* Sensory/Perceptual Alterations (auditory), related to hearing loss secondary to chronic middle-ear effusion
* Impaired Verbal Communication, related to the anatomic defect
* Risk for Altered Parenting, related to the birth of a child with altered facial appearance and special care needs
* Altered Nutrition: Less than body requirements, related to feeding difficulties

planning and implementation

* Special feeding methods before and after surgery may be required, such as a Brecht feeder (Fig. 34-8). Weigh

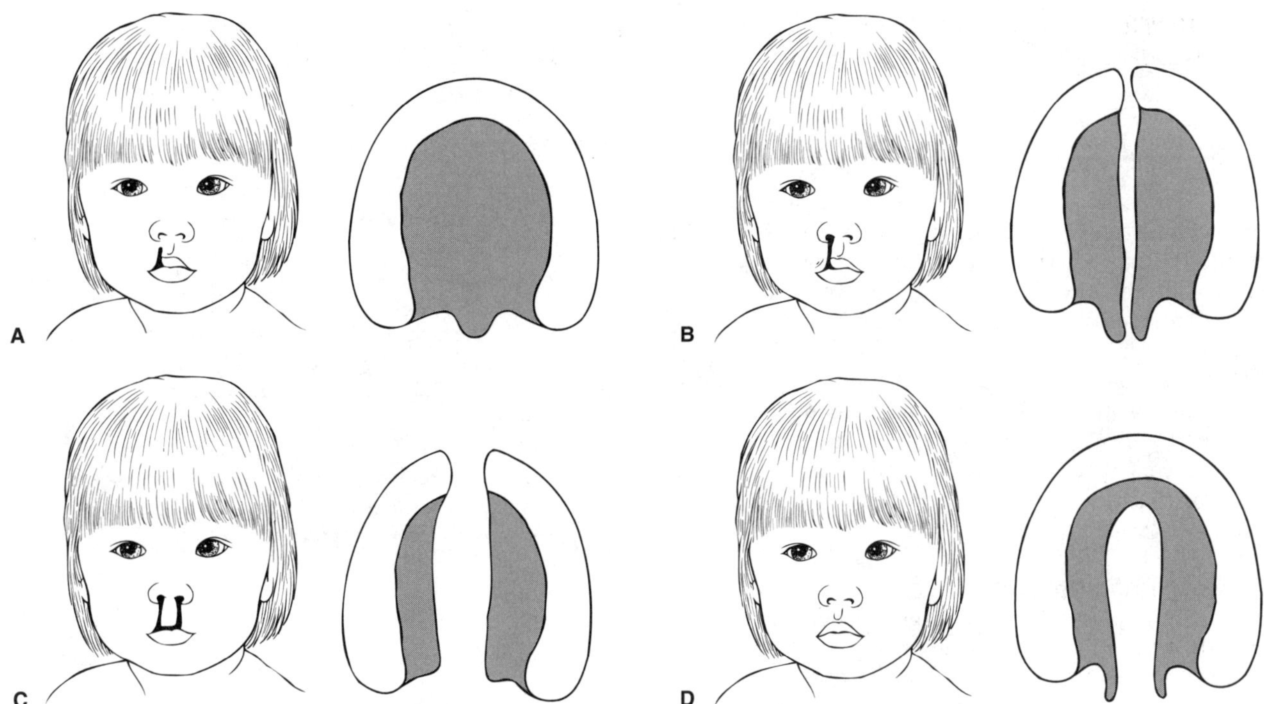

figure 34-7 *(**A**) Cleft lip. (**B**) Cleft lip and cleft palate. (**C**) Bilateral cleft lip and cleft palate. (**D**) Cleft palate.*

daily. Teach breast-feeding mothers to extend the nipple as far as possible into the infant's mouth, creating a tight seal. Feed infant slowly in an upright position, and burp frequently. Assess the caregiver's understanding and ability to use a special nipple or administer feedings through a tube.

- Prevent aspiration of secretions by positioning on the side, elevating head, or placing in an infant seat; avoid positioning on the abdomen. Use gentle bulb syringe suctioning.
- Encourage caregivers to verbalize concerns about the infant's appearance. Family members may need time to grieve. The nurse can help caregivers by listening to their feelings in a nonjudgmental manner. Encourage holding and cuddling of the infant. Provide factual information about available medical or surgical procedures to correct the disorder.

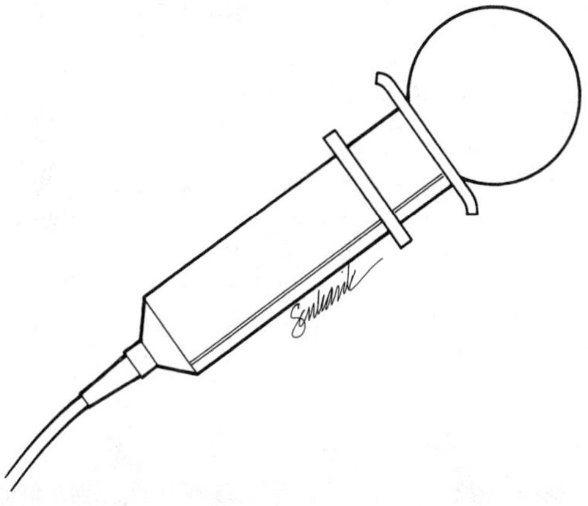

figure 34-8 *Feeding apparatus for cleft palate, known as Brecht feeder, consists of a rubber catheter on a large syringe.*

postoperative care

- Maintain suture line integrity by placing the infant in elbow restraints and assessing placement of a plastic bridge known as a Logan bow as a protection for the incision.
- Promote comfort and reduce crying by releasing elbow restraints every hour, changing body position every 2 hours, holding and cuddling the infant.
- Feed infant with a rubber-tipped medicine dropper or bulb syringe to reduce the risk of putting pressure on the suture line during feedings.
- Caregiver instructions include surgical wound care, proper feeding and positioning, long-term follow-up, increased risk of speech problems and the need for therapy, correction of dental abnormalities, and importance of annual hearing evaluations because of the increased risk of ear infections.

evaluation

- Caregivers demonstrate correct and effective feeding techniques.
- Caregivers and infant demonstrate affection with physical closeness.
- Suture line is clean and free from infection.

abdominal wall defects (hernias and hydrocele)

Common abdominal wall defects considered to be congenital anomalies include umbilical and inguinal hernias and hydrocele. *Hernia* is described as weak spot of the muscle, which allows part of the bowel to slip through. *Herniogram* is an x-ray that determines the presence of a hernia. The procedure involves placing a needle into the suspected hernia site and injecting dye through the needle into the stomach area. After x-rays are taken, the needle is removed.

Hydrocele involves the presence of abdominal fluid in the infant's scrotal sac. Most hernias do not require surgical intervention; however, if the protruding bowel becomes twisted, resulting in an inadequate blood supply to the intestinal segment, emergency laparotomy is performed to restore a normal blood flow.

teaching guidelines
home care of the child with hernia surgery

* Keep the dressings as clean and dry as possible. Dressings are frequently clear plastic or Steri-strips (a special tape) or both.
* You will not be able to see the stitches because they are under the skin and will dissolve on their own.
* Notify the surgeon if any of the following occur:
  The child develops a fever of 101°F.
  Incision line becomes red, swollen, or starts to drain.
  Child is irritable, fussy, and appears to be in pain that is unrelieved by rocking, holding, or administering prescribed analgesic.
  Infant has not urinated in 8 hours.

diaphragmatic hernias

The diaphragmatic hernia is a congenital hernia occurring when the abdominal contents are displaced upward into the thoracic cavity. Treatment must be immediate to repair the opening and replace the abdominal contents.

The repair may be complicated if there is not enough room in the abdomen. Stretching the muscle and skin to close the cavity or placing protective silicone over the contents may be necessary initially to close the cavity.

hiatal hernias

A hiatal hernia in a newborn is usually sliding; the herniation permits the cardiac sphincter to slide above the diaphragm, allowing contents from the abdominal cavity to reflux into the esophagus and precipate regurgitation.

When palliative treatment is not successful, the child will need a surgical intervention to reduce the size of the esophageal opening. The Nissen fundoplication is a common corrective procedure.

umbilical hernia

An umbilical hernia results from a protrusion of intestine and omentum through a weakness or opening of the umbilical ring in the abdominal wall around the umbilicus. A soft swelling or protrusion is noted around the umbilicus, which becomes more pronounced with crying. If the fascial ring is 2 cm or less, the hernia usually closes spontaneously. If the fascial ring is larger than 2 cm, the child will need surgical intervention. Umbilical hernias are more common in African American children.

inguinal hernia

Inguinal hernia is described as a weak spot in the muscle in the groin area, allowing part of the bowel to slip through into the inguinal ring. Inguinal hernias frequently produce painless inguinal swelling. On assessment, a lump can be detected in the inguinal area. The effect is more noticeable with coughing or crying. Inguinal hernias are more common in boys.

A major complication of this type of hernia occurs when the descended portion of bowel becomes caught in the hernia sac, compromising the blood flow (incarcerated). Inguinal hernias require surgical intervention known as *inguinal herniorrhaphy*, usually performed on an outpatient basis.

hydrocele

Hydrocele involves an abnormal accumulation of fluid in the scrotum. Hydroceles are described as communicating or noncommunicating. A *communicating* hydrocele is frequently seen with an inguinal hernia. The serous membrane covering the front and sides of the testis and epididymis remains open from the scrotum to the abdominal cavity, allowing fluid to circulate into the scrotum. A communicating hydrocele requires surgical intervention if it does not spontaneously disappear by 1 year. The surgical procedure involves excision of the hydrocele, referred to as *hydrocelectomy*.

A *noncommunicating* hydrocele occurs when excess peritoneal fluid is trapped in the lining of the testes or along the spermatic cord, causing the scrotum to enlarge. The scrotal sac is visibly large and pendulous, with a shiny appearance and absent normal folds. The fluid seen in a noncommunicating hydrocele usually is absorbed during the first months after birth and requires no treatment.

meckel's diverticulum

Meckel's diverticulum is a sac that protrudes from the wall of the ileum due to an incomplete closure during fetal development. It is a common cause of rectal bleeding in children. Meckel's diverticulum places the child at risk for intussusception and bowel obstruction. Diagnosis is made by a nuclear scintiscan. Surgical resection is the treatment of choice.

pyloric stenosis

Pyloric stenosis is a narrowing of the pyloric sphincter at the lower end of the stomach. The cause of pyloric stenosis is unknown. Incidence is higher in white boys.

pathophysiology

The pyloric sphincter narrows because of a gradual enlargement of the circular pyloric muscle. The enlargement leads to obstruction of the pyloric sphincter, preventing the stomach from emptying properly. The delay in emptying creates gastric distention and projectile vomiting. Excessive vomiting predisposes to metabolic alkalosis because acidic gastric contents are lost to the body. The child loses weight and is excessively hungry and dehydrated.

Ultrasonography and radiographic examination of the upper GI tract reveal delayed gastric emptying and an elongated, thin pylorus. Laboratory findings include increased serum pH and bicarbonate levels (indicating metabolic alkalosis), increased hematocrit and hemoglobin values (reflecting hemoconcentration), and decreased serum chloride, sodium, and potassium levels (typically seen in excessive vomiting).

medical–surgical management

Medical intervention for mild pyloric stenosis involves giving cereal-thickened formula. Surgical intervention is typically required to correct pyloric stenosis. Preoperatively, fluid and electrolyte balance are established, the infant is kept NPO, and a nasogastric tube is inserted to provide gastric decompression. The surgical procedure is known as a *pyloromyotomy* and involves making an incision along the anterior pylorus to split the muscle and relieve the obstruction.

preoperative nursing care

nursing assessment

* Monitor explosive projectile vomiting episodes. Usually emesis contains no bile, and the infant is eager to refeed immediately after vomiting.
* Assess bowel sounds. Gastric peristaltic waves can be seen moving from left to right across the epigastrium (Fig. 34-9).
* Assess the infant's abdomen during sleep by slipping the index and middle fingers of both hands under the child; using the thumbs for control on the back, gently lift the child and palpate the epigastrium just to the right of the umbilicus. If a pyloric stenosis is present, an olive size mass can be felt.

nursing diagnoses

* Risk for Fluid Volume Deficit, related to vomiting
* Altered Nutrition: Less than body requirements, related to inability to retain feedings
* Risk for Altered Respiratory Function, related to potential for aspirating vomitus

planning and implementation

* Monitor output (urine, emesis, nasogastric tube drainage, and stools), weigh daily, and monitor IV fluids.
* Assess skin turgor, fontanels, sputum, and tear production for signs of dehydration.
* Place infant on the side or with head elevated to reduce the risk of aspirating vomitus.
* Monitor patency of nasogastric tube.

evaluation

* Infant appears well hydrated; electrolytes are within normal range.
* Normal respiratory status is maintained with clear breath sounds, and respiration rate is within normal range according to age.

postoperative nursing care

nursing assessment

* Monitor vital signs, skin color, and level of consciousness to determine infant's reaction to the anesthetic.
* Assess incision for signs of bleeding.

nursing diagnoses

* Risk for Infection, related to surgical incision
* Ineffective Breathing Patterns, related to anesthesia
* Knowledge Deficit, Parental or Caregiver, related to feeding procedures and dressing changes

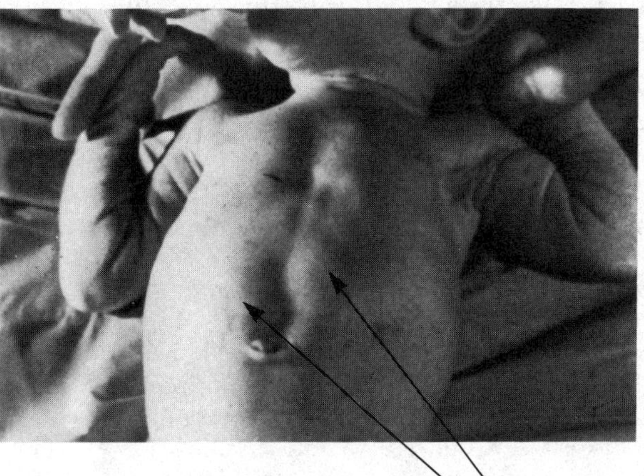

figure 34-9 *Assessment for pyloric stenosis includes listening to bowel sounds and taking note of peristaltic waves.*

planning and implementation

* Maintain NPO status for up to 8 hours after surgery; initiate clear liquid feedings advancing to formula according to surgeon's orders.
* Provide caregiver instructions concerning home care relative to dressing changes, feedings, and postfeeding positioning.

evaluation

* Child is free of signs of infection.
* Vital signs are within normal range.
* Caregiver verbalizes understanding of home care procedures.

inflammatory and infectious disorders

esophagitis

Esophagitis is an acute or chronic inflammation of the esophagus. The backward flow of stomach contents seen in gastroesophageal reflux is associated with inflammation of the esophagus. *Corrosive esophagitis* is common in young children following the ingestion of highly acidic or alkaloid materials.

pathophysiology

Burns are present on the mouth and in the stomach if acid is swallowed. Alkaloid substances rapidly cause second- and third-degree burns on the skin and in the mouth and esophagus. During the first 48 hours after ingestion, tissue edema occurs, compromising eating, swallowing, and breathing. Two to four days later, necrotic tissue at the burn sites begins to slough, and edema decreases. Esophageal healing occurs in approximately 2 weeks, resulting in stricture formation.

medical management

Immediate intervention is aimed at neutralizing the ingested chemical. Forced vomiting is contraindicated because regurgitation of the chemical would increase esophageal injury and increase the risks of aspiration. The treatment of choice is to aspirate the stomach contents, administer cool-water lavage, begin IV fluid therapy, and keep the child NPO. Endoscopy is performed to evaluate the degree of esophageal injury. Children with first-degree burns are usually hospitalized for close observation. Antibiotics and steroids are administered to prevent or minimize stricture formation at the burn site.

nursing care A major consideration during the acute phase of caring for children with corrosive esophagitis is to assess for signs of shock reflected by vital sign changes. Some of the anxiety experienced by children and caregivers can be reduced by careful explanation of procedures and treatments. After the acute phase, the child's hydration status must be evaluated by monitoring weight, intake and output, and IV fluid administration. When the child is allowed to eat, feeding tolerance must be observed because difficult swallowing and vomiting may be signs of stricture formation.

Caregiver teaching is a critical factor in discharge planning. Caregivers must understand normal growth and development patterns. Toddlers have a natural curiosity and a short attention span; thus, telling the toddler not to get into cupboards where cleaning supplies are kept will not guarantee the child's safety. Constant attention must be given to the safety of the child through close supervision and "child-proofing" the house.

inflammatory bowel disease (ulcerative colitis and crohn's disease)

Ulcerative colitis and *Crohn's disease* are classified as inflammatory bowel diseases (IBD). Their cause is unknown, and there is no known association between the incidence of IBD and environmental factors, viral agents, or immunologic disorders. This disease affects children between 15 and 20 years. White children are diagnosed with IBD more often than African Americans, with a higher incidence among American Jewish people.

pathophysiology

Ulcerative colitis is a recurrent inflammatory and ulcerative disease of the large intestine. Ulcerative colitis lesions are continuous and cause vascular congestion, capillary dilation, edema, and hemorrhage in the superficial mucosa of the bowel.

Crohn's disease is an inflammatory and ulcerative disease affecting any portion of the intestines. The inflammation and ulcers affect the deep walls of the bowel. The lesions are scattered, with normal tissue found between lesions. Fissures, fistulas, and thickened intestinal walls are part of the disease process.

Symptoms of ulcerative colitis and Crohn's disease are similar: diarrhea, rectal bleeding, abdominal pain, fever, malaise, anorexia, weight loss, malnutrition, electrolyte imbalances, delay in sexual maturation, growth retardation, and anemia (Table 34-9). Periods of remission and exacerbation are seen with both disorders. Ulcerative colitis predisposes the child to cancer, hemorrhage, and sepsis. Crohn's disease may be complicated by liver abscess and liver disease.

medical–surgical management

Antidiarrheal drugs, such as Lomotil, are used to control diarrhea. Anti-inflammatory drugs, such as Solu-Medrol, are used to control inflammation. The child is placed on a high-protein, high-calorie, low-fat, low-fiber diet. If the child does not respond to medical management, surgical intervention often involves a colostomy or ileostomy procedure.

Ileostomy is a surgical opening into the ileum to allow drainage of body wastes. Ileostomy usually accompanies total colon and rectum removal, making the surgical correction permanent. Ileostomy drainage is liquid or

table 34-9 characteristics of inflammatory bowel syndrome

	Ulcerative Colitis	*Crohn's Disease*
SITE AFFECTED	Originates in rectum and distal colon and spreads proximally to entire colon; unknown cause	Most common in right colon (terminal ileum); can affect any part of the GI tract; unknown cause
DISEASE COURSE	Abrupt onset; remissions and exacerbations	Slow, progressive; periods of remission and exacerbation
DESCRIPTION OF MUCOSA	Ulceration, bleeding, congestion, abscess formation with pus drainage; scarring, pale, flattened	Peyer's patches (circular or oval nodules), edema, ulceration, fissures, abscesses; thick bowel wall with rigid fibers that narrow bowel lumen
ABDOMINAL PAIN	Rare; may have tenderness in lower left quadrant	Common; lower right quadrant pain, cramps, spasms
NATURE OF STOOL	Bloody, mucopurulent diarrhea	Soft or semiliquid, foul-smelling, fatty stools
RECTAL BLEEDING	Rare	Common
COMPLICATIONS	Stricture of colon, nutritional deficiencies, anal fissures, perirectal abscess	Anal fistula, perianal abscess, internal fistulas to the bladder or vagina, small bowel obstruction.
NURSING CONSIDERATIONS	Assess tolerance to bland diet high in protein, calories, vitamins, and minerals and low in fats and fiber. Encourage small, frequent feedings; avoid lactose; monitor hyperalimentation.	Same as for ulcerative colitis
DRUG THERAPY	Sulfasalazine, antidiarrheal medications, cortisone, and antibiotics	Same as for ulcerative colitis
SURGICAL INTERVENTION	Total proctocolectomy with ileostomy. Kock pouch or ileal pouch—anal anastomosis.	Bowel resection

semisolid and continuous because the child no longer has a colon to absorb water.

nursing assessment

Objective assessment of the child with inflammatory bowel disease includes the following:

* Assess for weight loss or failure to gain as expected, small for age, lack of subcutaneous fat, inadequate intake and concentrated urine output, vitamin deficiencies, delayed sexual development, dry scaly skin, and fever.
* Assess child's response to changes in body function and appearance. Encourage child to verbalize fears and perceived limitations. Encourage child and parent to focus on strengths and abilities.
* Assess bowel sounds, abdominal pain.
* Assess child and caregiver compliance with dietary management aimed at decreased intake of gas-forming foods; elimination of "natural laxatives," such as caffeinated foods and drinks; and fiber and lactose reduction (if lactose intolerant).

nursing diagnosis

* Altered Nutrition: Less than body requirements, related to impaired intestinal absorption, anorexia, pain, increased nitrogen and fluid loss through diarrhea, and blood loss from damaged intestinal mucosa
* Body Image Disturbance, related to delayed sexual maturation, side effects of steroids (moon face), delays in growth and development compared with peers, and frequent bouts of diarrhea, pain, and surgical interventions
* Fear, related to loss of control

planning and implementation

* Teach child and caregivers about drugs, such as antispasmodics, steroids, and sulfasalazine, and their side effects.
* Assess child and caregiver knowledge of ileostomy care, including use of appliances (if applicable).
* Assess adolescent's fears concerning disfigurement related to surgical ileostomy. Provide written materials, detailed books, and diagrams.

evaluation

* Child and caregiver will describe foods appropriate for the diet and foods to be avoided.
* Child will maintain stable body weight with normal fluid and electrolyte balance.
* Child will verbalize acceptance of bodily changes and speak in a positive way about self.
* Child and caregiver will demonstrate appropriate care of external ileostomy.

See the Nursing Care Plan.

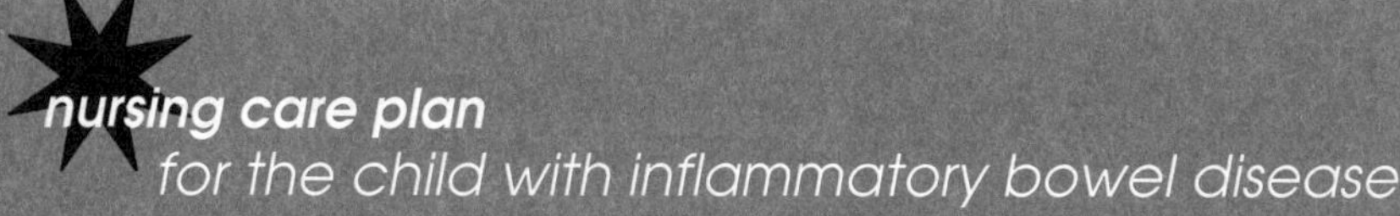

nursing care plan for the child with inflammatory bowel disease

NURSING DIAGNOSIS

Altered Nutrition: Less than body requirements, related to impaired intestinal absorption, anorexia, and increased nitrogen fluid loss through diarrhea

GOAL: Child will receive adequate nutrition

NURSING INTERVENTIONS	RATIONALE	EVALUATION
Educate the family on the use of TPN as ordered, when necessary.	With severe IBD symptoms, weight loss, and nutritional deficits, TPN is the treatment of choice.	The family and child will understand the importance of TPN and accept it when necessary.
Monitor daily weight	Weight loss is an important indicator of fluid status and nutritional status.	The child will maintain a stable weight.
Monitor electrolyte levels.	Deficient oral intake and chronic diarrhea can exhaust electrolyte supplies.	The child's electrolytes will be monitored and maintained within normal range.
Assess stool for amount, consistency, and odor. Administer antidiarrheal agents as necessary.	Stool evaluation provides information on fat absorption and the success of anti-diarrheal agents.	Stool will be assessed, and there will be less incidence of diarrhea episodes.
Coordinate a meeting with the dietitian and the family.	A plan for adequate dietary regime is necessary for the family and child to understand.	The family/child will be involved in planning necessary dietary supplements.

NURSING DIAGNOSIS

Chronic Pain, related to the inflammatory nature of the disease

GOAL: The child will relate an improvement in pain

NURSING INTERVENTIONS	RATIONALE	EVALUATION
Establish the presence of pain experienced by the child.	This will validate the pain and may help reduce the child's anxiety and pain.	The child's pain will be assessed on an objective scale.
Determine if a relationship exists between intake of solids or fluid and the pain.	Determine if the child associates food with pain and is therefore limiting oral intake.	Relationships of the onset of pain and oral intake will be discussed.
Assist child in finding optional pain remedies including a change in body position, relaxation exercises, and diversional activities.	Repositioning may help move gas through the bowel, therefore decreasing pain; realization enhances the effect of pain medication, diversion can help distract the child.	The child will use various measures to manage pain.
Teach the family and the child about antispasmodics and pain medications.	Antispasmodics can help relieve cramping, narcotics are discouraged secondary to the masking of life-threatening symptoms associated with obstruction.	The child will obtain pain relief as assessed on an objective scale and as evidenced by increasing ADLs.

appendicitis

The *appendix*, a small dead-end tube of lymphatic tissues attached to the cecum, is a common site for infection requiring surgical intervention in the school-age child. Appendicitis is the most common cause of abdominal surgery in school-age children.

pathophysiology

Appendicitis is an inflammation of the appendix resulting from bacterial infection or obstruction. Obstructions can occur from a *fecalith* made up of hard, formed fecal mass; a tumor; foreign body; kinks; or stenosis. *Peritonitis*, inflammation of the peritoneum produced by bacteria introduced into the abdominal cavity, is a common complication of a ruptured appendix.

Although appendicitis in adults usually begins with sharp abdominal pain, in children, pain is a late symptom. Other symptoms of appendicitis include loss of appetite for 12 to 24 hours, disinterest in play, fatigue, and nausea and vomiting. Early complaints of abdominal pain are often unclear, gradually localizing to the right lower quadrant. Until the pain localizes, it is sometimes difficult to distinguish appendicitis from gastroenteritis.

surgical management

Treatment of appendicitis is surgical removal of the appendix before it ruptures. Often, the condition warrants emergency surgery, allowing little preparation time for the child or caregivers. Diagnosis is often based on clinical findings, elevated white blood count, and child's complaints. If perforation has not occurred, recovery is typically rapid and uneventful. However, if rupture and peritonitis have occurred, surgery may be delayed temporarily. Treatment is based on fluid and electrolyte management, systemic antibiotics, nasogastric suction, and NPO status until bowel function returns.

nursing care

Care of the child with appendicitis and appendectomy follows the principles outlined in the section, Nursing Care of the Child Having GI Surgery, page 584.

hepatitis

Hepatitis is a viral inflammation of the liver. Three common viruses are causative factors: hepatitis A, hepatitis B, and non-A, non-B hepatitis (also referred to as hepatitis C; Table 34-10).

Hepatitis A virus is often referred to as *infectious hepatitis*. It is excreted in the stool and transmitted to the child by oral–fecal contact related to inadequate handwashing. Symptoms include fever, jaundice, anorexia, nausea, malaise, abdominal pain, and headache. Infants and preschool children are asymptomatic or have mild cases without jaundice. Hepatitis A is endemic in many developing countries where children are exposed to raw sewage wastes. Children in day care centers are at increased risk for hepatitis A unless handwashing is frequent and thorough for children and day care workers.

Hepatitis B virus is often referred to as *serum hepatitis* because the major mode of transmission is through blood. It can be transmitted through other body fluids, such as saliva, breast milk, vaginal secretions, and semen. Hepatitis B patients are often asymptomatic. This virus can cause a severe form of hepatitis known as *fulminant hepatitis,* which is almost always fatal.

The risk of hepatitis B virus is increased in children receiving blood transfusions or blood components (children with hemophilia), children who are sexually abused, dialysis patients, transplant patients, IV drug abusers, and children with leukemia or lymphoma.

Non-A, non-B hepatitis is transmitted similar to hepatitis B. Most children contracting hepatitis from blood transfusions have the non-A, non-B type (see Table 34-10).

pathophysiology

The hepatitis virus infects the liver cells, causing inflammation. In most cases, the disease is self-limiting with complete regeneration of liver tissue without permanent damage. Some forms of hepatitis lead to degeneration and necrosis of the liver cells. Chronic hepatitis puts the child at risk for liver failure and cirrhosis.

The child infected with hepatitis will excrete dark amber urine due to an increase in excreted bilirubin. An alteration in normal liver function is seen from the infection. The secretion of bile is diminished, causing the child's stools to be light or clay colored. Older children often experience jaundice due to the increased destruction of red blood cells and an elevation of bilirubin.

medical management

No specific treatment is available for hepatitis. Care of the child with hepatitis centers around support, education of

table 34-10 incubation, symptoms, transmission, and immunization for hepatitis

	Hepatitis A	*Hepatitis B*	*Non-A, Non-B Hepatitis*
INCUBATION PERIOD	1–2 mo	50–180 d; average of 120 d	2–12 wk
CONTAGION PERIOD	1–3 mo, 2 wk preceding jaundice	10% become carriers; immunization available	Unknown
USUAL; ONSET	Acute	Insidious	Insidious
MODE OF TRANSMISSION	Fecal–oral route (can be transmitted through contaminated food or water)	Blood and blood products, sexual contact, vaginal secretions, breast milk, saliva, and perinatal contact	Blood or blood products; possible risk through sexual contact; fecal–oral acquired from contaminated drinking water or person-to-person contact.

the child and caregivers about preventing transmission of the disease, rest, and proper nutrition.

nursing care

The child with hepatitis may have flulike symptoms at the onset of the infection. A diagnosis of hepatitis is suspected when the child displays jaundice. Many children with mild or uncomplicated hepatitis receive care at home. Preventing further spread of hepatitis is important and can be achieved with good handwashing techniques; proper disposal of soiled diapers, used needles, and blood; isolation measures (usually enteric); and active or passive immunization.

Perinatal transmission of hepatitis B increases the risk of hepatitis in newborns. It is important to wear gloves when handling the infant and suctioning secretions from the mouth and nose.

For newborns with mothers who are negative for hepatitis B surface antigen, the recommended hepatitis B immunization schedule is to give the first dose of the vaccine during the first 2 days of life, the second at 1 to 2 months, and the third at 6 to 18 months. If the mother is positivie for hepatitis B surface antigen, the immunization schedule is more aggressive with the first dose given as soon as possible after birth, the second at 1 month, and the third at 6 months. Good handwashing techniques are important; soiled diapers and needle should be handled cautiously to prevent disease transmission.

table 34-11 myths and facts about failure to thrive (FTT)

Myth	*Fact*
FTT is an emotional disorder.	FTT is diagnosed on physical growth.
FTT children are from poor or developing countries and tend to be genetically small, making the standard growth charts inaccurate.	Children born of immigrants from developing countries tend to grow taller than their parents. Growth standards are appropriate during the child's first 5 years of life.
FTT is either organic or nonorganic in origin.	Categorizing the disorder in either organic or nonorganic terms depicts opposite extremes. Undernutrition creates biologic and psychological complications that require treatment. Children with FTT may lack an organic diagnosis but have innate temperamental traits that make feeding difficult.

other gastrointestinal disorders

failure to thrive

Failure to thrive is a syndrome in which the child experiences delayed growth and development from an inability to obtain or use calories. Growth falls below the fifth percentile in weight. This is a complex ailment with medical and psychosocial causes. It is not an emotional disorder nor is it limited to low-income families (Table 34-11).

pathophysiology

The three types of failure to thrive include *organic failure to thrive*, resulting from physical causes, such as congenital heart disease and occurring more often in newborns; *nonorganic failure to thrive* (NOFT), described as a decrease in weight gain unrelated to an organic cause but often resulting from psychosocial factors, such as deficient parenting skills and impaired infant–parent attachment; and *idiopathic failure to thrive,* unrelated to organic or nonorganic factors.

The majority of failure to thrive cases have NOFT; these infants appear listless, slow to respond to stimulation, below normal in weight and height, and unresponsive to cuddling and nurturing. Poverty, family stress, and parental confusion about proper infant nutrition are contributing factors to NOFT. This condition is seen more often in boys than girls.

Characteristics of the NOFT child include fussiness, higher reactivity, disturbed sleep patterns, disturbed eating, vomiting, and diarrhea. Many times a NOFT child does not exhibit stranger anxiety when separated from the caregiver and may become stiff and unresponsive to cuddling.

medical management

Medical intervention includes adequate food intake to ensure weight gain. Vitamin supplements are ordered. Parents are referred to a family therapist, social worker, and public health nurse for education on effective parenting skills.

nursing care

Growth failure may start with intrauterine growth retardation influenced by premature delivery or the mother's personal habits, such as cigarette smoking. To determine appropriate weight for premature infants, the nurse subtracts the weeks of prematurity from the infant's age to determine growth parameters. For example, if a child was born 1 month premature, the expected weight at 6 months would be equivalent to a 5-month-old infant. Daily monitoring of the child's weight, intake, and output allows for direct evaluation of the nutritional status and developmental progress. Parenting skills may be lacking in the caregivers, based on how they were treated as children. Counseling may be needed to improve caregivers' parenting skills. Parents should be supported by encouraging daily care of the child, including providing unhurried meals and frequent nutritious snacks. Follow-up home care is important.

gastroesophageal reflux

Gastroesophageal reflux (GER) is a backflow of gastric contents into the esophagus due to relaxation or incompetence of the lower esophageal (cardiac) sphincter. The exact cause is unknown but is often seen when lower esophageal neuromuscular function is immature. It is the most common esophageal problem in infants and it frequently disappears by 1 year.

pathophysiology

Gastroesophageal reflux occurs when the lower esophageal sphincter relaxes and fails to contract. The increase in gastric or abdominal pressure results in a backward flow (reflux) of gastric contents. Some reflux is normal in infants and is described as *regurgitation.*

Gastroesophageal reflux is regarded as pathologic when it is severe, persists into late infancy, or is associated with complications such as esophagitis. It is common in premature infants, children with neurologic problems, and those with cystic fibrosis. The following findings are common: delay in growth and development, recurrent respiratory infections from aspiration of stomach contents, and guaiac-positive stools.

medical–surgical management

Traditional noninvasive treatment for infants with uncomplicated GER includes upright positioning at a 45- to 60-degree angle, using infant seats or other suitable means, and giving small, frequent, thickened feedings (Fig. 34-10). Pharmacologic management includes administration of medication to produce a cholinergic effect in the stomach, Maalox to coat the stomach and produce an antacid effect, bethanechol to increase the muscle tone of the lower esophageal sphincter, and metoclopramide (Reglan) to promote gastric emptying.

Surgical intervention is recommended for the more severe GER cases or for infants failing to respond to medical intervention. The surgical procedure for GER is called *fundoplication* and involves wrapping the gastric fundus around the distal esophagus. Children with GER are at higher risk for aspiration and sudden infant death syndrome. Caregivers are encouraged to learn cardiopulmonary resuscitation.

intussusception

Intussusception is a frequent cause of intestinal obstruction in children between 3 months and 5 years, affecting boys more often than girls. The cause is unknown. There tends to be a strong relationship between intussusception and viral infections. Intestinal polyps, Meckel's diverticulum, lymphoma, and foreign body obstruction contribute to a small percentage of intussusceptions.

pathophysiology

Intussusception is a telescoping of one portion of the intestine into an adjacent distal portion, usually at the ileocecal valve (Fig. 34-11). The hyperactive peristalsis pulls the telescoped portion of intestine along the bowel; the two walls of the intestine press against each other, causing edema and obstruction. The blood supply to the area is diminished, resulting in bowel strangulation, necrosis, hemorrhage, perforation, peritonitis, and shock.

Diagnosis is based on a history of sudden onset of vomiting with severe cramping, abdominal pain, and jelly-like stools (blood and mucus). Physical examination of the abdomen often reveals a palpable, sausage-shaped mass that crosses the right upper and middle quadrants of the abdomen.

medical–surgical management

Barium enema is often ordered and is frequently therapeutic and diagnostic. The continuous pressure exerted by the barium enema is usually sufficient to reduce or push back the telescoped intestine into normal position.

Tracheasophageal Fistula (TEF)
S/s drooling, aspiration into lungs.
pouch fills + then they drool it out end up c̄ Gtube.

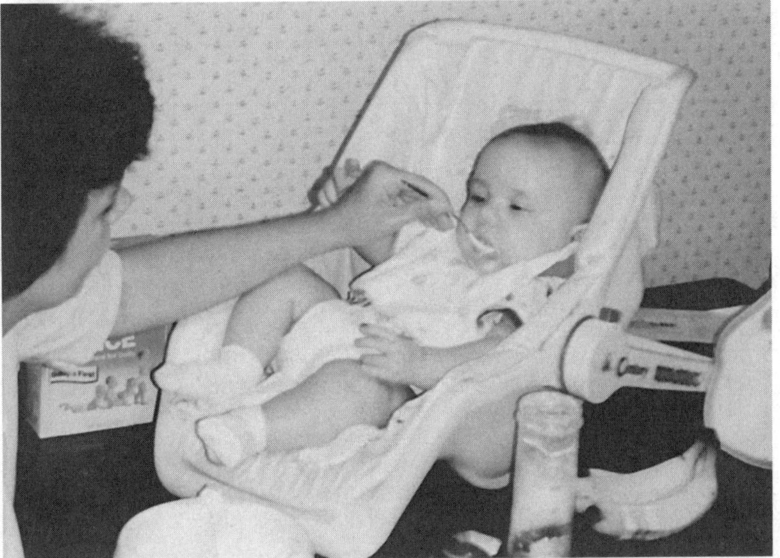

figure 34-10 *Treatment for gastroesophagel reflux is often as simple as properly positioning the child during feedings and offering small amounts of thickened food.*

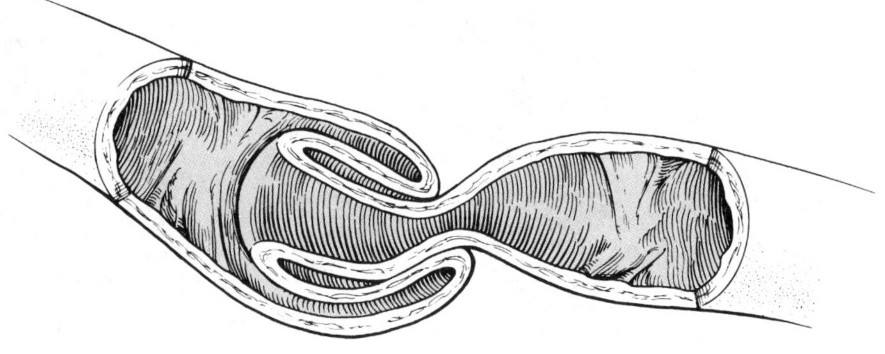

figure 34-11 *Intussusception.*

If a barium enema is not successful in reducing the intussusception, surgery is necessary. An abdominal incision is made, and the bowel is manipulated in place manually; nonviable portions of the bowel are removed. Serious complications or death is rare if the condition is diagnosed and treated as quickly as possible.

nursing care

* Assess degree of discomfort, and administer analgesics with follow-up regarding effectiveness. The child with intussusception often experiences severe abdominal pain and responds by screaming and drawing the knees to the abdomen. The child may have a nasogastric tube to decrease distention. Offer support to parents; monitor vital signs, bowel sounds, and general condition.
* Monitor vital signs every 4 hours and intake and output every 8 hours.
* Assess bowel sounds; note abdominal distention, patency of nasogastric tube, and color and amount of nasogastric tube drainage.
* Assess hydration status. Encourage intake of clear liquids after surgery, and advance diet as ordered.
* Monitor bowel elimination status for return to normal function. "Currant jelly" stools are replaced by normal brown stools when the intussusception has reduced itself.

what would you do?

Jane is a 3-year-old brought to the clinic by her mother for complaints of stomach pain, diarrhea, nausea, and vomiting for the past 3 days. She has herpes simplex lesions on her mouth. She has a dirty, unkempt appearance and a noticeable odor. She is small for her age. She displays stranger anxiety and whines when you look at her. When questioning the mother, you learn the family is homeless. They have been staying at a local shelter for the last 2 nights, planning to move on, and hoping to find employment as soon as Jane is well enough to travel. Their main food supply is from soup kitchens. The mother appears anxious about Jane's condition and her own inability to pay for services needed.

key points

* Alteration in GI function affects ingestion, digestion, absorption, and elimination, interfering with the child's ability to process food effectively and disrupting growth and development. This alteration may be related to congenital, hereditary, functional, or psychological influences or bacterial or viral infections.
* A mother's responsibility for providing the child's nutritional needs begins in pregnancy and continues throughout the growing years, reinforcing physiologic and psychosocial growth, fostering infant–caregiver attachment, and supporting eating habits that last into adult years.
* Caregiver responses to children with GI disorders include strong feelings of inadequacy or guilt when the child refuses to eat or symptoms require hospitalization; fear about the safety of the food supply related to pesticides and other cancer-causing chemicals and food additives; knowledge deficit concerning use of home remedies and changes in a "colicky" infant's behavior, indicating a GI disorder; and inability of caregivers to provide the child with adequate nutrition due to knowledge deficit or poverty.
* Fad dieting and fast food diets are common among adolescents, contributing to nutritional imbalances that can be harmless unless extended for a long time, resulting in eating disorders, such as anorexia nervosa, bulimia, and obesity.
* Nursing care of children with GI disorders is based on knowledge about nutrition and age-related nutritional factors; consideration of cultural dietary customs that affect a child's nutritional well-being; provisions for continued breast-feeding when infants are hospitalized; knowledge of child and caregiver needs when caring for a child with congenital defects, such as cleft lip and palate; and ability to give age-appropriate explanations to children concerning dietary restrictions and medical or surgical procedures.
* Diagnostic tests for GI disorders include stool analysis for the presence of blood, worms, bacteria, and fat; endoscopy examination; imaging studies, such as fluoroscopy or x-ray of upper and lower GI tract and

gastric-emptying nuclear scan; bowel and liver biopsy; and other laboratory tests.

* The digestive tract begins with the mouth, where ingestion takes place and digestion starts. Teeth break down food, making it easier to swallow. Food travels to the stomach, where digestion continues. Peristalsis moves the nutrients through the small and large intestines where absorption occurs. The GI tract ends with the rectum, where elimination of undigested and unabsorbed food from the body takes place. The child's GI tract has a smaller stomach capacity than that of an adult, lacks certain digestive enzymes, and empties faster than that of the adult.
* Gagging and swallowing reflexes present at birth do not become strong until about 6 months, increasing the risk for aspiration pneumonia during regurgitation or vomiting.
* Nursing assessment in altered GI function includes observation of the child's appearance, behavior, and growth and of caregiver–child interactions; color and condition of skin; hydration status, especially in children with diarrhea and vomiting; condition of mouth and teeth; abdominal tenderness, bruising, scarring, or presence of congenital anomaly, such as hernia; presence or absence of bowel sounds; pattern of vomiting and amount, consistency, color, and smell of emesis; and presence of pain.
* Dehydration results from excessive loss of body water and is common in infants and small children with diarrhea and vomiting because large, liquid stools can deplete the infant's water volume. Infants and children have a higher metabolic rate than adults; their body surface is larger when compared to weight, and immature kidney function impairs their ability to conserve water.

review questions

1. Jerry is a 2-month-old admitted to the pediatric unit for severe diarrhea and vomiting. Your initial assessment of Jerry must include
   a. weight, length, head circumference, and hydration status.
   b. skin coloring, presence of hernia, and crying pattern.
   c. type of diet, eating patterns, abdominal tenderness, and parental reactions to child's diet.
   d. family history, ability to sit without support, condition of hair and nails.
2. Maria Amidone is a 3-year-old clinic patient suspected of having pinworms. Maria's mother is instructed to collect a specimen for laboratory evaluation and asks why the specimen must be collected while Maria sleeps. An appropriate nursing response would be,
   a. "If Maria is awake, she will not allow you to put tape on her rectum."
   b. "The worms lay their eggs at night while the child sleeps."
   c. "It probably does not make any difference when you collect the specimen."
   d. "The laboratory policy is to collect pinworm specimens while the child sleeps."
3. Latisha is a 5-year-old clinic patient with excoriation noted around her G tube insertion site. Latisha's caregiver voices concern about having to change the G tube dressing twice a day. An appropriate nursing intervention includes
   a. suggesting that Latisha change her own dressing once a day.
   b. asking the doctor to discontinue the dressing changes.
   c. observing Latisha's caregiver changing the stoma dressing and offering encouragement and information.
   d. asking the doctor to order a consultation with the social services department.
4. Zachary is a 15-year-old boy admitted to the pediatric unit with complaints of abdominal tenderness, small petechiae noted over the body, jaundice of the skin and sclera, and clay-colored stools. An appropriate nursing intervention includes
   a. administering a tap water enema.
   b. using universal precautions when handling urine, stool, and body secretions.
   c. wearing a mask and gown while bathing Zachary.
   d. encouraging Zachary to ingest foods high in protein and fat and low in carbohydrates.
5. Children diagnosed with a malabsorption disease are at an increased risk for experiencing
   a. obesity.
   b. vitamin deficiencies.
   c. allergies.
   d. constipation.

references

Chung, K., Olson, R., & Vinson, J. (1996). *Lippincott's pediatric nursing review*. Philadelphia: Lippincott–Raven.

Sackor, A. (1994). "Healthy" or "fat"? *RN, 57*(12), 40–42.

bibliography

Bartholmey, S. (1994). Infant rice cereal: A simple oral rehydration treatment solution. *Pediatric Basics, 67*, 1.

Beckert, B., & Heyman, M. (1993). Comparison of two skin-level gastrostomy feeding tubes for infants and children. *Pediatric Nursing, 19*(4), 351–354.

Carpenito, L. (1996). *Nursing diagnosis application to clinical practice.* (6th ed.). Philadelphia: Lippincott–Raven.

Castiglia, P., & Harbin, R. (1992). *Child health care.* Philadelphia: J.B. Lippincott.

Eisenberg, P. (1994). Nasoenteral tubes. *RN, 57*(10), 62–69.

Fischbach, F. (1995). *Quick reference to common laboratory and diagnostic tests.* Philadelphia: J.B. Lippincott.

Frank, D., Needlman, R., & Silva, M. (1994) What to do when a child won't grow. *Patient Care, March*, 107–135.

Gulanick, M., Knoll, M., & Gradishar, D. (1994). *Ambulatory pediatric nursing.* Albany, NY: Delmar Publishers.

Hofland, S., & Dardis, P. (1992). Bulimia nervosa associated physical problems. *Journal of Psychosocial Nursing, 30*(2), 23–27.

Holmgren, C. (1992). Abdominal assessment. *RN, March*, 28–33.

Jackson, D., & Saunders R. (1993). *Child health nursing.* Philadelphia. J.B. Lippincott.

Kleinman, R., Sack, D., & Dale, C. (1994). Diarrhea management with oral rehydration therapy. *Pediatric Basics, 67*, 10–16.

Marks, M. (1994). *Introductory pediatric nursing.* Philadelphia: J.B. Lippincott.

Mayers, M. (1991). *Clinical care plans. Pediatric nursing.* Philadelphia: Markham-McKenzie Publishers.

Memmler, R., Cohen, B., & Wood, D. (1996). *The human body in health and disease* (8th ed.). Philadelphia: Lippincott–Raven.

Natural Resources Defense Council (1993) *Questions and answers on pesticides and food.* New York: National Resources Defense Council.

Shannon, R. (1994). Gastroesophageal reflux in infancy: Review and update. *Journal of Pediatric Health Care, 7*(2), 71–76.

Staab, B. (1992). Antecedents to nonorganic failure-to-thrive. *Pediatric Nursing, 18*(6), 579–582.

Sterling, C., Schaffer, S., & Jolley, S. (1993). Home management related to medical treatment for chilhood gastresophageal reflux. *Pediatric Nursing, 19*(2), 167–173.

Suddarth, D. (1996). *The Lippincott manual of nursing practice* (6th ed.). Philadelphia: Lippincott–Raven.

Thomas, C. (1993). *Taber's medical dictionary* (17th ed.). Philadelphia: F.A. Davis.

Thompson, M. (1995). *Pediatric nursing concepts and activities.* Springhouse, PA: Springhouse Corporation.

outline ✳

the child with an alteration in neurologic or sensory function

35

objectives ✳

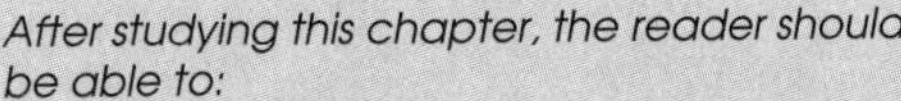

After studying this chapter, the reader should be able to:

- ✳ Discuss the anatomy and physiology of the nervous and sensory systems, acknowledging age-specific differences.
- ✳ Identify no fewer than five family considerations concerning neurologic and sensory disorders.
- ✳ Discuss the nursing process related to the promotion of normal neurologic and sensory functioning and the promotion of optimal growth and development.
- ✳ Describe at least four diagnostic tests pertinent to neurologic function.
- ✳ Describe appropriate nursing interventions for a child following a lumbar puncture.
- ✳ Compare the nursing care of children experiencing congenital anomalies and trauma to the central nervous system, spinal cord, and sensory system.
- ✳ List at least five symptoms specific to neurologic infections.
- ✳ Describe the impact of hearing loss on the child's emotional and cognitive development.
- ✳ List at least four measures necessary for home care of a child with surgical insertion of Teflon tubes in the middle ear.
- ✳ List at least four difficulties experienced by a child with hearing or vision impairments.

key terms ✳

aura
concussion
contusion
dyslexia
encephalopathy
increased intracranial pressure
level of consciousness
lumbar puncture
opisthotonos
otitis media
Rhomberg test
seizure
status epilepticus
Tay-Sachs disease
tripod posturing

Neurologic maturation is evident in the grace and beauty of child development. Sensory function, particularly the sense of vision and hearing, enables children to discover and respond to the world around them. Sensory disorders are rarely life-threatening, but they can have a major impact on the quality of a child's life and the ability to achieve normal growth and development. Therefore, when neurologic or sensory function is impaired, the impact can devastate families. Neurologic and sensory disorders may be acute or chronic, may result from a variety of causes, and may be manifested in many body systems. Many of these disorders have disabling and even life-threatening consequences, making early diagnosis and intervention essential. By understanding the causes, nature, and systemic effects of neurologic and sensory disorders, nurses are better able to provide optimal care for affected children and their families.

Neurologic disorders often require care administered by a specialist called a *pediatric neurologist.* Vision problems involve examination by an *optometrist*, a person specifically trained and licensed to examine the eyes and prescribe and adapt lenses to correct vision problems, or a *pediatric ophthalmologist*, a physician who specializes in the treatment of disorders of the eye in children.

Nursing care of children with neurologic and sensory disorders is based on understanding age-related anatomy and physiology of neurologic and sensory systems. This chapter discusses anatomy and physiology of the neurologic and sensory systems, age-related differences, common diagnostic tests, parental and nursing considerations, specific disease information, and procedures pertinent to pediatric neurologic and sensory care.

anatomy and physiology of the nervous system

The nervous system consists of three main divisions: the *central nervous system* (CNS), the *peripheral nervous system*, and the *autonomic nervous system* (ANS). The major CNS structures include the cerebrum, thalamus, hypothalamus, cerebellum, brain stem, and spinal cord (Fig. 35-1). The *cerebrum* is the center for consciousness, thought, memory, sensory input, and motor activity. It consists of two hemispheres (left and right) and four lobes, each with its specific functions:

* The *frontal lobe* controls voluntary muscle movements and contains motor areas, including the area for speech. It is the center for personality, behavioral, and intellectual functions; autonomic functions; and emotional and cardiac responses.
* The *temporal lobe* is the center for taste, hearing, and smell and is the brain's dominant hemisphere, which interprets spoken language
* The *parietal lobe* coordinates and interprets sensory information from sensory receptors in the skin and joints.
* The *occipital lobe* interprets visual stimuli.

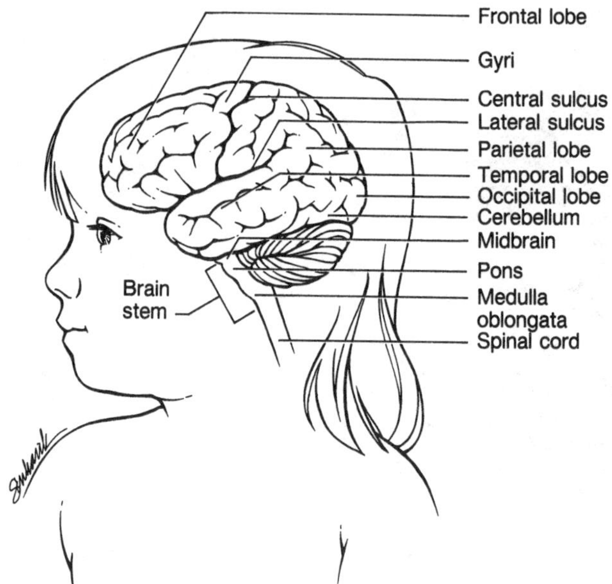

figure 35-1 *External surface of the brain showing major lobes of the cerebrum, the cerebellum, and divisions of the brain stem.*

The *thalamus* further organizes cerebral function by sending impulses to and from the cerebrum. It also is responsible for primitive emotional responses, such as fear, and for distinguishing between pleasant and unpleasant stimuli. Lying beneath the thalamus, the *hypothalamus* is an autonomic center that regulates blood pressure, temperature, libido, appetite, breathing, sleeping patterns, and peripheral nerve discharges associated with certain behaviors and emotional expression. It also helps control pituitary secretion and stress reaction.

The *cerebellum*, or *hindbrain*, controls smooth muscle movements, coordinates sensory impulses with muscle activity, and maintains muscle tone and equilibrium. The *brain stem*, which includes the *mesencephalon*, *pons*, and *medulla oblongata*, relays nerve impulses between the brain and spinal cord. With the thalamus and hypothalamus, it makes up the *reticular formation*, a nerve network that acts as an arousal mechanism.

The *peripheral nervous system* (Fig. 35-2) is composed of the cranial nerves that travel to or from the brain stem and the spinal nerves that travel to or from the spinal cord. These may be *motor (efferent)* or *sensory (afferent)*. The spinal cord forms a two-way conductor pathway between the brain stem and peripheral nervous system. It also is the reflex center for motor activities that do not involve brain control. Consisting of 31 pairs of spinal nerves and their intricate branches, the peripheral nervous system connects the CNS to remote body regions and conducts signals to and from these areas and the spinal cord.

The ANS is composed of the sympathetic and parasympathetic systems, which provide automatic control of vital functions. The ANS regulates body functions, such as digestion, respiration, and cardiovascular function.

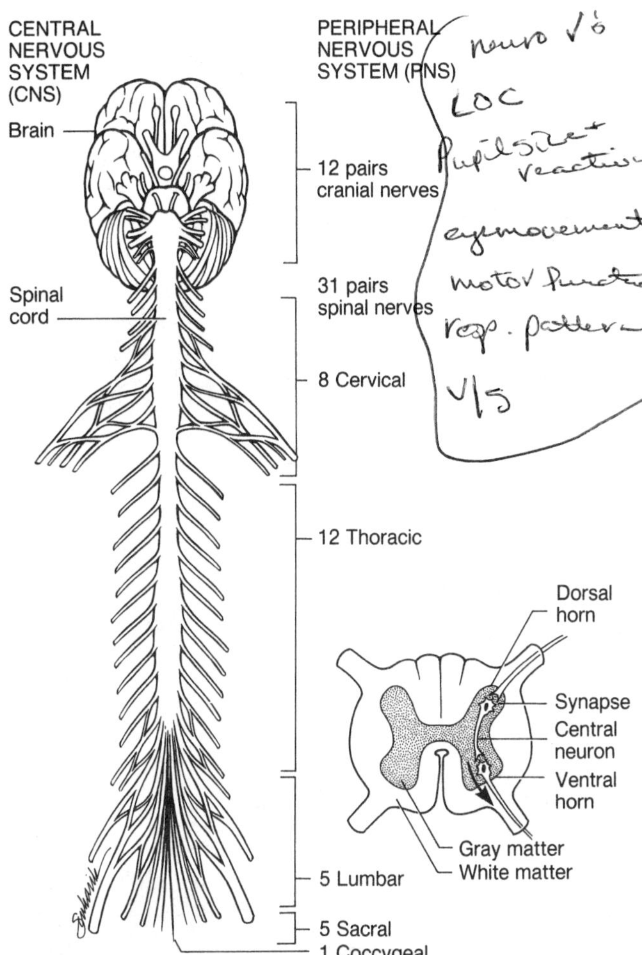

figure 35-2 *The spinal cord and vertebral column showing location of spinal nerves and vertebrae. Enlarged vertebrae showing gray and white matter and horns. (After Memmler, R. L. Cohen, B. J., & Wood, D. L. [1992].* Structure and function of the human body *[5th ed.]. Philadelphia: J. B. Lippincott, reprinted by permission.)*

age-specific considerations

The CNS arises from the neural tube during embryonic development. The neural tube develops by the fourth week of gestation; by the 8th to 12th week, the cerebrum and cerebellum begin to develop. In the first year of extrauterine life, the number of brain neurons increases rapidly.

Normally comprising 25% of the body weight at birth, the brain doubles in weight by the child's first birthday. Nerve *myelinization* in the CNS, the formation of myelin sheaths around nerve fibers, enables neuromuscular function to develop with time. Myelinization follows the cephalocaudal and proximodistal sequence, accelerating rapidly after birth.

The brain and spinal cord are among the first recognizable organs in the fetus and the last to finish significant development after birth. The development of motor skills depends on the maturation and myelinization of the nervous system; the process cannot be sped up by any type of special training. Nurses familiar with child development can better understand neurologic development and vice versa.

✳ family considerations

The manifestations, disabling consequences, and life-threatening nature of neurologic and sensory disorders create intense anxiety within the family. Many of the acute problems are rapid and aggressive, allowing little time for the family to adapt to the crisis situation. Chronic neurologic and sensory problems may be disabling, taking a heavy toll on the family's psychosocial, physical, and financial resources. Some of these disorders are genetic, adding to the guilt that families may have about their child's illness.

Families exert a tremendous influence on their members' physical, mental, spiritual, and social health through role modeling, verbal and nonverbal communications, customs, and values. A child's disabilities from traumatic injury or chronic illness affect the whole family.

Well-being and health dilemmas tend to appear and reappear in families over generations, and family members frequently engage in lifestyles promoting health, such as exercise, nutrition, and safety concerns, or engage in lifestyle patterns increasing health risks, such as poor nutrition (especially obesity), alcoholism, abuse, and chronic illness.

Families adjust to a diagnosis of a neurologic or sensory disorder in individual ways, especially to those that are disabling or life-threatening. Factors that affect a family's adjustment include available support systems, perception of the child's disorder and level of disability, coping mechanisms, available resources (such as finances), and other family stressors (such as divorce).

Families need to be educated about normal growth and development, and ways to allow their child to reach his or her own optimal level of development. They also need to develop coping skills and the ability to set realistic goals for their child and themselves.

✳ nursing considerations

Nurses need to know that neurologic and sensory disorders stem from many sources, including congenital defects, ingestion, infections, hereditary disorders, and trauma. Neurologic and sensory disorders affect many systems and may compromise the child's development and safety. Thus, the nurse needs to promote optimal functioning in a safe environment.

Many of the specialized tests for neurologic or sensory function can be threatening to children and frightening to parents. Pictures of special equipment and explanations about treatments are helpful to the older child. Dolls and puppets are helpful for preschoolers, and young children should be allowed to have personal objects with them whenever possible during procedures. Adequate preparation with time for questions and ventilation of feelings is necessary for the parents.

Nurses assist families in developing coping skills to promote positive adaptation and develop realistic goals. Nurses may assist in referrals to appropriate agencies for genetic counseling and financial assistance. Referrals can be made to organizations and self-help groups specific for the child's disorder (Display 35-1).

Rehabilitation of the child includes prevention of future problems, such as orthopedic deformities occurring in children with paralysis. Proper positioning, range of motion exercises, and effective use of splints help prevent foot drop and contracture.

A child's level of independence in mobility, bowel and bladder care, and social skills has an impact on the child's sense of initiative, industry, and self-concept. Age-appropriate information about sexuality is important to the child experiencing a neurologic or sensory problem.

Some studies have associated birth defects, disability, and chronic illness with an increased frequency of child abuse. Nurses working with disabled children must become aware of the risk factors and signs of abuse, such as unexplained injuries, such as spiral fractures and burns (see Chap. 37).

When neurologic disorders become life-threatening, parents must cope with the issues of death and dying. The primary nursing goals are to help the family and child understand and confront the possibility of the child's death (see page 452) and work through the grieving process. The nurse needs to allow the child to discuss his or her feelings about death (see page 454) and to determine ways to offer comfort and security to the child and family, using customs and rituals whenever possible. Families are encouraged to verbalize their feelings and to move through the grieving process at their own pace. Clergy are called as needed.

display 35-1
self-help groups and organizations for neurologic disorders

Epilepsy Foundation of America
4351 Garden City Drive
Landover, MD 20785

March of Dimes Foundation
1275 Mamaroneck Avenue
White Plains, NY 10605

National Association of Mothers of Special Children
9079 Arrowhead Court
Cincinnati, OH 45231

National Easter Seal Society
70 East Lake Street
Chicago, IL 60601

National Head Injury Foundation
333 Turnpike Road
Southboro, MA 01772

The National Tay-Sachs and Allied Diseases Association
385 Elliot Street
Newton, MA 02164

United Cerebral Palsy, Inc.
66 East 34th Street
New York, NY 10016

diagnostic tests

Diagnosis of neurologic and sensory disorders is usually based on a complete history, physical examination, and pertinent laboratory tests and imaging procedures. These tests and procedures may be noninvasive or invasive, and children and parents need to be prepared for them.

x-ray examinations

X-rays of the skull and spinal column allow for detection of traumatic fractures and bony changes associated with space-occupying lesions and malformations. The machinery is usually frightening to the small child who needs to be adequately prepared and comforted.

myelography

Myelography is an x-ray examination used to determine if the spinal cord is normal. The test requires a spinal tap followed by injection of a radiopaque dye or air into the subarachnoid space of the spinal canal and x-rays to outline the contents of the canal. If an oil-based dye is used, it is completely removed following the procedure, and the child is kept flat for up to 12 hours according to agency's policy.

Water-soluble contrast material, such as Omnipaque, is frequently used and does not require aspiration because it is absorbed by the blood and excreted by the kidneys. Following the procedure, the child's head and thorax are elevated 30 to 50 degrees for about 6 to 8 hours, with bed rest for 24 hours.

magnetic resonance imaging

Magnetic resonance imaging is a magnetic field study that provides information about the body's biochemistry by viewing the head, spinal cord, face, neck, heart, liver, bone and joints, and soft tissues.

electroencephalography

Electroencephalography (EEG) is a procedure that records amplified brain activity from several different points. It is used to analyze focal (localized) or generalized abnormalities of brain function.

The absence of brain wave activity is used to determine *brain death*. Brain death is used to sanction discontinuing life support systems.

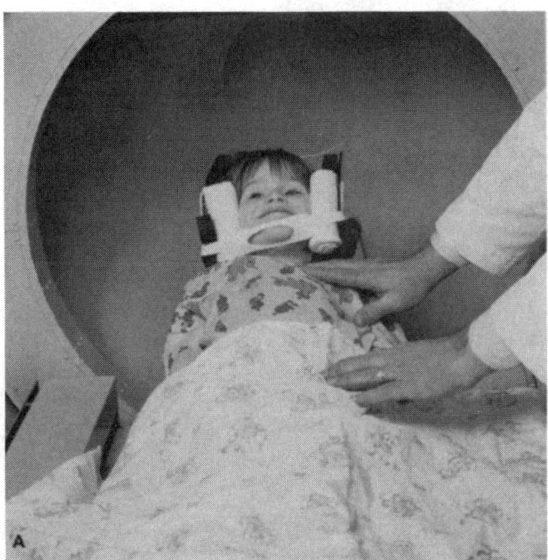

figure 35-3 *Computed tomography scan.*

This procedure takes about 1 hour and requires that electrodes be attached to the child's head. The hair must be washed before and after the EEG, and the child may be required to be "sleep deprived" the night before. Sedation also may be required during the test.

computed tomography

Computed tomography (CT) is a combination of x-ray and computer technology used to obtain a series of pictures of different tissue densities. The child must remain still on a large table that moves through a tubelike structure (Fig. 35-3); therefore, adequate preparation and possible sedation are required.

brain scans

Brain scans use a radioisotope substance that is injected intravenously, after which the brain is scanned for lesions. The child should be prepared for the injection and the scan.

lumbar puncture

In a lumbar puncture, also called a spinal tap, a needle is introduced into the subarachnoid space in the lower spinal canal. It is used to detect the presence of infection and increased pressure and can be used to introduce medications (intrathecal administration). One of the most important roles in performing a lumbar puncture belongs to the nurse who is holding and monitoring the child. The child is placed in a sitting or side-lying position with the knees and head flexed to cause the back to bow out and open the lumbar vertebral spaces (Fig. 35-4). Immobility in this position is critical to ensure a safe and accurate

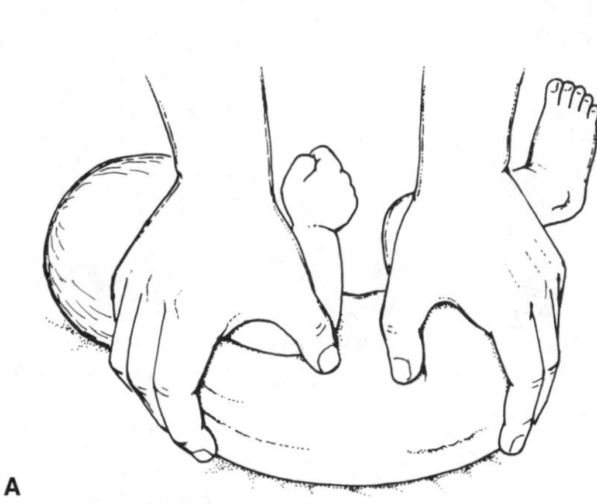

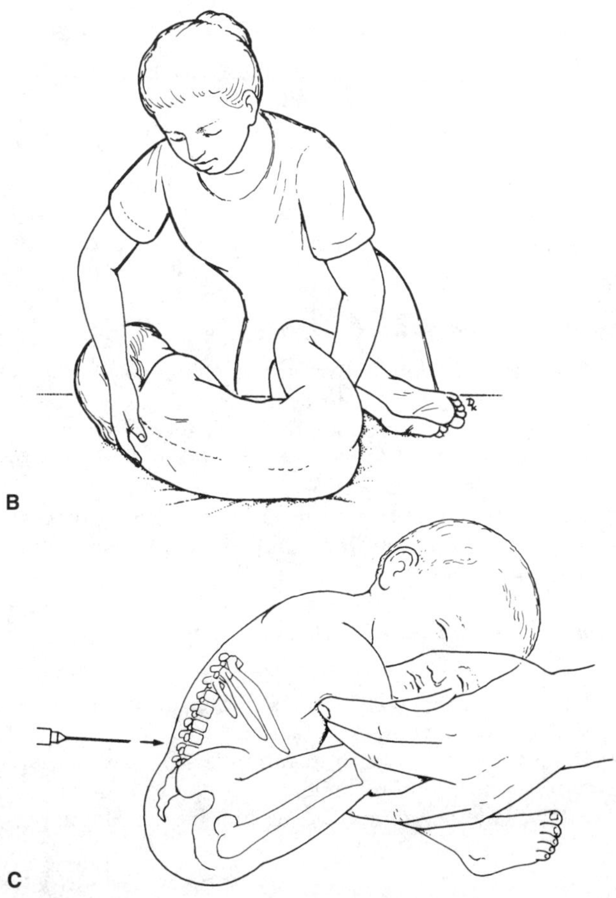

figure 35-4 *Positions for lumbar puncture.* ***(A)*** *The nurse places the child in the knee–chest position, either seated or reclining with neck flexed toward the knee.* ***(B)*** *The nurse restrains the patient by placing one arm under the fixed knee and grasps the child's wrists. The other arm is placed posteriorly around the patient's neck and shoulders.* ***(C)*** *The older child may sit voluntarily on the table, with elbows resting on knees and back arched. A pillow can be placed in front of the chest and the child instructed to grasp it. The small infant must be held in a sitting position by the assistant. By flexing the thighs on the abdomen, the assistant is able to grasp the elbow and knees in both hands, thus flexing the spine in the appropriate angle.*

puncture. Neonates have less distress in the side-lying position; however, they are still more susceptible to cardiorespiratory changes than older children and must be more carefully monitored. The sitting position may be used as an alternate with the child's buttocks at the edge of the table and the head flexed to the chin. Immobility is still critical.

Following the procedure, the child must remain flat or in a side-lying position (without a pillow) for 8 to 12 hours, depending on health care agency's protocol, to avoid a severe headache from unequal spinal fluid pressure or development of a subdural hematoma. The child's vital signs and level of consciousness (LOC) must be monitored, and the puncture site checked for drainage. Cerebrospinal fluid (CSF) specimens are carefully labeled and sent immediately to the laboratory.

✳ nursing process in neurologic and sensory disorders

assessment

Neurologic assessment of children is based on the developmental level of the child and helps to determine if problems are acute or chronic, diffuse or focal, and stable or progressive. Most of the neurologic assessment (Display 35-2) is nonintrusive and can even be fun if the nurse incorporates play, such as "Simon Says."

Subjective data to be assessed include the following:

health perception and health management

* Developmental history may point to lags in development or loss of important milestones.
* The child's ability to perform age-appropriate hygienic tasks is important.
* Question the family and child about the occurrence of seizure activity, such a loss of concentration, excessive day dreaming, facial "tics," muscle jerks, foot movement, rocking.

self-perception and self-concept

* Children with conditions such as spinal cord injuries, cerebral palsy (CP), and deafness may have negative feelings about their bodies and their sexuality.
* Children may be fearful of procedures and may cry or become withdrawn, anxious, or restless and agitated.
* Poor self-concept contributes to decreased positive interactions with peers, especially in the school-age child and adolescent.

family and peer relationships

* Neurologic or sensory disorders can affect the child's family and peer relationships due to impaired cognitive, sensory, and motor function.
* Determine what type of communication patterns are used for deaf or blind children.
* Sibling interaction may be impaired if the sibling perceives that the parents are devoting a greater amount of time to the ill child than they are to the siblings.
* The adolescent may have altered sexuality patterns, especially with spinal cord injuries.

Regardless of a child's age, neurologic objective data must include observing the child's grasping ability. An infant between 10 to 13 months uses a pincer grasp, while an older child can grasp and stack blocks or hold a crayon or pencil (Fig. 35-5). Objective data to be assessed include the following:

vital signs

* Temperature, blood pressure, pulse, and respiration provide information regarding circulation adequacy and LOC.
* Body temperature may be elevated from acute infec-

display 35-2
neurologic assessment

There are two general types of neurologic assessment: the initial assessment and the intermittent assessment. The initial assessment is comprehensive, while the intermittent assessment varies with the severity of the child's condition.

Initial assessment should include the following:

HISTORY

* Complete developmental history
* Any learning problems, clumsiness, coordination problems
* Febrile seizures, any other seizure activity
* Headaches, fainting, dizziness, head trauma
* Tremors and tics
* Memory loss, speech problems, unusual habits
* Sensory and motor problems
* Recent infections or ingestions of possible toxins

PHYSICAL ASSESSMENT

* General: general appearance, affect, interactions, speech
* Developmental: cognitive, psychosocial, gross and fine motor skills
* Mental status: level of consciousness, orientation, reasoning ability, memory
* Head circumference and fontanel assessment in infants
* Cranial nerve function
* Sensory status: vision, hearing, taste, tactile, olfactory
* Motor function: muscle tone and strength, posture
* Cerebellar status: balance and coordination
* Reflexes: infantile, later reflexes (eg, parachute); deep tendon reflexes

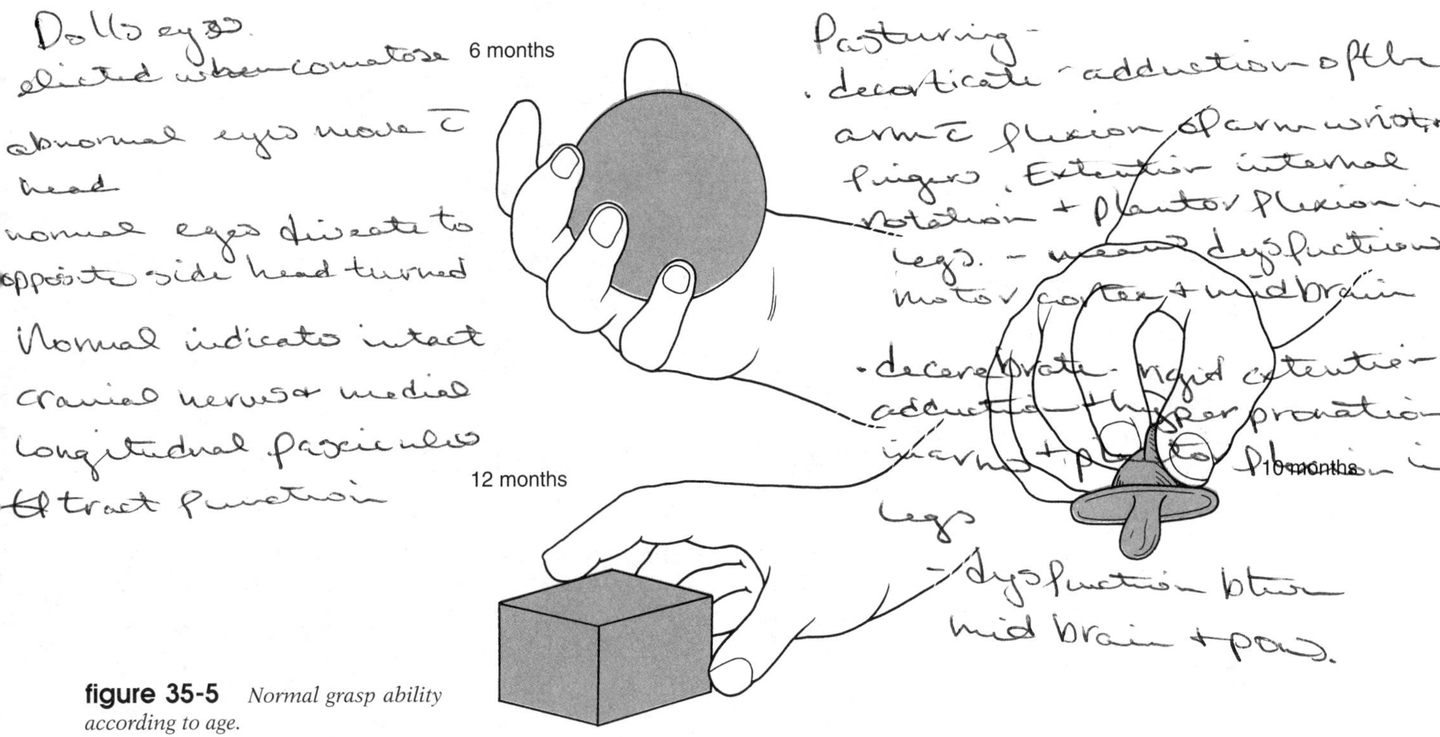

figure 35-5 *Normal grasp ability according to age.*

tious processes, toxic ingestion, or intracranial hemorrhage.

* Blood pressure may be normal, decreased, or increased. An increase in blood pressure signifies increased intracranial pressure (ICP), which may result from head trauma or tumors. A decrease in blood pressure may be due to excessive bleeding, causing hypovolemic shock symptoms, or to an extreme allergic response noted in anaphylactic shock.
* Pulse may be rapid, slow and bounding, or weak. The pulse rate decreases in increased ICP. The heart rate increases in response to cell oxygen deprivation.
* Respirations may be slow, deep, and irregular with increased ICP or increased with shock.
* Assess arterial blood gases.

head circumference, symmetry, eyes, and ears

* Assess head circumference (at birth, normal range is about 33–35 cm or 12–14 in), with increases of 2.6 cm (1 in) between 1 and 2 years. Significant decreases in head size indicate *anencephaly* (absence of both cerebral hemispheres or the entire brain) or *microcephaly* (small head measuring 2 standard deviations below average circumference size for age), predisposing the infant to inadequate brain growth and mental retardation. The cause of these two conditions is unknown but is linked with genetic disorders; intrauterine infections, such as rubella; and maternal alcoholism.
* The symmetry of the head is important because asymmetry is characteristic of *craniosynostosis*, described as premature closing of skull sutures, increasing a child's risk of poor brain development and mental retardation. When head asymmetry is noted, it is important to carefully assess for unequal eyes, low-set ears, and other body areas because when asymmetry appears in one area, it is frequently seen in others.
* Assess shape of eyes to detect slanted eyes (not specific for race), noted in Down syndrome, or "sunset eyes" (sclera is exposed above the iris), seen in advanced hydrocephalus or in brain stem lesions. Note eye movement, size of pupils, pupil response to light (darken the room, shine a penlight across the pupil, and observe the degree of constriction).
* Assess ear for signs of infection, such as drainage from ear canal or child pulling on ear. Low-set ears or misshapen ears can indicate neurologic problems.

orientation, mental status, speech, and language development

This assessment must be keyed to the child's developmental status. The Denver Developmental Screening Test may be used as a guide for children younger than 6 years (see Appendix). Concrete thinking begins during the school-age years, and speech is fairly well developed by 7 years; therefore, older children are somewhat easier to assess.

* Observe for memory deficit, disorientation, inaccurate interpretation of the environment, and distractibility.
* The child's LOC is assessed according to age and must be adapted to the traditional assessment of time, place, and person used in adult care. Infant assessment includes alertness, ability to recognize parents or caregivers, ability to follow sound with eyes, presence of a strong sucking reflex, strength of cry and ability to quiet when cuddled. Alteration of LOC in infants in-

cludes no response to parents or caregivers, lethargy, poor sucking response, shrill cry, persistent irritability, and "floppy," or "flaccid" muscle tone. A toddler's LOC is assessed by similar observations made in the infant.

* Toddlers are asked to point to their nose, mouth, or other body parts. Alert toddlers are able to reach or point to their parents, to self when asked, and will point to a light made by either a flashlight or penlight. Steadiness of gait can be assessed in an older toddler if ambulation is permitted.
* Preschool and school-age children are assessed similar to an adult. Although preschool and young school-age children have limited understanding of the concept of time, they have the ability to respond to questions about their age and recent holidays. School-age children are asked to state their address or telephone number and grade in school.
* Recent and remote memory may be tested by questioning the child about his or her first day of school and what he or she did recently in school. Children are considered *comatose* when they respond only to painful stimulation. *Coma* is described as an abnormally deep stupor resulting from trauma (especially concerning the head); illness, such as diabetic coma seen in insulin-dependent diabetes mellitus; or ingestion of drugs, such as nervous system depressants.
* Speech should be clear and not slurred. Preschoolers have a normal tendency to stutter (physiologic dysfluency). Observe for inappropriate or absent speech, decreased comprehension, and confusion. Cultural influences must be considered when evaluating speech patterns.

gross and fine motor control

* For the infant, observe the activity level, mobility, coordination of spontaneous movements, hand–eye coordination, grasp, resting position, and muscle tone.
* For the older child, observe the activity level, symmetry of posture, ability to walk and balance during walking, gait, hand grip, and muscle tone.
* For the adolescent, observe the gait, coordination, grip, and muscle tone.

coordination and balance

* For the infant, observe the coordination of spontaneous movements, hand–eye coordination, and coordination of rising from supine position to sitting.
* For the older child, observe gait, finger-to-nose coordination, heel-to-shin coordination, and Romberg test. This test is used to detect cerebellar dysfunction. The client is asked to stand with feet together, eyes open, and arms at the side while the nurse observes client's balance. The nurse then asks the client to close the eyes, and again the nurse observes the client's balance. As a safety precaution, the nurse holds outstretched arms on either side of the client to provide support if client sways to one side or the other. The test is considered positive if the client falls to one side.
* For the adolescent, observe the gait, finger-to-nose and heel-to-shin coordination, and Romberg test (Fig. 35-6).
* Neurologic disorders may result in absent, diminished, or unequal coordination.

sensation

* The infant normally withdraws from painful stimuli and grimaces.
* The child and adolescent normally have intact pain perception and the ability to perceive light touch, temperature, and vibration.

sleep and rest

* Neurologic disorders may interfere with the child's sleep and rest pattern. The child may be agitated, awaken frequently during the night, complain of interrupted sleep, or be increasingly listless and lethargic.

infant reflexes

* Infantile reflexes are checked to evaluate CNS integrity. See Chapter 16 for more information on infant reflexes.

nursing diagnoses

* Altered Health Maintenance, related to judgmental impairment or decreased motor functioning
* Impaired Skin Integrity, related to immobility
* Constipation, related to immobility
* Reflex Incontinence, related to neurologic impairment

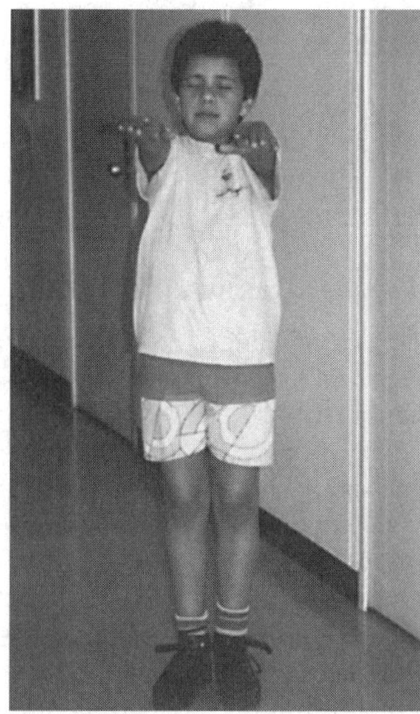

figure 35-6 *Romberg test: Have the child close eyes and stand with both feet together and arms raised in front for several seconds. Note any drift in arms or tendency to "list" to one side. (Courtesy of Dr. Donna Deanne, Wright State University, Dayton, OH.)*

* Impaired Physical Mobility, related to motor impairment
* Sleep Pattern Disturbance, related to interrupted sleep
* Pain, related to injury
* Impaired Verbal Communication, related to altered LOC
* Altered Thought Processes, related to altered LOC
* Sensory/Perceptual Alterations, related to altered LOC
* Fear and Anxiety, related to hospitalization and procedures
* Powerlessness, related to chronic illness
* Body Image Disturbance, related to altered mobility, hearing, and vision
* Parental Role Conflict, related to frequent or prolonged hospitalizations of the child
* Social Isolation, related to hospitalization and sensory deprivation
* Altered Sexuality Patterns, related to disabilities
* Risk for Ineffective Individual Coping, related to chronic illness
* Altered Nutrition: Less than body requirements, related to altered LOC

planning and implementation

promotion of orientation and speech

* Monitor child's orientation status and speech.
* Orient child to time, place, and person with frequent reminders and the use of helpful objects, such as calendars and clocks.
* Encourage normal speech patterns by encouraging child to speak for himself or herself.

promotion of fine and gross motor development

* Monitor child's fine and gross motor development.
* Encourage age-appropriate play activities that enhance fine and gross motor skills.

promotion of movement and safety factors

* Keep the crib or side rails up to prevent falls.
* Pad hard surfaces on beds and bony prominence on child to prevent injury due to involuntary movement.
* Perform passive range of motion exercises to prevent contracture.
* Reposition every 2 hours; if needed, place rolled pad in palms and use foot board and splint joints to prevent deformities.
* Provide skin care to maintain skin integrity. Use pressure-reducing mattress; protect pressure points on body, and inspect skin frequently for breakdown.

promotion of sensory stimulation

* Provide appropriate visual, auditory, and tactile stimulation through the use of crib mobiles, games, music, and touch.
* Encourage parents to bring in objects and toys from home that will enhance sensory stimulation, and encourage parents to participate in sensory stimulation.
* Assess for pain, and medicate as needed. Plan play periods when child's pain is lessened.
* Recommend respite care to allow parents and caregivers a break from child care and provide child stimulation from another source.

promotion of normal nutrition

* Provide adequate nourishment as indicated by the child's condition; consult nutritionist whenever possible.
* Monitor intravenous, nasogastric, and gastric feedings as indicated.
* Weigh daily, if possible, and monitor accurate intake.

promotion of normal growth and development

* Teach parents about normal growth and development patterns and what is expected for their child.
* Provide toys and play activities that are appropriate for the child's developmental level, which may not necessarily be the same as the child's chronologic age.

promotion of home care

* Recognize parental anxiety.
* Encourage parents to verbalize their feelings about caring for the child at home.
* Assist family in identifying available support systems.
* Observe parents' involvement with child and their ability to meet the child's needs.
* Answer parents' discharge concerns regarding reaching primary care provider 24 hours per day, reaching emergency services, monitoring child's neurologic status, detecting signs of deterioration, maintaining a safe environment to protect child from injuries, providing necessary treatments for child at home, promoting normal growth and development, and handling possible negative social reactions toward child's condition.
* Emphasize the importance of keeping follow-up appointments.

promotion of family and peer communications

* Encourage child and family to verbalize their concerns about interactions.
* Assist child and family in alternate methods of communication when necessary, with assistance from appropriate personnel, such as speech and physical therapists.

evaluation

* The child reaches and maintains optimal neurologic and sensory functioning.
* The child is free of complications from neurologic and sensory disorders.
* The child and family verbalize an understanding of diagnosis, treatment, home care, and follow-up care.
* The family system remains intact.

inherited disorders of the central nervous system

tay-sachs disease

Tay-Sachs disease is an inherited disorder that leads to mental retardation, paralysis, blindness, and death before 5 years of age. It is an autosomal recessive disorder usually noted in the Jewish Ashkenazi population.

pathophysiology

Tay-Sachs disease is characterized by the lack of an enzyme required to metabolize lipids (fats). The absence of this enzyme, hexosaminidase A, causes the lipids to accumulate in the cells of the body.

Infants with Tay-Sachs show an exaggerated startle response to noise and lose interest in the environment between the ages of 2 and 6 months. Mental retardation develops, along with progressive loss of vision, motor function, and control. Spasms and seizures occur as the disease progresses. Feeding becomes difficult, resulting in emaciation.

medical management

Because there is no cure for Tay-Sachs disease, care of the child and family is palliative.

Tay-Sachs can be prevented through genetic testing and counseling. Because the gene that causes the disease is recessive, both parents must be carriers for the disease to appear in their offspring. People who carry the recessive gene can be identified by a blood test. Tay-Sachs can be detected prenatally through amniocentesis, offering couples the opportunity to decide whether to continue a pregnancy if the fetus is affected by Tay-Sachs.

Prevention of Tay-Sachs through preconception counseling or prenatal testing may not be acceptable to the population most affected by this disorder, however. Strict Jewish laws forbid abortion and permit contraception only under special circumstances. In addition, most ultra-orthodox Jews choose not to take the blood test that identifies carriers, because it limits their marriageability. Confidential screening programs available in most major cities in the United States have been successful for the population involved, a group that follows the custom of arranged marriages. In these screening programs, individuals are assigned a number, and no names are recorded. Those who are identified as carriers are notified only if the proposed marriage partner also is a carrier. Families can thus report that the match has failed and seek a new marriage partner for their child.

nursing care

The nurse provides physical and psychosocial comfort measures for the child and teaching and emotional support for the grieving family. Genetic counseling is suggested if the couple plan to have other children.

injuries to the central nervous system

Injury accidents are the leading cause of death in children 1 year and older and the primary cause of CNS injuries. These injuries inflict a heavy psychological toll as well. Parents may feel guilty for not being able to protect their child, and children may feel that the injury is punishment for wrongdoing.

head injuries

Head injury is one of the most common causes of disability and death in children and can include anything from a mild bump to severe damage, such as skull fractures, brain injury, and subdural and epidural hematomas, concussion, and contusions. The common causes of head injuries vary with age and include birth trauma, abuse, falls, and motor vehicle accidents (see Chap. 20).

skull fractures

The type, extent, and accompanying symptoms of skull fracture depend on the speed, force, and weight of the object hitting the skull, the area of skull involved, and the age of the child. The younger the child, the more fragile the skull and the more delicate the soft tissue.

brain injury

Signs and symptoms depend on location and severity of the impact. Post-traumatic syndromes can include seizures, hydrocephalus, focal neurologic deficits, and metabolic complications (diabetes insipidus, hyponatremia or hypernatremia, hyperglycemic, or hyperosmolar states), and may occur as long as 2 years after the injury.

subdural and epidural hematomas

A *subdural hematoma* is formed by venous bleeding between the dura and arachnoid layer of the skull (Fig. 35-7*A*); this is the most common type of hematoma and can occur in neonates due to excessive molding of the skull during birth. An *epidural hematoma* is formed by bleeding (usually arterial) between the skull and the dura and subdural layers (see Fig. 35-7*B*), generally caused by severe head trauma; it is rarely seen in newborns. Subdural hematomas occur within 48 hours of injury and are characterized by headache, agitation, confusion, drowsiness, decreased LOC, and increased ICP (refer to page 611). Epidural hematomas have a rapid onset and are life-threatening; characteristic signs and symptoms include rapid deterioration, headache, seizures, coma, and brain herniation with compression of the brain stem.

cerebral concussions and contusions

A *concussion* is a head injury that produces a brief loss of consciousness, lasting from a few seconds to several hours, followed by amnesia. It is the most common type of head injury, particularly in contact sports, such as football. A *cerebral contusion* is a more severe injury that

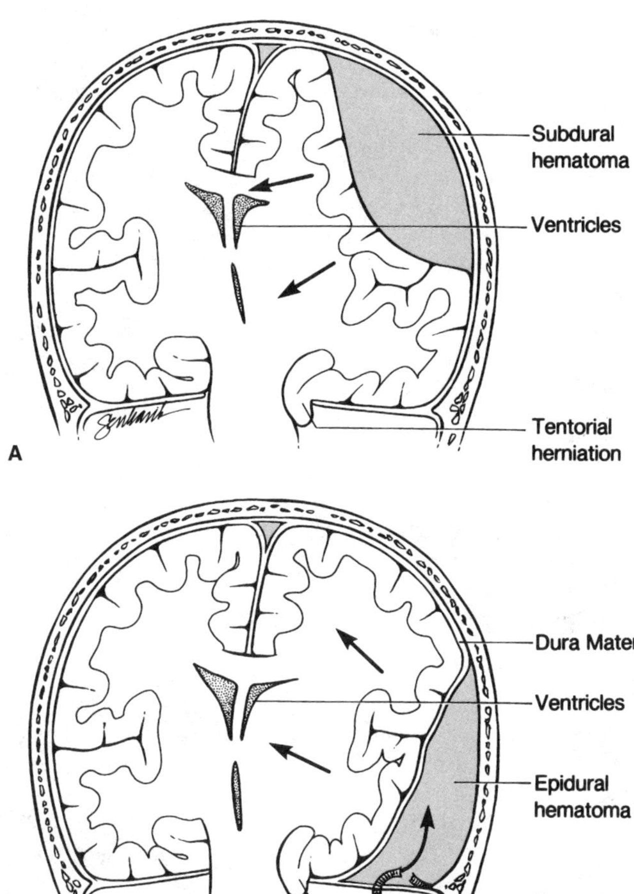

figure 35-7 *Epidural and subdural hematomas **(A)** Subdural hematoma. **(B)** Epidural hematoma. Note the broken blood vessel and the shift in the midline structures of the brain.*

bruises the brain tissue. Contusions cause loss of consciousness and other neurologic symptoms ranging from weakness and lethargy to coma or paralysis. Contusions in an infant or young child can be caused by violent shaking, called "shaken baby syndrome."

Diagnosis of concussion or contusion is based on the signs and symptoms, plus the history of the injury. If contusion is suspected, a CT scan is used to locate the bleeding lesion.

pathophysiology Concussions are often caused by a blunt force striking the skull hard enough to cause temporary unconsciousness but usually not hard enough to fracture the skull. Contusions bruise the brain when it strikes the rough inner surface of the skull, causing hemorrhaging. The bruising can occur at the site of the impact, called a *coup* injury, or opposite the site of the impact, called a *contrecoup* injury. Contusions occur more often in the occipital lobe than in the frontal lobes of the brain.

medical–surgical management Intervention is based on the extent of the injury. Children with mild concussions are simply monitored for complications. Children with more severe injuries are managed according to the amount of neurologic damage suffered.

nursing care The nurse carefully assesses the child for any signs of neurologic damage. This includes monitoring behavior, LOC, vital signs, pupils, mental status, movement, and coordination. Any signs of bleeding and increased ICP are reported immediately (Display 35-3).

increased intracranial pressure

pathophysiology

Increased ICP is excessive pressure within the rigid cranial vault that disrupts neurologic function. Normal intracranial pressure (ICP) ranges are from 0 to 15 mm Hg; ICP above 15 mm Hg is considered a medical emergency.

Increased ICP can result from any factor that increases tissue or fluid volume within the cranium, including tumors or other space-occupying lesions; accumulation of CSF in the ventricular system of the brain; intracranial bleeding; and edema of the cerebral tissues. Conditions that produce increased ICP include head injuries, birth trauma or asphyxia, hydrocephalus, brain tumor, meningitis, encephalitis, and intracerebral hemorrhage; many of these are related to the age of the child (Table 35-1).

The skull or cranium encloses and protects the brain, which is surrounded by CSF. Once the sutures of the infant skull fuse, any significant increase in the volume of the cranial contents (brain, CSF, and blood) can cause a life-threatening increase in ICP. Only two mechanisms can relieve increasing ICP: displacement of CSF to the

display 35-3
signs of increased intracranial pressure in infants and children

INFANTS

* Irritable, lethargic behaviors
* Increased head circumference
* Bulging fontanels
* Widening suture lines
* "Sunset" eyes
* High-pitched cry

OLDER CHILDREN

* Change in level of consciousness
* Irritability
* Vomiting
* Headache
* Elevated blood pressure
* Motor dysfunction
* Unequal pupil response
* Seizures

table 35-1 age-related causes of increased intracranial pressure

Newborn	*Infant and Preschooler*	*Older Child and Adolescent*
Birth trauma	Brain tumors	Brain tumors
Hemorrhage	Central nervous system infections	Diabetic ketoacidosis
Hydrocephalus	Diabetic ketoacidosis	Guillain-Barré syndrome
Perinatal asphyxia	Head trauma	Head trauma
	Hydrocephalus	Vascular disorders
	Hypercapnia	
	Hypoxia	
	Reye's syndrome	

spinal subarachnoid space and increased CSF absorption. If the increased volume exceeds the capacity of these mechanisms to relieve the ICP, brain damage can occur.

As ICP rises, it triggers a dangerous cycle: decreasing cerebral blood flow, increasing edema, and further increasing ICP. Unchecked, this cycle can result in complete loss of cerebral blood flow and brain cell death. Brain stem compression secondary to herniation (displacement of tissue) can cause life-threatening deterioration of vital functions.

Early signs and symptoms of increased ICP are usually subtle. Infants younger than 18 months have open fontanels and sutures that allow for limited expansion in response to ICP, but older children do not. Initial symptoms in infants and young children are irritability and restlessness and a tense, bulging anterior fontanel. Early, intermediate, and late symptoms in infants and older children are summarized in Table 35-2.

medical–surgical management

Treatment of increased ICP focuses on reducing intracranial volume and treating the underlying disorder. The physician may restrict fluids and order diuretics to reduce intracranial volume. Blood pressure control is critical because hypotension can further reduce oxygen supply to the brain, and hypertension can increase cerebral edema. Corticosteroids are often ordered to help reduce cerebral edema. Surgery may be necessary if acute subdural or epidural hematomas have formed.

nursing care

The nurse can assist in reducing ICP by elevating the head of the bed 15 to 45 degrees. The nurse assesses for early changes in ICP by monitoring vital signs (increased systolic blood pressure, wide pulse pressure, and bradycardia indicate increased ICP), noting alteration of LOC, respiratory status, motor activity, behavior, and pupil size and reactivity.

The nurse assists with treatments and supportive measures as ordered, such as mechanical ventilation, fluid re-

table 35-2 early, intermediate, and late symptoms of increased intracranial pressure

Early Symptoms	*Intermediate Symptoms*	*Late symptoms*
Irritability	Decrease in pulse and increase in systolic blood pressure	Decreased level of consciousness
Restlessness	Seizures	Decreased reflexes
Lethargy	Sluggish, unequal pupillary response	Decreased respiration or change in pattern
	Papilledema	Elevated temperature
	Projectile vomiting	Herniation of optic disc
		Dilated pupils
		Decorticate and decerebrate posturing
Poor feeding	Tense, bulging fontanel in child younger than 18 mo	Prominent scalp veins
Increased pitch of cry	Shrill cry	Enlarged head (prominent frontal portion over the eyes)
Full scalp veins	Increased head circumference	Sunset eyes
Tense fontanel		
Rubbing head		
Headache	Severe headache	
Anorexia	Blurred vision	
Nausea or vomiting	Diplopia	
Unsteady gait		

striction, and temperature control. It is important to help the child avoid positions or activities that increase ICP, such as activities that could cause neck vein compression (eg, flexion or extension of the neck, turning the head from side to side); painful or stressful stimuli, and respiratory suctioning or percussion.

> **nursing insight**
> *Activities such as coughing, straining, turning, or being suctioned causes an increase in intracranial pressure.*

The nurse promotes regular bowel elimination to prevent straining during defecation. Small, frequent feedings help prevent weight loss; however, intravenous nutrients may be needed. Gastrostomy tube feedings are used if the child remains unconscious or not alert enough to take foods by mouth. Normal growth and development should be promoted without overstimulating the child. The nurse prevents skin breakdown by placing the child on a sheepskin or other resilient mattress appliance. When surgical intervention is necessary to relieve increased ICP; procedures may include subdural tap, ventriculostomy, epidural evacuation, placement of ventricular shunt, decompressive craniectomy, or tumor resection.

cerebral palsy

Cerebral palsy is a nonspecific term used to describe a group of disabilities involving impaired motor function and posture. The most common childhood physical disability, CP is nonprogressive and not inherited but is closely associated with low birth weight and prematurity. About 25,000 new cases of CP are reported annually.

pathophysiology

Injury or insult to the brain before or during birth or in early infancy is the cause of CP. Risk factors include prematurity, asphyxia, ischemia, perinatal trauma, congenital and perinatal infections, and perinatal metabolic problems, such as hyperbilirubinemia and hypoglycemia. Infection, trauma, or tumors can cause CP in early infancy, and some cases remain unexplained.

Disabilities usually result from injury to the cerebellum, the basal ganglia, or the motor cortex. However, it is often difficult to identify the exact location of the lesion or the cause because CP varies widely in its clinical manifestations.

Delayed gross motor development is the most universal sign of CP. The child often shows a poor ability to suck and persistent tongue thrusting, creating feeding problems. Crawling is delayed and asymmetric. Alterations of muscle tone are common: increased or decreased resistance to passive movements, stiffness when being handled or dressed, and opisthotonos (exaggerated arching of the back). Abnormal posturing includes scissoring legs and persistent infantile positions, such as flexed elbows and fisted hands. Primitive reflexes, such as the tonic neck, Moro, and plantar, which normally disappear by 6 months, persist in CP.

Associated disabilities include mental retardation, seizures, attention deficit disorder, and sensory impairment. However, not all children with CP are mentally retarded; some have average or near-average intelligence. Each child with CP must assisted to achieve his or her full potential.

medical–surgical management

Although CP is nonprogressive, it may become more apparent as the child grows older. Severe cases may be detected at birth, but mild and moderate cases are not usually detected until the child is 1 or 2 years old. Failure to achieve developmental milestones may be the first sign of CP. There is no specific test to determine CP. Diagnosis is based on prenatal, birth, and postnatal history; neurologic examination; and assessment of muscle tone, behavior, and abilities. Other disorders such as degenerative disorders need to be ruled out.

There is no cure, but the child can be assisted to reach his or her highest potential. As with many neurologic disorders, treatment involves a multidisciplinary team of physician, nurse, physical therapist, social worker, and others. The goals of treatment are to promote mobility, communication skills, and self-care; correct associated problems as effectively as possible; offer educational opportunities appropriate to the individual child's needs and abilities; and provide support and health teaching to the child and caregivers.

Mobility in the child with CP can be promoted with braces and wheeled mobilization devices that allow self-propulsion, such as walkers, go-carts, scooter boards, and wheelchairs. Safety devices, such as helmets and body pads, are recommended for children with poor head and body control.

Orthopedic surgery may be needed to correct deformities and decrease spasticity. Surgery needs to be followed with physical therapy and regular exercises at home.

Medications are not helpful for spasticity. However, seizure medications, such as phenytoin, may be prescribed.

nursing care

The goals of nursing care include prevention of physical injury and physical deformity, promotion of mobility and self-care, and continuation of the rehabilitation treatment plan at home. The nurse administers prescribed medications and provides the child with a safe environment, appropriate toys, and a protective helmet if needed. Prescribed braces and other devices and range of motion

> **nursing insight**
> *Feeding children with cerebral palsy involves the following:*
>
> * *Slow pace to prevent aspiration*
> * *Upright position*
> * *Support of lower jaw*

exercises help prevent physical deformity. The nurse encourages the child to perform age-appropriate and condition-appropriate motor activities. A high-protein, high-calorie diet helps children with CP meet their increased energy needs. The nurse promotes relaxation and general health by providing rest periods.

The child is encouraged to participate in activities of daily living, using age- and condition-appropriate utensils and implements. Talking to the child deliberately and slowly and using pictures to reinforce speech facilitates communication. Speech therapy and physical therapy may be warranted. Electronic devices, such as computers, may help children with severe articulation problems. As necessary, encourage parents to seek referrals for corrective lenses and hearing devices to decrease sensory deprivation related to visual and hearing loss.

The nurse helps promote a positive self-image by praising the child's accomplishments, setting realistic and attainable goals, encouraging an appealing physical appearance, and encouraging peer group activities. Encouraging family members to express anxieties, frustrations, and concerns and to explore support networks, such as the United Cerebral Palsy Association, helps families cope with this permanent disability.

spinal cord injuries

Spinal cord injury is damage to the vertebral column, the spinal cord itself, or the spinal cord nerves. It is more common in adults than in children, but adolescents are at increased risk due to motor vehicle accidents, gunshot and knife wounds, and diving accidents. Spinal cord injury can cause paraplegia (loss of function in the lower extremities) or quadriplegia (loss of function below the shoulder area).

pathophysiology

Spinal cord injury may result from internal or external factors. Internal injuries are the most common, caused by fractures, dislocations of vertebrae, or violent agitation of the cord. External injuries are caused by an object, such as a bullet or knife, penetrating the cord.

Manifestations of spinal cord injury depend on the location and extent of the injury. Signs and symptoms are divided into three phases: *First recovery phase* occurs immediately after injury and results in spinal shock syndrome, also called *diaschisis*. Spinal shock syndrome causes loss of reflexes and sensory and motor functions at or below the level of injury; loss of temperature and vasomotor control, including ability to sweat; loss of bowel and bladder function; and flaccid paralysis of the affected muscles.

During *second recovery phase,* flaccid paralysis changes to spastic paralysis, which may be mistaken for normal movement. The bowel and bladder also may become spastic (hypertonic), causing forceful evacuation of feces and urine.

Neurologic signs stabilize in the *third recovery phase*, and the prognosis for recovery of function becomes clearer. Permanent disabilities depend on the location of the injury; the higher the injury, the greater the loss of function (Fig. 35-8). The diagnosis is based on a careful history and physical and by x-ray examination and possible CT scan.

> **nursing alert**
> *Spinal cord injury must be suspected any time a child has received a trauma with any degree of force.*

During initial emergency care, it is essential to stabilize the child's head and trunk to prevent further damage. Medical management typically includes steroids and possibly diuretic administration to prevent or reduce cerebral edema, artificial ventilation if respiratory function is compromised, and cervical traction to stabilize and maintain vertebral alignment. Long-term management is aimed at restoration of function and involves a multidisciplinary rehabilitation team to enable the child to reach his or her maximum potential.

Prognosis depends on extend and location of spinal cord damage. Thoracic lesions usually result in loss of motor function and life in a wheelchair. Cervical injuries are variable. Clients with *incomplete lesions* may have some level of function below the level of injury; those with *complete lesions* have no function below the level of injury.

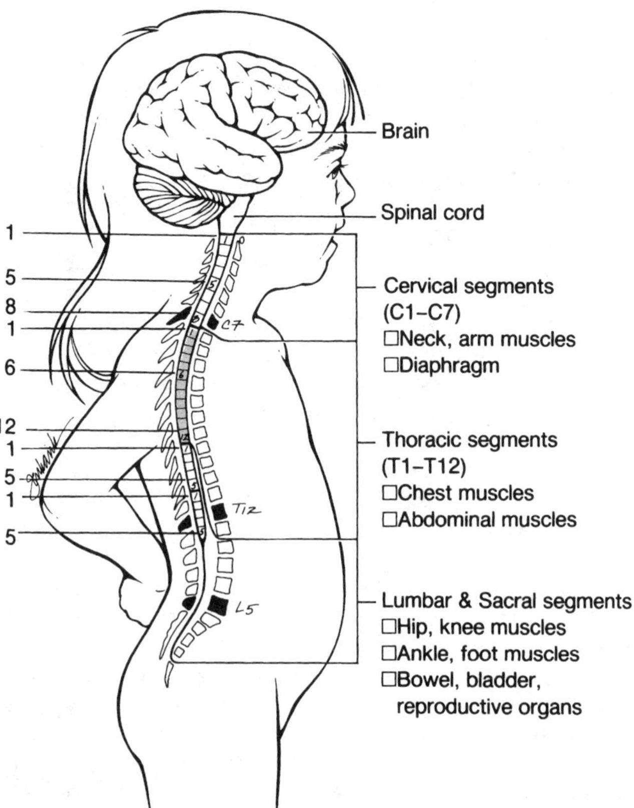

figure 35-8 *The level of a spinal cord injury determines the degree of function that can ultimately be regained.*

Many require artificial maintenance of respirations. Lumbar lesions involve partial or complete loss of function in the lower extremities and loss of bladder function.

nursing care

recovery phases Initial nursing care is supportive and focused on preventing complications and maintaining vital functions. The nurse assists with intravenous fluids, oxygen therapy, medication management, urethral catheterization, and nasogastric suctioning. To prevent aspiration, the client takes nothing by mouth.

During the second phase, care is aimed at rehabilitation and preparing the child and family for discharge. Medications may include nitrofurantoin to prevent bladder infection, diazepam or baclofen to control muscle spasms, and analgesics to relieve pain.

respiratory care Children with injuries above the fourth cervical vertebra (C4) require continuous respiratory support. Oral or a nasotracheal intubation will later be replaced with a tracheostomy tube. Children with lesions below C4 can breathe on their own but are usually unable to cough and deep breath properly, making breathing exercises and assistive devices essential to prevent respiratory infections.

temperature control Dysfunction of the ANS can disrupt the body's temperature regulation mechanisms. Because the child with spinal cord injury cannot sweat, hyperthermia can develop if dressed or covered too warmly. If covered inadequately, the child can lose heat. Therefore, the temperature of the room and of the child need to be monitored frequently and regulated carefully.

immobilization and safety Children with spinal cord injury are usually immobilized for prolonged periods with cervical traction devices. The appearance of these devices and the nature of the procedures can cause child and parents great fear and anxiety unless the nurse helps them understand what to expect and why the procedures are important. Extreme caution is used when positioning the child to avoid further injury.

Passive range of motion during bathing and a minimum of once a shift is effective in preventing contracture. The use of foot boards and tennis shoes helps prevent foot drop. Muscle spasms are a common occurrence and can be severe enough to cause bruising of the soft tissue or bone fracture as the extremity swings out of control. Nursing interventions aimed at care of the child with frequent muscle spasticity include padding crib sides or side rails, applying splints as ordered, handling extremities with gentle yet firm control, and using safety devices, such as seat belts, when child is in a wheelchair or chair.

skin care Prolonged bed rest, inability to change positions, and decreased sensation and peripheral circulation put children with spinal cord injury at high risk for pressure sores. Special beds and mattresses can be used, such as water beds, alternating pressure mattresses, foam rubber mattresses, and sheepskin, to prevent skin breakdown. Assessment of the skin, especially in prime breakdown areas, such as the sacrum, scapulae, heels, and occiput when supine; the trochanter and lateral aspects of the ankles, heels, and knees when sidelying; and the ischial tuberosities when sitting, helps identify problems and promotes early intervention. The skin must be kept clean and dry, and the use of foam protectors is encouraged. Children are turned every 2 hours, using a log-rolling technique to keep the spine in straight alignment (See Teaching Guidelines).

nutritional management To promote healing and continued growth and development, the child with spinal cord injury requires a diet rich in protein, calories, and vitamins. Vitamin C may be administered to acidify the urine and help prevent the formation of renal calculi. The nurse monitors the child's weight and intake and output.

bladder and bowel training Restoring bladder function after spinal cord injury requires urologic evaluation. Nursing care is aimed at preventing skin breakdown and infection and educating the child and family in bladder training. Bladder training involves strengthening the bladder muscle to promote retention and interventions aimed at promoting elimination. Loss of bladder tone can lead to urinary retention. During the initial treatment phase, the child may have an indwelling catheter, replaced by an intermittent catheterization program during rehabilitation. Intermittent catheterization is performed by the child if age appropriate or by the caregiver and involves self-catheterization to drain the bladder at least every 4 hours. Clients are taught to use a mirror to view the urinary meatus, wipe the meatus with betadine, and insert the catheter using aseptic technique as opposed to sterile technique. The frequent catheterization can lead to chronic cystitis, requiring prophylactic urinary antibiotic administration and urine cultures. Repeated infections can lead to renal failure, a frequent cause of death in spinal injury patients. Unless edema is a problem, forcing fluids, such as cran-

teaching guidelines
log rolling

Log rolling is a way of moving a person so the spine is kept straight.

* This requires two or more people, depending on the child's size.
* The child is carefully moved on a "lift" pad or sheet to the side of the bed away from where he or she is to be turned (eg, if moving to the left, child would face the right).
* Turn the child in a synchronized motion (log rolled), supporting the spine in a straight line.
* Place pillows between the child's legs, to the back, and in other areas for support and comfort, taking care to maintain a straight position.

berry juice, and encouraging compliance to proper catheterization technique and medication administration helps prevent urinary tract infections.

Collection devices for boys, such as condom catheters, and incontinent pants or diapers may be necessary because dribbling occurs if the bladder sphincter lacks muscle tone. Older children are often anxious about urine odors and require careful incontinence monitoring to prevent embarrassment and skin breakdown.

Bowel training is usually simpler and more successful than bladder training. A high-fiber diet is recommended. Regularly scheduled use of suppositories, such as glycerin or bisacodyl (Dulcolax), helps establish a pattern for bowel movements. Stool softeners and digital stimulation may be required.

activity promotion Active and passive range of motion exercises are planned in collaboration with the physical therapist. Antispasmodic medications, such as diazepam, are helpful for children who are spastic. A number of adaptive devices and appliances are available to help children with mobility and activities, including play.

psychosocial support Spinal cord injuries are usually sudden and represent a devastating loss for the child and family. This loss triggers a grief reaction that includes denial and shock in the acute phase. The nurse needs to provide psychological support for the child and family and physical care of the child. Losing control over body functions and becoming dependent on others can have a dramatic effect on the child's self-concept and body image.

The grieving process continues in later stages of treatment, as both child and family express anger, anxiety, and depression in trying to cope with immobility and learning new skills. The nurse can help by explaining the child's condition, procedures, and skills needed for self-care and by allowing the child and family to verbalize their feelings. The financial and emotional impact of the child's condition is so great, however, that many families will need a more experienced counselor and referral to support groups.

rehabilitation The family may need assistance in selecting a rehabilitation facility, and referrals need to be made for home health when indicated. The nurse discusses the possibilities with the family and encourages them to ask questions and visit the site whenever possible. Quality rehabilitation centers are accredited by the Commission on Accreditation of Rehabilitation Facilities.

neurologic infections

meningitis

Meningitis is an infection of the meninges caused most frequently by bacterial invasion (bacterial meningitis) and less frequently by viruses (aseptic meningitis). Infants between 6 and 12 months are at greatest risk of developing meningitis.

pathophysiology

Haemophilus influenzae, *Neisseria meningitides*, and *Streptococcus pneumonia* are the most common organisms responsible for bacterial meningitis in children 2 months or older. Group B streptococci and *Escherichia coli* are the most common causative organisms for neonatal meningitis. Bacterial meningitis is fatal if not treated immediately. Viral meningitis is a self-limiting disease that lasts 7 to 10 days.

In bacterial meningitis, the bacteria enter the meninges through the bloodstream and spread through the CSF. The infection may occur directly through trauma or neurosurgery. The pathogen acts as a toxin, triggering an inflammatory response of the meninges, leading to release of purulent exudate, which quickly spreads the infection. Vascular congestion and inflammation lead to cerebral edema, which may produce increased ICP and hydrocephalus. Necrosis of brain cells can cause permanent damage and death.

In children younger than 2 years, assessment of symptoms includes nuchal rigidity (stiff neck), poor feeding, frequent regurgitation, irritability and lethargy, high-pitched cry, bulging fontanel, fever or low temperature, and a resistance to being held. Later in the disease, they may exhibit *opisthotonus* (hyperextension of the neck and spine).

> **✱ nursing insight**
>
> *Assess neck (nuchal) rigidity in older children with suspected meningitis by asking them to kiss their knees while keeping their legs extended; neck rigidity will prevent them from completing the task.*

Older children with meningitis may show initial symptoms of respiratory or gastrointestinal problems and then nuchal rigidity. A petechial (pinpoint hemorrhage under the skin) type rash may be present, and vomiting can indicate increased cranial pressure.

Diagnosis is based on examination of CSF obtained through lumbar puncture and blood tests. The fluid is typically cloudy with protein values increased and glucose levels decreased. Blood tests include an elevated white blood cell count and blood cultures to identify the causative organism.

medical management

Bacterial meningitis is treated with intravenous antibiotics. Corticosteroid and mannitol may be used to treat cerebral edema. Careful monitoring is necessary up to 24 hours following antibiotic administration because bacterial toxins are released as the antibiotic destroys the bacteria, predisposing the child to septicemia, purpura, and seizure activity.

nursing care

The child with meningitis can deteriorate rapidly. Nursing interventions include monitoring vital signs every 15 minutes to 1 hour until the child has stabilized; assessing behavior, LOC, signs of increased cranial pressure, seizure activity, and posturing; monitoring intake and output every 2 hours or as ordered (fluid intake may be limited to prevent cerebral edema); assessing specific gravity every 8 hours; and measuring head circumference and assessing fontanels every 8 hours.

> **nursing alert**
> *Children with diminished consciousness receive nothing by mouth to prevent aspiration pneumonia.*

The nurse administers prescribed intravenous antibiotics, such as gentamicin, and assesses the intravenous site for redness and edema. The type of antibiotic depends on the causative organism. Steroids may be ordered to decrease cerebral edema.

The nurse provides a quiet environment with minimal environmental stimuli. Elevating the head of the bed slightly usually makes the child more comfortable. Because seizures can occur, it is important to pad the side rails and keep them elevated and maintain oxygen and suction equipment in the room.

isolation A child is placed in isolation as soon as meningitis is suspected and remains in isolation until the causative organism is identified. Children with bacterial meningitis require respiratory isolation until they have completed 24 hours of antibiotic therapy. Children with viral meningitis require excretion precautions throughout their hospitalization. Nurses must observe universal precautions when taking care of all patients.

encephalitis

Encephalitis is an acute inflammation of the brain, usually caused by a virus. Because it can lead to coma, encephalitis is also called *sleeping sickness.* Viral encephalitis is an acute and sometimes fatal disease, with mortality rates of 5% to 20%.

pathophysiology

Arboviruses carried by mosquitoes and ticks can cause encephalitis, as can the herpes simplex virus. Most deaths result from herpes simplex-related encephalitis. Chronic or nonepidemic encephalitis may follow measles, chickenpox, or mumps. Viral encephalitis can cause diffuse damage to the nerve cells of the brain and increase cerebral edema.

Characteristics are similar to meningitis but have a more gradual onset. Seizures, high fever, headache, and altered LOC are the most common characteristics. Diagnosis is made by history and physical assessment and assessment of blood and CSF.

medical–surgical management

Treatment is symptomatic and includes treatment of cerebral edema when indicated. Treatment for herpes encephalitis includes acyclovir administration, which is started before diagnosis is confirmed due to increased risk of mortality.

nursing care

Nursing care is the same as for the child with meningitis or ICP. Key assessments include monitoring LOC, vital sign changes, and signs of increased cranial pressure.

reye's syndrome

Reye's syndrome is an acute, multisystem disorder that follows a mild viral infection, usually influenza or varicella. The cause of Reye's syndrome is not known; however, it has been linked to use of aspirin during a viral illness. Since 1980, the number of cases reported has declined 91% in children younger than 5 years and 75% in children older than 5 years.

pathophysiology

Reye's syndrome is characterized by encephalopathy and fatty degeneration of the liver, kidneys, heart, skeletal muscle, and pancreas. Impaired liver function causes hypoglycemia and increased levels of ammonia and lactic acid in the blood and brain.

Laboratory findings include elevated serum glutamic-oxaloacetic transaminase, serum glutamic-pyruvic transaminase, and lactic dehydrogenase; elevated ammonia levels; and prolonged prothrombin time. Acid–base imbalance occurs with both respiratory alkalosis and metabolic acidosis. White blood cell count may be as high as 20,000/μL. Liver biopsy establishes definitive diagnosis.

stages of reye's syndrome Reye's syndrome progresses in stages (Table 35-3). Children who are diagnosed and treated while in stage I have a good prognosis. Those who are beyond stage II when admitted to the hospital have a poor prognosis. Nearly half of children in stage III or beyond die; those who do recover may have major neurologic dysfunction. Deterioration to coma and death from Reye's syndrome can occur in 24 to 48 hours.

table 35-3 stages of Reye's syndrome

Stage	Characteristics
Stage I	Vomiting, lethargy, confusion, rhythmic slowing of electroencephalogram, liver dysfunction
Stage II	Disorientation, combativeness, hyperventilation, hallucinations, appropriate responses to painful stimuli, liver dysfunction
Stage III	Coma, decorticate rigidity, hyperventilation, preservation of pupillary and ocular reflexes
Stage IV	Deepened coma, decerebrate rigidity, loss of "doll's eye" reflexes, large fixed pupils, evidence of brainstem dysfunction
Stage V	Seizures, flaccidity, respiratory arrest, loss of deep tendon reflexes

medical management

The most important aspect of treatment is to diagnose the disorder early and to treat it aggressively, particularly increased ICP and fluid and electrolyte imbalance. Children are treated in an intensive care setting; arterial and central venous lines are inserted to monitor hemodynamics, and fluid restriction and mechanical ventilation may be needed. Hypoglycemia is controlled with hypertonic glucose and NaCl; vitamin K may be given to increase blood clotting ability.

The priority intervention for Reye's syndrome is prevention: children with viral infections are not to be given aspirin. Early identification of Reye's syndrome is essential for a positive outcome.

nursing care

Altered respirations is a common problem in children with Reye's syndrome; this requires careful monitoring of respiratory status, including airway patency, respiration rate, and presence of dyspnea, cyanosis, sternal retractions, and nasal flaring.

The child in a comatose state is totally dependent on caregivers to satisfy all biologic needs. The nurse provides sensory stimulation and ensures adequate nutritional intake, usually through intravenous or nasogastric tube, until the child can tolerate oral feedings.

It is important to support the family, provide information about the disease process and treatment, and allow the family to verbalize their concerns and fears. Parents may feel guilty if they administered aspirin to the child.

rabies

Children exposed to wild animals or household pets that have not been immunized against rabies are at risk for contracting rabies if bitten. This infection can be fatal if not treated.

pathophysiology

Rabies is an acute infection of the CNS caused by a virus and transmitted to humans through the bite (and sometimes scratch) of an infected mammal. Cats are the most common domesticated animal to carry the rabies virus; bats are the most common carriers among wild animals. Skunks, raccoons, and foxes also are potential carriers. Any child bitten by a wild animal is considered exposed and must be treated promptly to avoid infection.

The incubation period is usually from 1 to 3 months. Early signs and symptoms include general malaise, fever, sore throat, and irritability, followed by an excitement phase with hypersensitivity and increased reaction to external stimuli, seizures, confusion, combative behavior, and choking. Severe spasms of the respiratory muscles cause apnea, cyanosis, and anoxia. Diagnosis is based on history and physical findings.

medical management

Treatment for a bite or scratch from an animal thought to carry rabies includes prompt, thorough wound cleansing and passive immunization with human rabies immunoglobulin (HRIG). The HRIG injection provides only short-term immunity. Long-term immunity involves a series of injections of the human diploid cell rabies vaccine. The first dose is administered with the passive vaccine, followed by doses at 3, 7, 14, and 28 days after the first dose. The World Health Organization recommends an additional dose 3 months after the 28-day injection.

nursing care

Animal bites, the threat of rabies, and treatment involving multiple injections make this a frightening emergency for children and parents. The nurse can provide emotional support, explanations, and the reassurance that the therapy is effective. Nurses encourage prevention by teaching children and caregivers not to approach wild or unfamiliar animals and by encouraging people to obtain rabies vaccinations for their cats, dogs, and other pets.

neurologic tumors

neuroblastoma

Neuroblastoma is a tumor coming from cells in the adrenal medulla or sympathetic ganglia extending from the neck to the pelvis. It is the most common solid tumor formation of children with better survival rates in children younger than 1 year. The tumor is staged from I to IV according to chest x-ray, chest CT scan, skeletal survey, bone scan, and magnetic resonance imaging (Table 35-4).

pathophysiology

Children with neuroblastoma typically have a palpable abdominal mass at about 2 years. They often complain of bone and back pain and experience weight loss, weakness, urinary and stool retention, and fever. Anemia and thrombocytopenia (decreased platelets) are often noted.

medical–surgical management

Treatment of neuroblastoma involves the combined use of surgery, radiation therapy, and chemotherapy. The size of

table 35-4 neuroblastoma staging

Stage	*Description*
Stage I	Tumor is limited to the initial organ site.
Stage II	Tumor expands beyond the initial organ site, may involve lymph nodes on affected side but does not cross the midline.
Stage III	Tumor expands from the initial organ site, beyond the midline, affecting lymph nodes on both sides of the body.
Stage IV	Tumor affects bones, soft tissue, and distant lymph nodes.
Stage V	Tumor expands from the initial organ site to one or more of the following sites: liver, skin, and bone marrow.

the tumor dictates the initial form of treatment. If possible, surgical removal is the first choice of treatment, followed by radiation and chemotherapy.

nursing care

Nursing care involves providing age-appropriate explanations to the child and parents. Palliative treatment during radiation and chemotherapy is aimed at providing comfort, proper nutrition, and safety.

brain tumors

Brain tumors are the second most common cancer in children (leukemia is the most common). Most pediatric brain tumors are situated close to vital structures, making them difficult to excise. Gliomas are the most common childhood brain tumor.

nursing care

Headache, especially when awakening, is the most common presenting symptom of a brain tumor. Vomiting without nausea usually occurs in the morning. Assessment of the child reveals a loss of coordination and vision problems when the head is tilted. Widening of sutures with increasing frontal occipital circumference is seen in infants.

Child and parents must be supported during diagnostic work-up and treatment. If surgery is the treatment, the nurse provides preoperative teaching, including information about the child's head being shaved and the protocol for the intensive care unit. Postoperatively, the nurse monitors intravenous fluids and output every 2 to 4 hours (overhydration can cause cerebral edema and increased ICP). Steroids and diuretics are administered as ordered.

other disorders

seizure disorders

A seizure is a disturbance in normal brain function that can lead to loss of consciousness, uncontrolled body movements, loss of bowel and bladder control, and changes in behaviors and sensation.

pathophysiology

Seizures result from overly active and hypersensitive neurons in the brain, which cause abnormal electrical discharges. Seizures can be caused by many different diseases and disorders, such as prenatal or perinatal hypoxia, infections, congenital malformations, metabolic disturbances, lead poisoning, head injuries, drug abuse, alcohol misuse, tumors, medications, and toxins (Table 35-5). Most seizures are idiopathic (of unknown origin).

✳ nursing insight

Seizures are more common in children younger than 2 years due to the immaturity of the central nervous system.

table 35-5 origin of seizures based on age

Age	*Cause*
Infancy	Prenatal trauma, hypoxia, infections, congenital factors such as hydrocephalus
Childhood	Central nervous system infections, ingestion of poison (especially lead), and head trauma typical of falls, bicycle accidents
Adolescence	Drug and alcohol abuse or misuse, intracranial pressure (brain tumors, trauma), and toxins

Adapted from Castiglia, P., & Harbin, R. (1992). *Child health care: Process and practice* (p. 668). Philadelphia: J.B. Lippincott.

phases of a seizure

Seizure activity is described in three phases: prodromal, ictal, and postictal.

prodromal phase The *prodromal* phase precedes the seizure by several hours to several days; during this time, the child experiences warning signs (prodromes), such as changes in mood or behavior or the appearance of an *aura*. An aura is a particular sensation that a child experiences before the onset of a seizure, such as a flash of light or a strange smell. An aura gives the child and caregivers an alert so that seizure precautions can be implemented. The nature of the aura also can suggest where the abnormal electrical activity originates. For example, an aura involving an unusual taste or smell likely originates in the temporal lobe of the brain.

ictal phase The seizure is the *ictal* phase, characterized by muscle contractions, unusual eye movements, and possible loss of consciousness.

postictal phase The *postictal* phase immediately follows the seizure, and behavior in this stage varies. The child may be sleepy, confused, or uncoordinated, with loss of feeling or movement in parts of the body.

classification of seizures

Seizures are classified as *generalized*, *partial* or *focal*, and *unclassified*. This classification was established by the International League Against Epilepsy.

Generalized seizures involve both hemispheres of the brain, are bilateral and symmetric, and may or may not involve prodromal syndromes. Partial or focal seizures involve a limited area of the cerebral cortex where damage of brain tissue has occurred, either through surgery, trauma, malformation, or a space-occupying lesion. Unclassified seizures include seizures that do not fit the criteria of the International Classification of Seizures for partial or generalized seizures, such as febrile seizures.

There are four types of generalized seizures:

* Tonic–clonic (grand mal) seizures: *Tonic* behaviors include rigidity, extension of extremities, fixed jaw, respiratory cessation, dilated pupils; *clonic* behaviors include rhythmic jerking of extremities, autonomic symptoms, and possible incontinence.
* Myoclonic seizures: *Myoclonic* behaviors include generalized short muscle contractions, with distinctive movements in individual children. *Infantile spasms* are a type of myoclonic seizures and involve brief flexion of the neck, trunk, or legs but with no loss of consciousness. These seizures are most common in infants between 3 and 12 months and disappear by 5 years. Nearly 90% of children who develop infantile spasms will suffer severe mental retardation.
* Absence seizures (petite mal): These are episodes of unconsciousness lasting only a few seconds, with intervals of blinking or staring. The affected child may experience hundreds of these episodes each day.
* Atonic seizures: Sometimes called *drop attacks,* atonic seizures involve sudden loss of muscle tone followed by postictal confusion. Myoclonic behaviors also may appear. As with absence seizures, the child may experience hundreds of atonic seizures daily. Mental retardation and impaired motor function often accompany atonic seizures.

There are three types of partial (focal) seizures:

* Psychomotor (complex) seizures: This type of seizure involves *automatism*, involuntary behaviors, such as drooling, lip smacking, grimacing, or chewing, followed by postictal confusion or sleep. Affecting children between 3 years and adolescence, complex seizures are often preceded by an aura, particularly an unusual taste or smell. Complex seizures most commonly are related to temporal lobe foci.
* Motor seizures: This type of seizure begins in the head or face and spreads to a larger area of the body, sometimes affecting an entire side of the body. It can include tonic–clonic movements, drooling, and impaired speech.
* Sensory-motor seizures: Most common in children 8 years and older, this type of seizure includes numbness, tingling, prickling, or burning, followed by tonic–clonic movements.

Unclassified seizures include febrile seizures, pseudoseizures, and status epilepticus:

* Febrile seizures: This type of seizure is most common in children between 6 months and 6 years and is associated with a high fever. The precise cause is incompletely understood, but the seizures generally occur when the temperature is rising rapidly, often within the first 24 hours of a respiratory or gastrointestinal infection. Other possible causes, such as CNS infections, fluid and electrolyte imbalance, and space-occupying lesions, must be ruled out.
* Pseudoseizures: This seizure-like behavior is most common in children and adolescents. Although pseudoseizures include abnormal motor activity, no abnormal electrical impulses are evident on EEG testing. Neither tongue-biting, incontinence, nor postictal confusion occurs.
* Status epilepticus: This condition involves recurrent, continuous, generalized seizure activity with the danger of cardiac arrest and brain damage. It is a medical emergency that requires rapid, early diagnosis and treatment. Mortality may be as high as 50%, and as many as 15% to 20% of affected children suffer permanent neurologic impairment.

medical–surgical management

An EEG is performed to document abnormal activity. Other testing, such as complete blood count and blood chemistries, may be done to seek underlying causes of seizure activity. Once the child is on anticonvulsant medications, serum levels of medications may be ordered. Treatment often includes anticonvulsant medications (phenobarbital, phenytoin, diazepam, carbamazepine). The dose is adjusted as the child grows.

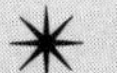 **nursing insight**

The most frequent reason for increased seizure activity is medication noncompliance.

If seizure behavior is not controlled by medications, surgery may be required to remove the lesion; sometimes this can be done without causing further deficit. Surgery involves a *craniotomy* (surgical opening of the skull) with removal of a small area of brain tissue, a lobe, or a complete brain hemisphere.

In some children, a ketogenic diet (high-fat, low-carbohydrate, low-protein diet that induces ketosis) may help control seizures, but this is difficult to maintain.

nursing care

The nurse obtains a thorough family and medical history (birth trauma, medications, injuries, illnesses, family history), including a history of seizure behavior.

Protecting the child from injury during the seizure and educating the family on how to take precautionary measures while at home are the nurse's primary roles (see Teaching Guidelines). In addition, the nurse carefully observes and documents events, including any known or suspected trigger factor, behavior prior to the seizure, any aura, the time the seizure began and ended, clinical manifestations of the seizure, and postseizure behavior and symptoms.

Client and caregiver teaching includes helping to prevent seizures by avoiding exposing the child to known or suspected trigger factors, such as emotional stress or blinking lights. Staying with the child during attacks helps minimize the child's anxiety. The nurse provides reassur-

teaching guidelines
seizure precaution measures

* If necessary, have the child wear a helmet.
* If seizure occurs:
    Do not restrain child during seizure.
    Remove harmful objects.
    Do not place anything in child's mouth.
    Hyperextend neck to maintain airway.
    Have child lie on the side to allow secretions to drain from mouth.
    Loosen child's clothing.
    Observe, time, and document all seizure activity.

ance and explanations of all procedures and treatments. The child needs to be allowed to participate in normal activities as much as possible.

medication therapy

The nurse administers anticonvulsant medications as ordered, maintains safety precautions due to sedation and possible seizure activity, and monitors blood levels as ordered. Children are reevaluated periodically to readjust their medication levels.

dyslexia

Dyslexia is a condition in which a child with normal vision is unable to comprehend written grammar. The learning disability affects the child's ability to comprehend basic language skills, including reading, writing, and spelling. The exact cause is unknown; however, it is associated with a CNS defect limiting the ability to organize graphic symbols. There tends to be a familial tendency, often affecting several children in one family.

Children with dyslexia have trouble figuring out words, lose their place when reading, and have difficulty listening, speaking, and concentrating. They observe words differently from the average child and frequently reverse letters when writing.

Dyslexic children are sometimes mistaken as being mentally retarded when they are often intelligent. Children with dyslexia benefit from special school programs designed to identify their distinctive learning limitations.

headache

Headache can be described as a pain anywhere in the head. Headaches are a frequent complaint in pediatrics and occur from a variety of causes, such as tension, sinusitis, or fever, and usually responds to rest and acetaminophen administration.

Frequent and continuous headaches requiring evaluation can be secondary to conditions such as hypertension; trauma; vomiting; migraine; infections, such as dental caries and meningitis; or brain tumor.

the child with an alteration in vision or hearing

anatomy and physiology of the eye and ear

The eye includes external and internal structures. The *external eye* contains the sclera, iris, pupil, lens, ciliary body, retina, and vitreous chamber (Fig. 35-9). The *retina* is the innermost layer of the eye and includes the *optic disk,* the *macula,* and the *retinal vessels.* The retina is composed of *rods,* necessary for night vision and visual field movement, and *cones,* necessary for color distinction.

Eyelids and eyelashes protect the eyes. The conjunctiva lines the lids and is the site for inflammation known as *conjunctivitis.*

Aqueous humor is the clear fluid produced in the eye located between the iris and the cornea. *Vitreous humor* is the transparent gel located behind the lens and in front of the retina.

Refraction is the process by which light rays bend as they pass through the lens and fall on the retina. Most visual defects are caused by *refractive errors,* such as *myopia* and *hyperopia.* Myopia (nearsightedness) occurs when light rays focus in front of the retina; the condition in which light rays focus behind the retina is called *hyperopia* (farsightedness).

The ear is divided into three compartments: the *external ear, middle ear,* and *inner ear* (Fig. 35-10). The *external ear* includes the auricle, external auditory canal, and *tympanic membrane* (eardrum). The *middle ear* is positioned between the tympanic membrane and the inner ear. The *eustachian tube* connects the middle ear and the nasopharynx and helps equalize pressure between the middle ear and the atmosphere. The inner ear contains the *cochlea* and the *semicircular canal.* The semicircular canal helps maintain balance and regulate body position.

age-specific considerations

Eye development begins in the first 4 weeks of gestation and is completed by the first trimester of pregnancy. Maternal infections, especially rubella during the first trimester, affect the lens of the eye, contributing to childhood cataracts.

A significant difference between a child's ear and an adult's involves the eustachian tube. In young children, the eustachian tube is wide, short, and straight, compared with the longer, more narrow and angled tube found in adults. The shape and position of the child's eustachian tube leads to an increased incidence of middle-ear infections, called *otitis media.* Vision and hearing impairments are sometimes accompanied by below average intelligence or mental retardation. The Fagan Tests of Infant Intelligence are used with infants up to 1 year who are at risk for cognitive deficits (Display 35-4).

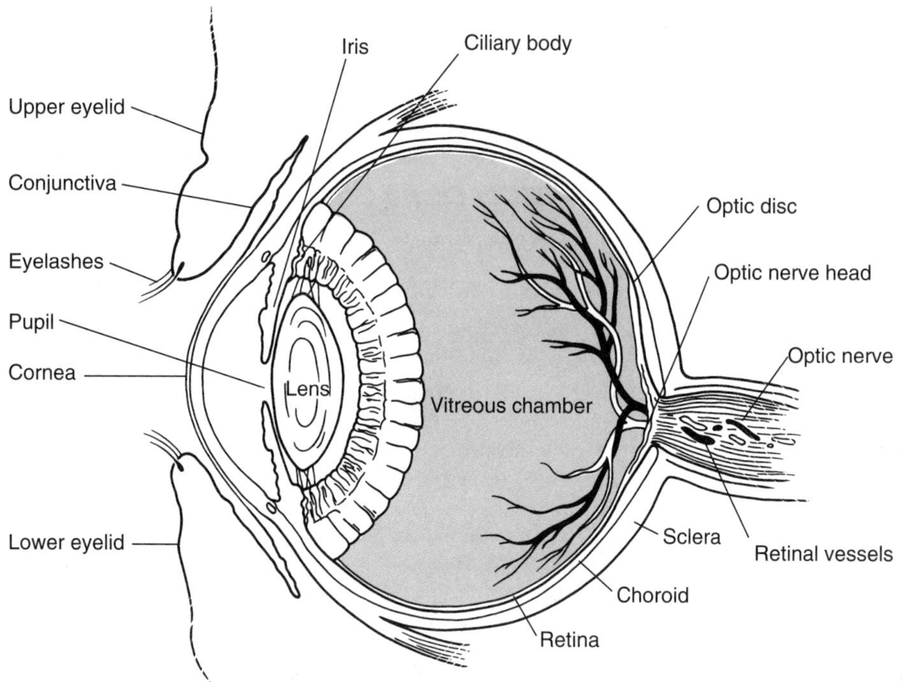

figure 35-9 *Cross-section of the eye.*

✳ family considerations

One of the joys of parenthood involves communicating with a baby by watching the infant's eyes brighten in recognition of a parent's voice, followed by "baby talk" sounds. Vision or hearing impairment limits this type of interaction. Hearing screening of newborns has greatly increased early detection of hearing deficits and appropriate intervention.

Hearing impairment affects the ability to learn language, develop intelligence, and interact with others. During the first year, a child acquires two thirds to three fourths of all basic language needed for life.

Parents are typically the first to suspect a hearing or vision problem in the child. Lack of language development symbolizes a severe handicap. Confusing words and sounds are noted in children with mild hearing impairment but may be overlooked until the child is older (Table 35-6).

✳ nursing considerations

Discovery of a hearing loss places stress on the entire family system because 90% of deaf children are the first hearing impaired person in the family. Nursing care that pro-

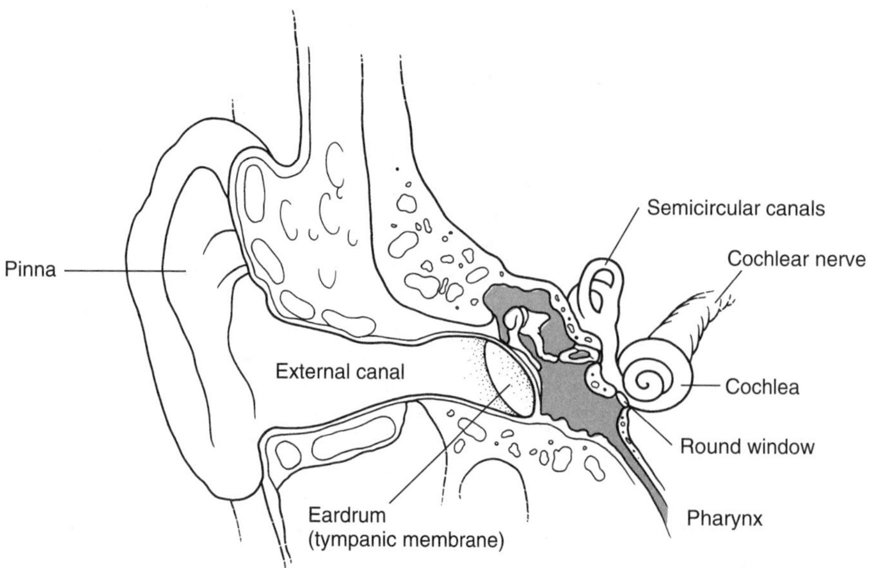

figure 35-10 *Structure of the middle ear.*

display 35-4
fagan test of infant intelligence

- The Fagan test is a screening device for detection of visual attention in infants at risk for learning problems.
- The test is easy to administer and takes about 15 minutes.
- During the test, you will hold the infant on your lap.
- A variety of visual image will be displayed on a rotating stage.
- The Fagan testor determines the direction of the infant's visual attention by watching the infant's eye reflections through a small opening in the back of the testing machine.

motes an understanding and respect for an alterative way of communicating encourages parents to be more positive. "Deafness" is not always viewed as being "disabled" in the deaf culture. People experiencing deafness have a sense of pride in sharing a culture and a common language.

The best medicine for a hearing impaired or visually impaired child is love and support from parents, caregivers, nurses, and all others involved with the child. The nurse provides information to the family about available community support groups and other resources.

Low–birth-weight infants are at risk for visual impairment, related to high concentrations of oxygen administration and immature eye muscle development. Early, periodic vision screening of very low–birth-weight children is important because even minor vision problems can interfere with learning and development.

table 35-6 development of normal hearing

Age	*Reaction to Sound*
Birth–2 wk	Startled by loud sounds; soothed by parent's voice
2 wk–mo	Cries at loud noises; eyes search for a sound; aware of voices
3–6 mo	Turns eyes toward the speaker or sound; enjoys musical toys
6–9 mo	Finds the source of a sound; will turn head when called from behind; noise awakens child from sleep; smiles in response to hearing name
9–12 mo	Turns toward soft sound or name spoken softly; imitates simple sounds
By 2 y	Can point to at least one part of the body; accurately point to a picture of an animal or house; and select a toy on command without seeing speaker's lips

diagnostic examinations

Ear examination includes the use of an otoscope, an instrument used to examine the ear, providing visual inspection of the tympanic membrane (eardrum, normally a light translucent, pearly-gray), detection of ear wax build-up, and drainage.

Tympanometry shows the dynamics of the tympanic membrane, middle ear, and auditory canal system.

Acoustic emittance measurements test determines conductive hearing loss.

Auditory acuity estimates the child's ability to hear a whispered phrase or a ticking watch.

Audiogram is a machine that measures the ability of sound based on decibels (pressure exerted by sound).

Culture and sensitivity of ear, eye, shunt drainage, blood, and spinal fluid determine bacteriologic factors.

Snellen's E chart or alphabet chart is used to determine visual acuity in children.

otitis media

Otitis media is an inflammation of the middle ear. *Otitis media with effusion* is a condition in which there is fluid behind the eardrum, occurring with or without infection.

Bacterial or viral agents cause purulent exudate to collect in the space of the middle ear behind the tympanic membrane. Otitis media is one of the most common treatable infections of childhood and can be acute or chronic.

Acute otitis media usually follows viral upper respiratory infection. Half of all children have an episode of otitis media by 1 year. More than 75% of all children will have had at least one episode by the time they are 5 years old. The earlier the first episode of otitis media, the greater the risk of subsequent recurrent otitis media and chronic otitis media with effusion.

Suppurative (producing pus) otitis media is more common in children younger than 5 years; the highest incidence occurs before 2 years of age. Nonsuppurative otitis media is seen more often in school-age children. There is an increased incidence of otitis media during fall, winter, and early spring.

Environmental factors that favor the transmission of upper respiratory pathogens, such as crowding and poor ventilation in housing, increase the risk of acute and chronic otitis media. Infants subjected to second-hand or passive smoke have an increased incidence of acute and chronic otitis media. Bottle feeding an infant in the supine position promotes pooling of formula in the pharyngeal cavity and increases the risk of otitis media. Several studies have shown that breast-feeding offers an infant some protection against the development of otitis media.

pathophysiology

The eustachian tube is an open airway between the middle ear and mouth. The tube's main function involves the in and out movement of air in the middle ear spaces. A swollen eustachian tube impairs air movement. Fluid can accumulate in the middle ear space, providing an opportune environment for bacterial growth. Blockage of the eustachian tube can result from one or a combination of factors, including large adenoids, allergies, or bacterial or fungal throat infections.

Allergic acute otitis media and otitis media with effusion involve one or more of the following mechanisms: Middle ear is a target organ for allergens; inflammatory reaction to the allergen causes edema of the eustachian tube and nose; bacteria-laden allergic nasopharyngeal secretions are aspirated into the middle ear cavity; and allergic influences affect the mucous membrane-lined cavity of the middle ear.

diagnostic tests

Examination of the ear with an otoscope reveals a red and bulging eardrum. If the eardrum has ruptured, the presence of drainage may prevent visual inspection of the drum. Culture and sensitivity of the drainage determines bacteriologic factors.

medical–surgical management

The medical treatment of this condition is twofold: Remove the fluid to improve hearing, and if possible, relieve the cause. Treatment of allergies includes identifying allergens and desensitization (see Chap. 32).

Surgical intervention involves myringotomy, myringotomy with tube insertion, or a tonsillectomy or adenoidectomy later in the toddler years if chronic or recurrent infections occur.

myringotomy *Myringotomy* involves making a small delicate opening in the eardrum membrane (tympanic membrane). Collected fluid is drawn off with tiny suction instruments. The actual procedure lasts about 15 minutes. Because of the short duration of surgery, problems during and after surgery are rare. The infant spends time in the recovery room postoperatively.

myringotomy with tube insertion When tube insertion is necessary, a small, plastic (Teflon aeration) tube is placed in the opening of the eardrum to keep fluid from collecting in the middle ear. The tiny aeration tube has an opening of about 1/25″ in diameter. Infants are unaware of the presence of ear tubes because they are painless after insertion. Tubes stay in place for several weeks to months and sometimes for 1 year or more; they gradually and painlessly work their way out of the ear. It is seldom necessary for the surgeon to remove tubes. Tubes can be inserted as many times as necessary.

Colds and sore throats can cause ear infections after tube insertion; however, there is less pain and fever because the tubes prevent the accumulation of pus and pressure in the ear.

Antibiotics are used to treat otitis media. Amoxicillin is often prescribed because it is active against *S. pneumoniae* and most strains of *H. influenzae*, two common causative organisms. Antibiotic therapy is given for 10 days. Ordinarily, infants improve significantly within 48 to 72 hours of receiving antibiotics. The effectiveness of antihistamines and decongestants in the treatment of acute otitis media has not been proven; however, these drugs can be effective in relieving the nasal congestion that accompanies otitis media.

✳ nursing process in otitis media

assessment

Subjective data to be assessed include the following:

- Infant's cry associated with discomfort when the infected ear is examined or touched. Pain in the ear (otalgia) may be evident by ear tugging, turning head from side to side, irritability, and sleeplessness. A decrease in hearing may be noted.
- Parental report of onset of symptoms.

Objective data to be assessed include the following:

- Careful assessment of temperature elevation, increase in heart rate, and increased respirations, indicating infectious process.
- Nasal congestion of white to yellow purulent nasal discharge and thick, tenacious drainage and crusting in nares may be present. Infant's refusal to suck may indicate nasal congestion and blockage.
- Presence, color, and odor of drainage in the external ear canal are visible with or without an otoscope.
- Coughing, vomiting, and diarrhea are present.

nursing diagnoses

- Pain, related to accumulation of fluid causing pressure on eardrum
- Risk for Infection to brain
- Altered Skin Integrity, related to drainage from infected ear
- Sensory/Perceptual Alterations, related to impaired hearing
- Risk for Altered Growth and Development, related to inability to respond effectively to sounds in the environment
- Parental Knowledge Deficit, related to disease condition and treatment protocol

planning and implementation

- Relieve pain by administering prescribed analgesics. Place infant in a side-lying position with the infected ear down. This position facilitates comfort and drainage. Responding to the infant in a positive way by rocking and holding him helps give comfort and establish trust.
- Administer antibiotics as prescribed according to sensitivity of organism. Usual course of treatment is 10 to 14 days (loose stools and fungal diaper rash are common adverse effects). Keep head of bed elevated in a low to semi-Fowler's position. Use universal precautions for handling drainage. Always wash hands before and after contact with the infected ear.

* Instill nose drops as prescribed prior to bottle feeding so that infant's suck response is uninhibited. Saline nose drops are ordered as needed and are effective in softening nasal crusts and cleaning the nares prior to feedings. Hold infant in an upright position for feedings.
* Ear drops are frequently prescribed to soften cerumen (triethanolamine polypeptide oleate [Cerumenex], carbamide peroxide [Debrox], or hydrogen peroxide) and to ease pain or control infection (antibiotics, Auralgan). Ear drops are instilled at room temperature. To straighten the ear in a child younger than 2 years and promote the placement of medication in the ear canal, the pinna is pulled down and back. For children older than 2 years, the pinna is pulled up and back.
* Cleanse drainage from the area around the ear with hydrogen peroxide to prevent skin breakdown. Zinc oxide or petrolatum can be applied to protect the skin around the ear. Hair must be kept clean and away from the infected ear.
* Following tube insertion, water must not enter the ear as long as tubes are in place. Swimming is permitted only with special fitted custom ear molds that plug the ears. Avoid getting water in the ear canal when bathing or washing the hair. Cotton mixed lightly with vaseline can be placed in the ear canal prior to bathing and removed immediately afterwards as a precaution. All other ordinary activities, including flying, are permitted.
* Alert parents about signs of hearing loss and the importance of audiology testing.

evaluation

* Recovery from otitis media is evident by the absence of symptoms, specifically pain and fever.
* Client and caregivers comply with medication regimen, preventive measures, and postoperative care if myringotomy with tube insertion is performed.

hearing loss

Hearing loss is described as *conductive* when an external ear disorder, such as impacted cerumen (ear wax) or otitis media, prevents the transmission of sound by air to the inner ear. *Sensorineural* or *perceptive* hearing loss involves damage to the eighth cranial nerve or a disorder of the inner ear. This type of hearing loss is due to heredity; infection of the brain, meninges, or spinal cord; exposure to intrauterine infections, such as rubella, cytomegalovirus, and herpes simplex virus; exposure to loud sounds; and use of ototoxic medications, such as gentamicin, neomycin, erythromycin, furosemide (Lasix), and aspirin.

Treatment for conductive hearing loss involves diagnosing the cause and medical or surgical intervention to correct the blockage. Sensorineural hearing loss is a permanent loss. Intervention involves assisted hearing through the use of a hearing aid.

hearing aids

Hearing aids are instruments that act as microphones to amplify sounds. A hearing aid makes speech louder, sometimes distorting the clarity. A new form of amplification is the cochlear implant, a disk-shaped receiver implanted under the skin behind the ear with wires surgically inserted into the inner ear to transmit electrical impulses that are interpreted by the brain.

care of hearing aids Hearing aid care requires washing the ear mold with soap and water daily, cleansing the small cannula with a small applicator or pipe cleaner, and checking the batteries weekly or after 100 to 150 hours of wear. Care must be taken to turn the hearing aid off when it is not being used. Hearing aids must be kept away from household pets because animals seem to be attracted to the wax on the ear piece and will chew on the hearing aid. Heat and moisture also damage hearing aids.

sign language

Young, deaf children exposed to sign language develop language in a like manner and on a similar timetable as hearing children exposed to spoken language. When deaf children are exposed primarily to spoken language, they acquire language much more slowly.

cognitive and psychosocial development

Cognitive development in deaf children is similar to hearing children, with a slight decrease in the ability to conserve and use transitive thinking. Deaf children tend to be less socially mature than hearing children, and data suggest they may have fewer positive self-concepts.

nursing care

The nurse encourages parents of deaf children to explore their feelings and reactions. Hearing parents may feel overwhelmed with recommended interventions, such as sign language. The nurse can suggest that hearing parents connect with deaf parents for general support and useful communication tips.

The nurse needs to establish the most effective way to communicate with the child and parents when administering care. It is important to communicate the child's special needs with others involved with the care by using care indicators in the chart, on the bed, and in the bathroom.

The nurse assesses the child's development, especially relative to language. If the child uses sign language but has an arm or hand restricted by a dressing, intravenous line, or cast, alternative communication methods need to be used. The nurse devotes full attention to what the child is saying and speaks directly at the child in a normal tone of voice to facilitate lip reading.

See the Nursing Care Plan.

primary congenital glaucoma

Glaucoma is a condition that results when fluid in the eyes does not drain properly. Hereditary factors are thought to play a role with most cases diagnosed before 1 year.

pathophysiology

Pressure builds up within the eye, causing optic nerve damage or nearsightedness and vision loss. Primary con-

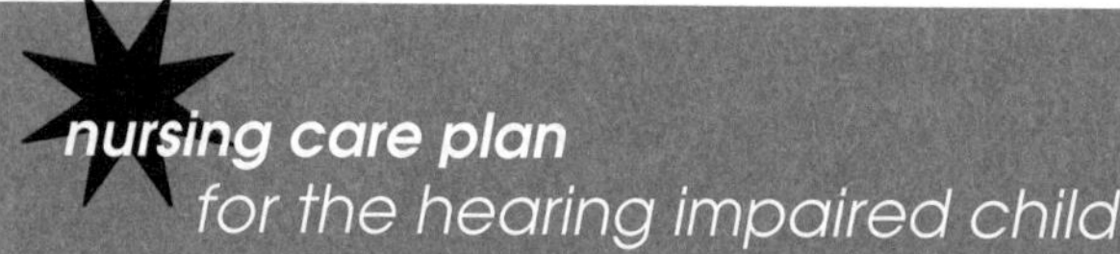

nursing care plan for the hearing impaired child

NURSING DIAGNOSIS

High Risk for Sensory Alteration, related to new diagnosis of hearing impairment and insufficient alternate methods of communication

GOAL: The family and the child will state an understanding of an effective alternate mode of communication

NURSING INTERVENTIONS	RATIONALE	EVALUATION
Educate family and child on alternative methods of communication, such as sign language.	The sadness and lack of control associated with a diagnosis of hearing impairment can be offset by learning about available options.	The family and the child will openly discuss their feelings and understand their options.
Advise the parents on the use of hearing aids.	Children with conductive hearing losses can have an improvement of hearing with hearing aids.	The family and the child will state an understanding of hearing aids with the various types of hearing loss.
Discuss school options and special programs for the hearing impaired with parents of children with hearing impairment.	Early exposure to speech and hearing therapy is recommended as soon as hearing loss is discovered.	The child will receive adequate sensory stimulation as evidenced by his increasing involvement with his environment.

genital glaucoma occurs when a child's drainage channels are incompletely or incorrectly formed. Symptoms include loss of visual field and visual acuity, cloudy or abnormally large eyes, sensitivity to light or shying away from light, and excessive tearing.

medical–surgical management

Surgery is recommended for children because typical drugs used for adults are generally ineffective. The major goal of treatment is to keep intraocular pressure within normal limits by increasing the flow of aqueous humor. Surgery may be needed several times to accomplish the goal.

nursing care

Nursing care centers on age-appropriate explanations about surgery. Administration of eye medication in young children is usually easier for two people and requires instructing both parents or two caregivers. Medications used to open the tear ducts are put in the inner corner of the eye; antibiotics are administered in the center of the eye so that the solution will bathe the eye before going down into the tear ducts.

Visually impaired infants enjoy meaningful auditory and tactile stimulation, such as listening to family talk or being stroked. The best interventions are personal one-to-one interactions.

congenital cataracts

A *cataract* is described as clouding of the lens. Congenital cataracts result from viral, metabolic, hereditary, or unknown mechanisms before birth. Surgical removal of the cataracts immediately after birth is the recommended treatment. Following surgery, the child has no lens and is unable to focus at close range. Corrective contact lenses or glasses are necessary after surgery.

nursing insight

Before buying a young child prescription glasses, suggest to the caregivers that they buy an inexpensive pair of sunglasses and remove the lenses. Encourage the child to wear the "rehearsal glasses" for a couple of weeks to encourage compliance.

Suggest to the caregivers that before buying a young child prescription glasses, they buy an inexpensive pair of sunglasses and remove the lenses. Encourage the child to wear the "rehearsal glasses" for a couple of weeks to encourage compliance.

Contact lens care includes cleanliness, insertion, and removal. It is vital to stress good handwashing before touching the contact lenses. Children and parents need to understand that redness, excessive tearing, and pain are symptoms of inflammation and must be reported immediately.

vision impairments

Vision impairments frequently seen in children include amblyopia, strabismus, and myopia. *Amblyopia* (also called lazy eye) is thought to develop due to an imbalance of the eye muscles. The child's vision is distorted because the images received from either eye cannot be focused together, causing "double vision." The child often displays no outward signs of amblyopia. The most common treatment involves placing an eye patch over the stronger eye, forcing the muscles of the weak eye to strengthen.

Strabismus (cross-eye) occurs when there is an imbalance of the eye muscles, causing uncoordinated eye movements. Usually only one eye is affected and is apparent because the eye tends to turn inward or outward. Treatment of strabismus includes surgical correction, patching the unaffected eye, and eye exercises.

Myopia (nearsightedness) is common among school-aged children. Children with myopia see close objects but have poor distant vision. Squinting is a common behavior as the child attempts to focus on distant objects. Corrective lenses are the common method of treatment.

Early discovery of vision impairments enhances a child's possibility of rapid and successful treatment. Eye examinations are recommended for infants beginning at 3, 6, and 12 months and yearly thereafter.

blindness

Children are considered legally blind if their visual acuity is 20/200 or less. Many children who are legally blind have some remnants of vision. Blindness occurs in 1 out of every 2,500 school children in the United States.

nursing care

Assessment of how the visually impaired child perceives self, family, and peer relationships provides the nurse with information on the child's adjustment to the condition. Self-care, self-esteem disturbances, follow-up care, educational planning, and use of visual aids, such as large-print books, audio tapes of class materials, or braille materials, must be included in home care planning.

key points ✳

- **The neurologic assessment is based on the child's developmental level.**
- **Family caregivers of children with neurologic disorders experience anxiety and concern about the diagnosis, hospitalizations, the disease process, care of well siblings, costs, medications, equipment, monitoring for complications, possible lifestyle changes, transmission of communicable diseases to others, and potential threat to the child's life.**
- **Nurses caring for children with neurologic disorders need to be aware of normal growth and development behaviors because some of these disorders may start with subtle changes and then rapid deterioration, requiring careful and accurate assessment skills.**
- **The anatomy and physiology of the nervous system in children differ significantly from that of the adult with development following a cephalocaudal and proximodistal pattern.**
- **The nurse's role in the monitoring and holding a child for a lumbar puncture is critical to prevent trauma to the child during the procedure.**
- **Children with neurologic problems may be more prone to accidents, such as falls, then other children and therefore must be more carefully monitored, especially for signs of increased ICP.**
- **Seizures result from overly active and hypersensitive neurons in the brain, which cause abnormal electrical discharges and are caused by many different diseases and disorders, such as prenatal or perinatal hypoxia, infections, congenital malformations, metabolic disturbances, lead poisoning, head injuries, drug abuse, alcohol misuse, tumors, medications toxins, and unknown origin.**
- **Cognitive development in deaf children is similar to hearing children, although deaf children are less socially mature than hearing children, and studies suggest they may have a lower self-concept; hearing impairment affects the ability to learn language, develop intelligence, and interact with others. During the first year, a child acquires two thirds to three fourths of all basic language needed for life.**
- **Discovery of a hearing loss places stress on the entire family system, placing importance on nursing care that promotes an understanding and respect for an alterative way of communicating; deafness is not always viewed as being "disabled" in the deaf culture.**
- **Vision impairments include glaucoma, a condition that results when fluid in the eyes does not drain properly; congenital cataracts resulting from clouding of the lens; and eye muscle weakness seen in amblyopia and strabismus.**

review questions ✳

1. Which of the following is the chief cause of disability and death in children?
   a. Head injury
   b. Meningitis
   c. Spinal cord injury
   d. Neuroblastoma
2. A major concern of adolescents after a spinal cord injury is
   a. schooling.
   b. body image.
   c. death.
   d. parental response.
3. Seizure activity is typically diagnosed by doing what procedure?
   a. CT scan
   b. Electroencephalogram
   c. Blood test
   d. X-ray of the head
4. A common symptom of acute otitis media in infants includes
   a. headache.

b. pulling on the affected ear.
c. pharyngitis.
d. dyspnea.

5. A common noninvasive method of treating vision impairments involving the eye muscles includes
a. surgical intervention.
b. placing a patch over the unaffected eye.
c. administering eye drops.
d. wearing prescription glasses.

bibliography

Alfaro-LeFevre, R., et al. (1992). *Drug handbook: A nursing process approach*. Redwood City, CA: Addison-Wesley.

Betz, C. L., Hunsberger, M. M., & Wright, S. (1994). *Family centered nursing care of children* (2nd ed.). Philadelphia: W.B. Saunders.

Castiglia, P. T., & Harbin, R. B. (1993). *Child health care: Process and practice.* Philadelphia: J.B. Lippincott.

Engel, J. (1989). *Pocket guide: Pediatric assessment.* St. Louis: Mosby–Year Book.

Jackson, D. B., & Saunders, R. B. (1993). *Child health nursing: A comprehensive approach to the care of children and their families.* Philadelphia: J.B. Lippincott.

Kravitz, L., & Selekman, J. (1992) Understanding hearing loss in children. *Pediatric Nursing, 18*(6), 591–594.

Luerssen, T. G. (1991). Head injury in children. *Neurosurgical Nursing Clinics of North America, 2*(2), 399–410.

Marhoefer, P., & Vadnais, L. (1992). *Caring for the developing child* (2nd ed.). Albany, NY: Delmar Publishing.

(1994). *Mosby's medical, nursing and allied health dictionary* (4th ed.). St. Louis: C.V. Mosby.

(1996). Lippincott review series: *Pediatric nursing* (2nd ed.). Philadelphia: Lippincott–Raven.

Ray, J., Booth, J., & Rojeski, T. (1990) *Medical and surgical interventions, parental instructions, myringotomy and teflon tube insertion*. Zanesville, OH: Southeastern Ohio Otolaryngology.

Schilling, L., & Dejesus, E. (1993). Developmental issues in deaf children. *Journal of Pediatric Health Care*, 7(4), 161–166.

Sizer, F., & Whitney, E. (1994). *Nutrition: Concepts and controversies* (6th ed.). Minneapolis/St. Paul: West Publishing.

Skale, N. (1992). *Manual of pediatric nursing procedures.* Philadelphia. J.B. Lippincott.

Speer, K. (1990) *Pediatric care plans.* Springhouse, PA: Springhouse Corporation.

(1996). *The Lippincott manual of nursing practice* (6th ed.). Philadelphia: Lippincott–Raven.

Wong, D. L. (1993). *Whaley and Wong's essentials of pediatric nursing* (4th ed.). St. Louis: Mosby–Year Book.

Wong, D. L. (1995). *Whaley and Wong's nursing care of infants and children* (5th ed.). St. Louis: Mosby–Year Book.

the child with an alteration in musculoskeletal function

36

outline ✳

objectives 

After studying this chapter, the reader should be able to:

* Discuss the role of bones, joints, and muscles in the musculoskeletal system.
* List three types of traction.
* Describe three diagnostic tests used to screen for musculoskeletal disorders.
* Discuss medical–surgical management for the child with congenital dislocation of the hip.
* Discuss nursing care for the child with Duchenne's muscular dystrophy.
* Compare and contrast the three types of spinal curves.
* List three types of juvenile arthritis.
* Identify the types of fractures most common in children.
* Define strain and sprain.
* Discuss the two most common forms of bone cancer in children.

key terms 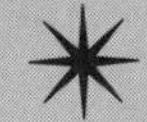

abduction
adduction
amphiarthrosis
atrophy
diarthroses
contractures
kyphosis
lordosis
pathologic fracture
scoliosis
subluxation
synarthrosis
torticollis

Neff C & Spray M. *Introduction to Maternal and Child Health Nursing,*

Most disorders of the musculoskeletal system cause some degree of movement limitation causing temporary or permanent restriction on motion and support. Children with disorders of the musculoskeletal system often receive care from an *orthopedic* specialist, who is a physician specializing in the preservation and restoration of skeletal system function.

anatomy and physiology

bones

The bones of the body are the organs of the skeletal system and are arranged to provide support and protection for the entire body. Bones are made of living cells and nonliving intracellular material and they are the storage site for calcium and marrow. Bones can be grouped into four categories according to their shape: long, short, irregular, and flat. The structure of the long bone is seen in Figure 36-1.

joints

Bones are held together at joints by tough connective tissues known as ligaments and tendons. Ligaments connect bones to bones; tendons connect muscles to bones. Joints require daily use to maintain function. If movement has been limited for some reason, ankylosis (fixation of a joint with permanent loss of motion) may develop. This can be prevented by performing daily range-of-motion exercises.

Joints provide flexibility of movement. The shape of the joint determines the type of movement.

- Synarthroses (fibrous) joints have no movement, as in the skull.
- Amphiarthoses (cartilaginous) joints have little movement, such as intervertebral joints.
- Diarthroses (synovial) joints have free movement, such as the knee, elbow, shoulder, and hip.

muscles

Muscles are clusters of red contractible fibers that are capable of movement when stimulated by a nerve. When a muscle fiber receives a stimulus, it contracts completely and becomes shorter and fatter. Muscles can not partially contract. Muscle tissue can also be stretched. It will return to its normal resting length once the stretching force is removed. The role of muscles in the body is to move, stabilize and support body parts.

Loss of muscle tone (*atrophy*) results in flabby, weak muscles. Atrophy occurs when an extremity is immobilized, for example, cast application for a fracture. Following removal of the cast, physical therapy treatment is necessary to restore muscle strength.

Muscle tone is maintained by active exercise (voluntary movements) or passive exercise. *Passive exercise* is performed by the nurse when the child is paralyzed or when movement is restricted. The goal is to maintain muscle function. Lack of normal muscle movement can result in *contractures*, which are shortened skeletal muscles and permanent loss of muscle elasticity.

age-specific considerations

Children's bones are more porous than adult bones. Therefore, they can absorb more energy before breaking. The epiphyseal growth plate, found at the end of long bones, is a weak point in the bones of children. If this area

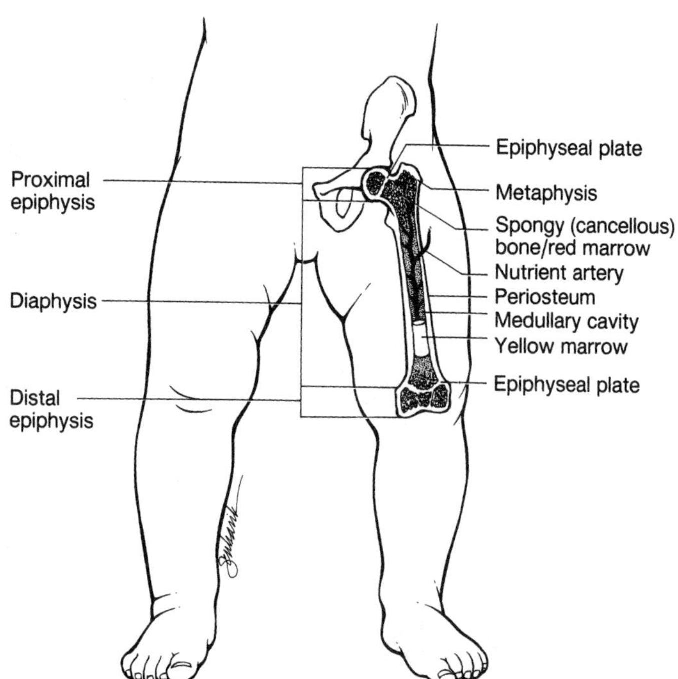

figure 36-1 *Portions of the long bone.*

of growing cells is damaged, the length of the developing bone may be shortened. Bone healing follows the same pattern in both adults and children.

Increased musculoskeletal development is seen during the preschool years. The child takes a more upright stance as the abdominal muscles strengthen. Increased dexterity and ambulation skills are noted. Knock-knees (genu valgus) is frequently seen in the preschooler and disappears with increased growth in the length of long leg bones. Preschoolers have a high bone cartilage content, which enables them to heal quickly when trauma occurs.

✳ family considerations

Patient, family, and peer support is important when dealing with either short- or long-term alterations in musculoskeletal function. Families need to understand the management of the injury as well as how to deal with its psychological effects and activity restraints. Social contact with peers is important with any injury. It is very helpful to maintain as normal a daily routine as possible for all involved.

Immobilization can be difficult and can cause frustrating effects when prolonged. Regressive behavior is common. Children often think they are being punished for something they have done.

Orthopedic appliances, such as braces, splints, and crutches, are expensive and can cause financial concerns, especially when the child's growth requires frequent updating of equipment. Most hospital appliance businesses are knowledgeable about insurance coverage for such devices. Crippled Children's Foundation, American Red Cross, and social service agencies can offer family assistance.

A typical family concern involves normal physical and social growth of the child. Anticipatory family grief or anxiety may be noted concerning the child's potential for altered height or the increased risk of being "teased" or "bullied" about body size and shape.

Family energy can be a concern, especially if the primary care giver is required to carry or handle an infant with a heavy cast or brace. Encouraging all members of the family to assist in the child's care is important. For example, young children can bring the immobile child something to eat, drink, play with, or read.

Prolonged hospitalization and/or housebound status increases the child's risk of depression and feelings of isolation. Encouraging the school-age child to keep a diary or scrapbook with get-well cards or to record events on a computer helps pass the time. Encourage parents to involve family and friends in care of the child.

Mysterious bone or muscle pain in children should not be dismissed simply as the child's imagination. The pains may signal normal changes in the child's bones and muscles, referred to as *growing pains*. However, they may be signalling a serious disease or disorder. Parental concern often centers on what is considered normal development. Common developmental disorders such as flat feet, pigeon toes, and knock knees are usually outgrown (Table 36-1).

table 36-1 musculoskeletal developmental conditions and considerations

Toeing in (pigeon toes); medical term—metatarsus varus. Feet toe in from the middle of one or both feet (shaped like kidney beans), probably due to curled-up position before birth.	Stretching the infant's feet helps them turn out. Place one hand on the heel and the other one near the big toe; gently push the big toe toward the little toes. This can be done with every diaper change. Casting or corrective shoes (or both) for about 1 mo may be necessary in severe cases. Reversing the child's shoes makes little impact on direction of feet.
Turning in from the knees. One or both feet may toe in from the knee, caused by position before birth and prolonged if child sleeps curled up.	This may require intervention, but usually the child outgrows the condition. Encourage child to sleep on back. If extreme, doctor may have infant wear a brace or splint at night for several months.
Feet turn in from the thigh or hip.	This is caused by position before birth. Child usually outgrows it. Encourage the child to sit cross-legged to help gently turn the hips outward.
Flat feet; failure of arch development when "baby fat" disappears due to loose arch-supporting ligaments.	Flat feet do not limit the child's ability to play sports. If the child has painful flat feet, doctor may suggest arch supports; for extreme cases, surgery may be necessary.
Bowlegs; curvature of legs outward.	Child usually outgrows it. The way a child's legs are shaped is similar to the shape of the parents legs.

Providing accurate information enables parents to alert the pediatrician about abnormal growth patterns so that early interventions can be initiated.

✳ nursing considerations

Children with musculoskeletal alterations are at increased risk for disorders such as anemia and increased bleeding because erythrocytes, platelets, and lymphocytes are manufactured in bone marrow. The child's complaints of fatigue may be caused by anemia in addition to painful movement.

Age-appropriate explanations are important to reduce the child's fear of body mutilation and permanent disfigurement. Anger is common in children with traumatic injuries to the bones. They often have difficulty understanding "why it happened?" Assigning age-appropriate tasks to promote the child's sense of control is essential. For example, allow a school-age child to apply a sling, adjust their crutches, or elevate their cast on pillows.

Administration of pain medication approximately 30 minutes before performing painful procedures is important to help the child endure discomfort. Age-appropriate explanations and teaching aides to promote understanding help reduce anxieties. Children must be given permission to cry when they feel pain and then must be praised for their courage when the painful experience is over.

Trauma to the musculoskeletal system frequently occurs from motor vehicle accidents, play, and sports injuries. Parents often feel a degree of guilt or blame themselves with these types of accidents. It is important for the nurse to listen in a nonjudgmental manner as parents express concern. Special documentation may be necessary (depending on agency policy) if legal factors exist.

diagnostic tests

x-rays

X-rays are the most common diagnostic procedures for altered musculoskeletal functioning. Serial x-rays may be necessary to monitor the healing process. The nurse should encourage the child to lie still during the procedure so that an accurate picture is obtained.

bone scan

Radioactive material is injected intravenously to determine uptake in areas of higher metabolic activity, such as tumors, infection, and inflammation. The injection site should be monitored for signs of infection following the procedure.

computed tomography scan

This procedure consists of an x-ray and computer to scan individual bone layers to visualize density details. The nurse should make sure that the child follows any food or fluid restriction policies prior to the test. Positioning for the test should be explained to the child.

arthroscopy

This is a surgical procedure performed with a scope to visualize the inside of a joint. A properly signed and witnessed consent form must be obtained. Food and fluid restrictions must be followed before the test. The nurse should explain the procedure to the child and the parents. Following the procedure, the nurse should monitor vital signs, perform neurovascular checks of the affected extremity, administer pain medication, and provide discharge information.

 **nursing alert**

Elevate the entire leg following an arthroscopy procedure to avoid flexion contracture of the knee, and do not massage the area because there is an increased risk of blood clot formation.

electromyography (emg)

This is performed to detect neuromuscular abnormalities by using skin and needle electrodes that measure and record nerve and muscle control and electrical movement. The nurse should explain the procedure and alert the older child that a small wire needle is inserted under the skin and produces a bit of discomfort. The nurse should administer the ordered sedation or analgesics and instruct the child not to get out of bed without assistance.

joint aspiration

Fluid is withdrawn from the joint under study for analysis. The aspiration site should be assessed following the procedure for signs of infection such as edema, redness, and tenderness.

other common procedures

Angiography—introduction of radiopaque medium to study vascular structures

Ultrasound—high-frequency vibration of sound wave echoes, producing a visual image

Complete blood count—determines if the child is anemic and determines the ability of the bone marrow to produce blood cells.

Erythrocyte sedimentation rate (ESR)—indicates the presence of an inflammatory reaction somewhere in the body

Latex agglutination test (latex fixation)—detects the presence of IgM version of rheumatoid factor present in rheumatoid arthritis

Synovial fluid aspiration—determines presence of joint inflammation

Synovial membrane biopsy—used to determine rheumatoid arthritic changes in the joint

traction procedure used for musculoskeletal disorders

Traction involves the application of pull to a body part. It can be used to align and stabilize bone fragments, allow an extremity to rest, correct a deformity, immobilize an area, or reduce muscle spasms. Three components to traction management are traction (forward force), countertraction (backward force), and friction (the patient's contact with the bed). These forces work together to align or correct parts of bones. Weights may be added to adjust the amount of forward force. Elevation of the extremity will increase countertraction.

types of traction

There are three types of traction. These include:

Manual traction—applied by hand distally to the fracture
Skin traction—applied directly to the skin by adhesive material or elastic bandage
Skeletal traction—applied by pin, wire, or tongs inserted directly into the diameter of the bone distal to the fracture.

These types of traction can be used in a variety of ways. Figure 36-2A-C shows the different types of traction.

> ✳ **nursing insight**
> *Braces used for scoliosis treatment do not correct a scoliosis curve but will slow the progression.*

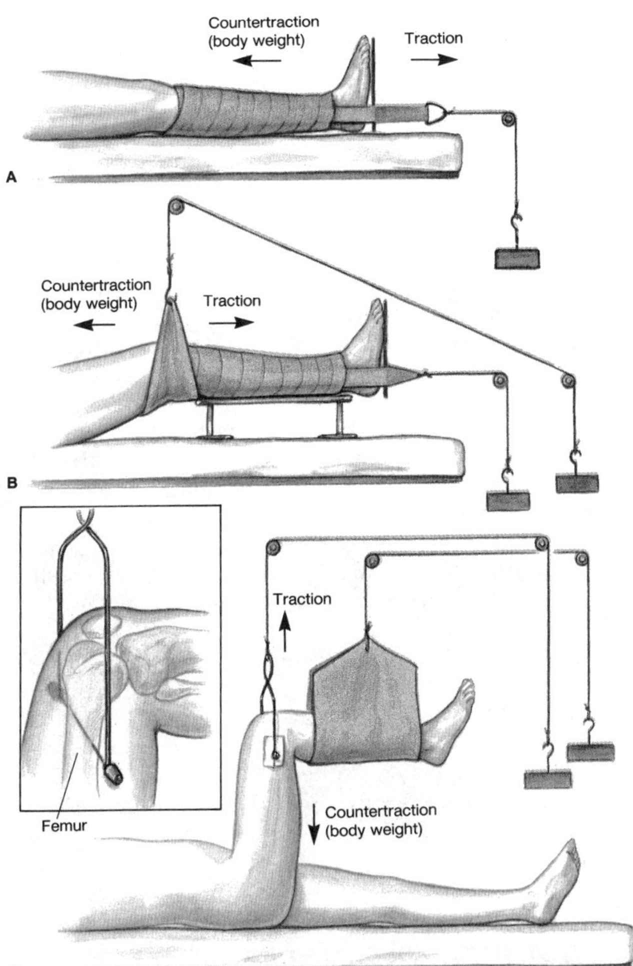

figure 36-2 *Types of traction.* **(A)** *Buck's extension, a form of skin traction.* **(B)** *Russell traction, a type of skin traction. Two lines of traction (one horizontal and one vertical) allow for good bone alignment for healing.* **(C)** *90 degree (skeletal) traction. A wire pin is inserted into the distal femur.*

nursing care

Traction may be ordered as continuous or intermittent. Nursing care of children in traction requires expertise in understanding the principles of traction. The nurse should assess the correct alignment and placement of equipment every 2 to 4 hours. Marking the bed to see where the parts of the patient's body should be will make the process quicker, easier and more reliable. Note the position of pulleys, amount and position of the weights, and the correct angle of the body part in traction.

Assessment for signs of complications also should be done every 2 to 4 hours. Note color, sensation, and temperature of the body part in traction. The nurse should use techniques to prevent skin breakdown. These include using clean, wrinkle-free sheets, keeping the skin clean and dry, and performing range-of-motion exercises for unaffected joints. Assessment for signs of complications should continue.

Wire and pin site care for patients in skeletal traction is important. This involves careful, on-going assessment for signs of infection. The site should be cleaned with an appropriate antibacterial agent, such as Betadine, every 8 hours.

✳ nursing process for the child with a musculoskeletal disorder

assessment

Subjective data to be assessed include the following:

* Question the child (if age-appropriate) and parents about recent trauma, delays in walking, or other musculoskeletal system deformities, such as clubfoot or hip dysplasia; need for mobility aids, such as crutches, braces, or splints; and presence of discomfort, including degree, frequency, and relief measures.

Objective data to be assessed include the following:

* Weight and height compared with age-appropriate values plotted on growth grid, limb lengths and spinal deformities affecting posture and gait such as *kyphosis* (an increase in the curve of the spine at the lumbar region) and *scoliosis* (an S curvature of spine), muscle development and strength, and neurovascular assessment of extremities.

nursing diagnosis

Nursing diagnoses are determined from the assessment data and must be individualized for each child and condition. Diagnoses might include the following:

* Body Image Disturbances, related to alteration of musculoskeletal system
* Ineffective Individual/Family Co*scoliosis* (an S curvature of spine), muscle development and strength, and neurovascular assessment of extremities.

* Risk for Disuse Syndrome, related to musculoskeletal maturity
* Diversional Activity Deficit, related to immobility
* Altered Family Process, related to child's condition
* Altered Growth and Development, related to disease process
* Risk for Injury, related to altered balance and gait
* Acute Pain, related to trauma and disease process
* Situational Low Self Esteem
* Impaired Skin Integrity, related to trauma and immobility
* Knowledge Deficit, related to technical procedures, diagnostic tests, home care

nursing interventions

* Promote positive body image: Evaluate child's level of understanding and parental knowledge of condition such as fractured bone requiring cast or use of crutches. Encourage child to describe self and then how others would describe him or her. Note ethnic and/or cultural perceptions. Recognize child's behavior indicating overconcern with body. Observe interactions of child with peers and family members. Discuss concerns about fears of mutilation, interventions, and prognosis. Help the child use clothing to minimize body changes and enhance appearance.
* Strengthen client and family coping skills: Encourage child and parents to assist in planning the client's daily activities. Encourage the school-age child to continue schoolwork, with parents serving as a link between the school and the hospital. Provide the child and parents with a daily update on the condition, progress, expected treatments, and medication changes or additions. Provide diversional activity through age-appropriate play therapy, music, videos, and television.
* Promote skin integrity, regular bowel patterns, and respiratory, circulatory, and urinary system function: Encourage child and parents to change body position every 2 hours (if unable, schedule nurse to reposition), cough, and deep breathe every 2 hours. Use pressure-reducing devices such as egg crate/water mattress and cushions. Monitor nutritional status and encourage balanced diet high in fiber and fruit juices. Monitor intake and output and force fluids unless otherwise ordered. Monitor bowel elimination and evaluate need for stool softeners. Monitor breath sounds and characteristics of respiratory secretions. Assess skin integrity every shift. Assess pressure points every 2 hours. Check neurovascular status of affected extremity every 4 hours, noting changes in sensation, circulation, general color, presence of swelling, and complaints of pain when cast, splint, ace wrap, or other type of support device is being used. Monitor vital signs, including temperature.
* Promote the family process: Note components of family and family developmental stage, such as marriage or birth of a child. Identify patterns of communication in the family, who visits child, and emotional connections. Identify and encourage use of previous successful coping behaviors. Assess role expectations of family members, identify parenting skills and expectations, assess energy direction and task sharing, and assess available support systems.
* Promote safety: Evaluate developmental level, decision-making ability, and level of competence. Assess mood, coping abilities, and knowledge of safety needs. Review parents' expectations of children. Discuss concerns about child care and discipline practices. Practice safe nursing by keeping siderails up, bed position at lowest level, call light within reach, and assistance if needed when client ambulates.
* Promote comfort: Assess pain location, presence of inflammation, stability of support devices, and body position. Demonstrate use of self-administration or patient-controlled analgesia (PCA). Encourage rest periods to prevent fatigue. Administer prescribed analgesia.
* Promote home care: Determine level of knowledge and child's and parent's ability to learn. Determine blocks to learning, such as language barriers. Determine client's method of accessing information, such as visual or auditory learning styles. Begin teaching by giving information the client already knows and providing for feedback and questions. Involve client in procedures required at home and provide encouragement and praise.

evaluation

* Child demonstrates improved body image by verbalizing acceptance of self and by using adaptive devices or prosthesis appropriately.
* Child and parents verbalize awareness of coping abilities and meet psychological needs by appropriate expression of feelings.
* Child displays intact skin, reestablishes effective elimination patterns, is free of infection, demonstrates adequate peripheral perfusion, and maintains optimal level of functioning.
* Family members interact in a positive manner, demonstrating individual involvement in problem-solving, and directing energies in a purposeful manner to resolve family problems.
* Child and parents verbalize an understanding of individual factors that contribute to risk of injury; child remains free of injury.
* Pain is controlled or relieved, demonstrated by child's willingness to play and interact socially.
* Child and parents participate in learning process, exhibiting increased interest and ability to perform assigned tasks.

congenital disorders

congenital muscular torticollis

Torticollis (wryneck) is a congenital or acquired condition resulting in limited range of motion of the neck. Acute torticollis sometimes follows an upper respiratory infection or trauma.

pathophysiology

Torticollis results from injury or shortening of the sternocleidomastoid muscle. The child's neck is flexed and the head turned to one side. On inspection, a tender mass is often felt in the midportion of the muscle. The neck appears short, with skin folds between the head and shoulders. Asymmetry of the head and face are related to impaired blood supply to the area. Torticollis is often seen with congenital deformities of the cervical spine.

medical management

Without treatment, torticollis will result in permanent limitation of neck movement and unsightly facial asymmetry. Treatment consists of gentle stretching exercises. Surgical release or division of the sternocleidomastoid muscle may be necessary if the exercises are unsuccessful in the first year of life.

nursing care

Parental instructions about the importance of exercises are necessary to encourage compliance. The nurse may suggest ways to play with and feed the child that encourage head turning away from the affected side (eg, mobiles placed in crib to encourage head movement). Follow-up care is essential.

congenital dislocation of the hip

Congenital dislocation of the hip or hip dysplasia, an instability of the hip, is usually noticed during the newborn period. It is often referred to as "loose hip." Hip dysplasia is more common in girls, possibly because female hips flare more, or because the pelvic ligaments are more relaxed due to the hormone relaxin and the femur is not able to efficiently press into the acetabulum.

pathophysiology

True hip dysplasia is noted when the femoral head slides completely out of the acetabulum. The supporting structures that hold the femoral head in the acetabulum are too loose to support the hip. In a subluxed (incomplete dislocation) hip, the femoral head is in the acetabulum but tends to slide laterally and "slips."

The primary cause of dislocation or dysplasia is thought to be prenatal or postnatal positioning. This condition is associated with breech positioning and small uterine size. It is also seen when an infant is held for long periods with legs extended and adducted, such as in the Native American culture when infants are carried in a papoose. It is therefore important to have several hip examinations throughout the first year of life.

medical/surgical management

Treatment begun in the first 2 months of life is most successful. The severity of the deformity increases with delayed treatment. Treatment varies but is directed at relocation and stabilization of the femoral head in the acetabulum. Protection of the local blood vessels and nerves is accomplished by keeping the joint immobilized.

In infancy, the Pavlik harness (Figure 36-3) is the most commonly used immobilization device. It is worn fulltime for 3 to 6 months. Skin traction and hip spica casts are used with **adduction** (draw toward the body) contractures or when there is difficulty maintaining a stable reduction. These require longer use but are usually successful within 1 year. When the condition is not recognized until older infancy, traction followed by casting is necessary because of limb shortening with apparent contractures. In an older child, treatment is difficult due to secondary adaptive changes that have taken place. Traction with operative reconstructive procedures is necessary and must be followed by physical therapy.

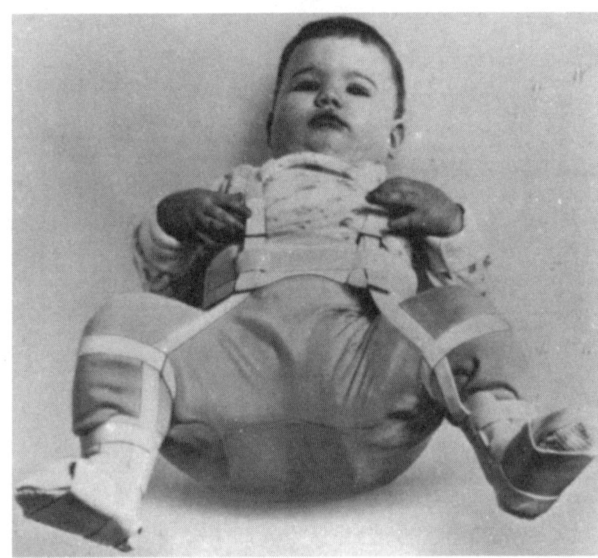

figure 36-3 *Pavlik harness. (From Mulley, D. A.* Harnessing babies dysplastic hip. *American Journal of Nursing, 84, 1006. Courtesy of Durr-Fillauer Medical, Inc.)*

✳ nursing process for the child with hip dislocation or dysplasia

assessment

Assess for the following signs of hip dislocation or dysplasia:

* Shortened limb on affected side
* Positive Ortolani test, clicking with abduction
* Restricted hip abduction (movement of limb away from midline) on affected side
* Unequal folds of skin on buttocks and thighs
* Lordosis (older infant/child)
* Waddling gait or limp (older infant/child)

nursing diagnosis

* Impaired Physical Mobility, related to hip displacement

teaching guidelines
for parental teaching concerning application of the Pavlik harness for CHI

* Harness is placed over clothing, and care must be taken to secure the straps without tightness. Straps must be kept off the abdomen.
* Harness can be removed for bathing unless contraindicated by the doctor.
* When the harness is removed for short time periods, use 2 to 3 diapers or a receiving blanket to keep the legs apart.
* Conventional car seats can not be used, but infant carriers can. Backpacks and grocery-cart seats can be used.
* Check the child's skin for redness, chafing, or irritation and report findings to the nurse or doctor.
* Feed the child in an upright position if possible.
* Wash the harness with mild soap, air dry or machine dry on low heat.
* Keep follow-up appointments (often scheduled weekly) so doctor can monitor the child's progress, evaluate the effectiveness of treatment, and intervene if complications occur. Keep emergency and doctor's office phone numbers posted for quick access.

* Parental Knowledge Deficit, regarding home care related to cast care
* Potential for Impaired Skin Integrity, related to immobility, traction or spica cast
* Diversional Activity Deficit, related to immobility secondary to traction or spica cast application

nursing interventions

promotion of immobilization

* Keep legs abducted by following recommended treatment plan. For mild problems, use a double-diapering technique to provide the abduction necessary to keep hips stable. Pavlik harness, braces, traction, or a spica cast are necessary for more severe cases.
* Bryant's traction involves keeping the child's hips in a 90 degree flexion. The buttocks are elevated off the bed.

nursing alert
Monitor circulation to feet when a child is in traction.

providing home instructions

* Teach parents home care, including the application and removal of splint or harness.
* Child's skin must be inspected for redness at least once every 4 hours if spica cast or traction is being used. Irritation, especially over the bony prominences, must be kept clean and dry. Application of A&D ointment is helpful for irritated skin. Turn child every 2 hours.
* Cast care includes padding with plastic wrap or wrapping the edges of the cast with strips of waterproof tape or Op-Site in the perianal area to keep it clean and dry. Stress the importance of observing the skin above and below the cast for signs of impaired circulation, such as cold skin, complaints of tingling or pain, presence of swelling, and inability to move foot.
* Inform the parents about the importance of providing the child with a diet high in calories, calcium, protein, and fiber.
* Encourage the parents to provide stimulation by placing the child's bed near a window, moving the bed into

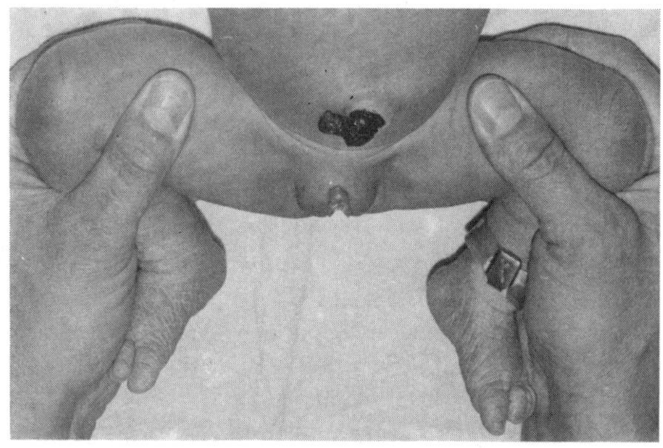

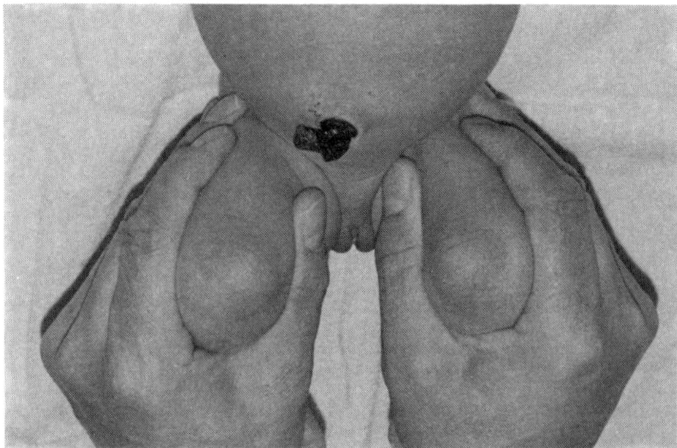

figure 36-4 **(A)** *Ortolani's sign. The fingers are on the trochanter and the thumb grips the femur as shown. The femur is lifted forward as the thighs are abducted. If the head was dislocated, it can be felt to reduce.* **(B)** *The thighs are adducted, and if the head dislocates, it will be felt and seen as it suddenly jerks over the acetabulum. (Avery G. F.: [1987].* Neonatology: Pathophysiology and Management of the Newborn *(3rd ed.). Philadelphia: J. B. Lippincott.)*

different rooms, providing toys and games appropriate for age, and placing objects on the walls.

postoperative care for child requiring surgical intervention

* ✳ Assess vital signs, including temperature, according to agency protocol, usually done every 1/2 X 4, and, if stable, every 2 to 4 hours.
* ✳ Assess cast for drainage and bleeding. If drainage is noted on the cast, draw a circle around the site with ink, and mark the time and date and your initials to evaluate progression of drainage.
* ✳ Perform neurovascular assessment of extremities, checking for pulselessness, pallor, puffiness, pain, and paresthesia (numbness and tingling).
* ✳ Assist the child in turning, coughing, deep breathing, and using the incentive spirometer.
* ✳ Administer analgesics as ordered. When morphine sulfate is ordered, check respirations before giving since drug acts as a respiratory depressant.

evaluation

* ✳ child's legs are maintained in an abducted state.
* ✳ parents verbalize understanding of home care and demonstrate proper handling and movement of the child with a spica cast.
* ✳ child's skin remains intact, exhibited by warm, pink skin.
* ✳ child engages in play activities.

osteogenesis imperfecta

Osteogenesis imperfecta (OI) is an inherited disorder characterized by multiple fractures. The prognosis is poor.

pathophysiology

Bones fracture easily because of their brittle nature. There are four classifications of OI, from class I with mild bone fragility to class IV with multiple intrauterine or perinatal fractures, severe deformity, and early death. Bone deformities and growth retardation are common. The shafts of long bones are thin. The child usually has blue scleras, thin skin, hearing loss, and deformed teeth.

management

Treatment is primarily supportive. The goal is to prevent and treat fractures and deformities. Braces and splints may help support the limbs, aid in ambulation, and help prevent fractures. Physical therapy is aimed at improving bone density and strengthening muscles. Surgery may be done to correct deformities. Insertion of intermedullary rods can provide stability to the bones but require replacement as the child grows.

nursing care

In addition to careful handling to prevent fractures, educating parents is the goal of nursing. Parents must be taught how to diaper, caress, position, and feed their child without causing injury. Education is essential to promote optimum infant development. Parents should be given information on the Osteogenesis Imperfecta Foundation, Inc., which will lend support through education and contact with other families with an OI child.

muscular dystrophy

Muscular dystrophy is a group of progressive, hereditary disorders involving loss of muscle strength. The disorder is characterized by age of onset, rate of progression, inheritance patterns, and muscle group affected. The most common type is Duchenne's muscular dystrophy.

duchenne's muscular dystrophy

Duchenne's muscular dystrophy is an X-linked recessive disorder that affects only boys. Initial symptoms in childhood involve difficulty running, riding a bike, and climbing stairs. Parents may report that the child has difficulty rising from a sitting position to a supine position and is extremely clumsy. Diagnosis is made by clinical examination, with careful assessment of gait, muscle weakness, and sensation. Age of onset is usually between 2 and 6 years of age.

pathophysiology

The skeletal muscle of children with Duchenne's muscular dystrophy is missing a protein product called dystrophin. A muscle biopsy will reveal degeneration of muscle cells with loss of fiber and variation in fiber size. As the disease progresses, there is profound muscular atrophy, contractures, and joint deformities. Wheelchair confinement is usually necessary by adolescence. Facial, oropharyngeal, and respiratory muscles are often spared until the terminal stages of the disease. There is no cure for Duchenne's muscular dystrophy and 75% of children die by age 20 years (Hathaway, Hay, Groothuis, & Paisley, 1993).

medical management

Treatment for muscular dystrophy includes managing symptoms and maintaining functional capabilities as long as possible through physical therapy, range-of-motion exercises, bracing, wheelchair use, and weight control. Surgical intervention involves cutting tendons to correct contractures.

nursing care

Nursing care involves supportive therapy with progression of symptoms. Assisting the child to maintain independence as long as possible is a primary goal. Another goal is to prevent injury. Emotional support, considering the fatal nature of the disease, must be offered to the patient and family. Careful assessment of respiratory function is important because children have an increased risk of pneumonia, which often proves fatal. The Muscular Dystrophy Association of America, Inc. can provide consistent support and assistance.

nursing care plan
osteogenesis imperfecta (OI)

NURSING DIAGNOSIS:
Risk for injury, related to neuro/skeletal effects of OI

GOAL: *The child will have no new fractures.*

NURSING INTERVENTIONS	RATIONALE	EVALUATION
Use careful handling: * Avoid sharp movements. * Cushion movements with pillows. * Pad crib, tub, hard surfaces. * Lift buttocks, not legs, with diaper changes.	Improves environmental safety.	New injuries are prevented.

NURSING DIAGNOSIS:
Risk for altered nutrition: Less than body requirements, related to increased need for bone healing and decreased stomach capacity.

GOAL: *The child will ingest appropriate amounts of protein and minerals for bone healing.*

NURSING INTERVENTIONS	RATIONALE	EVALUATION
Encourage well-balanced diet: * Allow food choices high in protein and minerals. * Allow favorite foods. * Offer small, frequent meals.	Improves nutritional status, increases weight and bone strength.	Child's weight will increase.

NURSING DIAGNOSIS:
Parental knowledge deficit
Altered parenting

GOAL: *The child will show signs of bonding and attachment through increased parental knowledge of disease and ability to care appropriately for child.*

NURSING INTERVENTIONS	RATIONALE	EVALUATION
Encourage parent-child interaction: * Assist with care routines as needed to increase parenting ability. * Assess support systems. * Refer to OI Foundation for assistance.	Parenting is a learned behavior.	Parents engage in childcare activities.
Encourage questions and expression of feelings: * Offer positive feedback about condition. * Allow quiet time with parents to encourage discussion.	Parents need positive feedback to build confidence.	

musculoskeletal growth disorders

Legg-Calve-Perthes disease

Legg-Calve-Perthes disease is an aseptic, avascular necrosis of the femoral head. The disease is self-limiting and prognosis is excellent. Although the duration of the disease is unpredictable, it follows a predictable pattern to recovery. It is primarily a disease of white boys between the ages of 4 and 8, but it can affect any child between 3 and 12 years.

pathophysiology

The blood supply to the femoral head becomes interrupted for no clear reason. Necrosis may follow trauma, infection, or during growth spurts. Complete replacement of the epiphysis is seen as necrotic tissue is replaced by normal bone cells.

management

Treatment goals include allowing the femoral head to develop normally while maintaining its shape with full range of motion. Initially, rest is prescribed with or without traction. Non–weight-bearing support devices, such as braces or cast, may be necessary when the child becomes more active. Surgery may be needed to keep the femoral head in the acetabulum.

nursing care

Most care for Legg-Calve-Perthes disease is done on an outpatient basis. The primary nursing responsibility is initial education of the child and parents, with follow-up for specific areas of treatment and complaints. The nurse should assist the family with coping strategies, play therapy, and an understanding that although the treatment may be a long process, there is a good prognosis for complete recovery.

acquired disorders

curvature of the spine

Most spinal abnormalities seen in children are related to spinal curvature. They can cause pain, disfigurement, and respiratory difficulties if untreated. There are three types of spinal curves: kyphosis, lordosis, and scoliosis (Figure 36-5).

kyphosis

Kyphosis is curvature of the thoracic spine. It can occur as a result of tuberculosis, chronic arthritis, osteodystrophy, or compression fractures of the thoracic spine.

management

Postural exercises to strengthen the shoulders and abdominal muscles can help correct kyphosis. Emphasizing the cosmetic value of these exercises may help children to perform the exercises. In addition, encouraging desirable activities such as track running, weight lifting, swimming, and dancing may also aid in compliance.

lordosis

Lordosis is a curvature of the cervical or lumbar spine. It can be idiopathic or result from trauma or disease. Lordosis may also be seen in varying degrees during growth spurts, especially in girls.

management

Treating the predisposing cause when possible is the primary goal of management. Postural exercises and support garments can help decrease pain.

scoliosis

Scoliosis, the most common spinal deformity, is a lateral curvature of the spine. It occurs more frequently in adolescent girls, but it can occur at any age.

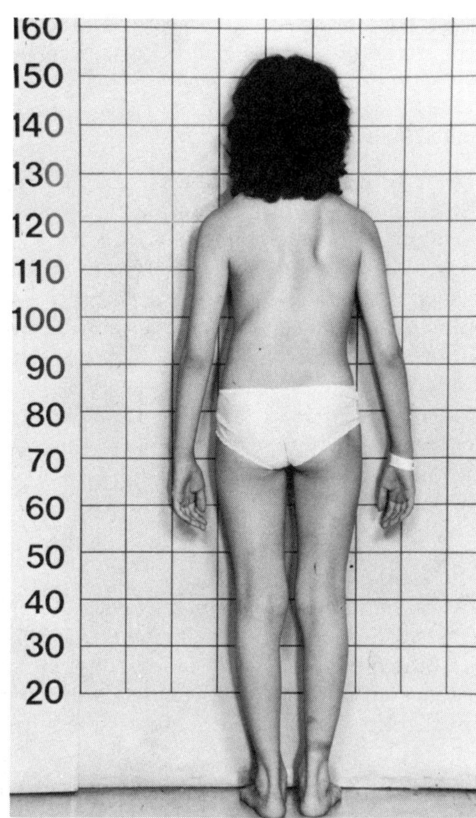

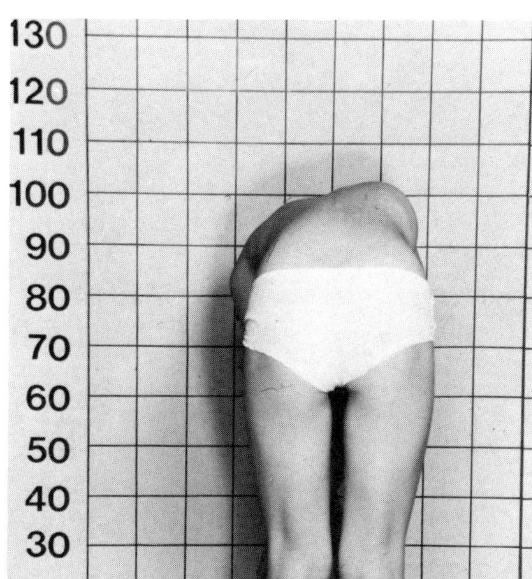

figure 36-5 **(A)** *When examining for scoliosis, asymmetry of the trunk (shoulders, scapular height, waist area, pelvic height) should be noted carefully.* **(B)** *The forward-bending examination will detect even small curvatures.*

pathophysiology

A sideway curve of 10 degrees or more is considered scoliosis. Diagnostic assessment is done by physical examination. See Display 36-1 for a simplified scoliosis screening technique.

Scoliosis can be **functional** or **structural**. Functional scoliosis is caused by a deformity, such as unequal leg length, and can be treated by treating the underlying cause. Structural scoliosis is characterized by changes in the spine that cause loss of flexibility. Structural scoliosis can be congenital or secondary to disorders such as neuromuscular disease.

management

Therapeutic management primarily involves bracing and surgery. Bracing will not correct the curve but will stop its progression. Low-profile braces, such as the Boston or Wilmington brace, are used for low thoracic and lumbar curves. These braces can be hidden by clothing. A high-profile brace, such a the Milwaukee brace, is used for high thoracic curvatures. This brace extends up to the chin and therefore is more noticeable. All braces must be worn 20 to 22 hours a day.

display 36-1
scoliosis screening procedure

Observe from front while child is standing erect:

* **Shoulder asymmetry**
* **Anterior rib asymmetry**
* **Breast asymmetry**
* **Hip asymmetry**

Observe from side and back while child is standing erect:

* **Shoulder asymmetry**
* **Scapular asymmetry**
* **Rib cage asymmetry**
* **Waist asymmetry**
* **Tape measure from occiput to floor; note if it does not pass through gluteal fold**

Observe from back while child bends or back parallel to floor:

* **Thoracic asymmetry**
* **Hip asymmetry**

Measuring tape from anterior superior iliac spine to medial malleolus at ankle:

* **Leg length asymmetry**

Abnormal symptoms with simple scoliosis screening procedure

Surgical correction involves spinal realignment and fusion using a metal rod. This stabilizes the spine and prevents progression of the curve.

nursing care

* Body image disturbance can be distressing to children and adolescents experiencing scoliosis.
* Child and parental education must be done to enhance compliance and prevent complications.
* Adolescent children, especially girls, must be screened during "growth spurts." Have the child bend forward and note the presence of a rib hump.
* Prepare the child and family for conservative treatment such as use of a brace. T-shirt is worn under the brace to decrease the risk of skin irritation and/or breakdown.
* Assess skin for signs of skin irritation or breakdown.

✳ nursing insight

Children may deny pain for fear of getting a "shot." Assess body language, activity, and irritability factors in determining discomfort.

* Prepare child and parents for surgical intervention when necessary. Teach child and family log-rolling technique (See Teaching Guidelines)
* Practice respiratory exercises such as coughing and deep breathing.
* Orient child and parents to the intensive care unit.
* Discuss postoperative dressings and tubes. Describe postoperative pain control and explain the use of a patient-controlled analgesic (PCA).

postoperative care

* Perform neurologic assessments, including level of consciousness, pupillary reaction to light, extremity strength and movement, and vital signs.
* The child usually needs to be log rolled for at least 5 days, depending on surgeon's orders.
* Administer IV fluids and analgesics as ordered.
* Monitor bowel sounds.
* Assist with ambulation.
* Encourage parents to arrange for continuation of school work. Encourage child to participate in self care to promote self-esteem and activities, such as games, video games, and peer interaction.

home care instructions

Instruct child and parents about cast care (if applicable), use of braces or other posture aides, and signs of infection, such as elevated temperature, weakness, and pain, redness and drainage around incision site. Stress the importance of keeping follow-up appointments so the surgeon can monitor the child's progress.

infectious or inflammatory disorders

juvenile rheumatoid arthritis (jra)

The word *arthritis* refers to *inflammation of joints* characterized by edema, heat, and pain especially with activity. Rheumatoid arthritis is a systemic disease affecting many organ systems, such as the lungs, heart, blood vessels, muscles, eyes, and skin. Juvenile rheumatoid arthritis generally occurs between the ages of six months and 16 years, with peak onsets at 1 to 3 years and 8 to 12 years. Girls are usually more susceptible than boys. There is no known cause of JRA, although it is thought to be an autoimmune disorder. There are several different types of JRA. The major types are systemic, polyarticular, and pauciarticular onset.

types of jra

Systemic onset is defined as the presence of recurrent, intermittent high fever (103°F or more) with or without rash and organ involvement (10%–20% of cases)

Polyarticular onset involves 5 or more joints (15%–25% of cases)

Pauciarticular onset involves 4 or less joints and is the most common type (69%–75% of cases) (White & Ansell, 1992).

pathophysiology

Symptoms of JRA vary widely. Attacks of joint pain and swelling (usually in the large joints) often have a sudden onset and remission. The most notable feature of JRA is chronic inflammation of the synovial membrane of affected joints (**synovitis**).

Synovitis has the potential to cause pain and cripple the joint. A measles-like rash, an elevated temperature with readings above 102°F, and growth disturbances are common in JRA. Diminished vision and blindness can occur but they are not common experiences. Up to 40% of patients have increased disability and require long-term therapy. The disease can continue into adulthood.

The prognosis depends on the type of disease. The prognosis is best for pauciarticular arthritis and worst for polyarticular arthritis (Wallace and Levinson, 1991).

medical management

Therapy for JRA is aimed at relieving pain, reducing inflammation, and preventing permanent deformities and blindness. Children usually benefit from physical therapy and other measures such as heat and splints. Pharmacologic treatment includes nonsteroidal antiinflammatory drugs (NSAIDs), antirheumatic drugs, corticosteroids, and cytoxic drugs (Table 36-2).

Physical or occupational therapy may preserve function and/or prevent deformity of the joint. Therapy is directed at muscle strengthening, freeing restricted joints, and prevention/ correction of deformities. Surgical intervention may be needed for joint replacement after bone growth is complete, usually in late adolescence (Witt et al, 1991).

nursing care

Nursing care includes planning a home health program of prescribed exercise, activity, and splinting. Children and parents must be knowledgeable about the drugs being used and their side effects. Encourage periodic eye exams for early detection of visual problems.

Parents must be encouraged to allow their child age-appropriate independence to promote normal growth and development. Children with JRA may be able to run, play sports, swim, and do lots of things, regardless of their diagnosis. They quickly learn what bothers them and can simply stop doing that activity. Children may need help in selecting a substitute activity for one in which they are not able to participate.

The nurse should stress what the child **can do** rather than dwell on limitations. Children must be encouraged to go to school. Teachers and school officials should know about the child's condition. National, state, and local organizations such as the Arthritis Foundation and American Juvenile Arthritis Foundation can offer support and counseling to children and their families.

table 36-2 drug therapy for juvenile rheumatoid arthritis (JRA)

Drug	*Action*	*Special Considerations*
Aspirin	Analgesic and anti-inflammatory	Platelet fragility increases risk of bleeding. Aspirin use in children linked with Reye's syndrome. Risk of gastrointestinal upset is increased.
Gold salts	Antirheumatic drug used to treat JRA that is unresponsive to salicylates	Gastrointestinal reactions, hematologic changes, metallic taste, hematuria, and dermatitis are common.
Corticosteroids	Anti-inflammatory agent	These are used short term in low doses during exacerbations. Long-term use is avoided due to side effects and adverse effect on growth.

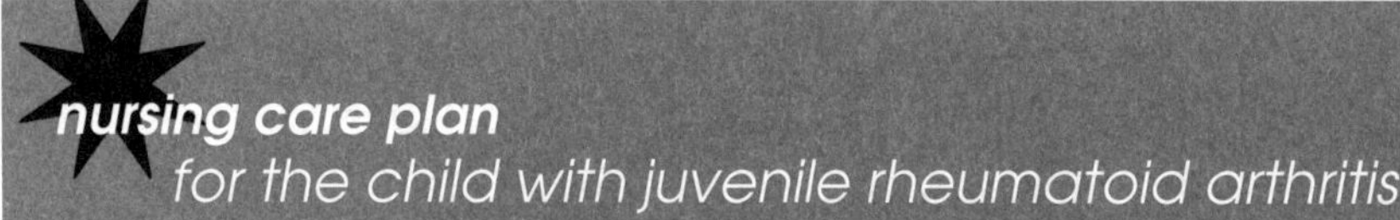

nursing care plan
for the child with juvenile rheumatoid arthritis

NURSING DIAGNOSIS

Risk for Activity Intolerance, related to inflammation and pain

GOAL: Maintenance of mobility and joint function and control symptoms.

NURSING INTERVENTIONS	RATIONALE	EVALUATION
Discuss disease and supportive treatment with the family and the child.	An understanding of the disease and how to prevent symptoms will help the family and the child adapt to this chronic disease.	The family and the child will state treatments that will promote mobility.
Educate the parents and the child to follow drug therapy.	To decrease inflammation and pain, aspirin or NSAIDs will be prescribed. Corticosteroids are indicated for a child with severe complications.	The child will comply with drug regimen and symptoms will be controlled, allowing the child to maintain self-care activities.
Teach the parents and the child about the application of dry or moist heat.	Application of heat to stiff joints will reduce stiffness.	Prevention of pain and stiffness will occur, and the child will participate in maximal activities.
Encourage recreational activities, such as swimming.	Regular physical activities will promote maintenance of mobility and preserve joint function, as well as increase the child's self-esteem.	The child will engage in regular physical activity.

NURSING DIAGNOSIS

Body image Disturbance, related to deformity of joints, effects of corticosteroids

GOAL: The child will communicate feelings regarding appearance

NURSING INTERVENTIONS	RATIONALE	EVALUATION
Educate the child on the temporary side effects of corticosteroids.	This can reduce the child's fear of permanent changes and maintain self-concept.	The child will state an understanding of the side effects of corticosteroids.
Encourage recreational acitivties.	This can help to preserve joint functioning and also decrease social isolation.	The child will be involved with appropriate recreational activities.
Encourage the child to express feelings about the disease.	Verbalization will allow the child to express frustrations and feelings.	The child will trust the caregiver and share feelings related to the disease.
Recommend a support group for the child.	This will help the child to deal with the consequences of living with a chronic and crippling disease.	The child will join a support group or state the availability of support groups to join when needed.

osteomyelitis

Osteomyelitis is an infectious process of the bone that occurs more frequently in boys between 5 and 14 years of age. The most common causative organism is *Staphylococcus aureus*. Other organisms include pneumococci and streptococci. The disease spreads as a result of direct penetrating wounds, open fractures, surgical contamination, preexisting impetigo, upper respiratory infections, acute otitis media, abscessed teeth, or infected burns.

pathophysiology

Bones most commonly affected include the distal femur and proximal and distal tibia. Bone-producing cells called osteoblasts are destroyed in the infected bone. Osteoclasis, which destroy bone, begin to accumulate at the infection site. A pus-filled abscess usually forms under the periosteum.

medical—surgical management

Therapeutic management involves prompt, rigorous antibiotic therapy. The appropriate antibiotic is continued for approximately 3 to 4 weeks, depending on the symptoms. Bed rest is also advocated. Surgical options may include incision and drainage of the infected bone to prevent abscess formation or removal of the dead bone (sequestrectomy).

nursing care

Nurse care involves decreasing the child's pain, supporting the affected limb, administering antibiotics and performing skin care. Universal precautions are necessary when providing nursing care. Intake and output are monitored every 8 hours. If casts are used for immobilization, appropriate cast care is implemented (see page 645). Attention to nutrition is important because the child often experiences an initial period of anorexia. Maintaining optimal functioning of the affected limb is essential. This is often accomplished through physical therapy.

skeletal tuberculosis

Tuberculosis of the bones is acquired through blood dissemination from a primary source. The carpals, phalanges, and bones of the feet are the most common sites in infants and young children. In the older child, the infection is often located in the spine area and causes kyphosis. If joint involvement is present, the hip is most commonly affected and the femoral head is destroyed. Clinical symptoms include irritability, body splitting at the affected site, limping, pain, swelling, and avoidance of movement that causes discomfort.

management

Immobilization with a splint or cast, antibiotic therapy, and rest are most often prescribed for tuberculosis of the bone. With tuberculosis of the spine, spinal fusion may be necessary. Hip fusion may be done when the disease affects that area.

nursing care

Nursing care involves providing support measures for an immobilized, young patient and educating the patient and family. Assisting the child with movement helps to minimize pain, and play may be helpful to assist with compliance. Administering prescribed antibiotic therapy is essential. The process of healing is slow, so the patient and family should be encouraged to stick to the prescribed plan of treatment.

traumatic injuries

fractures

Fractures in children are common and often the result of everyday, physical activities, such as running, jumping, and climbing. A fracture is a break in the continuity of the bone that occurs when the bone is subjected to more stress than it can withstand. The patterns of fractures in children are not specific. This leads to problems of diagnosis and treatments that are different from standard adult treatments.

Fractures are either complete or incomplete and the fracture line is either transverse, oblique or spiral (Figure 36-6). Fractures may also be either **simple** (closed) or **compound** (open). A simple (closed) fracture does not protrude through the skin. If it protrudes through the skin, it is compound (open). When a bone is broken into pieces and causes damage to organs or tissue, it is called a **comminuted** fracture.

When a fracture occurs, the surrounding muscle tightens and acts like a splint. The examiner may notice a deformity produced when the muscle tightness pulls the bone out of alignment. (See Display 36-2)

bone healing

Fractures in children heal more rapidly than in adults. For example, a femoral shaft fracture in a neonate will usually heal in 2-3 weeks, in an older child in 6 weeks, and in an adolescent in 8-10 weeks. When a bone is fractured, osteoblasts are immediately stimulated to form large quantities of new bone cells. Deposits of calcium form a callus, which repairs the integrity of the fracture.

management

The goals of fracture management include realignment of the bones (reduction–either open or closed), retaining alignment (immobilization), and restoring function to the area. Most fractures heal easily using traction and immobilization. An open reduction requires surgery. Casting is required with most fractures. There are four types of casts used for fractures: upper extremity casts to immobilize the wrist or elbow; lower extremity casts to immobilize the ankle or knee; spinal and cervical casts to immobilize the spine; and spica casts to immobilize the hip and knee.

nursing care

Goals of nursing care are individualized depending on the type of fracture and medical management. The nurse should assess for pain and anxiety and provide prescribed pain relief medications, counseling, and education. Therapeutic play activities help distract the child from boredom of inactivity. The nurse should assess for signs of complications such as neurovascular compromise, self-care deficits, and impaired skin integrity on a frequent, regular schedule—usually at least every four hours. Parents and peers should be encouraged to be supportive and actively involved will to help decrease anxiety and boredom. Good nutrition for appropriate healing is vital.

> **nursing alert**
>
> *The injured extremity must be checked for color and capillary refill because compromised circulation can cause death of tissue and pressure against nerves can cause permanent damage.*

cast care

Different types of casts require specialized care. However, the Teaching Guideline discusses the important care guidelines for all types of casts that the nurse should discuss with the child and the family.

sprains and strains

A **strain** is the stretching of a muscle or tendon beyond its capacity. The involved muscle or tendon is often microscopically torn. A **sprain** is the tearing if ligaments around a joint.

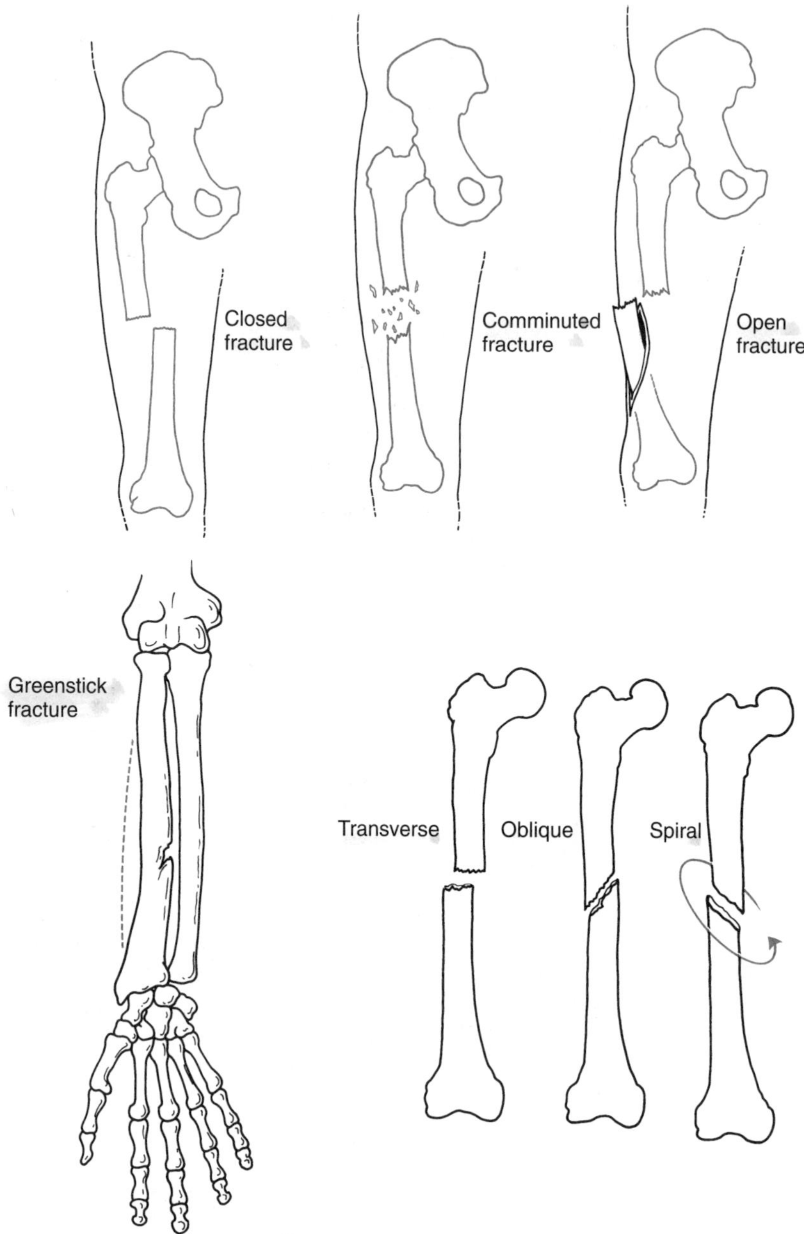

figure 36-6 *Types of fractures.*

Strains and sprains are common soft tissue injuries in children. They often result from play activities or sports. Pain, swelling, inflammation, stiffness, and disability in the affected area are common symptoms for strains and sprains.

management
Therapeutic management for soft tissue injuries is important in the first 6 to 12 hours after occurrence. Basic principles to use can be remembered in the acronym RICE: rest, ice, compression, elevation. Immobilization for torn ligaments may be necessary.

nursing care
Nursing care involves prevention of further injury, education for compliance, analgesic administration and promotion of optimal mobility. Safety factors must be addressed if the patient will require appliances to aid in ambulation.

bicycle injuries

Bicycle riding is a common childhood activity. The number of bicycle related injuries and deaths is increasing. Nearly one fourth of all significant head injuries in children younger than 14 years are caused by bicycle injuries.

display 36-2
clinical signs of a fracture

Generalized swelling
Pain or tenderness
Sensory motor deficits
Bruising
Crepitus
Diagnostic x-ray for confirmation

Mechanical defects, inappropriate frame size, reckless riding, and failure to wear a helmet often result in bicycle accidents. Injuries vary from simple cuts and scrapes to head, trunk, and limb trauma.

management

Medical and nursing care should include safety education in prevention strategies to decrease the number of bicycle-related injuries. Bicycle safety courses are available and teach the child proper riding techniques and use of safety helmets. These helmets can reduce the risk of serious head injury by 85 per cent. However, less than 5% of the at-risk population wear helmets (Pendergrast, Hay, Groothuis, & Paisley, 1992). Education that will enhance the child's role in compliance is essential for continued reduction of bicycle-related injuries.

bone cancer

Neoplastic disease can occur in any tissues involved with bone growth. Until puberty, both boys and girls are affected equally. After puberty, boys are twice as likely to be affected. Peak age of onset is between 15 and 18 years. About 85% of primary malignant tumors in children are osteogenic sarcoma and Ewing sarcoma.

osteogenic sarcoma

Osteogenic sarcoma is the most frequently encountered malignant bone tumor in children (Cancer Facts and Figures, 1990). The primary tumor sites are in the long bones near the epiphyseal growth plate. More than half occur in the femur.

Localized pain increasing in intensity is the primary symptom of osteogenic sarcoma. Swelling at the site is considered a late sign. X-rays, bone scans, and surgical biopsy will help confirm the diagnosis. Sometimes trauma to the tumor site may initially draw attention to the area. In addition, if the tumor is advanced, it may cause a fracture in the bone (**pathologic fracture**). Because bones are vascular, metastasis occurs quickly. The most common site of metastasis associated with osteogenic sarcoma is the lungs.

management

Therapeutic management usually begins with chemotherapy to shrink the primary tumor and treat micrometastases. After several weeks of chemotherapy, surgical removal of the tumor is necessary, after which chemotherapy will begin again. The 5-year survival rates are more than 50% if the tumor is detected early and a rigorous treatment plan is followed.

ewing's sarcoma

Ewing's sarcoma is a malignant tumor that primarily occurs in older children and adolescents. The primary site is in the bone marrow of the midshaft of long bones. Metastasis to the bones and lungs is common. The tumor initially causes sporadic pain that may be attributed to an injury. When pain is severe and the child and parents seek help, metastasis has already occurred. The bones and the lungs are common sites of metastasis. As with osteogenic sarcoma, care must be taken to avoid the occurrence of a pathologic fracture.

management

Treatment usually involves initial chemotherapy to shrink the tumor site(s) followed by surgical removal of all tu-

teaching guidelines
cast care to prevent complications associated with altered skin integrity

* Keep cast dry (to protect skin from breakdown and irritation).
  - Give sponge bath if cast is placed other than on an arm.
  - Protect cast in all cases by plastic wrap or a bag.
* Do not poke inside cast with any object, and do not apply liquid or powder inside cast (to protect from damaging skin or creating a source of irritation).
  - An antihistamine may be used to ease itching.
  - A blow dryer on cool air may be blown into edge of cast to soothe and decrease itching.
* Protect cast edges (will help decrease irritation from rubbing and protect from urine and feces if near perineal area).
  - Use waterproof tape to petal edges (covers sharp areas).
  - Use waterproof pad gently tucked into edges when using the bathroom.
* Observe for signs of complications.
  - Assess extremity for color, sensation, and temperature (initially every 2 hours, increasing to every 8 hours).
  - Assess for swelling or increased pain.
  - Assess for foul smell.
  - Report any deviations from normal to physician.

mors. Another round of chemotherapy is usually administered. The prognosis for Ewing's sarcoma is the same as for osteogenic sarcoma.

key points ✳

- ✳ Bones provide support and protection for the entire body. Joints hold bones together, provide flexibility of movement, and require daily use to maintain function. Muscles move, stabilize, and support body parts.
- ✳ Traction can be used to align and stabilize bone fragments, allow an extremity to rest, correct a deformity, immobilize an area, or reduce muscle spasms. Three types of traction used include manual, skin, and skeletal.
- ✳ Common diagnostic tests used to detect musculoskeletal disorders are x-rays, bone scans, arthroscopy, electromyography (EMG), joint aspiration, and CAT scans.
- ✳ Treatment for congenital dislocation of the hip is designed to relocate or stabilize the femoral head in the acetabulum. Techniques used to accomplish this include the Pavlik harness, skin traction, hip spica casts, surgical reconstruction, and physical therapy.
- ✳ Nursing care for the child with Duchenne's muscular dystrophy includes assisting the child to maintain independence for as long as possible, preventing injury, providing emotional support, and carefully assessing respiratory function.
- ✳ Three types of spinal curves include kyphosis (curvature of the thoracic spine), lordosis (curvature of the cervical or lumbar spine), and scoliosis (a lateral curvature of the spine).
- ✳ Juvenile rheumatoid arthritis (JRA) can be one of three types: systemic onset, polyarticular onset, and pauciarticular onset.
- ✳ Fractures in children can be complete, incomplete, transverse, oblique, spiral, simple, compound, or comminuted.
- ✳ A strain is the stretching of a muscle or tendon beyond its capacity. A sprain is the tearing of ligaments around a joint.
- ✳ Osteogenic sarcoma and Ewing's sarcoma cause about 85% of primary malignant tumors in children. The 5-year survival rate for both types of cancers is greater than 50% if the tumor is detected early and a rigorous treatment plan is followed.

review questions ✳

1. Scoliosis is defined as a sideways curve of at least
   a. 10 degrees.
   b. 15 degrees.
   c. 25 degrees.
   d. 30 degrees.
2. The *primary* therapeutic management of osteomyelitis is
   a. maintaining bed rest.
   b. administrating antibiotics.
   c. improving nutrition.
   d. maintaining limb functioning.
3. The deformity often produced when a fracture occurs is primarily the result of
   a. a compound fracture.
   b. the break in bone continuity.
   c. surrounding muscle tightness.
   d. scattered bone fragments.
4. Children with juvenile rheumatoid arthritis must be encouraged to
   a. exercise by swimming, walking, or running.
   b. maintain good nutrition by eating foods high in carbohydrates.
   c. conserve their energy by using wheelchairs, crutches, and splints.
   d. prevent recurring streptococcal infections by having routine serum evaluations.
5. The component of traction management that involves backward force is called
   a. traction.
   b. countertraction.
   c. friction.
   d. pull.

references ✳

Cancer facts and figures 1990, Atlanta, GA., 1990, American Cancer Society.

Hathaway, W., Hay, W., Groothuis, J., & Paisley, J. (1993). *Current pediatric diagnosis and treatment* (11th ed.). East Norwalk, CT: Appleton & Lange.

Pendergrast, R. A., Ashworth, C. S., DuRant, R. H. & Litaker, M. (1992). Correlate of children's bicycle helmet use and short-term failure of school level interventions. *Pediatrics, 90*(3), 354–358.

Wallace, C.A. & Levinson, J.E. (1991). *Juvenile rheumatoid arthritis: outcome & treatment for the 1990's*. Rheumatic Disease Clinics of North America, 17:891–905.

White, P. H. & Ansell, B. M. (1992). Methotrexate for juvenile rheumatoid arthritis. *New England Journal of Medicine, 326*(16): 1077–1078.

Witt, J. D., Swann, M. & Ansell, B. M. (1991). Total hip replacement for juvenile chronic arthritis. *Journal of Bone and Joint Surgery, 73*(6), 770–773.

bibliography ✳

Barrett, J. B. & Bryant, B. H. (1990). Fractures: Types, treatment, perioperative implications. *AORN Journal, 52*(4), 755–771.

Betz, L. B., Hunsberger, M. M. & Wright, S. (1994). *Family centered nursing care of children* (2nd ed.). Philadelphia: W.B. Saunders.

Brosnan, H. (1991). Nursing management of the adolescent with idiopathic scoliosis. *Nursing Clinics of North America, 26*(1), 17–31.

Gagliardi, B. (1991). The impact of Duchenne muscular dystrophy on families. *Orthopaedic Nursing, 10*(5), 41–49.

Gulanick, M., Puzas, M. K. & Wilson, C. R. (1992). *Nursing care plans for newborns and children–acute and critical care.* St. Louis: Mosby–Year Book.

Jackson, D. B. & Saunders, R. B. (1993). *Child health nursing–a comprehensive approach to the care of children and their families.* Philadelphia: J.B. Lippincott.

Jones-Walton, P. (1991). Clinical standards in skeletal pin site care. *Orthopaedic Nursing, 10*(2), 12–17.

Martinez, A. G., Weinstein, S. L., & Dietz, F. R. (1992). The weight bearing abduction brace for treatment of Legg-Perthes disease. *The Journal of Bone and Joint Surgery*, 74A, 12–21.

Mason, K. J. (1991). Congenital orthopaedic anomalies and their impact on the family. *The Nursing Clinics of North America, 26* , 1–16.

Morrissy, R. T. & Selman, S. (1991). Slipped capital femoral epiphysis. *Orthopedic Nursing, 10*(1), 11–20.

Rockwood, C. A., Wilkins, K. F., & King, R. E. (Eds.) (1991). *Fractures in children* (3rd ed.). Philadelphia: J.B. Lippincott.

Thompson, D. C., Thompson, R. S., & Rivara, F. P. (1990). Incidence of bicycle-related injuries in a defined population. *American Journal of Public Health, 80*, 1388–1389.

Whaley, L. F. & Wong, D. L. (1991). *Nursing care of infants and children* (4th ed.). St. Louis: Mosby–Year Book.

Wong, D. L. (1993). *Whaley and Wong's Essentials of pediatric nursing* (4th ed.) St. Louis: Mosby–Year Book.

outline

the child with an alteration in integumentary function

37

objectives

After studying this chapter, the reader should be able to:

* Name the components of the integumentary system.
* Describe at least three differences between infant and adult skin characteristics.
* Describe cultural differences related to white, African American, and Asian people, focusing on skin color, presence of sweat glands, and mongolian spots.
* Discuss the impact of skin lesions on the child's physical and psychosocial well-being.
* Discuss nursing measures to prevent discomfort associated with pain and pruritus.
* Define vitiligo, seborrheic dermatitis, diaper dermatitis, and acne vulgaris.
* Discuss the treatment for scalded skin syndrome and impetigo.
* Compare and contrast the following disorders: pediculosis, scabies, herpes simplex, and tinea infections.
* Describe the four degrees of burn trauma and appropriate nursing measures for each.

key terms

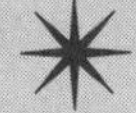

alopecia
apocrine glands
colloid
comedone
débridement
dermis
eccrine sweat glands
epidermis
erythema
eschar
homograft
infestations
keloid
kerion
macule
papule
pruritus
sebum
septic shock
vesicle

Neff C & Spray M. *Introduction to Maternal and Child Health Nursing,*

The integumentary system is a protective covering for the body. The major parts of the integumentary system include the skin, hair, and nails.

The skin is the body's natural barrier against infection. Any break in the skin provides a means for pathogens to enter the body, producing local and systemic infections. Skin disorders are associated with pruritus (itching), which increases the child's risk of secondary skin infectious disorders.

This chapter covers common skin disorders affecting children. A brief review of anatomy and physiology is provided, emphasizing major differences between children and adults. Cultural skin characteristics are presented to assist the nurse in making appropriate assessments of children from different racial groups.

> **display 37-1**
> *skin color related to disease factors*
>
> Areas of darkly pigmented brown skin may be caused by the sun or may indicate pituitary tumors, Addison's disease, or liver disease in light skin.
>
> Areas of black skin in children with light complexions indicate tissue death; these areas may be localized in the case of gangrene or generalized due to burns.
>
> Blue skin in children with light complexions can be caused by anxiety or a cold environment. Circumoral pallor may indicate cardiovascular or pulmonary disease.
>
> Reddish-blue skin in children with a light complexion may indicate increased amounts of hemoglobin, reduced hemoglobin (containing decreased amounts of oxygen), capillary stasis, or polycythemia.
>
> Red skin in children with a light complexion is caused by dilation of blood vessels or increased blood flow, as seen in fever, alcohol intake, viral exanthems, hives, local inflammation, or blushing.
>
> Localized areas of white skin may result from decreased or absent melanin, as seen in vitiligo or some rashes in dark-skinned children. Generalized white skin results from albinism (in African American children) or decreased oxygenated red blood cells, as seen in anemia (light skin)
>
> Jaundice in dark-skinned children is detected by examining the hard palate. Yellowing of the skin in children with a light complexion can be caused by accumulation of hardened tissue, as seen in calluses on the palms of the hands or soles of the feet.
>
> Flushing is best noted at the tips of the ears in dark-skinned children.

✳ family considerations

Home care of skin problems ranges from first aid treatment for skin lacerations and burns to reducing the itching experienced in many infectious disorders of children. The majority of disorders involving the skin are not life-threatening, but because skin is so visible, skin lesions alter the child's appearance. Changes in skin color can indicate health problems (Display 37-1).

Flawless skin is recognized as a personal beauty asset in our society. Children with skin lesions or scars can suffer rejection and humiliation from others. Peer rejection and social isolation increase the child's risk for emotional distress.

Bathing and grooming a young child is a parental or caregiver role. When a young child has a soiled and unkempt appearance (other than during play time), he or she may be neglected or abused.

It is important to keep cleanliness in perspective when children are busy playing. Children tend to attract dirt. Getting dirty is an important part of discovering the world. Rolling and tumbling on the ground are a meaningful part of play that promotes growth and development.

Young children have a limited understanding about being "clean." Personal hygiene routines are established early in childhood and include washing hands before eating and after using the bathroom. Making soap, water, and towels accessible to young children contributes to their taking responsibility for handwashing. Children with clean, intact skin are less likely to experience an infection if a skin break occurs.

✳ nursing considerations

Although skin lesions are typically not life-threatening, they can produce anxiety about appearance. The nurse needs to be prepared to reassure and provide information to child and parents. It is important for the nurse to show concern and accept the child. Any hesitation on the nurse's part to touch the child can be misinterpreted as rejection based on appearance. Parental rejection of the child may be reflected by negative comments about the skin lesions.

emergencies

Emergency measures may be necessary if the child's rash results from a systemic infection or allergic response. Incidence of *septic shock* increases with systemic bacterial infections. Serious allergic responses contribute to increased risk of *anaphylactic shock.*

Symptoms of septic shock include petechiae (pin-point hemorrhages), purpura (large purple hemorrhages), increased heart rate, decreased blood pressure, diminished level of consciousness, and cool, mottled skin. Major concerns with anaphylactic shock include breathing difficulties progressing to respiratory arrest and death (see Chap. 20).

children at special risk

Children with human immunodeficiency virus or acquired immunodeficiency syndrome are at increased risk for skin disorders because they are immune suppressed (see Chap. 32).

behavioral considerations

Care of children with altered skin integrity involves measures to prevent discomfort and reduce anxiety. Young children tend to believe that they may lose everything inside their body if a hole is made in their skin. Consequently, most toddlers and preschoolers think bandages will keep their body intact. Colorful bandages and happy face stickers over sterile dressings act as distractors.

> **nursing alert**
>
> *Before removing tape from a child's skin, apply mineral oil to the tape to help it come off more easily.*

Dressing changes are not always understood by young children. They often cry from fear, rather than pain. Providing age-appropriate explanations and allowing caregivers to stay during procedures help reduce the child's fear.

Preschool and school-age children appreciate nursing explanations about procedures that include drawings, dolls, teddy bears, or toys. Dressing change fears can be reduced if the child is given the opportunity to handle supplies and put dressings on a favorite toy.

Young children are not able to understand the concept of sterile and contaminated. Care must be taken to secure dressings with adequate tape and keep children from taking the dressing off, scratching the skin underneath, or putting the soiled dressings in their mouths.

Clean technique and universal precautions are used when providing care for children who have skin rashes without skin breakdown. Sterile technique must always be used when providing care to open skin areas. Hospital protocol must be followed when performing specific sterile and clean dressing procedures. Care must be taken when warm compresses are used to avoid burning sensitive skin.

teaching guidelines
maintaining healthy skin

* Maintain cleanliness to reduce number of bacteria on the skin.
* Avoid sun (ultraviolet light) exposure to reduce the risk of skin cancer. Use hats, clothing, and sunscreen with a sun-protection factor (SPF) of 15 or higher to protect the skin.
* Keep skin covered when playing in cold weather to prevent chapping and cracking of skin and freezing of exposed areas.

chronic care considerations

Any skin disorder that lasts more than 6 months is considered chronic. Care for these types of problems is usually provided by nurses on an outpatient basis, although some acute episodes may require hospitalization. Chronic skin conditions, such as eczema, may have periods of remission and exacerbation, which can be frustrating for children, parents, and nurses.

Skin problems can reflect disorders in other body systems. For example, spots of patchy light brown pigmentation, called café-au-lait spots, may resemble vitiligo but instead indicate *neurofibromatosis,* an inherited disease characterized by the development of tumors in bone and soft tissue at the onset of puberty. See the Teaching Guidelines for maintaining healthy skin.

anatomy and physiology of the integument

The skin is the largest component of the integumentary system and can be described as follows:

* A thin layer of tissue covering the entire body, containing sweat and oil glands
* An important indicator of alterations of other body systems (especially cardiovascular, respiratory, gastrointestinal, endocrine and urinary; see Display 37-1)

The skin of the adult varies in thickness and consists of three major layers: the *epidermis,* the *dermis*, and the *hypodermis* or subcutaneous layer (Fig. 37-1). The subcutaneous layer includes fat deposits and supports the two outer layers.

The *dermis* contains blood vessels, nerves, and glands, including the *eccrine* (which regulate body heat), *apocrine* (sweat glands in the axillary and pubic areas), and *sebaceous* glands. The secretions of the apocrine glands produce the characteristic odor of perspiration. *Sebaceous glands* (oil glands) usually contain a hair follicle and secrete *sebum*, an oily substance that helps the skin retain water.

pediatric factors

Infant skin, especially in premature infants, is thin, and the cells are loosely attached to each other. Infant skin contains more water and less oil than adult skin. These characteristics contribute to skin sensitivity and decreased heat regulation. In addition, infants are at increased risk for skin reactions from absorbing harmful topical products, such as soaps and sprays, which are normally nontoxic in adults.

Infants readily exhibit signs of alterations in skin integrity, especially blistering, as a reaction to trauma. Because an infant's skin contains more water than an adult, dehydration is easily detected by loss of skin turgor.

A toddler's skin becomes tougher as the epidermis and dermis fuse together. The fused skin provides more protection from fluid loss, infection, and irritation.

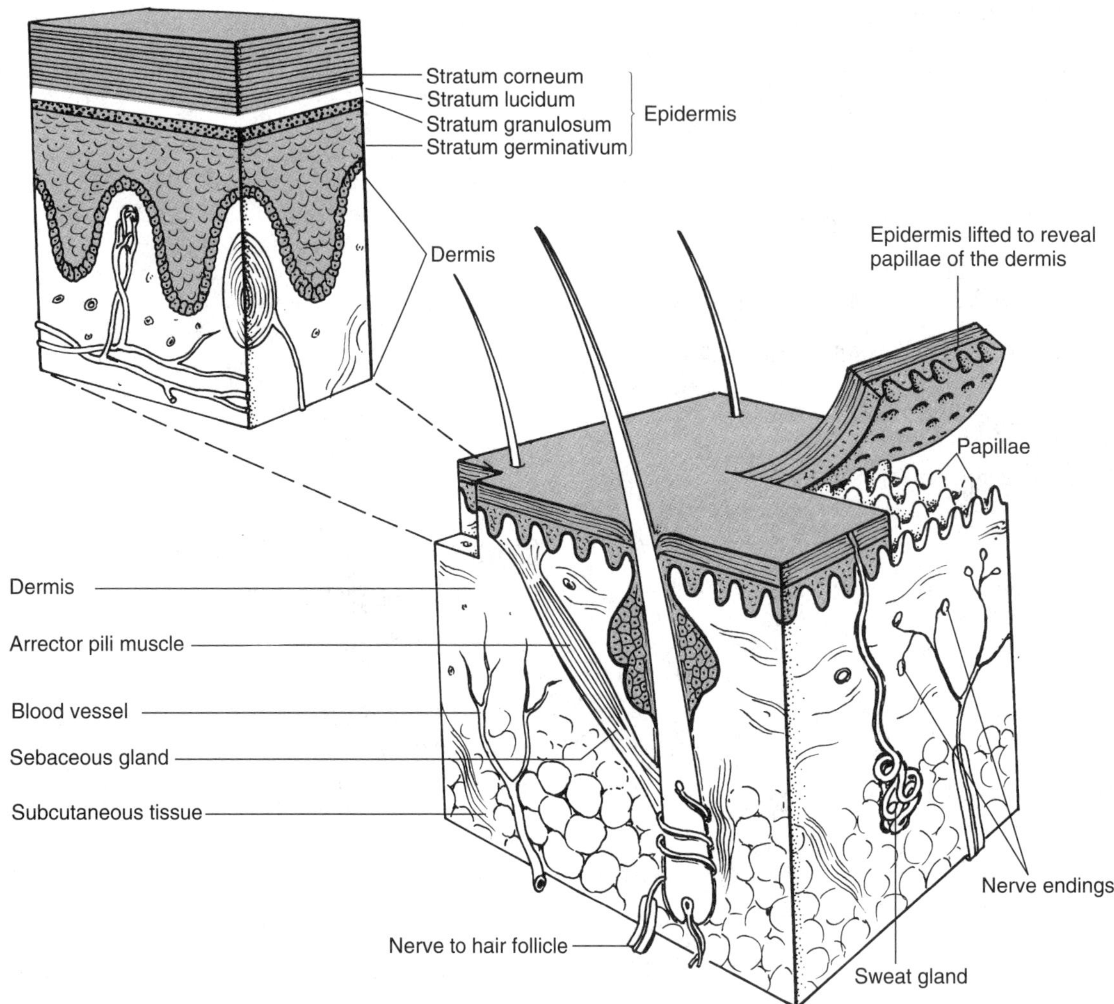

figure 37-1 *Layers of the skin. (Chafee, E. E., & Lytle, L. M. [1980].* Basic physiology and anatomy. *Philadelphia: J. B. Lippincott, p. 72.)*

Skin structures are stable during the school-age period. However, the school-age child is exposed to many different kinds of skin problems, such as scabies, impetigo, and fungal infections.

The skin is fully mature at puberty. The increase in size and secretion of the oil (sebaceous) glands during adolescence increases the risk of acne on the face, back, and chest. During adolescence, increased eccrine and apocrine sweat gland activity contributes to a strong body odor.

hair

The entire body, except the palms of the hands and soles of the feet, contains hair follicles. Loss of hair, called alopecia, may result from infections, endocrine disorders, drug reactions, chemotherapy, and various hair products. "Cornrowing" (making small tight braids in the hair) or using a hair pick may cause temporary or permanent bald spots.

Hair loss influences a child's perception of body image. It is important for the child and family to understand the underlying cause of hair loss. Most alopecia in children is reversible, and hair growth resumes once the cause is eliminated. Children should be encouraged to think about alternative ways to cope with the loss, such as the use of scarfs, wigs, and hats.

nails

Hard, hornlike nail plates are formed from the epidermis at the tips of the fingers and toes. They protect the soft tip of the fingers and aid in grasping. The nails are pink from underlying blood vessels, and they have a contoured shape.

Children with nutritional deficiencies often have split, thin, easily broken nails. Alterations in heart and lung functioning cause nailbeds to be *cyanotic* (bluish) and blunt (*clubbed*) on the ends. Anxious and emotional children tend to bite and tear their nails until the nailbeds bleed.

table 37-1 cultural variations of skin coloring

	Asian	African American	Hispanic	Native American	White
Skin type and color	Light pigment Brown to pale at birth; skin darker white with yellowish tinge, peaks at 6–8 wk	Increased melanin protects against sun Outer layer of skin more compact with more cell layers	Varying degrees of pigmentation Large percentage have tan to dark brown skin	Varying degrees of pigmentation	Skin color variations (eg, sallow, pink, olive)

cultural differences

Skin color, texture, and characteristics differ according to the child's race. An understanding of the basic differences enables the nurse to be more accurate when assessing the child's skin (Table 37-1).

Pallor is best detected in nail beds, conjunctivae, mouth, and tongue in children with dark skin, especially African Americans. Nail beds are darker than in children with light skin. Skin rashes may be difficult to see in children with dark skin. Cyanosis can appear black, and ashen skin may indicate pallor.

African American children have an increased amount of melanin that protects against solar radiation. The outermost layer of skin is compact, tends to be dry, has more cell layers, and provides increased protection from injury. African American hair has more sebaceous secretions than the hair of white children. Common skin manifestations in African American children include skin pits, extra nipples in females, and *keloid* scar formation (hyperplastic scar tissue).

mongolian spots

Mongolian spots are blue or blue-black patches on the lower back or buttocks. They are a collection of pigment cells in children of Asian, Southern European, African, and Native American descent. They tend to fade as the skin becomes thicker; however, pigmentation can be seen throughout the lifespan in some individuals.

Mongolian spots should be documented to prevent being mistaken for bruises. Parents need reassurance that mongolian spots are normal in some races.

sweat gland differences

Asian and Native American children have fewer apocrine sweat glands than white or African American children. They have mild to absent body odor and sparse body hair. Eskimo children also have a decreased number of apocrine sweat glands on the body trunk and extremities.

✳ nursing process in integumentary disorders

Most indications of a skin disorder involve rashes or other lesions. Childhood rashes can be caused by a variety of pathogens, including bacteria, parasites, allergens, and viruses. Universal precautions must be used when direct contact is made with skin lesions because they may be contagious.

nursing assessment

Subjective data to be assessed include the following:

- Information about the child's developmental level, general health status, ethnic background, and cultural practices pertinent to hygiene. Activities of daily living, such as bathing; routines used to cleanse the diaper area; laundering practices (changing soap or laundry detergent); daily habits, such as dietary practices, constant pulling of the hair, scratching, or nail-biting; and contact with animals provide important information. The following questions should be answered: When was the rash first noticed? Did an event, such as playing outdoors, precede it? Is the child scratching the rash or complaining about it? Has the child been exposed recently to an animal or a child with a similar rash? What is the child's immunization status? When and what was the last vaccine received? What medications, including over-the-counter drugs, such as vitamins and cough syrup, does the child take? Have there been any changes or additions to the medication regimen recently?
- Medical history information includes childhood diseases, known allergies, diet, environmental hazards, and possible exposure to infectious diseases (important for children who attend day care centers). Medical history for school-age children and adolescents includes information about the use of alcohol, drugs, and sexual activity.
- Family history information includes allergies, familial hair loss, and genetic patterns or predispositions for skin problems.

Objective data to be assessed include the following:

* Determine location, size, color, other characteristics (eg, flat or raised) of skin lesions; presence of drainage; and signs of scratching and secondary infection.
* Assess type and amount of clothing worn; type of diapers used (disposable or cloth); and whether the child wears plastic pants.
* Vital sign data indicate temperature elevation as a response to infection. Fever can increase the sensation of pruritus and child's irritability.

nursing diagnosis

Nursing diagnoses related to alteration in integumentary function include the following:

* Altered Comfort, related to pruritus
* Impaired Skin Integrity, related to lesions and inflammatory response
* Risk for Infection, related to impaired skin integrity
* Risk for Self Esteem Disturbance, related to appearance of lesions and response of others
* Risk for Altered Health Maintenance, related to insufficient knowledge of condition, topical agents, and contraindications
* Parental Anxiety, related to child's disorder, treatments, and uncertainty of outcome

planning and implementation

promotion of comfort

* Assess factors that cause pruritus. Administer prescribed medications, such as antipyretic drugs (Tylenol), skin lotions, and creams. Administer special baths known as colloid (oatmeal) soaks or compresses as ordered for itching. Soaking in a tub of tepid water without bubbles or oils may help. Avoid putting powders or oils on affected skin. A cold water humidifier is recommended to combat dryness. Avoid overdressing because perspiration intensifies itching. Explain to the child how it will feel when cool compresses are applied. Monitor and document the effectiveness of medications and treatments. Maintain cool room temperature, and promote ventilation. Apply loose clothing that will not constrict or irritate affected skin.

promotion of skin integrity

* Inspect skin often; document skin condition, and report any status changes. Keep skin clean and dry. Avoid use of irritating soap; rinse skin well. Keep bed linen dry, clean, and free of wrinkles. Supervise patient and family in skin care measures to promote healing and prevent recurrence.
* Perform prescribed treatment regimen for skin condition involved; monitor and document progress. Apply bed cradle to protect lesions from bed covers. Apply mittens to prevent young children from scratching the skin. Provide diversional play activities, such as games, stories, and interactive television watching. Cotton pajamas and nightgowns are less likely to cause pruritus than nylon or rayon. Avoid using heavy blankets (especially wool) to cover the child.
* Clip the child's fingernails to reduce the risk of scratching and tearing the skin. The parents must understand why the child's nails need to be cut.
* Monitor nutritional status. Maintain adequate fluid intake. Monitor intake and output.

infection control

* Maintain infection control standards (especially universal precautions) to reduce the risk of spreading disease. Observe skin lesions for changes in color, presence, amount, and odor of drainage. Warn against tampering with wound or dressings to reduce the risk of secondary infection.
* Supervise older children and parents in skin care management, and provide feedback. Explain the significance of using prescribed medications, side effects, and expected reactions.
* Monitor vital signs every 4 hours, noting any changes in pulse, respirations, or body temperature. Monitor white blood count. Culture drainage from open lesions.

promotion of self-concept

* Allow child and caregivers an opportunity to express feelings regarding skin problem to reduce anxiety. Encourage the child to focus on strengths, such as school success and athletic skills.

promotion of home care

* Explain therapy to child (if age appropriate) and caregivers to encourage compliance with treatment regimen and reduce anxiety. Make appropriate referrals to social service or support groups as indicated by child's condition.

evaluation

* Child exhibits signs of diminished discomfort with decreased irritability, increased willingness to play, and effective rest periods.
* Child exhibits improved or healed skin lesions with no skin breakdown. Adequate nutritional and fluid intake are maintained. Child is afebrile with no signs of infection. When skin condition is a secondary problem, primary problem (ie, infection or allergy) is controlled.
* Child and parents express feelings about body image changes.
* Children (age-appropriate) and parents understand and demonstrate skin integrity regimen, preventive skin care measures, and risk factors associated with skin condition.

types of skin lesions

Skin lesions are commonly classified as primary and secondary. *Primary lesions* erupt from previously normal skin in the form of macules, papules, or vesicles. *Secondary le-*

table 37-2 types and descriptions of skin lesions

Skin Lesion	Description
Crusts	Dried residue of exudate (scab)
Desquamation	Areas of flaking
Excoriation	An abrasion of the outer layer of the skin (floor burn)
Fissure	Crack in the skin
Macules	Flat, discolored spots on the skin that are not depressed or raised (eg, freckle)
Maculopapular	Multiple lesions consisting of macules and papules
Papules	Solid elevations of the skin that do not contain fluid (eg, wart)
Nodule	Small node
Petechiae	Tiny hemorrhagic spots on the skin
Pustules	Vescicules that contain pus
Scales	Thin flakes of skin
Ulcer	Open skin area with loss of skin resulting in a crater-type lesion
Vesicle	An elevation that contains serous, seropurulent, or bloody fluid
Wheals	Raised lesions often accompanied by severe itching (hives)
	Wheals may or may not itch.

sions result from changes in primary lesions. Secondary lesions are described as erosions, ulcers, fissures, crusts, and scales (Table 37-2).

diagnostic tests

Several different diagnostic tests can be used to determine the causes of integumentary problems. The most common tests follow:

* Potassium hydroxide test determines the presence of fungal infection on the skin or hair.
* Tzanck smear distinguishes viral diseases from nonviral diseases (eg, herpes simples, varicella, or herpes zoster).
* Wood's light (ultraviolet light) helps diagnose selected fungal, bacterial, and pigmentary disorders.
* Skin cultures confirm and characterize pathogens. They are usually limited to fungi and bacterial infections because viral cultures are less available.
* Complete blood count provides a thorough evaluation of blood components. For example, an elevated white blood count establishes presence of infection, decreases in red blood cells and hemoglobin count indicate anemia, and an elevated eosinophil level indicates the body's response to allergies.
* Patch test identifies responses to contact allergens.
* Skin biopsy provides information about skin nodules, such as presence of cancer cells.
* Tuberculin tests (PPD, Mantoux, and Tine), determine whether the child has been exposed to infection with the tubercle bacillus (see Chap. 30).

Prior to any of these tests, the nurse explains the procedure to the child and caregivers. During the procedure, the nurse helps the child hold still. After the specimen is obtained, the nurse performs any wound care necessary and comforts the child.

inflammatory skin disorders

Inflammatory disorders of the skin include atopic dermatitis (eczema), seborrheic dermatitis, diaper dermatitis, contact dermatitis, and acne vulgaris. These disorders cause erythema (redness) and rashes, and may be complicated by secondary bacterial infections.

atopic dermatitis (eczema)

There is no known cause of atopic dermatitis. It is believed to be inherited and is often associated with asthma and hay fever. In the infant, it appears between 2 months and 2 years and is more common in infants who are formula fed. Symptoms worsen in cold weather. The childhood phase occurs between 4 and 10 years and is characterized by more scattered lesions than seen in the infant.

pathophysiology

Symptoms of infantile eczema include a raised red papular rash with blisters. Ruptured vesicles secrete yellow sticky drainage that dries and forms crusts on the skin.

Atopic dermatitis affects the face, scalp, neck, chest, back of the arms, and front of the legs. The palms of the hands and soles of the feet are unaffected. Dry skin accompanies eczema and leads to scratching and inflammation. The pruritic lesions are uncomfortable and cause children to be fussy and irritable.

medical management

Medical management is aimed at reducing the amount of allergen exposure (if identified) and control of pruritus. Eliminating certain foods from the diet may be necessary because milk, eggs, wheat, citrus fruits, and tomatoes are common allergens in infants.

Reducing pruritus and preventing secondary infection from scratching is accomplished by applying wet dressings and topical steroids, such as 1% hydrocortisone cream. As lesions heal, emollients and moisturizers are used to lubricate the skin.

seborrheic dermatitis

Seborrheic dermatitis in infants is often called *cradle cap*. It is most common before 6 months of age. Seborrheic dermatitis may occur in adolescents and affects the eyebrows, face, and scalp.

pathophysiology

Seborrheic dermatitis involves a thick, scaly, mildly pruritic and oily yellowish crust formation on the scalp. Infants with dry, sensitive skin may develop crusts on the eyelids, external ear canals, and groin.

medical management

Diagnosis of seborrheic dermatitis is based on history and examination of the skin. No laboratory tests are used to diagnose this disorder, and it is often confused with other skin conditions like psoriasis or atopic dermatitis.

Medical management includes daily shampooing of the hair and scalp using an antiseborrheic shampoo containing selenium. Salicylic acid or tar shampoos and topical steroids (except on the face) may be used. Severe cases may require the administration of systemic antibiotics. Gentle removal of the scales from the scalp using a comb or brush also is helpful.

nursing care

The nurse assesses the child's and caregiver's understanding of the condition and their ability and motivation to follow the treatment regimen. If the client is an adolescent, the social implications of seborrheic dermatitis can be severe, leading to diminished self-esteem and isolation. The nurse encourages the client and caregiver to express concerns about the condition and teaches them precautions to prevent infection of lesions.

contact dermatitis

Contact dermatitis is an inflammatory reaction triggered by contact with a natural or synthetic substance to which the skin is sensitive. Poison ivy, poison oak, topical medications, soaps, chemicals, clothing (especially wool), and jewelry made with nickel are common irritants.

pathophysiology

The onset, severity, and duration of contact dermatitis varies, depending on the allergen. The affected skin has a faint, transient, erythematous rash. Some children have localized patches of raised red papules or vesicles confined to the exposed area.

medical management

Treatment of contact dermatitis requires identifying and removing the child from the irritant. Medication (usually topical) is administered to control the itching, and antibiotic ointments are prescribed if the skin is broken. Treatment of contact dermatitis is similar to eczema.

diaper dermatitis

Diaper dermatitis (diaper rash) is a type of contact dermatitis that results primarily from prolonged exposure to wet or soiled diapers. As urine decomposes, it produces ammonia, which irritates the infant's delicate skin. The skin may be further irritated by use of plastic or rubber pants or diapers that have been washed with strong laundry detergents and inadequately rinsed.

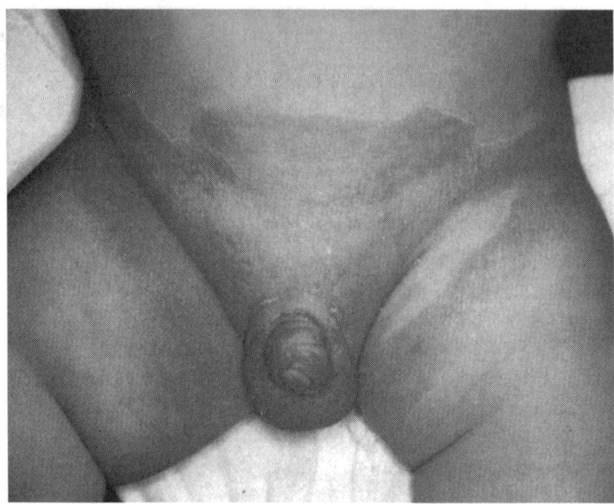

figure 37-2 *Diaper dermatitis. (Sauer, G. C. [1991].* Manual of skin diseases *[6th ed.]. Philadelphia: J. B. Lippincott.)*

pathophysiology

Chafing dermatitis is the most common type of diaper dermatitis. Reddened, inflamed skin is seen on the buttocks, medial thighs, mons pubis, or scrotum where the skin has touched the diaper (Fig. 37-2).

Yeast (*Candida albicans*), bacterial (streptococcal or staphylococcal), and fungal infections can further complicate diaper dermatitis. Vesicles and erosions, red papules with drainage, and ulceration are signs of secondary infection. Diaper dermatitis may exist with an underlying skin disorder, such as eczema.

> **nursing alert**
> *Infants taking antibiotics are at increased risk for developing a yeast infection (Candida albicans) diaper rash.*

medical management

Diagnosis of diaper dermatitis is based on the pattern and color of the rash and lesions and the history of its onset, duration, and treatment.

Bacterial infections are treated with a topical antibiotic cream or ointment, such as polymyxin B sulfate (Neosporin or Polysporin). Mild inflammation is treated with a topical corticosteroid, such as triamcinolone (Aristocort or Kenalog). Fungal infections, such as *C. albicans*, are treated with topical nystatin or other antifungal drugs. Clioquinol and iodoquinol are contraindicated because of their neurotoxicity.

nursing care

Parental education is essential for preventing diaper dermatitis. Caregivers are instructed to change diapers frequently and cleanse the diaper area with warm water. If soap is necessary, the diaper area needs to be thoroughly rinsed and completely dry before a clean diaper is applied. Parents need to know that commercially available wet wipes may further irritate infant skin.

Protective ointments, such as zinc oxide, can be used for diaper dermatitis. However, it should not be used on severely inflamed areas because it increases sweat retention and may make the condition worse. Mineral oil is effective in removing zinc oxide without irritating the infant's genitalia. Desitin is a protective ointment used for mild inflammation.

It is important to evaluate the type of diaper being used because some infants are allergic to disposable diapers. When cloth diapers are used, laundry methods should be determined to rule out the risk of irritation from soap residue in the diaper. Plastic or rubber pants used with cloth diapers trap heat and wetness, increasing the infant's risk of skin breakdown.

Some parents use baby powder before putting on a clean diaper on their infant. Many physicians question this practice because of the risk of aspiration if the powder contains talc, a known carcinogen (Hollinger, 1990). Powder containing cornstarch is not recommended because it can be metabolized by microorganisms. If powder has been used, all traces of powder residue must be removed because wet powder holds ammonia next to the infant's skin.

acne vulgaris

Approximately 80% to 90% of adolescents experience acne at some point and to some degree. It can begin as early as 9 or 10 years and most often reaches a peak in late adolescence.

pathophysiology

The cause of acne is not fully understood. However, endogenous (within the person) and exogenous (outside the person) factors are believed to play a role. Endogenous factors include increased sebum production, resulting from androgenous hormone production at puberty; bacterial colonization; the individual host immune response; and obstruction of the pores (the opening of the oil follicles) with keratinous and sebaceous debris. Exogenous factors include hot, humid climates; cosmetics; hair spray; and medications, such as corticosteroids and lithium. Diet is not believed to be a major factor in the development of acne.

Although the site of the disease involves the oil follicles, the oil gland (sebaceous gland) is normal. Inflammation results when the oil follicle ruptures, spreading follicle contents into the skin. Acne lesions occur primarily on the face and upper trunk. Types include comedones, also called blackheads; papules; and inflamed lesions or pustules (Fig. 37-3). Acne is graded according to severity using the criteria in Table 37-3.

medical management

Treatment of acne depends on its severity and whether bacterial infection is present. Mild cases of acne can be managed with improved hygiene and patient education.

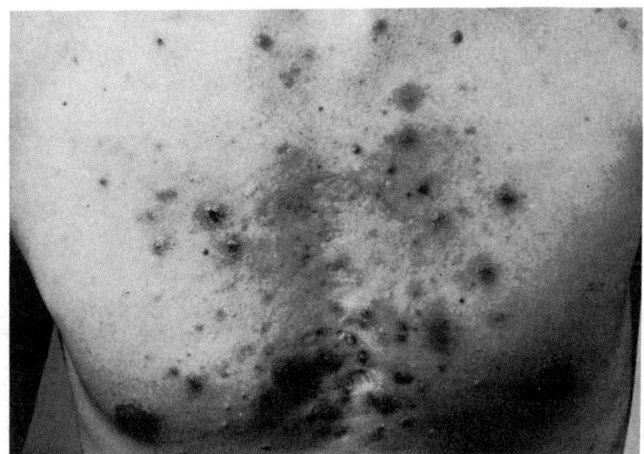

figure 37-3 *Acne vulgaris. (Sauer, G. C. [1991].* Manual of skin diseases *[6th ed]. Philadelphia: J.B. Lippincott.)*

More severe cases can damage the adolescent's self-esteem and lead to withdrawal and social isolation. In these instances, medical management may include topical benzoyl peroxide, tretinoin (retinoic acid, Retin-A), and systemic antibiotics, such as erythromycin, clindamycin, or tetracycline. Adolescent girls may be treated with oral contraceptive pills that contain poorly androgenic progestins. The most severe cases may require systemic retinoids, such as isotretinoin 13-cis-retinoic acid (Accutane). However, caution must be used when prescribing these agents because of numerous side effects. Accutane must never be given to pregnant women or women who are likely to become pregnant because it causes birth defects.

nursing care

Teaching children and caregivers about acne vulgaris is an important nursing role. The nurse can dispel myths about the causes of acne and stress healthy lifestyle practices, such as balanced diet, adequate rest, and daily exercise. Although diet has often been mentioned as a cause of acne, there is no scientific evidence linking acne with certain foods. Some teenagers believe that acne is caused by dirty skin and therefore use harsh soaps and vigorous scrubbing. These practices may make the condition worse.

table 37-3 grading scale for acne

Grade I (mild): Comedones, occasional papules
Grade II (moderate): Comedones, papules, occasional pustules
Grade II (severe): Comedones, papules, pustules, abscesses
Grade IV (congloblate): Comedones, papules, pustules, abscesses, widespread scarring

From Castiglia, P.T. & Harbin, R.E. (1992). *Child health care: Process and practice.* (p. 976). Philadelphia: J. B. Lippincott.

teaching guidelines
skin care of acne vulgaris

Wash gently with mild soap.
Dry the skin.
Avoid oil-based cosmetics.
Never leave cosmetics on the face overnight.
Avoid over-the-counter skin preparations that cause excessive drying.
Follow instructions carefully concerning application of ointment and creams.
The following medications are used for acne vulgaris:

* Benzoyl peroxide comes in gel, liquid, or cream and has an antibacterial action. The medication is applied in a thin layer and is left on all day. It tends to have a drying effect on the skin.
* Topical antibiotic creams are used when benzoyl peroxide treatment fails. Antibiotics kill bacteria on the skin.
* Oral contraceptive pills containing poorly androgenic progestins have been known to improve acne problems in adolescent girls.
* Retin-A acts by preventing blackhead (comedone) formation, opening closed comedones, and increasing blood flow to the skin. Topical Retin-A is applied at night and has a drying effect on the skin. Sun exposure must be avoided while using the cream. Oral Retin-A (Accutane) is a powerful agent used in the most severe cases of acne. It is important to prevent pregnancy while using oral Retin A because it can cause severe fetal malformations or fetal death.

The nurse discourages adolescents from squeezing or picking blackheads because this can damage tissue and increase the risk of secondary infection. Consistent, correct use of prescribed or recommended treatments can improve the skin condition gradually; however, adolescents may be impatient for results.

The adolescent's psychosocial needs are an important consideration. Any noticeable lesion can be a crisis to teenagers, especially in terms of peer relationships, dating, and sexual intimacy. Isolation and depression need immediate intervention. Early intervention and effective treatment of acne reduce the risk of scarring associated with acne lesions. See skin care Teaching Guidelines.

disorders of pigmentation

vitiligo

Vitiligo is a disorder in which areas of the skin completely lack melanin pigmentation. Although vitiligo affects all races, it is more common in African Americans because the lack of pigment is more noticeable and can affect self-image.

pathophysiology

The cause of vitiligo is unknown. The condition is usually progressive and is associated with a dominantly inherited predisposition. It has been speculated that autoimmune mechanisms are involved. Depigmented white patches may be surrounded by a hyperpigmented border. Depigmentation of the iris occurs in some cases.

medical management

Treatment of vitiligo is prolonged, tedious, expensive, and not always successful. In highly motivated clients with less than 20% of skin involved, topical methoxsalen, 0.1% Acid Mantle cream, or Unibase is used. People undergoing this treatment should apply the ointment, avoid exposure to long-wavelength ultraviolet light, thoroughly wash the ointment off the skin, and apply a sunscreen with a sun protection factor of 15. Cosmetics such as Dermablend designed to cover birthmarks offer a practical solution to vitiligo.

infectious diseases of the skin

Infectious skin diseases are most often caused by bacterial infections (*Staphylococcus*, *Streptococcocus*), viral, or fungal pathogens. The infections are contagious and can be easily spread by lesion drainage.

Most bacterial skin infections are caused by *Staphylococcus aureus* or group A, beta-hemolytic streptococci. *S. aureus* can colonize on the skin and enter through damaged skin or a hair follicle. Group A streptococci usually enter damaged skin by scratches, insect bites, and so forth.

scalded skin disease

Scalded skin disease is a staphylococcal infection seen in children younger than 2 years, primarily newborns. Affected children develop a rough-textured skin and general erythema.

pathophysiology

Scalded skin disease is caused by a toxin produced by staphylococci. It often begins as a lesion around the nose and mouth that becomes bright red and spreads rapidly. Large bullae (vesicles) filled with clear fluid form. The epidermis separates and peels off in large sheets, leaving a red, glistening, scalded-looking surface.

medical management

The child with scalded skin disease is hospitalized and given intravenous antibiotics, such as methicillin, and intravenous fluids to combat this extreme infection. Antipyretics are used for fever. In the newborn, silver sulfadiazine or another burn therapy may be used. Topical therapy is unnecessary in older children.

nursing care

Care of the child with scalded skin disease includes maintaining isolation procedures, administering medications as ordered, and maintaining hydration and nutrition. Educating caregivers to prevent future infection is essential, and scrupulous infection control procedures are vital in the newborn nursery.

impetigo

Impetigo is a bacterial infection of the upper epidermis that affects newborns and older children. It is highly contagious, and the lesions are pruritic.

pathophysiology

Impetigo in the newborn is usually caused by *Staphylococcus aureus* and can quickly reach epidemic proportions in a hospital nursery. Impetigo begins as small vesicles, usually on the face, that rupture and form a honey-colored crust bordered by an area of clear fluid.

Impetigo in the older child is generally caused by group A, beta-hemolytic *Streptococcus*, sometimes in combination with *S. aureus*. Because of the contagious and pruritic nature of the crusts and lesions, it is easily spread to all parts of the body or to other children. On rare occasions, rheumatic fever or acute glomerulonephritis may follow impetigo, and caregivers need to be aware of that possibility.

medical management

Impetigo in the newborn is treated with oral dicloxacillin or topical antibiotics, such as Neosporin or bacitracin. Topical or oral corticosteroids and antihistamines are used to reduce inflammation and provide relief from itching.

Impetigo in the older child is usually treated at home with oral penicillin and topical mupirocin. Oral antihistamines help reduce inflammation and relieve itching. Typically, the lesions are superficial. However, if the lesions are left untreated, impetigo can cause scarring. Children who have impetigo may return to school 24 hours after they begin antibiotic therapy.

nursing care

The hospitalized newborn with impetigo is isolated, and strict precautions are followed, including wearing a cover gown and gloves. The lesions are cleaned with mild soap or half-strength hydrogen peroxide twice a day. Warm soaks can help loosen thick crusts, followed by application of antibiotic ointment. The infant's hands must be covered or elbow restraints applied to prevent scratching.

Because the older child with impetigo is treated at home, the nurse teaches family members how to care for the lesions and prevent further spread of infection on the child or to other family members. The infected child and the caregivers should never share towels or washcloths. Caregivers need to be reminded to follow the physician's treatment plan and to avoid overusing creams and ointments because they may produce toxic effects.

cat-scratch disease

Cat-scratch disease (CSD), or cat scratch fever, is an acute illness, also known as benign lymphoreticulosis. The cause of this infection is not clearly understood, although recent studies suggest it may be due to a previously unknown bacterium related to the rickettsia *Rochalimaea quintana* (Tortora, Funke, & Case, 1995). This disease is most common in children between 5 and 14 years of age; 80% of patients are younger than 20 years. Family outbreaks have been known to occur, but not all family members are always symptomatic.

pathophysiology

Apparently healthy cats can transmit CSD through a scratch, puncture, abrasion, or directly through mucous membranes. The first symptom of CSD is a papule at the infection site, appearing within 3 to 10 days after contact with a cat. In a few days, the papule progresses to a fluid-filled vesicle and forms a crust. Within 2 to 4 weeks, the lymph nodes become enlarged, inflamed, and tender; large areas of redness appear over the body; and prolonged low-grade fever and malaise occur. The skin lesion tends to be nonpruritic and heals within several months without scars.

Complications include conjunctivitis associated with inoculation on the face, encephalopathy (brain involvement), osteomyelitis, thrombocytopenia, and erythema multiforme.

medical–surgical management

The diagnosis of CSD is based on a history of cat scratch, bite, or other contact with a cat or other animal; positive skin test; and laboratory data to rule out other causes of lymph node enlargement.

Antibiotics are the treatment of choice for children with CSD, and rifampin has proved particularly effective. Children and caregivers need to know that rifampin turns urine, sweat, and tears orange. Therefore, contact lenses should not be worn while taking rifampin because they can be permanently stained. Children with CSD are usually managed as outpatients, but some may require hospitalization. Activity is limited to prevent trauma to the affected node(s). Analgesics and bed rest may be indicated if fever is present. Isolation is not necessary. Local heat and moist soaks may be helpful for primary lesions. In severe cases, surgical removal or needle evacuation of the pus-filled lymph node may be necessary.

nursing care

Care of the child with CSD is similar to that for impetigo or other bacterial infections. The nurse maintains strict infection control procedures, gives antibiotics as prescribed, applies local heat and moist soaks, and performs other comfort measures. Caregivers need to be taught home care measures, possible side effects of treatment, and precautions to avoid future infection.

infestations

Infestation disorders are caused by animal parasites that invade the human body and suck blood to survive. Parasitic infestations cause intense itching, are difficult to diagnoses, and can result in secondary bacterial infections that may become more serious than the original infestation.

pediculosis

Pediculosis is infestation by lice. There are three types of pediculosis: Head lice (*Pediculus capitis*) infest the hair of the head and the eyelashes. Body lice (*Pediculus corporis*) are found in the seams of clothing or in bedding. Pubic or crab lice *(Pediculosis pubis)* infest the hairs of the genital area but may extend to other hairy areas of the body, such as the axilla. Sexually active adolescents are at increased risk for pubic lice infestation. Pubic lice also may be found in the eyelashes of the newborn. Pubic lice infestation in young children suggests possible sexual abuse. Head lice are most common, particularly among school-age children or those in day care.

pathophysiology

Itching of the scalp, especially around the ears, is a common complaint of the child infested with head lice. The head louse is microscopic (2–3 mm) and has a lifespan of 40 to 50 days. The female lays an egg encased in a gelatinous (jelly-like) nit. The nits attach to the hair shaft near the scalp and are more visible on dark hair. Immature nits have a clear white appearance, while mature nits are darker brown. Within 7 to 10 days, the egg matures and hatches, and the cycle begins again unless interrupted by treatment. Once removed from the human host, the head louse survives less than 24 hours.

The principal hazard of lice infestation is the dangerous diseases they can transmit to the infested person. These include endemic typhus, murine typhus, trench fever, and louse-borne relapsing fever (Taplin & Menking, 1988).

medical management

Management of lice infestation includes shampooing, bathing, combing hair with a metal comb to remove nits, and decontaminating inanimate objects, such as clothing, headgear, bedding, and mattresses. A solution of 50% vinegar and 50% water applied to the hair for 1 hour before shampooing can help loosen nits. Secondary bacterial infections are treated with topical antibiotics, such as Neosporin or mupirocin.

Until recently, lice infestations were treated with Kwell shampoo and other products containing lindane (gamma-benzene-hexachloride). However, Kwell was taken off the market in 1993 following a class action suit filed by more than 300 people following reports of neurologic damage associated with lindane. Lindane also has been labeled a carcinogen by the World Health Organization, the Environmental Protection Association, and the Department of Health and Human Services. Other products containing lindane are still being marketed but should not be used because of their neurotoxicity and carcinogenicity (Moses, 1995; Olkowski, Daar, & Olkowski, 1991).

For infants and children whose eyelashes are infested, petrolatum is applied two to five times daily for 8 days to suffocate and kill the lice.

nursing care

Client and caregiver education is a principal nursing role in the care of the child with pediculosis. The nurse explains why it is essential to follow the treatment regimen, including combing the hair with a fine-tooth comb to remove nits, frequent shampooing and bathing, and decontaminating household items, such as bedding, clothing, and headgear. Washable items are washed in hot water (above 125°C) and dried in a hot dryer. Other clothing should be dry-cleaned and pressed. Mattresses, furniture, and other items that cannot be cleaned should be sealed in plastic for 10 days and then vacuumed. Floors and carpeting need to be thoroughly vacuumed. Harmful pesticide sprays should be avoided.

Treatment for pediculosis must include all close personal contacts of the infected child: siblings, other family members, playmates, and schoolmates.

Caregivers may feel guilty and ashamed that their child has been infested with lice. By helping them understand treatment and hygiene practices to prevent future infestation, the nurse can assist them in dealing with those feelings.

scabies

Scabies results from infestation by a mite called *Sarcoptes scabiei*. Scabies is often called "the itch." Scabies is highly contagious and can be spread through direct or indirect contact. It is most common in school-age children, and many authorities believe that the incidence is rising dramatically. Animals infected with canine scabies, also known as *sarcoptic mange*, can cause local irritation in humans but will not cause infestation.

pathophysiology

"Itch mites" burrow under the skin to lay their eggs, create tunnel-like lines of skin lesions or bumps 5 to 15 mm long, and cause intense itching, particularly at night. Scratching often leads to secondary bacterial infections and is easily confused with other skin disorders. Scabies is transmitted by intimate contact, including sexual contact, and is seen in children of all ages and in adults. Scabies is noticeable on the hands as the mite burrows between the fingers and causes redness and flaking of the skin. It also can be found at the wrists, elbows, navel, and around the waist.

medical management

The most critical issue in treatment of scabies is accurate diagnosis. Scabies can easily be confused with other skin conditions. Therefore, it is essential that the physician perform microscopic examination of scrapings from a burrow to confirm the presence of mites or eggs. Multiple scrapings may be required for definitive diagnosis. The physician may prescribe a *scabicide* product containing topical 5% permethrin or a 10% precipitated sulfur in an aquasol base. Permethrin products can cause serious side effects in children with allergies or asthma. If secondary infection is present, antibiotic therapy may be used. Products containing lindane should not be used (see previous discussion of pediculosis). Treatment must include the infested person and all other members of the household, playmates, schoolmates, and baby sitters. Itching may continue for 2 or 3 weeks after treatment. This is normal and not a reason to reapply the scabicide product. Personal and household articles must be decontaminated (see discussion of pediculosis).

nursing care

As with pediculosis, client or caregiver education is central to care and prevention of future infestation. Clients and caregivers need to understand the importance of carefully following product instructions to reduce the risk of side effects and unnecessary overtreatment. The school or day care center must be notified that a child has been diagnosed with scabies. Educational materials can be obtained from the National Pediculosis Association.*

viral infections

Viral infections of the skin include herpes simplex (fever blisters, genital herpes) and verruca (warts).

herpes simplex

Herpes simplex virus type 1 causes oral and facial lesions called fever blisters or cold sores (gingivostomatitis). It is the most common herpetic infection in children. Until children have contracted a primary form of the disease, they do not form antibodies against the herpesvirus. Children between 1 and 4 years have a higher incidence of primary herpes. Some children become permanent carriers of herpes simplex.

Herpes simplex type 2 virus is associated with genital herpes (see Chap. 9). This condition can be life-threatening when transmitted from mother to newborn during delivery.

pathophysiology

Herpesvirus has an incubation period of 1 to 26 days. It is transmitted by direct contact. Immunity to a primary herpes response occurs after one infection. There is no immunity to recurrent herpes infections because the virus lies dormant in the body until it is activated by stress, sun exposure, fever, menstruation, and other factors. Herpesvirus is considered an opportunistic infection because the virus remains inactive until the immune system is compromised.

Lesions of herpes type 1 appear on or in the mouth (Fig. 37-4). Lesions along the gum line cause edema, redness, and bleeding. Children may have few other symptoms or may present with high fever (>104°F, 40.0°C.), restlessness, and anorexia. The cervical lymph nodes may be enlarged and tender.

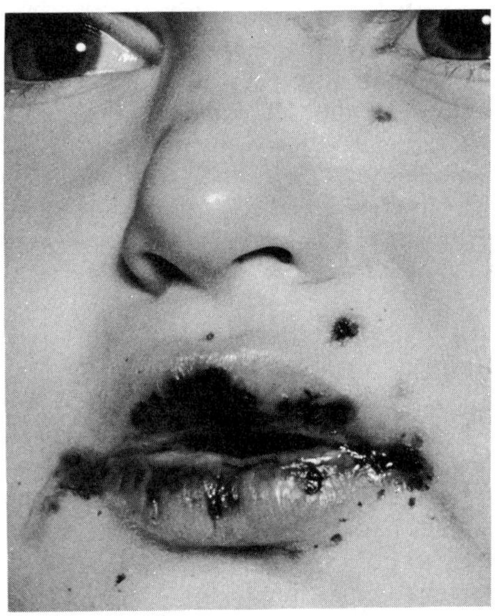

figure 37-4 *Primary herpes simplex in a 2-year-old child.*

medical management

There is no specific treatment for herpes simplex type 1 except to treat the symptoms. The disease runs its course in 5 to 7 days. Antipyretics are given for high fever. Some physicians recommend administration of anesthetic mouthwashes, such as viscous lidocaine, before meals. Avoiding hot or spicy foods is important.

warts (verruca)

Warts are skin-colored, often dirty-looking benign growths with irregular (verrucous) surfaces. Warts can appear anywhere on the body and are most common in children between 12 and 16 years. There are four types of warts: *common*; *plantar*, found on the soles of the feet; *flat*; and *genital*, known as condyloma accuminatum or venereal warts, a sexually transmitted disease. Genital warts are discussed in Chapter 9.

pathophysiology

Warts are caused by infection with one of the more than 50 types of human papillomavirus. The virus causes the cells in the epidermis to proliferate, resulting in the warty growth. Depending on the strength of the virus, the growth may be small, as in a flat wart, or great, as in the common wart (verruca vulgaris). The virus is transmitted directly (by contact with a wart on another person) and indirectly (by inanimate objects, such as a locker room floor). Like many viral diseases, warts tend to recur.

medical–surgical management

Flat warts usually disappear within 6 to 9 months without treatment. Common warts are generally frozen with an

*P.O. Box 149, Newton, MA, 02161.

application of liquid nitrogen. It is important not to apply pressure during the treatment process because it can cause ulceration and scarring. Plantar warts are treated only when they become large and painful. Treatment involves application of 40% salicylic acid paste to the lesion, taping it securely, and leaving it in place for 5 days. When the plaster is removed, necrotic tissue is gently rubbed off and a new plaster applied. This process is repeated every 5 days for 2 to 4 weeks until the wart has disappeared.

fungal infections

Fungi are a group of microorganisms that include yeasts and molds. Fungal infections can invade skin, subcutaneous tissue, mucous membranes, and bone. Fungi that affect the hair, nails, and outer epidermis are called *dermatophytes.* The two most common fungal infections in infants and children are tinea (ringworm) and *C. albicans* (yeast infection or thrush). *C. albicans* is discussed in Chapter 16.

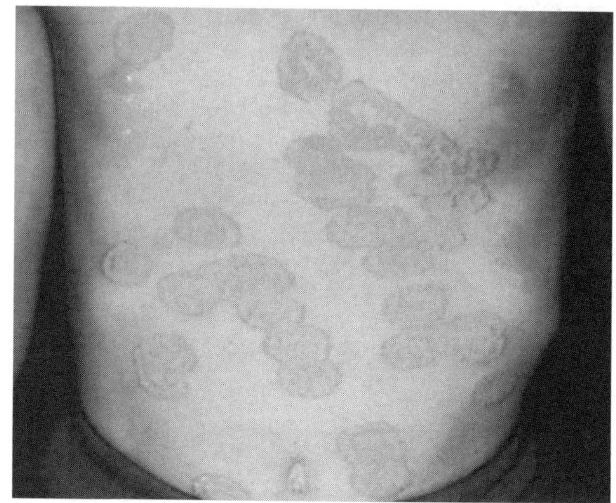

figure 37-5 *Tinea corporis. (Sauer, G. C. [1991].* Manual of skin diseases *[6th ed.]. Philadelphia. J. B. Lippincott.)*

tinea

Tinea is a fungal infection of the outer layer of the epidermis. Common examples of tinea in children include tinea capitis (head), tinea corporis (body), tinea cruris ("jock itch"), and tinea pedis (athlete's foot).

pathophysiology

When dermatophytes invade the superficial layer of the epidermis, nails, or hair, they begin to grow, release toxins, and cause a variety of lesions. The most common are round, red, scaly papules, plaques, and patches with a "wormlike" border, hence the name "ringworm."

Transmission of tinea can occur directly or indirectly through combs, brushes, barber scissors, headgear, or other clothing. It also can be transmitted by contact with an infected dog or cat. *Tinea capitis,* ringworm of the scalp, is common in school-age children. Hair thickens and breaks off, revealing a red scaly scalp. Pustule formation is followed by development of a red, boggy, fluid-filled mass called a *kerion.* Fungal culture is performed to confirm the diagnosis.

Tinia corporis, ringworm of the body (Fig. 37-5), is most commonly the result of exposure to infected pets. Lesions are round papules with a thin scale and a clear center or a circular area with no distinct lesions. The diagnosis is made by microscopic examination of scrapings using a potassium hydroxide solution.

Tinea pedis, ringworm of the feet, commonly called athlete's foot, is unusual in children younger than 10 years. Atopic or contact dermatitis is much more likely to cause similar symptoms. Tinea pedis is more common in boys after puberty and manifests as blisters on the instep. Cracking between the toes sometimes occurs. Microscopic examination of scales or blister covering is necessary to confirm the diagnosis.

Tinea cruris, "jock itch," is common in athletes, obese people, and those who perspire heavily. Lesions are red macules with sharp margins and clear centers surrounded by spreading scaly areas. They appear in the groin and the gluteal cleft (between the buttocks), and cause severe itching. Microscopic examination or fungal culture is necessary to confirm the diagnosis.

medical management

Tinea capitis is treated with oral griseofulvin. If hair is involved, the drug is given for a minimum of 6 weeks. If there is nail involvement, the drug is given for 3 months. Taking the drug with whole milk or ice cream increases absorption. If a kerion forms, prednisone is administered daily for 10 to 14 days to reduce inflammation.

Tinea corporis and tinea cruris may be treated with topical antifungals, such as clotrimazole cream, powder, or solution applied twice a day to all lesions for 3 to 4 weeks.

Tinea lesions of the feet can be effectively treated with an antifungal powder and keeping the area dry. Warm soaks two to four times a day are recommended for acute lesions that are blistered and oozing. White cotton socks help absorb moisture on the feet. It is important not to overtreat.

nursing care

The nurse teaches the client and caregiver about treatment measures and hygiene practices to avoid future infection. The full course of treatment must be completed. Headgear and shoes should not be shared, rubber or wooden sandals should be worn in community showers and on public beaches, hair should be shampooed after haircuts, and the area between the toes should be dried thoroughly after bathing or showering. In addition, contact with infected or unknown pets should be avoided.

acute integumentary problems

burns

Burn injuries can be physically life-threatening and emotionally devastating. If the child was responsible for whatever action led to being burned, he or she may feel guilty. Caregivers may feel guilty about not having prevented the burn injury.

Natural curiosity of preschool and school-age children can lead them to play with matches, touch hot burners and grab hot pots, or experiment with fire. Most burns in adolescents are the result of combustible fuels or other solvents. Although hot liquid and flame burns are the most common cause of childhood burns, chemicals and electricity also cause burns.

At least 75% of burn injuries are preventable. Teaching children what to do in case of fire can help reduce injury and death related to burns. Unless children have been taught to stop, drop, and roll when clothing is on fire, fear will cause them to run, making the fire burn faster. Fire safety is discussed in Chapter 20.

Most burn accidents injure much more than the skin. Burn injuries often involve structures below the skin, including muscles, bones, nerves, and blood vessels. Burns can injure the eyes and respiratory system structures and involve every body system. Burns can cause severe emotional and psychological problems that may last a lifetime.

Age is a major factor in the outcome of burn injuries. The younger the child, the more devastating the effects of a major burn. Immature body systems and regulatory mechanisms make it difficult for infants and children to maintain fluid and electrolyte balance and resist secondary infections. Children younger than 5 years have more severe body reactions to burns and different healing patterns when compared with other age groups. They have a greater surface area in proportion to total body size when compared with the older child and adult. Because of this difference, the "rule of nines" method for determining size or percentage of the body burned in adults is not accurate for children.

Using the adapted charts in Figure 37-6, the percentage of burned body surface is determined by estimating what percentages of limbs, trunk, and head are burned and adding the percentages. These assessments aid in determining medical treatment and in anticipating scarring and healing time.

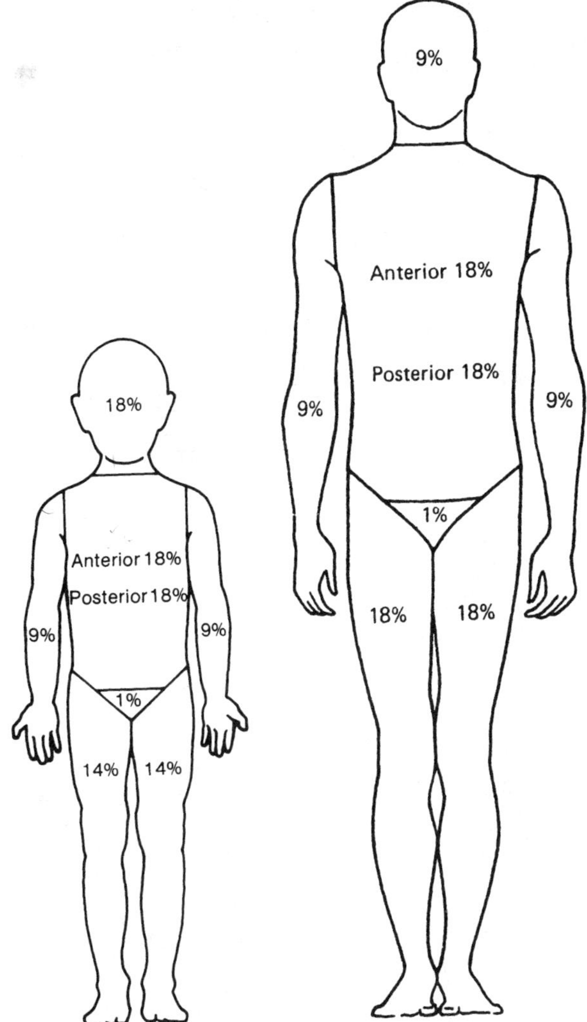

figure 37-6 *Adaptation of the "rule of nines" for estimating body surface area in burned children. (Adapted from Scherer, J. C. [1986].* Introductory medical surgical nursing *[4th ed]. Philadelphia: J.B. Lippincott, p. 687.)*

classification

Burns are classified and evaluated by agent and source, by degree, and by severity (Table 37-4). Burn agents include thermal, chemical, electricity, intense light (including sunlight), and radiation.

degree The degree of skin burns can be classified as superficial, partial thickness, and full thickness. First-degree burns are the least serious, while fourth-degree burns are the most serious.

severity The severity of burns depends on the burn agent. A burn caused by ionizing radiation may produce a minor skin burn but may be considered major because of the effects of radiation on the body. Chemical burns may remain on the skin and continue to burn for hours or even days, eventually entering the bloodstream. Any burn to the face is considered severe because it may injure the airway or eyes.

Burns of the hands and feet may cause loss of movement of fingers or toes, which may require amputation. When the groin, buttocks, or medial thighs are burned, bacterial contamination can be serious. Burns that encircle the body or a body part are considered serious because they constrict the skin and can impair circulation.

table 37-4 classification of burns

Classification	*Depth*	*Characteristics*
First degree (partial thickness)	Injury to epidermis (outer skin layer) Superficial	Painful, pink or red; may be edema Heals completely in a few days (eg, sunburn) No scarring
Second degree (partial thickness)	Injury to epidermis and dermis May heal in 3–4 weeks; burns may become deeper from ischemia and infection	Blister formation; pain and some scarring Heals in 14–17 d
Third degree (full thickness)	Epidermis and dermis destroyed; hair follicles and nerve endings destroyed	Color varies from white, tan, black, brown, bright red; surface may be wet or dry; leathery covering (eschar) present No pain; can heal only with graft Scarring
Fourth degree (full thickness)	Total destruction of skin with injury to fat, muscle, or bone	Blackened, depressed surface; no pain; scarring occurs Needs grafting

pathophysiology

Major burns create devastating changes in a child's fluid and electrolyte balance. Tissue damage, increased capillary permeability and changes in capillary pressure cause fluid to shift from the vascular system to the interstitial spaces, resulting in edema. Fluid and protein are lost through the burn wound. Loss of protein causes more fluid to shift to the interstitial spaces.

complications

shock Shock is a major problem during the first 24 to 48 hours after a major burn. Shock can result from pain or massive fluid loss (hypovolemia). Decreased blood flow to tissues from hypovolemia leads to tissue hypoxia.

Heat from the burn shortens the half-life of red blood cells and causes the child to become anemic. However, the anemia is not evident until 4 to 7 days after the injury because fluid loss raises the hematocrit.

smoke inhalation Inhalation injury is the leading cause of complications and death in burned children. Modern building materials and furniture contain plastics and other materials that release toxic fumes when burned. Smoke, carbon monoxide, and other toxic fumes can cause rapid development of pulmonary obstruction and edema. Nasotracheal intubation needs to be performed quickly to establish and maintain an open airway. Respiratory status of the child is assessed carefully and frequently to determine the need for ventilatory support.

infection When skin protection is burned away, the child is at high risk for infection. An increased risk of septicemia (systemic sepsis) occurs because the immune system is immature, decreased protein levels reduce the ability to fight infection, and germs invading the body and feeding on dead skin create a favorable environment for sepsis. Septicemia is a catastrophic illness that can quickly lead to circulatory collapse, clotting disorders, and death.

musculoskeletal involvement Burns can have critical effects on the child's musculoskeletal system. Contracture and scar formation are especially troublesome in the burned child.

Because scar tissue is less elastic than normal tissue, the new cells forming the scar pull on surrounding tissues. Scar tissue reduces the size of the skin covering the wound. The child is at increased risk for developing *contractures* (shortening of the muscle) when tissue over joints is burned. Contractures limit joint movement.

To minimize scar formation and preserve joint function, treatment includes positioning, exercise, and splinting. Splinting is used to immobilize a body part. Full-thickness burns must be splinted within 24 hours.

medical–surgical management

phases of burn care Care of burn injuries is organized into three phases: resuscitative, acute, and rehabilitative. The *resuscitative* or *emergent phase* includes the first 72 hours after the burn. The *acute phase* can last from several weeks to several months, depending on the degree and severity of the burn. The *rehabilitative phase* occurs several months to years after the initial trauma (Table 37-5).

resuscitative phase Emergency care of a burn injury addresses the ABCs of emergency care: airway patency, breathing effectiveness, and circulatory status. When inhalation injury or carbon monoxide poisoning is suspected, humidified 100% oxygen is provided.

Treatment to stop the burning process includes washing or soaking the wound gently with clean, cold water. Ice

table 37-5 phases of burn care

Phase	*Duration*	*Priorities*
Resuscitative	Onset of burn	First aid; airway, breathing and circulation; pain and shock prevention
Acute and intermediate	48–72 h following the burn	Maintaining respiratory and circulatory status; burn wound care; infection prevention; fluid and electrolyte balance; gastrointestinal function
Rehabilitation and long-term care	Wound closure to highest level of physical and social function	Prevention of scars and contractures Physical, occupational, and vocational rehabilitation Psychosocial counseling Functional and cosmetic reconstruction

should not be used because it can cause further tissue damage.

Fluid replacement is given during the first 24 hours to restore fluid and electrolyte imbalances and maintain perfusion of vital organs. An intravenous infusion of lactated Ringer's solution, isotonic saline, or plasma is given to replace lost fluids and maintain blood volume. Careful monitoring of vital signs, urine output, level of consciousness, and laboratory data is essential to detect possible fluid overload. Urine output of 1= mL/kg per hour indicates adequate hydration. Output that exceeds 1.5 to 2.0 mL/kg per hour signals fluid overload and needs to be reported to the registered nurse.

A tetanus booster is administered to prevent tetanus, and intravenous antibiotics are ordered to prevent infection. Sedatives and analgesics are given to relieve pain and restlessness. However, the child must be observed carefully because these drugs can lead to respiratory depression.

To prevent vomiting, a nasogastric tube is inserted. A urinary catheter is inserted for critical monitoring of urinary output. The child usually receives nothing by mouth for at least 24 hours.

acute phase. After the immediate resuscitative phase, care focuses on wound care; prevention and treatment of complications, such as infections; and prevention of scarring and contractures. Fluid and electrolyte balance continues to be a critical issue and requires careful monitoring until wounds close. Depending on the burn site and the physician's preference, wounds may be bandaged or remain open to air (Table 37-6).

rehabilitative phase Care of the burned child and the caregivers in the rehabilitative phase centers on maintaining and promoting function, helping the child develop coping mechanisms for living with disfigurement, and promoting normal growth and development. Rehabilitative care requires a multidisciplinary team of nurses, physicians, physical therapists, psychologists, and social workers who work with the child and the caregivers.

table 37-6 comparison of open and closed method of burn treatment

Method	*Advantages*	*Disadvantages*
Open	No dressings are used, which allows for continual observation of wound Burns are visible and easily assessed Allows for easier movement of extremities It is less expensive Exposure to air reduces risk of *Pseudomonas* infection	A greater degree of discomfort is experienced Burns are visible to child, increasing emotional anxieties Increased risk of hypothermia Isolation is necessary to reduce the risk of infection
Closed	Wounds are covered with dressings Dressings promote comfort and reduce evaporation and heat loss Isolation is not required	More expensive in terms of materials, nursing care hours Risk of *Pseudomonas* infection is increased

medications used in burn care Silver sulfadiazine (Silvadene) is an effective antimicrobial cream used to control infection. It is applied with a sterile glove to the burn site about 1/16 of an inch in thickness twice a day. It can be used with open and closed techniques. It does not sting and effectively covers the wound without staining.

Mafenide acetate (Sulfamylon) is a sulfonamide and broad-spectrum antimicrobial that penetrates *eschar*, the crust that forms over the burn wound. It is the topical agent of choice in electrical burns because of its ability to penetrate the thick eschar associated with this type of burn. The cream is applied in a thin layer once or twice daily. It may cause metabolic acidosis if used for an extended time. It causes burning pain for a few minutes following application and is usually used with open technique.

Silver nitrate (0.5%) solution is an antimicrobial that inhibits bacterial growth. It is an effective agent in preventing eschar contamination. Burn wounds are covered with gauze dressings soaked in silver nitrate, and the dressings are kept wet. Silver nitrate turns black in sunlight and stains clothing, hands, floors. Silver nitrate treatment increases the risk of electrolyte imbalances (especially sodium and potassium).

Travase is a proteolytic enzyme used for débridement of wounds. It dissolves dead protein and exudate but causes discomfort when applied. There is no systemic toxicity noted with the drug's use.

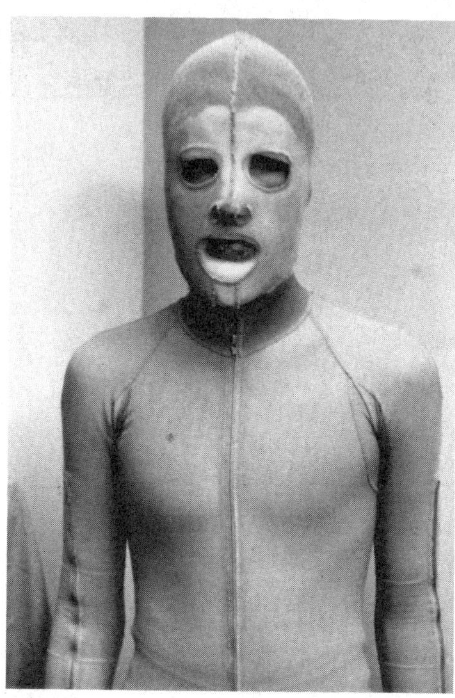

figure 37-7 *Use of pressure garments to avoid contractures and scar formation.*

débridement Débridement removes contaminated and dead tissue. *Natural débridement* occurs when dead tissue spontaneously separates from living tissue. For example, soaking and washing burn wounds in a large whirlpool such as a Hubbard tank, shower, or whirlpool softens dead tissue (*eschar*) for easy removal.

Mechanical débridement involves the use of surgical scissors and forceps to separate and remove eschar. Wet-to-dry dressings are an example of débridement. Dead tissue is removed when the dry dressing is pulled loose. The débridement procedure causes the child extreme pain and fear. Pain medication prior to the treatment and periodic breaks to give the child relief can be helpful.

Surgical débridement is an operative procedure that excises dead tissue down to living tissue, a procedure called an *escharotomy*. Surgical débridement followed by prompt skin grafting results in shorter hospital stays and decreases risk of infection from the build-up of eschar. Eschar prevents healing and provides an ideal environment for bacteria to grow.

elastic pressure dressings Elastic pressure dressings are used to prevent hypertrophic burn scarring (Fig. 37-7). Applying elastic pressure garments induces the loosening of *collagen* (protein found in connective tissue) bundles and encourages a restructuring of collagen.

skin grafts (biologic dressings) Full-thickness burns require skin grafts to heal. Skin grafts are biologic dressings and include autografts, homografts, allografts, and heterografts.

* *Autografts* are skin from the burned child's body; almost any unburned area can be a donor site.
* *Homografts* are skin from another person; unless it is from an identical twin, this is only a temporary graft because it will eventually be rejected by the child's tissue. Although temporary, homografts help reduce pain, infection risk, and fluid and heat loss.
* *Allografts* are cadaver skin, also used as a temporary covering.
* *Heterografts* are skin from another species (such as a pig). They are temporary but often life-saving.

The surgeon harvests skin from the donor site using a *dermatome* (an instrument that cuts thin slices of skin). The skin is then meshed and stretched to cover as large an area as possible. The grafted areas are covered with dressings that are generally left in place for at least 72 hours. Postgraft dressings are changed by the surgeon. Ideally, the skin graft attaches to underlying tissue and functions like normal skin. However, many grafts may be needed to cover the burned area.

biosynthetic and synthetic wound coverings The use of autografts may not be possible if the child has extensive burns. The cost of homografts and heterografts has prompted a search for synthetic skin substitutes. Synthetic wound dressings include Biobrane.

Biobrane is a wound covering made of a nylon, Silastic membrane combined with a collagen derivative. It is semitransparent, sterile, and less costly than homograft or pigskin. Biobrane dressings adhere to wounds, and within

nursing care plan for the child with a burn injury

NURSING DIAGNOSIS

Risk for Infection, related to impaired skin integrity

GOAL: *The child will remain free of infection*

NURSING INTERVENTIONS	RATIONALE	EVALUATION
Use aseptic techniques when caring for the child and maintain isolation precautions.	The child has lost integumentary defenses against infection and will have decreased protein levels, which reduce the body's ability to fight infection. Prevention is essential and can be maintained with both aseptic technique and isolation precautions.	The child will receive safe care and remain free of infections.
Monitor the child's temperature, WBC, and differential.	These are indicators of infection and may necessitate a change in treatment.	Signs of infection will be monitored and changes in treatment instituted, as necessary.
Apply antimicrobial agents when performing wound care.	The break in skin integrity has provided an open portal for attack by microorganisms, which can be treated prophylactically with antimicrobial agents.	The health care professional caring for the child will use antimicrobial topical agents with dressing changes as prescribed.
Obtain wound cultures with signs of infection.	This will provide information early as to the type of microorganism requiring treatment.	The child's bacterial infection will be identified early and specific treatment instituted to prevent further complications, such as sepsis.
Administer systemic antibiotics as prescribed for known infection.	Use of specific antibiotics directed at the infecting organism is beneficial for eradicating it.	The child will be treated with appropriate antibiotics, and signs of the infection will abate.

NURSING DIAGNOSIS

Body Image Disturbance, related to limited physical mobility and burn scars

GOAL: *The child will maintain functional ability, verbalize frustrations regarding injury and self-image, and participate in self care*

NURSING INTERVENTIONS	RATIONALE	EVALUATION
Urge family to visit and participate in care.	The child will need the support of his family to sustain a positive self-image.	The family will visit and learn about the child's care, showing the child their support.
Encourage family and the child to verbalize feelings.	An open and nonjudgmental environment will facilitate expression of feelings.	The family and the child will feel nonthreatened in sharing their frustrations.
Explain all procedures to the child and allow the child choices.	This will serve to increase the child's control of the environment.	The child will understand the rationale for all the treatments and how they can help to prevent further scarring.
Use a primary nurse.	A primary nurse provides consistency in care and promotes a trusting relationship for the child.	The child will be assigned a primary nurse and will be involved in decisions regarding his or her plan of care.
Promote the child in participation of self-care.	This will serve to increase the child's self-esteem by showing the child what he or she is capable of doing while increasing functional capacity.	The child will continue to increase physical mobility and participation in self-care.
Refer the child and family to appropriate resources.	Continued support will be necessary to help the child to continue adapting to emotional and physical trauma of the burn injury.	The child and family will state an understanding of available resources and know how to access them.

5 days, cells migrate into the nylon mesh. The dressing is left in place for 3 to 4 weeks.

nursing care

Nursing care of the burn patient includes considering the severity of the burns and body areas involved, creating a treatment plan, and educating and giving psychosocial support for the child and family. The nurse collaborates with other members of the multidisciplinary care team, including the child and caregivers.

resuscitative phase In the resuscitative phase, the child is monitored for decreased blood pressure and increased pulse and respiration rate, which are signs of shock. In addition, the child must be assessed for pain, fluid and electrolyte imbalance, and respiratory complications. Intravenous fluids may be given, and ventilatory support may be necessary. A catheter is usually inserted to measure urinary output.

acute phase During the acute phase, nursing care addresses the child's pain related to tissue damage, increased risk for infection, and fluid and electrolyte imbalance. These are monitored by careful intake and output records, daily weights, and skin turgor. As the edema begins to reabsorb, there is increased urinary output (diuresis), which leads to potassium loss. Sodium and protein are lost through the open wound. Potassium, albumin, and packed red blood cells may be given to replace these losses and prevent cardiac arrhythmias.

comfort measures The nurse administers analgesics and sedatives as ordered and carefully monitors the child's respiratory status for any signs of respiratory depression. Explaining what to expect during treatment procedures can help relieve the child's anxiety. Maintaining an environmental temperature of 24.4° to 28.8°C (76°–84°F) helps ensure warmth and comfort.

wound care Burned areas may be left open to the air (open method) or covered with dressings (closed method), depending on the physician's preference. Heated bed cradles are recommended when burns are treated with the open method. Preventing infection is vital when caring for burned children, and sterile procedures are followed for all dressing changes. Graft sites must be supported and free of pressure.

The nurse is often responsible for cleansing to remove dead tissue. Dreft baths may be used to soften dead tissue. For this procedure, ½ cup of Dreft is added to a tub containing about 6 in of luke warm water.

nutrition Calories are used to maintain normal temperatures; therefore, changes in body temperature increase nutritional demands. Children with extensive burns have a greatly increased metabolism—their energy needs may increase as much as 200%. The child requires a high-calorie, high-protein diet, rich in vitamins and minerals to help rebuild body tissue, replace lost fluids and protein, and fight infection. The nurse collaborates with the dietitian and caregivers to interest the child in eating foods that are essential to healing and growth. Total parenteral nutrition or tube feedings are often necessary to meet the child's increased nutritional requirements. Painful procedures should be scheduled after meals.

If a nasogastric tube is inserted, placement is assessed before administering feedings to prevent instilling food into the lungs. Bowel sounds are checked every 4 hours, and stool is monitored for diarrhea or constipation.

Burns cause decreased gastrointestinal motility, which can lead to a stress ulcer (Curling's ulcer). This gastric or duodenal ulcer occurs during the first 6 weeks after a burn injury. Symptoms include vague abdominal discomfort and blood in the stool. Treatment includes a bland diet, antacids, and antispasmodic food.

The child's weight is monitored daily at the same time and with the same clothing or dressings. Intake and output are measured and documented.

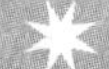

nursing alert

Banana peelings can be a source of Pseudomonas *infection in burn children.*

rehabilitative phase Nursing care during the rehabilitative phase includes skin care, nutritional support, and promotion of function. Education and emotional support of the child and caregivers take on new importance as responsibility for care shifts to home and family caregivers. The nurse encourages the child and family to express their concerns and feelings. These feelings may include guilt about the accident, fear and anxiety about returning to school, and diminished self-esteem due to scarring and disfigurement. Referring the family to peer support groups and other health and social service professionals can help the child and family continue the long and difficult healing process. See the Nursing Care Plan and the Teaching Guidelines for more information on the child with a burn injury.

teaching guidelines

skin care of healed burn areas

Care of healed burn areas includes the following:

* Providing moisture to the skin by gently rubbing lotion (such as cocoa butter cream) on the site.
* Avoiding sun exposure to the burn site for at least 1 year
* Keeping fingernails short to reduce the risk of tissue damage from scratching
* Putting 2 cups of cornstarch in the bath water to reduce itching

what would you do?

Augie is a 7-year-old boy who is in the rehabilitation stage of burn care. He has scarring on his face and upper extremities. He refuses to go to school because he doesn't like the way he looks. He refuses to eat and has scratched the scar areas until they are bleeding. Augie's mother works from 11 PM to 7 AM. Augie is allowed to play inside while his mother sleeps.

key points

* **The integumentary system includes skin, hair, and nails. Skin, the largest component, consists of a layer of tissue covering the entire body. It contains sweat and oil glands, is a natural barrier against infection, and is an important indicator of alterations of other body systems (especially cardiovascular, respiratory, gastrointestinal, endocrine, and urinary).**
* **Infant skin (especially premature infants) is very thin. Cells are loosely attached to each other, and it contains less oil and more water than adult skin. These characteristics contribute to skin sensitivity, decreased heat regulation, and alterations in skin integrity. Skin reaches maturity at puberty.**
* **Cultural differences of the integumentary system include color, texture, and characteristics. Skin color varies between and within ethnic groups. Asians tend to have darker white skin with a yellowish tinge; African Americans have increased amounts of melanin and thus dark brown skin; and Hispanics generally have tan to dark brown skin. Native Americans vary in the degree of pigmentation, and white skin can be sallow, pink, or olive tinged. Dark skin tends to be dry and compact with more cell layers to protect against injury. Mongolian spots, blue or blue-black patches, are commonly found on the lower back and buttocks of Asian, Southern European, African, and Native American children. Skin pits, extra nipples in women, and keloid scar formation are common in African American children.**
* **Skin lesions typically are not life-threatening but produce great anxiety about appearance in children and caregivers.**
* **Emergency measures may be necessary if a child's rash is due to a systemic infection or allergic response and results in septic or anaphylactic shock.**
* **Care of children with altered skin integrity involves measures to reduce pain or pruritus, promote skin integrity, prevent infection, promote self-concept, and reduce anxieties.**
* **Burns can be classified as superficial, partial thickness, and full thickness and range from a somewhat mild first-degree burn to a life-threatening fourth-degree burn.**

review questions 

1. Jimmy, age 8 years, is brought to the clinic for complaints of itching of the scalp, especially around the ears. Select the condition that the symptoms indicate.
   a. scabies
   b. tinea pedis
   c. pediculosis capitus
   d. vitiligo
2. Mrs. Ramero, an African American, is concerned about a large bruised area on her 5-day-old daughter's back, just above the coccyx. She thinks a nurse might have been abusive. Select the most appropriate response to Mrs. Ramero's concern.
   a. "The child has a mongolian spot that is typically seen in children of Asian, Southern European, African, and Native American descent."
   b. "The nurses working with children are not in the habit of abusing children; there must be a mistake."
   c. "Children who are dark skinned often have various discolorations that can look like a bruise."
   d. "I will check on your complaint and talk to the nurse who was in charge of your baby."
3. Ali Mae is a 3-month-old with severe diaper dermatitis. Select the most significant comment made by Ali's mother during subjective data collection pertinent to the condition.
   a. "Ali's skin is usually flawless."
   b. "I recently changed from cloth to disposable diapers."
   c. "Ali doesn't drink water but nurses well."
   d. "Ali's Apgar scores were 8 and 9."
4. Select the most appropriate nursing intervention for a toddler experiencing pruritus.
   a. Apply a generous amount of powder to affected areas.
   b. Permit the child to take a bubble bath when itching begins.
   c. Layer the child's clothing to prevent hypothermia and decrease itching.
   d. Place mittens on the hands.
5. Kerry is a 5-year-old burn patient admitted through the emergency department after he ignited charcoal fuel. His face and hands have second- and third-degree burns. Select the most appropriate nursing concern for the first 24 to 48 hours following a burn.
   a. Scar tissue formation
   b. Infection
   c. Shock
   d. Contractures

references

Hollinger, M. A. (1990). Pulmonary toxicity of inhaled and intravenous talc. *Toxicology Letters, 52*, 121–127.

Moses, M. (1995). *Designer poisons: How to protect your health and home from toxic pesticides.* San Francisco: Pesticide Education Center.

Olkowski, W., Daar, S., & Olkowski, H. (1991). *Least toxic solutions for your home, garden, pets and community.* Newtown, CT: Taunton Press.

Taplin, D., & Menking, T. (1988). Infestations. In L. A. Schachner & R. C. Hansen (Eds.), *Pediatric dermatology* (p. 1465). New York: Churchill Livingstone.

Tortora, G. J., Funke, B. R., & Case, C. L. (1995) *Microbiology: An introduction.* Redwood City, CA: Benjamin Cummings Publishing.

bibliography

Anastasi, J., & Rivera, J. (1992). Skin manifestations of HIV. *Nursing 92, 22*(11), 58–61.

Campbell, L. (1993). Assessing pediatric rashes. *RN, 56*(4), 58–64.

Carpenito, L. (1995). *Handbook of nursing diagnosis* (6th ed.). Philadelphia: J.B. Lippincott.

Castiglia, P. (1995). Hemangiomas. *Journal of Pediatric Health Care, 8*(3), 130–131.

Castiglia, P., & Harbin, R. (1992). *Child health care.* Philadelphia: J.B. Lippincott.

Farrington, E. (1992). Diaper dermatitis. *Pediatric Nursing, 18*(1), 81, 82.

Fischbach, F. (1995). *Quick reference to common laboratory and diagnostic tests.* Philadelphia: J.B. Lippincott.

Gulanick, M., Gradishar, D., & Puzas, M. (1994). *Ambulatory pediatric nursing.* Albany, NY: Delmar.

Lynch, M. (1992). Special children, special needs: The ectodermal dysplasias. *Pediatric Nursing, 18*(3), 212–216.

Nativio, D., & Belz, C. (1990). Childhood neurofibromatosis. *Pediatric Nursing, 16*(6), 575–580.

Pillitteri, A. (1995). *Maternal and child health nursing* (2nd ed.). Philadelphia: J.B. Lippincott.

Smeltzer, S., & Bare B. (1996). *Brunner and Suddarth's textbook of medical-surgical nursing.* Philadelphia: Lippincott.

Stevenson, L., & Brooke, D. (1994). Tinea capitis. *Journal of Pediatric Health Care, 8*(4), 189.

Wong, D., Brantly, D., Clutter, L., DeSimone, D., Lammert, D., Nix, K., Perry, C., Smith, D., & White, K. (1992). Diapering choices: A critical review of the issues. *Pediatric Nursing, 18*(1), 41–53.

the child with an alteration in endocrine function

38

outline

objectives

After studying this chapter, the reader should be able to:

* Discuss the importance of normal hormone secretion to growth and development.
* Name at least three endocrine glands, their hormones, and the disease condition resulting from hormone deficiency or excess.
* List and discuss stressors experienced by children and their caregivers when endocrine disorders are suspected.
* Discuss why preschool children diagnosed with endocrine disorders often perceive their problem as a form of punishment.
* Discuss the importance of assessing a child's weight and height on routine examinations.
* Compare and contrast the symptoms of hypothyroidism with hyperthyroidism and the respective treatment of each.
* Define type I insulin-dependent diabetes.
* List symptoms of ketoacidosis.
* Discuss appropriate nursing measures for insulin reaction or shock.
* Describe the symptoms of diabetes mellitus.

key terms

ambiguous genitalia
carotenemia
exopthalmia
glucagon
glycosuria
Graves' disease
Hashimoto's thyroiditis
hormones
hypoglycemia
hypophysectomy
hypopituitary dwarfism
insulin reaction
ketones
ketoacidosis
polyphagia
polydipsia
polyuria
tetany
thyroid storm
thyroxine hyperglycemia

The endocrine system is the master regulatory system of the body. It involves the endocrine (ductless) glands, which secrete chemicals called *hormones* directly into the blood, lymph, and extracellular fluids. Hormones help regulate metabolic processes and coordinate body activities. Hormones control growth, energy production, fluid and electrolyte balance, stress responses, personality, and sexual development.

Alteration in endocrine function can result in any of a variety of disorders with long-term implications for normal growth and development. Endocrine disorders include deficiencies of growth hormones (GHs), thyroxin, and insulin, which are controlled with lifelong hormone replacement therapy.

This chapter focuses on three specific alterations in endocrine function. Alteration in growth related to pituitary GH, dysfunction of the thyroid gland, and diabetes mellitus. Anatomy and physiology include an overview of all the endocrine glands and hormones. Patient and caregiver teaching is emphasized because appropriate home care is an essential part of the long-term care needed for the child with an alteration in endocrine function. Procedures specific to diabetes mellitus are included.

✳ family considerations

Alteration in endocrine function is not easily diagnosed and often requires extensive testing before a diagnosis is made. Many kinds of endocrine dysfunction are rare and require a medical specialist known as an *endocrinologist*.

Medical services needed for diagnosis and treatment of rare endocrine problems may not be available in smaller communities. When the child is referred to a specialist outside the community, the family must cope with the expense and stress of traveling, a new doctor, and unfamiliar surroundings.

Endocrine testing usually involves blood analysis obtained from venipuncture or subcutaneous sticks that are painful to children. Caregivers who question the need for frequent blood testing may fear the child will blame them for the discomfort.

Caregivers may grieve over a perceived loss of the child's being "normal." They may express anger and self-blame for the child's condition and fear having additional children. A diagnosis such as diabetes mellitus becomes a crisis for the entire family. Children with diabetes, their caregivers, and siblings may wonder if the illness is punishment for wrongdoing.

Siblings often have difficulty understanding the endocrine disorder and may fear that they will contract the disease. Siblings may feel left out because of the increased attention focused on the sick child. The caregiver may resent dietary restrictions necessary in the care of diabetes mellitus.

Most endocrine dysfunctions require hormone replacement throughout the lifespan of the child. Many of the hormone replacement regimens require hormone injections. Caregivers of younger children are expected to give the prescribed injections. Caregivers of older children must provide supervision to ensure the child is giving the correct dosage and using safe injection technique.

These new responsibilities are time consuming and add stress to the family's life. The chronic nature of endocrine disorders requires caregiver and patient education (and re-education) to help the family maintain a normal lifestyle. Caregivers need to balance encouragement for the child during the uncomfortable procedures and responsibility for carrying out the procedures to keep the child healthy. Health agency services and community, state, and national chapters of such organizations as the American Diabetes Association provide support for children and their caregivers.

The family's coping abilities influence the newly diagnosed child's psychological adjustment and compliance to prescribed treatments. Dysfunctional family relationships pose a threat to the child's compliance.

✳ nursing considerations

Delays in growth and development frequently are seen in children with alteration in endocrine function and can be readily detected by plotting weight and height measurements on a growth grid. For example, sudden unexplained growth increases may indicate thyroid or pituitary gland dysfunction. Children with congenital endocrine conditions show persistent growth deviations, whereas those with an acquired endocrine problem reflect normal values for a time, followed by a sudden deviation at the onset of the problem.

A complete history of the child's physical, emotional, and social growth helps to assess growth and development within normal age limits. Information about a typical day in the child's life provides significant clues as to play, rest, and temperament. Decreased or increased activity patterns reflect thyroid dysfunction; however, care must be taken to distinguish between disease process and normal temperament. A quiet child may desire rest and reading after school compared with an active child who desires more play and activity. The activity level of these children differs but does not reflect an abnormality.

> **✳ nursing insight**
> *A quiet child will lie down to read or watch television, compared with an ill child who lies down to sleep.*

A comprehensive family history may reveal a genetic predisposition to endocrine dysfunction. For example, although the exact cause of diabetes mellitus is not known, genetic factors play a role. If one child in a family has diabetes, the possibility of a sibling acquiring the illness is higher than normal.

The social effects of an often highly visible condition must be approached with concern and support. Providing caregivers with factual information about the disease condition helps alleviate some of the fear of the unknown. Establishing caregiver rapport enables the nurse to evaluate the need for disease information, genetic counseling, medication administration information, help with home care, and financial assistance. Compliance with long-term treatment tends to improve when nurse-patient or nurse-caregiver rapport is present.

Teaching complex procedures needed for home care requires thorough instructions (verbal, written, and if appropriate, demonstrated), practice time, and return demonstrations enabling the nurse to evaluate the child's or caregiver's abilities. Praise and encouragement given by the nurse help bolster confidence.

The capacity for assuming self-care responsibilities differs greatly from one child to another. When caregivers and children share responsibilities, such as diabetic care, compliance is better and errors with diet and injections are fewer.

Understanding age-specific developmental concerns helps the nurse prepare children for invasive testing and procedures. A young child may perceive the injections and frequent venipuncture as punishment for wrongdoing. Adolescents may rebel against the procedures, taking an "I don't care" attitude about future consequences.

anatomy and physiology of the endocrine system

The endocrine system includes the *pituitary gland, thyroid gland, parathyroid gland, adrenal gland, pancreas, testes*, and *ovaries* (Table 38-1). The location of the endocrine glands is shown in Figure 38-1.

pituitary gland

The pituitary gland also is called the *hypophysis*. It is a small but powerful gland located at the base of the brain. It consists of two lobes: *anterior* and *posterior*. The pituitary gland is often called the *master gland* because it releases hormones that affect the other endocrine glands. Pituitary hormones are not released from the gland until chemical messengers indicate they are needed; thus, they operate on a supply and demand basis.

The posterior lobe of the pituitary gland stores two hormones that are produced by the hypothalamus and released when hypothalamic nerve impulses are stimulated.

table 38-1 endocrine glands, their hormones, and major functions

Gland	*Hormone*	*Major Function*
Anterior pituitary	GH, TSH, ACTH, prolactin, FSH, and LH	Regulates growth, secretion of thyroxine and T_3, secretion of cortisol
		Stimulates milk production
		Initiates growth of ova in women
		Initiates sperm production in the testes
		Causes ovulation in women and increases secretion of testosterone in men
Posterior pituitary	Antidiuretic hormone	Regulates water loss
	Oxytocin	Promotes contraction of uterus during labor
		Promotes release of milk
Thyroid	Thyroxine (T_4) and triiodothyronine (T_3)	Regulates body metabolism
Parathyroid	Parahormone	Regulates serum calcium
Adrenal cortex	Cortisol, ACTH	Regulates serum sodium
	Glucocorticoids	
Adrenal medulla	Norepinephrine, epinephrine	Secreted in stress situation
		Helps body with "fight or flight" reactions
Islets of Langerhans	Insulin	Regulates blood sugar
	Glucagon	Stimulates liver to change glycogen to glucose
Ovaries	Estrogen	Promotes ovum maturation in the ovarian follicle
	Progesterone	Stimulates build-up of endometrium in pregnancy
Testes	Testosterone	Promotes sperm production
	Inhibin	Decreases the secretion of FSH by the anterior pituitary gland

GH, growth hormone; TSH, thyroid-stimulating hormone; ACTH, adrenocorticotropic hormone; FSH, follicle-stimulating hormone; LH, leuteinizing hormone.

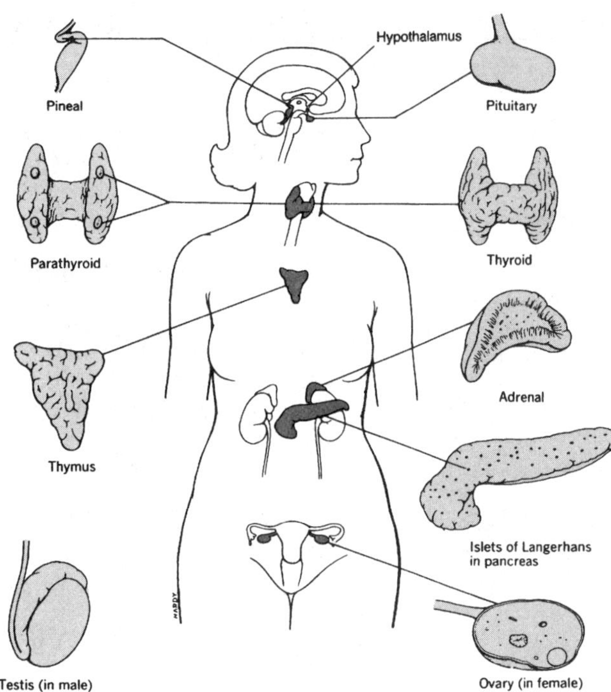

figure 38-1 *Location of the major endocrine glands in the body.*

Posterior pituitary hormones consist of an antidiuretic hormone, responsible for reabsorption of water by the kidneys, and oxytocin hormone, responsible for uterine contraction and release of milk from the mammary glands.

The anterior lobe of the pituitary gland is similar to the posterior because it responds to hypothalamus impulses to secrete hormones. The anterior lobe releases six hormones, as shown in Table 38-1. These hormones control metabolic functions of the body. Dysfunction of the pituitary gland directly affects the child's growth. A hypoactive (underactive) pituitary gland results in short stature and hypopituitary dwarfism, whereas a hyperactive (overactive) pituitary gland results in giantism (hyperpituitarism).

thyroid gland

The thyroid gland is the largest of the endocrine glands and is located in the neck. The two lobes of the thyroid are found on either side of the voice box, resembling a bow tie against the windpipe. The thyroid gland needs dietary iodine to manufacture its hormones. Hormones produced by the thyroid gland regulate the metabolic rate of the entire body.

The main hormone produced by the gland is *thyroxine*. Overproduction or underproduction of thyroxine can occur for various reasons, including tumor growth affecting the gland and surgical removal. Thyroid hormone secretions stimulate the growth of cells. Alteration in the amount of thyroid hormone secreted greatly influences the child's growth because it regulates cell metabolism.

pancreas

Pancreatic tissue contains small groups of specialized cells called islets of Langerhans. The islet cells function as an endocrine gland and are independent from the rest of the pancreas. The most important hormone secreted by the islets of Langerhans is insulin. Insulin is needed to transport sugar into cells to be used as energy; thus, it plays a major role in regulating blood glucose levels.

Glucagon is the second hormone produced by the islet of Langerhans and works with insulin to regulate blood sugar levels. A lack of insulin production results in a condition known as diabetes mellitus (refer to page 680 for additional information).

adrenal glands

The adrenal glands are located on top of each kidney. Each gland has two parts: the adrenal cortex and the adrenal medulla. The cortex and medulla have two distinct functions and act as two different organs.

The adrenal cortex secretes steroid hormones known as mineralocorticoids, glucocorticoids, and sex hormones (see Table 38-1). The sex hormones estrogen and androgen are produced in small amounts by the adrenal cortex.

ovaries

The ovaries are located in the pelvic cavity on either side of the uterus. The hormones produced by the ovaries are estrogen and progesterone. Secondary sex characteristics in women develop in response to estrogen. Progesterone promotes the growth of blood vessels in the endometrium during pregnancy.

testes

The testes are located in the scrotum and secrete testosterone and inhibin hormones. Testosterone is responsible for secondary sex characteristics in the man. Inhibin inhibits the secretion of luteinizing hormone from the anterior pituitary gland. Inhibin, testosterone, and the anterior pituitary hormones maintain a continuing supply of mature sperm.

age-specific considerations

Endocrine glands are better organized than other systems. Most endocrine glands develop during the first trimester of gestation. Disorders of the glands are often related to hormonal problems in the mother. Inadequate iodine intake and maternal diabetes are the two most common problems.

A rare but disturbing neonatal occurrence is ambiguous genitalia (*hermaphroditism*), resulting from chromosomal and hormonal influences. Ambiguous genitalia occurs when the child has male and female sex characteristics. Additional information about this condition is given in Chapter 32.

diagnostic tests

Many tests are used to diagnose alteration in endocrine function. These include analysis of blood and urine, imaging studies, ultrasound, and genetic karyotyping.

Blood chemistry studies include tests to determine thyroid function, levels of hormones, calcium, phosphorus, alkaline phosphatase, electrolytes, and glucose. For example, when diabetes mellitus is suspected, a glucose tolerance test is ordered. Prior to the test, the child is required to eat a high-carbohydrate diet to stimulate an insulin response.

Urine studies include sodium, calcium, phosphorus, ketone and glucose levels, and specific gravity. For example, an excess amount of glucose and ketones in the urine is usually associated with poorly controlled diabetes.

Imaging studies include x-rays, usually of the hand and wrist, to determine skeletal maturation; these help determine bone age and density. The x-ray reveals the degree of epiphyseal separation from the main portion of long bones and whether epiphyseal fusion has occurred. Children suspected of having hypopituitary dwarfism will have delayed epiphyseal closure of long bones. Computed tomography (CT), magnetic resonance imaging (MRI), and nuclear medicine scans are used to study the brain if pituitary abnormalities are suspected.

Ultrasound is often used to identify the size and placement of thyroid tissue.

Genetic studies, including karyotyping (microphotography of the chromosomes), can confirm genetic syndromes known to affect growth.

✳ nursing process in endocrine disorders

nursing assessment

Subjective data to be assessed include the following:

* Detailed history of genetic disorders in the family; prenatal care; mother's description of the labor and birthing process, including length of labor and any known problems with delivery; child's developmental progress; general health and nutritional status
* Exercise and rest patterns relative to changes involving strength and stamina
* Reported excessive hunger and thirst
* Reported headache and impaired vision
* Reported pruritus of the skin or genitalia

Objective data to be assessed include the following:

* Assess size. Note weight and height measurements that are less than or more than normal ranges on a standardized growth chart. Notice abnormalities of bone development and body proportions expected for the child's age and stage of development. For example, the child with excessive production of adrenal cortex hormones (Cushing's syndrome) will have abnormal fat distribution in the face, neck, upper back, and trunk; muscle wasting; and osteoporosis.

> **✳ nursing insight**
> *Cloth or plastic measuring tapes should not be used to obtain lengths on children from birth to 2 to 3 years because they can stretch, producing inaccurate readings.*

* Assess facial characteristics. Note the presence of such characteristics as round face, flattened nasal bridge, large protruding tongue, bulging eyes (*exophthalmos*) seen in hyperthyroidism, low anterior hairline, delayed dentition, dental caries, fruity odor to the breath typical of diabetic ketoacidosis, and visual disturbances.
* Assess genitalia. Check their appearance for signs of ambiguous genitals. Note the presence of undescended testicles, an inability to retract tight foreskin over the penis (*phimosis*), or a urinary opening on the underside of the penis (*hypospadias*) or on the upper side or top of the penis (*epispadias*). These disorders are discussed in Chapter 32. Note any abnormal appearance of the labia and size of the clitoris in girls. Vaginal discharge or odor and the presence of masses in the inguinal canals are considered abnormal. Note the presence or absence of secondary sex characteristics, such as breast development and pubic and axillary hair in girls and penis size and pubic and axillary hair in boys.
* Assess vital signs. Obtain baseline temperature, pulse, respirations, and blood pressure readings. Vital sign readings are typically lower than the normal range in hypothyroidism and higher in hyperthyroidism.
* Assess hydration status reflected by dry skin, scant tear and urine production, sunken fontanel in infants, poor skin turgor, and thick mucus, indicative of dehydration.
* Assess skin. Note the presence of thick, dry, coarse skin typically seen in hypothyroidism. Observe the skin for hair distribution, hyperpigmentation, flushing, skin rashes, jaundice, mottling, and perspiration.
* Assess emotional status. Note behaviors such as quieting after crying, irritability, flat affect, shakiness, and lethargy. In the older child, evaluate peer relationships by questioning about friends, social activities, and group memberships.

nursing diagnoses

* Altered Growth and Development, related to chronic illness
* Self-Esteem, related to abnormal growth
* Risk for Altered Nutrition: Less than body requirements, related to inability to metabolize glucose; increased metabolism
* Fluid Volume Deficit, related to excessive urination
* Knowledge Deficit, related to treatment needs
* Altered Family Processes, related to child's chronic illness
* Ineffective Family Coping, related to additional responsibilities, stress, and financial concerns
* Grieving, related to acceptance of long-term illness
* Fear, related to illness outcome

* Pain, related to tests, procedures, and treatments
* Altered Nutrition: More than body requirements, related to decreased metabolism

planning and intervention

* To promote growth, praise the child and caregivers for progress made toward goal weight. If nutrition is a problem, teach the patient or caregiver how to keep a 24-hour dietary history. Encourage patient and caregiver compliance with the restrictive diet plans often necessary in the care of diabetic patients. Promote compliance by using reminder charts for special meals, snacks, and medications.
* To promote development, evaluate the child's school status in regard to absenteeism and inappropriate demands on the child. Teachers need to be aware of a student's health status, treatment plan, and potential barriers to learning. A diagnosis of insulin-dependent diabetes puts the school-age child at risk for hypoglycemia if not dismissed from class on time for lunch. Teach parents appropriate age-related developmental tasks affecting the child's involvement with the disorder. (see Display 38-6 later in this chapter.)
* To promote self-concept, encourage child to express personal feelings. Encourage child to ask questions about health problems, treatment, progress, and prognosis. Clarify any patient or caregiver misconceptions about the disease. Praise the child's compliance with treatment plan. Avoid negative criticism.
* To promote hydration, assess child's likes and dislikes; provide favorite fluids within dietary restrictions; provide diabetic child with fruit juices.
* To promote family coping, assist the family in evaluating the situation and options available. Encourage parents to verbalize their fears and concerns. Involve family members in the care of an ill child whenever possible. Provide home care instructions. Provide information about prescribed medications, possible side effects, and expected outcomes. Teach parents and children (if age appropriate) how to draw up insulin, select injection site, prepare site, and give the injection. Assist the family to set priorities to maintain family integrity and reduce stress. Acknowledge family strengths.

evaluation

* The child demonstrates an increase in growth reflected by weight and height. Child's actions and interactions reflect increases in age-appropriate developmental behaviors in personal, social, language, cognition, and motor activities.
* The child verbalizes positive self-attributes and realistic perceptions of self.
* Normal hydration status is maintained, demonstrated by absence of signs and symptoms of dehydration.
* Family members verbalize feelings, participate in the care of the child, maintain functional system of mutual support for each other, seek appropriate external resources, and comply with medication administration.

alteration in pituitary function

hypopituitary dwarfism

Hypopituitary dwarfism occurs as a result of growth hormone deficiencies (GHD). Increased pressure on the pituitary gland from nonmalignant cystic tumors formed in the embryo stage is linked with the decrease of GH production. In most children, the cause of the defect is unknown.

pathophysiology

These children are usually normal weight and height at birth, but within the first few years of life, they fall below the third percentile on growth charts. Children with untreated GHD will not reach a height of more than 3 or 4 ft. Typically, they are well children with a proportionally normal physical appearance except for the abnormal lack of growth.

Diagnosis of GHD includes neurologic testing to detect the presence of a pituitary lesion or tumor. Monitoring blood levels of GH relative to the child's sleep and play is important when making the diagnosis because GH levels rise after a period of sleep or activity. When GH levels remain low after sleep or activity periods, insulin injections are used to artificially stimulate the hormone (unless contraindicated because of existing diabetes mellitus). Healthy children respond to insulin administration by becoming hypoglycemic. Hypoglycemia stimulates the release of circulating GH. Children with GHD will not have an increase in the level of GH.

medical–surgical management

Surgical removal of a pituitary tumor is the treatment of choice. The surgeon may be able to remove the tumor while leaving functional pituitary tissue intact. Surgical removal of the pituitary gland is called total *hypophysectomy*. Hormonal therapy following removal of the pituitary gland involves maintaining thyroid, adrenal, and gonadal function.

The medical management of hypopituitary dwarfism involves the administration of intramuscular human GH injections two or three times a week. Because GH is destroyed by the gastric juices in the stomach, it must be given subcutaneously or intramuscularly. Children who are treated with GH will grow at faster than normal speed for 2 to 4 years.

nursing care

Careful assessment of a child's height and weight helps determine potential growth problems and allows early intervention (Table 38-2). Size is determined by many factors, including heredity, diseases affecting body size, and eating a well-balanced diet.

Reassure children with short stature that the most important thing to remember is that people are special because of what they feel inside, not how short or tall they are on the outside. Children with small stature are often the

table 38-2 growth rates and guidelines for monitoring growth

Age	*Normal Growth Rate Expectations*	*Nursing Considerations*
Birth to 12 mo	23–28 cm (9–11 in)/y	Rapid growth influenced by genetics, nutrition, psychosocial causes. Growth hormone secretion influences growth late in the first year. Weigh, measure, plot on growth charts. Measure lying down with mounted measuring tape or yardstick. Requires two people; one holds infant on the back with heels, backs of knees, buttocks, shoulders, and the back of the head secure against the measuring device. Second person stretches infant.
12–36 m	7.5–13 cm (3–5 in)/y	Decline then steady, consistent growth pattern. Weigh, measure, and plot on growth chart two times per year.
3 y to puberty	5–6 cm (2–2.5 in)/y	Decline then steady, consistent growth pattern. Weigh, measure, and plot on growth chart two times per year.
Puberty +	Puberty growth spurt varies with each child	Growth spurt begins after first sign of puberty and continues for about 4 y. Growth spurt preceded by a small but measurable decline in growth rate.

target for aggressive behaviors and malicious teasing from other children. High anxiety and the child's inability to cope with peer teasing may require counseling interventions. Involvement in a sports activity in which size has little or no bearing on success can help build self-confidence (eg, track, golf, gymnastics, karate).

Administration of GH is less painful when given subcutaneously. An injection schedule including days of the week and specific times enables the child to develop a routine. Children feel more in control when they have input in making the schedule. Some suggestions for explaining this procedure to the pediatric population are explained in the following Teaching Guidelines display.

teaching guidelines
growth hormone testing

"Your doctor told me that you need to have a test called a growth hormone test. This test helps the doctor find out if your body is making enough growth hormone. Hormones are chemicals that come from specific glands to help your body grow. There are special ways to get ready for this test, but the good news is you don't have to study! This is what will happen on the day of the test:

* You won't be allowed to eat or drink anything for several hours before and after the test.
* You may need to wear a gown or pajamas that belong to the hospital instead of your own clothes.
* You will lie on a table.
* You will have a pinch in your arm or hand when the nurse starts an IV (that stands for intravenous). You can cry or yell OUCH!
* A small amount of blood will be taken through the IV (The IV gets pinched—not you!) This may happen several times during the test. Your body is so smart it makes new blood all the time, and you won't miss the small amount needed for the test.
* You may feel dizzy, warm, or sick to your stomach during the test. Be sure you tell the nurse if you do. These feelings are ok and will soon go away.
* You can sleep or read stories during the test because it takes a little longer than three cartoon shows (90 minutes).
* After the test, you can eat, and the IV comes out! Hurray!"

alteration in thyroid function

hypothyroidism

Hypothyroidism in children can be either congenital or acquired. *Congenital hypothyroidism* occurs when the infant is born with insufficient or dysfunctional thyroid tissue. Neonates born with congenital hypothyroidism experience bone growth retardation. *Acquired hypothyroidism* is related to neck radiation or neck surgery that damages the gland. Thyroiditis is a cause of acquired hypothyroidism and may result from tuberculosis, mumps, or an autoimmune process called *Hashimoto's thyroiditis*. Hypothyroidism occurs in 1 in 4,000 live births, is seen twice as often in girls as in boys, and is associated with chromosomal abnormalities, such as Down syndrome.

Maternal thyroid hormones maintain adequate levels in the fetus during pregnancy. When thyroid growth is altered during fetal development, a reduced amount of thyroxine (T_4) and triiodothyronine (T_3) is produced.

pathophysiology

Thyroid tissue may be completely absent (*aplasia*) or partially absent (*hypoplasia*). If some of the gland is present, small amounts of thyroid hormone are produced, and severe symptoms of hypothyroidism are not always apparent until 3 to 6 months after birth.

Symptoms become obvious because increases in growth and development require greater amounts of thyroid hormone production. The lack of adequate thyroid hormone production can cause serious physical and mental delays. Infants who remain untreated until 6 months of age will be mentally retarded. Most states require a mandatory screening test for congenital hypothyroidism at birth.

nursing insight

Low serum thyroxine levels at birth may not result in permanent hypothyroidism. Many pediatricians recommend that children diagnosed as having congenital hypothyroidism at birth be evaluated and retested at 3 to 4 years of age.

Affected infants have feeding difficulties, seldom cry, sleep more than usual, have slow pulse rates and low body temperatures, and tend to be constipated. The child's extremities are short in comparison to the body. Bone development is slowed, muscles are weak, tooth development is delayed and abnormal, and skin is dry and scaly. The skin may be discolored with a yellow tinge as a result of the liver's decreased ability to metabolize vitamin A. The yellow discoloration is called *carotenemia*. An abnormally large or small head circumference can indicate hypothyroidism.

nursing alert

Neonates with pronounced open posterior fontanels are at increased risk for congenital hypothyroidism.

In acquired hypothyroidism, the child's thyroid gland functions normally for several years but as the child's growth accelerates, the gland is unable to produce enough hormone. Onset of acquired hypothyroidism is typically seen in older children.

Symptoms of acquired hypothyroidism include growth arrest with weight gain, decreased activity levels and hair growth, and a drop in pulse rate, respirations, and blood pressure. Adolescent girls experience irregular menstrual cycles.

Diagnosis of hypothyroidism is made by laboratory tests, including serum T_4, T_3, thyroid-stimulating hormone (TSH) levels, and cholesterol levels. A complete history and physical examination help the pediatrician determine growth and development delays. Pulse, respirations, and blood pressure readings are below normal limits according to age. Enlarged heart and respiratory infections occur frequently in children with hypothyroidism.

medical management

Thyroid replacement therapy is used to initiate normal growth and development. The drug of choice is synthetic sodium levothyroxine (T_4) given orally for the duration of the child's life. Periodic examinations, including serum thyroxine levels, help the pediatrician to maintain a proper dosage of thyroid hormone producing an euthyroid (normal thyroid) level. The effectiveness of thyroid hormone administration is measured by the child's growth rate and bone age.

nursing care

Nurses working with new mothers in well baby clinics are in a good position to identify hypothyroidism. Caregiver descriptions of infants who feed poorly, maintain an open mouth with a protruding tongue, suffer constipation, and are easily fatigued need referral to a pediatrician to rule out the possibility of hypothyroidism.

Thyroid administration helps prevent physical and mental growth delays. The nurse must emphasize the importance of giving the medication on a daily schedule. Caregiver instructions concerning thyroid administration are included under Teaching Guidelines.

The nurse must warn caregivers that an overdose of T_4 can have a toxic effect on the child, primarily affecting the nervous system. Nurses must stress the important of follow-up examinations to monitor effectiveness of drug therapy. Thyroid function tests are performed at least yearly and sometimes more often. Children may experience par-

teaching guidelines
thyroid administration

Your child needs to take thyroid pills because the thyroid gland is not producing enough thyroid hormone. Giving thyroid pills is a treatment that helps prevent further physical and mental growth delays.

* Give the thyroid medicine according to the pediatrician's directions.
* Give the pill at the same time each day.
* The medication is best given in the morning.
* Do not skip a dose. If a dose is missed, give it as soon as remembered unless it's almost time for the next dose. If your child is unable to take the pill because of nausea or vomiting or has missed two to three doses, notify the pediatrician's office.
* Do not discontinue giving the medication without consulting the pediatrician.
* Write a schedule to help avoid missing a dose or giving your child an extra dose of medication.
* Do not change brands of medication because some generic brands may not be as effective.
* Watch for changes in your child's behavior about 1 to 3 weeks after starting him or her on thyroid medication.

tial hair loss as a temporary condition when first placed on thyroid therapy.

Side effects of thyroid therapy include headache, nervousness, diarrhea, excessive sweating, heat intolerance, chest pain, increased pulse rate, and heart palpitations. Signs of thyroid effectiveness include diuresis, weight loss, increased sense of well-being, increased energy, increased pulse rate, increased appetite, normal skin texture and hair, and regular bowel movements.

hyperthyroidism

Hyperthyroidism occurs when an increased level of thyroid hormone stimulates increased metabolic function throughout the body. Graves' disease is the most common type of hyperthyroidism. This condition is rare in infants and young children, and the incidence is higher in girls than boys. There tends to be a high familial frequency of Graves' disease.

pathophysiology

Hyperthyroidism is often caused by an autoimmune process within the thyroid gland that stimulates the secretion of an excessive amount of thyroid hormone. The increase in thyroid hormone acts as a stimulant, producing heightened energy. The child is thin, fails to gain weight in spite of a robust appetite, and experiences sleeplessness, restlessness, flushed skin, fever, staring eyes, jaundice, irritability, and constant body movement.

Symptoms of neonatal hyperthyroidism are present at birth and are treated as an emergency because of the potential for severe brain damage. The onset of symptoms in older children is usually gradual. Bulging eyes (exophthalmos) and enlargement of the thyroid gland referred to as goiter are common in older children. Hyperactive behavior often results in poor academic achievement and discipline problems.

Diagnosis of Graves' disease is based on history, physical examination, and serum blood levels of TSH, T_4, and thyroid antibodies. In Graves' disease, blood studies show normal to low TSH levels with high levels of T_4 and thyroid antibodies. The elevation of antibodies results from destruction of the gland by autoimmune processes. Radionuclide scans show a rapid and diffuse concentration of the radioactive material in an enlarged thyroid gland. A low cholesterol level is typically seen in Graves' disease.

medical–surgical management

The medical management of Graves' disease is to administer an antithyroid drug, such as oral propylthiouracil (PTU), that collects in the thyroid gland, preventing the production of excessive thyroid hormone. PTU can be given by suppository. PTU is administered daily, and dosage varies with the weight of the child.

Clinical improvement is noted during the first 2 weeks of treatment. Children need to wear a medical alert bracelet describing their medication regimen (Fig. 38-2). Medication is usually given for 1 year, at the end of which, the thyroid gland is reevaluated, and if normal, medication is stopped. Thyroid function studies are monitored monthly during initial therapy and every 2 to 3 months throughout drug treatment.

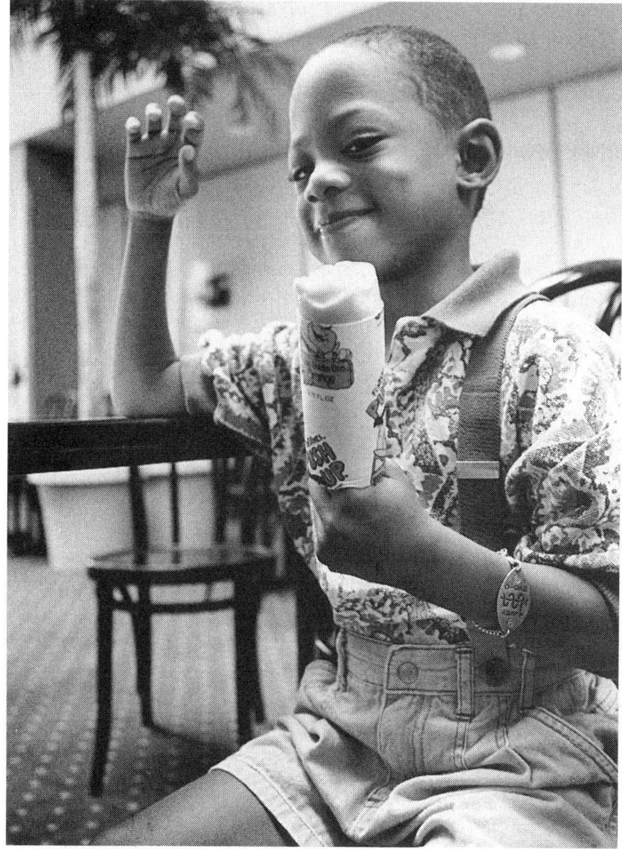

figure 38-2 *Medical alert tags may be worn for a variety of conditions that require specific care in case of injury or emergencies. (Photo by Kathy Sloane.)*

Side effects of PTU include headache, drowsiness, vertigo, diarrhea, nausea, vomiting, loss of taste, fever, skin rash, itching, joint pain, sore throat, and short-term decrease in white cells, called *leukopenia*. The effectiveness of the drug is evaluated by lowered pulse rate and weight gain, increased attention span, and more normal activity levels. Surgical intervention for Graves' disease is partial or total removal of the thyroid gland (*thyroidectomy*). Before surgery, an iodine preparation called Lugol's solution is given to reduce the vascularity and function of the thyroid gland. Administration of the solution involves diluting the medication in juice to reduce the bitter taste and giving the medication through a glass straw to avoid dental staining.

"Thyroid storm" can occur within the first postoperative day, resulting from excessive thyroid hormone being released into the bloodstream during surgery. Symptoms include irritability, vomiting, abdominal cramping, diarrhea, and convulsions.

Tetany is a condition characterized by cramps, convulsions, and twitching of the muscles, especially in the hands and feet. Tetany occurs in response to low serum calcium levels (*hypocalcemia*) resulting from accidental damage or removal of the parathyroid glands during a thyroidectomy. Treatment of tetany is aimed at increasing the serum calcium level by calcium administration. A solution of 10% calcium chloride can be given orally to infants who can suck. Calcium gluconate is given intravenously to children with poor muscle coordination who might choke and aspirate on oral medication. Symptoms of tetany and thyroid storm are reported to the charge nurse immediately because early intervention is necessary to prevent serious consequences, including death.

radiation therapy

When medical or surgical treatment is not possible, radioactive iodine can be used to destroy the thyroid gland. Although the exposure to radiation is low, the treatment poses some risks to the child, including thyroid carcinoma, leukemia, and genetic mutations.

nursing care

Children with Graves' disease become fatigued from their overactive behavior yet have difficulty resting. The child has no control over the excessive amount of thyroid hormone, resulting in rapid and constant movement even when disciplined. Instruct parents to maintain a quiet, nonstimulating environment during rest periods. A cool quiet environment free of stimulating television shows, video games, and large numbers of visitors helps promote rest. Active play is minimized, while quiet games, such as age-appropriate puzzles, short stories, and coloring, are encouraged.

The child's ability to focus on a puzzle, story, or game tends to be limited, regardless of age expectations. The child with Graves' disease is like a compact car with a large truck engine. Both have small exteriors, tremendous energy, and are difficult to manage at a normal speed.

The child's increased metabolic rate increases daily nutritional requirements. Small, frequent nutritional meals are recommended. Carbohydrate intake is increased to provide additional calories.

postoperative nursing care

Close observation for signs of bleeding, throat edema, and tetany is required following thyroidectomy. Oxygen and suctioning equipment are placed in the room for emergency use in case respiratory obstruction occurs from edema at the surgical site. An emergency tracheotomy set is kept close to the bedside for emergency use. Calcium gluconate is readily available in case tetany occurs.

Children and their caregivers are given information about prescribed medications, postoperative care, and symptoms of hypothyroidism, which can occur because thyroid hormone production is decreased.

alteration in pancreatic function

diabetes mellitus

Diabetes mellitus is a chronic disorder characterized by a lack of sufficient insulin to produce normal carbohydrate, protein, and fat metabolism. The outstanding disease trait is a fluctuating blood glucose level relative to lack of insulin production that creates specific warning signals (Display 38-1).

> **display 38-1**
> *warning signals of diabetes*
>
> **Drowsiness**
> **Itching**
> **A family history of diabetes**
> **Blurred vision**
> **Excessive appetite with weight loss**
> **Tingling, numbness, pain in extremities**
> **Easy fatigue**
> **Skin infections; slow healing of cuts and scratches, especially on the feet**

Insulin is a hormone that regulates the metabolism of glucose, lowers blood glucose levels, and boosts the transport and entry of glucose into tissue cells. When there is not enough insulin to support these tasks, the condition is called diabetes mellitus.

The two major classifications of diabetes are type 1 insulin-dependent diabetes mellitus (IDDM) and type 2 non–insulin-dependent diabetes mellitus (NIDDM). A common, serious disease of childhood and adolescence, IDDM affects approximately 1 in 600 children between the ages of 5 and 15 years (Marks, 1994). The incidence is higher at approximately 6 years of age and around the time of puberty. The child with IDDM requires insulin injections as part of the treatment plan. IDDM is often called juvenile onset, ketosis-prone, or brittle diabetes (hard to control). About 5% to 10% of people with diabetes have IDDM (Brunner & Suddarth, 1992).

The exact cause of IDDM is unknown. Type 1 IDDM can be intensified by a number of factors:

- *Genetic predisposition*—IDDM is not inherited; however, there appears to be a genetic tendency to develop the disease. For example, if one child in a family has diabetes, the chance of a sibling developing the illness is higher than normal.
- *Environmental agents*—Viral infections and toxins have been linked with beta cell damage of the pancreas.
- *Autoimmune mechanisms*—These create an abnormal response whereby antibodies are directed against normal tissue.

Non–insulin-dependent diabetes mellitus is commonly found in adults who are overweight. This type of diabetes is called adult-onset, maturity-onset, ketosis-resistant, or stable diabetes. Age of onset is between 40 and 65 years. Management of type 2 NIDDM includes restricted diet, weight control, and administration of either insulin or oral hypoglycemic agents. Insulin injections are not always necessary, and some patients can control their diabetes through dietary measures alone.

pathophysiology

The child with IDDM lacks an adequate supply of insulin to move glucose from the blood into body cells. Some children with IDDM show a resistance to insulin in peripheral tissues, further diminishing the body's ability to use whatever insulin is produced by the beta cells.

Children without diabetes release stored insulin within 10 minutes of a meal and then produce and secrete new insulin as needed. Children with IDDM secrete little or no insulin. These children require insulin administration throughout their lifetime.

the role of insulin in maintaining normal blood glucose levels Insulin is a major hormone that converts simple substances into more complex compounds within the body and maintains a normal level of blood glucose (blood sugar). Stress hormones, secreted in response to physical illness, infections, and emotional upsets, interfere with the action of insulin.

The normal actions of insulin to support blood glucose levels are explained in Figure 38-3. Insulin secretion increases after food is ingested. The increased amount of insulin moves glucose from the blood into muscle, liver, and fat cells. In those cells, insulin stimulates the storage of glucose in the form of glycogen and speeds up the transport of amino acids into body cells to be used for energy. When children are fasting or sleeping, insulin release is decreased but continuous. Because the body must maintain a constant blood sugar level even though there is no food ingested during fast and sleep (remember how hard the body works to maintain homeostasis), a pancreatic hormone called *glucagon* is released. Glucagon is secreted by the alpha cells of the islets of Langerhans. Glucagon stimulates the conversion and release of *glycogen*, a major carbohydrate formed from glucose and stored in the liver. Normal blood sugar levels are maintained.

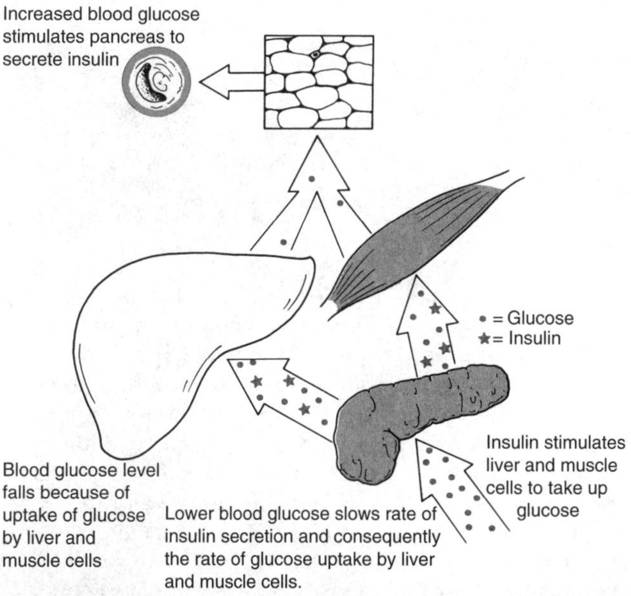

figure 38-3 *Normal metabolism of glucose.*

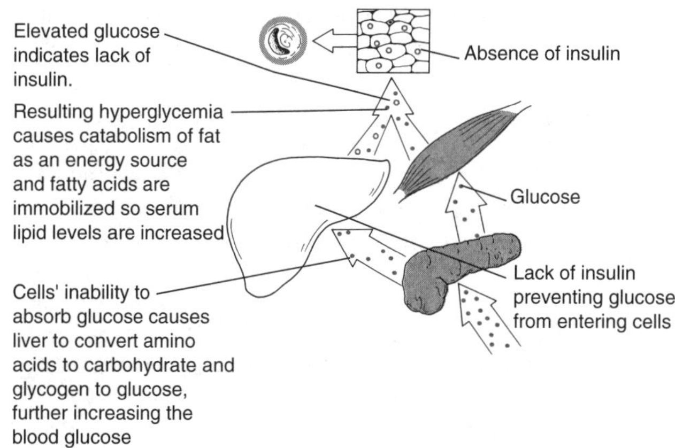

figure 38-4 *Abnormal metabolism of glucose in diabetic patients*

body responses to inadequate insulin production Glucose is unable to enter body cells without insulin. Carbohydrates taken into the body and converted into glucose remain in the bloodstream, causing abnormal increases in blood glucose levels (*hyperglycemia*; Fig. 38-4).

The body's attempt to rid the excess blood glucose stimulates the excretion of abnormally large amounts of urine (*polyuria*). Children may begin to be incontinent as a response to frequent and excessive urination. The excreted urine contains sugar. *Glycosuria* is the medical term for an increased amount of sugar in the urine. Glycosuria increases the child's risk for urinary infections and vaginal irritation.

Because of the increased amount of fluid lost through urination, the child complains of thirst and drinks a lot of water (*polydipsia*). Because the extra water is excreted in larger amounts through the urine, polydipsia does not correct the problem; rather, it puts the child at risk for dehydration.

Also, water loss contributes to loss of electrolytes, especially potassium and phosphate, and increases the child's risk of electrolyte imbalance. Insulin deficiency impairs the metabolism of proteins and fats, resulting in weight loss. In response to a decreased storage of calories, an increase in appetite, known as *polyphagia*, occurs.

As the insulin deficiency persists, the body cells remain unable to use glucose for energy. In response, the cells begin to break down protein and fat (see Fig. 38-4). Fat breakdown causes an increased production of ketone bodies or acetones (waste product of fat metabolism).

Ketone bodies are acids. When they accumulate in large amounts, the body creates an acid–base imbalance known as *diabetic ketoacidosis*. Ketoacidosis, also called diabetic coma, is a life-threatening condition.

medical management

Diagnosis of IDDM is based on history and physical examination, presence of symptoms, and blood glucose readings, including an oral glucose tolerance test. Major symptoms of diabetes include hyperglycemia, glycosuria, and the three Ps, polyuria, polydipsia, and polyphagia (Display 38-2).

An *oral glucose tolerance test* consists of giving high-carbohydrate meals for 3 days before the test. Following an overnight fast, a blood sample is drawn; a simple carbohydrate solution, such as a carbonated sugar beverage (Glucola), is then given. Water may be given during the test but nothing else. Blood samples are drawn 2 hours after the ingestion of Glucola. Blood values according to age are given in Table 38-3. Acceptable blood glucose readings are between 80 and 150 mg/dL before eating and between 80 and 180 mg/dL 2 hours after eating (Castiglia, 1992).

Management of IDDM centers around insulin administration, diet, and exercise, with the major focus on maintaining normal blood glucose levels. Diet and exercise are adjusted to potentiate the effects of insulin and promote overall growth and development. Dietary management involves guidelines established by the American Diabetes Association. Treatment of the child with diabetes involves the family, child, nurse, pediatrician, nutritionist, pharmacist, and diabetic nurse educator. Management of diabetes requires a team approach to prevent complications associated with the disease.

Complications of IDDM include diabetic ketoacidosis, insulin shock, infections, atherosclerosis, blindness related to retinal edema or hemorrhage and cataracts, and nerve dysfunction (neuropathy). Adequate insulin therapy removes the problem of growth failure among children with diabetes.

Insulin therapy requires careful monitoring of blood glucose levels with the goal of maintaining normal values. Insulin is injected into subcutaneous tissue, rather than taken orally, because it would be digested as a protein and eliminated from the body without benefitting the patient.

display 38-2
major symptoms of diabetes

Inadequate insulin production in the diabetic child results in five cardinal symptoms of diabetes described as follows:

- **Hyperglycemia—elevated blood sugar resulting from an inability of glucose to enter body cells**
- **Glucosuria—increased sugar in the urine resulting from the kidneys' inability to reabsorb all of the filtered glucose from the blood**
- **Polyuria—increased urination resulting from the body's attempt to eliminate the excess sugar through the urine.**
- **Polydipsia—increased thirst resulting from the body's attempt to replace the fluid lost during polyuria**
- **Polyphagia—increased appetite in response to cell starvation resulting from an inability to convert sugar for cell use; accompanied by weight loss**

table 38-3 age-specific blood glucose levels

Age	*Blood Glucose Level*
Full-term newborn	20–110 mg/dL
1 wk to 16 y	60–105 mg/dL
Over 16 y	70–115 mg/dL

Some diabetics use insulin pumps. They deliver a steady low dose of insulin through a polyethylene tube connected to a small-gauge subcutaneous cannula implanted in the abdomen. The tubing is connected to an insulin-filled syringe inside the pump. When extra insulin is needed, the child can push a button on the pump to release additional insulin.

The pump is about the size of a transistor radio and can be worn strapped to the waist or shoulder. Careful glucose monitoring is necessary to adjust insulin dosages because the pump only administers insulin and is unable to sense glucose levels.

The cannula site must be carefully observed for signs of inflammation, and it must be cleaned daily and covered with sterile gauze. The site is changed every 24 to 48 hours to ensure optimum absorption. The pump, cannula, and syringe must be removed for bathing. Children who fear needles may respond more positively to insulin injections using an automatic injection device, such as the Autojector. The device pushes the needle into the skin and injects the medication into the patient. Once loaded, the entire syringe is hidden from view (Fig. 38-5).

✳ nursing alert

Children using insulin pumps require a 2 AM blood glucose test to reduce the risk of hypoglycemia associated with the continuous delivery of insulin in the absence of food ingestion.

Commercial insulin is derived from the pancreas of pork and beef animals and from synthetic chemicals. Insulin is available as pork and beef, purified pork, purified beef, and laboratory-manufactured human (*Humulin*) insulin. Insulins are divided into three groups with respect to peak and duration of hypoglycemic action.

Regular insulin, when given subcutaneously, begins to lower glucose ½ hour to 1 hour after administration. Regular insulin is soluble and clear. Regular insulin may be mixed with an intermediate-acting insulin to provide an early insulin peak and increase an early hypoglycemic ef-

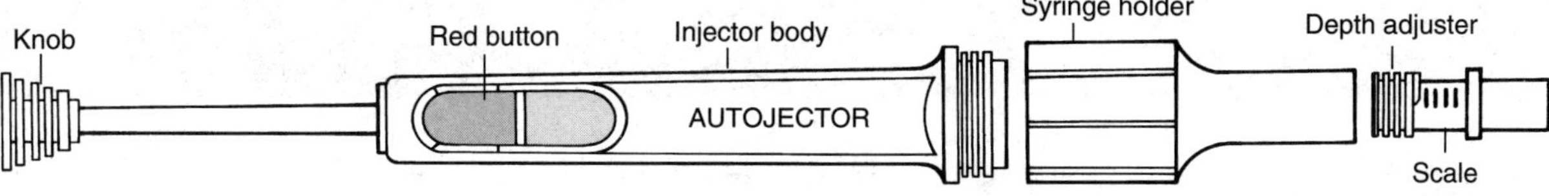

figure 38-5 *The Autojector*

fect. Regular insulin is used for fast-acting coverage of the following patients:

* Elevated blood glucose levels before meals and at bedtime
* Emergencies, such as ketoacidosis
* Conditions requiring surgery

Neutral protamine Hagedorn (NPH) and Lente are insulins used for customary "day-long" control. Both are zinc insulins modified so that insulin absorption from a subcutaneous injection site is delayed. They are classified as intermediate-acting insulins (Table 38-4).

Protamine zinc insulin (PZI) and ultralente insulin are long-acting preparations. They typically have late-onset action with a major hypoglycemic effect during the night (see Table 38-4).

Complications of insulin administration include allergic reactions, insulin hypoatrophy, fibrous swelling at injection sites, and insulin resistance (Table 38-5). Researchers are studying other routes of insulin administration, such as inhalation therapy in an attempt to reduce some of the risks associated with injections. Currently, however, only injectable insulin is available.

diabetic ketoacidosis The child with diabetes mellitus may go without medical intervention until the advancement of the disease causes diabetic ketoacidosis. This life-threatening condition is characterized by hyperglycemia, metabolic acidosis, dehydration, and altered level of consciousness ranging from lethargy to coma. Additional symptoms include air hunger, called Kussmaul respirations; acetone breath; abdominal discomfort; nausea and vomiting; blurred vision; and dry, flushed skin (Display 38-3). Diabetic ketoacidosis remains the most important cause of death in children with diabetes (Rosenbloom, 1994).

table 38-4 types of insulin: onset, peak, duration

Action	*Preparation*	*Onset*	*Peak*	*Duration*
Rapid acting	Regular iletin Pork, beef	½–1 h	2–4 h	6–8 h
	Humulin R Human (Lilly)	½–1 h	2–4 h	6–8 h
	Novolin Human (Squibb)	½ h	2½–5 h	8 h
	Semilente	½–1 h	5–10 h	12–16 h
Immediate acting	NPH Pork, beef	1½–2 h	6–12 h	24 h
	Humulin Human (Lilly)	1–2 h	6–12 h	18–24 h
	Novolin N Human (Squibb)	1½ h	4–12 h	24 h
	Lente Beef, pork	2–4 h	6–12 h	18–26 h
	Humulin 70/30 70% N, 30% R	½ h	4–8 h	24 h
	Novolin 70/30 70% N, 30% R	½ h	4–8 h	24 h
Long acting	Protamine zinc Beef, pork	4–8 h	14–24 h	28–36 h
	Ultralente Beef, pork	4–8 h	14–24 h	28–36 h

table 38-5 compliactions of insulin administration

Complication	*Physical Characteristic*	*Medical Management*	*Nursing Considerations*
Allergic reactions at injection site	Red and edematous lesions developing within 2 h after the injection Occasionally systemic allergic reaction with the development of hives	Change from beef–pork insulin to pork insulin. Give small doses of insulin, gradually increasing the amount until a tolerated dose is reached and child is desensitized, or add corticosteroid in small doses to insulin injected.	Assess injection sites, and document findings. Allergy is often seen in patients who have previously taken insulin.
Insulin shock/hyperinsulinism	Hypoglycemia (<60) Glycosuria depending on type of insulin and time taken Normal breath odor Pale, diaphoretic, cold, and clammy Mental confusion, nervousness, bizarre behavior, loss of consciousness C/O hunger, double vision	Rapid onset requires immediate attention to increase blood sugar level and maintain brain function. If unconscious, IV glucose is given. Diet, exercise, and insulin prescribed must be evaluated.	FSBS, give 10–15 g of glucose, such as 4 oz nondiet cola, 2 tbsp of cake icing, half cup of sweetened orange juice
Insulin resistance	Produced by numerous factors that include obesity, endocrine disturbances, antibodies to insulin, and abnormalities within the cell	Patients requiring more than 200 U of insulin per day are described as being insulin resistant	Assess child for symptoms of diabetes, and document findings. Assess blood glucose levels in response to insulin administration.
Insulin lipoatrophy	Complete disappearance of subcutaneous fat in and around the injection sites Common in children	Cosmetic surgery	Rarely seen in children using human insulin More common with beef/pork insulins Rotate injection sites

Medical treatment of diabetic ketoacidosis is aimed at maintaining a normal pH balance (7.35–7.45), lowering the blood sugar levels to within normal limits for child's age, and providing hydration. Medical intervention includes intravenous electrolyte fluid infusion, regular insulin given subcutaneously or intravenously, oxygen therapy, and blood and urine testing to evaluate the degree of acidosis. Gastric lavage may be performed to relieve abdominal distention and decrease the risk of aspiration.

honeymoon period Following a confirmed diagnosis of diabetes mellitus and treatment with insulin injections, some children experience a "honeymoon period." The honeymoon period is characterized by glucose regulation with minimal or no insulin administration. The presence of administered insulin stimulates the islet cells to produce natural insulin. Patients and caregivers are convinced that the diagnosis is not correct or the child has been cured. The honeymoon period may last 1 month to 1 year before the islet cells begin to fail and diabetic symptoms recur.

nursing care

Managing the child's stress associated with diabetes is crucial to health and normal development. Painful procedures, such as blood glucose monitoring and insulin injections, can interfere with formation of trust necessary in infant development (Table 38-6). Distraction is a useful intervention for painful procedures. Infants can be distracted with a toy while blood glucose tests are taken and insulin injections given. Tips about insulin are given in Display 38-4.

patient and caregiver teaching The nurse spends a significant amount of time providing clear, current information about diabetic care to children and their caregivers and reinforcing what they already know. Insulin injection technique can be simulated by substituting normal saline for insulin (normal saline is more cost effective to use for practice) and injecting a laboratory mannequin (Display 38-5).

An older child's capacity for assuming self-care responsibilities differs greatly from one child to another. When

display 38-3
comparison of insulin reaction and diabetic coma

INSULIN REACTION	***DIABETIC COMA***
Rapid onset	Slow onset
Pale face	Flushed face
No odor to breath	Fruity odor to breath
Moist tongue	Dry tongue
Normal, shallow, or rapid breathing	Labored prolonged breathing (Kussmaul respirations)
Perspiration	Frequent urination
Weakness	Drowsiness
Hunger	Lack of energy
Tingly and numb fingers, feet, or tongue	Thirst
Nervousness	Nausea
Shakiness	Sometimes vomiting
Headache	Later stupor and coma
Urine negative for sugar and acetone	Urine positive for sugar and acetone
CAUSES:	***CAUSES:***
Too much insulin	Too little insulin
Not eating enough food	Failure to follow diet
	Infection, fever
	Emotional stress
WHAT TO DO:	***WHAT TO DO:***
Take B-D glucose tablets or food containing sugar (orange juice, cola, candy).	Call doctor immediately.
Do not give fluid if patient is not conscious.	Give patients fluids without sugar if able to swallow.
Call doctor.	Test urine frequently for sugar and acetone.

caregivers and children share diabetic care responsibilities, there tends to be better compliance and fewer errors with diet and insulin injections. The child's readiness for diabetes management includes an assessment of cognitive, emotional, and physical development and present self-care status (Display 38-6).

Insulin injections may be given in areas that have a thick layer of fat and are free from large blood vessels and nerves. The arms, abdomen, thighs, and buttocks can be used. It is important to rotate sites to avoid a build-up of scar tissue in a site, which would prohibit insulin absorption. Intrasite rotation is the most popular rotation method and involves the use of one body area for as long as possible, spacing the injections at least 1 in apart. This technique enables a more consistent insulin absorption rate (Fig. 38-6).

nursing insight

Cover the injection site with a small spot Bandaid to identify the area so the next injection can be spaced 1 in from the previous site.

nursing alert

Type 1 diabetes in children younger than 1 year is rare; by the time the disease becomes obvious, infants are often seriously ill with hyperglycemia, metabolic acidosis, or dehydration.

infections common to diabetes mellitus The child with diabetes is easy prey for skin infections. Skin breakdown from cuts, scrapes, and blisters can become a major health concern. Children and caregivers must inspect the skin daily, treat small breaks in the skin, and seek medical attention at the first indication that infection is present. Daily bathing is encouraged. The skin must be dried thoroughly and kept free of irritating perfumes, lotions, and powder.

Foot care is important. Shoes worn without socks can put the child at risk for athlete's foot. The dye in colored socks may be an irritant. Going barefoot increases the child's risk of a foot infection. Care must be taken to trim toenails straight across.

Areas of high moisture, such as the axilla, groin, or other skin folds, are prone to fungus infections. Girls ex-

table 38-6 special concerns and considerations for care of the infant with diabetes

Concern	Caregiver Considerations
Infants have small area size, making rotation of insulin injection sites difficult.	Map out suitable areas for injections using upper arms, thighs, abdomen, and buttocks to rotate sites.
Small insulin dose contributes to increased risk of inaccurate measurement.	Use a conversion chart to measure smaller doses when using a U-100 syringe, and refer to lines of insulin (eg, 0.1 U = 1 line on the syringe when using U-10 insulin dosage).
Blood glucose monitoring is difficult on small fingers.	To rest the fingers, toes can be used if the baby is not walking. Small-gauge lancets are used for infants.
Infant hypoglycemic reactions are common.	Watch for hunger, lethargy, irritability, night terrors, apnea, cyanosis, and hypothermia.
Ketone testing is necessary.	Place a cotton ball in the diaper to absorb enough urine to test for ketones.
Dietary management is important.	Provide an unmeasured diet with one to three snacks per day to maintain blood sugar level. Infant formula is given if younger than 12 mo. If older than 12 months, whole milk is used (not 2% or skim). Night bottle may need to be water instead of formula depending on blood sugar range.

periencing vaginitis from *Candida albicans* benefit from wearing cotton panties rather than nylon. Urinary infections are more common with diabetes, and children need to know that burning on urination must be reported to the caregiver.

Fatty accumulation beneath the skin may form with repeated injections in the area. Children may tend to use the same site because the skin becomes fibrous and insensitive to needle insertion, causing less discomfort or because the site is convenient for the injection. Insulin will be absorbed poorly from these sites, and these areas are at risk for becoming infected.

"Shin spots" or brownish discoloration of the shins may be seen in the diabetic child. The brownish color is considered to be from iron-containing substances that remain after small hemorrhages in the skin. The shin is subject to more trauma than most other areas of the body. The brown spots are harmless but are a clue to widespread blood vessel changes.

dietary management

Children with diabetes need a sound nutritional program that provides them with adequate nutrition for normal growth needs. To accommodate the varying peak action of insulin, the child should have food distributed throughout the day, changing in relation to increased or decreased ex-

display 38-4
tips about insulin

- **Absorption of insulin depends on the insulin's quality, concentration, amount injected, blood flow to injection site, and whether or not the insulin's date of expiration has passed.**
- **Do not draw insulin up ahead of time to store it for use because insulin tends to cling to plastic and glass, increasing the risk of getting an inaccurate dose.**
- **If unsure about the patency of insulin, check its color. Regular and globin insulins are clear; others are cloudy and free of clumps.**
- **Insulin must be stored in a cool place away from sunlight; it does not require refrigeration. Do not inject cold insulin because the action may be delayed. A practical tip is to store unopened insulin in the refrigerator, and keep opened bottles in a purse, locker, or drawer. Extreme cold and heat must be avoided.**
- **Human insulin manufactured synthetically by a special DNA technique tends to have fewer side effects, especially lipoatrophy.**
- **When combining regular and NPH insulin for one injection, inject air equal to the dose of insulin required into each vial. Regular insulin must be drawn into the syringe first. If the vial of regular insulin is contaminated with a small drop of NPH, the action time will be altered. However, if the vial of NPH insulin is exposed to a small drop of regular insulin, the action time basically remains the same. The amount of regular or NPH insulin would not be correct. It is important to be careful when mixing insulins.**
- **When mixing two types of insulin, if bubbles or too much insulin has been drawn, it is necessary to start all over again, because a bubble or portion of the mixture cannot be removed without risking an inaccurate dose.**

display 38-5
insulin injection technique

* Select correct site (see Fig. 38-6). Intrasite rotation is recommended because insulin absorbs differently in various parts of the body. For example, if the morning dose of insulin is given in the child's thigh, the subsequent morning injections are given to the same thigh, making sure the site is 1 in away from the previous site. No injection site should be used before 1 month.
* Wipe site with alcohol and allow to dry.
* Grasp fold of skin, and insert needle at 90-degree angle (4 degrees recommended for thin patients and small children).
* Release folds of skin.
* Aspirate for blood before injecting insulin in children because they may have superficial blood vessels at the injection site. (Aspiration is not always necessary for adult insulin injections.)
* Inject insulin, and then remove needle at the same angle.
* Observe for leakage; estimate the amount of insulin lost; apply gentle pressure to injection site. Do not massage.
* Record amount, time, location, and condition of injection site.
* Carefully dispose of needle and syringe.

ercise. Young children tend to tolerate three meals and three between-meal snacks because they have proportionately smaller stomachs. See the Nursing Care Plan for the Child With Diabetes Mellitus.

One of the greatest difficulties in dietary management of children with diabetes is the need for increased calories during exercise. The child with diabetes absorbs glucose after exercise with less dependence on insulin, increasing the need for extra food before and during the activity. Many times, children and parental caregivers find out the right balance by trial and error (Display 38-7).

procedures specific for diabetes mellitus

ketones in urine Ketone detection in urine indicates fat metabolism. Urine testing involves detecting acetone using Acetest tablets or Ketostix. Urine test strips are affected by humidity and sunlight. Urine testing for ketones is recommended for children during illness and if the finger stick blood sugar (FSBS) reading is greater than 240 mg/dL.

The procedure involves the following:

* Collect a double-voided specimen to ensure accuracy.
* Place a drop of urine on the Acetest tablet or dip the Ketostix into the urine; wait 15 to 30 seconds according to manufacturer's guidelines.

display 38-6
growth and development considerations for children with insulin-dependent diabetes mellitus

PRESCHOOL YEARS

Autonomy issues are important. Child's feelings of control and autonomy are reinforced when allowed to help select snack items, determine fingers to be pricked for FSBS, and gather testing equipment. Preschool child cannot understand restrictions in food intake, may fantasize about body parts and function, and fear harm from injections.

EARLY SCHOOL YEARS

Children engage in the developmental tasks of industry versus inferiority, tend to solve problems by trial and error, follow rules to avoid punishment, and begin to expand socially. Children between 6 to 8 years are able to deal with symbols and manipulate things mentally rather than physically. Their ability to tell time helps them to remember snack times. Participation with blood glucose testing helps reinforce learning according to rules when the procedure is performed consistently each time. Praise helps build self-esteem.

LATE SCHOOL YEARS

Children between 9 to 12 years have an increasing interest in body and appearance. They may voice disgust at having to take insulin injections. They have an understanding about time and events, such as insulin action and timing of food intake. They have knowledge about performing daily glucose testing but may forget to do so.

EARLY ADOLESCENT YEARS

Children between 13 and 15 years may understand explanations of potential diabetic complications but are more concerned with "now" rather than "future" events. Lectures from adults about taking responsibility for diabetes self-care are not accepted by this age group, making continued support and guidance necessary to ensure correct technique for FSBS testing and insulin injections.

LATE ADOLESCENT YEARS

Older adolescents between 16 and 18 years are establishing a sense of identity with "adult" privileges and responsibilities, such as employment, driving, and dating. Many older adolescents begin to show more responsible attitudes toward diabetes self-care. They can use abstract reasoning, show concern about potential diabetic complications, and have the cognitive and fine and gross motor skills to manage FSBS testing, insulin injections, and diet plans. Need continuous support and guidance from caregivers.

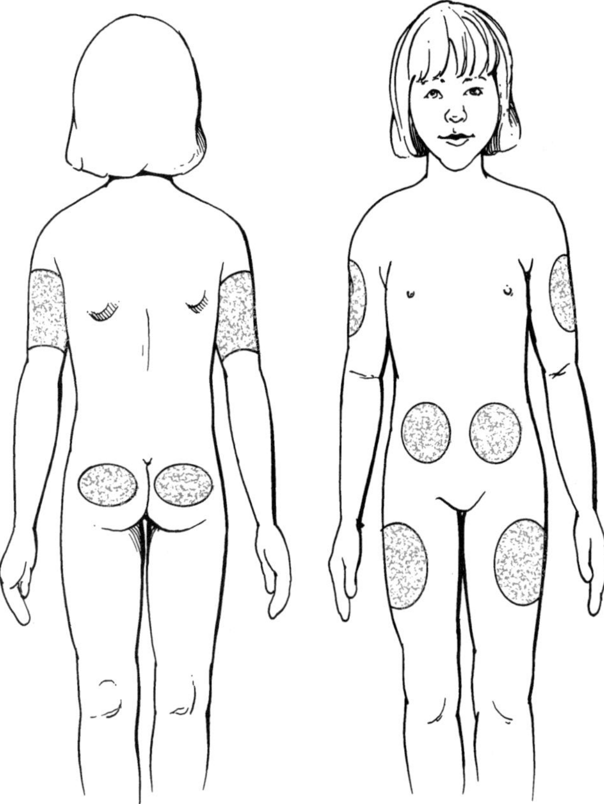

figure 38-6 *Subcutaneous injection sites. (From Castiglia, P. T., Harbin, R. E. (1992) Child health care [p. 904]. Philadelphia: J. B. Lippincott.)*

* Use the color chart provided by the manufacturer to interpret the results. The tablet or strip turns a purple color when acetone is present. A positive reaction results when the concentration of acetone is greater than 5 mg/dL.
* Notify the pediatrician if the child's urine contains acetone because normally no ketones are present in the urine. The presence of ketones indicates excess fat metabolism and increases the child's risk for metabolic acidosis.

nursing alert

Acetest tablets are poisonous and must be kept away from young children.

blood glucose meters Blood glucose monitoring, also called finger stick blood sugar, must be individualized for each patient by the health care team, child, and caregiver. The goal of blood glucose monitoring is to maintain blood glucose at normal or near-normal levels. Patients on insulin are usually required to test their blood glucose four times daily—before each meal and at bedtime—to evaluate the effectiveness of insulin dosages. However, children may find this schedule difficult because of school, sports, and so forth. Testing twice a day at alternating times will reveal the blood glucose levels at all four times of the day in a 2-day period. Children are encouraged to test before exercise and whenever they experience signs of hypoglycemia or hyperglycemia.

The many blood glucose meters on the market provide accurate measurements if used according to manufacturer's guidelines. Equipment malfunction and human error can affect the accuracy of the readings.

A quality control test must be done once a week and each time a new vial of strips is opened. This quick and easy test helps determine the accuracy of the meter.

Human error is a major factor for inaccurate glucose readings. Failing to obtain a large drop of blood on the strip and a delay in setting the appropriate timing device are common errors. The Teaching Guidelines display suggests ways to get a more accurate finger stick blood sugar reading.

display 38-7
diabetic food plan

1. **Plan well-balanced meals that are appealing to the child and age appropriate, such as finger foods for the toddler.**
2. **Be positive with children when discussing foods allowed on the diabetic diet; explore alternative foods and substitutions.**
3. **Space three meals and three snacks throughout the day. Do not skip meals. Daily caloric intake is divided to provide 20% at breakfast, 20% at lunch, 30% at dinner, and 10% at each of the snacks.**
4. **When NPH or Lente insulin is used, an insulin reaction is most likely to occur in the late afternoon when the insulin is peaking. Stress the importance of the afternoon snack, and alert the child to the increased risk of an insulin reaction at this time.**
5. **Calories are made up of 50% to 60% carbohydrates, 15% to 20% protein, and not more than 30% fat.**
6. **Avoid concentrated sweets, such as jelly, syrup, pie, candy bars, and cola. Dietetic candies and other foods labeled as such contain some calories and must be included in the calorie count prescribed by the pediatrician. Many of these foods contain artificial sweeteners.**
7. **Foods containing dietary fiber, such as whole grains, cereals, fruits, and vegetables, help prevent hyperglycemia.**
8. **The American Diabetes Association diet plan and exchange list provides a variety of food choices.**

nursing care plan
for child with diabetes mellitus

NURSING DIAGNOSIS

Altered Nutrition: Less than body requirements, related to reduction in insulin production

GOAL: *The child will have adequate nutrition and stable glucoses*

NURSING INTERVENTIONS	***RATIONALE***	***EVALUATION***
Educate the child and the family on the disease process, its treatment, and the importance of following a prescribed nutritional program.	If the child and family understand the relationship between glucose and insulin in diabetes mellitus, then they will be better able to make informed nutritional decisions and see the importance of them.	The child and the family will describe appropriate diets and understand the importance of regular meals.
Inform the family and child of the need to be prepared to give a complex carbohydrate and protein snack if a meal is late.	Since children and life can be unpredictable, the family must be cognizant of necessary impromptu snacks and their importance.	The family and the child will state appropriate high carbohydrate and protein snacks which they will always have available.
Teach the child to avoid excessive or concentrated sugars.	This will assist in lessening insulin requirements and pevent long-term complications.	The child will state what concentrated and excessive sugars are and understand the importance of monitoring them.
Encourage the family and the child to meet with the dietitian to plan meals at home and social settings.	Teaching the importance of a balanced diet and obtaining facts from a dietitian for all eating scenarios will be beneficial to the entire family.	The family and the child will list various food options for different eating situations.

NURSING DIAGNOSIS

Knowledge Deficit, associated with new diagnosis of diabetes mellitus and it's management

GOAL: *Improve child and family's knowledge base and control of blood glucoses*

NURSING INTERVENTIONS	***RATIONALE***	***EVALUATION***
Explain the disease and its treatment to the parents and to the child in terms understood by all.	Understanding the disease can maximize the effect of treatment.	Family and child will state they have an understanding of the disease process.
Teach the importance of insulin and blood glucose monitoring.	Urine testing and blood glucose monitoring will be necessary.	The family and the child will demonstrate blood glucose and urine testing procedures.
Help the family and child understand that the child's metabolism and insulin needs will continue to change with age, stress, and exercise.	The changing needs of the child must be addressed to stress the potential for increased carbohydrate or insulin in certain situations.	The family and child will list situations which will affect their metabolism and insulin requirements.
Educate the family and the child on about the action and side effects on insulin and the signs and symptoms of hypoglycemia and hyperglycemia.	Effects of insulin and signs of hypoglycemia and hyperglycemia can alert the child to serious symptoms and help to prevent fluctuations in blood glucoses.	The family and the child will report the action of insulin and understand the side effects.
Ensure the family and the child understand the dangerous complications that will occur with uncontrolled diabetes mellitus.	Long-term complications can be controlled if glucoses are well regulated.	The family and the child will state potential complications and understand the importance of good glucose control.
Demonstrate insulin injection technique and monitor the child's injection technique.	Monitoring technique will ensure that the child understands appropriate technique, thereby avoiding complications of poor technique.	The family and child will demonstrate adequate subcutaneous injection technique and state and realize the importance of rotating sites.

teaching guidelines
blood glucose monitoring

You can get a more accurate finger stick blood sugar reading by doing the following:

* Wash hands with warm water.
* Hang hands down below the level of the heart for several minutes.
* Prick the side of the finger to make it easier to get a full drop of blood. Also there are fewer nerve endings and less pain.
* Avoid smearing blood on the strip or trying to add an extra drop because this will result in an incorrect reading.

what would you do?

Alisa is a 13-year-old diabetes mellitus patient diagnosed 2 years ago. Recently, she has been noncompliant with diet and insulin administration. She refuses to wear a medical alert bracelet. She has been treated twice in the last 2 months for a yeast infection of the vagina. She talks back in an angry tone when her parents try to talk about the need to balance diet, insulin, exercise, and rest. Her mother has asked that the nurse talk to her.

key points

* **Endocrine disorders affect glands known as "ductless" glands because they secrete chemicals called hormones directly into the blood, lymph, and extracellular fluids. These hormones influence the regulation of metabolic processes, such as growth, energy production, fluid and electrolyte balance, and coordination of body activities, such as stress responses, personality, and sexual development.**
* **Alteration in endocrine function results in a variety of disorders with long-term implications for normal growth and development, including deficiencies of GH, thyroxin, and insulin, requiring lifelong hormone replacement therapy.**
* **The endocrine system includes the pituitary gland, also called the hypophysis, thyroid gland, parathyroid gland, adrenal gland, pancreas, testes, and ovaries.**
* **Endocrine disorders are not easily diagnosed, are rare, and need the services of an endocrinologist; this requires families to cope with the expense and stress of a new doctor, traveling, unfamiliar surroundings, blood tests, fear about the child's ability to live a normal life, and concern about abilities to learn required procedures, such as giving injections at home.**
* **Growth and development alterations are frequently seen in children with endocrine system disorders and are readily detected by plotting weight and height measurements on a growth grid. Persistent growth deviations are seen in congenital endocrine disorders, whereas normal growth followed by a sudden deviation is seen at the onset of an acquired endocrine problem.**
* **Nursing assessment of endocrine disorders includes a complete history of the child's physical, emotional, and social growth; activity patterns; familial genetic predisposition to endocrine disorders; and physical signs of increased or decreased hormone secretions based on data concerning size, facial characteristics, genitalia, vital signs, hydration, skin, and emotional status.**
* **Diagnostic testing for endocrine disorders includes blood chemistry studies to determine thyroid function, hormone levels, calcium, phosphorus, alkaline phosphatase, electrolytes, blood glucose, GH; urine studies to determine sodium, calcium, phosphorus, glucose, cortisol, and specific gravity; imaging studies to determine skeletal maturation, bone age and density, the degree of epiphyseal separation from the main portion of long bones, occurrence of epiphyseal fusion, ultrasound, and CT and MRI studies; and genetic studies to determine karyotype.**
* **Hypopituitary dwarfism results from deficiencies of GH resulting from unknown causes or from increased pressure on the pituitary gland by nonmalignant cystic tumors formed in the embryo stage.**
* **Dysfunction of the thyroid gland can result in hypothyroidism or hyperthyroidism and can be congenital or acquired, causing symptoms of physical and mental delays.**
* **Diabetes mellitus is a chronic disorder characterized by a lack of sufficient insulin to produce normal carbohydrate, protein, and fat metabolism, causing fluctuating blood glucose levels relative to the lack of insulin production, and it occurs as type I IDDM in children with symptoms of hyperglycemia, glycosuria, polyphagia, polydipsia, polyuria, and weight loss despite a robust appetite.**

review questions

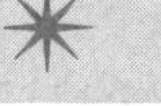

1. Shane is 3 months old and is being seen in the clinic for a routine examination. What nursing intervention would be significant in screening infants for growth delays?
   a. Weight
   b. Weight and head circumference
   c. Length
   d. Weight and length plotted on a growth grid
2. The endocrine gland known as the hypophysis is the
   a. thyroid.
   b. pancreas.
   c. pituitary.

   d. islets of Langerhans.
3. Mrs. Gaitors' son has been recently diagnosed as having hypothyroidism. Mrs. Gaitors asks the nurse what the thyroid gland does for the body. An appropriate response includes,
   a. "The thyroid gland is responsible for your son's ability to use sugar from the blood."
   b. "The thyroid gland is responsible for breaking down food that is used for body energy."
   c. "The thyroid gland controls many other glands and is responsible for your child's growth."
   d. "Children with hypothyroidism must be treated with medication to avoid being physically and mentally retarded."
4. Ms. Chen complains that her 5-year-old son who was diagnosed with diabetes 1 year ago cannot correctly give his own insulin injections. Select the most appropriate explanation for the child's behavior.
   a. A 5-year-old is typically contrary and rebellious.
   b. Most 5-year-old children are eager to please adults. This child lacks the ability to comprehend the complexity of giving an insulin injection.
   c. Ms. Chen must continue to encourage her child to learn independence.
   d. Ms. Chen needs to use firm but fair discipline measures to impress on her child the importance of correct injection technique.
5. Select the most accurate statement about endocrine disorders.
   a. Endocrine disorders are curable if diagnosed early.
   b. Endocrine disorders are never life-threatening.
   c. Endocrine disorders typically require lifetime hormone therapy.
   d. Endocrine disorders are always hereditary.

references

Castiglia, P., & Harbin, R. (1992). *Child health care*. Philadelphia: J.B. Lippincott.

Marks, M. (l994) *Broadribb's Introductory pediatric nursing* (3rd ed.). Philadelphia: J.B. Lippincott.

Rosenbloom, A. (l994). Diabetes in childhood and adolescence. *Pediatric Annals*, *23*(6), 282–283.

Smeltzer, S. & Bare, B. (1995). *Brunner and Suddarth's Textbook of Medical–Surgical Nursing*, 7th ed. Philadelphia: J.B. Lippincott.

bibliography

Amer, K., August G., & Robnett, M. (1992). *The nursing perspective: Monitoring and evaluation of growth. Califon,* New Jersey: Synermed.

Brandt, P., & Magyary, D. (1993). The impact of a diabetes education program on children and mothers. *Journal of Pediatric Nursing: Nursing Care of Children & Families*, *8*(1), 31–40.

Campbell, R. (1991). Preventing diabetic eye disease. *U.S. Pharmacist Diabetes Supplement*, November, 2–15.

Chung, K., Olson, R. & Vinson, J. (1992). *Lippincott's pediatric nursing review*. Philadelphia: J.B. Lippincott.

Clarke, W., Vance, M., & Rogol, A. (1993). Growth and the child with diabetes mellitus. *Diabetes Care*, *16*(3), 101–104.

Deglin, J., & Vallerand, A. (l993). *Davis drug guide for nurses* (4th ed.). Philadelphia: F.A. Davis.

(1993). Diabetes update. *Nursing 93, August*, 59–61.

Drass, J. (1992). Insulin injections. *Nursing 92, November*, 40–43.

Fischback, F. (1995). *Quick reference to common laboratory and diagnostic tests*. Philadelphia: J.B. Lippincott.

Fisher, D. A. (l990). The thyroid. In S. A. Kaplan (Ed.), *Clinical pediatric endocrinology*. Philadelphia: W.B. Saunders.

Giordano, V., Petrila, A., Banion, C., & Neuenkirchen, G. (1993). The challenge of transferring responsibility for diabetes management from parent to child. *Journal of Pediatric Health Care*, *6*(5), 235–239.

Grant, H., Murray, R., & Bergeron, J. (1994). *Brady emergency care* (6th ed.). Englewood Cliffs, New Jersey: Prentice Hall.

Grey, M., Cameron, M., Lipman, T., & Thurber. F. (1994). Initial adaptation in children with newly diagnosed diabetes and healthy children. *Pediatric Nursing*, *20*(1), 17–22.

Hathaway, E., Hay, W., Groothuis, J., & Paisley, J. (1993). *Current pediatric diagnosis and treatment* (11th ed.). Norwalk, CT: Appleton & Lange.

Jackson, D., & Saunders. R. (1993). *Child health nursing*. Philadelphia: J.B. Lippincott.

Kestel. F. (1993). Using blood glucose meters. *Nursing 93, March*, 33–41.

Martin, R., Kupis, B., Novak, P., & Kushion, W. (1994). The infant with diabetes mellitus: a case study. *Pediatric Nursing*, *20*(1), 27–34.

Memmler, R., Cohen, B., & Wood, D. (1996). *The human body* (2nd ed.). Philadelphia: J.B. Lippincott.

Nettina, S. (1996). *The Lippincott manual of nursing practice* (6th ed.). Philadelphia: Lippincott–Raven.

Rose-Savinett, B. (1994). Developmental issues in managing children with diabetes. *Pediatric Nursing*, *20*(1), 11–15.

Thomas, P. (l992). Poised for progress in diabetes. *Harvard Newsletter*, *17*(12), 3–4.

appendices

appendix a
NANDA approved nursing diagnoses—1994

Activity Intolerance

Risk for Activity Intolerance

Adjustment, Impaired

Ineffective Airway Clearance

Altered Family Process: Alcoholism

Anxiety

Risk for Aspiration

Body Image Disturbance

Risk for Altered Body Temperature

Effective Breastfeeding

Ineffective Breastfeeding

Interrupted Breastfeeding

Ineffective Breathing Pattern

Caregiver Role Strain

Risk for Caregiver Role Strain

Impaired Verbal Communication

Potential for Enhanced Community Coping

Ineffective Community Coping

Acute Confusion

Chronic Confusion

Constipation

Colonic Constipation

Perceived Constipation

Decisional Conflict (Specify)

Decreased Cardiac Output

Defensive Coping

Ineffective Denial

Diarrhea

Risk for Disuse Syndrome

Diversional Activity Deficit

Dysreflexia

Energy Field Disturbance

Impaired Environmental Interpretation Syndrome

Ineffective Family Coping: Compromised

Ineffective Family Coping: Disabling

Family Coping: Potential for Growth

Altered Family Processes

Fatigue

Fear

Fluid Volume Deficit

Risk for Fluid Volume Deficit

Fluid Volume Excess

Impaired Gas Exchange

Anticipatory Grieving

Dysfunctional Grieving

Altered Growth and Development

Altered Health Maintenance

Health-Seeking Behaviors (Specify)

Impaired Home Maintenance Management

Hopelessness

Hyperthermia

Hypothermia

Bowel Incontinence

Functional Incontinence

Reflex Incontinence

Stress Incontinence

Total Incontinence

Urge Incontinence

Ineffective Individual Coping

Ineffective Infant Feeding Pattern

Risk for Disorganized Infant Behavior

Disorganized Infant Behavior

Potential for Enhanced Organized Infant Behavior

Risk for Infection

Risk for Injury

Decreased Adaptive Capacity, Intracranial

Knowledge Deficit (Specify)

Risk for Loneliness

Impaired Memory

Noncompliance (Specify)

Altered Nutrition: Less than body requirements

Altered Nutrition: More than body requirements

Altered Nutrition: Potential for more than body requirements

Altered Oral Mucous Membrane

Pain

Chronic Pain

Parental Role Conflict

Altered Parenting

Risk for Altered Parenting

Risk for Altered Parent/Infant/Child Attachment

Personal Identity Disturbance

Risk for Peripheral Neurovascular Dysfunction

Risk for Perioperative Positioning Injury

Impaired Physical Mobility

Risk for Poisoning

Post-Trauma Response

Powerlessness

Altered Protection

Rape-Trauma Syndrome

Rape-Trauma Syndrome: Compound Reaction

Rape-Trauma Syndrome: Silent Reaction

Relocation Stress Syndrome

Altered Role Performance

Bathing/Hygiene Self-Care Deficit

Feeding Self-Care Deficit

Dressing/Grooming Self-Care Deficit

Toileting Self-Care Deficit

Chronic Low Self-Esteem

Situational Low Self-Esteem

Self-Esteem Disturbance

Risk for Self-Mutilation

Sensory/Perceptual Alterations (Specify) (Visual, auditory, kinesthetic, gustatory, tactile, olfactory)

Sexual Dysfunction

Altered Sexuality Patterns

Impaired Skin Integrity

Risk for Impaired Skin Integrity

Sleep Pattern Disturbance

Impaired Social Interaction

Social Isolation

Spiritual Distress (distress of the human spirit)

Potential for Enhanced Spiritual Well Being

Risk for Suffocation

Impaired Swallowing

Ineffective Management of Therapeutic Regimen: Families

Ineffective Management of Therapeutic Regimen: Community

Ineffective Management of Therapeutic Regimen: Individual

Ineffective Thermoregulation

Altered Thought Processes

Impaired Tissue Integrity

Altered Tissue Perfusion (Specify Type) (Renal, cerebral, cardiopulmonary, gastrointestinal, peripheral)

Risk for Trauma

Unilateral Neglect

Altered Urinary Elimination

Urinary Retention

Inability to Sustain Spontaneous Ventilation

Dysfunctional Ventilatory Weaning Response

Risk for Violence: Self-directed or directed at others

(Nursing Diagnoses: Definitions & Classification 1995–1996, Philadelphia: North American Nursing Diagnoses Association, 1994)

appendix b
conversion tables

temperature conversion table (centigrade to fahrenheit)

Celsius (C°)	*Fahrenheit (F°)*	*Celsius (C°)*	*Fahrenheit (F°)*
34.0	93.2	38.6	101.4
34.2	93.6	38.8	101.8
34.4	93.9	39.0	102.2
34.6	94.3	39.2	102.5
34.8	94.6	39.4	102.9
35.0	95.0	39.6	103.2
35.2	95.4	39.8	103.6
35.4	95.7	40.0	104.0
35.6	96.1	40.2	104.3
35.8	96.4	40.4	104.7
36.0	96.8	40.6	105.1
36.2	97.1	40.8	105.4
36.4	97.5	41.0	105.8
36.6	97.8	41.2	106.1
36.8	98.2	41.4	106.5
37.0	98.6	41.6	106.8
37.2	98.9	41.8	107.2
37.4	99.3	42.0	107.6
37.6	99.6	42.2	108.0
37.8	100.0	42.4	108.3
38.0	100.4	42.6	108.7
38.2	100.7	42.8	109.0
38.4	101.0	43.0	109.4

Conversion of Celsius (Centigrade) to Fahrenheit: 9/5 × temperature) + 32
Conversion of Fahrenheit to Celsius (Centigrade): (Temperature − 32) × 5/9
(Used with permission from May, K.A. & Mahlmeister, L.R. (1994). *Maternal and neonatal nursing* (3rd ed.). (Philadelphia: J.B. Lippincott.)

pounds and ounces to grams conversion table

Pounds	Ounces 0	1	2	3	4	5	6	7	8	9	10	11	12	13	14	15
0	—	28	57	85	113	142	170	198	227	255	283	312	340	369	397	425
1	454	482	510	539	567	595	624	652	680	709	737	765	794	822	850	879
2	907	936	964	992	1021	1049	1077	1106	1134	1162	1191	1219	1247	1276	1304	1332
3	1361	1389	1417	1446	1474	1503	1531	1559	1588	1616	1644	1673	1701	1729	1758	1786
4	1814	1843	1871	1899	1928	1956	1984	2013	2041	2070	2098	2126	2155	2183	2211	2240
5	2268	2296	2325	2353	2381	2410	2438	2466	2495	2523	2551	2580	2608	2637	2665	2693
6	2722	2750	2778	2807	2835	2863	2892	2920	2948	2977	3005	3033	3062	3090	3118	3147
7	3175	3203	3232	3260	3289	3317	3345	3374	3402	3430	3459	3487	3515	3544	3572	3600
8	3629	3657	3685	3714	3742	3770	3799	3827	3856	3884	3912	3941	3969	3997	4026	4054
9	4082	4111	4139	4167	4196	4224	4252	4281	4309	4337	4366	4394	4423	4451	4479	4508
10	4536	4564	4593	4621	4649	4678	4706	4734	4763	4791	4819	4848	4876	4904	4933	4961
11	4990	5018	5046	5075	5103	5131	5160	5188	5216	5245	5273	5301	5330	5358	5386	5415
12	5443	5471	5500	5528	5557	5585	5613	5642	5670	5698	5727	5755	5783	5812	5840	5868
13	5897	5925	5953	5982	6010	6038	6067	6095	6123	6152	6180	6209	6237	6265	6294	6322
14	6350	6379	6407	6435	6464	6492	6520	6549	6577	6605	6634	6662	6690	6719	6747	6776
15	6804	6832	6860	6889	6917	6945	6973	7002	7030	7059	7087	7115	7144	7172	7201	7228
16	7257	7286	7313	7342	7371	7399	7427	7456	7484	7512	7541	7569	7597	7226	7654	7682
17	7711	7739	7768	7796	7824	7853	7881	7909	7938	7966	7994	8023	8051	8079	8108	8136
18	8165	8192	8221	8249	8278	8306	8335	8363	8391	8420	8448	8476	8504	8533	8561	8590
19	8618	8646	8675	8703	8731	8760	8788	8816	8845	8873	8902	8930	8958	8987	9015	9043
20	9072	9100	9128	9157	9185	9213	9242	9270	9298	9327	9355	9383	9412	9440	9469	9497
21	9525	9554	9582	9610	9639	9667	9695	9724	9752	9780	9809	9837	9865	9894	9922	9950
22	9979	10007	10036	10064	10092	10120	10149	10177	10206	10234	10262	10291	10319	10347	10376	10404

(Used with permission from May, K.A. & Mahlmeister, L.R. (1994). *Maternal and neonatal nursing* (3rd ed.). (Philadelphia: J.B. Lippincott.)

appendix c
cervical dilatation

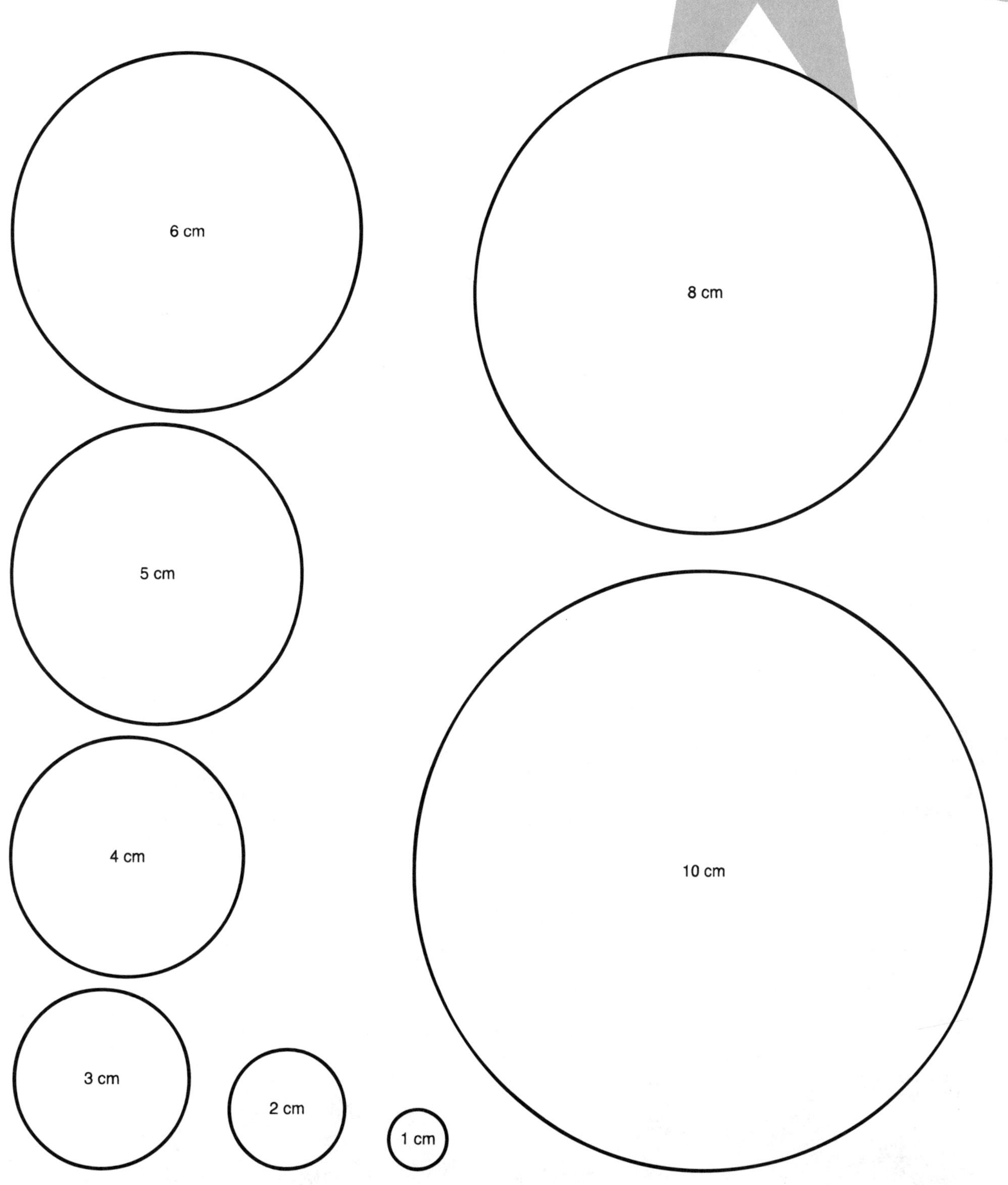

appendix d
recommended dietary allowances (RDAs)

food and nutrition board, national academy of sciences—national research council recommended dietary allowances, revised 1989*

Category	Age (yr) or Condition	Weight† (kg)	Weight† (lb)	Height† (cm)	Height† (in)	Protein (g)	Fat-Soluble Vitamins: Vitamin A (μgRE)‡	Fat-Soluble Vitamins: Vitamin D (μg)§	Fat-Soluble Vitamins: Vitamin E (mg α-TE)
Infants	0.0–0.5	6	13	60	24	13	375	7.5	3
	0.5–1.0	9	20	71	28	14	375	10	4
Children	1–3	13	29	90	35	16	400	10	6
	4–6	20	44	112	44	24	500	10	7
	7–10	28	62	132	52	28	700	10	7
Male	11–14	45	99	157	62	45	1000	10	10
	15–18	66	145	176	69	59	1000	10	10
	19–24	72	160	177	70	58	1000	10	10
Females	11–14	46	101	157	62	46	800	10	8
	15–18	55	120	163	64	44	800	10	8
	19–24	58	128	164	65	46	800	10	8
Pregnant						60	800	10	10
Lactating									
1st 6 months						65	1300	10	12
2nd 6 months						62	1200	10	11

* The allowances, expressed as average daily intakes over time, are intended to provide for individual variations among most normal persons as they live in the United States environmental stresses. Diets should be based on a variety of common foods to provide other nutrients for which human requirements have been less well defined.
† The use of these figures does not imply that the height-to-weight ratios are ideal.
‡ Retinol equivalents. 1 retinol equivalent = 1 μg retinol or 6 μg β-carotene.
§ As cholecalciferol. 10 μg cholecalciferol = 400 IU of vitamin D.
|| α-Tocopherol equivalents. 1 mg d-α tocopherol = 1 α-TE.
¶ NE (niacin equivalent) is equal to 1 mg of niacin or 60 mg of dietary tryptophan.
Adopted from Recommended Dietary Allowances, 10th edition, © 1989 by the National Academy of Sciences. Published by National Academy Press, Washington, DC.

Water-Soluble Vitamins							Minerals						
Vitamin C (mg)	Thiamin (mg)	Riboflavin (mg)	Niacin (mg NE)¶	Vitamin B (mg)	Folate (μg)	Vitamin B_{12} (μg)	Calcium (mg)	Phosphorus (mg)	Magnesium (mg)	Iron (mg)	Zinc (mg)	Iodine (μg)	Selenium (μg)
30	0.3	0.4	5	0.3	25	0.3	400	300	40	6	5	40	10
35	0.4	0.5	6	0.6	35	0.5	600	500	60	10	5	50	15
40	0.7	0.8	9	1.0	50	0.7	800	800	80	10	10	70	20
45	0.9	1.1	12	1.1	75	1.0	800	800	120	10	10	90	20
45	1.0	1.2	13	1.4	100	1.4	800	800	170	10	10	120	30
50	1.3	1.5	17	1.7	150	2.0	1200	1200	270	12	15	150	40
60	1.5	1.8	20	2.0	200	2.0	1200	1200	400	12	15	150	50
60	1.5	1.7	19	2.0	200	2.0	1200	1200	350	10	15	150	70
50	1.1	1.3	15	1.4	150	2.0	1200	1200	280	15	12	150	45
60	1.1	1.3	15	1.5	180	2.0	1200	1200	300	15	12	150	50
60	1.1	1.3	15	1.6	180	2.0	1200	1200	280	15	12	150	55
70	1.5	1.6	17	2.2	400	2.2	1200	1200	300	30	15	175	65
95	1.6	1.8	20	2.1	280	2.6	1200	1200	355	15	19	200	75
90	1.6	1.7	20	2.1	260	2.6	1200	1200	340	15	16	200	75

appendix e
excretion of drugs in breast milk

drugs that appear to pose little or no risk when used during lactation

Some Drugs Excreted in Human Milk but Without Apparent Clinical Significance		*Some Drugs Not Excreted in Human Milk*
Acetaminophen	Meperidine	Amitriptyline
Ampicillin	Mesoridazine	Cephalosporins, first and second generation
Antihistamines	Morphine	Chloroquine
β_2-Agonists	Nitrofurantoin	Desipramine
Caffeine	Novobiocin	Dextroamphetamine
Codeine	Propranolol	Heparin
Colchicine	Propantheline	Imipramine
Digoxin	Quinidine	Oxacillin
Diphenhydramine	Quinine	Pentazocine
Guanethidine	Scopolamine	Phenylbutazone
Hydroxyphenbutazone	Thyroid hormones	
Insulin	Tolmetin	
Lidocaine	Tranylcypromine	
Mefanimic acid		

(Swonger, A. K., & Matejski, M. P. [1991]. *Nursing pharmacology: An integrated approach to drug therapy and nursing practice* [2nd ed.] Philadelphia: J.B. Lippincott.).

drugs requiring close observation of infant when administered to nursing mothers

Drug	*Comment*
Alcohol	OK in small amounts; large amounts depress infant and inhibit lactation
Antimicrobials	
Cephalosporins, 3rd generation	Possible enterocolitis
Erythromycin	Concentrated in milk. Possible jaundice.
Isoniazid	Concentration is the same in milk as in serum; monitor child for possible toxicity
Kanamycin	Monitor child for toxicity
Nalidixic acid	Possible hemolytic anemia
Penicillin G or V	Possible hypersensitivity reactions
Barbiturates	Induce liver enzymes in infant
Benzodiazepines	Possible drowsiness
Carbamazepine	Possible tiredness, vomiting, or poor sucking
Chloral hydrate	Possible sedation in infant
Decongestants	May decrease milk volume
Diuretics (thiazides, spironolactone)	Avoid use during lactation; they decrease milk production and appear in milk
Glucocorticoids	Growth suppression; suppression of infant's production of glucocorticoids; retarded sexual development
Indomethacin	Convulsions reported in one breast-fed infant
Lithium	Monitor child for lithium toxicity
Meprobamate	Concentrated in milk 2 to 4× plasma level; monitor child for depressive effects
Methyldopa	Possible depression of respirations, blood pressure, and alertness
Minoxidil	Monitor for hypertrichosis
Neuroleptics	May cause galactorrhea in mother; not present in significant amounts in milk
Nicotine	Nicotine effects in infant occur if rate is greater than 20 cigarettes per day
Oral contraceptives	Gynecomastia in male infants
Phenytoin	One case of methemoglobinemia reported; induces liver enzymes
Primidone	Somnolence or drowsiness may occur in infant
Reserpine	Nasal stuffiness and lethargy in infant; galactorrhea in mother
Salicylates	Cause bleeding tendency; mother should take after feedings, not before. Possible skin rash
Vitamin D	Possible hypercalcemia in infant

(Swonger, A. K., & Matejski, M. P. [1991]. *Nursing pharmacology: An integrated approach to drug therapy and nursing practice* [2nd ed.]. Philadelphia: J.B. Lippincott.)

drugs contraindicated in nursing mothers

Drug	*Comment*
Antimicrobials (some)	
Amantadine	Possible vomiting, urinary retention, skin rash
Chloramphenicol	Infant's capacity to metabolize this drug is underdeveloped
Metronidazole	Avoid breastfeeding for 3 days after a single dose
Sulfonamides	Possible allergic skin reactions, jaundice, or hemolysis in G6PD-deficient infants
Streptomycin	Accumulates in liver of infant
Tetracyclines	Possible discoloration of teeth of infant
Antineoplastics	Nursing should be discontinued
Antithyroid drugs	May cause goiter or myxedema
Atropine	May cause atropine intoxication
Bromides	Cause rash and drowsiness
Cathartics	Diarrhea in infant
Cimetidine	Induces liver enzymes, suppresses gastric secretions, and stimulates the central nervous system in the infant
Ergot alkaloids	Vomiting, diarrhea, weak pulse, unstable blood pressure in the infant
Heavy metals	Mercury and lead poisoning can occur in infants if mother's milk is contaminated
Iodides	May cause thyroid impairment in infant
Narcotics	May cause addiction in infant
Oral anticoagulants (especially phenindione)	Cause hypocoagulation in the infant
Oral hypoglycemics	Tolbutamide achieves high concentration in milk; possible adverse effect on pancreas of infant
Radioactive drugs	Contraindicated in nursing mothers

(Swonger, A. K., & Matejski, M. P. [1991]. *Nursing pharmacology: An integrated approach to drug therapy and nursing practice* [2nd ed.]. Philadelphia: J.B. Lippincott.)

appendix f
pulse, respiration, and blood pressure values for children

normal pulse ranges in children

Age	Normal Range	Average
0–24 h	70–170 beats/min	120 beats/min
1–7 d	100–180 beats/min	140 beats/min
1 mo	110–188 beats/min	160 beats/min
1 mo–1 y	80–180 beats/min	120–130 beats/min
2 y	80–140 beats/min	110 beats/min
4 y	80–120 beats/min	100 beats/min
6 y	70–115 beats/min	100 beats/min
10 y	70–110 beats/min	90 beats/min
12–14 y	60–110 beats/min	85–90 beats/min
14–18 y	50–95 beats/min	70–75 beats/min

From Skale, N. (1992). *Manual of pediatric nursing procedures* (p. 35). Philadelphia: J.B. Lippincott.

normal blood pressure ranges

Age	Systolic (mm Hg)	Diastolic (mm Hg)
Newborn—12 hr (Less than 1000 g)	39–59	16–36
Newborn—12 hr (3000 g)	50–70	24–45
Newborn—96 hr (3000 g)	60–90	20–60
Infant	74–100	50–70
Toddler	80–112	50–80
Preschooler	82–110	50–78
School-age	84–120	54–80
Adolescent	94–140	62–88

From Skale, N. (1992). *Manual of pediatric nursing procedures* (p. 46). Philadelphia: J.B. Lippincott.

variations in respirations with age

Age	Rate per Minute
Newborn	40–90
1 y	20–40
2 y	20–30
3 y	20–30
5 y	20–25
10 y	17–22
15 y	15–20
20 y	15–20

Lowrey, G. H. (1973) *Growth and development of children* (6th ed). Chicago: Year Book Medical Publishers. Used by permission.

appendix g
growth charts

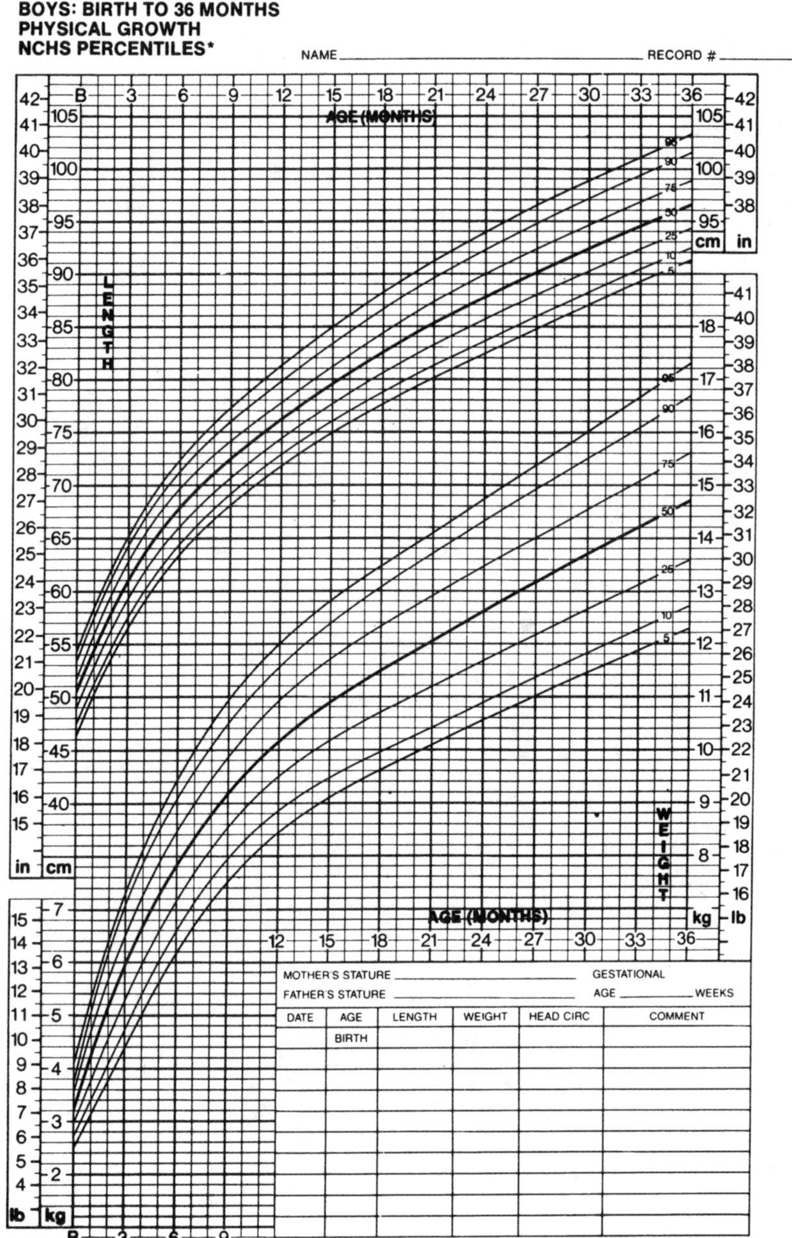

Source: *Adapted from Hamill, P. V. V., et al. (1979). Physical growth: National Center for Health Statistics percentiles.* American Journal of Clinical Nutrition, 32, 607. *Data from the Fels Research Institute, Wright State University School of Medicine, Yellow Springs, OH. Courtesy of Ross Laboratories.*

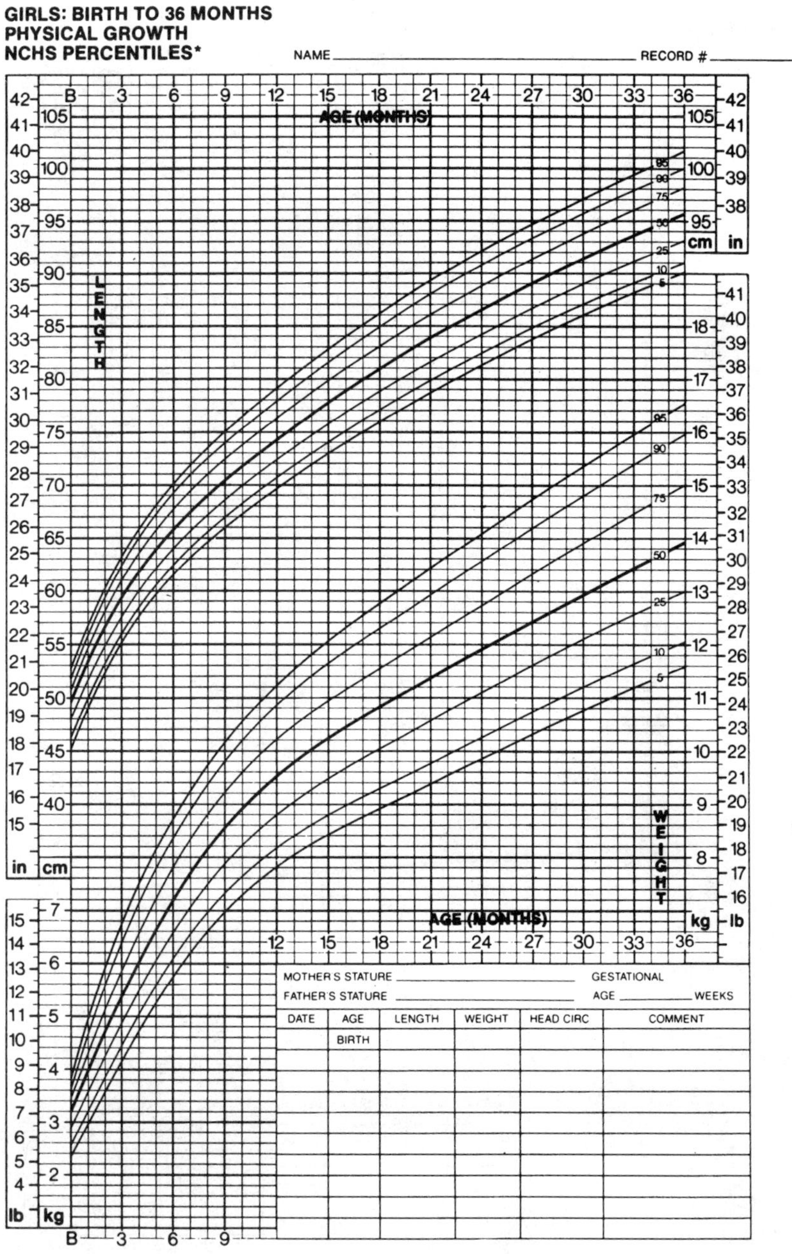

Source: *Adapted from Hamill, P. V. V., et al. (1979). Physical growth: National Center for Health Statistics percentiles.* American Journal of Clinical Nutrition, 32, 607. *Data from the Fels Research Institute, Wright State University School of Medicine, Yellow Springs, OH. Courtesy of Ross Laboratories.*

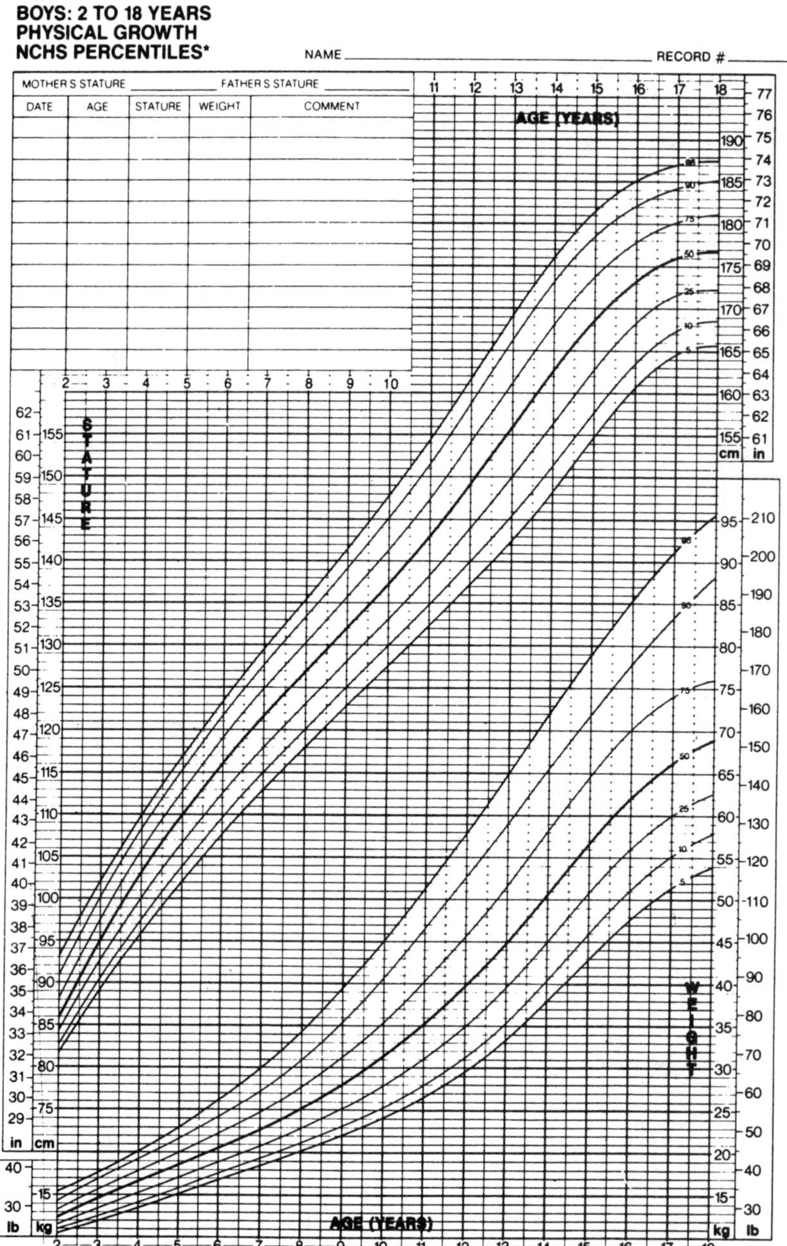

Source: *Adapted from Hamill, P. V. V., et al. (1979). Physical growth: National Center for Health Statistics percentiles.* American Journal of Clinical Nutrition, 32, 607. *Data from the Fels Research Institute, Wright State University School of Medicine, Yellow Springs, OH. Courtesy of Ross Laboratories.*

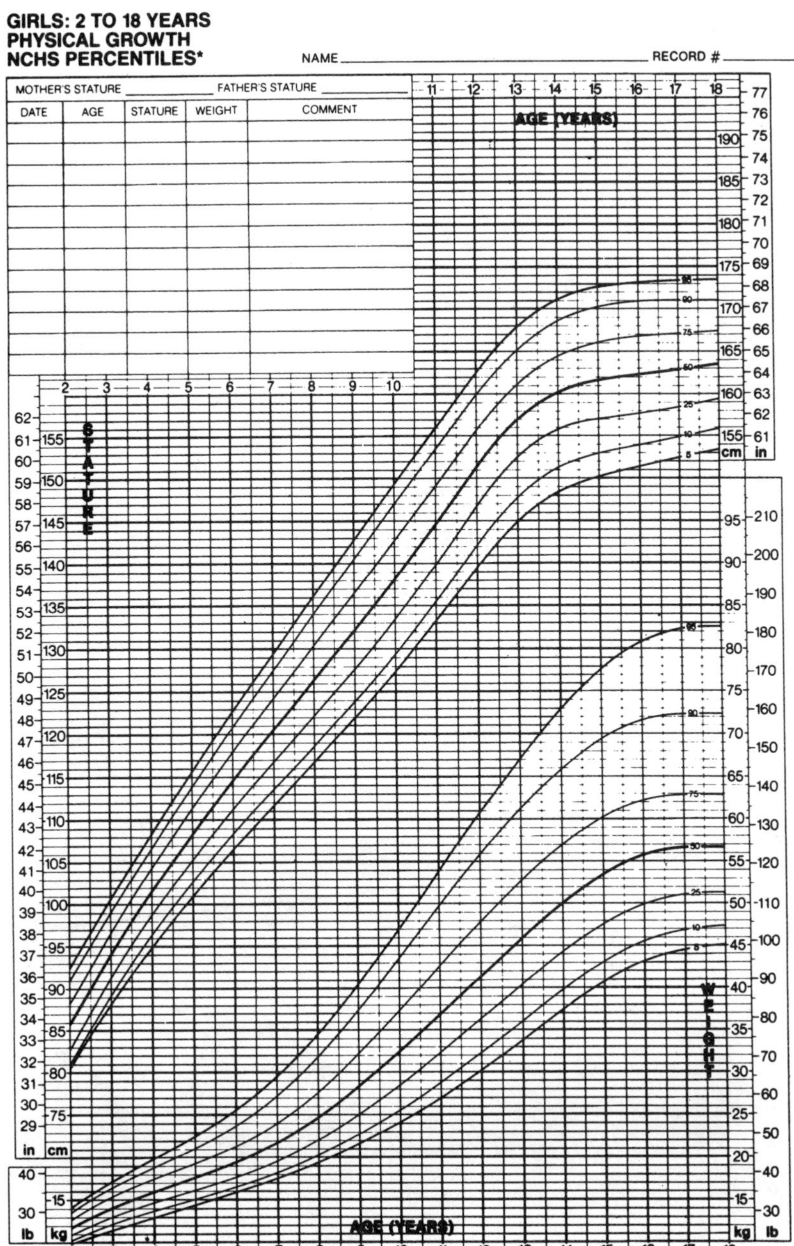

Source: *Adapted from Hamill, P. V. V., et al. (1979). Physical growth: National Center for Health Statistics percentiles.* American Journal of Clinical Nutrition, 32, 607. *Data from the Fels Research Institute, Wright State University School of Medicine, Yellow Springs, OH. Courtesy of Ross Laboratories.*

appendix h
teaching considerations for maternal-newborn care

✳ complications of pregnancy

symptoms to report

vaginal bleeding
May indicate threatened abortion, ectopic pregnancy in first pregnancy in first trimester, placenta previa or abruptio placentae in second or third trimester.

leakage of fluid from vagina
May indicate premature rupture of membranes.

dizziness or pelvic uterine pain
May indicate ectopic pregnancy (especially with shoulder pain), or abruptio placentae.

uterine/pelvic cramping or low backache
May indicate preterm labor, especially when associated with rhythmic tightening of uterus or leakage of fluid from vagina.

epigastric pain
May indicate severe preeclampsia, especially if associated with headache or visual disturbances.

decrease or absence of fetal movement
May indicate fetal distress or death, or be the effects of maternal medication.

decrease in or difficulty in urination
May indicate oliguria associated with pregnancy-induced hypertension or dysuria associated with urinary tract infection.

persistent vomiting
May indicate hyperemesis gravidarum or infection.

✳ early postpartum care

The lining of the uterus is a perfect site for infection to occur following delivery. Meticulous hygienic care is imperative.

bathing

Daily baths or showers should be taken and perineal area washed with soap and water and patted dry.

perineal pads

Pads should be applied from front to back, being careful not to touch the side of the pad that covers the perineum. Pads should be changed with each voiding, defecation, or when soiled with lochia. Lochia is usually a moderate flow with small clots (6–8 pads used daily on average). If clots larger than a quarter are passed, they should be saved and the health care provider notified. Any foul odor to lochia should be reported to the health care provider.

lochia changes

Lochia rubra lasts 1–3 days and looks and smells like menstrual blood. Lochia serosa is light pink to brownish color and last 2–3 days. Lochia alba is a whitish discharge, which may last for several weeks.

episiotomy care

Peri-bottle spray should be used with each voiding or defecation, patting perineum dry with toilet paper or disposable wash cloth.

episiotomy discomfort

Apply ice packs to perineum for first 24 h to decrease swelling. Use Sitz bath or whirlpool tube for 20 min, 3–4 time daily. Heat lamp placed 12–18 inches from perineum for 20 min, 2–3 times daily. Keep perineum clean and free of lochia. Perineal analgesic spray may be used.

hemorrhoidal discomfort

Increase fluid and fiber intake to ease defecation. Use of Sitz bath (as above) or topical hemorrhoidal preparation as ordered.

bladder distention

Encourage early and frequent voidings, increased fluid intake. Painful urination and ability to urinate only small amounts should be reported to health care provider.

postpartum uterine cramping

Walking, lying on abdomen, requesting medication should be encouraged.

nipple soreness or cracking

Air dry nipples, and avoid use of soap on nipples. Change wet breast pads frequently. Break suction with finger in infant's mouth when removing infant from breast. Consider use of breast shields as necessary.

✳ postpartum complications

symptoms to report

infection
Temperature of 100.4°F(38°C) for 2 consecutive days may indicate uterine infection.

lochia changes
When lochia changes from alba to serosa or rubra or has foul odor, uterus may be relaxed or infection present.

uterine tenderness
Indicative of uterine infection.

breast engorgement
If breastfeeding, encourage feeding on demand, warm showers, and breast massage. Warm moist heat before nursing will facilitate emptying of breasts. If not breastfeeding, apply ice packs PRN, wear tight bra or binder for 24 h and avoid breast stimulation. Take analgesics as needed.

sore nipples
Air dry breasts. Start feeding on least affected side. Change nursing position and encourage infant to suckle from a different angle for each feeding. Massage each breast before breastfeeding to promote ease in let-down of milk once infant begins to suckle.

mastitis
If tenderness, redness, and warmth are noted in breasts, and general malaise with fever is present, woman should notify health care provider. Antibiotic therapy may be needed. Woman should continue to breastfeed, starting on unaffected breast first.

continued tenderness of episiotomy
May be indicative of infection, especially if swelling, redness, or discharge at episiotomy site is noted.

swelling, tenderness, or warmth in leg
May be indicative of deep vein thrombosis or thrombophlebitis. Woman should elevate leg, avoid massage of affected area, and contact health care provider immediately.

urinary tract infection
Burning on urination, frequency, fever, malaise, chills, and flank pain are indicative of urinary tract infection. Woman should contact health care provider immediately.

✳ signs of newborn illness

symptoms to report

significant signs and symptoms of illness

* Lethargy—Listless behavior or difficulty rousing newborn
* Loss of appetite—Refusal of two feedings in a row
* Fever—Axillary temperature above 100°F (37.3°C) or below 97°F (36.1°C), or rectal temperature above 101°F (38.3°C) or below 98°F (36.6°C)
* Vomiting—Spitting up large amount of feeding two or more times
* Diarrhea—Three or more green, liquid stools in succession
* Fewer than 6 wet diapers a day

procedure for taking axillary and rectal temperature

* Shake thermometer down (away from neonate or crib in case thermometer is accidentally broken) until mercury falls below 95°F.
* Place neonate on back.
* For rectal temperature, lubricate thermometer; hold neonate's legs with one hand and insert thermometer 1/2 inch into anus with other hand. (Rectal temperature is not recommended during the first 3 months of life because of risk of perforating rectal mucosa.
* For axillary temperature, place in fold of axilla.
* Hold thermometer firmly in place for 5 min.
* *Never* leave neonate unattended while taking temperature.

avoiding newborn illness

To cut down on possibility of infections, wash hands frequently, especially after changing diaper. Limit number of people who handle neonate. Avoid contact with anyone who is ill. Avoid taking neonate into large crowds.

✳ newborn safety factors

importance

Accidents are the leading cause of death in children from age 1 mo until adolescence. Accident prevention should be discussed in detail with parents.

infant car seat

All states have mandated child restraint laws. Parents should be instructed to purchase a car seat, and use it *every time* infant is in the car. Car seats should be placed on the back seat and turned toward the rear of the car with the seat belt attached to the car seat. Used car seats should be carefully inspected to ensure the restraint device works properly.

poisoning

Second leading cause of death in older infants and children. Teach parents to "childproof" their home. Electrical outlets should have covers. Cleaning solutions, medications, and toxic substances should be in locked cabinets or cabinets where doors cannot be opened by infants or children. Household plants may be poisonous. Poison control center and ER numbers should be posted near telephone. Keep ipecac in household medicine cabinet for use as directed by poison control or ER professionals.

falls

Infants should never be left alone on an unguarded surface. Belts and straps on infant seats and strollers should always be fastened.

choking and aspiration

Infants should never be left with bottles propped. All objects small enough to fit in infant's mouth should be kept out of reach. Avoid toys with sharp edges, buttons, or small pieces that could come off and be swallowed or aspirated.

sleep hazards

Do not use pillows in infant's crib; may cause suffocation. Slats of bed should be appropriately distanced and painted with nonlead paint. Parents who choose to have infant sleep with parents should be encouraged to put infant in a soft crib or basket to avoid parent rolling over on infant and causing suffocation. Infant should be positioned on side, using rolled diaper at infant's back; should not be positioned on abdomen or back to sleep.

May, K. A. & Mahlmeister, L. R. (1994). *Maternal and neonatal nursing* (3rd ed.). Philadelphia: J.B. Lippincott.

glossary

Glossary

abdominal girth measurement of the abdominal circumference, a waist measurement

abduction lateral movement away from the midline of the body

abortion the termination of pregnancy before fetal viability

abruptio placentae early detachment of the placenta after 20 weeks gestation

absorption the taking in of a substance into the body through a membrane surface

acculturation embracing another culture to be accepted into that culture

acme the time of greatest intensity

acrocyanosis bluish coloration of the hands and feet that can occur in a normal newborn

acupuncture pain treatment from the Far East that uses thin needles inserted through the skin at certain points, producing regional anesthesia

acute illness any illness that is of short duration and impairs normal functioning

adduction lateral movement toward the midline of the body

adolescence a period of development between the onset of puberty and adulthood in which the individual goes through tremendous changes physically, mentally, socially, and spiritually.

adoptive family a family who assumes the responsibility of rearing another child who is not of the same blood relation

aggression forceful behavior, which can be demonstrated in verbal, nonverbal, or symbolic activity

Alateen an international organization for children of alcoholics, which provides support, counseling, and guidance.

albumins one group of proteins widely found in body tissues

alopecia loss or absence of hair

amblyopia dimming of vision in one or both eyes without any pathology to the eye; lazy eye

amniocentesis aspiration of amniotic fluid via a transabdominal puncture for chemical and cytology studies

amnion the inner fetal membranous sac that holds the fluid and baby in the first trimester

amniotomy artificial rupture of the amniotic sac to accelerate labor

amphiarthrosis cartilaginous joint having slight movement in all directions; for example, vertebrae

analgesia decreased or absent sense of pain

anaphylactic shock sudden, severe, and sometimes fatal systemic hypersensitivity (allergic) reaction to a substance

androgen any steroid hormone that increases male characteristics in the body

anesthesia surgical analgesia; loss of sensation with or without loss of consciousness

angioedema acute painless swelling of the face, neck, lips, hands, feet, genitalia, or viscera seen in allergic reaction, infection, or emotional stress; if severe, can cause respiratory obstruction; also called angioneurotic edema

anorexia nervosa an eating disorder characterized by a fear of obesity and starvation results; most often seen in adolescent girls

anovulation ovaries fail to produce, mature, or release eggs

antagonist any drug or muscle that exerts an opposite effect

antibodies an immunoglobulin produced by lymphocytes that are specific to an antigen

anticholinergic of or pertaining to blocking acetylcholine receptors that results in blocking or parasympathetic nerve impulses

antigen substance (usually a protein) found on the cell surface, which triggers formation of antibodies

anuria absence of urine produced

apnea absence of external breathing

apocrine glands sweat glands located in the axillary, anal, genital, and mammary areas that become functional after puberty and having a characteristic odor

appendicitis inflammation of the vermiform appendix, usually caused by an obstruction in the lumen of the appendix; pain is usually felt in the right lower quadrant, accompanied with low-grade fever and vomiting; occurs more often in teenagers and young adults and more often in males than females

ascites abnormal accumulation of fluid in the abdominal cavity containing a large amount of proteins and electrolytes

asphyxia suffocation due to lack of breathable oxygen in the environment, with no airway obstruction

aspiration anything other than air going into the bronchial tree; can cause bronchospasm and pneumonia

assessment evaluation or appraisal of a condition or data

atelectasis abnormal condition causing part of the lung tissue to collapse, preventing air exchange

atrophy wasting away of tissues in the body

attention deficit disorder a disease of infancy and childhood demonstrating inappropriate inattention, impulse activity, and hyperactivity. Symptoms noted in school are an inability to keep to task; difficulty in organizing; and sloppy, hurried school work filled with omissions, insertions, or misinterpreted easy items. Hyperactive component may or may not be present. Also called hyperactive child syndrome or minimal brain dysfunction

attitude body posturing behavior demonstrating conscious or unconscious feelings developed from life's experiences

aura a subjective sensation occurring before a sudden attack; usually affecting the person's sensorium or psyche

autonomy state of self direction or self-governing behavior

autosome any of the chromosomes except the X and Y sex chromosomes

azotemia increased nitrogenous compounds in the blood, especially urea

barium enema a fluoroscopic and x-ray exam of the colon using radio-opaque barium sulfate as an enema; also called lower GI series

basophil a type of WBC that carries granules of anticoagulants into an area of inflammation during the healing phase or chronic inflammation; it stains readily for identification

behavior modification a conscious use of reinforcement to change behavior

biotransformation the amount of the active drug absorbed, distributed, and chemically changed in the body

birth rate the number of live births per 1000 in a year

birth trauma Otto Rank's term to describe the source of any anxiety in a person that comes from the birth process

birthing room a hospital labor room that can be transformed into a delivery room without moving the mother

blended family divorced people remarrying and forming a new family unit; stepfamilies

bottle caries tooth decay in an infant caused by having prolonged feedings; for example, sleeping with a bottle of formula in the mouth

brachial plexus a network of cervical nerves passing under the clavicle and into the axilla

Braxton Hicks contractions irregular tightening of the uterus during pregnancy, which increases in frequency, duration, and intensity as pregnancy progresses

brittle diabetic a type of childhood diabetes demonstrating a varying insulin response and tendency to develop ketosis

bruit an adventitious venous or arterial sound with auscultation

bulb syringe a type of syringe used for gentle suction or irrigation; it has a rubber squeezable bulb on one end and a nozzle tip on the other and can hold 60 to 90 cc of fluid

bulimia an eating disorder, characterized by periods of binge followed by purging the digestive system with laxatives, enemas, and fasting. Psychologic counseling recommended.

Candida albicans yeastlike fungus that is part of the normal flora of the mouth, skin, intestinal tract, and vagina; can cause yeast infections when allowed to flourish; also called Monilia

caput suddedaneum swelling in the presenting part of the head during labor; subsides in 2 to 3 days

cardinal movements in labor, typical sequence of positions of the fetus descending through the pelvis; engagement, flexion, descent, internal rotation, extension, and external rotation

cardiomegaly abnormal enlargement of the heart

caries tooth decay; cavities

carotenemia a benign yellowing of the skin from too much carotene in the body; sclera do not have the yellow color

case management assignment of a health care provider to assist the patient in obtaining health and social services needed

catch-up growth accelerated growth occurring after a period of growth retardation until normal growth pattern is established

caustic that which is irritated or eaten away by chemicals

centration a tendency to remain in or at the center

cephalocaudal pertaining to the long axis of the body

cephalhematoma swelling on the head caused by subcutaneous bleeding brought on by trauma during labor or forceps

cephalopelvic disproportion (CPD) a condition in which either the baby's head is too large or the mother's pelvis too small to allow normal delivery

cervical ripening the softening and effacing of the cervix that occurs late in the ninth month of pregnancy

Chadwick's sign early sign of pregnancy; a violet coloration of the vulva and vagina

chalasia relaxation of the cardiac sphincter of the stomach allowing gastric reflux to occur

chemical barrier method use of spermicides for birth control

childhood mortality death rate of children over 1 year old

chloasma hyperpigmentation of the face seen during pregnancy or use of oral contraceptives; mask of pregnancy

chorea a condition characterized by involuntary twitching, grimacing, or shoulder shrugging; may also have emotional discord and muscle weakness with the involuntary movements

chorion the outermost extraembryonic membrane that develops as the placenta, and the membrane containing amniotic fluid

chorionic villi tiny vascular extensions of the chorion that implant the placenta into the endometrial wall of the uterus

chromosome all the genes of an organism contained in the nucleus of the cell

chronic illness disease of lingering symptomology but usually not severe; may have relapses of acute phases

closed adoption adoption papers are sealed so biologic information is not revealed

clostridium botulism anaerobic bacteria that produce a powerful toxin if allowed to grow in food

cohabitation family unmarried couple provide the support and nurturing commitment as a nuclear family

coitus sexual intercourse

colic spasm in any hollow organ causing pain; infantile colic occurs in the first few months after birth

collagen protein bundles of inelastic fibrils found in the tendons, ligaments, and fascia

colloid a type of solution that is thick enough to keep disperse particles suspended; jellylike substance found in thyroid follicles

colonoscopy visual examination of the upper rectum using a speculum or flexible scope

comedo comedones (pl), blackhead; lesion of acne vulgaris

commissurotomy a surgical division of a fibrous band connecting parts of a body structure; commonly performed to separate a sclerosed mitral valve

communal family unrelated persons living together to provide a family situation

compensated heart failure treatment regimen designed to relieve symptoms of heart failure and improve heart function

complete breech abnormal birth presentation when legs are flexed on the thighs and thighs are flexed on the abdomen, allowing the buttocks and feet to present first

concussion sudden violent jarring or shaking of soft tissues caused by trauma or explosion such as a brain concussion

conditioning in psychology, to subject a person to a stimulus so that a specific response will always occur

congenital malformation defect present at birth

conservation a stage in concrete operations when the concept that liquids and solids can be transformed in shape but not change in amount

contracture abnormal permanent condition of flexion and fixation of a joint that occurs from muscular atrophy or loss of elasticity from scarring

contraception the technique of preventing pregnancy

contusion trauma to the skin that causes swelling, discoloration and pain but does not break the skin; bruise or ecchymosis

convalescent pertaining to the recovery phase of an illness or injury

copulation the sexual union of two people of the opposite sex

cor pulmonale pulmonary hypertension causing right ventricular enlargement; some diseases that contribute to this condition are cystic fibrosis, pulmonary arteritis, and myasthenia gravis

counselor a support person who uses therapeutic technique to facilitate improved communication among a family or group

couvade a custom whereby the husband goes through mock labor while his wife is giving birth

cradle cap seborrheic dermatitis of an infant's head

craniostosis congenital deformity from premature closure of the sutures between the cranial bones; impaired brain growth may or may not occur depending on the extent of sutures involved

creatinine a waste product produced by the body that is an indicator of kidney function

crepitus abnormal subcutaneous air trapping from air leakage of the lung; crackly like Rice Krispies when palpated; subcutaneous emphysema

crowning term used to describe visualization of the fetus's head during delivery

cultural diversity many cultural backgrounds represented in a society

cultural bias a prejudiced outlook toward another's culture

culture set of beliefs and customs shared by a group of individuals

cyanosis bluish coloration of the skin, indicating lack of oxygen

debridement removal of dead tissue and debris from a wound

decenter the ability to focus on views other than your own

decidua epithelial layer of the endometrium lining the uterus

decompensated heart failure not complete response to treatment regiment for heart failure, residual failure prevalent

decrement decrease or decline

delusion a persistent aberrant belief held by a person even after it is proven to the contrary

dentition teething; growth of teeth

dermis true layer of skin located between the epidermis and subcutaneous layer

developmental sequence the order of change in growth and development of an organism

deviant behavior actions that involve failure to comply with usual limits of normal behavior

diagonal conjugate radiographic measurement between the inferior border of the symphysis pubic to the sacral promontory; measurement averages 12.5 cm

dialysate the solution used in dialysis

dialysis medical procedures using diffusion to remove toxins from the body

diaphoresis sweating

diarthrosis synovial joint

digestion the mechanical and chemical breakdown of food in the gastrointestinal tract to absorbable substances

dilatation dilation; expansion of an organ or orifice

discipline control gained by enforcing order

disseminated intravascular coagulation (DIC) a pathologic diffused coagulation disorder associated with incomplete abortion and some types of surgery

diuretic any agent that causes the body to release more water in the form of urine

doll's eye reflex normal response of the newborn to keep eyes stationary when the head is moved back and forth; this reflex disappears as ocular fixation occurs

ductus arteriosus the connection between the main pulmonary artery and the aorta in the fetus

ductus venosus the smaller of the two branches of the umbilical vein as it empties into the inferior vena cava

duration the average length of time

dyscrasia old term meaning bad mixture of the four humors; now used as a synonym for disease

dyslexia impaired interpretation of the written word; a disorder found in children with reading difficulties who are able to recognize letters but unable to spell or write words

dyspnea difficulty in breathing

dysrhythmia any irregular heart rhythm; can be benign or lethal; may or may not be felt in the pulse

dystocia difficult labor from either a too large fetus or too small pelvic outlet

dysuria painful urination

eccrine sweat glands secrete sweat to cool the body and are all over the skin

ectoderm the outer layers of cells in the developing embryo

ectopic pregnancy implantation of a fertilized egg outside the uterus

effacement thinning of the cervix

egocentrism self centered in thought and action

elective abortion termination of pregnancy at the request of the mother

electrocution act of destroying life with electric current

electronic fetal monitoring electrical monitoring device used during labor to detect early signs of fetal distress

emancipated minor released from parental care before legal age is reached

embolus free-floating mass in the blood or lymphatic vessel; may be solid, liquid, or gaseous

emotional abuse damaging a person's self esteem verbally; chronic browbeating of a person to control him or her

empathy caring of a person's feelings

encephalopathy any dysfunction of the brain

endocarditis inflammation of the lining of the heart and valves

endoderm the inner layer of cells of the developing embryo

endometriosis endometrium located outside the uterus in the abdominal and pelvic cavities

engagement lightening; the entrance of the fetus into the pelvic strait

enuresis incontinence occurring after the age of 5 years when bladder control should have been accomplished

eosinophil granular leukocyte that increases count in response to allergic or parasitic disorders

epidermis the outer layers of the skin that do not contain nerve endings and blood vessels

epidural anesthesia regional anesthesia of the pelvic, abdominal, and genital area by analgesic injection into the epidural space of the lumbar spine

episiotomy surgical incision made in the perineum during delivery to prevent vaginal wall tearing into the rectum

Epstein's pearls small white cysts that normally occur on the hard palate of the newborn and disappear within a few weeks

Erb's paralysis caused by traumatic injury, commonly from forcible traction during childbirth, to the upper brachial plexus

erythema redness of the skin or mucosa

erythema toxicum neonatorum pink papular rash commonly appearing 24 to 48 hours after birth mainly on the trunk and spontaneously disappears; papular smear shows eosinophils instead of neutrophils

eschar black dead tissue found in wounds and gangrene

esophagogastroduodenoscopy fiberoptic exam of the esophagus, the stomach, and the duodenum; pictures and biopsies can be taken and minor ulcer repair or dilation can be done during the exam

estrogen a female hormone that regulates secondary sex characteristics

ethnic group a population sharing a common cultural origin

exophthalmus an abnormal protrusion of the eyeballs caused by tumor, fluid collection, or endocrine disorder

extended family a family group consisting of biologic or adoptive parents, children, grandparents, and other family

extinction a process of eliminating a conditioned response by not reinforcing it

extrusion abnormal external positioning, such as a tooth being pushed out of bite occlusion

false pelvis the portion of the pelvis above the iliopectineal line; also called the pelvis major

family a group of people bound by blood or friendship to provide long-term emotional and physical commitment to the group

febrile convulsion high fever in the infant triggering a convulsive episode

fertilization union of the male and female sex cells

fertility rate number of live births per 1000 women between the ages of 15 and 44

fetal mortality rate fetal death per 1000 births

fetal alcohol effects set of congenital abnormalities causing a degree of psychological, cognitive, or physical retardation seen in babies born to a mother who used alcohol during the pregnancy; characteristic wide-set eyes, cardiovascular defects, and retarded development. There is no known lower limit of alcohol use during pregnancy to prevent malformations

fetal alcohol syndrome birth defects in babies born of alcoholic mothers; babies exhibit alcohol withdrawal shortly after birth

fibrinogen clotting factor of the blood

fluorosis chronic exposure to fluorine at high levels, often causing tooth enamel mottling

fontanel unossified space between cranial bones, commonly called soft spots

foramen ovale opening between the atria in the fetal heart that closes after birth

forceps obstetric instrument that looks like scissors with spoon blades to cup the baby's head during delivery

frank breech legs are extended against the abdomen and chest, with feet to the shoulders and buttocks presentation

frequency a pattern of repetitions of a behavior or phenomenon during a certain period of time

functional a term to describe a problem with no organic origin

funic souffle a purring sound of rushing umbilical cord blood heard over the pregnant uterus

gamete a mature female or male sex cell

gene a section of DNA (deoxyribonucleic acid)

genetic abnormality flaw in the genetic code

genetic counseling providing advice about the possibility of hereditary defects to couples

genogram a diagram of family structure depicting interactive roles that exist in the family

genu valgum knock-knees; inward curving at the knees

gestational diabetes diabetic condition that is present in the mother only during pregnancy

gifted child a child who demonstrates rapid development in cognitive and language abilities, above average curiosity, long concentration span and independence

globulins protein molecules involved with immunity activities

glucagon a hormone secreted by the pancreas to stimulate conversion of glycogen to glucose when blood sugar is low

glycosuria glucose found in urine; abnormal finding

Goodell's sign presumptive sign of pregnancy; cervical softening

Grave's disease thyroid hypersecretion, thought to be autoimmune disorder

gravida term referring to pregnancy

gray syndrome or gray baby syndrome appearance of abdominal distention and vomiting, cyanosis, and rapid respirations in newborns treated at birth with chloramphenicol. Loss of suckling, flaccidness, and ashen color are present within 24 hours. Mortality rate of this syndrome is about 40%.

grief mourning process involving predictable emotional phases

guaiac a reagent used on feces and urine to detect occult blood

Hashimoto thyroiditis autoimmune thyroid dysfunction where lymphocytes replace thyroid structures; has hereditary pattern; more common in women than men; most frequently occurs in ages 30 to 50 yrs

Hegar's sign probable sign of pregnancy; softening of the lower part of the uterus early in gestation

Heimlich maneuver emergency procedure for dislodging a foreign object from the windpipe

HELLP syndrome a type of hypertension occurring in pregnancy with common symptoms of hemolysis, elevated liver enzymes, and low platelet count

hemolytic anemia low RBC count due to cell loss greater than cell growth

hemangioma vascular tumors of the skin; commonly called port wine stain or strawberry birthmarks

hemarthrosis bloody effusion into a joint cavity

hematoma a bruise; a confined swelling of blood caused a break in a blood vessel

hematuria blood in the urine; abnormal finding

hormonal method using oral contraceptives for birth control hormones (protein or steroid) molecules manufactured in the body's various gland affecting the function of the body

human chorionic gonadotropin (HCG) the first hormone to be produced by the chorionic villi of the placenta; this hormone produces estrogen and progesterone to keep the endometrial lining from being sloughed

hydatiform mole multiple cysts that rapidly grow from the chorionic villi causing hemorrhage

hydronephrosis distended kidney pelvis due to an obstruction of urine outflow

hyperbilirubinemia excessive level of bilirubin in the blood

hyperemesis gravidarum excessive and severe vomiting during pregnancy that causes electrolyte imbalance, dehydration, and weight loss

hyperglycemia elevated blood glucose level

hyperthermia unusually high fever; hyperpyrexia; induced fever as a form of treatment

hypoglycemia lower than normal blood glucose level

hypophysectomy surgical removal of the pituitary gland

hypopituitary dwarfism stunted growth from deficient secretion of growth hormone from the pituitary gland

hypoplastic kidneys underdeveloped kidneys

hypovolemic shock circulatory impairment leading to collapse, caused by loss of circulating volume of fluids

hypoxemia decreased oxygen in the blood

hypoxia decreased oxygen in inspired air

icterus neonatorum mild hemolytic jaundice of the newborn not requiring treatment

immune deficient lacking ability to respond to antigen exposure effectively

implantation attachment of the embryo in the uterine wall

implementation enacting a plan to reach a goal
impotence inability to obtain and sustain an erection
increased cranial pressure caused by increased fluid collection inside the cranium
increment the amount or degree in which something changes
incubation stage a period of time maintaining an embryo during its development
induction the act or process of initiating labor
infant mortality rate number of infant deaths per 1,000 live births
infection control methods of breaking the chain of infection to stop the spread of a disease
inferiority the sense of feeling less worthy when comparing oneself to others
infertility inability to conceive a child; lower number of sperm or lack of sperm in the male; no release of egg or blocked passage of the egg in the female
infestations disease caused by parasitic insects
informed consent voluntary and competent permission for a health-related procedure
ingestion to take into the body via the GI tract
initiative the ability to self motivate
insulin reaction rapid low blood sugar occurring when too much insulin is active at one time; rapid onset of hypoglycemic symptoms can cause coma and death if not treated
internal electronic monitoring most reliable method of fetal monitoring by which a scalp electrode is attached to the fetus when cervix is 3 mm and membranes have ruptured
isolation the fear of other people; method of limiting contact with a contagious person to prevent the spread of disease
karyotype visual presentation of the chromosome pattern
keloid scar tissue buildup
kernicterus bilirubin infiltrating the brain and spinal cord of the newborn; if untreated, has poor prognosis
ketoacidosis abnormal drop in body pH from accumulation of ketone acids when diabetes is out of control; can cause coma and death if untreated
ketone waste product from fat metabolism
kyphosis abnormal curvature of the spine
labor physiologic process of the body expelling the fetus from the uterus; childbirth
lactose intolerance inability to digest milk and milk products
laminaria type of kelp seaweed used to dilate the cervix
lanugo fine hair on the fetus, more prominent when premature
latchkey child child who is left unattended by an adult for a time during each weekday
LDRP abbreviation used to describe maternity rooms: labor, delivery, recovery, postpartum
Leopold's maneuvers systemic method of palpation and observation to determine the fetal position, which is important to help the course of labor
leukocyte term given to white blood cells
level of consciousness sensory awareness of the environment and the ability to response to it
lie refers to the position of the fetus in the womb
lightening fetal descent into the pelvis about 3 weeks before onset of labor
linea nigra the darkened midline from navel to pubis symphysis that occurs during pregnancy
lordosis abnormal curvature of the lumbar spine
lumbar puncture invasive procedure performed to obtain cerebrospinal fluid for exam and diagnosis
macrophage white blood cell that engulfs invading pathogens and debris in the body
macule an unraised discoloration noted on the skin; may have varying shapes, sizes, or colors
mainstreaming federal law states that disabled children must receive equal education in the least restrictive situation referring to the regular classroom
maladaptive behavior negative behavior response to a stressor
malnutrition failing to receive daily required nutrients for a period of time, causing poor health
malposition faulty or abnormal position of body parts
malpresentation abnormal position of the fetus during labor and delivery
MAR abbreviation for medication administration record sheet
mast cell granulocyte that migrates into connective tissue and responds to injury and infection by releasing heparin and histamine as a defense response
mastitis inflammation of the breast commonly occurring in lactating women
mechanical barrier method contraception methods using condoms and diaphragms
meditation to project a thought in the mind
menarche the first menstrual cycle in a female, usually occurring around the age of 12 years
menopause the cessation of menses; usually occurs in women around the age of 50 years
menstrual cycle the four phases of changes in the uterus occurring over an average of 28 days
mesoderm embryonic tissue layer between the ectoderm and endoderm from which all connective tissues arise
methane colorless, flammable gas produced by putrefaction and fermentation of organic matter
middle school child a child attending fifth, sixth, seventh, or eighth grade
milia unopened sebaceous glands frequently found on the newborn's face
molding cervical tapering of the fetal head during birth; head shape returns to normal within a week after birth
molestation the act of sexually fondling or abusing
mongolian spots dark spots created by a collection of pigment cells on the buttocks or sacrum of the newborn; usually seen in children of Asian, African, and southern European origin; fades with age and requires no treatment
morals principles of right and wrong behavior

mucous plug blood-streaked thick vaginal discharge indicating the beginnings of labor; collection of mucus in the respiratory tract causing obstruction

multifactorial inheritance unpredictable genetic susceptibility because more than a single gene and environmental influences are involved

Munchausen syndrome by proxy type of mental disorder in which the mother will complain of sickness or injury in the child that is difficult to diagnose from history given

Nägele's rule prediction of length of pregnancy; count back 3 calendar months from first day of last menses and add 7 days

narcotics a classification of drugs derived from the opium poppy, used for severe pain control; its use is regulated by federal law

natural family planning use of rhythm method and temperature methods to plan pregnancies; methods approved by the Roman Catholic Church and Orthodox Judaism

neonate newborn baby

nephron the filtering structure in the kidney

neutrophil the most numerous of the white cells in the body

neva flammeus port wine stain; red discoloration of face or neck, not raised but large and deep-colored deformity

nocturnal enuresis incontinence during sleep after bladder control has been accomplished; first born and boys more often have this problem.

nonsteroidal anti-inflammatory drugs (NSAIDs) a classification of drugs used to control minor pain

nuclear family a mother, father, and children group

oblique lie diagonal position of the fetus to the mother's longitudinal axis

observational learning learning a complicated task by watching another perform it

occiput refers to the back of the head

oliguria less than 30 cc of urine produced hourly

open adoption the child knows of the adoption and biologic parents

opisthotonos a spasm of the back muscles causing the body to become arched, with head and heels pressed into the bed

orchiopexy surgical procedure to descend the testicle into the scrotum and suture it there

otitis media infection of the middle ear; can cause hearing loss and ear drum rupture

ovum egg cell containing 23 chromosomes

oxytocin hormone secreted by the pituitary gland that causes uterine contractions and milk letdown; can be given as IV drip to induce labor

papule firm, red, elevated area on the skin

para term referring to a pregnant woman who delivers an infant weighing at least 500 grams or over 20 weeks' gestation

parallel play children play by themselves but are in close proximity to each other

paracervical block transvaginal injection of anesthesia on each side of the cervix to relieve uterine contraction pain for about an hour

parent one who has long-term emotional and physical commitment to raising a child

pathologic fracture bone breakage occurring from disease, not trauma

pathologic jaundice also called congenital jaundice; jaundice in the newborn due to maldevelopment of biliary tract

pediatrician a physician who specializes in children's illnesses

pediatrics the study of children's illnesses

pedophile sexual disorder where an adult finds sexual gratification from sexual encounter with a prepubescent child

perception one's interpretation of a situation

percussion technique of tapping a body part to assess the condition within by the resulting sound

perinatal mortality rate perinatal period begins when the fetus has reached 500 g and ends 4 weeks after birth; mortality rate is the sum of fetal and neonate deaths

personality a unique combination of traits, characteristics, and behavior that defines a person as an individual

pesticide chemical that kills insects

pharmacokinetics study of the process in which the body absorbs, distributes, metabolizes, and excretes drugs

phimosis tightening of the foreskin making it unable to be retracted

phobia an anxiety disorder exhibiting extreme, irrational fear of an object or activity

physiologic leukorrhea normal white or yellowish mucous discharge from cervical canal or vagina; may be constant and increased flow before and after menses and during sexual stimulus

physiologic jaundice newborn jaundice lasting a few days and not requiring treatment

pincer reflex ability to bring thumb and first finger together; pinching grasp; ability obtained by 10 months of age

placenta previa placenta implants low in the uterus increasing risk of hemorrhage and abortion

placenta accreta placenta implanted deeply into the uterine musculature, making separation of the placenta impossible

play therapy a treatment modality used to assist child to express self through dolls or role playing

plumbism chronic lead poisoning

poison any substance that is toxic to the body to the extent that function is affected

polycythemia excess of red blood cells

polydipsia excess thirst

polyphagia gluttony; overeating

polyuria excessive urination

positive reinforcement recognition given for only accepted behavior

postpartum psychosis severe mental disorder triggered by the crisis of childbirth within 6 weeks' postpartum; about a third of these women may have had mental symptoms before pregnancy; woman appears sad and denies that pregnancy and childbirth ever occurred

postpartum blues due to hormonal changes after delivery, the woman experiences feelings of sadness and inadequacy, tearfulness, anorexia, and sleep disturbance; occurrence 80%

postpartum depression feeling of sadness that continues beyond the usual first few days' postpartum; extreme fatigue, inability to stop crying, heightened anxiety over child's health are also signs of more serious problem

postural drainage a technique of positioning the client to assist lung clearance of secretions

poverty the state of a person lacking sufficient resources; officially defined in terms of income and size of family, using an index originated by the Social Security Administration; figures are adjusted to reflect economic conditions

preadolescent the period of human development between the ages of 9 to 12 yrs

precipitous delivery rapid labor resulting in quick delivery within 3 hours; likely to occur with multiparity

precocious puberty development of breasts or pubic hair before the age of 8 yrs or menses before the age of 9 yrs; occurs more often in girls than boys

preconventional phase Kohlberg's first level of moral development in which punishment/obedience directs the child to do right; carries out action for own needs, not society's needs

pregnancy-induced hypertension (PIH) rarely apparent before 24 wks, hypertension associated with proteinuria and edema; toxemia

prejudice preconceived opinion

preterm labor labor occurring before the end of 37 weeks of gestation or before fetal weight reaches 2500 g

primary hypertension elevated blood pressure that occurs without apparent cause

prodromal stage premonitory stage of a disease before symptoms appear

progesterone hormone secreted by the ovaries and placenta that stimulates uterine growth

prolapsed cord cord is expulsed before the fetus during labor

prolactin a hormone produced by the pituitary gland that stimulates breast enlargement and milk production during pregnancy; stimulus for release is suckling. Stress can cause hypersecretion of prolactin, bringing on amenorrhea and male impotence.

prostaglandins a wide assortment of autocoids effect tissues locally where they are produced; increased production can cause dysmenorrhea

prothrombin a clotting factor in the blood

pruritus itching

pseudohermaphrodite ambiguous genitalia

puberty period of development when a person becomes sexually capable of reproduction, usually between the ages of 13 to 15 yrs for boys and 9 to 16 yrs for girls

pubescence becoming hairy; approaching or reaching puberty

pudendal block local anesthetic administered just before delivery and injected through the vagina; onset 2 to 10 minutes and duration up to 1 hour

puerperium the first 42 days after giving birth when generative organs return to normal

purulent containing pus

pyelonephritis inflammation of the kidney pelvis, usually due to bacterial infection

pyloromyotomy incision and suture of the pyloric sphincter

quickening first fetal movement felt by the mother

race a large group of people having similar physical characteristics and heredity

radiant warmer a bassinet with a warmer above to keep the baby warm after birth

reflux backward flow; regurgitation

regression resort to coping behavior used at an earlier stage of development in handling stress

reinforcement reward for appropriate response in learning

relaxin a hormone released by the corpus luteum that softens pelvic joints to facilitate birthing

respiratory distress syndrome (RDS) severe impairment demonstrated in the premature newborn; hyaline membrane disease

restitution making good for some injury; a defense mechanism that exaggerated the response

retained placenta placenta not discharged for 2 hours after the second stage of labor

ripening changes of the cervix just before labor and delivery

Romberg sign (test) evaluation of intact proprioreceptors by having the person stand with feet together and eyes closed; loss of balance indicates loss of the sense of position

Salmonella gram-negative rod bacteria that can cause mild to lethal food poisoning

scoliosis abnormal S-shaped curve of the spine

seborrheic dermatitis excessive secretion of sebum causing oily scaly patches

sebum fatty substance secreted by sebaceous glands

secondary hypertension high blood pressure resulting from another health condition

seizure a sudden onset of symptoms; epileptic episode

seminal fluid thick viscous fluid containing sperm released during ejaculation; semen

separation anxiety anxiety that appears in American infants about 10 to 12 months but disappears by 24 months when mother leaves the child

septic shock vascular collapse caused by bacterial toxins, causing the capillary beds to lose selective permeability

seriation ability to put a group of objects in order according to a specific shared property

sexually transmitted disease any pathogenic microorganism that can be given to another through sexual contact

sexual response cycle has four distinct stages (excitement, plateau, orgasm, resolution) leading to sexual gratification

shaken-baby syndrome a form of child abuse involving head and neck injuries; if repeated and severe can cause death

shoulder dystocia difficult labor of either a large fetus or small pelvic outlet involving shoulders that cause obstruction

shunt for hemodialysis, arteriovenous connection in the forearm; for hydrocephalus, polyethylene tube surgically placed from the cerebral ventricle into the abdomen to reduce fluid accumulation

single-parent family only one adult in the nuclear family

socialization the process by which an individual develops behavior patterns and beliefs that are valued by the individual's family and culture

sperm male sex cell carrying 23 chromosomes

spinal bifida failure of laminae of the vertebrae to occur in fetal development

spinal block type of regional anesthesia used during labor and delivery

station the relationship of the presenting part of the fetus with the level of ischial spine

status epilepticus state of continuous seizuring that can lead to death if not stopped

steatorrhea excess secretion of sebaceous glands; also fatty stools seen with pancreatic disease

sternal retractions ribcage drawn inward during inspiration; indication of respiratory distress in the newborn

stimulus anything occurring in the environment that will cause a response

strabismus disorder of the eye when optic axes do not coordinate focus; lazy eye

strain gauge a catheter inserted between baby and uterine wall that measures contraction pressure and is attached to the fetal monitor

striae gravidarum streak marks appearing on the sides of the abdomen; pink streaks change to silvery white after pregnancy

stridor high-pitched harsh breath sound caused by airway obstruction

stuttering speech defect of spasmodic repeat of a word or hesitant, repetitive sounds

subinvolution failure of the uterus to return to prepregnant size after birth

subluxation dislocation of a synovial joint without tearing the joint capsule

surfactant fluid secreted in the alveoli to prevent structure collapse

symbiotic play 2- to 3-year-olds combining objects to copy life experiences during play

synarthrosis cartilaginous bone joint with very little or absent movement; suture

tachypnea rapid rate of breathing

Tay-Sachs disease inherited disease depicting neurologic deterioration, physical and mental retardation; exaggerated startle reflex; death usually occurs by the age of 4 years

telangiectatic nevi vascular lesion forming a birthmark

temperament an individual's emotional, intellectual, and ethical expression

teratogen anything that causes abnormal development of the fetus

testosterone principal hormone secreted by the testes

tetany intermittent spasms seen in extremities

thelarche beginning of breast development

thyroid storm a crisis in uncontrolled hyperthyroidism characterized by high fever, rapid pulse, respiratory distress, restlessness, and prostration. The patient can become delirious, comatose, and die of heart failure.

thyroxine (T_4) a hormone secreted by the thyroid gland to regulate metabolism

tocolytic agent any drug used to suppress premature labor

TORCH infections a group of pathogens that can infect the fetus or newborn, causing stillbirth, abortion, intrauterine growth retardation, and premature labor; an abbreviation for *toxoplasmosis, other, rubella virus, cytomegalovirus, herpes simplex viruses*

torticollis abnormal contraction of neck muscles on one side; wryneck

TPAL classification of a woman by the number of pregnancies, followed by the number of full-term deliveries, the number of premature infants, the number of miscarriages or abortions, and the number of living children at present

transductive reasoning a type of problem-solving in which an idea or experience is related to a similar situation

transverse lie when the fetus is horizontal to the cervix

tripod posturing seen in children with poliomyelitis, unable to sit up without arms behind to support themselves

true pelvis the lower portion of the pelvis defined by an oblique plane from the sacrum to the pubic symphysis

tubal ligation surgical lysis of the fallopian tubes producing sterility

urea nitrogenous waste product of the body

uremia abnormal state in which uric acid accumulates in the blood, usually due to significant kidney impairment

uremic frost uric acid crystals that are formed (usually across the brow) from diaphoresis in a person with endstage kidney failure

urethral "stents" instruments used to dilate strictures of the urethra and allow improved bladder emptying

urticaria irregular wheals seen on the skin as an allergic reaction; commonly called hives

uterine inversion uterus turns inside out

uterine souffle blowing sound caused by blood in the uterine arteries in the last months of pregnancy

vacuum extraction when the fetal head is at the perineum, the vacuum extractor is used instead of forceps to deliver the fetus

valvuloplasty plastic or restorative surgery on a heart valve
variability capable of changing form, behavior, or structure
vasectomy surgical lysis of the vas deferens producing sterility
vernix caseosa waxy covering of the fetus in utero; most abundantly found in skin creases of the newborn
vertex top of the head
vesicle a blisterlike elevation of the skin
vesicoureteral reflux back flow of urine from the bladder into the ureter
weaning substitution of other nourishment for breast milk
Wharton's jelly jellylike intracellular substance found in the umbilical cord
zygote a fertilized ovum until it implants into the uterine wall

answer key

unit I
issues and trends in maternal-child health nursing

1 nursing care of the family

1. A 2. B 3. C 4. A 5. D

2 issues and trends in maternity care

1. C 2. B 3. A 4. C 5. B

3 issues and trends in child health care

1. D 2. B 3. A 4. D 5. C

unit II
reproductive health

4 reproductive function and sexuality

1. C 2. D 3. B 4. B 5. C

5 family planning

1. D 2. B 3. C 4. A 5. B

unit III
the expectant family

6 embryology and fetal development

1. B 2. C 3. A 4. B 5. C

7 physiologic and psychosocial changes during pregnancy

1. B 2. B 3. C 4. B 5. B

8 needs and care of the expectant family

1. A 2. C 3. C 4. B 5 D

9 nursing care during pregnancy at risk

1. A 2. B 3. C 4. C 5. B

unit IV
the family during childbirth

10 the process of labor

1. A 2. B 3. D 4. C 5. C

11 analgesia and anesthesia

1. C 2. C 3. B 4. C 5. D

12 nursing care of the family during childbirth

1. D 2. C 3. D 4. B 5. A

13 complications and emergencies during childbirth

1. A 2. B 3. B 4. B 5. B

unit V
the postpartum family

14 nursing care of the postpartum family

1. A 2. B 3. B 4. B 5. D

15 complications and emergencies of the postpartum period

1. B 2. C 3. B 4. C 5. C

16 nursing care of the normal newborn

1. C 2. B 3. B 4. B 5. C

17 nursing care of the newborn at risk

1. B 2. D 3. B 4. C 5. A

unit VI
growth and development

18 theories of growth and development

1. A 2. C 3. D 4. B 5. D

19 health maintenance and health promotion

1. A 2. B 3. C 4. D 5. C

20 health protection and safety

1. D 2. C 3. B 4. C 5. B

21 the infant

1. B 2. D 3. D 4. A 5. D

22 the toddler

1. D 2. C 3. A 4. C 5. A

23 the preschool child

1. B 2. C 3. C 4. B 5. A

24 the school-age child

1. B 2. A 3. A 4. C 5. D

25 the adolescent

1. A 2. C 3. B 4. C 5. B

unit VII
the child and family during illness

26 nursing administration of medications and management of pain

1. D 2. A 3. B 4. B 5. D

27 nursing care of the child and family during acute illness

1. C 2. A 3. D 4. B 5. B

28 nursing care of the child and family during chronic, life-threatening, or terminal illness

1. A 2. A 3. C 4. B 5. B

29 nursing care of the child and family with a mental health problem

1. C 2. B 3. A 4. C 5. A

unit VIII
the child with specific alterations in health status

30 the child with an alteration in respiration

1. B 2. A 3. B 4. A 5. D

31 the child with an alteration in cardiovascular function

1. C 2. D 3. C 4. A 5. A

32 the child with an alteration in hematologic or immune system function

1. A 2. C 3. C 4. B 5. B

33 the child with an alteration in urinary or reproductive system function

1. B 2. C 3. C 4. A 5. A

34 the child with an alteration in gastrointestinal function

1. A 2. B 3. C 4. B 5. B

35 the child with an alteration in neurologic or sensory function

1. A 2. B 3. B 4. B 5. B

36 the child with an alteration in musculoskeletal function

1. A 2. B 3. C 4. A 5. B

37 the child with an alteration in integumentary function

1. B 2. A 3. B 4. D 5. C

38 the child with an alteration in endocrine function

1. D 2. C 3. B 4. B 5. C

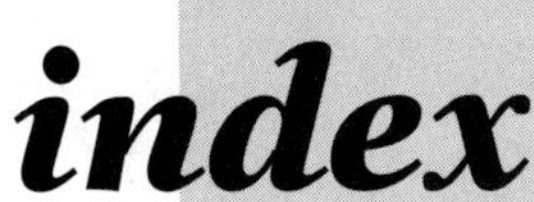

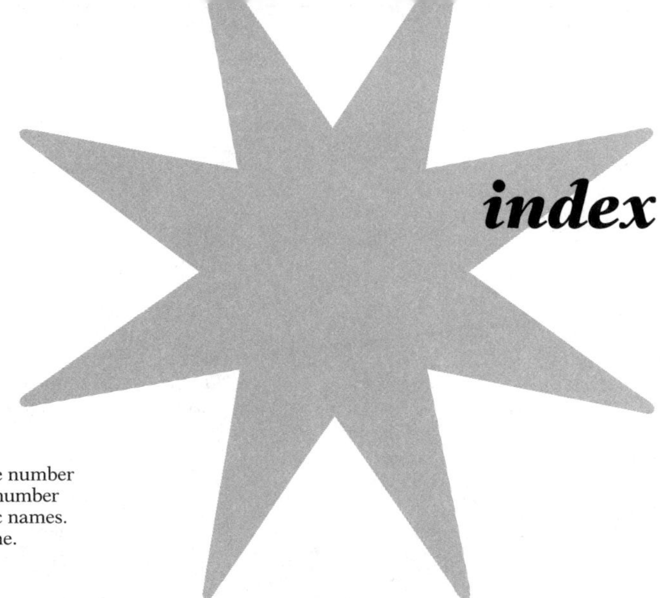

index

NOTE: A *t* following a page number indicates a table; an *f* following a page number indicates a figure, an *i* indicates a nursing insight, and a *d* following a page number indicates a display. Insofar as possible, drugs are listed under their generic names. When a drug trade name is listed, the reader is referred to the generic name.

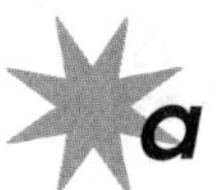

a

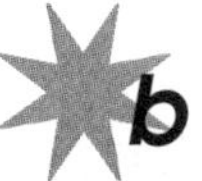
b

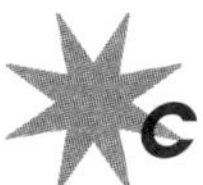

d

e

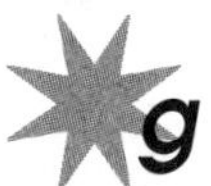

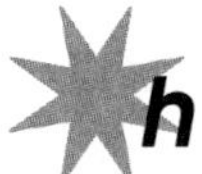

I

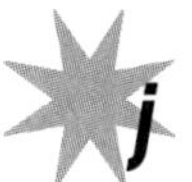

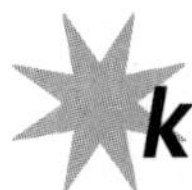

L

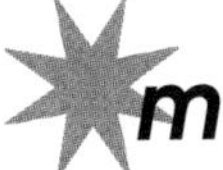

m

n

O

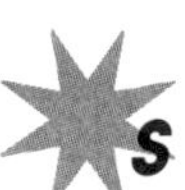

U

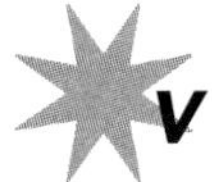

V

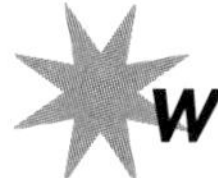

W

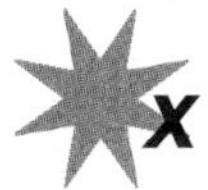

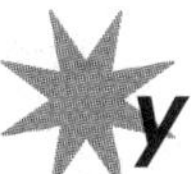

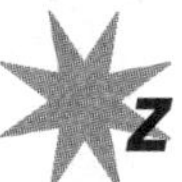